Perinatal Nursing

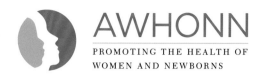

AWHONN
PROMOTING THE HEALTH OF
WOMEN AND NEWBORNS

Perinatal Nursing

FIFTH EDITION

Editors

Kathleen Rice Simpson, PhD, RNC, CNS-BC, FAAN
Perinatal Clinical Nurse Specialist
Editor-in-Chief
MCN The American Journal of Maternal Child Nursing
St. Louis, Missouri

Patricia A. Creehan, MSN, RNC
Manager of Clinical Operations, Labor and Delivery
Advocate Christ Medical Center
Oak Lawn, Illinois

Nancy O'Brien-Abel, MN, RNC
Perinatal Clinical Nurse Specialist
Perinatal Consulting, LLC
Affiliate Instructor
School of Nursing
University of Washington
Seattle, Washington

Cheryl K. Roth, PhD, WHNP-BC, RNC-OB, RNFA
Nurse Practitioner, Labor and Delivery/Couplet Care
HonorHealth Scottsdale Shea/Osborn Medical Centers
Scottsdale, Arizona

Annie J. Rohan, PhD, RN, NNP-BC, CPNP-PC, FAANP
Chair of Graduate Studies & Director of Doctor of
Nursing Practice Program
Associate Professor & Director of Pediatric Research
College of Nursing
SUNY Downstate Health Sciences University
Brooklyn, New York

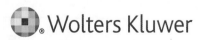
Wolters Kluwer

Philadelphia • Baltimore • New York • London
Buenos Aires • Hong Kong • Sydney • Tokyo

Acquisitions Editor: Nicole Dernoski
Development Editor: Maria M. McAvey
Editorial Coordinator: Cody Adams
Production Project Manager: Sadie Buckallew
Design Coordinator: Teresa Mallon
Manufacturing Coordinator: Kathleen Brown
Marketing Manager: Linda Wetmore
Prepress Vendor: Absolute Service, Inc.

5th edition

9 8 7 6 5 4 3 2 1

Printed in China

978-1-9751-7453-8
Library of Congress Cataloging-in-Publication Data available upon request

shop.lww.com

To all perinatal nurses and the mothers and babies
they care for every day

&

To my parents, William and Dorothy; my husband,
Dan; and my children, Daniel, Katie, Michael,
John, and Elizabeth

—KRS

To Patrick, Sean, Melissa, and Kelly Mitchell

—PAC

To my husband, Mike, and my son, Thomas

—NOA

To my parents, Glenn and Ardis Egli; my husband,
Marty; and my children, Katie, Mike, Kyle,
and Rebecca

—CR

To Alexa, Jack, Arielle . . . and Faith

—AJR

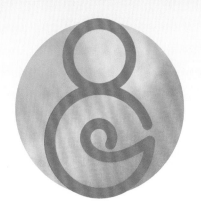

Contributors

Ellise D. Adams, PhD, CNM
Associate Professor, College of Nursing
Doctor of Nursing Practice Program Coordinator
University of Alabama in Huntsville
Huntsville, Alabama
Chapter 4: Antenatal Care

Julie Arafeh, MSN, RN
Director of Simulation
Clinical Concepts in Obstetrics
Brentwood, Tennessee
Chapter 9: Cardiac Disease in Pregnancy

Susan Tucker Blackburn, RN, PhD, FAAN
Professor Emerita
School of Nursing
University of Washington
Seattle, Washington
Chapter 3: Physiologic Changes of Pregnancy

Nancy A. Bowers, BSN, RN, MPH
Perinatal Education Consultant
Birmingham, Alabama
Chapter 11: Multiple Gestation

Adriane Burgess, PhD, RNC-OB, CCE, CNE
Clinical Research Specialist
Women and Children Service Line
WellSpan Health
York, Pennsylvania
Chapter 5: Hypertensive Disorders of Pregnancy

Carol Burke, MSN, APRN, CNS, RNC-OB, C-EFM
Perinatal Clinical Nurse Specialist
Chicago, Illinois
*Chapter 16: Pain in Labor: Nonpharmacologic and
    Pharmacologic Management*

Lynn Clark Callister, PhD, RN, FAAN
Professor Emerita
Brigham Young University
Provo, Utah
*Chapter 2: Integrating Cultural Beliefs and Practices
    When Caring for Childbearing Women and Families*

Debbie Fraser, MN, CNEON(C), RNC-NIC
Associate Professor
Director, Nurse Practitioner Program
Faculty of Health Disciplines
Athabasca University
Athabasca, Alberta, Canada
*Chapter 18: Newborn Adaptation to
    Extrauterine Life*

Dotti C. James, PhD, RNC-OB
St. Louis, Missouri
Chapter 17: Postpartum Care

Jill Janke, PhD, RN, WHNP
Professor
School of Nursing
University of Alaska
Anchorage, Alaska
Chapter 20: Newborn Nutrition

Mary Ann Maher, MSN, RNC-OB, C-EFM
St. Louis, Missouri
Chapter 12: Obesity in Pregnancy

Nancy O'Brien-Abel, MN, RNC
Perinatal Clinical Nurse Specialist
Perinatal Consulting, LLC
Affiliate Instructor
School of Nursing
University of Washington
Seattle, Washington
Chapter 14: Labor and Birth
Chapter 15: Fetal Assessment during Labor

Sheryl E. Parfitt, MSN, RNC-OB
Clinical Educator—Obstetrics Department
HonorHealth Scottsdale Shea/Osborn Medical Centers
Scottsdale, Arizona
Chapter 7: Preterm Labor and Birth

Annie J. Rohan, PhD, RN, NNP-BC, CPNP-PC, FAANP
Chair of Graduate Studies & Director of Doctor of
    Nursing Practice Program
Associate Professor & Director of Pediatric Research
College of Nursing
SUNY Downstate Health Sciences University
Brooklyn, New York
Chapter 19: Newborn Physical Assessment
Chapter 21: Common Neonatal Complications

Cheryl K. Roth, PhD, WHNP-BC, RNC-OB, RNFA
Nurse Practitioner, Labor and Delivery/Couplet Care
HonorHealth Scottsdale Shea/Osborn Medical Centers
Scottsdale, Arizona
Chapter 8: Diabetes in Pregnancy
Chapter 10: Pulmonary Complications in Pregnancy

Jean Salera-Vieira, DNP, PNS, APRN-CNS, RNC-OB, C-EFM
Perinatal Clinical Nurse Specialist
Newport Hospital
Newport, Rhode Island
Chapter 6: Bleeding in Pregnancy

Kathleen Rice Simpson, PhD, RNC, CNS-BC, FAAN
Perinatal Clinical Nurse Specialist
Editor-in-Chief
*MCN The American Journal of Maternal Child
    Nursing*
St. Louis, Missouri
Chapter 1: Perinatal Patient Safety and Quality
Chapter 14: Labor and Birth
Chapter 15: Fetal Assessment during Labor

Patricia D. Suplee, PhD, RNC-OB
Divisional Chair, Center of Academic Excellence
Division of Baccalaureate Nursing Practice
Associate Professor
Rutgers University—Camden
Camden, New Jersey
Chapter 17: Postpartum Care

Judy Wilson-Griffin, MSN RNC-OB, C-EFM
Perinatal Clinical Nurse Specialist
Family Birth Place
SSM St. Mary's Health Center
St. Louis, Missouri
Chapter 13: Maternal–Fetal Transport

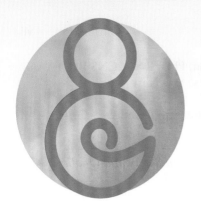

Reviewers

Mary Lee Barron, PhD, APRN, FNP-BC, FAANP
Associate Professor
School of Nursing
Southern Illinois University Edwardsville
Edwardsville, Illinois

Debra Bingham, DrPH, RN, FAAN
Perinatal Consultant
Founder and Executive Director
Institute for Perinatal Quality Improvement
Associate Professor for Healthcare Quality and Safety
Department of Partnerships, Professional Education
    and Practice
University of Maryland School of Nursing
Baltimore, Maryland

Mary C. Brucker, CNM, PhD, FACNM, FAAN
Editor
Nursing for Women's Health
Faculty
School of Nursing and Health Sciences
Georgetown University
Washington, DC

Terri A. Cavaliere, DNP, NNP-BC, FAANP
Clinical Associate Professor
Graduate Department School of Nursing
Stony Brook University
Stony Brook, New York

Nancy Cibulka, PhD, WHNP-BC, FNP-BC, FAANP
Associate Professor and FNP Program Coordinator
Saint Louis University
St. Louis, Missouri

Kimberly Dishman, MSN, WHNP-BC, RNC-OB
OB/NICU Nurse Manager
Saint Luke's Health System
Kansas City, Missouri

Carmen Giurgescu, PhD, RN, FAAN
Associate Professor
Martha S. Pitzer Center for Women, Children
    and Youth
College of Nursing
The Ohio State University
Columbus, Ohio

Sandra L. Hering, MSN, RNC-OB, CPHIMS
Specialist—Informatics Support, Obstetrics
HonorHealth Scottsdale Shea/Osborn Medical Centers
Scottsdale, Arizona

Halsey Hill, MSN, RNC-OB, C-EFM
Perinatal Specialist
Arizona Mother-Baby Care, Dignity Health, and
    Phoenix Children's Hospital
Phoenix, Arizona

Carol J. Huston, RN, MSN, MPA, DPA, FAAN
Professor Emerita, School of Nursing
California State University
Chico, California

Valerie Yates Huwe, MS, RNC-OB, CNS
Perinatal Outreach Educator
UCSF Benioff Children's Hospital
University of California, San Francisco
San Francisco, California
Direct Care Nurse, Labor and Delivery
El Camino Hospital
Mountain View, California

Molly Killion, RN, MS, CNS
High-Risk Obstetric Program Nurse Coordinator
University of California, San Francisco Medical Center
San Francisco, California

Cheryl Larry-Osman, RN, MS, CNM, CNS
Perinatal Clinical Nurse Specialist
Labor & Delivery, High Risk Antepartum,
    Postpartum
Henry Ford Hospital
Detroit, Michigan

Terrie Lockridge, MSN, RNC-NIC
Staff Nurse
Neonatal Intensive Care Unit
Swedish Medical Center
Seattle, Washington

Mary Ann Maher, MSN, RNC-OB, C-EFM
St. Louis, Missouri

Lisa Miller, CNM, JD
President
Perinatal Risk Management and Educational Services
Portland, Oregon

Kathleen Murray, MN, RNC-EFM
Regional Educator for Women's Care
CHI Franciscan Health
Tacoma, Washington

Loraine M. O'Neill, RN, MPH
System Chief Patient Safety Officer
Department of Obstetrics and Gynecology
The Mount Sinai Health System
New York, New York

Sheryl Parfitt, MSN, RNC-OB
Clinical Educator—Obstetrics Department
HonorHealth Scottsdale Shea/Osborn Medical Centers
Scottsdale, Arizona

**Elizabeth Li Sharpe, DNP, APRN, NNP-BC, VA-BC,
    FAANP**
Associate Professor Clinical Nursing
College of Nursing
The Ohio State University
Columbus, Ohio

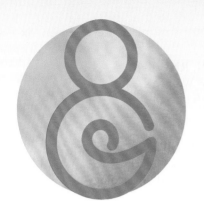

Previous Edition Contributors

Julie Arafeh, RN, MSN

Suzanne McMurtry Baird, DNPc, MSN, RN

Mary Lee Barron, PhD, APRN, FNP-BC

Susan Tucker Blackburn, RN, PhD, FAAN

Nancy A. Bowers, BSN, RN, MPH

Carol Burke, MSN, RNC, APN

Lynn Clark Callister, RN, PhD, FAAN

Annette Carley, RN, MS, NNP-BC, PNP-BC

Julie M. Daley, RN, MS, CDE

Debbie Fraser, MN, RNC-NIC

Dotti C. James, PhD, RNC-OB, C-EFM

Jill Janke, RN, WHNP, PhD

Betsy B. Kennedy, MSN, RN

Audrey Lyndon, PhD, RNC

Mary Ann Maher, MSN, RNC-OB, C-EFM

Nancy O'Brien-Abel, MN, RNC

Judith H. Poole, PhD, MBA/MHA, RNC-OB,
    C-EFM, NEA-BC

Nancy Jo Reedy, RN, CNM, MPH, FACNM

Joan Renaud Smith, PhD, RN, NNP-BC

Mary Ellen Burke Sosa, RNC, MS

Kathleen Rice Simpson, PhD, RNC, CNS-BC, FAAN

Lyn Vargo, PhD, RN, NNP-BC

Judy Wilson-Griffin, RN-C, MSN

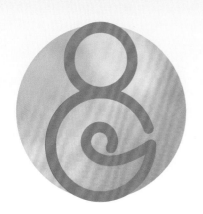

Previous Edition Reviewers

Susan Bakewell-Sachs, PhD, RN, PNP-BC

Ocean Berg, RN, MSN, CNS

Mary Campbell Bliss, RN, MS, CNS

Cathy Collins-Fulea, MSN, CNM, FACNM

Phyllis Lawlor-Klean, MS, RNC, APN/CNS

Audrey Lyndon, PhD, RNC

Mary Ann Maher, MSN, RNC-OB, C-EFM

Nancy O'Brien-Abel, MN, RNC

Mary Ellen Burke Sosa, RNC, MS

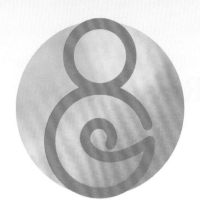

Preface

The fifth edition of *AWHONN Perinatal Nursing* represents over 25 years of collaboration between Kathleen Simpson and Patricia Creehan and new partnership with Nancy O'Brien-Abel, Cheryl Roth, and Annie Rohan to produce this textbook. As with all important projects, working as a team offers an opportunity for contribution, innovation, and insight not possible with individual efforts. We have assembled expert nurses from across the country who were willing to volunteer their considerable time and talent to contribute to the book. It is only through their collective generosity that this book was possible. Expert reviewers offered their feedback as the work was underway and enhanced the content. We offer suggestions for clinical practice based on the most recent evidence, standards, and guidelines. Our goal is to provide a practical resource for perinatal nurses, and we hope we have succeeded.

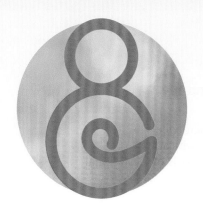

Contents

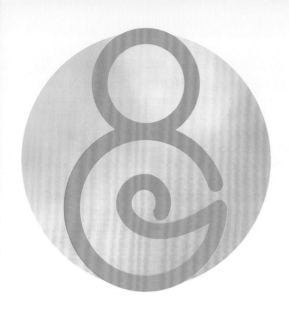

CHAPTER 1

Perinatal Patient Safety and Quality

Kathleen Rice Simpson

INTRODUCTION

In the 1990s, a number of health scientists and leaders conducted a critical evaluation of the health system in the United States and found numerous opportunities to provide better care and avoid preventable adverse outcomes (Institute of Medicine [IOM], 1999). The landmark initial IOM publication and its follow-up report with additional detailed recommendations (IOM, 2001) were catalysts to what is now a more widely accepted view of the importance of patient safety as an essential element of high-quality care. The framework and recommendations in these seminal publications are still useful 20 years later and are worth reviewing periodically to get a sense of what has been accomplished and how much more needs to be done (IOM, 1999, 2001).

The focus on perinatal patient safety was advanced by recommendations for adopting the principles of high reliability in the maternity care setting (Knox, Simpson, & Garite, 1999). Attributes of perinatal units at high and low risk for preventable adverse outcomes were identified by applying high-reliability science to the review of hundreds of medical records involving adverse outcomes and professional liability claims. Key suggestions were made for making care safer for mothers and babies during the childbirth hospitalization. Minimizing risk of preventable adverse outcomes and decreasing professional liability were the main objectives (Knox et al., 1999; Knox, Simpson, & Townsend, 2003). Important recommendations were using evidence-based national standards and guidelines as the foundation for clinical practice, reducing unnecessary variations in practice, working together as a clinical team, mutual respect, professional behavior, accountability, speaking up in the context of unsafe practices, measurement, and highlighting the interests of mothers and babies as

first priority (Knox & Simpson, 2011). Although initially some clinicians and leaders felt that these recommendations threatened physician autonomy and would not be practical in a hierarchical health system, they eventually have been adopted and enhanced by many patient safety scientists and leaders in the perinatal setting through multiple hospital, healthcare system, state, and national safety and quality collaboratives.

As the perinatal patient safety initiative has matured over the last two decades, there has been more emphasis on quality of care rather than liability exposure; however, these concepts are complementary. A number of healthcare systems have found that providing high-quality perinatal care based on the most recent evidence-based standards and guidelines has led to decreased liability costs (Clark, Belfort, Byrum, Meyers, & Perlin, 2008; Pettker et al., 2014; Simpson, Kortz, & Knox, 2009). A basic premise of perinatal patient safety and quality care is emphasizing "what is best for mothers and babies" over other issues when considering unit operations and clinical practices. Without this focus, often what is best (or more convenient or less costly) for hospitals, healthcare systems, leaders, and clinicians can be inappropriately prioritized at the expense of mothers and babies.

In the past few years, professional associations such as the Association of Women's Health, Obstetric and Neonatal Nurses (AWHONN), American College of Nurse-Midwives (ACNM), American Academy of Nursing (AAN), American College of Obstetricians and Gynecologists (ACOG), American Academy of Pediatrics, and Society for Maternal-Fetal Medicine (SMFM), among others, have taken major steps in promoting perinatal safety and have been working with organizations and advocacy groups led by childbearing women and their families to seek realistic solutions to the current state of

1

perinatal healthcare. Participation in perinatal quality improvement projects has become common practice. Perinatal quality care collaboratives have been established in almost all states. Perinatal safety has been expanded beyond the focus of the inpatient setting. Heightened awareness of the poor standing of the United States on quality markers of maternity care, including maternal and infant mortality, when compared to other developed countries has fueled some of these changes. Our maternal mortality rate should be one of the lowest among developed countries in the world given our resources. Maternal and infant health status should reflect other measures of prosperity. We can and must do better for childbearing women and babies in the United States.

Many of the "traditional" but outdated ways of providing care to childbearing women are being replaced with partnerships. The patriarchal culture that involves telling women what to do, expecting them to follow without questions, and treating them disrespectfully when they are unable or unwilling to "comply" is being slowly transformed to include women and their families as true partners in care. The extent of the concerns and dissatisfaction with perinatal healthcare by many childbearing women, clinicians, and healthcare leaders can be measured in part by the wide coverage of the problems by the lay media including *ProPublica*, *USA Today*, *The New York Times*, *The Washington Post*, and *Consumer Reports*. There has been a rapid growth in advocacy groups for safe maternity care (Display 1–1), many led by women who have experienced complications during childbirth and by families of women who did not survive childbirth.

In previous editions of AWHONN's *Perinatal Nursing*, this chapter has covered a variety of processes and systems focused on clinicians and individual hospitals and healthcare systems with suggestions for how to make care safer for mothers and babies and reduce professional liability (Simpson, 2014). Those recommendations, tools, and resources are still useful. In this edition, the focus is on the current state of maternity care in the United States and some of the projects and programs that have the most likelihood of achieving better outcomes on a large scale. National policies and national organization leadership have made a significant difference in widespread acceptance of the need for following the best evidence, reducing unnecessary variations in care, and working together as a collaborative team as ways to improve maternity care in our country. The resistance to these ideas that was prevalent 20 years ago (Knox et al., 1999) has been diminished, although not universally. It is anticipated that every state will eventually have a robust perinatal quality care collaborative, a maternal mortality review committee, and an active role in the Alliance for Innovation on Maternal Health (AIM) program. Every birthing hospital must be an active participant so the childbirth process for every mother and baby is as safe as it can be. Each of these processes requires perinatal nurse-leaders as vital participants. Nurses are in an ideal position to take a leadership role in improving maternity care in the United States and reducing risk of preventable adverse outcomes.

MATERNAL–INFANT OUTCOMES IN THE UNITED STATES

Data Sources and Definitions

The National Center for Vital Statistics at the Centers for Disease Control and Prevention (CDC) is the source of the majority of natality and mortality data in the United States. The Pregnancy Mortality Surveillance System of the CDC (2019b) collects data on maternal mortality. Data are based on death certificates of women on which there is a notation of recent pregnancy via a checkbox and links to fetal or infant death certificates from the prior year. Using vital statistics data as the main measure of maternal mortality has limitations, as there is minimal information from the death certificate to determine if the death was related to pregnancy. These events are likely underreported. Maternal mortality review committees are used to provide detailed information and analysis of each maternal death, including potential causative or associated factors; however, they have not been convened in every state. Various definitions are used to identify maternal deaths and other measures of maternal and infant health. Each definition has specific criteria and time frames (Display 1–2). It is important to be aware of these definitions when evaluating reports on the ongoing maternity care crisis in the United States.

Although other developed countries have shown improvement (World Health Organization, 2014),

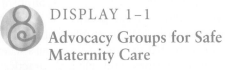

DISPLAY 1–1

Advocacy Groups for Safe Maternity Care

4Kira4Moms

Association of Maternal & Child Health Programs

Black Mamas Matter Alliance

Childbirth Connection

Effie's Grace

Every Mother Counts

March for Moms

Maternal Near-Miss Survivors

MomsRising

National Accreta Foundation

National Association to Advance Black Birth

National Partnership for Women & Families

Preeclampsia Foundation

Save The Mommies

SisterSong

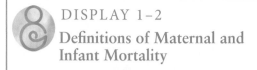

DISPLAY 1–2
Definitions of Maternal and Infant Mortality

World Health Organization

Maternal mortality is defined as death of a woman while pregnant or within 42 days of termination of pregnancy, irrespective of the duration and site of the pregnancy, not from accidental or incidental causes.

Pregnancy-related death is defined as the death of a woman while pregnant or within 42 days of termination of pregnancy, irrespective of the cause of death. This category was introduced to facilitate identification of maternal deaths in circumstances in which cause of death attribution is inadequate.

Centers for Disease Control and Prevention

Maternal mortality. National Vital Statistics System uses *International Statistical Classification of Diseases and Related Health Problems*, 10th revision (ICD-10), diagnosis codes and a pregnancy checkbox on death certificates to identify maternal deaths up to 42 days postpartum.

Pregnancy-related death is defined as the death of a woman while pregnant or within 1 year of the end of a pregnancy, regardless of the outcome, duration, or site of the pregnancy—from any cause related to or aggravated by the pregnancy or its management but not from accidental or incidental causes. The Centers for Disease Control and Prevention requests the 52 reporting areas (50 states, New York City, and Washington, DC) to voluntarily send copies of death certificates for all women who died during pregnancy or within 1 year of pregnancy, and copies of the matching birth or fetal death certificates, if they have the ability to perform such record links. All of the information obtained is summarized, and medically trained epidemiologists determine the cause and time of death related to the pregnancy.

Pregnancy-related mortality ratio is an estimate of the number of pregnancy-related deaths for every 100,000 live births.

Severe maternal morbidity is defined as including unexpected outcomes of labor and birth that result in significant short- or long-term consequences to a woman's health.

Infant mortality rate (IMR) is the number of infant (aged under 1 year) deaths per 1,000 live births. The IMR is the ratio of infant deaths to live births in a given year.

Neonatal infant deaths are deaths occurring within the first 28 days from birth.

Postneonatal infant deaths are deaths occurring after 28 days from birth to under 1 year of age.

Available at https://www.who.int/healthinfo/statistics/indmaternalmortality /en/; https://www.cdc.gov/reproductivehealth/maternalinfanthealth/pregnancy -mortality-surveillance-system.htm?CDC_AA_refVal=https%3A%2F%2Fwww .cdc.gov%2Freproductivehealth%2Fmaternalinfanthealth%2Fpmss.html; https://www.cdc.gov/nchs/data/databriefs/db285.pdf

data from the United States indicate a continued rise in maternal deaths. Each year in the United States, it is estimated that 700 to 900 women die from pregnancy or complications related to pregnancy (Building U.S. Capacity to Review and Prevent Maternal Deaths, 2018). For each maternal death, there are likely 70 to 100 other women who suffered severe maternal morbidity (ACOG, 2019; Ellison & Martin, 2017).

The most recent data on pregnancy-related deaths in the United States from the CDC (2019b) are reported in Figure 1–1. Unfortunately, there is a significant lag time between events and reporting; however, despite not yet including data from 2016 to 2019, the increasing trend in deaths from 1987 to 2015 is apparent. Of the 7,208 deaths within a year of the end of pregnancy that occurred during 2011 to 2014 and were reported to CDC, 2,726 were found to be pregnancy related. The pregnancy-related mortality ratios were 17.8, 15.9, 17.3, 18.0, and 17.2 deaths per 100,000 live births in 2011, 2012, 2013, 2014, and 2015, respectively. Considerable racial disparities in pregnancy-related mortality were noted. During 2011 to 2015, the pregnancy-related mortality ratios were (CDC, 2019b):

- 42.8 deaths per 100,000 live births for Black non-Hispanic women
- 32.5 deaths per 100,000 live births for American Indian/Alaskan Native non-Hispanic women.
- 14.2 deaths per 100,000 live births for Asian/Pacific Islander non-Hispanic women
- 13.0 deaths per 100,000 live births for White non-Hispanic women
- 11.4 deaths per 100,000 live births for Hispanic women

Figure 1–2 shows causes of pregnancy-related deaths in the United States during 2011 to 2015 (CDC, 2019b):

- Cardiovascular diseases (15.1%)
- Noncardiovascular diseases (14.3%)
- Infection (12.4%)
- Hemorrhage (11.2%)
- Cardiomyopathy (10.8%)
- Thrombotic pulmonary embolism (9.2%)
- Cerebrovascular accidents (7.6%)
- Hypertensive disorders of pregnancy (6.8%)
- Amniotic fluid embolism (5.5%)
- Anesthesia complications (0.3%)
- Unknown (6.7%)

A recent report from nine states' maternal mortality review committees highlights the need for more scrutiny for each maternal death and offers insight on causative factors and potential strategies for prevention (Building U.S. Capacity to Review and Prevent Maternal Deaths, 2018). In a review of 237 deaths, they found that 63% were likely preventable. Some clinical factors have been suggested as associated with increased risk of maternal death. They include maternal age, maternal morbidities, and cesarean birth. These factors have also been associated with adverse neonatal outcomes. Opportunities

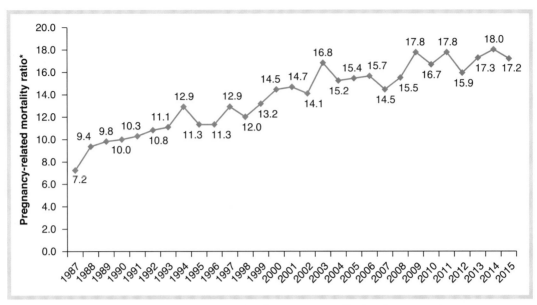

FIGURE 1–1. Trends in pregnancy-related mortality in the United States: 1987–2015. *Number of pregnancy-related deaths per 100,000 live births per year. (From Centers for Disease Control and Prevention. [2019b]. *Pregnancy Mortality Surveillance System*. Atlanta, GA: Author.)

for improvement in care of pregnant women have been identified in several large studies of severe maternal morbidity (near-miss maternal mortality) and maternal deaths (Building U.S. Capacity to Review and Prevent Maternal Deaths; Creanga, 2018; Ozimek et al., 2016). Suggestions for how to conduct a rigorous case review have been published (ACOG & SMFM, 2015) as well as measurement techniques (Main et al., 2016).

Maternal Age

Maternal age has increased over the past three decades (Martin, Hamilton, Osterman, Driscoll, & Drake, 2018). Figure 1–3 illustrates that trend from 1990 to 2017. In 2017, the mean age of mothers at first birth was 26.8 years, a record high for the United States (Martin et al., 2018). As births to

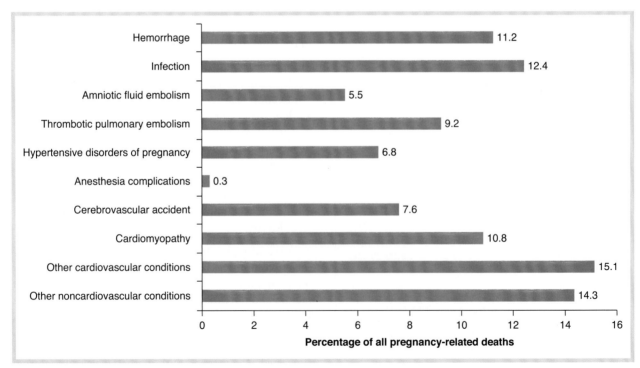

FIGURE 1–2. Causes of pregnancy-related death in the United States: 2011–2015. Note: The cause of death is unknown for 6.7% of all pregnancy-related deaths. (From Centers for Disease Control and Prevention. [2019b]. *Pregnancy Mortality Surveillance System*. Atlanta, GA: Author.)

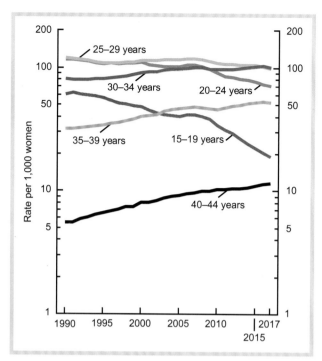

FIGURE 1–3. Births by age of mother from 1990 to 2017. Note: Rates are plotted on a logarithmic scale. (From Martin, J. A., Hamilton, B. E., Osterman, M. J. K., Driscoll, A. K., & Drake, P. [2018]. Births: Final data for 2017. *National Vital Statistics Reports, 67*[8], 1–50.)

Healthcare Research and Quality (AHRQ), severe maternal morbidity was highest among women aged ≥40 years and lowest for those aged 20 to 29 years (248 and 136 per 10,000 births, respectively) (Fingar, Hambrick, Heslin, & Moore, 2018). Figure 1–4 shows the increase in maternal morbidity from 2006 to 2015. Rate of severe maternal morbidity at birth increased 45% from 2006 to 2015, from 101.3 to 146.6 per 10,000 hospitalizations for birth (Fingar et al., 2018). Age of mother is a factor in the outcome of the baby. Figure 1–5 shows the differences in infant, neonatal, and postnatal mortality based on maternal age (Ely, Driscoll, & Matthews, 2018). The highest rates of adverse outcomes were at the extremes of maternal age. Babies of teen mothers and women aged ≥40 years had worse outcomes.

Cesarean Birth

Cesarean birth is an often-mentioned factor in the rise in maternal morbidity and mortality, mainly due to hemorrhage and placental abnormalities in subsequent pregnancies (Korb, Goffinet, Seco, Chevret, & Deneux-Tharaux, 2019). Cesarean births have risen from 4.5% in 1965 to 31.9% in 2018—more than a 600% increase (Fig. 1–6) (Hamilton, Martin, Osterman, & Rosen, 2019). Figure 1–7 shows the most common types of maternal morbidity based on method of birth including blood transfusion, ruptured uterus, unplanned hysterectomy, and admission to the intensive care unit (Curtin, Gregory, Korst, & Uddin, 2015).

teenage mothers decreased during this period, births to women from 35 to 39 years and 40 to 44 years increased significantly. Maternal age is associated with more morbidity including diabetes, hypertension, and heart disease. In a recent report from the Agency for

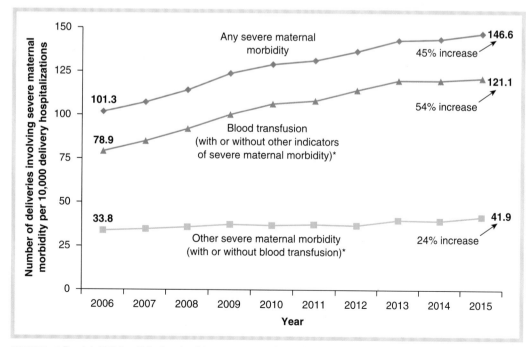

FIGURE 1–4. Trends in birth hospitalizations involving severe maternal morbidity from 2006 to 2015. *If a birth involved blood transfusion and 1 of the other 20 types of severe maternal morbidity, the birth was counted in both categories. (From Fingar, K. F., Hambrick, M. M., Heslin, K. C., & Moore, J. E. [2018]. *Trends and disparities in delivery hospitalizations involving severe maternal morbidity, 2006–2015* [Statistical Brief No. 243]. Rockville, MD: Agency for Healthcare Research and Quality.)

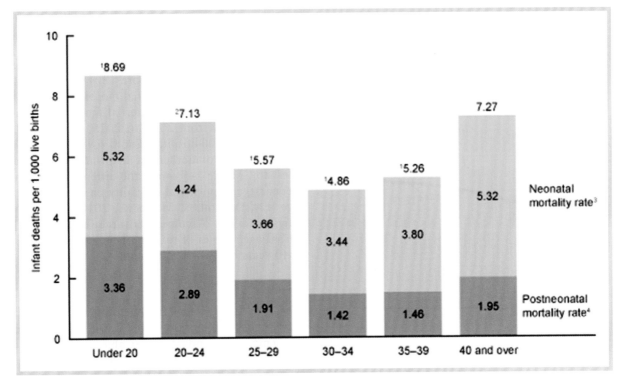

FIGURE 1–5. Infant, neonatal, and postnatal mortality rates by maternal age in 2016. [1]Significantly different from all other maternal age groups ($p < 0.05$). [2]Significantly different from all other maternal age groups except aged 40 and over ($p < 0.05$). [3]Significant difference between all age groups except between those under age 20 and aged 40 and over, and between those aged 25–29 and 35–39 ($p < 0.05$). [4]Significant difference between all age groups except between those aged 25–29 and 40 and over, and between those aged 30–34 and 35–39 ($p < 0.05$). Notes: Total neonatal and postneonatal mortality rates may not sum to totals due to rounding. (From Ely, D. M., Driscoll, A. K., & Matthews, T. J. [2018]. *Infant mortality by age at death in the United States, 2016* [NCHS Data Brief, No. 326]. Hyattsville, MD: National Center for Health Statistics.)

Racial and Ethnic Disparities

Similar to data reported by the CDC (2019b; Petersen et al., 2019), the report based on the nine states' maternal mortality review (Building U.S. Capacity to Review and Prevent Maternal Deaths, 2018) found wide variations in adverse outcomes based on race and ethnicity of the mother and baby. Non-Hispanic White women and non-Hispanic Black women differed in cause of death. Cardiovascular and coronary conditions (15.5%), hemorrhage (14.4%), infection (13.4%),

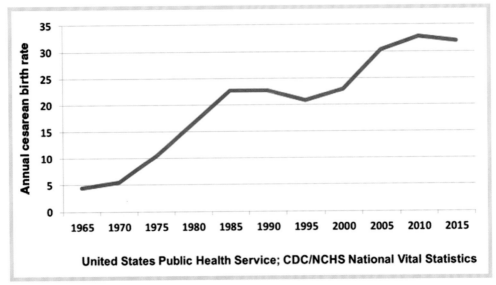

FIGURE 1–6. Trends in cesarean birth in the United States from 1965 to 2015. (From Centers for Disease Control and Prevention/National Center for Health Statistics, National Vital Statistics System.)

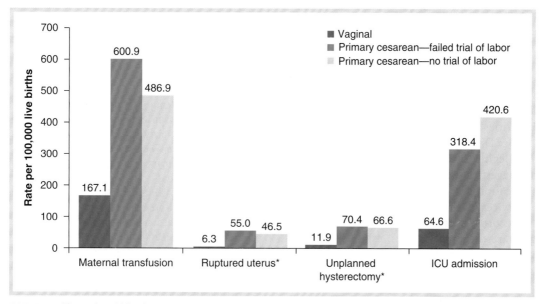

FIGURE 1–7. Maternal morbidity for women without a prior cesarean birth by method of birth and trial of labor (41 states and District of Columbia in 2013). Note: The birth certificate reporting area represented 90% of all U.S. births in 2013. ICU, intensive care unit. *Difference in rates between Primary cesarean–failed trial of labor and Primary cesarean–no trial of labor is statistically significant. (From Curtin, S. C., Gregory, K. D., Korst, L. M., & Uddin, S. F. [2015]. Maternal morbidity for vaginal and cesarean deliveries, according to previous cesarean history: New data from the birth certificate, 2013. *National Vital Statistics Reports*, 64[4], 1–13.)

mental health conditions (11.3%), and cardiomyopathy (10.3%) were leading causes for White women, whereas cardiomyopathy (14%), cardiovascular and coronary conditions (12.8%), preeclampsia and eclampsia (11.6%), hemorrhage (10.5%), and embolism (9.3%) were leading cause for Black women (Building U.S. Capacity to Review and Prevent Maternal Deaths, 2018).

The AHRQ report on maternal morbidity found that although on average Black mothers were younger than White mothers, the rate of severe maternal morbidity was 112% to 115% higher for Black mothers than for White mothers in 2006 (164 vs. 76) and 2015 (241 vs. 114) (Fingar et al., 2018). Although deaths decreased for all races/ethnicities from 2006 to 2015, in-hospital mortality was 3 times higher for Black mothers than for White mothers in 2015 (11 vs. 4 per 100,000 births). Infant mortality is likewise associated with maternal race and ethnicity. Outcomes for babies differ by race and ethnicity (CDC, 2019a). Figure 1–8 shows infant mortality rates by race and ethnicity for 2016. Non-Hispanic Black babies had worse outcomes than those of other races and ethnic groups.

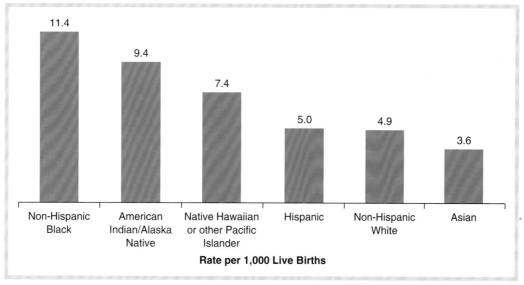

FIGURE 1–8. Infant mortality rates by race and ethnicity, 2016. (From Centers for Disease Control and Prevention/National Center for Health Statistics, National Vital Statistics System.)

It is important to note that instead of race as a factor, racism and racial inequity in how healthcare is available, accessed, and provided are more likely causative (Howell et al., 2018). Race and ethnicity are factors that cannot be modified; however, racism must be acknowledged, addressed, and eliminated. A patient safety bundle "Reduction of Peripartum Racial and Ethnic Disparities" was recently published (Howell et al., 2018). See Display 1–3 (Council on Patient Safety in Women's Health Care, 2016). The bundle offers a number of suggestions on topics such as patient and caregiver education; making sure everyone who needs interpreter services gets them; easier patients' access to their health records; promoting shared decision making; being aware of implicit biases; establishing ways for patients, families, and caregivers to report care that is not respectful or equitable; enhancing discharge teaching including warning signs of potential postpartum complications; offering better coordinated care after hospital discharge for childbirth; and examining care processes and operations for disparities based on race or ethnicity. These recommendations have now been supplemented by a conceptual framework and consensus statement prepared by the bundle workgroup, which details many of the issues behind the racial and ethnic disparities in care and outcomes for minority women in the United States (Howell et al., 2018). The focus is on modifiable causes and potential solutions to promoting safe and equitable healthcare during childbirth (Howell et al., 2018).

Underlying factors in racial and ethnic disparities in healthcare include challenges in knowing the full scope of the problem because issues involving healthcare disparities are not well studied; lack of recognition or awareness of inequitable care; lack of appreciation of the social determinants of health, poverty, and long-standing disadvantages; fragmented care through pregnancy, birth, and postpartum; miscommunication; poor communication; language and cultural barriers to understanding health information; and general misconception of etiologies and potentially successful strategies for improvement (Howell et al., 2018). Bundle workgroup experts offer suggestions for improvement including learning about personal, institutional, and system implicit biases and ways to tackle each of these problems (Howell et al., 2018). Mindfulness and applying the just culture framework to equitable care may be beneficial. Advocating for processes to identify, report, and remedy instances of bias and inequitable healthcare has merit. Implicit bias can be addressed with self-awareness, a focus on concern for others (a characteristic of the vast majority of caregivers in all disciplines), and leadership support from the top of the organization and all others. Eliminating racism in the healthcare system has the potential to reduce the disparity between women and babies of different races and ethnicity and promote healthier outcomes.

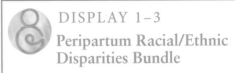

DISPLAY 1–3
Peripartum Racial/Ethnic Disparities Bundle

Readiness

Every Health System

- Establish systems to accurately document self-identified race, ethnicity, and primary language.
  - Provide system-wide education and training for all clinicians and team members on how to ask demographic intake questions.
  - Ensure that patients understand why race, ethnicity, and language data are being collected.
  - Ensure that race, ethnicity, and language data are accessible in the electronic medical record.
  - Evaluate non-English language proficiency (e.g., Spanish proficiency) for providers who communicate with patients in languages other than English.
  - Educate all clinicians and team members (e.g., inpatient, outpatient, community based) on interpreter services available within the healthcare system.
- Provide education for all clinicians and team members on
  - Peripartum racial and ethnic disparities and their root causes
  - Best practices for shared decision making
- Engage diverse patient, family, and community advocates who can represent important community partnerships on quality and safety leadership teams.

Recognition and Prevention

Every Patient, Family, and Staff Member

- Provide education for all clinicians and team members on implicit bias.
- Provide convenient access to health records without delay (paper or electronic), at minimal to no fee to the maternal patient, in a clear and simple format that summarizes information most pertinent to perinatal care and wellness.
- Establish a mechanism for patients, families, and staff to report inequitable care and episodes of miscommunication or disrespect.

Response

Every Clinical Encounter

- Engage in best practices for shared decision making.
- Ensure a timely and tailored response to each report of inequity or disrespect.
- Address reproductive life plan and contraceptive options not only during or immediately after pregnancy but at regular intervals throughout a woman's reproductive life.
- Establish discharge navigation and coordination systems after childbirth to ensure that women have appropriate follow-up care and understand when it is necessary to return to their healthcare provider.
  - Provide discharge instructions that include information about what danger or warning signs to look out for, whom to call, and where to go if they have a question or concern.
  - Design discharge materials that meet patients' health literacy, language, and cultural needs.

From Council on Patient Safety in Women's Health Care. (2016). *Reduction of peripartum racial/ethnic disparities.* Washington, DC: American College of Obstetricians and Gynecologists.

DISPLAY 1-4

Never Events in the Perinatal Setting

- Infant abduction
- Infant death or serious disability (kernicterus) associated with failure to identify and treat neonatal hyperbilirubinemia
- Infant discharged to the wrong person
- Maternal or infant death or serious disability associated with a hemolytic reaction resulting from the administration of ABO-incompatible blood or blood products
- Maternal death or serious disability associated with labor and birth in a low-risk pregnancy in a healthcare facility
- Maternal or infant death or serious disability associated with a medication error, for example, errors involving the wrong drug, wrong dose, wrong patient, wrong time, wrong rate, wrong preparation, or wrong route of administration (includes overdose of oxytocin, misoprostol, and magnesium sulfate)
- Death or serious injury of a neonate associated with labor or birth in a low-risk pregnancy
- Wrong surgical procedure performed on a mother or infant (e.g., circumcision, tubal ligation)
- Retention of a foreign object in a mother or infant after surgery or other procedure
- Artificial insemination with the wrong donor sperm or procedure involving wrong egg

Suggested Additions
- Infant breastfed by wrong mother or breast milk given to wrong infant
- Death or serious disability of a fetus/infant with a category II fetal heart rate (FHR) pattern on mother's admission for labor,

that was not acted on in a timely manner, barring any acute unpredictable event
- Prolapsed umbilical cord after elective rupture of membranes with the fetus at high station
- Prolonged periods of untreated uterine tachysystole during oxytocin or misoprostol administration
- Prolonged periods of a category II or III FHR pattern during labor unrecognized and/or untreated with the usual intrauterine resuscitation techniques
- Fundal pressure during birth involving shoulder dystocia
- Ruptured uterus following prostaglandin administration for cervical ripening/labor induction to a woman with a known uterine surgical scar
- Missed administration of RhoGam to a mother who is an appropriate candidate
- Circumcision without pain relief measures
- Neonatal group B streptococcus or HIV infection after missed intrapartum chemoprophylaxis
- Infant death or disability after multiple attempts with multiple instruments to attempt an operative vaginal birth
- Infant death or disability after prolonged periods of sustained coached second-stage labor pushing efforts without intrauterine resuscitation measures during a category II or III FHR pattern
- Death or serious injury of an infant during the first 2 hours postpartum when the mother or baby has been left unattended
- Death or serious injury of an infant while breastfeeding or being held in the arms of the new mother when the mother has been told that 24/7 rooming-in is the only option in the maternity unit

Adapted from National Quality Forum. (2011). *List of serious reportable events.* Washington, DC: Author; Simpson, K. R. (2006). Obstetrical "never events." *MCN: The American Journal of Maternal/Child Nursing, 31*(2), 136.

THREATS TO PATIENT SAFETY

In 2002, the National Quality Forum published a list of serious reportable events, also known as *never events*. They have been updated over the years, with the last update in 2011 (NQF, 2011). Suggestions have been made for additional events specific to the perinatal setting (Display 1–4) (Simpson, 2006). Recent data on sentinel events reported to The Joint Commission (2019b) from 2015 to 2018 indicate that these issues still require attention. There are numerous threats to patient safety and high-quality maternity care. Each participant and stakeholder bring factors, preferences, and considerations to the process and outcome of childbirth.

Clinicians working in a flawed system are often challenged to provide safe, high-quality care (Simpson, 2018a). Dedicated clinicians in these conditions are at risk for stress, burnout, and involvement in a preventable adverse outcome. There has been an appropriate focus on systems as major contributing factors to adverse outcomes instead of blaming individual clinicians. Clinicians involved in an error or adverse event

often suffer negative consequences for months and years after. Clinicians have responsibilities for speaking up when they see an unsafe situation; keeping up on the latest evidence, standards, and guidelines; supporting colleagues; and not participating in disruptive behavior. Partnering with patients, respecting their autonomy, and making sure they have enough information and in a format that they understand for decision making are responsibilities of individual clinicians (Simpson, 2019). Display 1–5 lists some common threats and risks and offers potential solutions. The list is not all inclusive.

EVOLVING SOLUTIONS

Collaboration Using Best Evidence

Adopting clinical guidelines based on rigorous evidence can occur by a variety of strategies. Individual hospitals and healthcare systems can initiate change or they can be part of participation in statewide quality improvement collaboratives. Within either framework,

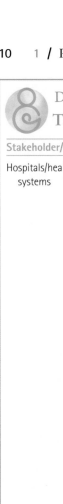

DISPLAY 1–5

Threats to Perinatal Patient Safety and High-Quality Maternity Care

Stakeholder/setting	Threat/risk	Recommendations/potential strategies for improvement
Hospitals/health care systems	Prioritizing cost, convenience, or provider preferences over what is best for mothers and babies	Each unit operation should be based on the answer to the question "What is best for mothers and babies?" Cost, convenience, and provider preferences should be secondary considerations in a high-quality healthcare system.
	Prioritizing graduate medical education over what is best for mothers and babies	Administrative and clinical leaders must acknowledge that quality evidence-based patient care, patient safety, and optimal patient outcomes are the primary goals of hospital and healthcare system. Graduate medical education is a secondary and compatible goal. Proper supervision of trainees and patient consent are essential as part of the process.
	Failure to hold leaders accountable for adopting evidence-based national standards and guidelines	Evidence-based national standards and guidelines are the hallmark of safe, high-quality perinatal care. Establish processes in which new standards and guidelines promulgated by professional associations and other pertinent bodies are reviewed on monthly basis and plans made for adoption in a timely manner.
	Failure to financially and administratively support clinician leaders in participating in perinatal quality care collaboratives and quality improvement initiatives	Participation in quality care collaboratives and other similar quality improvement processes often meet with resistance. Active participation requires support including a person designated to lead the project, persons to monitor practices, allocation of times for lead participants, and resources for data collection.
	Failure to hold leaders accountable for professional behavior and not acting in the context of disruptive clinician behavior including sexual harassment	Zero-tolerance polices similar to those recommended by The Joint Commission (2016) and professional organizations such as ACOG (2017) and American Nurses Association (ANA, 2015b) should be in place.
	Failure to support and protect clinicians who speak up in the context of threats to patient safety	The ANA *Code of Ethics for Nurses* details nursing responsibilities for speaking up to advocate for the rights, health, and safety of patients and the nurse's primary commitment to the patient. Administrative and clinical leaders must support the nurse in these efforts and protect them from retaliation if it occurs (ANA, 2015a).
		ACOG (2009) committee opinion on patient safety outlines how all clinicians have responsibility of speaking up and should be able to do so without fear of retribution.
		A joint publication from AWHONN, ACNM, ACOG, and SMFM offers further guidance on effective professional communication and support of those who speak up as needed to promote and protect patient safety (Lyndon et al., 2015).
	Failure to financially support following the AWHONN (2010) and AAP and ACOG (2017) nurse staffing guidelines for safe, quality care during hospitalization for childbirth	Administrative team leaders should review, budget for, and support following the nurse staffing guidelines (AAP & ACOG, 2017; AWHONN, 2010).
	Failure to financially support offering continuing education for the clinical team, including a nurse responsible for orientation and continuing nursing education	The importance of education, training, and competence validation care is critical to the provision of safe, high-quality care. Accreditation bodies require evidence of this process.
Perinatal services	Failure to have policies, procedures, protocols, and algorithms based on national standards and guidelines	*Guidelines for Perinatal Care* (AAP & ACOG, 2017) detail the need for perinatal services to have these types of resources available. AWHONN, ACNM, AAP, ACOG, ASA, and SMFM each offer numerous publications and clinical guidelines available on their Web site. Some require membership to access; most do not.
	Failure to make sure all clinicians are competent in knowledge and skills for the responsibilities they are assigned	AWHONN (2013) offers details of knowledge and skills required to care for childbearing women. *Guidelines for Perinatal Care* (AAP & ACOG, 2017) detail the need for all clinicians to be competent in their area of practice.

(continued)

DISPLAY 1–5

Threats to Perinatal Patient Safety and High-Quality Maternity Care *(Continued)*

Stakeholder/setting	Threat/risk	Recommendations/potential strategies for improvement
	Failure to follow the AWHONN (2010) and AAP and ACOG (2017) nurse staffing guidelines for safe quality care during hospitalization for childbirth. Specific areas of concern include one nurse to no more than three patients for OB triage; one nurse for each woman in labor with complications; one nurse for each woman in labor receiving IV oxytocin; at least two nurses at every birth (one for mother and one for baby), a full 2-hour recovery after every birth with a nurse in attendance and no other patient assignment; no more than three mother–baby couplets per nurse; a nurse and a nursery available to care for newborns as per the mother's choice; and a nurse with knowledge and skill to help women achieve their breastfeeding goals.	Review, budget for, and support following the nurse staffing guidelines (AAP & ACOG, 2017; AWHONN, 2010).
	Inflexible, restrictive policies and practices and unit operations that inhibit the choices of childbearing women and families including visitors/support persons, 24-hour mandatory rooming-in, and video recording	Support women in their choices for childbirth. Respect their autonomy. Offer information that is comprehensible, literacy level appropriate, and in a language they understand (provide interpretive services as necessary). If patient safety precludes granting their requests, thoroughly explain rationale and offer alternatives (National Quality Forum, 2018).
Clinicians	Failure to keep up with evidence, standards, and guidelines specific to their area of clinical practice	Membership in professional organizations specific to area of practice such as AWHONN, ACNM, ACOG, ASA, AAP, and SMFM is an essential aspect of keeping up with current evidence, standards, and guidelines. Develop processes to actively seek information about new evidence, standards, and guidelines as they are published. Seek certification in specific area of practice such as electronic fetal monitoring and inpatient obstetrics.
	Failure to follow national standards and guidelines	National standards and guidelines are available; unit policies, procedures, practices, protocols, and algorithms should offer details. Safe, high-quality care is based on standardized evidence-based national standards and guidelines. AWHONN, ACNM, AAP, ACOG, ASA, and SMFM each offer numerous publications and clinical guidelines available on their Web site. Some require membership to access; most do not.
	Disruptive behavior	Each clinician has a personal responsibility to act in a professional manner in all professional interactions. These resources can be helpful in offering review of behaviors and expectations (ACOG, 2009; ANA, 2015a, 2015b). A joint publication from AWHONN, ACNM, ACOG, and SMFM offers further guidance on effective professional communication and support of those who speak up as needed to promote and protect patient safety (Lyndon et al., 2015).
	Attitudes and care practices that do not respect autonomy of childbearing women	Be open; listen to women. Support women in their choices for childbirth. Respect their autonomy. Offer information that is comprehensible, literacy level appropriate, and in a language they understand (provide interpretive services as necessary). If patient safety precludes granting their requests, thoroughly explain rationale and offer alternatives (National Quality Forum, 2018).

AAP, American Academy of Pediatrics; ACNM, American College of Nurse-Midwives; ACOG, American College of Obstetricians and Gynecologists; ASA, American Society of Anesthesiologists; AWHONN, Association of Women's Health, Obstetric and Neonatal Nurses; SMFM, Society for Maternal-Fetal Medicine.

the change is initially led by innovative leaders trying to make a positive difference in outcomes for mothers and babies. Their efforts are often initially met with resistance. Comprehensive perinatal patient safety initiatives that are based on adopting evidence-based standardized clinical protocols and guidelines, promoting professional collaboration through improving teamwork and unit culture, and measuring outcomes have shown promise in reducing adverse obstetric events and professional liability, including number of claims and costs of claims (Clark et al., 2008; Pettker et al., 2014; Pettker et al., 2009; Pettker et al., 2011; Simpson et al., 2009). As perinatal patient safety and quality improvement have become widespread, and measures have been initiated by accrediting bodies and regulatory agencies, acceptance and participation have increased. Hospitals accredited by The Joint Commission (2018) with at least 300 live births per year are required to report on the perinatal care core measures listed in Display 1–6.

The Joint Commission released information in August 2019 about new standards to keep mothers safe during childbirth that will be effective July 1, 2020 for their accredited hospitals. The focus of the new standards for maternal safety are to reduce likelihood of harm related to maternal hemorrhage and severe hypertension and preeclampsia (The Joint Commission, 2019a). For postpartum hemorrhage, the standards involve establishing written clinical protocols, a postpartum hemorrhage supply kit, education of clinicians, hemorrhage drills, case reviews, and patient education on signs and symptoms of postpartum hemorrhage and when and how to seek care for these symptoms after hospital discharge (The Joint Commission). The standards for severe hypertension and preeclampsia include accurate and timely blood pressure measurement, clinician education, case reviews, severe hypertension drills patient education on signs and symptoms of severe hypertension and preeclampsia, when and how to seek care for these symptoms after hospital discharge, and when to schedule follow-up postpartum care (The Joint Commission).

The AIM program of the Council on Patient Safety in Women's Health Care (2016), which has partnered with most of the leading professional organizations for maternal health in the United States including AWHONN, ACNM, ACOG, SMFM, the American Academy of Family Physicians, and the Health Resources and Services Administration Maternal and Child Health Bureau of the U.S. Department of Health and Human Services, is a coalition working to collectively promote safe maternity care for all women through maternal patient safety research, programs and tools, education, dissemination, and promotion of a culture of respect, transparency, and accountability. The goal is to decrease the number of severe maternal morbidity events by 100,000 and to avoid at least 1,000 maternal deaths (AIM, 2016). As of April 2019, 26 states are participating, with more expected soon (ACOG, 2019). The AIM program has collaboratively developed various maternal safety bundles including obstetric hemorrhage; severe hypertension/preeclampsia; maternal prevention of venous thromboembolism; safe reduction of primary cesareans/support for intended vaginal birth; reduction of peripartum racial disparities; postpartum care basics for maternal safety; and patient, family, and staff support after a severe maternal event (AIM, 2016). Each bundle is formatted similarly with key aspects of readiness, recognition and prevention, response, and reporting/systems learning and focuses on giving the best care to every woman in every setting whenever an event occurs (AIM, 2016). Each aspect of the framework includes key points for every woman, care giver and provider, and birthing facility as applicable. References to supportive evidence are likewise organized in this framework (Council on Patient Safety in Women's Health Care, 2016).

DISPLAY 1–6

The Joint Commission Perinatal Care Core Measures Effective January 2019

Measure	Brief definition
Elective Delivery	Women with elective vaginal birth or elective cesarean birth at ≥37 and <39 completed weeks of gestation
PC-02: Cesarean Birth	Nulliparous women with a term, singleton baby in a vertex position born by cesarean
PC-03: Antenatal Steroids	Women at risk for preterm birth at ≥24 and <34 weeks' gestation receiving antenatal steroids prior to giving birth to preterm newborns
PC-04: Health Care- Associated Bloodstream Infections in Newborns	Staphylococcal and gram-negative septicemias or bacteremias in high-risk newborns
PC-05: Exclusive Breast Milk Feeding	Exclusive breast milk feeding during the newborn's entire hospitalization
PC-06: Unexpected Complications in Term Newborns	The percentage of babies with unexpected newborn complications among full-term newborns with no preexisting conditions

From The Joint Commission. (2018). New perinatal care measure. *Perspectives, 38*(8), 7–8.

DISPLAY 1–7
Patient Safety Bundles and Tools

- Maternal Mental Health: Depression and Anxiety
- Maternal Venous Thromboembolism (+AIM)
- Obstetric Care for Women with Opioid Use Disorder (+AIM)
- Obstetric Hemorrhage (+AIM)
- Postpartum Care Basics for Maternal Safety
  - From Birth to the Comprehensive Postpartum Visit (+AIM)
  - Transition from Maternity to Well-Woman Care (+AIM)
- Prevention of Retained Vaginal Sponges After Birth
- Reduction of Peripartum Racial/Ethnic Disparities (+AIM)
- Safe Reduction of Primary Cesarean Birth (+AIM)
- Severe Hypertension in Pregnancy (+AIM)
- Severe Maternal Morbidity Review (+AIM)
- Support After a Severe Maternal Event (+AIM)

AIM, Alliance for Innovation on Maternal Health.
Available at https://safehealthcareforeverywoman.org/patient-safety-bundles/

DISPLAY 1–8
California Maternal Quality Care Collaborative Toolkits

- Improving Health Care Response to Maternal Venous Thromboembolism, 2018
- Improving Health Care Response to Cardiovascular Disease in Pregnancy and Postpartum, 2017
- Toolkit to Support Vaginal Birth and Reduce Primary Cesareans and Implementation Guide, 2016
- Improving Health Care Response to Obstetric Hemorrhage, V2.0, 2015 (V1.0 released in 2010)
- Improving Health Care Response to Preeclampsia, 2014
- Elimination of Non-medically Indicated (Elective) Deliveries Before 39 Weeks Gestational Age, 2010 (Licensed to March of Dimes)

Available at https://www.cmqcc.org/resources-tool-kits/toolkits

The council also offers a Maternal Early Warning Signs (MEWS) Protocol and a toolkit for Implementing Quality Improvement Projects. There are abundant evidence-based resources available at no charge from the council and from other organizations. Nurses and other members of the multidisciplinary team that provide maternity care should be familiar with these bundles, tools, and references. Display 1–7 lists some of the AIM patient safety bundles.

Although individual hospitals can make a significant difference, working with a multidisciplinary team in a variety of clinical settings in many states has the potential to raise the impact of these collective efforts exponentially. This premise is the foundation of the National Network of Perinatal Quality Collaboratives sponsored by the CDC (Henderson et al., 2018; Simpson, 2018b). The program was initiated in 2016 by the CDC and the March of Dimes Foundation. The main goal is to assist statewide perinatal quality collaboratives in their work to improve care and outcomes for mothers and babies (Gupta, Donovan, & Henderson, 2017). Many states have perinatal quality collaboratives, although there are a variety of organizational structures, clinical goals, funding, and leadership teams. The CDC offers a resource guide on how to develop and sustain a perinatal quality collaborative.

Some state programs, such as the one in California, have been in operation for many years and have robust data collection processes, widespread participation, and developed a number of helpful resources. The California Maternal Quality Care Collaborative (CMQCC) has multiple well-developed toolkits for maternal patient safety as well including topics such as obstetric hemorrhage, promoting vaginal birth, reducing

primary cesareans and preeclampsia, and elimination of nonmedically indicated births before 39 weeks' gestation. Display 1–8 lists some of the CMQCC toolkits. They describe current evidence and suggest strategies for promoting best practices on each topic. California is the only state where maternal mortality rates have decreased over the past 14 years (MacDorman, Declercq, Cabral, & Morton, 2016). The difference between California and the rest of the United States is likely due to intensive team efforts between hospitals, healthcare systems, professional organizations, and public health agencies to address some of the major complications from obstetric hemorrhage and preeclampsia, via encouragement to adopt evidence-based protocols sponsored by CMQCC. This work was not easy, and there were many ongoing challenges, but by perseverance and working together as an interprofessional team, adoption and implementation have been successful in many participating hospitals (Lyndon & Cape, 2016).

Perinatal quality collaboratives have produced excellent results including a decrease in healthcare-associated bloodstream infections in newborn babies (Gupta et al., 2017), fewer elective births before 39 completed weeks of gestation (Kacica, Glantz, Xiong, Shields, & Cherouny, 2017; Simpson, Knox, Martin, George, & Watson, 2011), a lower cesarean birth rate (Main et al., 2019), and a decline in severe pregnancy complications (Main et al., 2017). Success in part is due to the team approach. These efforts are not led by individual physicians, nurses, or hospital administrators; rather, they are initiated by clinicians, researchers, and public health experts with a stake in perinatal outcomes such as midwives, perinatal and neonatal nurses, obstetricians, maternal–fetal medicine specialists, neonatologists, pediatricians, and family medicine physicians. New mothers are an essential part of the group, and their voices are highly valued. The ongoing results of perinatal quality collaboratives provide evidence that clinicians from many professional disciplines can work together for a common goal.

Mothers and babies can benefit from standardized clinical protocols for the most common maternity care situations. When everyone has reviewed the evidence, practiced using drills, knows the step-by-step plan in an emergent situation, and works as a team in a culture of safety with mutual respect and collaboration, there is the best chance for healthy outcomes. Many aspects of maternal morbidity and mortality are preventable (Council on Patient Safety in Women's Health Care, 2016). Standardized clinical protocols for maternity care may offer an opportunity to reduce risk of preventable harm.

Partnering with Patients and Families for Shared Decision Making during Childbirth

Childbearing women have the most vested interest in their pregnancy and outcome, and they know their bodies and their preferences, concerns, and fears best. Safe, high-quality care begins with listening to women, followed by making efforts to meet their needs and desires. Choice of prenatal care setting, care provider, and birth place all have significant implications for the process and outcome of childbirth. It is important to consider that some women do not have these choices because they are in situations based on where they live, their socioeconomic status, and insurance coverage in which access to care is challenging and continuity of care is minimal.

When a woman presents in labor, often, she goes along with directions from nurses, midwives, and physicians during the childbirth process, trusting that they know best (Sakala, Declercq, Turon, & Corry, 2018; Simpson, Newman, & Chirino, 2010). Some women have a birth plan, but most do not. In a study that included 14,630 births, only 12% of women had a birth plan and less than one third had attended prepared childbirth classes (Afshar et al., 2017). Women often seek childbirth information online, but not all sites offer accurate data (English, Alden, Zomorodi, Travers, & Ross, 2018; Sakala et al., 2018).

During childbirth hospitalization, many clinical events involve choice (Display 1–9). The list is not all inclusive. Most allow ample time for detailed conversation and patient consent. Information should be provided at the appropriate literacy level and language. Interpreter services should be used as needed. Women should be treated as true partners in their care. Shared

DISPLAY 1–9

Events and Options during the Childbirth Process that Warrant Confirming Patient Knowledge or Offering Additional Information so She and Her Family Can Make an Informed Decision

Whether or not to be admitted based on labor status and maternal–fetal condition

Cervical ripening, induction, or augmentation of labor (if any, what type)

Intravenous line placement and oral intake

Type of fetal assessment (intermittent auscultation, continuous or intermittent electronic fetal monitoring; external or internal)

Evaluation of labor progress

Hydrotherapy via shower or tub

Pain relief measures including epidural analgesia

Ambulation; use of the peanut ball; positioning

Artificial rupture of membranes

When to begin pushing during second stage labor and type of pushing method

Method of birth

Episiotomy

Skin-to-skin contact with the newborn after birth

Method of newborn feeding

Routine newborn care and rooming-in

Circumcision

Participation of trainees in their care including nursing, midwifery, or medical students or resident physicians in training

Support persons in attendance

From Simpson, K. R. (2019). Partnering with patients and families during childbirth: Confirming knowledge for informed consent. *MCN: The American Journal of Maternal/Child Nursing, 44*(3), 180. doi:10.1097/NMC.0000000000000527

decision making involves communication between clinicians and patients to make healthcare decisions that are consistent with key patient preferences (NQF, 2018). Information should be evidence based, unbiased, and individualized and include potential benefits and risks (NQF, 2018). Choice goes beyond clinical decisions. Women's preferences for support persons in her room during labor, birth, and postpartum should be respected. Restrictive policies about "visitors" including who, when, how many, must be immediate family, and so forth need careful scrutiny; in some hospitals (but not most), concerns about space and security limit options. At times, contagious diseases limit options. The woman decides how "family" is defined. Restrictive policies about video recording are outdated. Nurses are ideally positioned as part of the healthcare team to facilitate shared decision making during childbirth.

Maternal Mortality Review Committees

All cases of severe maternal morbidity and maternal mortality should be reviewed by an interdisciplinary quality committee. Criteria for identifying cases for review of severe maternal morbidity have been offered by ACOG and SMFM (2016) and include transfusion of four or more units of blood and admission of a pregnant or postpartum woman to an intensive care unit.

By evaluating processes involved in near-miss cases, lessons can be learned that can potentially avoid maternal deaths. Thorough review of the process of care, such as timely and appropriate diagnosis and treatment, can be extremely useful in developing plans for improvement and potentially preventing a subsequent similar case.

Findings from the nine states' maternal mortality review committees suggest that there are common contributing factors (Building U.S. Capacity to Review and Prevent Maternal Deaths, 2018). They include patients' lack of knowledge on warning signs and the need to seek care, healthcare provider misdiagnosis and ineffective treatments, and systems of care factors such as lack of coordination between providers. Based on these data, the review committees offered a number of recommendations specific to common causes of death. Overall recommendations included adopting levels of maternal care (ACOG & SMFM, 2019), enhancing prevention initiatives, enforcing policies and procedures on obstetric hemorrhage, and improving policies about patient management. Participating in reviews of severe maternal morbidity and maternal mortality at the facility level and as part of a state review committee are opportunities for nurses to be involved as active members in significant efforts to understand causation and develop prevention strategies. Together, we must do better in preventing these types of adverse events.

SUMMARY

On a national level, recommendations for improving the state of maternity care in the United States to reduce maternal mortality include establishing maternal mortality committees in each state, participation in perinatal quality care collaboratives, adoption of standardized practices such as those in the bundles published by the AIM project, expansion of Medicaid for all states, making sure women receive the appropriate care in a facility capable of providing that care including patient transfer as necessary, providing more comprehensive and timely postpartum care, and better reporting of vital statistics data about women and newborns including data stratified by race and ethnicity (ACOG, 2019; SMFM, 2019). Local and national policies must be revised to improve access to maternity care and access to health insurance benefits, reduce healthcare disparities, eliminate racism, and standardize data collection on maternal morbidity and mortality (ACOG, 2019; SMFM, 2019).

In the hospital setting and for each clinician, when the focus of care is putting safety of mothers and babies first, practice based on the cumulative body of science and national standards and guidelines is a natural and obvious conclusion. Partnering with childbearing women and making sure they have enough information to make informed decisions about their care is essential. Keeping current is critically important for perinatal nurses to maximize safe care for mothers and babies and to minimize the risk of patient injuries and professional liability. Effective leadership and interdisciplinary collaboration are essential. When there is mutual respect and professional behavior among all members of the perinatal team, a safe care environment is enhanced. Practice in a perinatal setting where patient safety is the number one priority is professionally rewarding and personally fulfilling.

REFERENCES

Afshar, Y., Wang, E. T., Mei, J., Esakoff, T. F., Pisarska, M. D., & Gregory, K. D. (2017). Childbirth education class and birth plans are associated with a vaginal delivery. *Birth, 44*(1), 29–34. doi:10.1111/birt.12263

Alliance for Innovation on Maternal Health. (2016). *Maternal safety bundles.* Washington, DC: Author. Retrieved from http://www.safehealthcareforeverywoman.org/aim.php

American Academy of Pediatrics & American College of Obstetricians and Gynecologists. (2017). *Guidelines for perinatal care* (8th ed.). Elk Grove Village, IL: Author.

American College of Obstetricians and Gynecologists. (2009). *Patient safety in obstetrics and gynecology* (Committee Opinion No. 447; Reaffirmed, 2019). Washington, DC: Author.

American College of Obstetricians and Gynecologists. (2017). *Behavior that undermines a culture of safety.* (Committee Opinion No. 683). Washington, DC: Author

American College of Obstetricians and Gynecologists. (2019). *How ACOG is combating maternal mortality.* Washington, DC; Author.

American College of Obstetricians and Gynecologists & Society for Maternal-Fetal Medicine. (2019). Levels of maternal care (Obstetric Care Consensus No. 9). *Obstetrics and Gynecology, 134*:e41–e55. doi.org/10.1016/j.ajog.2019.05.046

American College of Obstetricians and Gynecologists & Society for Maternal-Fetal Medicine. (2016). Severe maternal morbidity: Screening and review. *American Journal of Obstetrics and Gynecology, 215*(3), B17–B22. doi:10.1016/j.ajog.2016.07.050

American Nurses Association. (2015a). *Code of ethics for nurses with interpretive statements.* Silver Spring, MD: Author.

American Nurses Association. (2015b). *Incivility, bullying, and workplace violence.* Silver Spring, MD: Author.

Association of Women's Health, Obstetric and Neonatal Nurses. (2010). *Guidelines for professional registered nurse staffing for perinatal units.* Washington, DC: Author.

Association of Women's Health, Obstetric and Neonatal Nurses. (2013). *Basic, high-risk, and critical care intrapartum nursing: Clinical competencies and education guide* (5th ed.). Washington, DC: Author.

Building U.S. Capacity to Review and Prevent Maternal Deaths. (2018). *Report from nine maternal mortality review committees*. Retrieved from http://reviewtoaction.org/Report_from_Nine_MMRCs

Centers for Disease Control and Prevention. (2019a). *Infant mortality*. Atlanta, GA: Author.

Centers for Disease Control and Prevention. (2019b). *Pregnancy mortality surveillance system*. Atlanta, GA: Author.

Clark, S. L., Belfort, M. A., Byrum, S. L., Meyers, J. A., & Perlin, J. B. (2008). Improved outcomes, fewer cesarean deliveries, and reduced litigation: Results of a new paradigm in patient safety. *American Journal of Obstetrics & Gynecology*, 199(2), 105. e1–105.e7. doi:10.1016/j.ajog.2008.02.031

Council on Patient Safety in Women's Health Care. (2016). *Reduction of peripartum racial/ethnic disparities*. Washington, DC: American College of Obstetricians and Gynecologists.

Creanga, A. A. (2018). Maternal mortality in the United States: A review of contemporary data and their limitations. *Clinical Obstetrics and Gynecology*, 61(2), 296–306. doi:10.1097/grf.0000000000000362

Curtin, S. C., Gregory, K. D., Korst, L. M., & Uddin, S. F. (2015). Maternal morbidity for vaginal and cesarean deliveries, according to previous cesarean history: New data from the birth certificate, 2013. *National Vital Statistics Reports*, 64(4), 1–13.

Ellison, K., & Martin, N. (2017). *Severe complications for women during childbirth are skyrocketing—and could often be prevented*. New York: NY: ProPublica.

Ely, D. M., Driscoll, A. K., & Matthews, T. J. (2018). *Infant mortality by age at death in the United States, 2016* (NCHS Data Brief, No. 326). Hyattsville, MD: National Center for Health Statistics.

English, C. L., Alden, K. R., Zomorodi, M., Travers, D., & Ross, M. S. (2018). Evaluation of content on commonly used web sites about induction of labor and pain management during labor. *MCN: The American Journal of Maternal/Child Nursing*, 43(5), 271–277. doi:10.1097/NMC.0000000000000455

Fingar, K. F., Hambrick, M. M., Heslin, K. C., & Moore, J. E. (2018). *Trends and disparities in delivery hospitalizations involving severe maternal morbidity, 2006-2015* (Statistical Brief No. 243). Rockville, MD: Agency for Healthcare Research and Quality.

Gupta, M., Donovan, E. F., & Henderson, Z. (2017). State-based perinatal quality collaboratives: Pursuing improvements in perinatal health outcomes for all mothers and newborns. *Seminars in Perinatology*, 41(3), 195–203. doi:10.1053/j.semperi.2017.03.009

Hamilton, B. E., Martin, J. A., Osterman, M. J. K., & Rosen, L. M. (2019). *Births: Provisional data for 2018* (Vital Statistics Rapid Release Report No. 007). Hyattsville, MD: National Center for Health Statistics.

Henderson, Z. T., Ernst, K., Simpson, K. R., Berns, S. D., Suchdev, D. B., Main, E., . . . Olson, C. K. (2018). The National Network of State Perinatal Quality Collaboratives: A growing movement to improve maternal and infant health. *Journal of Women's Health (Larchmt)*, 27(3), 221–226. doi:10.1089/jwh.2018.6941

Howell, E. A., Brown, H., Brumley, J., Bryant, A. S., Caughey, A. B., Cornell, A. M., . . . Grobman, W. A. (2018). Reduction of peripartum racial and ethnic disparities: A conceptual framework and maternal safety consensus bundle. *Obstetrics and Gynecology*, 131(5), 770–782. doi:10.1097/AOG.0000000000002475

Institute of Medicine. (1999). *To err is human: Building a safer health system*. Washington, DC: National Academies Press.

Institute of Medicine. (2001). *Crossing the quality chasm: A new health system for the 21st century*. Washington, DC: National Academies Press.

Kacica, M. A., Glantz, J. C., Xiong, K., Shields, E. P., & Cherouny, P. H. (2017). A statewide quality improvement initiative to reduce non-medically indicated scheduled deliveries. *Maternal and Child Health Journal*, 21(4), 932–941. doi:10.1007/s10995-016-2196-5

Knox, G. E., & Simpson, K. R. (2011). Perinatal high reliability. *American Journal of Obstetrics and Gynecology*, 204(5), 373–377. doi:10.1016/j.ajog.2010.10.900

Knox, G. E., Simpson, K. R., & Garite, T. J. (1999). High reliability perinatal units: An approach to the prevention of patient injury and medical malpractice claims. *Journal of Healthcare Risk Management*, 19(2), 24–32. doi:10.1002/jhrm.5600190205

Knox, G. E., Simpson, K. R., & Townsend, K. E. (2003). High reliability perinatal units: Further observations and a suggested plan for action. *Journal of Healthcare Risk Management*, 23(4), 17–21.

Korb, D., Goffinet, F., Seco, A., Chevret, S., & Deneux-Tharaux, C. (2019). Risk of severe maternal morbidity associated with cesarean delivery and the role of maternal age: A population-based propensity score analysis. *Canadian Medical Association Journal*, 191(13), E352–E360. doi:10.1503/cmaj.181067

Lyndon, A., & Cape, V. (2016). Maternal hemorrhage quality improvement collaborative lessons. *MCN: The American Journal of Maternal/Child Nursing*, 41(6), E24–E25. doi:10.1097/NMC.0000000000000277

Lyndon, A., Johnson, M. C., Bingham, D., Napolitano, P. G., Joseph, G., Maxfield, D. G., & O'Keefe, D. F. (2015). Transforming communication and safety culture in intrapartum care: A multi-organization blueprint. *Journal of Obstetric, Gynecologic, and Neonatal Nursing*, 44(3), 341–349. doi:10.1111/1552-6909.12575

MacDorman, M. F., Declercq, E., Cabral, H., & Morton, C. (2016). Recent increases in the U.S. maternal mortality rate: Disentangling trends from measurement issues. *Obstetrics and Gynecology*, 128(3), 447–455. doi:10.1097/aog.0000000000001556

Main, E. K., Abreo, A., McNulty, J., Gilbert, W., McNally, C., Poeltler, D., . . . Kilpatrick, S. (2016). Measuring severe maternal morbidity: Validation of potential measures. *American Journal of Obstetrics & Gynecology*, 214(5), 643.e1–643.e10. doi:10.1016/j.ajog.2015.11.004

Main, E. K., Cape, V., Abreo, A., Vasher, J., Woods, A., Carpenter, A., & Gould, J. B. (2017). Reduction of severe maternal morbidity from hemorrhage using a state perinatal quality collaborative. *American Journal of Obstetrics & Gynecology*, 216(3), 298.e1–298.e11. doi:10.1016/j.ajog.2017.01.017

Main, E. K., Chang, S.-C., Cape, V., Sakowski, C., Smith, H., & Vasher, J. (2019). Safety assessment of a large-scale improvement collaborative to reduce nulliparous cesarean delivery rates. *Obstetrics & Gynecology*, 133(4), 613–623. doi:10.1097/AOG.0000000000003109

Martin, J. A., Hamilton, B. E., Osterman, M. J. K., Driscoll, A. K., & Drake, P. (2018). Births: Final data for 2017. *National Vital Statistics Reports*, 67(8), 1–50.

National Quality Forum. (2011). *List of serious reportable events*. Washington, DC: Author.

National Quality Forum. (2018). *National Quality Partners Playbook™: Shared decision making in healthcare*. Washington, DC: Author.

Ozimek, J. A., Eddins, R. M., Greene, N., Karagyozyan, D., Pak, S., Wong, M., . . . Kilpatrick, S. J. (2016). Opportunities for improvement in care among women with severe maternal morbidity. *American Journal of Obstetrics and Gynecology*, 215(4), 509.e1–509.e6. doi:10.1016/j.ajog.2016.05.022

Petersen, E. E., Davis, N. L., Goodman, D., Cox, S., Mayes, N., Johnston, E., . . . Barfield, W. (2019). Vital signs: Pregnancy-related deaths, United States, 2011–2015, and strategies for prevention, 13 States, 2013–2017. *MMWR Morbidity and Mortality Weekly Report*, 68(18), 423–429. doi:10.15585/mmwr.mm6818e1

Pettker, C. M., Thung, S. F., Lipkind, H. S., Illuzzi, J. L., Buhimschi, C. S., Raab, C. A., . . . Funai, E. F. (2014). A comprehensive obstetric patient safety program reduces liability claims and payments. *American Journal of Obstetrics & Gynecology*, 211(4), 319–325. doi:10.1016/j.ajog.2014.04.038

Pettker, C. M., Thung, S. F., Norwitz, E. R., Buhimschi, C. S., Raab, C. A., Copel, J. A., . . . Funai, E. F. (2009). Impact of a comprehensive patient safety strategy on obstetric adverse events. *American Journal of Obstetrics & Gynecology*, 200(5), 492. e1–492.e8.

Pettker, C. M., Thung, S. F., Raab, C. A., Donohue, K. P., Copel, J. A., Lockwood, C. J., & Funai, E. F. (2011). A comprehensive obstetrics patient safety program improves safety climate and culture. *American Journal of Obstetrics & Gynecology, 204*(3), 216.e1–216.e6. doi:10.1016/j.ajog.2010.11.004

Sakala, C., Declercq, E. R., Turon, J. M., & Corry, M. P. (2018). *Listening to mothers in California: A population-based survey of women's childbearing experiences.* Washington, DC: National Partnership for Women & Families.

Simpson, K. R. (2006). Obstetrical "never events." *MCN: The American Journal of Maternal/Child Nursing, 31*(2), 136.

Simpson, K. R. (2014). Perinatal patient safety and professional liability issues. In K. R. Simpson & P. A. Creehan (Eds.), *AWHONN's Perinatal nursing* (4th ed., pp. 1–40). Philadelphia, PA: Lippincott Williams & Wilkins.

Simpson, K. R. (2018a). Emerging trends in perinatal quality and risk with recommendations for patient safety. *Journal of Perinatal & Neonatal Nursing, 32*(1), 15–20. doi:10.1097/jpn .0000000000000294

Simpson, K. R. (2018b). The National Network of Perinatal Quality Collaboratives: Opportunity to enhance the care and outcomes for mothers and babies. *MCN: The American Journal of Maternal/Child Nursing, 43*(3), 125. doi:10.1097/nmc .0000000000000433

Simpson, K. R. (2019). Partnering with patients and families during childbirth: Confirming knowledge for informed consent. *MCN: The American Journal of Maternal/Child Nursing, 44*(3), 180. doi:10.1097/NMC.0000000000000527

Simpson, K. R., Knox, G. E., Martin, M., George, C., & Watson, S. R. (2011). Michigan Health & Hospital Association Keystone Obstetrics: A statewide collaborative for perinatal patient safety in Michigan. *Joint Commission Journal on Quality and Patient Safety, 37*(12), 544–552.

Simpson, K. R., Kortz, C. C., & Knox, G. E. (2009). A comprehensive perinatal patient safety program to reduce preventable adverse outcomes and costs of liability claims. *The Joint Commission Journal on Quality and Patient Safety, 35*(11), 565–574.

Simpson, K. R., Newman, G., & Chirino, O. R. (2010). Patient education to reduce elective labor inductions. *MCN: The American Journal of Maternal/Child Nursing, 35*(4), 188–194. doi:10.1097/NMC.0b013e3181d9c6d6

Society for Maternal-Fetal Medicine. (2019). *Progress toward reducing maternal mortality.* Washington, DC: Author.

The Joint Commission. (2016). *Behaviors that undermine a culture of safety* (Sentinel Event Alert No. 40). Oakbrook Terrace, IL: Author.

The Joint Commission. (2018). New perinatal care measure. *Perspectives, 38*(8), 7–8.

The Joint Commission. (2019a). *Provision of care treatment, and services standards for maternal safety* (R3 Report: Requirement, Rational, Reference, 24, 1–6). Oakbrook Terrace, IL: Author.

The Joint Commission. (2019b). *Summary data of sentinel events reviewed by The Joint Commission.* Oakbrook Terrace, IL: Author.

World Health Organization. (2014). *Trends in maternal mortality: 1990 to 2013. Estimates by WHO, UNICEF, UNFPA, the World Bank and the United Nations Population Division.* Geneva, Switzerland: Author.

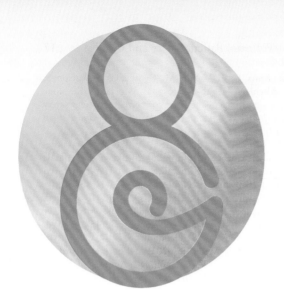

CHAPTER 2

Integrating Cultural Beliefs and Practices When Caring for Childbearing Women and Families

Lynn Clark Callister

INTRODUCTION

All women desire and deserve respectful maternity care that is affirming of their cultural beliefs and practices. Nurses are ideally positioned to make sure all childbearing women receive this type of high-quality care. Being knowledgeable or aware of various culture-specific childbirth practices can be challenging as the United States is quite diverse, with many cultural and ethnic groups that comprise the total population (US Census Bureau [USCB, 2019). In 2019, the USCB estimated that 13.5% of those living in the United States were not born in the United States and 21.5% of those over the age of 5 live in households where a language other than English is spoken at home (USCB, 2019). An overview of select examples of various childbirth practices are presented. While nurses cannot be expected to be familiar with each one, they can apply the framework of respectful maternity care as discussed here to meet the needs of childbearing women.

Clinical examples in this chapter represent only a fraction of the possible cultural beliefs, practices, and behaviors the perinatal nurse may see in practice. It is beyond the scope of this chapter to thoroughly discuss in detail each cultural group. Although generalizations are made about cultural groups, a stereotypical approach to the provision of perinatal nursing care is not appropriate. Cultural beliefs and practices are dynamic and evolving, requiring ongoing exploration. In any given culture, each generation of childbearing families perceives pregnancy, childbirth, and parenting differently. Each individual woman should be treated as such—an individual who may or may not espouse specific cultural beliefs, practices, and behaviors.

Cultures are not limited to the obvious traditional ethnic or racial groups. Examples of other "cultures" include refugees and immigrants, poverty-stricken women, women who have experienced ritual circumcision, adolescent childbearing women, women with disabilities, and deeply spiritual women such as those espousing their religious beliefs. Perinatal nursing units may also be considered a culture, for some women a "foreign country."

Maria, a Mexican American woman having her first baby, attended a childbirth education class where the expectant fathers learned labor support techniques. She declined to lie on the floor surrounded by other men while her husband massaged her abdomen. Inaam, a Muslim Arabic woman experiencing her first labor, was attended by her mother and mother-in-law. As the labor slowly progressed and Inaam began to be more uncomfortable, the two mothers alternated between offering her loving support, chastising her for acting like a child, and praying loudly that mother and baby will be safe from harm. Nguyet, a primiparous Vietnamese immigrant, had been in the United States only a short time when she went into labor. She arrived at the birthing unit in active labor dilated to 5 cm. Nguyet and the father of the baby, Duc, spoke very limited English. Her labor was difficult, but she did not utter a sound. Duc entered the birthing room only when the nurses asked him to translate for Nguyet. After 20 hours of labor, a cesarean birth was performed. On the mother–baby unit, Nguyet cooperated with the instructions from the nurse to cough and deep breathe, but she did not want to have a bed bath when the nurse offered. When she was encouraged to walk, she shook her head and refused. She also did not drink the chilled apple juice the nurse brought to her. Because of abdominal distention and dehydration, a nasogastric tube was inserted, and intravenous fluids were restarted. No one could understand why she appeared to be uncooperative.

Because of a concerning fetal heart rate tracing, Koua Khang needed an emergent cesarean birth. The nurse told her she would need to remove a nondescript white string bracelet from her wrist before surgery. Koua became upset, gesturing and trying to convey the message that the bracelet would protect her during the birth from evil spirits. Michelle, a certified nurse midwife, cared for a Mexican immigrant mother who finally confided in her that during her postpartum hospitalization she went in the shower and turned on the water but was very careful not to get wet. She was following instructions from her nurse while trying to practice her own cultural traditions. Mei Lin, a Chinese woman in graduate school in the United States, promised her mother she would follow traditional Asian practices after her son was born, including "doing the month" and subscribing to the hot/cold theory. Even though this woman was intellectually aware these practices had little scientific basis, she demonstrated her respect for her mother and her culture by honoring her mother's request. Sameena was having a scheduled cesarean birth. Her family had a tradition that the newborn be placed immediately in a blanket that had been in the family for generations but were concerned that since it was a surgical birth, the tradition would not be followed. The nurses accommodated this cultural tradition, and the blanket was placed inside the hospital receiving blanket when their child was born. The grandmother was pleased and grateful.

Childbirth is a time of transition and social celebration in all cultures (Callister, 1995). A Wintu child living in Africa, in deference to his mother, refers to her as, "She whom I made into mother." Culture also influences the experience of perinatal loss because the meaning of death and rituals surrounding death are culturally bound. Healthcare beliefs and health-seeking behaviors surrounding pregnancy, childbirth, and parenting are deeply rooted in cultural context. Culture is a set of behaviors, beliefs, and practices, a value system that is transmitted from one woman in a cultural group to another (Lauderdale, 2011). It is more than skin color, language, or country of origin. Culture provides a framework within which women think, make decisions, and act. It is the essence of who a woman is. The extent to which a woman adheres to cultural practices, beliefs, and rituals is complex and depends on acculturation and assimilation into the dominant culture within the society, social support, length of time in the United States or Canada, generational ties, and linguistic preference. Even within individual cultural groups, there is tremendous heterogeneity. Although women may share a common birthplace or language, they do not always share the same cultural traditions.

The United States has a diverse population (Napier et al., 2014; USCB, 2019). Nurses provide care to immigrants, refugees, and women from almost everywhere in the world, many of whom are of childbearing age. Nurses are finding the profile of childbearing women in their practice are increasingly culturally diverse (Callister, 2016). More than 30% of the U.S. population now consists of individuals from culturally diverse groups other than non-Hispanic Whites, whereas only 9% of registered nurses come from racial or ethnic minority backgrounds. It is projected that by the year 2050, minorities will account for more than 50% of the population of the United States. Each year, nearly 1 million immigrants come to the United States, half of whom are immigrant women of childbearing age. Since 1980, more than 200,000 refugees have resettled in the United States (United States Bureau of Population, 2016). Approximately 13.5% of people living in the United States are foreign-born. Twenty-seven percent of women living in the United States are women of color. One of the challenges for healthcare in this century is that members of racial and ethnic minorities make up a disproportionately high percentage of persons living in poverty, which in turn has a negative effect on health outcomes. See Figures 2–1 and 2–2 for differences in maternal and infant mortality rates in the United States based on racial and ethic identity (Ely & Driscoll, 2020; Hoyert & Minuno, 2020).

Poverty brings many challenges in healthcare delivery (USCB, 2015, 2019; U.S. Department of Health and Human Services [USDHHS], Office of Minority Health, 2017). Approximately 11.8% of the US population is living in poverty (USCB, 2019). Women and families in poverty can be considered a culture associated with health disparities and increased vulnerability in childbearing women.

Poverty is often caused by disadvantages and structural racism that disproportionately affects women in minority groups such as those who are Black, Hispanic, and Native American (McLemore, 2019). Access to equitable maternity care before, during, and after pregnancy is an important issue in promoting the health of all mothers and babies in the United States. When women access healthcare, they are not always treated with respect, and in some cases, healthcare workers do not listen to their concerns or act on them appropriately (Callister, 2020; Simpson, 2019). Disrespectful care is physical, sexual, or verbal abuse; stigma and discrimination; failing to meet professional standards of care; poor communication between women and their providers; and health system conditions and constraints (Bohren et al., 2019). Lack of respectful maternity care is an ongoing issue in the United States and around the world. Recent studies highlight disrespectful maternity care based on ethnicity, cultural group, racial identity, or health insurance status (Declercq, Sakala, & Belanoff, 2020; Hennegan, Redshaw, & Miller, 2014; McLemore et al., 2018; Shakibazadeh et al., 2018; Sigurdson, Morton, Mitchell, & Profit, 2018; Vedam et al., 2019). A comprehensive report by the

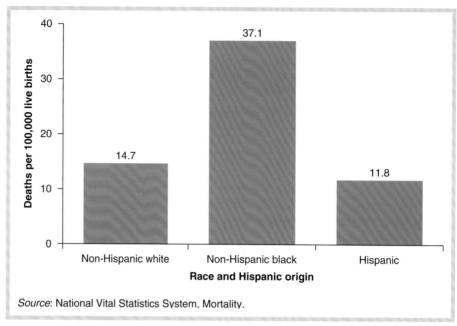

FIGURE 2–1. Maternal mortality in the United States: Changes in coding, publication, and data release, 2018. (From Hoyert, D. L, & Miniño, A. M. [2020]. Maternal mortality in the United States: Changes in coding, publication, and data release, 2018. *National Vital Statistics Reports, 69*[2], 1–18. Hyattsville, MD: National Center for Health Statistics.)

World Health Organization (WHO, 2018) covering the respectful maternity care spectrum ranging from neglect to overuse of medical interventions noted a *good birth goes beyond having a healthy baby*. Respectful maternity care is a human right. Women should be able to routinely experience respectful maternity care as part of high-quality clinical services and not be expected to be happy simply to have survived the process (Callister, 2020; National Academies of Sciences, Engineering, and Medicine [NASEM], 2020).

Nurses must advocate for respectful maternity care and make sure each woman is treated appropriately

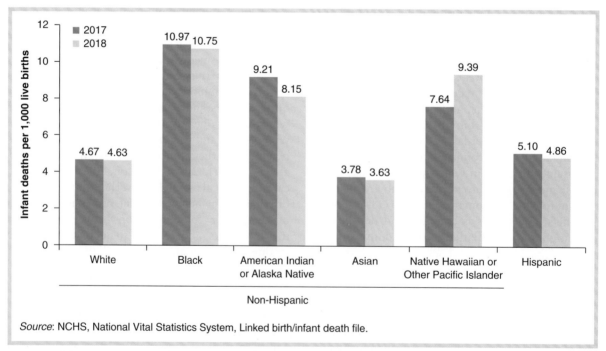

FIGURE 2–2. Infant mortality in the United States, 2018: Data from the period linked birth/infant death file. (From Ely, D. M., & Driscoll, A. K. [2020]. Infant mortality in the United States, 2018: Data from the period linked birth/infant death file. *National Vital Statistics Reports, 69*[7], 1–18. Hyattsville, MD: National Center for Health Statistics.)

DISPLAY 2–1

Essential Aspects of Respectful Maternity Care

- Is based on listening to women, hearing their concerns, and acting on them in a timely and appropriate manner
- Treats all women equally, regardless of age, race, ethnicity, religion, ability, or other subgroups
- Shares information in understandable language at the appropriate literacy level
- Involves effective communication, including the use of interpreters when needed
- Respects women's choices that strengthen their capabilities to give birth
- Offers quality and type of information that promotes informed consent

- Makes sure the woman and her family are true partners in their care
- Is free from harm and mistreatment, rather promotes, encourages, and supports them
- Maintains privacy and confidentiality
- Preserves women's dignity
- Ensures continuous access to family and community support
- Enhances the quality of the physical labor and birth environment and resources
- Involves competent and motivated maternity care providers including nurses, midwives, physicians, doulas, and other members of the healthcare team
- Provides effective and efficient care
- Ensures continuity of care

Adapted from National Academies of Sciences, Engineering, and Medicine. (2020). *Birth settings in America: Outcomes, quality, access, and choice.* Washington, DC: The National Academies Press. Retrieved from https://www.nap.edu/catalog/25636/birth-settings-in-america-outcomes-quality-access-and-choice
Shakibazadeh, E., Namadian, M., Bohren, M. A., Vogel, J. P., Rashidian, A., Nogueira Pileggi, V., . . . Gülmezoglu, A. M. (2018). Respectful care during childbirth in health facilities globally: A qualitative evidence synthesis. *British Journal of Obstetrics and Gynaecology, 125*(8), 932–942. doi:10.1111/1471-0528.15015

(Callister, 2017; Simpson, 2019). Essential aspects of respectful maternity care are listed in Display 2–1. This list is not all-inclusive. Respectful maternity care that is equitable for all women cannot be accomplished without commitment of multiple stakeholders to make fundamental changes including policy makers, payers, healthcare institutions including those that educate healthcare providers and those that give care, and all healthcare workers (Callister, 2017; Council on Patient Safety in Women's Health Care, 2016; Howell et al., 2018; Morton & Simkin, 2019; WHO, 2018). See Display 1–3 in Chapter 1. Nurses and all healthcare workers must make sure that the care they give to all women is respectful, supportive, and based on current evidence (NASEM, 2020).

Figure 2–3 illustrates a conceptual model of high-quality, respectful maternity care across the spectrum that involved access, choice, and risk assessment with the mother and the baby as the central focus with systems, caregivers, and settings around them (NASEM, 2020). The social, clinical, financial, and structural factors that contribute to access, informed choice, quality of care, and outcomes and displayed. They represent opportunities for interventions to improve individual and population health, well-being, and health equity (NASEM, 2020).

CULTURAL FRAMEWORKS AND CULTURAL ASSESSMENT TOOLS

Cultural frameworks and cultural assessment tools have been developed to guide perinatal nursing practice. The Sunrise Model is based on culture care theory (McFarland & Wehbe-Alamah, 2015) (Fig. 2–4). The Transcultural Assessment Model (Giger, 2016) includes variables such as communication, space, social organization, time, environmental control, and biologic variations (Fig. 2–5). Others have identified the dimensions of culture, including values, worldview, disease etiology, time orientation, personal space orientation and touch, family organization, and power structure (Purnell & Paulanka, 2013). The Transcultural Nursing Model is illustrated in 16 considerations in caring for childbearing women (Andrews & Boyle, 2015) (Fig. 2–6). Mattson (2015) has conceptualized specific ethnocultural considerations in caring for childbearing women (Fig. 2–7). Four assumptions define the influence culture has on pregnancy, childbirth, and parenting (Display 2–2). Models should focus on the person, the processes, the environment, and the outcomes. Recently, a model has been proposed for person, family, and culture-centered nursing care (Lor, Crooks, & Tluczek, 2016).

Cultural Competence

The process of cultural competence in the delivery of healthcare includes cultural awareness, skills, encounters, and knowledge (Campinha-Bacote, 2014). Cultural competence is more than a nicety in healthcare. Cultural competence has become imperative because of increasing health disparities and population diversity; the competitive healthcare market; federal regulations on discrimination; complex legislative, regulatory, and accreditation requirements; and our litigious society (deChesnay, Hart, & Branan, 2016; Rorie & Brucker, 2015; The Joint Commission, 2019) (Fig. 2–8).

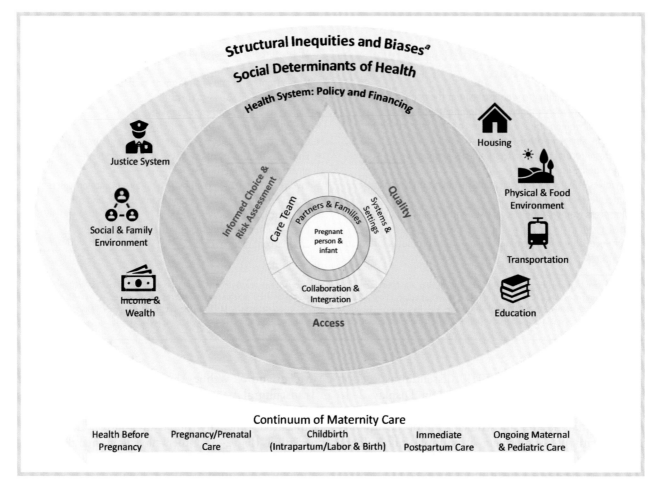

FIGURE 2–3. Interactive continuum of maternity care: A conceptual framework. (From National Academies of Sciences, Engineering, and Medicine. [2020]. *Birth settings in America: Outcomes, quality, access, and choice.* Washington, DC: The National Academies Press. Retrieved from https://www.nap.edu/catalog/25636/birth-settings-in-america-outcomes-quality-access-and-choice.) Used with permission.

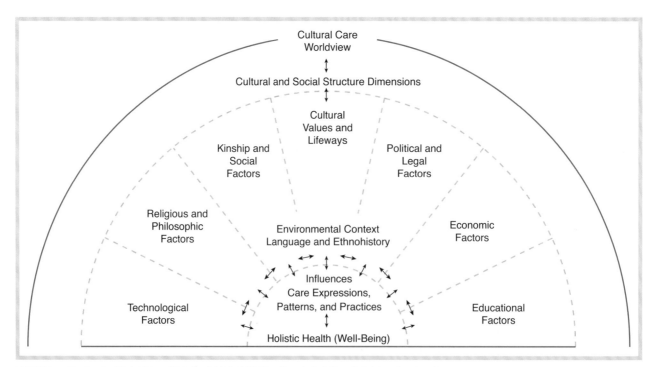

FIGURE 2–4. The Sunrise Model. (From McFarland, M. R., & Wehbe-Alamah, H. B. [2015]. *Leininger's cultural care diversity and universality: A worldwide nursing theory* [3rd ed.]. Sudbury, MA: Jones & Bartlett.)

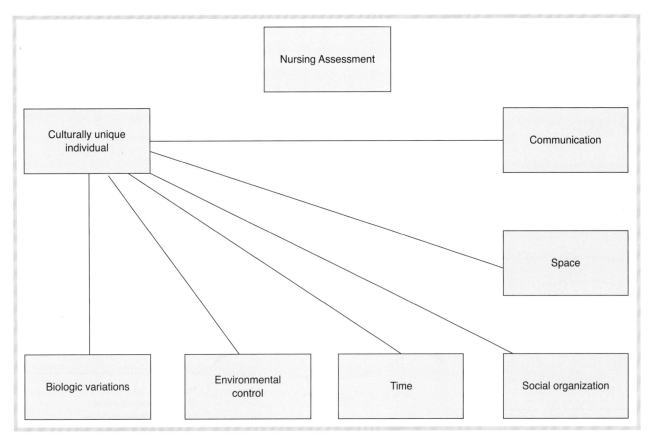

FIGURE 2–5. Transcultural Model. (From Giger, J. N. [2016]. *Transcultural nursing: Assessment and intervention* [7th ed.]. St. Louis, MO: Elsevier.)

Acculturation is a complex variable that is challenging to measure, and current measures need to be refined. Acculturation can be at a cultural or group level and a psychological or individual level (Beck, 2006). Anderson and associates (2010) have identified conducting cultural health assessment.

A framework for acculturation has been identified by Berry (1980). Acculturation may be characterized by (1) assimilation; (2) establishment of relationships in the host society at the expense of the patient's native culture; (3) integration, in which cultural identity is retained and new relationships are established in the host society; (4) rejection, in which one retains cultural identify and rejects the host society; and (5) deculturation, in which one values neither. Nurses will encounter immigrant and refugee women who fall into different categories of acculturation.

The General Acculturation Index scale can be used to assess level of acculturation, and it includes items such as written and spoken language, the country where the childhood was spent, the current circle of friends, and pride in cultural background (Balcazar, Peterson, & Krull, 1997). Other instruments include the Short Acculturation Scale, the Acculturation Rating Scale for Mexican Americans (ARSMA), the ARSMA-II, and the Bidimensional Acculturation Scale for Hispanics (Beck, 2006).

What constitutes a positive and satisfying birth experience varies from one culture to another (Callister, Eads, & Yeung Diehl, 2011; Corbett, Callister, Gettys, & Hickman, 2017; Reed, Callister, Kavaefiafi, Corbett, & Edmunds, 2017). For example, within the Japanese culture, there is the belief in a process called "education of the unborn." A happy mother is thought to ensure joy and good fortune because the unborn child learns, communicates, and responds in utero. The individual personality is formed before birth. Such a belief about the fetus is reflected in many cultures, with concern during pregnancy about evil spirits and birthmarks. Other cultural considerations include fertility rites and beliefs about what determines the gender of the unborn child.

Rich meaning may be created by women espousing traditional religious beliefs and also influence healthy promoting behaviors (Callister & Khalaf, 2010; Murray & Huelsman, 2009). An Orthodox Jewish mother gives silent thanks in the ancient words of the Psalms following the birth of her firstborn son. She believes that by birthing a son she has fulfilled the reason for her creation in obedience to rabbinical law. The creation of life and giving birth represent obedience to religious law and the spiritual dimensions of the human experience.

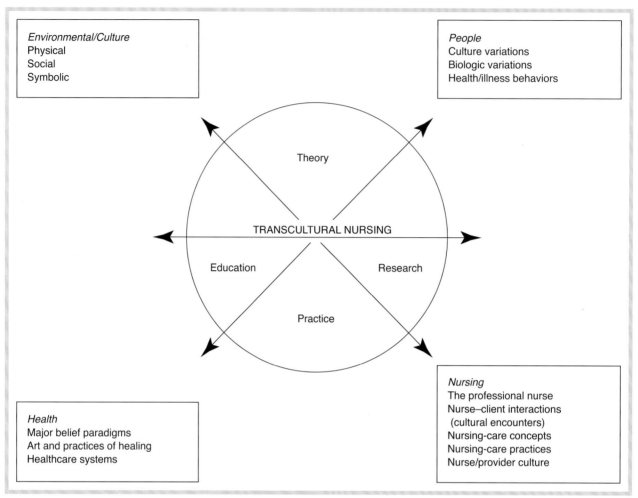

Environmental/Culture
Physical
Social
Symbolic

People
Culture variations
Biologic variations
Health/illness behaviors

Theory

TRANSCULTURAL NURSING

Education   Research

Practice

Nursing
The professional nurse
Nurse–client interactions
  (cultural encounters)
Nursing-care concepts
Nursing-care practices
Nurse/provider culture

Health
Major belief paradigms
Art and practices of healing
Healthcare systems

FIGURE 2–6. Transcultural Nursing: assessment and intervention. (From Anderson, N. L. R., Boyle, J. S., Davidhizar, R. E., Giger, J. N., McFarland, M. R., Papadopoulos, I., . . . Wehbe-Alamah, H. (2010). Cultural health assessment. *Journal of Transcultural Nursing, 21*(4 Suppl.), 307S–336S. doi:10.1177/1043659610377208)

Giving birth is a significant life event, a reflection of a woman's personal values about childbearing and child rearing and the expression and symbolic actualization of the union of the parents. For Muslim women, giving birth fulfills the scriptural injunctions recorded in the Quran. Muslim women may be asked soon after getting married, "Do you save anything inside your abdomen?" meaning, "Are you pregnant yet?" Pregnancy in a traditional Asian family is referred to as a woman having "happiness in her body." In Latin America, if you were to ask an expectant mother when her baby is due, the direct translation from Spanish to English is "When are you going to give light?"

PRACTICES ASSOCIATED WITH CHILDBEARING

There are many diverse cultural rituals, customs, and beliefs associated with childbearing. Some American Indian mothers believe tying knots or weaving will cause birth complications associated with cord accidents. Some Navajo expectant mothers do not choose a name or make a cradleboard because doing so may be detrimental to the well-being of the newborn. Some Arabic Muslim women do not prepare for the baby in advance (such as no baby showers, layette accumulation, or naming the unborn child) because such planning has the potential for defying the will of Allah regarding pregnancy outcomes. Similarly, some Eastern European women may not make prenatal preparations for the newborn, believing such actions would create bad luck. Some Filipino women believe that daily bathing and frequent shampoos during pregnancy contribute to having a clean baby. Some Asian American women may not disclose their pregnancy until the 120th day, when it is believed the soul enters the fetus. In many cultures, girls are socialized early about childbearing. They may witness childbirth or be present when other women repeat their birth stories, especially extended female family members. In the Sudan, a pregnant woman is honored in a special

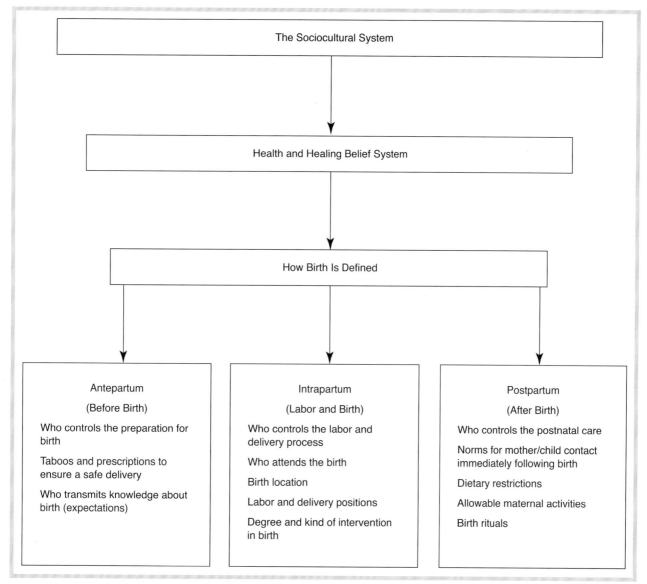

FIGURE 2–7. The sociocultural system, health and healing belief system, and how birth is defined. (From Mattson, S. [2015]. Ethnocultural considerations in the childbearing period. In S. Mattson & J. E. Smith [Eds.], *Core curriculum for maternal-newborn nursing* [5th ed., pp. 66]. St. Louis, MO: Elsevier.)

ceremony, as extended female family members rub her belly with millet porridge, a symbol of regeneration, empowering her to give birth. Because of the importance of preserving modesty, some Southeast Asian women tie a sheet around their bodies like a sarong during labor and express a preference to squat while giving birth. An Italian maternal grandmother may request permission to give her newborn grandson his first bath. After the bath, she dresses him in fine, white silk clothing that she stitched by hand for this momentous occasion. When women in Bali hear the first cries of a newborn, they lavish the new mother with gifts such as dolls, fruit, flowers, or incense to bless, honor, purify, and protect the new child.

The placenta is called *el compañero* in Spanish, translated to mean "the companion of the child." And there are a variety of cultural rituals associated with the disposal of the placenta, including having it dried, burned, or buried in a specific way. Although disposing of the placenta must meet with standard infection control precautions, individual family preferences should be honored as much as possible.

A variety of cultural practices influence postpartum and newborn care. Many Laotian women stay home the first postpartum month, near a fire or heater in an effort to "dry up the womb." The traditional postpartum diet for Korean women includes a soup made from beef broth and seaweed that is believed to cleanse the body of lochia and increase breast milk production. In Navajo tradition, a family banquet is prepared following the baby's first laugh because this touches the hearts of all those who surround the baby.

DISPLAY 2-2
Influence of Culture on Pregnancy, Childbirth, and Parenting

- Within the framework of the *moral and value system*, cultural groups have specific *attitudes* toward childbearing and the meaning of the birth experience.
- Within the framework of the *ceremonial and ritual system*, cultural groups have specific *practices* associated with childbearing.
- Within the framework of the *kinship system*, cultural groups prescribe *gender-related roles* for childbearing.
- Within the framework of the *knowledge and belief system*, cultural groups influence *normative behavior* in childbearing and the *pain experience* of childbirth.

From Callister, L. C. (1995). Cultural meanings of childbirth. *Journal of Obstetric, Gynecologic, and Neonatal Nursing, 24*(4), 327–331. doi:10.1111/j.1552-6909.1995.tb02484.x

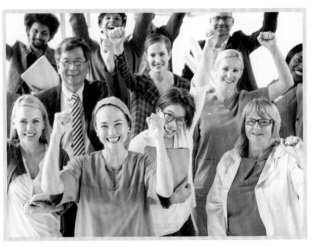

FIGURE 2–8. Cultural competence is a necessity in the delivery of healthcare. (Figure credit: Shutterstock/Rawpixel.com.)

Care of the newborn's umbilical cord includes the use of a binder or belly band, the application of oil, or cord clamping, and then sterile excision. A Southeast Asian woman may not bring her newborn to the pediatrician during the first month after birth because this is considered to be a time for confinement and rest.

Postpartum cultural rituals are important for women of different cultures. Culturally diverse women may experience postpartum depression, with an increased risk related to the gender of the child, related to higher valuing of sons in some societies (Callister, Beckstrand, & Corbett, 2010).

GENDER ROLES

Many cultural groups show strong preference for a son. For example, according to Confucian tradition, only a son can perform the crucial rites of ancestor worship. A woman's status is closely tied to her ability to produce a son in many cultures including Asian Indian families (Goyal, 2016).

Some Mexican immigrant women may prefer that their mother or sister be present during her childbirth rather than the father of her child. In some cultures, fathers may prefer to remain in the waiting room until after the birth. Some Vietnamese fathers may not participate in the birth of their children. Only after the newborn is bathed and dressed may the father see him or her. In cultures in which the husband's presence during birth is not thought to be appropriate, nurses should not assume this denotes lack of paternal involvement and support.

Modesty laws and the law of family purity found in the Torah prohibit the Orthodox Jewish husband from observing his wife when she is immodestly exposed and from touching her when there is vaginal bleeding. Depending on the specific religious sect, observance of the law varies from the onset of labor or bloody show to complete cervical dilation. Some Jewish husbands present at birth stand at the head of the birthing bed or behind a curtain in the room and do not observe the birth or touch their wives. Although cultural factors may limit a husband's ability to physically support or coach his wife during labor and birth, Jewish women still feel supported. Husbands praying, reading Psalms, and consulting with the rabbi represent significant and active support to these women.

For immigrant women living far from extended family support, there may be a shift to an emerging dominance of the nuclear family. For example, in Arab cultures, the extended family is primary, and with migration, fathers may assume more responsible very different than traditional roles. One mother, Fatima, said, "In my country I did not see my husband much . . . Here we are always with each other . . . When he is home he is with me and my son" (Bawadi & Ahmad, 2017, p. 104).

CHILDBIRTH PAIN AND CULTURE

A major pain experience unique to women is that associated with giving birth. Many cultural differences related to the perception of childbirth pain have been identified (Callister, 2011). Some women feel that pain is a natural part of childbirth and that the pain experience provides opportunity for important and powerful growth. Others see childbirth pain as no different from the pain of an illness or injury, that it is inhumane and unnecessary to suffer.

Words used to describe the pain associated with childbirth vary. Labor pain has been described as horrible to excruciating, episiotomy pain described as discomforting and distressing, and postpartum pain described as mild to very uncomfortable. Korean women described pain with words such as "felt like dying" or the "the sky was turning yellow," or the sense of "tearing apart." Mexican American women may view pain as a physical experience, composed of personal, social, and spiritual dimensions. One Australian woman viewed birth as symbolic of the challenges of life, "[Giving birth] makes you more resilient. You know you are able to handle things that you didn't think you could. I think it gives you strength because you know if you can through that, you can cope with a lot of other things" (Callister, Holt, & Kuhre, 2010, p. 133). Women's perceptions of personal control have been found to positively influence their satisfaction with pain management during childbirth.

Pain behaviors also are culturally bound. Some Hispanic laboring women may moan in a rhythmic way and rub their thighs or abdomen to manage the pain. During labor, some Haitian women may be reluctant to accept pain medication and instead use massage, movement, and position changes to increase comfort. Filipino women may believe that noise and activity around them during labor increases labor pain. Some African American women may be more vocally expressive of pain. American Indian women are often stoic, using meditation, self-control, and traditional herbs to manage pain. Puerto Rican women may be emotive in labor, expressing their pain vocally. There is disparity between the estimation of labor pain by caregivers and the pain the women reported they were experiencing. The Coping with Labor Algorithm is proving helpful in assessing pain in laboring women rather than use of the traditional pain scale (Fairchild, Roberts, Zelman, Michelli, & Hastings-Tolsma, 2017). Suggestions for communication skills related to pain assessment and management are included in Display 2–3. WHO (2018) has offered a series of recommendations for care to support a positive intrapartum experience including pain relief measures. A

summary of these recommendations are presented in Table 2–1.

MAJOR CULTURAL GROUPS

The major cultural groups in the United States include African American/Black (AA/B), American Indian/Alaska Native (AI/AN), Asian American/Pacific Islander (AA/PI), Hispanic/Latino (H/L), and White/Caucasian (W/C). Designation in one of these five categories is not equated with within-group homogeneity. The U.S. population by race and ethnic origin is shown in Figure 2–9 (USCB, 2015, 2019). The names used to identify these major U.S. cultural groups in this chapter are those used by the USCB, however some groups have preferences for other names and there is no consensus among groups on the best or most respectful name. For example, some prefer to use African-American women while others prefer to use Black women. Some people who identify as Hispanic prefer to use Latinx, a more gender neutral term than Latino or Latina. Native American, American Indian, and Indigenous People are all names used to describe people who are descendants of those living in the land now known as the United States before it was "discovered" and colonized. The following two modifications were made in the year 2000 census data. The AA/PI category was separated into two categories: AA or Native Hawaiian/PI, and Latino has been added to the Hispanic category (H/L).

African American or Black

According to 2019 census data estimates, this group constitutes 13.4% of the population in the United States (USCB, 2019). This heterogeneous group has origins in Black racial groups of Africa and the Caribbean Islands, including the West Indies, Dominican Republic, Haiti, and Jamaica. AA/B persons may speak French, Spanish, African dialects, and various forms of English. By 2050, the AA/B population is expected to nearly double its present size to 61 million. A disproportionate percentage of AA/Bs are disadvantaged because of poverty, racism, and low educational levels, and they are more likely to have only public insurance. AA/B women are less likely to use any contraceptive method and along with H/L are less likely to use a moderately or highly effective method (Dehlendorf et al., 2014). Comparative lifetime pregnancy rates for U.S. women between the ages of 15 and 44 years are 2.7 for W/Cs and 4.6 for AA/B and H/L women. Health disparities exist between W/C and AA/B women. The maternal mortality rate for non-Hispanic black women (37.1 deaths per 100,000 live births) is 2.5 times the rate for non-Hispanic white (14.7) and 3.1 times the rate for Hispanic women (11.8) (Hoyert

DISPLAY 2–3

Culture and Pain Communication

- Assess pain and cultural pain behaviors and practices.
- Accept the choices of the woman about pain control after providing available information about pain management.
- Demonstrate a willingness to listen to the woman's description of her pain.
- Learn about culturally appropriate pain management strategies.

From Callister, L. C. (2011). The pain of childbirth: Management among culturally diverse women. In K. H. Todd & M. Incayawar (Eds.), *Culture, brain, & analgesia: Understanding and managing pain in diverse populations* (pp. 231–239). New York, NY: Oxford University Press.

TABLE 2-1. Summary List of Recommendations on Intrapartum Care for a Positive Childbirth Experience

Care option	Recommendations
Respectful maternity care	Respectful maternity care, which refers to care organized for and provided to all women in a manner that maintains their dignity, privacy, and confidentiality; ensures freedom from harm and mistreatment; and enables informed choice and continuous support during labor and childbirth, should be the standard for all women and those who give birth.
Effective communication	Effective communication between maternity care providers and women in labor, using simple and culturally acceptable methods, is recommended. The communication should be at the appropriate literacy level and in a language the woman understands. Confirmation of understanding from the woman ensures effective communication.
Companionship during labor and childbirth	A companion of choice is recommended for all women throughout labor and childbirth. This may include the partner, father of the baby, family member, friend, or doula and often includes more than one of these types of support persons. The women should be able to have their support during labor, birth, and postpartum as they desire.
Continuity of care	Midwife-led continuity-of-care models, in which a midwife or small group of midwives supports a woman throughout the antenatal, intrapartum, and postnatal continuum, are recommended for pregnant women in settings with well-functioning midwifery programs. Appropriate risk assessment and transfer of care to an obstetrician, a family physician, or a maternal–fetal medicine physician as needed and per a woman's preferences
Analgesia for pain relief	If the woman desires pain relief during labor, her request should be honored. Epidural analgesia is recommended for healthy pregnant women requesting pain relief during labor, depending on a woman's preferences. Parenteral opioids are recommended options for healthy pregnant women requesting pain relief during labor, depending on a woman's preferences.
Relaxation techniques for pain management	Relaxation techniques, including progressive muscle relaxation, breathing, music, mindfulness, and other techniques, are recommended for healthy pregnant women requesting pain relief during labor, depending on a woman's preferences.
Manual techniques for pain management	Manual techniques, such as massage or application of warm packs, are recommended for healthy pregnant women requesting pain relief during labor, depending on a woman's preferences.
Oral fluid and food	For women at low risk, oral fluid and food intake during labor is recommended.
Maternal mobility and position	Encouraging the adoption of mobility and an upright position during labor in women at low risk is recommended.
Birth position (for women with and without epidural analgesia)	For women with and without epidural analgesia, encouraging the adoption of a birth position of the individual woman's choice, including upright positions, is recommended.
Method of pushing	Women in the expulsive phase of the second stage of labor should be encouraged and supported to follow their own urge to push.
Episiotomy	Routine episiotomy is not recommended

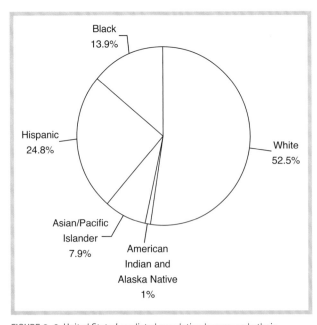

FIGURE 2-9. United States' predicted population by race and ethnic origin, 2050.

& Miniño, 2020) (see Fig. 2–1). There is a higher incidence of low-birth-weight and small-for-gestational-age infants in AA/B mothers, especially with advanced maternal age (Collins, Rankin, & Hibbs, 2015; Ely & Driscoll, 2020). Infant mortality rates for AA/Bs have consistently been twice those of the overall population (Ely & Driscoll, 2020; USDHHS, Office of Minority Health 2016).

Many AA/B families display resilience and adaptive coping strategies in their struggles with racism and poverty. They have a strong religious commitment, as observed in Southern Baptist, fundamentalist, and Black Muslim church communities, which helps to enhance their spiritual health and general well-being (Wehbe-Alamah, McFarland, Macklin, & Riggs, 2011). Fifty-one percent of AA/B families are headed by women, and more than 55% of all AA/B children younger than 3 years are born into single-parent families. AA/B families can have extensive networks of extended families, friends, and neighbors who participate in child rearing with a high level of respect for elders. Children are highly valued, and as a result of extended family networks, the "mothering" a child receives may come from many sources. AA/B women may be demonstrative; comfortable with touch, physical contact, and emotional sharing; and have an orientation toward the present. AA/B women demonstrate great strength and matriarchal leadership.

Some AA/B individuals do not want to be called African Americans because this does not represent their origin. Some AA/B people living in poverty may demonstrate a lack of respect or fear of public clinics and hospitals based on their previous experiences. They may seek prenatal care later than other women; e.g., after the first trimester.

American Indian and Alaskan Native

Descendants of the original peoples of North America (including AI, Eskimo, and Aleut), this group constitutes 1.3% of the population (USCB, 2019). Alaska has one of the largest AI/AN population in the United States, with 14.8% reporting a sole racial heritage (Dillard & Olrun-Volkheimer, 2014). There are over 500 federally recognized AI nations accessing healthcare from Indian Health Services and/or traditional healers.

AI/AN people have a higher unemployment and poverty rate than the general population. They average 9.6 years of formal education, the lowest rate of any major group in the United States. AI/AN living in urban areas have a much higher rate of low-birth-weight infants compared with urban W/Cs and rural AI/ANs and a higher rate of infant mortality than urban W/Cs (Raglan, Lannon, Jones, & Schulkin, 2015). AI/AN people have a high incidence of risk factors associated with poor birth outcomes, including delayed prenatal care, single marital status, adolescent motherhood, and use of tobacco and alcohol.

In general, AI/AN people have a strong spiritual foundation in their lives with a holistic focus on the circular wheel of life. It is important to live in complete harmony with nature. Values include oral traditions passed from generation to generation. Elders play a dominant role in decision making, and many AI/AN tribes are matrilineal (Palacios, Strickland, Chesla, Kennedy, & Portillo, 2014); involving maternal grandmothers in teaching young mothers is an important and culturally sensitive intervention. Because infant care may be multigenerational, Brooks, Holdtich-Davis, Docherty, and Theodorou (2016) note that visitation adjustment may be made when an AI/AN newborn is in the newborn intensive care unit.

Asian American and Pacific Islander

AA people have origins in the Far East, Southeast Asia, the Indian subcontinent, or the Pacific Islands. They constitute 5.9% of the population in the United States and are projected to make up 8.7% by 2050 (USCB, 2019). There is great diversity in the 28 AA/PI groups designated in the census. Asians comprise 95% of this population and are divided into 17 groups, speaking 32 different primary languages, plus multiple dialects. Major groups of AAs include Chinese, Japanese, Koreans, Filipinos, Vietnamese, Cambodians, and Laotians. The major groups, Chinese and Japanese, are the most long-standing groups of Asian immigrants.

PIs comprise 5% of AA/PIs, with specific groups including Hawaiian, Samoan, Guamanian, Tongan, Tahitian, North Marianas, and Fijian. There are more than 50 subgroups speaking at least 32 different languages. Approximately two thirds of Asians living in the United States are foreign-born. This group is culturally and linguistically heterogeneous. In the United States, AA/PIs are highly concentrated in the western states and in metropolitan areas.

There is a paucity of data on the health status of AA/PI people. Asian mothers have a 21% rate vaginal birth after cesarean (Cheng, Declercq, Belanooff, Iverson, & McCloskey, 2015). Because they are a small minority, AA/PI people are often overlooked in healthcare services planning and research. In relation to healthcare, AA/PI groups may comprise the most misunderstood, underrepresented, underreported, and understudied ethnic population. They are often mistakenly referred to as the healthy minority. Their educational attainment has a bimodal distribution, with 39% having college degrees and 5% assessed as functionally illiterate. They use primary and preventive care less often than non-Hispanic Whites. If they have limited English proficiency, barriers to healthcare include making an appointment, locating a health facility, communicating with healthcare providers, and acquiring health literacy. Post-traumatic stress syndrome is of concern in AA/PI refugee women, especially Hmong women, who may have suffered atrocities while living in their country of origin. Infant mortality rates are highest in Native Hawaiians (11.4/1,000 live births).

Values embody the philosophical traditions of Buddhism, Hinduism, and Christianity. Some believe events are predestined and strive for a degree of spirituality in their lives. Core values include cohesive families, filial piety and respect for the elderly, respect for authority, interdependence and reciprocity (group orientation), interpersonal harmony, and avoidance of disagreement and conflict. Motherhood is often viewed in some AA/PI cultures as the central role for women.

Traditional therapies are often employed concurrently with Western medicine, including acupuncture, herbs, nutrition, and meditation (Callister, Eads, et al., 2011).

Traditional Asian healthcare beliefs and practices are Chinese in origin, with the exception of Filipino beliefs and practices being based primarily on the Malaysian culture (Chin, Jaganathan, Hasmiza, & Wu, 2010). The yin/yang polarity is a major life force and focuses on the importance of balance for the maintenance of health. Yin represents cold, darkness, and wetness; yang represents heat, brightness, and dryness. For those who subscribe to the hot/cold theory (including women who are Asian and Hispanic), health requires harmony between heat and cold. Balance should be maintained for women to be in harmony with the environment. During pregnancy, women eat "cold" foods such as poultry, fish, fruits, and vegetables. Eating "hot" foods, such as red peppers, spicy soups, red meat, garlic, ginger, onion, coffee, and sweets, at this time is believed to cause abortion or premature labor. A designation of "hot" or "cold" does not necessarily refer to physical temperature but the specific effects the food is believed to have on the body (Li, Hsu, Chen, & Shu, 2017).

Because pregnancy is a "hot" condition, some expectant mothers may be reluctant to take prenatal vitamins, which are considered a "hot" medication. Encouraging the woman to take her prenatal vitamins with fruit juice may resolve the problem. Some pregnant Asian women believe that iron hardens bones and makes birth more difficult, and these women resist taking vitamin preparations containing iron.

Vaginal exams and an open hospital gown may be deeply humiliating and unnerving to Southeast Asian women who value humility and modesty. Giving birth is believed to deplete a woman's body of the "hot" element (blood) and inner energy. This places her in a "cold" state for about 40 days after birth, which is assumed to be the period for the womb to heal. Rice, eggs, beef, tea, and chicken soup with garlic and black pepper are foods high in "hotness" and are eaten by postpartum women. During postpartum, pericare and hygiene are considered important, but women are discouraged from showering for several days to 2 to 4 weeks. They believe that exposure to water cools the body and interrupts balance, which may cause premature aging. Differences between cultural traditions and the Western healthcare delivery system may cause cultural tension. One woman said, "American hospital workers don't really understand Chinese traditional customs and what may be important to a Chinese mother" (Callister, Eads, et al., 2011). Another Chinese woman noted,

> [The nurses] don't really know or understand. They just aren't aware. Right after birth, I told them I wanted to keep myself warm and I wanted more blankets but they said I didn't need blankets. As Chinese we are more afraid of the cold but the [nurses] didn't seem to think so. (Callister, Eads, et al., 2011, p. 390)

Many AA/PI women breast-feed for several years.

Chinese women focus on "doing the month" (*zuo yue zi*), with elaborate and specific restrictions for the first month following giving birth designed to promote the health and well-being of both mother and newborn (Saito & Lyndon, 2017). Sometimes, nurses assume that with acculturation and education, childbearing women will be less likely to practice traditional beliefs, but many educated Chinese childbearing women do indeed "do the month" and value other cultural practices (Callister, Eads, et al., 2011). Comprehensive lists of Asian Indian perinatal cultural practices and traditions have been generated (Goyal, 2016; Wells & Dietsch, 2014).

Hispanic and Latino

H/L women have ethnic origins from countries where Spanish is the primary language, including Mexico, Puerto Rico, Cuba, Spain, and South or Central America. They constitute 18.5% of the population in the United States and are the largest and fastest growing ethnic group (Centers for Disease Control and Prevention [CDC], 2015; USCB, 2019). Immigration is estimated at 1 million people per year, and census data does not include the significant number of undocumented H/Ls living and working in the United States. Spanish is the most common second language spoken in the United States. Sixty-seven percent of Hispanics are of Mexican origin. Assimilation is minimal, with strongly held cultural beliefs and behaviors. Traditional beliefs, values, and customs govern decision-making behaviors.

Significant increases in the H/L population are related to a natural increase (births over deaths) of 1.8%, high fertility rates, and immigration. It is estimated that by 2020, more than 13.8 million H/L women of childbearing age living in the United States (March of Dimes, 2014). Latino women are younger than non-H/L women at the age of first pregnancy. The fertility rate of H/L women is 84% higher than

White women and 31% higher than Black women. Although H/Ls are the most likely group of women to have children, they are the least likely to initiate early prenatal care. In a phenomenologic study of H/L childbearing women, emerging themes demonstrated that these women experienced anguish (*la angustia*) related to uncertainty and lack of knowledge, which leads to a yearning (*el anhelo*) to be educated without losing their native identity (*identidad*) (Fitzgerald, Cronin, & Bocella, 2016). Another study identified the importance of the development of trust so that H/L mothers feel comfortable and confident (*confianza*) (Jones, 2015).

Compared with women born in the United States, foreign-born H/L women are more likely to be economically disadvantaged and uninsured, factors usually associated with poor outcomes, and adjustments are made for maternal and healthcare factors (Ramos, Jurkowski, Gonzalez, & Lawrence, 2010). H/Ls make up over 21% of the uninsured population. With larger families and inadequate sources of income, more than 30% of H/L live below the poverty level.

Despite these factors, first-generation, or less acculturated, Mexican American women seem to have a perinatal advantage despite low levels of maternal education, low socioeconomic status, and less than adequate prenatal care. The infant mortality rate is lower in foreign-born Mexican-origin Latina women than those born to U.S.-born women (DeCamp, Choi, Fuentes-Afflick, & Sastry, 2015; Hessol & Fuentes-Afflick, 2014). Aspects of their culture that seem to protect them include nutritional intake, lower prevalence of smoking and alcohol consumption, extended family support, and spirituality and/or a religious lifestyle.

Cesarean birth rates in the border region have increased to 31.6% among U.S. Hispanics and to 27.9% among Hispanics living in the United States border region (McDonald, Mojarro Davilla, Sutton, & Ventura, 2015). H/Ls are at higher risk for diabetes (twice that in W/Cs—9.8% vs. 5%) (National Diabetes Information Clearinghouse, 2015), obesity, parasitic disease, and lactose intolerance (Spector, 2014). H/L people are not a homogenous group, with significant variations between Puerto Rican, Mexican, Peruvian, Chilean, and other H/Ls.

In the H/L community, there are strong family ties, large and cohesive kin groups, and a family decision-making process. It is believed that the family has a mediating effect on stress and depression. Family values include pride and self-reliance, dignity, trust, intimacy, and respect for older family members and authority figures. H/L women usually consult their husbands, significant others, or other important family members such as godparents about major health decisions.

Vitamins and iron are avoided by some women during pregnancy because they are thought to be harmful.

Women believe that walking during labor makes birth occur more quickly and that inactivity decreases the amount of amniotic fluid and causes the fetus to stick to the uterus, delaying the birth. Many Hispanic women prefer not to have epidural analgesia/anesthesia. Cesarean birth may be feared and viewed as life-threatening for the mother. Immigrant Hispanic women giving birth may exhibit "cultural passivity," demonstrating stoicism during labor and birth and deferring to healthcare providers for any decision making.

Avoiding foods such as chilies and beans is thought to protect the newborn from illness. In the early postpartum period, the maternal–newborn dyad is considered *muy delicados* (vulnerable or delicate) and stays at home for 7 to 15 days, and for some, up to 40 days postpartum (Spector, 2014). H/L women experiencing symptoms of postpartum depression may not seek mental health services because of the stigma attached to doing so (Callister, Beckstrand, et al., 2010). Traditionally, circumcision has not been practiced, but as acculturation occurs, this practice is becoming more acceptable. Some H/L families may want to keep and bury the placenta. Guidelines for providing culturally competent care for H/L families have been developed (Sobel & Metzler Sawin, 2016; USDHHS, Health Resources and Services Administration, 2016).

White or Caucasian

W/C people have origins in Europe, North Africa, or the Middle East and constitute 76.3% of the population of the United States (USCB, 2019). There are 53 ethnic groups classified as W/C living in the United States. W/C people are considered as being privileged by the advantages they have due to being white and not suffering the life-long effects of racism and all of its negative aspects. For example, there are substantial differences in sources of prenatal care, with 78% of W/C women receiving private care. W/C childbearing women had the lowest rate of vaginal births after cesarean than other racial/ethnic groups (Cheng et al., 2015). However, it should be noted that despite this perception, the median income of non-Hispanic White households declined by 1.7% between 2013 and 2014 with no significant changes in other racial or ethnic groups (USCB, 2015).

Immigrant and Refugee Women

Increasingly, the United States is becoming a global village. Immigrant women are coping with tremendous cultural differences and issues related to making transitions that may be extremely stressful (Missal, Clark, & Kovaleva, 2016). In addition to multiple challenges such as fear and isolation among childbearing women (Benza & Liamputtong, 2014), many demonstrate great resiliency and strength (deChesnay et al., 2016).

Immigrant and refugee women may embrace distinct culture practices such as Somali and Pakistani mothers (Hill, Hunt, & Hyrkäs, 2012; Qureshi & Pacquiao, 2013). Immigrant and refugee women are very heterogeneous.

Currently, there are unprecedented challenges in immigration policies and a global refugee crisis exists, with the vulnerable fleeing violence or persecution (https://www.refinery29.com/2015/09/93814/refugee-crisis-ways-to-help). Under the United States Resettlement Programs admits refugees from 79 countries, with over 70% coming from the Democratic Republic of the Congo, Syria, Burma, Iraq, and Somalia. Nearly 60,000 refugees come to the United States annually (CDC, 2014). Over 72% of refugees are women and children (United States Department of State Bureau of Population, Refugees, and Migration, 2017). Strategies have been identified to assist vulnerable refugee childbearing families (Callister, 2016).

As first-generation, less acculturated Americans, these women have stronger ties to cultural traditions and customs than second- or third-generation Americans. For instance, they may have given birth previously in their home attended by a traditional midwife and their mother or mother-in-law. In a phenomenologic study of Arab migrant women giving birth in the United Kingdom, the overriding theme was "displacement and reformation of self" (Bawadi & Ahmad, 2017, p. 101).

The biomedical and highly technologic environment of birthing units in the United States may be foreign and frightening (Winn, Hetherington, & Tough, 2017). There may be a deep sadness for these mothers as they give birth without the assistance of their own mothers. One Mexican immigrant mother explained her feelings, "When I had my baby I felt like crying. I called for my mother but she could not come to help. My mother was here in my heart because she could not come" (Callister, Beckstrand, & Corbett, 2011). Some immigrants and refugees are migrant farm workers, living in unsanitary, unsafe, and crowded conditions. Language, illiteracy, and cultural barriers have a negative impact on access to healthcare.

Beliefs about gender inequalities and intimate partner violence compromise the health of immigrant childbearing women. Some may be at risk for perinatal depression (Callister, Beckstrand, et al., 2011), and immigrant status may be a deterrent to seeking mental health services (Shellman, Beckstrand, Callister, Luthy, & Freeborn, 2014).

There are multiple barriers to Pap screening use among immigrant women. Among African immigrant women, these barriers include lack of knowledge about screening, cost, cultural beliefs such as modesty and privacy, fear, and communication issues (Adegboyega & Hatcher, 2017). For example, one woman felt her religious beliefs were protecting her, "Before I heard about all these cancers, who was taking care of me? It was God and He is still living. I believe God is still taking care of me" (Adegboyega & Hatcher, 2017, p. 482). Provider sensitivity, family support, and education may help to improve Pap screening use among immigrant women.

It is estimated that by 2025, there will be at least 15 million American Muslims, many of whom will be immigrants or refugees. Their beliefs include *shadadah* (monotheism), *salat* (prayer five times daily), *zakat* (purification), *sawm* (fasting during Ramadan), and *hajj* (a pilgrimage to Mecca). Islamic concepts include these five teachings, along with modesty, visiting the ill, and dietary and gender restrictions. The bride's status in the family is uncertain until she has proven fertility with the birth of her first child, and sons are highly valued. Seeking prenatal care is not considered important unless there are complications. Predictors of delayed healthcare seeking in Muslim women have been identified (Vu, Azmat, Radejko, & Padela, 2016). Childbirth education classes may be considered by H/L childbearing women to be excessive planning that may negatively affect the outcomes of pregnancy.

As conservators of family health, the role of immigrant women in health promotion is critical. Refugees are eligible for special refugee medical assistance during their first 18 months in the United States. After this initial coverage, those who cannot afford private health insurance and are ineligible for Medicaid benefits may become medically indigent. Limitations in literacy and language make it difficult to enter the healthcare system. Feelings of fear and paranoia create circumstances where these women are unwilling to access care. Like other childbearing women, immigrant women appreciate supportive and respectful care (Sheng, Le, & Perry, 2010).

Ritually Circumcised Women

It is estimated that at least 130 million women throughout the world have been ritually circumcised. Immigrants and refugee women from developing countries in Asia (including Malaysia, India, Yemen, and Oman) and 28 African countries may have experienced female genital mutilation. Among Somali women, more than 98% of the women have experienced female circumcision/female genital mutilation. Egypt has the highest incidence worldwide (Little, 2015). Genital mutilation may occur at any point between the newborn period and the time a woman gives birth to her first child. These women experience severe pain and complications during childbirth because the inadequate vaginal opening and scarring may prevent cervical dilatation and fetal passage. After giving birth in their native countries, some women experience

TABLE 2–2. Religious Dietary Prohibitions	
Religion	Dietary prohibitions
Hinduism	All meats are prohibited.
Islam	Pork and alcoholic beverages are prohibited.
Judaism	Pork, predatory fowl, shellfish, and blood by ingestion (e.g., blood sausage, raw meat) are prohibited. Foods should be kosher (i.e., properly prepared). All animals should be ritually slaughtered to be kosher. Mixing dairy and meat dishes at the same meal is prohibited.
Mormonism (Church of Jesus Christ of Latter-day Saints)	Alcohol, tobacco, coffee, and tea are prohibited.
Seventh-day Adventists	Pork, certain seafood (including shellfish), and fermented beverages are prohibited. A vegetarian diet is encouraged.

reinfibulation (i.e., suturing together of the labia). Because female circumcision is a culturally bound rite of passage, women may resent Western attitudes about this practice, which has strong social and cultural support but is illegal in the United States. Perinatal nurses need to create an environment of trust, establish rapport with male family members, ensure privacy, and be sensitive to the stoicism demonstrated toward childbirth pain. Cultural repatterning may occur with the acceptance of alternatives such as flattening of the clitoris and symbolic cutting of the pubic hair.

Deeply Religious Women

Many religious and spiritual beliefs and practices influence childbearing (Callister & Khalaf, 2010). Orthodox Jews have a rich body of traditions associated with childbearing and great reverence for childbearing and child rearing. Some Jewish women feel a moral responsibility to bring at least two children into the world because of the destruction of their progenitors during the Holocaust. Circumcision is a Jewish ritual based on a Hebrew covenant in the Old Testament of the Bible (Genesis 7:10–14) performed on all male children by a mohel on the eighth day of life.

For some Islamic women, creating an environment that honors traditional practices according to the precepts of Islam is important. Islamic women practice a cleansing process at the end of each menstrual period, and modesty is very important, which has an influence on cervical cancer prevention (Guimond & Salman, 2013). Some Palestinian refugee women feel a strong obligation to bear a significant number of children, especially sons, to continue the generations of the Arabic bloodline. A woman espousing the beliefs of the Church of Jesus Christ of Latter-day Saints (Mormon) may request her husband to lay his hands on her head and give her a blessing for strength, comfort, and well-being as she labors and gives birth. Mexican American women often speak in terms of a person's soul or spirit (*alma* or *espiritu*) when referring to one's inner qualities. Among Canadian aboriginal women, an elder provides one-on-one education about spiritual beliefs, including the role of the creator in conception, the valuing of life, and the blessings of motherhood (Di Lallo, 2014).

The sacred day of worship varies. Sunday is the Sabbath for most Christians. The Muslim's holy day is sunset Thursday to sunset Friday. Jews and Seventh Day Adventists celebrate the Sabbath from sunset on Friday to sunset on Saturday. For an Orthodox Jewish woman, honoring the Sabbath may mean not raising the head of the bed to breast-feed and not turning on the call light to request assistance because in the Orthodox culture, these acts would constitute work. Table 2–2 provides common religious dietary prohibitions.

There is a strong relationship between health status and spiritual well-being. Religiosity and a spiritual lifestyle have been found to be the source of powerful strength during childbearing, especially when complications such as fetal or neonatal demise occur. For example, in a study of the lived experience of Jordanian Muslim women having a critically ill neonate, such experiences are considered a test of faith, qualified by the phrase *inshallah* or "as God wills" (Obeidat & Callister, 2011). Spiritual beliefs and religious affiliations may represent effective coping mechanisms and act as sources of support.

BARRIERS TO CULTURALLY COMPETENT CARE

Culturally competent care is essential in the delivery of quality and safe care to childbearing women and their families. The new nursing scope and standards of clinical practice, specifically Standard 8, focuses on the importance of culturally competent nursing care, practicing "in a manner that is congruent with cultural diversity and inclusion principles" (American Nurses Association, 2016). Barriers to culturally competent care include values, beliefs, and customs; communication challenges; and the biomedical healthcare environment.

Differences in Values, Beliefs, and Customs

Ethnocentrism is the belief that one's ways are the only way. *Cultural imposition* is the tendency to thrust one's beliefs, values, and patterns of behaviors on another culture. Characteristics of caregivers that influence their ability to be culturally competent include educational level, multicultural exposure, personal attitudes and values, and professional experiences. Identifying and understanding the childbearing woman's attitudes, behaviors, values, and needs assists the perinatal nurse in identifying interventions that are culturally appropriate; are acceptable to healthcare providers, the women, and their families; have the potential to increase adherence to therapeutic regimens; and will over time result in constructive changes in perinatal healthcare delivery.

Cross, Brazon, Dennis, and Isaacs (1989) originally developed the cultural competence continuum, which moves incrementally across six stages: destructiveness, incapacity, blindness, precompetence, competence, and proficiency. Nurses demonstrate various levels of commitment when caring for culturally diverse women on a continuum from resistant care to generalist care to impassioned care. Nurses who are resistant judge behaviors, ignore client needs, and complain. Resistant nurses may ignore or resent culturally diverse women and their families. They may see culture as an inconvenience or problem. Nurses who provide generalist care are respectful and competent but do not differentiate cultural diversities. Culture, to them, is a nonissue. They may empathize with client experiences but don't feel empowered to bring about substantial change. Racist attitudes of colleagues are tolerated. Nurses who provide impassioned care have a high degree of personal commitment to provide culturally sensitive care. These nurses go beyond accommodation to an appreciation of cultural diversity. They are aware of the complexities of cultural competence and the variability of expressions within cultural groups. Creativity and flexibility are the hallmarks of the care they provide to culturally diverse clients. They feel empowered to make a difference through their clinical practice. Display 2–4 provides the characteristics of the culturally competent nurse. It is important for nurses to become culturally aware as the nurse becomes increasingly sensitive to multiple cultures in order to minimize health inequities (Horvat, Horey, Romios, & Kis-Rigo, 2014). Cultural knowledge involves gaining knowledge of the worldviews of others. Development of assessment skills to understand the values, beliefs, and practices of others means engaging in cross-cultural interactions rather than avoiding them.

It is essential that the nurse examines his or her own cultural beliefs, biases, attitudes, stereotypes,

DISPLAY 2–4

Characteristics of the Culturally Competent Nurse

- Moves from cultural unawareness to an awareness and sensitivity to his or her own cultural heritage
- Recognizes his or her own values and biases and are aware of how they may affect clients from other cultures
- Demonstrates comfort with cultural differences that exist between himself or herself and clients
- Knows specifics about the particular cultural groups he or she works with
- Understands the significance of historic events and sociocultural context for specific cultural groups
- Respects and is aware of the unique needs of specific women
- Understands the diversity that exists within and between cultures
- Endeavors to learn more about cultural communities through interactions with diverse women, participation in cultural diversity workshops and community events, readings on cultural dynamics, and consultations with community experts
- Makes a continuous effort to understand others' points of view
- Demonstrates flexibility and tolerance of ambiguity and is nonjudgmental
- Maintains a sense of humor
- Demonstrates willingness to relinquish control in clinical encounters, to risk failure, and to look within for sources of frustration, anger, and resistance
- Promotes cultural practices that are potentially helpful, tolerates cultural practices that are harmless or neutral, and works to educate women to avoid cultural practices that may be potentially harmful

and prejudice and asks, "Whose birth is it anyway?" The following story is told by Khazoyan and Anderson (1994, p. 226):

> Señor Rojas sat at the bedside of his laboring wife, held her hand, and spoke soft, encouraging words to her. This was the kind of support that she desired during her labor: his presence, his attention, and his affection. Following the birth of their child, Señora Rojas expressed contentment and proudly described the support that her husband had provided. He had met her expectations. The nurses, however, expected more. They had wanted Señor Rojas to participate more actively in his wife's labor by massaging her back and assisting her with breathing techniques.

Communication

Communication barriers include lack of knowledge, fear and distrust, racism, bias and ethnocentrism, stereotyping, nursing rituals, and language barriers (Ebanks et al., 2010). Communication (or lack of communication) between cultures occurs whenever a

DISPLAY 2–5

Standards for Medical Interpreters

- Confidentiality
- Accuracy: conveying the content and spirit of what is said
- Completeness: conveying everything that is said
- Conveying cultural frameworks
- Nonjudgmental attitude about the content to be interpreted
- Client self-determination
- Attitude toward clients
- Acceptance of assignments
- Compensation
- Self-evaluation
- Ethical violations
- Professionalism

From Commonwealth Fund. (2005). *National standards for medical interpreters.*

message produced in one culture must be processed into another culture. A study of African American expectant mothers concluded that high-quality patient–provider communication improved their experience with prenatal care (Dahlem, Villarruel, & Ronis, 2015).

A significant barrier to culturally competent care is language and the lack of bilingual personnel and staff with culturally diverse backgrounds (Koh, Gracia, & Alvarez, 2014). Hospitals frequently enlist nonprofessional employees of the client's ethnic background to act as interpreters. These individuals are often unfamiliar with English medical terminology and may not be able to translate accurately. Interpreters who are members of the client's cultural group may be of a different social class than the client or may be more acculturated and anxious to appear part of the dominant culture. In some cases, interpreters may be disdainful or dismissive of the client's belief system. Using children or other family members to interpret may also lead to problems. Interpretation may be based on the perceptions of the interpreter as to what is best to communicate, and they often may omit important information. According to the USDHHS, Office of Minority Health's (2016) *National Standards for Culturally and Linguistically Appropriate Services in Health Care*, interpreters should be provided by the healthcare facility (Display 2–5). The standards for culturally and linguistically appropriate services are described in Display 2–6. Interpreters may need the help of the nursing staff to feel comfortable and effectively provide services to the non–English-speaking patient. Guidelines for perinatal nursing staff as they work with a medical interpreter are reviewed in Display 2–7.

Healthcare Environment

This barrier includes bureaucracy (such as the inability of the dietary department to provide culturally appropriate foods), nonsupportive administration, lack of educational opportunities to promote cultural diversity, lack of translators, and rigid policies and protocols that do not support cultural diversity. Maternal child healthcare may be the first encounter immigrant women have with healthcare delivery systems in the United States. Consider how difficult it is for the woman who may be living in the United States without the support of extended family (especially female family members), speaking little or no English, having a limited understanding of the dominant culture, having little education, and working in a low-skills-level job without benefits. When this woman arrives at the birthing unit, the unfamiliar environment and procedures serve only to increase her stress. Being hospitalized means entering a new and foreign culture with a high level of technology, the necessity of conforming to unit policies and procedures and unfamiliar schedules, having one's privacy invaded, and behaving as a "patient." This may be very challenging for women.

Another issue is our birth language, which may not reflect how women feel about having a baby. For example, use of the term *delivery* versus *birth* diminishes what the woman's role really is, devaluing her accomplishment as a mother and de-emphasizing the important cultural and spiritual context of giving birth. The woman is not passively "delivered" by the omnipotent caregiver; she should be the central figure actively giving birth. Similarly, rather than "cesarean section," the focus should be on the woman giving birth rather than focusing on a surgical procedure, using the language "cesarean birth." These small but significant linguistic differences are important in the demonstration of respect.

TECHNIQUES TO INTEGRATE CULTURE INTO NURSING CARE

Understanding the cultural context in which patients live is important to fully appreciate their response to illness and is necessary for planning appropriate nursing and medical interventions. It is essential that culturally competent care be integrated into all standards of practice (Betancourt, Corbett, & Bondaryk, 2014; Douglas et al., 2014). Becoming culturally competent is a developmental process. In a recent study of cultural competence in obstetric and neonatal nurses, diversity training, the following variables were positively correlated with cultural competence: perceptions of cultural competence and years of practice in the specialty area (Heitzler, 2017). Neonatal intensive care nurses spoke of sometimes "fragile interactions"

DISPLAY 2–6

Standards for Culturally and Linguistically Appropriate Services (CLAS)

Standard 1. Healthcare organizations should ensure that the patients/consumers receive from all staff members effective, understandable, and respectful care that is provided in a manner compatible with their cultural health beliefs and practices and preferred language.

Standard 2. Healthcare organizations should implement strategies to recruit, retain, and promote at all levels of the organization a diverse staff and leadership that are representative of the demographic characteristics of the service area.

Standard 3. Healthcare organizations should ensure that staff at all levels and across all disciplines provide culturally competent care.

Standard 4. Healthcare organizations must offer and provide language assistance services, at no cost, to each patient/consumer with limited English proficiency at all points of contact in a timely manner during all hours of operation.

Standard 5. Healthcare organizations must provide to patients/consumers in their preferred language both verbal offers and written notices informing them of their right to receive language assistance services.

Standard 6. Healthcare organizations must ensure the competence of language assistance provided to limited English-proficient patients/consumers by interpreters and bilingual staff. Family and friends should not be used to provide interpretation services (except at the request of the patient/consumer).

Standard 7. Healthcare organizations must make available easily understood patient-related materials and post signage in the language of the commonly encountered group or groups represented in the service area.

Standard 8. Healthcare organizations should develop, implement, and promote a written strategic plan that outlines clear goals, policies, and operational plans and management accountability/oversight mechanisms to provide culturally and linguistically appropriate services.

Standard 9. Healthcare organizations should conduct initial and ongoing organizational self-assessments of CLAS-related activities and are encouraged to integrate cultural and linguistic competence-related measures into their internal audits, performance improvement programs, patient satisfaction assessments, and outcome-based evaluations.

Standard 10. Healthcare organizations should ensure that data on the individual patient's/consumer's race, ethnicity, and spoken and written language are collected in health records, integrated into the organization's management information systems, and periodically updated.

Standard 11. Healthcare organizations should maintain a current demographic, cultural, and epidemiologic profile of the community as well as a needs assessment to accurately plan for and implement services that respond to the cultural and linguistic characteristics of the service area.

Standard 12. Healthcare should develop participatory, collaborative partnerships with communities and utilize a variety of formal and informal mechanisms to facilitate community and patient/consumer involvement in designing and implementing CLAS-related activities.

Standard 13. Healthcare organizations should ensure that conflict and grievance resolution processes are culturally and linguistically sensitive and capable of identifying, presenting, and resolving cross-cultural conflict or complaints by patients/consumers.

Standard 14. Healthcare organizations are encouraged to regularly make available to the public information about their progress and successful innovations in implementing the CLAS standards and to provide public notice in their communities about the availability of this information.

From U.S. Department of Health and Human Services, Office of Minority Health. (2017). *Cultural competency.* Retrieved from https://www.minorityhealth.hhs.gov/

with cultural diverse families of vulnerable newborns. The importance of honoring diversity is essential in such settings (Hendson, Reis, & Nicholas, 2015).

Nurses who shared their experiences of caring for non–English-speaking patients identified the importance of an increased awareness of patient needs, professional development including more knowledge about other cultures, and more time and resources (Ian, Nakamura-Florez, & Lee, 2016). As nurses become more sensitive to the issues surrounding healthcare and the traditional health beliefs of the women they care for, more culturally competent healthcare will be provided. Examples of ways that perinatal nursing units might become more culturally competent are described in Display 2–8. Cooper, Grywalski,

Lamp, Newhouse, and Studlien (2007) have described a program in their hospital to increase the cultural competence of nurses.

When the cultural expectations of the nurse and the woman conflict, both are left feeling frustrated and misunderstood. The woman's adherence to traditional practices may be seen as strange and backward to the nurse, who responds by trying to "fit" the woman into the biotechnologic Western system. For example, an AI/AN mother may avoid eye contact and fail to ask questions or breast-feed in the presence of the mother–baby nurse. For many women, including Southeast Asian women, there is "loss of face" because they feel responsible for any confusion or cultural conflict with the nurse, who is perceived as a social superior. This

DISPLAY 2–7

Guidelines for Working with a Medical Interpreter

- Orient the interpreter.
- Request a female interpreter the approximate age of the woman.
- Be prepared prior to the interpreter coming and try to communicate with the woman prior to the interpreter arriving.
- Ask the interpreter the best way to approach sensitive issues such as sexuality or perinatal loss.
- Face the woman and direct your questions to the woman rather than the interpreter.
- Ask about one problem at a time, using concise questions and phrases.
- Look for nonverbal cues.
- After the interaction, review the woman's answers with the interpreter.

From Ebanks, R. L., McFarland, M. R., Mixer, S. J., Munoz, C., Pacquiao, D. F., & Wenger, A. F. Z. (2010). Cross cultural communication. *Journal of Transcultural Nursing, 21*(4 Suppl.), 137S–150S. doi:10.1177/104365961037432

DISPLAY 2–9

Cultural Assessment of the Childbearing Woman

- How is childbearing valued?
- Is childbearing viewed as a normal physiologic process, a wellness experience, a time of vulnerability and risk, or a state of illness?
- Are there dietary, nutritional, pharmacologic, and activity prescribed practices?
- Is birth a private intimate experience or a societal event?
- How is childbirth pain managed, and what maternal and paternal behaviors are appropriate?
- What support is given during pregnancy, childbirth, and beyond, and who appropriately gives that support?
- How is the newborn viewed, what are the patterns regarding care of the infant, and what are the relationships within the nuclear and extended families?
- What maternal precautions or restrictions are necessary during childbearing?
- What does the childbearing experience mean to the woman?

From Callister, L. C. (1995). Cultural meanings of childbirth. *Journal of Obstetric, Gynecologic, and Neonatal Nursing, 24*(4), 327–331. doi:10.1111/j.1552-6909.1995.tb02484.x

experience may discourage them from future contact with healthcare professionals. Assessment information should be accessed, including place of birth, how long the woman has lived in the United States, ethnic affiliation and the strength of that affiliation including ethnic communities, personal support systems, language and literacy, style of communication, religious practices, dietary practices, and socioeconomic status.

Display 2–9 provides the components of a cultural assessment of the childbearing woman.

Enhancing Communication Skills

Display 2–10 contains suggestions for communicating effectively with childbearing women and their families. It is important to remember that effective

DISPLAY 2–8

Changing Institutional Forces to Facilitate Culturally Competent Care

- Changing birthing room policies and unit protocols to promote individualized and family-centered care
- Lobbying for increased resources such as translation services and cultural mediators
- Designing continuing education opportunities to increase cultural competence
- Hiring a nursing staff reflecting the culture of the community
- Generating a pool of volunteer translators who meet women prenatally and follow them through their births and the postpartum period
- Increasing the availability of language line services
- Developing innovative programs addressing the unique needs of culturally diverse populations and integrating community and acute care services for childbearing women and their families

DISPLAY 2–10

Culturally Competent Communication

- Enhance communication skills (greet respectfully, establish rapport, demonstrate empathy, listen actively, provide appropriate feedback, demonstrate interest).
- Develop linguistic skills.
- Determine who the family decision makers are.
- Understand that agreement does not indicate comprehension.
- Use nonverbal communication.
- Use appropriate names and titles.
- Use culturally appropriate teaching techniques.
- Provide for sufficient time.

From Callister, L. C. (2016). *Developing and assessing culturally appropriate health education for childbearing women.* White Plains, NY: March of Dimes Foundation; Ebanks, R. L., McFarland, M. R., Mixer, S. J., Munoz, C., Pacquiao, D. F., & Wenger, A. F. Z. (2010). Cross cultural communication. *Journal of Transcultural Nursing, 21*(4 Suppl.), 137S–150S. doi:10.1177/104365961037432 communication requires a sincere desire to understand the other person's way of behaving and seeing the world. This allows for cultural reciprocity, when a woman feels that she has permission to share her cultural needs, concerns, and feelings. Respect and sensitivity characterize this kind of relationship. A perinatal nurse described the following experience:

> I cared for a Mexican-American woman in maternal/fetal testing. I was able to help her out by being her translator. Modesty was a big issue with her, and she was extremely uncomfortable with undoing her pants and showing her abdomen for the procedure. I felt that there was a unique bond and friendship that was created because of my understanding and sensitivity to her cultural values. It makes all the difference to the woman if she is able to communicate with you and you can convey that you really care.

Be considerate, be polite, and speak softly. Caring behaviors and personal attention from healthcare providers are important to individuals of all cultures. Spend a few minutes talking to the woman and her family as she is admitted to the birthing unit to build rapport. Just a greeting and knowing a few of the social words in the woman's language and use of culturally specific etiquette helps to establish rapport. It is essential to understand cultural communication patterns. For example, some Native Americans may maintain silence and not interrupt others. Some Hispanic women appreciate interactions that begin with personal conversation or small talk, which serves to promote trust. Informed consent should be obtained within the framework of culturally congruent care (Marrone, 2016).

Developing Linguistic Skills

Learning a second language is an excellent way to lower cultural barriers. A labor and delivery nurse described her experience caring for a Mexican immigrant woman:

> When I stepped into the room and began to speak in my high-school-level Spanish, her face brightened and she quickly responded in a rapid flow of unintelligible (to me) foreign syllables. Soon, we were able to communicate quite well, and I became comfortable with her. I translated the physician's words and vice versa. I rubbed her leg and stroked her hair when she cried out or moaned. I'd then ask her about the pain and reassured her as much as I could.

Pay attention to changing trends in language and incorporate them into your spoken and written language. Avoid using complex words, medical terms, and jargon that are difficult to understand in any language. Keep instructions simple and repeat as necessary. Saying "I understand" may be patronizing. Speak slowly, speak distinctly, and try to appear unhurried. State your message slowly, sentence by sentence. Find creative ways to convey information. One mother–baby nurse described caring for a woman who spoke no English:

> I was left with hand gestures and body language for communication. It was very difficult for her to understand my actions. Her assessment was especially hard because I was unable to assess her pain, bleeding, and nipple tenderness adequately. I finally found an English to Spanish dictionary, but this was of limited help to me because I was so bad at pronouncing the words that she still had a very difficult time understanding me. Finally, I just let her read the words from the dictionary. This was the most effective way of communicating that I could come up with. I know that she felt somewhat isolated because she had a difficult time communicating her needs to me also.

Determining Who Makes Family Decisions

Ask women whom they wish to include in their birth experience and make sure those persons are present for all discussions and participate in decision making. Families fulfill several roles for women, including providers of security and support, caregivers, advocates, and liaisons. Families should be treated respectfully with the goal of establishing trust. For some cultural groups, conversation should be directed toward a specific family member. It is important to identify a spokesperson in the family, often the family member most proficient in English. Ask about family roles and respect the preferences of the woman and her family.

Understanding That Agreement May Not Indicate Comprehension or the Ability to Adhere to Healthcare Recommendations

Maternal health literacy is an important consideration because it has an effect on the health of the childbearing woman and her child. Screening tools that may be useful include Rapid Estimate of Adult Literacy in Medicine (REALM), Test of Functional Health Literacy in Adults (TOFHLA), and the Newest Vital Sign (NVS) (Callister, 2016). The woman may pretend to understand in an effort to please the nurse and gain acceptance. The woman's smile may mask confusion, and her nod of assent or "uh-huh" may mean only that she hears, not that she understands or agrees. For example, a new mother who did not speak English was admitted to the mother–baby unit during the night shift. When asked if she was voiding sufficient amounts, she responded, "Yes." In the early morning hours, the mother began to complain of intense abdominal pain. She was catheterized and drained of more than 1,200 mL of urine. The nurse had incorrectly assumed the woman's understood.

The story is told of a 14-year-old AN new mother who was instructed to return to the hospital lab within 24 hours to have her newborn's bilirubin level drawn.

When the nurse inquired further, she learned that this young mother had only been in the city for 2 weeks and had never used public transportation and had no money. The nurse was able to assist with community resources to help this young mother rather than judging her as neglectful for not following discharge instructions (Ebanks et al., 2010).

Using Nonverbal Communication

Use eye contact, friendly facial expressions, and face-to-face positions. Do not assume the woman dislikes you, does not trust you, or is not listening to you because she avoids eye contact. Some consider direct eye contact rude and confrontational. Use touch to express caring and comfort. Nonverbal communication makes an important difference.

Use universally understood language, such as charades (acting out), drawings, and gestures, and repeat the message several times using different common words. Use of simple words that are easily translated serves to improve communication.

Using Names and Titles

Determine how the childbearing woman and her family wish to be addressed. Names and appropriate titles are often complex and confusing. It is important to learn how the woman wants to be addressed and to record it in the patient record so she won't have to answer the question over and over again.

Teaching Techniques

Use visual aids and demonstrations and assist with return demonstrations. Do not assume that the woman can read or write. Ensure that teaching or educational materials can be understood by the client and are appropriate for the woman's cultural group and educational level. Display 2–11 contains suggestions

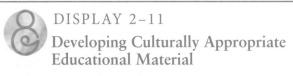

DISPLAY 2–11

Developing Culturally Appropriate Educational Material

- Be aware of your own assumptions and biases.
- Develop an understanding of the target culture, including core values.
- Work with a multicultural team.
- Develop materials in the native language rather than having materials translated.
- Have materials reviewed by members of the target cultural group.

for beginning the process of developing culturally appropriate patient education material. Appendix 2–A contains a sampling of culturally specific educational resources.

Accommodating Cultural Practices

Stereotypical generalization involves two dynamics: stereotyping and generalizing. Stereotyping, or believing that something is the same for everyone in a group, should be avoided. Generalizing, however, must be done to understand *potential* cultural beliefs and practices. The goal of individualizing care is to achieve a balance between what is indigenous to the culture and what may be specific to an individual woman. An experience that made one nurse sensitive to differences among women within the same culture was when she assumed that birth in H/L culture was exclusively a woman's experience, with little involvement by the father of the baby. She said,

> When I helped a Hispanic couple having their first baby, much to my surprise the father was right in there coaching his wife. So I supported his efforts and tried to make the birth experience what they wanted it to be.

If in doubt, ask. A culturally competent birthing nurse described the following experience with a Muslim family:

> I asked the father if there was anything I should know about their customs, and he told me that before anyone could handle the baby [besides the physician], the father had to hold the baby and whisper a prayer into the ear of the baby to protect the baby from evil. I told him that as long as there were no problems with the baby immediately after birth, I would hand him the baby, and if there were problems, he could "do his thing" while the baby was under the warmer and stabilized. He agreed to that. There were no problems, and the father got his wishes and I had the opportunity to attend a wonderfully rich cultural birth.

One Muslim husband stayed with his wife 24 hours a day during her hospitalization. The husband observed the tradition of prayers five times each day, which is a religious duty specified in the Holy Quran. It was challenging for the nurse who walked into the room while he was praying on the floor on his prayer mat, but she did all she could to support these religious rituals.

In many cultures, there is a gender preference for male children. For example, a Korean mother gave birth to a healthy baby girl. Her husband was an active, supportive coach during the labor and birth. When he saw the baby girl, however, his demeanor changed, and he shouted at his wife and started to cry. The mother also cried and refused to hold or look at her newborn daughter. The father left the room, and the mother became subdued but still refused to hold

TABLE 2–3. Perinatal Cultural Practices

Potentially helpful	Harmless or neutral	Potentially harmful
Postpartum diet, hygiene practices	Avoidance of sexual activity during menstruation	Avoiding iron supplements during pregnancy or lactation because of the belief that iron causes hardening of the bones and a hard labor
Carrying the infant close in a sling	Yarn tied around the middle finger to give hope and signify spiritual wholeness	
Breastfeeding on demand		Belief that colostrum is "dirty" or "old" and unfit for the newborn
Spacing of children by long-term breastfeeding	Keeping the mother's head covered at all times with a scarf or wig	Prolonged bed rest after birth
Remaining active throughout labor	Not allowing the newborn to see his or her image in a mirror	Placing a raisin on the umbilical cord to prevent a hernia
Giving birth in nonrecumbent position	Garlic charm around the baby's neck to offer protection from the "evil eye"	Use of abdominal binders to prevent umbilical hernia
	Eating garlic to prevent illness	

the baby. Later, the nurse commented about the beautiful infant, referring to her not as a "baby girl," but as "the baby." The mother asked to hold her newborn. The father came back into the room, and the nurse told him his baby was perfect and beautiful. This reinforcement seemed to appease the father, who then held his infant.

A perinatal nurse described caring for a 22-year-old Guatemalan woman whose pregnancy was a result of rape, "I believe I was meant to be there [with Teresa] that day . . . I learned about the power of presence, support, therapeutic communication, and collaboration" (Ierardi, 2013, p. 355).

It is important to respect the wisdom of other cultures. Healthcare beliefs and practices can be divided into three categories: potentially beneficial, harmless or neutral, and potentially harmful. Examples in each category are listed in Table 2–3. Preservation of potentially helpful beliefs or practices and harmless or neutral behaviors that respect the natural wisdom of the culture should be encouraged, valued, and celebrated. Beneficial as well as harmless or neutral practices and those of unknown efficacy may increase a woman's connection to her own historical and cultural roots.

Herbs commonly used in pregnancy include ginger, peppermint, chamomile, cinnamon, and red raspberry leaf for morning sickness; dandelion for constipation; field greens, dandelion, and red raspberry leaf for anemia; cranberry for urinary tract infections; and red raspberry leaf for prevention of preterm labor. Herbs should not be used in the first trimester of pregnancy, and some herbs, including blue or black cohosh, dong quai, ephedra chaste tree, and zinc, should never be used during pregnancy. Some nurse midwives recommend the use of black and blue cohosh for induction of labor in term women.

Focus energy on changing harmful practices. For example, the motivator for a pregnant woman to discontinue a harmful practice, such as the use of certain herbs or smoking, is to appeal to her protective instincts toward her unborn child. It is essential to show genuine interest and appreciation. The culturally competent nurse seeks to understand the woman's unique way of experiencing birth and expressing what birth means. Failure of the nurse to demonstrate interest and caring toward cultural practices she does not understand causes women to lose confidence in the nurse and the larger healthcare system and may decrease adherence with suggested health promotion strategies.

Reviews document there are relationships between cultural competency, improved healthcare provider/organizational behaviors, and patient outcomes (Truong, Paradies, & Priest, 2014). Changes are needed in nursing education, in healthcare delivery, and in nursing research to increase cultural competence in perinatal nursing practice. The Institute of Medicine (2002, 2009) has called for healthcare providers and the healthcare delivery system to confront and overcome their racial and ethnic disparities.

Nursing Education

Most nursing students have little knowledge about any culture other than their own. Changes in basic nursing education programs should begin to increase cultural competence. National nursing education standards require that educational programs prepare nurses to understand the effect cultural, racial, socioeconomic, religious, and lifestyle differences have on health status and responses to health and illness (American Association of Colleges of Nursing, 2010). Graduates need the knowledge and skills to provide holistic care to culturally diverse women and their families. Nursing education should expose students to diversity in a variety of settings, include theoretical and factual information about cultural groups, identify strategies and skills useful in providing nursing care to culturally diverse clients, allow students the opportunity to examine their own personal values and attitudes, and encourage

DISPLAY 2-12

Strategies Fostering Culturally Competent Care on Perinatal Nursing Units

- Educational offerings on ethnic, religious, cultural, and family diversity
- Educational offerings about available community resources
- Literature searches focused on the predominant cultural groups cared for, followed by development of a resource binder available on the unit
- Generating a culture database
- Establishing a task force to create culturally sensitive birth plans for the predominant cultural groups cared for
- Establishing cultural competencies that are part of the yearly staff evaluation
- Making cultural competence part of the interview process
- Supporting each other in frustrating situations
- Nursing grand rounds focusing on cultural issues
- Celebrating successes by peers in providing culturally competent care
- Sharing resources such as books and professional journal articles
- Discouraging negativism and discrimination on the unit
- Creating connections between community and acute care settings

DISPLAY 2-13

Communication in a Multicultural Healthcare Team

- Assess the personal beliefs of members.
- Assess communication variables from a cultural perspective.
- Modify communication patterns to enhance communication.
- Identify mannerisms that may be threatening and avoid using them.
- Understand that respect for others and the needs they communicate is central to positive working relationships.
- Use validating techniques when communicating.
- Be considerate of a reluctance to talk when the subject might involve culturally taboo topics, such as sexual matters.
- Use team members from a different culture as resources but do not support a dependency by the team on those members.
- Support team efforts to plan and adapt care based on communicated needs and cultural backgrounds of individual patients.
- Identify potential interpreters for patients whenever necessary in order to improve communication.

linguistic skills in a second language. Suggestions have been made for cultural competence curriculum in doctor of nursing practice students (Singleton, 2017).

Cross-cultural health education materials are available on many Web sites, and sources are listed in Appendix 2–A.

Healthcare Delivery

Most healthcare systems in the United States exhibit cultural blindness, ignoring differences as if they do not exist, but it is essential in moving toward a high-quality system of care for childbearing women that culture competence is a priority. Healthcare in the United States is a culture itself based on the dominant Western biomedical model of health beliefs and practices. In most hospitals, only American food is served, and there is a universal assumption that everyone seeking healthcare understands English. Nurses are in a position to challenge institutional forces that may inhibit culturally sensitive care. Effective strategies that have been used to reduce health disparities have been identified (Frieden, 2016). Display 2–12 provides examples of institutional changes and strategies that may facilitate culturally competent care. There are ethical issues related to caring for culturally diverse populations who do not speak English, including compromised

quality of care, increased risk of adverse events, lack of access to healthcare, and lack of informed consent. In addition to diversity in women and their families receiving care, there is also growing diversity within the healthcare work force. Display 2–13 describes how a multicultural healthcare team might improve communication between members.

Nursing Research

Culturally sensitive scholarship is essential in order for the delivery of culturally competent care to be evidence based. Many cultures are silent or invisible minorities because of the lack of research on their health needs, status, beliefs, behavior, and family roles. In cross-cultural comparative studies of childbirth, much of the information is medically or anthropologic oriented. Much of the current literature on how culture influences childbirth is descriptive or focuses on a case study approach. There is a need for qualitative approaches to research, with women as participants or coinvestigators, asking how sociocultural context and increasing technologic approaches to childbirth influence childbearing in different cultures. Qualitative research approaches include focus groups with a bilingual discussion leader or participative research in which results are returned rapidly to participants to improve service. Such approaches are empowering and give legitimacy to healthcare issues of culturally diverse women. The ideal research team includes both members from within the culture being studied as well as nonmembers (Nilson, 2017). Multidisciplinary research teams that include transcultural nurses, nurse anthropologists, sociologists, and others are effective. Cultural issues of specific interest to women have the potential to improve the quality of nursing care provided to women and their quality of life. One understudied area is the measurement of biologic and physiologic differences in cultural, ethnic, and racial groups of women. Studies on the sexual and emotional complications of female circumcision are also needed. Another important research priority is intervention studies designed to measure the effectiveness of strategies for providing healthcare to vulnerable populations of culturally diverse women.

SUMMARY

The story is told of a Native American childbearing couple who seemed like a typical mainstream American family but whose grandmother requested to take the placenta home. It would have been helpful if, on admission, the nurse had asked about their heritage and whether there were any cultural traditions that were important to them. The father would have perhaps responded that his mother was traditional and may want to take the placenta home. The nurse then would have had time to explain whether or not the request could be accommodated, demonstrating respect and providing culturally appropriate care (McFarland & Wehbe-Alamah, 2015). Nurses caring for childbearing women and their families should be respectful of women's cultural diversity and the societal context of their lives, balancing professional standards of care with attitudes, knowledge, and skills associated with cultural competence. Perinatal nurses should seek to create a healthcare encounter with childbearing women and their families that respects the sociocultural and spiritual context of life and moves beyond the superficial to understand the deeper meaning of childbearing. Perinatal nurses must never lose sight of the fact that a woman's childbirth experience is not only about making a baby but also about creating a mother—a mother who is strong and competent and who trusts her own capacities because she has been cared for by a culturally competent nurse. Giving birth has the potential to be a rich cultural, emotional, and spiritual experience facilitated by such a nurse.

REFERENCES

Adegboyega, A., & Hatcher, J. (2017). Factors influencing Pap screening use among African immigrant women. *Journal of Transcultural Nursing*, 28(5), 479–487. doi:10.1177/1043659616661612

Afiyanti, Y., & Solberg, S. M. (2015). "It is my destiny as a woman": On becoming a new mother in Indonesia. *Journal of Transcultural Nursing*, 26(5), 491–498. doi:10.1177/1043659614526243

American Association of Colleges of Nursing. (2010). *Cultural competency in baccalaureate nursing education*. Washington, DC: Author.

American Nurses Association. (2016). *Nursing: Scope and standards of practice* (3rd ed.). Silver Springs, MD: Author.

Anderson, N. L. R., Boyle, J. S., Davidhizar, R. E., Giger, J. N., McFarland, M. R., Papadopoulos, I., . . . Wehbe-Alamah, H. (2010). Cultural health assessment. *Journal of Transcultural Nursing*, 21(4 Suppl.), 307S–336S. doi:10.1177/1043659610377208

Andrews, M. M., & Boyle, J. S. (2015). *Transcultural concepts in nursing care* (7th ed.). Philadelphia, PA: Wolters Kluwer.

Balcazar, H., Peterson, G. W., & Krull, J. L. (1997). Acculturation and family cohesiveness in Mexican American pregnant women: Social and health implications. *Family and Community Health*, 20(3), 16–31.

Bawadi, H., & Ahmad, M. M. (2017). Childbirth and new mother experiences of Arab migrant women. *MCN: The American Journal of Maternal/Child Nursing*, 42(2), 101–107. doi:10.1097/NMC.0000000000000309

Beck, C. T. (2006). Acculturation: Implications for perinatal research. *MCN: The American Journal of Maternal/Child Nursing*, 31(2), 114–120.

Benza, S., & Liamputtong, P. (2014). Pregnancy, childbirth and motherhood: A meta-synthesis of the lived experiences of immigrant women. *Midwifery*, 30, 575–583.

Berry, J. W. (1980). Acculturation as varieties of adaptation. In A. M. Padilla (Ed.), *Acculturation: Theories, models and some new findings* (pp. 9–25). Boulder, CO: Westview Press.

Betancourt, J. R., Corbett, J., & Bondaryk, M. R. (2014). Addressing disparities and achieving equity: Cultural competence, ethics, and health-care transformation. *Chest*, 145(1), 143–148. doi:10.1378/chest.13-0634

Bohren, M. A., Mehrtash, H., Fawole, B., Maung, T. M., Balde, M. D., May, E., . . . Tunçalp, O. (2019). How women are treated during facility-based childbirth in four countries. *Lancet*, 394(10210), 1750–1763. doi:10.1016/S0140-6736(19)31992-0

Brooks, J. L., Holditch-Davis, D., Docherty, S. L., & Theodorou, C. B. (2016). Birthing and parenting a premature infant in a cultural context. *Qualitative Health Research*, 26(3), 387–398. doi:10.1177/1049732315573205

Callister, L. C. (1995). Cultural meanings of childbirth. *Journal of Obstetric, Gynecologic, and Neonatal Nursing*, 24(4), 327–331. doi:10.1111/j.1552-6909.1995.tb02484.x

Callister, L. C. (2012). The pain of childbirth: Management among culturally diverse women. In K. H. Todd & M. Incayawar (Eds.), *Culture, brain, & analgesia: Understanding and managing pain in diverse populations* (pp. 231–239). New York, NY: Oxford University Press.

Callister, L. C. (2016). *Developing and assessing culturally appropriate health education for childbearing women*. White Plains, NY: March of Dimes Foundation.

Callister, L. C. (2017). How are women giving birth in healthcare facilities treated? *MCN: The American Journal of Maternal/Child Nursing*, 42(1), 59. doi:10.1097/NMC.0000000000000295

Callister, L. C. (2020). Surviving and having a healthy baby are low bars for childbirth: Women have the right to expect much more. *MCN: The American Journal of Maternal/Child Nursing*, 45(2), 127. doi:10.1097/NMC.0000000000000607

Callister, L. C., Beckstrand, R. L., & Corbett, C. (2010). Postpartum depression and culture: Pesado Corazon. *MCN: The American Journal of Maternal/Child Nursing*, 35(5), 254–263. doi:10.1097/NMC.0b013e3181e597bf

Callister, L. C., Beckstrand, R. L., & Corbett, C. (2011). Postpartum depression and help-seeking behaviors in immigrant Hispanic women. *Journal of Obstetric, Gynecologic, and Neonatal Nursing*, 40(4), 440–449. doi:10.1111/j.1552-6909.2011.01254.x

Callister, L. C., Eads, M. N., & Yeung Diehl, J. P. (2011). Perceptions of giving birth and adherence to cultural practices in Chinese women. *MCN: The American Journal of Maternal/Child Nursing*, 36(6), 387–394. doi:10.1097/NMC.0b013e31822de397

Callister, L. C., Holt, S. T., & Kuhre, M. W. (2010). Giving birth: The voices of Australian women. *The Journal of Perinatal & Neonatal Nursing*, 24(2), 128–136. doi:10.1097/JPN.0b013e3181cf0429

Callister, L. C., & Khalaf, I. (2010). Spirituality in childbearing women. *The Journal of Perinatal Education*, 19(2), 16–24. doi:10.1624/105812410x495514

Campinha-Bacote, J. (2014). The process of cultural competence in the delivery of healthcare services: A model of care. *Journal of Transcultural Nursing*, 13(3), 181–184. doi:10.1177/10459602013003003

Centers for Disease Control and Prevention. (2014). *Immigrant and refugee health*. Atlanta, GA: Author.

Centers for Disease Control and Prevention. (2015). *Hispanic health*. Atlanta, GA: Author.

Cheng, E. R., Declercq, E. R., Belanoff, C., Iverson, R. E., & McCloskey, L. (2015). Racial and ethnic differences in the likelihood of vaginal birth after cesarean delivery. *Birth*, 42(3), 249–253. doi:10.1111/birt.12174

Chin, Y. M., Jaganathan, M., Hasmiza, A. M., & Wu, M. C. (2010). Zuo yuezi practice among Malaysian Chinese women: Traditional vs modernity. *British Journal of Midwifery*, 18(3), 170–175. doi:10.12968/bjom.2010.18.3.46918

Collins, J. W., Rankin, K. M., & Hibbs, S. (2015). The maternal age related patterns of infant low birth weight rates among non-Latino whites and African-Americans: The effect of maternal birth weight and neighborhood income. *Maternal and Child Health Journal*, 19(4), 739–744. doi:10.1007/s10995-014-1559-z

Commonwealth Fund. (2005). *National standards for medical interpreters*. New York, NY: Author.

Cooper, M., Grywalski, M., Lamp, J., Newhouse, L., & Studlien, R. (2007). Enhancing cultural competence: A model for nurses. *Nursing for Women's Health*, 11(2), 148–159.

Corbett, C. A., Callister, L. C., Gettys, J. P., & Hickman, J. R. (2017). The meaning of giving birth: Voices of Hmong women living in Vietnam. *The Journal of Perinatal & Neonatal Nursing*, 31(3), 207–215. doi:10.1097/JPN.0000000000000242

Council on Patient Safety in Women's Health Care. (2016). *Reduction of peripartum racial/ethnic disparities*. Washington, DC: American College of Obstetricians and Gynecologists.

Cross, T. F., Brazon, B. J., Dennis, K. W., & Isaacs, M. R. (1989). *Toward a culturally competent system of care*. Washington, DC: Child and Adolescent Service System Program Technical Assistance Center.

Dahlem, C. H. Y., Villarruel, A. M., & Ronis, D. L. (2015). African American women and prenatal care perceptions of patient-provider interaction. *Western Journal of Nursing Research*, 37(2), 217–235. doi:10.1177/0193945914533747

DeCamp, L. R., Choi, H., Fuentes-Afflick, E., & Sastry, N. (2015). Immigrant Latino neighborhoods and mortality among infants born to Mexican-origin Latina women. *Maternal and Child Health Journal*, 19(6), 1354–1363. doi:10.1007/s10995-014-1640-7

deChesnay, M., Hart, P. L., & Branan, J. (2016). Cultural competence and resilience. In M. deChesnay & B. A. Anderson (Eds.), *Caring for the vulnerable* (4th ed., pp. 33–48). Boston, MA: Jones & Bartlett.

Declercq, E., Sakala, C., & Belanoff, C. (2020). Women's experience of agency and respect in maternity care by type of insurance in California. *PLoS One*, 15(7), e0235262. doi:10.1371/journal.pone.0235262

Dehlendorf, C., Park, S. Y., Emeremni, C. A., Comer, D., Vincett, K., & Borrero, S. (2014). Racial/ethnic disparities in contraceptive use: Variation by age and women's reproductive experiences. *American Journal of Obstetrics & Gynecology*, 210(6), 526.e1–526.e9. doi:10.1016/j.ajog.2014.01.037

Di Lallo, S. (2014). Prenatal care through the eyes of Canadian aboriginal women. *Nursing for Women's Health*, 18(1), 38–46. doi:10.1111/1751-486X.12092

Dillard, D. M., & Olrun-Volkheimer, J. (2014). Providing culturally sensitive care for pregnant Alaska Native women and families. *International Journal of Childbirth Education*, 29(1), 62–66.

Douglas, M. K., Rosenkoetter, M., Pacquiao, D. F., Callister, L. C., Hattar-Pollara, M., Lauderdale, J., . . . Purnell, L. (2014). Guidelines for implementing culturally competent care. *Journal of Transcultural Nursing*, 25(2), 109–121. doi:10.1177/1043659614520998

Ebanks, R. L., McFarland, M. R., Mixer, S. J., Munoz, C., Pacquiao, D. F., & Wenger, A. F. Z. (2010). Cross cultural communication. *Journal of Transcultural Nursing*, 21(4 Suppl.), 137S–150S. doi:10.1177/1043659611037432

Ely, D. M., & Driscoll, A. K. (2020). Infant mortality in the United States, 2018: Data from the period linked birth/infant death file. *National Vital Statistics Reports*, 69(7), 1–18.

Fairchild, E., Roberts, L., Zelman, K., Michelli, S., & Hastings-Tolsma, M. (2017). Implementation of Robert's Coping With Labor Algorithm in a large tertiary care facility. *Midwifery*, 50, 208–218. doi:10.1016/j.midw.2017.03.008

Fitzgerald, E. M., Cronin, S. N., & Bocella, S. H. (2016). Anguish, yearning, and identity: Toward a better understanding of the pregnant Hispanic woman's prenatal care experience. *Journal of Transcultural Nursing*, 27(5), 464–470. doi:10.1177/1043659615578718

Frieden, T. R. (2016). Strategies for reducing health disparities—Selected CDC-sponsored interventions, United States, 2016. *Morbidity and Mortality Weekly Report*, 65(1), 1–70.

Giger, J. N. (2016). *Transcultural nursing: Assessment and intervention* (7th ed.). St. Louis, MO: Elsevier.

Goyal, D. (2016). Perinatal practices & traditions among Asian Indian women. *MCN: The American Journal of Maternal/Child Nursing*, 41(2), 90–97. doi:10.1097/NMC.0000000000000222

Guimond, M. E., & Salman, K. (2013). Modesty matters: Cultural sensitivity and cervical cancer prevention in Muslim women in the United States. *Nursing for Women's Health*, 17(3), 210–217. doi:10.1111/1751-486X.12034

Heitzler, E. T. (2017). Cultural competence of obstetric and neonatal nurses. *Journal of Obstetric, Gynecologic, and Neonatal Nursing*, 46(3), 423–433. doi:10.1016/j.jogn.2016.11.015

Hendson, L., Reis, M. D., & Nicholas, D. B. (2015). Health care providers' perspectives of providing culturally competent care in the NICU. *Journal of Obstetric, Gynecologic, and Neonatal Nursing*, 44(1), 17–27. doi:10.1111/1552-6909.12524

Hennegan, J., Redshaw, M., & Miller, Y. (2014). Born in another country: Women's experience of labour and birth in Queensland, Australia. *Women and Birth*, 27(2), 91–97. doi:10.1016/j.wombi.2014.02.002

Hessol, N. A., & Fuentes-Afflick, E. (2014). The impact of migration on pregnancy outcomes among Mexican-origin women. *Journal of Immigrant and Minority Health*, 16(3), 377–384. doi:10.1007/s10903-012-9760-x

Hill, N., Hunt, E., & Hyrkäs, K. (2012). Somali immigrant women's health care experiences and beliefs regarding pregnancy and birth in the United States. *Journal of Transcultural Nursing*, 23(1), 72–81. doi:10.1177/1043659611423828

Horvat, I., Horey, D., Romios, P., & Kis-Rigo, J. (2014). Cultural competence education for health professionals. *Cochrane Database of Systematic Reviews*, 5(5), CD009405. doi:10.1002/14651858.CD009405.pub2

Howell, E. A., Brown, H., Brumley, J., Bryant, A. S., Caughey, A. B., Cornell, A. M., . . . Grobman, W. A. (2018). Reduction of peripartum racial and ethnic disparities: A conceptual framework and maternal safety consensus bundle. *Obstetrics and Gynecology*, 131(5), 770–782. doi:10.1097/AOG.0000000000002475

Hoyert, D. L., & Miniño, A. M. (2020). Maternal mortality in the United States: Changes in coding, publication, and data release, 2018. *National Vital Statistics Reports*, 69(2), 1–18.

Ian, C., Nakamura-Florez, E., & Lee, Y. M. (2016). Registered nurses' experiences with caring for non-English speaking patients.

Applied Nursing Research, 30, 257–260. doi:10.1016/j.apnr.2015.11.009

Ierardi, J. A. (2013). With calm and steady hands. *Nursing for Women's Health, 17*(4), 354–356. doi:10.1111/1751-486X.12057

Institute of Medicine. (2002). *Unequal treatment: Confronting racial and ethnic disparities in health care.* Washington, DC: Author.

Institute of Medicine. (2009). *Race, ethnicity and language data: Standardization for health care quality improvement.* Washington, DC: Author

Jones, S. M. (2015). Making me feel comfortable: Developing trust in the nurse for Mexican Americans. *Western Journal of Nursing Research, 37*(11), 1423–1440. doi:10.1177/0193945914541519

Khazoyan, C. M., & Anderson, N. L. (1994). Latinas' expectations for their partners during childbirth. *MCN: The American Journal of Maternal/Child Nursing, 19*(4), 226–229.

Koh, H. K., Gracia, J. N., & Alvarez, M. E. (2014). Culturally and linguistically appropriate services—Advancing health with CLAS. *The New England Journal of Medicine, 371*(3), 198–201. doi:10.1056/NEJMp1404321

Lauderdale, J. (2011). Transcultural perspectives in childbearing. In M. M. Andrews & J. S. Boyle (Eds.), *Transcultural concepts in nursing care* (6th ed.). St. Louis, MO: Mosby.

Li, C. C., Hsu, K. L., Chen, C. H., & Shu, B. C. (2017). The impact of traditional health beliefs on the health practices of women from Southern Taiwan. *Journal of Transcultural Nursing, 28*(5), 473–478. doi:10.1177/1043659616660360

Little, C. M. (2015). Caring for women who have experienced female genital cutting. *MCN: The American Journal of Maternal/Child Nursing, 40*(5), 291–297. doi:10.1097/NMC.0000000000000168

Lor, M., Crooks, N., & Tluczek, A. (2016). A proposed model of person, family, and culture-centered nursing care. *Nursing Outlook, 64*(4), 352–366. doi:10.1016/j.outlook.2016.02.006

March of Dimes. (2014). *Maternal and infant health in US Hispanic populations: Prematurity and related health indicators.* White Plains, NY: Author.

Marrone, S. R. (2016). Informed consent examined within the context of culturally congruent care: An interprofessional perspective. *Journal of Transcultural Nursing, 27*(4), 342–348. doi:10.1177/1043659615569537

Mattson, S. (2015). Ethnocultural considerations in the childbearing period. In S. Mattson & J. E. Smith (Eds.), *Core curriculum for maternal-newborn nursing* (5th ed., pp. 66). St. Louis, MO: Elsevier.

McDonald, J. A., Mojarro Davila, O., Sutton, P. D., & Ventura, S. J. (2015). Cesarean birth in the border region: A descriptive analysis based on US Hispanic and Mexican birth certificates. *Maternal and Child Health Journal, 19*(1), 112–120. doi:10.1007/s10995-014-1501-4

McFarland, M. R., & Wehbe-Alamah, H. B. (2015). *Leininger's cultural care diversity and universality: A worldwide nursing theory* (3rd ed.). Sudbury, MA: Jones & Bartlett.

McLemore, M. R. (2019). *To prevent women from dying in childbirth, first stop blaming them.* Retrieved from https://www.scientificamerican.com/article/to-prevent-women-from-dying-in-childbirth-first-stop-blaming-them/

McLemore, M. R., Altman, M. R., Cooper, N., Williams, S., Rand, L., & Franck, L. (2018). Health care experiences of pregnant, birthing and postnatal women of color at risk for preterm birth. *Social Science and Medicine, 201,* 127–135. doi:10.1016/j.socscimed.2018.02.013

Missal, B., Clark, C., & Kovaleva, M. (2016). Somali immigrant new mothers' childbirth experiences in Minnesota. *Journal of Transcultural Nursing, 27*(4), 359–367. doi:10.1177/1043659614565248

Morton, C. H., & Simkin, P. (2019). Can respectful maternity care save and improve lives? *Birth, 46*(3), 391–395. doi:10.1111/birt.12444

Murray, M. L., & Huelsman, C. M. (2009). Psyche, spirituality, and cultural dimensions of care. In *Labor and delivery nursing: A guide to evidence-based practice* (pp. 195–205). New York, NY: Springer.

Napier, A. D., Ancarno, C., Butler, B., Calabrese, J., Chater, A., Chatterjee, H., . . . Woolf, K. (2014). Culture and health. *Lancet, 384*(9945), 1607–1639. doi:10.1016/S0140-6736(14)61603-2

National Academies of Sciences, Engineering, and Medicine. (2020). *Birth settings in America: Outcomes, quality, access, and choice.* Washington, DC: The National Academies Press. Retrieved from https://www.nap.edu/catalog/25636/birth-settings-in-america-outcomes-quality-access-and-choice

National Diabetes Information Clearinghouse. (2015). *National diabetes statistics 2014.* Washington, DC: National Institute of Diabetes and Digestive and Kidney Diseases.

Nilson, C. (2017). A journey toward cultural competence: The role of researcher reflexivity in indigenous research. *Journal of Transcultural Nursing, 28*(2), 119–127. doi:10.1177/1043659616642825

Obeidat, H., & Callister, L. C. (2011). The lived experience of Jordanian mothers with a preterm infant in the newborn intensive care unit. *Journal of Neonatal-Perinatal Medicine, 4*(2), 137–145. doi:10.3233/NPM-2011-2735

Palacios, J. F., Strickland, C. J., Chesla, C. A., Kennedy, H. P., & Portillo, C. J. (2014). Weaving dreamcatchers: Mothering among American Indian women who were teen mothers. *Journal of Advanced Nursing, 70*(1), 153–163. doi:10.1111/jan.12180

Purnell, L. D., & Paulanka, B. J. (2013). *Transcultural health care: A culturally competent approach* (4th ed.). Philadelphia, PA: F. A. Davis.

Qureshi, R., & Pacquiao, D. F. (2013). Ethnographic study of experiences of Pakistani women immigrants with pregnancy, birthing, and postpartum care in the United States and Pakistan. *Journal of Transcultural Nursing, 24*(4), 355–362. doi:10.1177/1043659613493438

Raglan, G. B., Lannon, S. M., Jones, K. M., & Schulkin, J. (2015). Racial and ethnic disparities in preterm birth among American Indian and Alaska native women. *Maternal and Child Health Journal, 20*(1), 16–24. doi:10.1007/s10995-015-1803-1

Ramos, B. M., Jurkowski, J., Gonzalez, B. A., & Lawrence, C. (2010). Latina women: Health and healthcare disparities. *Social Work in Public Health, 25*(3), 258–271. doi:10.1080/19371910903240605

Reed, S., Callister, L. C., Kavaefiafi, A., Corbett, C., & Edmunds, D. (2017). Honoring motherhood: The meaning of childbirth for Tongan women. *MCN: The American Journal of Maternal/Child Nursing, 42*(3), 146–152. doi:10.1097/NMC.0000000000000328

Rorie, J. L., & Brucker, M. C. (2015). *Varney's midwifery* (6th ed.). Sudbury, MA: Jones & Bartlett.

Saito, M., & Lyndon, A. (2017). Use of traditional birth practices by Chinese women in the United States. *MCN: The American Journal of Maternal/Child Nursing, 42*(3), 153–159. doi:10.1097/NMC.0000000000000326

Shakibazadeh, E., Namadian, M., Bohren, M. A., Vogel, J. P., Rashidian, A., Nogueira Pileggi, V., . . . Gülmezoglu, A. M. (2018). Respectful care during childbirth in health facilities globally: A qualitative evidence synthesis. *British Journal of Obstetrics and Gynaecology, 125*(8), 932–942. doi:10.1111/1471-0528.15015

Shellman, L., Beckstrand, R. I., Callister, L. C., Luthy, K. E., & Freeborn, D. (2014). Postpartum depression in immigrant Hispanic women: A comparative community sample. *Journal of the American Association of Nurse Practitioners, 26*(9), 488–497. doi:10.1002/2327-6924.12088

Sheng, X., Le, H. N., & Perry, D. (2010). Perceived satisfaction with social support and depressive symptoms in perinatal Latinas. *Journal of Transcultural Nursing, 21*(1), 35–44. doi:10.1177/1043659609348619

Sigurdson, K., Morton, C., Mitchell, B., & Profit. (2018). Disparities in NICU quality of care: A qualitative study of family and clinician accounts. *Journal of Perinatology, 38,* 600–607. doi:10.1038/s41372-018-0057-3

Simpson, K. R. (2019). Listening to women, treating them with respect, and honoring their wishes during childbirth are critical aspects of safe, high-quality maternity care. *MCN: The American Journal of Maternal/Child Nursing, 44*(6), 368. doi:10.1097/NMC.0000000000000578

Singleton, J. K. (2017). An enhanced cultural competence curriculum and changes in transcultural self-efficacy in doctor of nursing practice students. *Journal of Transcultural Nursing, 28*(5), 516–522. doi:10.1177/1043659617703162

Sobel, L. L., & Metzler Sawin, E. (2016). Guiding the process of culturally competent care with Hispanic patients: A grounded theory study. *Journal of Transcultural Nursing, 27*(3), 226–232. doi:10.1177/1043659614558452

Spector, R. E. (2014). *Cultural diversity in health and illness* (9th ed.). New York, NY: Pearson.

The Joint Commission. (2019). *Comprehensive accreditation manual for hospitals.* Chicago: Author.

Truong, M., Paradies, Y., & Priest, N. (2014). Interventions to improve cultural competency in healthcare: A systematic review of reviews. *BMC Health Services Research, 14,* 99. doi:10.1186/1472-6963-14-99

United States Bureau of Population. (2016). *Refugee admissions program fact sheet.* Washington DC: United States Department of State.

United States Census Bureau. (2015). *Income, poverty and health insurance coverage in the U.S.: 2014.* Washington, DC: Author.

United States Census Bureau. (2019). *QuickFacts.* Washington, DC: Author.

United States Department of State, Bureau of Population, Refugees, and Migration. (2017). *Fact sheet: Fiscal year 2016 refugee admissions.* Washington, DC: Author.

U.S. Department of Health and Human Services, Health Resources and Services Administration. (2016). *Quality health services for Hispanics: The cultural competency component.* Washington, CD: Author.

U.S. Department of Health and Human Services, Office of Minority Health. (2016). *National standards for culturally and linguistically appropriate services in health care.* Rockville, MD: Government Printing Office.

U.S. Department of Health and Human Services, Office of Minority Health. (2017). *Cultural competency.* Washington DC: Author.

Vedam, S., Stoll, K., Khemet Taiwo, T., Rubashkin, N., Cheyney, M., Strauss, N., . . . Declercq, E. (2019). The Giving Voice to Mothers study: Inequity and mistreatment during pregnancy and childbirth in the United States. *Reproductive Health, 16*(1), 77. doi:10.1186/s12978-019-0729-2

Vu, M., Azmat, A., Radejko, T., & Padela, A. I. (2016). Predictors of delayed healthcare seeking among American Muslim women. *Journal of Women's Health (2002), 25*(6), 586–593. doi:10.1089/jwh.2015.5517

Wehbe-Alamah, H., McFarland, M., Macklin, J., & Riggs, N. (2011). The lived experiences of African American women receiving care from nurse practitioners in an urban nurse-managed clinic. *Online Journal in Cultural Competence in Nursing and Healthcare, 1*(1), 15–26.

Wells, Y. O., & Dietsch, E. (2014). Childbearing traditions of Indian women at home and abroad: An integrative literature review. *Women and Birth, 27,* e1–e6. doi:10.1016/j.wombl.2014.08.006

Winn, A., Hetherington, E., & Tough, S. (2017). Systematic review of immigrant women's experiences with perinatal care in North America. *Journal of Obstetric, Gynecologic, and Neonatal Nursing, 46*(5), 764–775. doi:10.1016/j.jogn.2017.05.002

World Health Organization. (2018). *WHO recommendations for a positive childbirth experience.* Geneva, Switzerland: Author.

APPENDIX 2–A Culturally Competent Care Resources

al-bab.com (Arab topics)

https://www.al-bab.com

American Academy of Child & Adolescent Psychiatry

https://www.aacap.org/AACAP/Families_and_Youth/Facts_for_Families/FFF-Guide/FFF-Guide-Home.aspx (Spanish, French, German, Malaysian, Polish, and Icelandic translations available with links from the site)

American Diabetes Association

http://www.diabetes.org (English and Spanish)

American Immigration Resources on the Internet

https://immigration-usa.com/resource.html

Asian & Pacific Islander American Health Forum (Native Hawaiian and Pacific Islander Affairs)

https://www.apiahf.org (focuses on health status of AA/PI communities)

LanguageLine Solutions

https://www.languageline.com (800) 752-0093 Translation into over 140 languages. Subscribed interpretation (organizations, frequent use); membership interpretation (organizations, predictable need); personal interpreter (individuals, occasional use)

Center for Immigration Studies

https://cis.org (immigration issues)

Center for Reproductive Law and Policy

https://reproductiverights.org (global women's rights including reproductive rights)

Centers for Disease Control and Prevention

https://www.cdc.gov/epielective/ (Epidemiology Elective Program
https://www.cdc.gov/globalhealth (Office of Global Health)
https://www.cdc.gov/spanish (Spanish Web site)

Central Intelligence Agency (CIA) *The World Factbook*
https://www.cia.gov/library/publications/resources
/the-world-factbook/index.html

Culture and Health Care Program
(Cultural Competence Resources Guide)
https://www.cultureandlanguage.net/resources-culture
-and-cultural competence/

DiversityRx
https://www.diversityrx.org

EthnoMed
https://www.ethnomed.org (Amharic, Chinese,
Hmong, Karen, Khmer, Oromo, Somali, Spanish,
Tigrinya, Vietnamese)

Indian Health Service
https://www.ihs.gov

International Medical Interpreters Association
Videos available to improve patient–provider communication based on Joint Commission Standards and
federal laws:
Part 1: https://www.youtube.com
/watch?v=5mR0Vk2zHqs
Part 2: https://www.youtube.com
/watch?v=JJc6NQ4PzyM
Part 3: https://www.youtube.com
/watch?v=W7Labgs2GFw
Part 4: https://www.youtube.com
/watch?v=NFSwdUB88lU

MedlinePlus Health Information
https://medlineplus.gov/populationgroups.html

Multicultural Mental Health Australia
http://www.mhima.org.au/ (55 languages)

National Alliance for Hispanic Health
https://www.healthyamericas.org/

National Asian Women's Health Organization
https://www.nawho.org/

National Center for Complementary and
Integrative Health
https:/nccih.nih.gov

National Center for Cultural Competence
https://nccc.georgetown.edu/

National Institute on Minority Health and
Health Disparities
https://www.nimhd.nih.gov/

NOAH: New York Online Access to Health
http://www.noah-health.org/ (English and Spanish)

Oregon Health & Sciences University Patient
Education Resources for Clinicians
https://libguides.ohsu.edu/clinicalresources/patiented

Pan American Health Organization (PAHO)
https://www.paho.org/

Path Outlook
https://path.org/ (transcultural issues)

Population Reference Bureau (PRB)
https://www.prb.org (U.S. and international population trends)

Princeton University Office of Population Research
https://opr.princeton.edu/

Reproductive Health Outlook
http://www.rho.org/ (transcultural issues)

Safe Motherhood
http://www.safemotherhood.org

Transcultural C.A.R.E. Associates
http://transculturalcare.net

Transcultural Nursing Society
https://tcns.org/

UNICEF Statistical Data
https://www.unicef.org/reports

United States Census Bureau
https://www.census.gov/

U.S. Department of Health and Human Services
https://www.cdc.gov/nchs/data/hus/hus15.pdf

U.S. Department of Health and Human Services,
Office of Minority Health and Health Disparities
https://minorityhealth.hhs.gov

Utah Department of Health Office of
Health Disparities
https://health.utah.gov/disparities

World Health Organization
https://www.who.int/

World Population 2017
https://ww.prb.org/2017-world-population-data
-sheet/

Professional Journals

Birth

Journal of Cross-Cultural Psychology

International Journal of Cross Cultural Management

Culture, Health & Sexuality

Family and Community Health
Hispanic Health Care International (National Association of Hispanic Nurses)

Hmong Studies Journal

Journal of Cultural Diversity

Journal of Health Care for the Poor and Underserved

Journal of Immigrant and Minority Health

Journal of Multicultural Nursing and Health

Journal of Obstetric, Gynecologic & Neonatal Nursing (Association of Women's Health, Obstetric and Neonatal Nurses)

Journal of Transcultural Nursing (Transcultural Nursing Society)

Journal of Women's Health

MCN: *The American Journal of Maternal/Child Nursing*

Maternal and Child Health Journal

Nursing for Women's Health

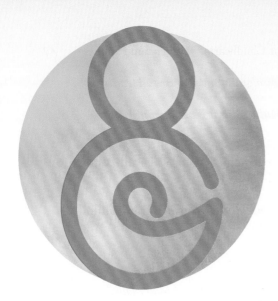

CHAPTER 3

Physiologic Changes of Pregnancy

Susan Tucker Blackburn

INTRODUCTION

The pregnant woman experiences dramatic physiologic changes to meet the demands of the developing fetus, maintain homeostasis, and prepare for birth and lactation. Maternal adaptations during pregnancy result from the interplay of multiple factors, including the influences of reproductive and other hormones, growth factors, cytokines, and other signaling proteins as well as mechanical pressures exerted by the growing fetus and enlarging uterus. An understanding of the normal physiologic changes of pregnancy is essential for discriminating between normal and abnormal states. Laboratory values and physical findings considered normal in the nonpregnant woman may not be normal for women during pregnancy. This chapter reviews physiologic changes during pregnancy to provide baseline information to guide the perinatal nurse in conducting an accurate and thorough assessment of the pregnant woman. A resource for normal reference ranges and laboratory values in the pregnant woman in each trimester is http://perinatology.com/Reference/Reference%20Ranges/Reference%20for%20Serum.htm (Abbassi-Ghanavati, Greer, & Cunningham, 2009).

HORMONES AND OTHER MEDIATORS

Many of the physiologic changes during pregnancy are mediated by hormones. Hormones are responsible for maintaining homeostasis, regulation of growth, and development and cellular communication. They are transported by the blood from the site of production to their target cells throughout the pregnant woman's body and are responsible for many physiologic adaptations to pregnancy. During pregnancy, the placenta serves as an endocrine gland, secreting many hormones, growth factors, and other substances. The major hormones produced by the placenta are human chorionic gonadotropin (hCG), human chorionic somatomammotropin (hCS) (also called human placental lactogen), estrogen, and progesterone. The placenta also produces pituitary-like and gonad-like hormones (i.e., placental corticotrophin, human chorionic thyrotropin, placental growth hormone), hypothalamus-like–releasing hormones (i.e., human chorionic somatostatin, corticotrophin-releasing hormone), gastrointestinal (GI)-like hormones (i.e., gastrin, vasoactive intestinal peptide), and parathyroid hormone–related protein (PTHrP) (Blackburn, 2018; Liu, 2014; Penn, 2017). The placental hormones are critical for many of the metabolic and endocrine changes during pregnancy. For example, PTHrP mediates placental calcium transport and fetal bone growth; corticotropin-releasing hormone (CRH) stimulates release of prostaglandins (PGs) and has a major role in initiation of myometrial contractility and labor onset.

The placenta, membranes, and fetus also synthesize peptide growth factors such as epidermal growth factor, nerve growth factor, platelet-derived growth factor, transforming growth factor beta (TGF-β), skeletal growth factor, and insulin-like growth factor 1 (IGF-1) and 2 (IGF-2) (Liu, 2014; Penn, 2017). These growth factors stimulate localized hormone release, regulate cell growth and differentiation, and enhance metabolic processes during pregnancy (Blackburn, 2018). For example, IGF-1 and IGF-2 enhance amino acid and glucose uptake and prevent protein breakdown, thus helping to regulate cell proliferation and differentiation to maintain fetal growth. TGF-β stimulates cell differentiation and is important in embryogenesis and neural migration and differentiation (Liu, 2014).

Human Chorionic Gonadotropin

hCG is a glycoprotein with alpha and beta subunits. In early pregnancy, the beta subunits predominate, whereas the alpha units are more prevalent in late pregnancy (Cole, 2010). Assessment of free beta subunits is a component of first and second trimester maternal serum screening for fetal genetic disorders (Carlson & Vora, 2017). hCG is secreted primarily by the placenta. The major function of hCG is to maintain progesterone and estrogen production by the corpus luteum until the placental function is adequate (about 10 weeks postconception). hCG may enhance uterine growth, maintenance of uterine quiescence, and immune function during pregnancy. hCG is also thought to have a role in fetal testosterone and corticosteroid production and angiogenesis (Fournier, Guidbourdenche, & Evain-Brion, 2015). hCG is found in the blastocyst prior to implantation and is detected in maternal serum and urine around the time of implantation (7 to 8 days after ovulation) (Liu, 2014). Levels increase to peak about 60 to 90 days after conception and then decrease rapidly after 10 to 12 weeks (when the placental becomes the main producer of estrogens and progesterone and the corpus luteum is no longer needed) to a nadir at 100 to 130 days (Liu, 2014). Maternal urine pregnancy testing assesses hCG levels, and positive results are found by 3 weeks after conception (about 5 weeks after the last normal menstrual period) (Moore, Persaud, & Torchia, 2015). hCG levels are elevated in multiple and molar pregnancies and low with ectopic pregnancy or abnormal placentation (Liu, 2014).

Human Chorionic Somatomammotropin

hCS, also known as human placental lactogen, is produced by the syncytiotrophoblast tissues of the placenta. Maternal serum hCS levels increase parallel to placental growth and peak near term. hCS is critical to fetal growth because it alters maternal protein, carbohydrate, and fat metabolism and acts as an insulin antagonist (Liu, 2014). This hormone increases free fatty acid availability for maternal metabolic needs and decreases maternal glucose uptake and use. Thus, glucose (the major fetal energy substrate) is reserved for fetal use, and free fatty acids are used preferentially by the mother (Blackburn, 2018). This preferred breakdown of free fatty acids increases levels of ketones and the risk of ketosis with significant decreased maternal food intake.

Estrogens

Estrogens (estrone, estradiol, and estriol) are steroid hormones secreted by the ovaries during early pregnancy and the placenta for most of pregnancy. Estrogen prevents further ovarian follicular development during pregnancy. Both luteinizing hormone (LH) and follicle-stimulating hormone (FSH) are inhibited by high concentrations of progesterone in the presence of estrogen. Estrogen affects the renin–angiotensin–aldosterone system and stimulates production of hormone-binding globulins in the liver during pregnancy. Estrogen also helps prepare the breasts for lactation, increases blood flow to the uterus, stimulates the growth of the uterine muscle mass, enhances myometrial activity, and is involved in the timing of the onset of labor (Cunningham et al., 2014).

Estriol is the primary estrogen produced by the placenta during pregnancy. Production of estriol involves interaction of the mother, fetus, and placenta. The mother provides cholesterol and other precursors, which are metabolized by placenta. These metabolites are sent to the fetus for further processing by the fetal liver and adrenal gland to produce dehydroepiandrosterone sulfate, which is sent back to the placenta to produce estriol. Maternal serum and urinary estriol levels increase throughout pregnancy, with a rapid rise during the last 6 weeks. This late increase in estriol alters the local (uteroplacental area) ratio of estrogens to progesterone, which is a factor in the onset of labor (Cunningham et al., 2014; Norwitz, Mahendroo, & Lye, 2014).

Progesterone

Progesterone is initially produced by the corpus luteum in early pregnancy and later primarily by the placenta. Progesterone maintains decidual secretory activities required for implantation and helps to maintain myometrial relaxation by acting on uterine smooth muscle to inhibit PG production and down-regulating contraction associated proteins such as gap junctions and PG and oxytocin receptors (Blackburn, 2018). Progesterone acts on smooth muscle in other areas of the body as well, especially in the GI and renal system; relaxes venous walls to accommodate the increase in blood volume; alters respiratory center sensitivity to carbon dioxide; mediates changes in immune function during pregnancy; and aids in the development of acini and lobules of the breasts in preparation for lactation (Cunningham et al., 2014).

Relaxin

Relaxin is secreted by the corpus luteum and later by the myometrium and placenta. Relaxin interacts with other mediators, such as PGs, to inhibit uterine activity, thereby maintaining myometrial quiescence during pregnancy and diminishing the strength of uterine contractions. Relaxin also plays a role in decidual development and implantation.

Prostaglandins

PGs are found in high concentrations in the female reproductive tract and in the decidua and fetal membranes during pregnancy. PGs are part of a family of substances called eicosanoids that are synthesized from arachidonic acid, which is present in plasma membrane phospholipids. This family includes PGs, prostacyclins (prostaglandin I2 [PGI$_2$]), thromboxanes, and leukotrienes. Eicosanoids are released quickly with plasma membrane stimulation and act near the site of release. PGs affect smooth muscle contractility. The interplay between thromboxanes and PGI$_2$ is believed to contribute to hypertensive disorders in pregnancy. PGI$_2$ release is mediated by nitric oxide, which regulates vascular tone and is an important mediator of reduced vascular resistance and myometrial relaxation during pregnancy (Blackburn, 2018).

PGs mediate the onset of labor, myometrial contractility, and cervical ripening. Throughout most of pregnancy, myometrial PG receptors are downregulated (Norwitz et al., 2014). Changes in receptor responsivity and increases in PG receptors and levels of stimulatory PG near the end of pregnancy are mediated by CRH, fetal cortisol, and uterine stretch (Norwitz et al., 2014). PGs play a critical role in labor onset via a variety of mechanisms, including formation of gap junctions (needed to transmit action potentials) and oxytocin receptors in the myometrium, increasing frequency of action potentials, stimulating myometrial contractility, and enhancing calcium availability (calcium is essential for smooth muscle contraction) (Norwitz et al., 2014). The physiologic roles of endogenous PGs have led to the use of various PGs for cervical ripening and induction of labor (Thomas, Fairclough, Kavanagh, & Kelly, 2014).

Oxytocin

Oxytocin is produced in the hypothalamus and released by the posterior pituitary and also produced by the myometrium, decidua, placenta, and fetal membranes. Circulating levels are stable until the intrapartum period when concentrations increase during the second stage of labor. Uterine oxytocin receptors increase 200- to 300-fold by term (Norwitz et al., 2014). Oxytocin enhances myometrial action potentials, intracellular calcium, and contractility.

Prolactin

Prolactin is released from the anterior pituitary. This hormone is responsible for the increase in and maturation of ducts and alveoli in the breasts and for initiation of lactation after birth. During pregnancy, there is a marked increase of prolactin secondary to the effects of angiotensin II, gonadotropin-releasing hormone, and arginine vasopressin (AVP) on the pituitary. However, the high estrogen levels throughout pregnancy inhibit initiation of lactation. After birth, this inhibition quickly disappears with removal of the placenta, the major source of estrogen during pregnancy. The anterior pituitary begins to produce larger amounts of prolactin, which stimulate the breast to begin lactation. The serum prolactin concentration begins to rise in the first trimester and by term may reach 10 times the nonpregnant concentration (Liu, 2014). After birth, prolactin levels rise rapidly, returning to prepregnancy levels by 7 to 14 days in non-breastfeeding mothers (Blackburn, 2018). In lactating women, baseline prolactin levels are elevated further during sucking; the baseline decreases over the first months of lactation.

CARDIOVASCULAR SYSTEM

The cardiovascular system undergoes numerous and profound adaptations during pregnancy (Table 3–1). Cardiovascular anatomy, blood volume, cardiac output, and vascular resistance are altered to accommodate the additional maternal and fetal circulatory requirements. Increased ventricular wall muscle mass, an increased heart rate, cardiac murmurs, and dependent peripheral edema are evidence of these anatomic and functional changes. Physical symptoms may occur during pregnancy in response to normal cardiovascular changes. Some women report palpitations, light-headedness, or decreased tolerance for activity. Cardiovascular adaptations have a significant impact on all organ systems. Women with normal cardiovascular function are generally able to accommodate the dramatic cardiovascular changes associated with pregnancy. Women with cardiovascular disease are at increased risk for complications during pregnancy, labor, or the immediate postpartum period, in part because of alterations in blood and plasma volume and cardiac output (Gandhi & Martin, 2015).

TABLE 3–1. Cardiovascular Changes during Pregnancy

Parameter	Change
Heart rate	Increases up to 15% to 20% (10 to 20 beats per minute)
Blood volume	Increases 30% to 50% (1,450 to 1,750 mL)
Plasma volume	Increases 45% (40% to 60%; an additional 1,200 to 1,600 mL)
Red cell mass	Increases 20% to 30% (250 to 450 mL)
Cardiac output	Increases 30% to 50% (average 30% to 45%)
Stroke volume	Increases 25% to 30%
Systemic vascular resistance	Decreases 20% to 30%
Colloid oncotic pressure	Decreases 20% (23 mm Hg)
Diastolic blood pressure	Decreases 10 to 15 mm Hg

Heart

The position, appearance, and function of the heart change during pregnancy. As the growing uterus exerts pressure on the diaphragm, the heart is displaced upward, forward, and to the left, to lie in a more horizontal position. The first-trimester increase in ventricular muscle mass and the second- and early third-trimester increase in end-diastolic volume cause the heart to undergo a physiologic dilation (Monga & Mastrobattista, 2014). The point of maximal impulse is deviated to the left at the fourth intercostal space. During the first few days postpartum, the left atrium also appears to be enlarged because of the increased blood volume that occurs with removal of the placenta.

Maternal heart rate increases progressively and peaks at 10 to 20 beats per minute above baseline by about 32 weeks (Monga & Mastrobattista, 2014; Sanghavi & Rutherford, 2014). Heart rate and atrial size return to normal prepregnancy values in the first 10 days postpartum, whereas left ventricular size normalizes after 4 to 6 months (Monga & Mastrobattista, 2014).

Between 12 and 20 weeks, a change in heart sounds and a systolic murmur is heard in approximately 90% to 95% of pregnant women because of the increased cardiovascular load (Cunningham et al., 2014; Monga & Mastrobattista, 2014). Ninety percent of pregnant women have a wider split in the first heart sound (which also becomes louder) and an audible third heart sound. Around 30 weeks' gestation, the second heart sound also demonstrates an audible splitting. Systolic murmurs are auscultated in 92% to 95% of pregnant women during the last two trimesters due to increased cardiac load. However, systolic murmurs greater than grade 2/4 and any type of diastolic murmur require further evaluation (Monga & Mastrobattista, 2014). Systolic murmurs can be best auscultated along the left sternal border and result from aortic and pulmonary artery blood flow. Murmurs from mammary vessels are heard in about 14% of pregnant women (Blackburn, 2018).

Blood Volume

Blood volume increases beginning as early as 6 to 8 weeks and peaking by 32 to 34 weeks at 1,200 to 1,600 mL higher (Monga & Mastrobattista, 2014). Blood volume then plateaus or decreases slightly to term, returning to prepregnancy values by 6 to 8 weeks postpartum or sooner (Monga & Mastrobattista, 2014). The increased blood volume is necessary to provide adequate blood flow to the uterus, fetus, and maternal tissues; to maintain blood pressure (BP); to assist with temperature regulation by increasing cutaneous blood flow; and to accommodate blood loss at birth (Blackburn, 2018). Failure of blood volume to increase is associated with altered fetal and placental growth. Blood volume is greater in multiple gestations and increases proportionally according to the number of fetuses (Monga & Mastrobattista, 2014).

Changes in blood volume are due to increases in both plasma volume and red blood cell (RBC) mass. Plasma volume increases approximately 45% (range, 40% to 60%) by term, and red cell mass increases 20% to 30% (250 to 450 mL) (Monga & Mastrobattista, 2014). The rapid increase in plasma volume and later rise in RBC volume result in relative hemodilution. Even with increased RBC production, there is a decrease in both hemoglobin and hematocrit values during pregnancy.

Hormonal stimulation of plasma renin activity and increases in the renin–angiotensin–aldosterone system components stimulate renal tubular reabsorption of sodium and a subsequent increase of 6 to 8 L in total body water (extracellular and plasma fluid volume) (Blackburn, 2018). Changes in systemic vascular resistance (SVR) decrease venous tone and increase the capacity of the blood vessels to accommodate the extra blood volume without overloading the maternal system.

The extra blood volume helps protect the woman from shock with the normal blood loss at birth. To prevent hemorrhage immediately after childbirth, the uterus contracts, shunting blood from uterine vessels into the systemic circulation and causing an autotransfusion of approximately 1,000 mL. Although up to 500 mL (10%) of blood may be lost with a vaginal birth and 1,000 mL (15% to 30%) with a cesarean birth, average loss is usually less. These changes are accompanied by a postpartum diuresis that further reduces the plasma volume during the first several days postpartum. Plasma volume returns to prepregnancy levels by 6 to 8 weeks or earlier.

Cardiac Output

Cardiac output is the product of heart rate times stroke volume, both of which increase during pregnancy. Cardiac output is also influenced by blood volume, cardiac contractility, vascular resistance, and maternal position. Cardiac output increases 30% to 50% during pregnancy when measured in the left lateral recumbent position. This increase begins early, with approximately half of the increase occurring by 8 weeks' gestation, peaks in the second trimester, and then plateaus until term (Monga & Mastrobattista, 2014). In early pregnancy, the increase in cardiac output primarily results from an increase in stroke volume. Stroke volume increases by as early as 8 weeks, peaks at 16 to 24 weeks, and then declines to term. The increase in cardiac output results initially from the increase in both heart rate and stroke volume but by late pregnancy is due primarily to the changes in heart rate, which continues increasing to term (Monga & Mastrobattista, 2014; Sanghavi & Rutherford, 2014). Cardiac output increases are greater in multiple pregnancies, especially after 20 weeks' gestation (Blackburn, 2018).

Maternal position can greatly influence cardiac output, most dramatically during the third trimester. Cardiac output is optimized in the lateral position, somewhat decreased in the sitting position, and markedly decreased in the supine position (Blackburn, 2018). In the supine position, pressure exerted on the inferior vena cava from the gravid uterus decreases venous return and results in decreased cardiac output. This position may lead to supine hypotension with diaphoresis and possible syncope.

Cardiac output rises progressively during labor. Changes in cardiac output during the intrapartum period depend on maternal position, type of anesthesia, and method of birth. During the first stage of labor, approximately 300 to 500 mL of blood are shunted from the uterus into the systemic circulation with each contraction (Harris, 2011; Monga & Mastrobattista, 2014). This results in a progressive and cumulative rise in cardiac output during the first and second stages. Epidural anesthesia causes a sympathectomy and a marked decrease in peripheral vascular resistance that may cause a decrease in venous return, resulting in decreased cardiac output. An intravenous fluid bolus before epidural placement may mitigate these effects.

Immediately after birth, cardiac output is 60% to 80% higher than during pre-labor levels, declining rapidly after 10 to 15 minutes to stabilize at pre-labor values after 1 hour (Monga & Mastrobattista, 2014; Sanghavi & Rutherford, 2014). As a result of these hemodynamic changes, the intrapartum and immediate postpartum periods are times of increased vulnerability in women with cardiovascular disease. Cardiac output remains higher than prepregnancy values for 24 to 48 hours after birth and then progressively decreases and returns to nonpregnant levels by 6 to 12 weeks postpartum in most women (Blackburn, 2018).

Distribution of Blood Flow

Most of the increase in blood volume during pregnancy is distributed to the uterus, kidneys, breasts, and skin. The uterus accommodates one third of the additional blood volume at term. The kidneys receive approximately 400 mL/min. Glandular growth, distended veins, and tissue engorgement reflect the increased blood flow to the breasts, which may lead to a sensation of heat and tingling. Hyperemia of the cervix and vagina is also evident. Blood flow to the maternal skin increases to facilitate dissipation of heat created by fetal and placental metabolism as well as increases in maternal metabolic rate. This increased blood flow can result in alterations in nail and hair growth, increased nasal congestion, rhinitis, increased risk of nosebleeds, and sensations of warm hands and feet (Blackburn, 2018).

Blood Pressure

Maternal position during BP measurement significantly affects BP values. Sitting or standing BP measurement shows minimal change in systolic BP, which is stable or decreases slightly during pregnancy. Diastolic BP, measured while in the sitting or standing positions, gradually decreases by approximately 10 to 15 mm Hg over the first-trimester values, with lowest values seen at 24 to 32 weeks followed by a gradual increase toward nonpregnant baseline values by term (Monga & Mastrobattista, 2014). Accurate comparison of BP values depends on consistent techniques of measurement and consistent maternal positioning. Changes in BP are thought to be related to the vasodilatory effects of nitric oxide, PGI_2, and relaxin that mediate a decrease in SVR (Monga & Mastrobattista, 2014).

Systemic Vascular Resistance

SVR decreases by 20% to 30% (Hegewald & Crapo, 2011). Changes in SVR are related to the increased capacity of the uteroplacental blood vessels; the effects of progesterone, nitric oxide, and PGI_2 on vascular smooth muscle and vasodilation; and softening of collagen fibers (Blackburn, 2018). The uteroplacental vascular system is a low-resistance network that accommodates a large percentage of maternal cardiac output. Uterine vascular resistance also decreases during pregnancy and enhances uterine blood flow. SVR decreases by 5 weeks' gestation, is lowest at 14 to 24 weeks' gestation, and gradually increases by term, when the mean SVR may approximate nonpregnant values (Monga & Mastrobattista, 2014).

HEMATOLOGIC CHANGES

To meet additional oxygen requirements of pregnancy, RBC volume increases approximately 20% to 30% (Monga & Mastrobattista, 2014). However, because plasma volume increases to a greater degree than the erythrocyte volume, the hematocrit decreases approximately 3% to 5%. This decrease is most obvious during the second trimester, after blood volume peaks.

Hemoglobin levels during pregnancy average 12.5 g/dL (range 11 to 13 g/dL) by term. With the increase in the number of RBCs, the need for iron for the production of hemoglobin also increases. Serum ferritin levels decrease, with the greatest decline seen at 12 to 25 weeks (Siu, 2015). Approximately 500 mg of iron is needed for the increases in maternal RBCs, 270 mg by the fetus and 90 mg by the placenta. Total iron needs during pregnancy, including replacement of losses are estimated at 1 g. Iron needs increases from 0.8 g/day in early pregnancy to 7.5 mg/day by term (Kilpatrick, 2014; Siu, 2015).

GI absorption of iron is increased during pregnancy, but additional iron supplementation is nonetheless necessary for most women to maintain maternal iron stores. If iron stores are initially low and supplemental iron is not added to enhance the diet, iron deficiency anemia may result (Kilpatrick, 2014). There is controversy surrounding the efficacy and benefit of prophylactic oral iron supplementation during pregnancy (Peña-Rosas, De-Regil, Garcia-Casal, & Dowswell, 2015; Siu, 2015). Thus, supplementation may not be needed to prevent iron deficiency anemia in a woman who has good iron stores prior to pregnancy and a diet during pregnancy that is high in bioavailable iron. However, many women of childbearing age have marginal iron stores (Monga & Mastrobattista, 2014). Iron supplementation does not prevent the normal fall in hemoglobin (due to hemodilution) but can prevent depletion of stores and onset of iron-deficiency anemia.

Leukocyte (especially neutrophil) production also increases in pregnancy. The average white blood cell (WBC) count in the third trimester is 5,000 to 12,000/mm^3 (Kilpatrick, 2014). Labor and early postpartum levels may reach 20,000 to 30,000/mm^3 without an infection. The increase in WBC count begins during the second month, and the level returns to the normal range for nonpregnant women by 6 days postpartum. Platelet counts range between 150,000/mm^3 and 400,000/mm^3, with perhaps a slight decrease in the third trimester (Anthony, Racusin, Aagaard, & Dildy, 2017).

Plasma proteins and other components are also altered during pregnancy. Serum electrolytes and osmolality decrease. Serum lipids, especially cholesterol (needed for steroid hormone synthesis) and phospholipids (needed for cell membranes), increase 40% to 60%. Total plasma protein decreases 10% to 14% due primarily to hemodilution, but with both absolute and relative decreases in serum albumin. This leads to decreased serum oncotic pressure that contributes to the dependent edema seen in many pregnant women. The decrease in albumin may increase plasma levels of unbound drugs or other substances such as calcium, this influencing the availability of free drug for the mother and placental transfer (Blackburn, 2018). Maternal pharmacokinetics may also be influenced by the elevated blood and plasma volume, cardiac output, total body water, and body mass in pregnancy, which increase the volume of distribution for some pharmacologic agents. This may lead to decreases in drug levels and alter the therapeutic effects of drugs taken for chronic conditions (Blackburn, 2018).

Coagulation and fibrinolytic systems undergo significant changes during pregnancy with alterations in coagulation (precoagulant) factors, coagulation inhibitors, and fibrinolysis. Pregnancy is considered a hypercoagulable state because of increased levels of many coagulation factors and a decrease in factors such as protein S that inhibit coagulation. The most marked increases occur in factors I (fibrinogen), VII, VIII, X, and von Willebrand factor (vWF) antigen (Anthony et al., 2017; Katz & Beilin, 2015). These changes are partially balanced by alterations in the plasminogen system that enhances clot lysis. Prothrombin time and activated partial thromboplastin time decrease slightly as the pregnancy comes to term; however, bleeding time and clotting time remain unchanged despite the increase in clotting factors (Blackburn, 2018). The net effect of these alterations places pregnant women at increased risk for thrombus formation and consumptive coagulopathies. After birth, coagulation is initiated to prevent hemorrhage at the placental site. Fibrinogen and platelet counts decrease as platelet plugs and fibrin clots form to provide hemostasis.

RESPIRATORY SYSTEM

Changes in the respiratory system are essential to accommodate increased maternal–fetal requirements and to ensure adequate gas exchange to meet maternal and fetal metabolic needs. The respiratory system must provide an increased amount of oxygen and efficiently remove carbon dioxide. Changes in the respiratory system are due primarily to a combination of mechanical forces (e.g., the enlarging uterus) and biochemical effects, especially the effects of progesterone and PGs on the respiratory center and bronchial smooth muscle. Table 3–2 summarizes the changes in respiratory function during pregnancy.

TABLE 3–2. Respiratory Changes during Pregnancy

Parameter	Change
Tidal volume	Increases 30% to 40% (500 to 700 mL)
Vital capacity	Unchanged
Inspiratory reserve volume	Unchanged
Expiratory reserve volume	Decreases 15% to 20%
Respiratory rate	Unchanged or slight increase
Functional residual capacity	Decreases 20% to 30%
Total lung volume	Decreases 5%
Residual volume	Decreases 20% to 25%
Minute ventilation	Increases 30% to 50%
pH	Slight increase to 7.40 to 7.45
P_aO_2 (first trimester)	104 to 108 mm Hg
P_aO_2 (by term)	101 to 104 mm Hg
P_aCO_2	27 to 32 mm Hg
Bicarbonate	18 to 21 mEq/L (base deficit of −3 to −4 mEq/L)

P_aCO_2, arterial partial pressure of carbon dioxide; P_aO_2, arterial partial pressures of oxygen.

Structural Changes

Pressure from the uterus shifts the diaphragm upward approximately 4 cm, decreasing the length of the lungs. To adjust to this decreased length, the anteroposterior diameter of the chest enlarges by 2 cm. Increased pressure from the uterus widens the substernal angle 50%, from 68 to 103 degrees, and causes the ribs to flare out slightly (Bobrowski, 2010; Whitty & Dombrowsky, 2014). The circumference of the thoracic cage may increase 5 to 7 cm, compensating for the decreased lung length (Bobrowski, 2010; Hegewald & Crapo, 2011). Many of these changes are probably caused by hormonal influence because they occur before pressure is exerted from the growing uterus. Despite the mechanical elevation of the diaphragm in pregnancy, most of the work of breathing remains diaphragmatic.

Lung Volume

Lung volumes are altered during pregnancy. Total lung volume (i.e., the amount of air in lungs at maximal inspiration) decreases slightly (5%). Residual volume (i.e., the amount of air in lungs after maximum expiration), expiratory reserve volume (i.e., the maximal amount of air that can be expired from the resting expiratory level), and functional residual capacity (i.e., the amount of air remaining in the lungs at resting expiratory level, permitting air for gas exchange between breaths) fall (Hegewald & Crapo, 2011; Whitty & Dombrowsky, 2014). Tidal volume (i.e., the amount of air inspired and expired with normal breath) increases 30% to 40% (500 to 700 mL/min) during pregnancy and compensates for decreases in expiratory reserve volume and residual volume. Vital capacity (i.e., the maximum amount of air that can be forcibly expired after maximum inspiration) and inspiratory reserve volume (i.e., the maximum amount of air that can be inspired at end of normal inspiration) remain unchanged. The net effect of these lung volume changes is that there is no change in maximum breathing capacity or work of breathing during pregnancy and enhancement of alveolar gas exchange. Spirometric measurements used for the diagnosis of respiratory problems do not change and remain useful evaluation tools.

Ventilation

Alveolar and minute ventilation increase. Minute ventilation (i.e., amount of air inspired in 1 minute) increases from the first trimester to values 30% to 50% higher by term. Minute ventilation is the product of the respiratory rate and the tidal volume. The increase in minute ventilation is caused by an increase in tidal volume because the respiratory rate remains unchanged or increases only slightly (Hegewald & Crapo, 2011). Progesterone stimulates ventilation by lowering the carbon dioxide threshold of the respiratory center and may also act as a primary stimulant to the respiratory center, independent of carbon dioxide sensitivity and threshold. For example, in the nonpregnant woman, an increase of 1 mm Hg in partial pressure of carbon dioxide in arterial blood (P_aCO_2) increases minute ventilation by 1.5 L/min, whereas in pregnancy, this same change in P_aCO_2 results in a 6 L/min change in minute ventilation (Whitty & Dombrowsky, 2014).

Oxygen and Carbon Dioxide Exchange

Oxygen consumption increases 20% to 40% by term to meet increasing oxygen demand in maternal, placental, and fetal tissues, with further increases during labor (Whitty & Dombrowsky, 2014). The increased oxygen demand during pregnancy is met by the increases in minute ventilation and cardiac output. Increased minute ventilation increases arterial partial pressures of oxygen (P_aO_2) and decreases alveolar carbon dioxide tension.

The P_aO_2 during pregnancy is mildly elevated to between 104 and 108 mm Hg during the first trimester and 101 and 104 mm Hg at term (Whitty & Dombrowsky, 2014). P_aCO_2 is decreased to between 27 and 32 mm Hg (Bobrowski, 2010). The decrease in P_aCO_2 is accompanied by a fall in plasma bicarbonate concentration to 18 to 21 mEq/L (base deficit of −3 to −4 mEq/L). Decreased carbon dioxide levels in the blood lead to higher pH values that are compensated for by renal excretion of bicarbonate, and the woman maintains a high normal pH in the range of 7.40 to 7.45. The result of these changes is mildly elevated P_aO_2 and decreased P_aCO_2 and serum bicarbonate levels compared with normal values for nonpregnant women (Blackburn, 2018). Thus, the acid-base status during pregnancy is that of a compensated respiratory alkalosis, which enhances movement of carbon dioxide from the fetus to the mother.

Up to 60% to 70% of pregnant women experience pregnancy-related dyspnea (Whitty & Dombrowsky, 2014). This is a physiologic dyspnea that occurs even at rest and with mild exertion (Blackburn, 2018). The exact cause of this dyspnea is unclear, but it may be due to the woman's sensation of hyperventilation, effects of progesterone, increased oxygen consumption, and decreased P_aCO_2 levels. Mechanical forces from pressure of the uterus on the diaphragm may increase the sensation of dyspnea, but these forces are not the primary cause because dyspnea usually begins during the first or second trimester. Symptoms of nasal stuffiness, rhinitis, and nosebleeds are also more common for pregnant women and are related to vascular congestion resulting from increased levels of estrogen (Caparroz, Gregorio, Bongiovanni, Izu, & Kosugi, 2016; Hegewald & Crapo, 2011). Changes in the upper respiratory tract may also increase snoring and risk of sleep disordered breathing during pregnancy (Blackburn, 2018; Sarberg, Svanborg, Wiréhn, & Josefsson, 2014). The respiratory system rapidly returns to the prepregnancy status within 1 to 3 weeks after birth.

RENAL SYSTEM

The renal system undergoes structural and functional changes during pregnancy (Table 3–3). Changes in renal function accommodate the increased metabolic and circulatory requirements of pregnancy. The renal system excretes maternal and fetal waste products. Pressure placed on the renal system and the relaxant effects of progesterone on vascular tissue enhance the ability of the renal system to accommodate the cardiovascular changes of pregnancy.

Structural Changes

Physiologic hydroureter and hydronephrosis develop. Increased renal blood flow, interstitial volumes, and hormonal influences increase renal volume by 30% and lengthen the kidneys by approximately 1 cm (Monga & Mastrobattista, 2014). The relaxing effects of progesterone on smooth muscle are probably primarily responsible for the dilation of the renal calyces, pelvis, and ureters (Blackburn, 2018). This muscular relaxation, coupled with increased urine volume and stasis, is associated with an increased risk of urinary tract infection.

TABLE 3–3. Renal Changes during Pregnancy

Parameter	Change
Renal blood flow	Increases 60% to 80%
Glomerular filtration rate	Increases 40% to 60%
Tubular function	Increased filtered load and excretion of amino acids, glucose, water-soluble vitamins, calcium
	Net retention of sodium, potassium, and water
	Decreased serum urea, blood urea nitrogen, and creatinine levels
Renin–angiotensin–aldosterone system	Increases in renin, angiotensin, aldosterone, and other system components
Structural changes	30% increase in renal volume
	1-cm increase in length
	Dilation of renal calyces, renal pelvis, and ureters
	Displacement of bladder in third trimester
	Increased risk of infection
Urodynamic changes	Increased urine output
	Increased frequency
	Increased incidence of stress and urgency incontinence

By late gestation, the growing uterus and the dilated ovarian vein plexus place pressure on and displace the ureters and bladder. The ureters become dilated, elongated, and more tortuous, primarily in portions above the pelvic rim. The urethra also lengthens. Dilation of the ureters on the right side is more pronounced than that on the left because of the cushioning that occurs on the left side and dextrorotation of the uterus by the sigmoid colon. The right ovarian vein crosses the pelvic brim and therefore experiences greater compression by the growing uterus than the left ovarian vein, which parallels the brim (Monga & Mastrobattista, 2014).

During the second trimester, hyperemia of pelvic organs, hyperplasia of muscles and connective tissues, and the gravid uterus elevate the bladder trigone and cause thickening of the interureteric margin. The bladder is displaced forward and upward in late pregnancy. Mechanical pressure placed on the bladder by the gravid uterus changes it from a convex to a concave organ. Urine output is increased primarily due to changes in sodium excretion. Urinary frequency (>7 daytime voidings) is common and begins in the first trimester, along with an increased stress and urge incontinence (Fiadjoe, Kannan, & Rane, 2010). Frequency develops due to hormonal changes, hypervolemia, increased renal blood flow and glomerular filtration, and, in the third trimester, uterine pressure. These changes regress after birth in most women. Nocturia is due to increased sodium and therefore water excretion, mediated by the effects of the lateral position at night, which decrease stasis and increase venous return renal blood flow and glomerular filtration rate (GFR) (Blackburn, 2018).

Pressure on the renal system can impair drainage of blood and lymph and impede urine flow, which increases risk of infection and trauma during pregnancy. Renal volumes normalize with the first week after birth. However, hydronephrosis and hydroureter may take 3 to 4 months or longer to return to normal (Monga & Mastrobattista, 2014).

Renal Blood Flow, Glomerular Filtration, and Tubular Function

Renal plasma flow (RPF) increases 60% to 80% by the second trimester due to increased blood volume and cardiac output and the lowered SVR caused by progesterone. RPF then progressively decreases by term to a level 50% greater than nonpregnant values (Monga & Mastrobattista, 2014). Women lying in the supine position can have decreased RPF in late pregnancy, compared with values obtained while in lateral positions. An increase in the GFR is seen as early as 3 to 4 weeks after conception. GFR peaks by the end of the first trimester, at 40% to 60% greater than nonpregnant levels or at an average of 110 to 180 mL/min

(Monga & Mastrobattista, 2014). This rise in GFR is thought to arise from the increased RPF and vasodilation of preglomerular and postglomerular resistance vessels without any alteration in glomerular capillary pressure (Blackburn, 2018). The increased GFR during pregnancy may alter renal excretion of drugs, especially water-soluble drugs, and shorten their half-lives.

The filtered load of many substances exceeds the tubular reabsorptive capacity. As a result, renal clearance of many substances is elevated during pregnancy, with increased excretion and a related decrease in serum levels of some substances. Amino acids, glucose (see "Glycosuria"), many electrolytes, and water-soluble vitamins are excreted in amounts higher than in nonpregnant women. Calcium excretion increases, but is balanced by increased intestinal absorption. Serum potassium values are influenced by both elevated plasma aldosterone levels, which promotes potassium excretion, and by progesterone, which promotes potassium retention (Monga & Mastrobattista, 2014). The net change favors potassium retention, with a net retention of 300 to 350 mEq/L. Because the extra potassium is used by maternal and fetal tissues, serum potassium is only slightly changed.

Protein excretion is also increased during pregnancy because the increased filtered load of protein exceeds the tubular reabsorptive capacity (see "Proteinuria"). Serum urea, blood urea nitrogen, and creatinine levels decline because of increased GFR. Serum uric acid levels decrease in early pregnancy and rise after 24 weeks. As a result, normal lab values during pregnancy and critical values indicating abnormality may be altered. Examples of critical values indicative of abnormal renal function during pregnancy include plasma creatinine >0.8 mg/dL, blood urea nitrogen >14 mg/dL, and urinary protein >300 mg/24 hours (Blackburn, 2018; Monga & Mastrobattista, 2014; Podymow, August, & Akbari, 2010).

Fluid and Electrolyte Balance

The kidneys play a significant role in the regulation of body sodium and water content. Renal sodium is the primary determinant of volume homeostasis. The filtered load of sodium increases from nonpregnant levels of 20,000 to approximately 30,000 mEq/day during pregnancy (Monga & Mastrobattista, 2014). Sodium balance is mediated by factors that promote sodium excretion versus those that promote sodium retention. Factors promoting sodium excretion during pregnancy include increased GFR, increased atrial natriuretic factor, decreased plasma albumin, elevated progesterone and PG levels, and decreased vascular resistance. The physiologic changes that cause excretion of sodium are accompanied by increases in tubular reabsorption of sodium to avoid sodium depletion. Increases in aldosterone, estrogen, and cortisol all contribute to sodium

reabsorption (Blackburn, 2018). The end result favors sodium retention, with a net retention of 900 to 950 mg of sodium or an additional 2 to 6 mEq of sodium reabsorbed each day for fetal and maternal stores (Monga & Mastrobattista, 2014).

Sodium retention (and thus water retention because as sodium is reabsorbed from the tubule back into the blood, it pulls water with it) is mediated by the changes in the renin–angiotensin–aldosterone system. Aldosterone acts on the distal tubule and cortical collecting ducts to enhance sodium reabsorption. Aldosterone release is controlled by a specialized region of the kidney, which secretes the peptide hormone renin in response to decreases in BP, or sodium contents of the renal tubules, and stimulation of the sympathetic nervous system. Renin converts angiotensinogen to angiotensin I. Angiotensin I is cleaved in the lungs by angiotensin-converting enzyme (ACE) to form angiotensin II. Angiotensin II is a potent stimulator of aldosterone secretion and a potent vasopressor. Angiotensinogen, plasma renin activity, plasma renin, angiotensin II, and aldosterone levels are all increased in pregnancy (Lindheimer, Conrad, Ananth Karumanchi, 2013; Lumbers & Pringle, 2014).

During pregnancy, renin is produced by the uterus, placenta, and fetus as well as the kidney. Release is stimulated by estrogen, changes in BP, PGs, and progesterone (an aldosterone antagonist). Increased plasma levels of aldosterone promote water and sodium retention, which results in the natural volume-overload state of pregnancy. Despite the elevated levels of angiotensin II, BP is not elevated in normal pregnancy due to a 60% decrease in sensitivity of the blood vessels to the vasoconstrictor effects of angiotensin II. This decreased sensitivity is thought to be due to decreased responsiveness of angiotensin II receptors and the relaxant effects of vasodilatory PGs and endothelial factors such as nitric oxide. Women with preeclampsia do not maintain this reduced sensitivity to angiotensin II, and BP rises (Cheung & Lafayette, 2013; Lindheimer et al., 2013). In healthy pregnant women, the net effect of these changes is the establishment of a new equilibrium that the women sense as normal. From this new baseline, she responds to changes in fluid and electrolytes in a manner similar to a nonpregnant woman (Blackburn, 2018). The postpartum period is characterized by a rapid loss of the accumulated fluid and sodium, especially on postpartum days 2 to 5, with restoration of prepregnancy values by 21 days or sooner (Blackburn, 2018).

Glycosuria

During pregnancy, the amount of glucose that is filtered by the kidneys increases 10- to 100-fold due to the increased RPF and GFR. The renal tubules increase reabsorption of glucose from the tubules back into the blood but are unable to match the dramatic increase in filtered glucose. The glucose that cannot be absorbed is lost in the urine; therefore, glycosuria is common. The glucose tolerance test is normal with most pregnant women with glycosuria, suggesting that this glycosuria is secondary to altered renal function and not abnormal carbohydrate metabolism (Blackburn, 2018). Clinical management of the woman with diabetes requires serum glucose evaluation rather than urine glucose evaluation during pregnancy.

Proteinuria

Protein excretion is also increased during pregnancy because the increased filtered load of protein exceeds the tubular reabsorptive capacity. Thus, urinary protein measurements should not be considered abnormal until 24-hour urine values greater than 300 mg are reached. Levels higher than 300 mg/24 hours may indicate renal disease, preeclampsia, or urinary tract infection (Monga & Mastrobattista, 2014; Podymow et al., 2010).

GASTROINTESTINAL SYSTEM

Nutritional requirements during pregnancy increase, and changes in the GI system meet these demands. The GI tract is altered physiologically and anatomically during pregnancy. Many of the common discomforts of pregnancy (e.g., heartburn, gingivitis, constipation, nausea, and vomiting) can be attributed to the GI system. Pregnancy is associated with increased appetite and consumption of food. Many women experience food cravings and avoidances, sometimes mediated by alterations in sensitivity to taste and smell.

Mouth and Esophagus

Pregnant women often experience gingival edema and hyperemia, which usually begins in the second month and peaks in the third trimester. Gingival changes are probably related to increased vascularity and blood flow, changes in connective tissue, and the release of inflammatory mediators. Tooth enamel is not altered, but increases in dental plaques and calculus have been reported. Existing periodontal disease may be exacerbated by pregnancy. Three percent to 5% of women develop an angiogranuloma (epulis) between their upper, anterior maxillary teeth. Epulis regresses postpartum but may recur with subsequent pregnancies (Blackburn, 2018).

Lower esophageal sphincter (LES) muscle tone and pressure decrease due to the effects of progesterone. LES function is further altered after the uterus is large enough to change the positioning of the stomach and intestines and to move the LES into the thorax (Cunningham et al., 2014; Kelly & Savides, 2014). These changes increase the risk of reflux and heartburn.

Nausea and Vomiting

Nausea with or without vomiting affects over 70% to 80% of pregnant women (Bustos, Venkataramanan, & Caritis, 2017). The exact mechanism for nausea and vomiting of pregnancy (NVP) is unclear. Theories have focused on mechanical, endocrinologic, allergic, metabolic, genetic, and psychosomatic etiologies (Blackburn, 2018; Bustos et al., 2017). The most frequent hormones linked with NVP are estrogens and especially hCG, whose secretion patterns parallel the appearance and disappearance of NVP in most women. Many studies have examined this link; however, data are inconsistent and inconclusive. NVP usually begins between 4 and 6 weeks and peaks at 8 to 12 weeks but may begin earlier or last longer in some women (Blackburn, 2018). Treatment is supportive and involves suggesting that the woman avoid foods that trigger nausea and to eat frequent, small meals. Hyperemesis gravidarum is a more severe and persistent form of nausea and vomiting and is associated with weight loss, electrolyte imbalance, ketosis, and dehydration. Any underlying illness should be excluded; hospitalization for fluid and electrolyte replacement may be necessary.

Stomach

Progesterone decreases stomach gastric smooth muscle tone and motility, whereas the gravid uterus displaces the stomach. Gastric emptying is probably unchanged in early pregnancy but may be delayed with a tendency toward reverse peristalsis later in gestation. Relaxation of the LES permits reflux of gastric contents into the esophagus, causing heartburn. Gastric reflux is more common later in pregnancy. Decreased gastric acidity may reduce symptoms in women with peptic ulcer (Kelly & Savides, 2014).

Small and Large Intestines

The intestines are pushed upward and laterally by the growing uterus. The appendix is displaced superiorly, reaching the right costal margin by term, which, along with milder guarding and rebound tenderness due to cushioning by the uterus, may delay diagnosis of appendicitis during pregnancy. Increased progesterone levels relax GI tract tone and decrease intestinal motility, allowing time for increased absorption from the colon. Increased height of the duodenal villi and activity of brush border enzymes also increase nutrient absorptive capacity (Kelly & Savides, 2014). As a result, absorption of substances such as calcium, amino acids, iron, glucose, sodium, chloride, and water are increased. The alterations in intestinal transport may lead to sensations "bloating" and abdominal distension (Blackburn, 2018). Reduced motility, mechanical obstruction by the uterus, and increased water absorption from the colon increase the risk of constipation. Hemorrhoids may develop when there is straining during bowel movements related to constipation and from the increased pressure exerted on the vessels below the level of the uterus.

Liver

Liver size and morphology do not significantly change during pregnancy, but liver production of many proteins is altered primarily due to the effects of estrogen. Hepatic blood flow increases during pregnancy, but the percentage of circulating blood volume reaching the liver remains unchanged. Plasma proteins, serum enzymes, and serum lipids produced by the liver are altered during pregnancy (Blackburn, 2018). Some tests of liver function during pregnancy produce values that would suggest hepatic disease in nonpregnant women. For example, fibrinogen levels increase by 50% by the end of the second trimester. Plasma albumin concentration decreases, which in nonpregnant patients could indicate liver disease, but is an expected change during pregnancy. Serum alkaline phosphatase activity and serum cholesterol concentration can be twice the normal range or even higher in multiple gestations (Blackburn, 2018). On the other hand, serum bilirubin, aspartate aminotransferase, and alanine aminotransferase are unchanged or slightly lower in normal pregnancy and therefore can be used to evaluate liver function during pregnancy. Hepatic changes during pregnancy can alter biotransformation of drugs by the liver and clearance of drugs from the maternal serum. Some liver enzymatic processes may be slowed during pregnancy, delaying drug metabolism and degradation (Blackburn, 2018). Liver enzymes generally return to prepregnancy levels by 3 weeks postpartum.

Gallbladder

Gallbladder size and function are altered during pregnancy. Elevated progesterone levels cause the gallbladder to be hypotonic and distended. Gallbladder smooth muscle contraction is impaired and may lead to stasis. Emptying time is slow after 14 weeks' gestation. In the second and third trimesters, fasting and residual volumes are twice as large as in the nonpregnant woman. As a result of these changes, cholesterol may be sequestered in the gall bladder, increasing the risk of gall stones (Blackburn, 2018). The gall bladder generally returns to the prepregnancy status by 2 weeks postpartum.

Weight Gain

Prenatal care, socioeconomic factors, and adequate nutrition influence pregnancy outcome. Women who are underweight before conception and women who have inadequate weight gain during pregnancy are at greater risk for having a low-birth-weight infant. The risk is greatest for women with both factors (Stotland, Bodnar, & Abrams, 2014). Maternal obesity and excessive weight gain during pregnancy have been associated with fetal macrosomia (Chen et al., 2015). A nutritional assessment should be made at the initial prenatal visit, with referral to a registered dietitian as needed.

The woman's prepregnancy height and weight determine her actual caloric intake needs. On average, the increased demands of pregnancy require an additional 300 to 340 kcal each day to meet maternal and fetal energy needs. Women who are pregnant with twins or higher order multiples need an additional 300 kcal per fetus each day. There are differences in suggested weight gain based on prepregnancy weight and body mass index (BMI). The Institute of Medicine guidelines on weight gain during pregnancy assume a 1.1- to 4-lb weight gain during the first trimester. Recommended weight gain during the second and third trimester varies with BMI: 0.8 to 1 lb/week in women with a normal BMI, 1 to 1.3 lb/week in underweight women, 0.6 to 0.7 lb/week in overweight women, and 0.4 to 0.6 lb/week in obese women (Rasmussen et al., 2010).

METABOLIC CHANGES

Profound metabolic changes occur throughout pregnancy to provide for the development and growth of the fetus. Adequate maternal weight gain and changes in maternal glucose, protein, and fat metabolism are important factors in normal fetal growth and development. During the course of pregnancy, approximately 3.5 kg of fat is deposited, approximately 30,000 kcal of energy is stored, and 900 g of new protein is synthesized to meet maternal and fetal needs (Blackburn, 2018). Estrogens, progesterone, and hCS influence metabolic processes during pregnancy by altering glucose utilization, fat metabolism and use, protein homeostasis, and insulin action. These changes meet fetal growth needs by increasing the availability of glucose and amino acid for transfer to the fetus while providing increased availability of fatty acids as an alternative energy substrate to meet maternal needs and maintain homeostasis (Blackburn, 2018). "The changes in carbohydrate and lipid metabolism parallel the energy needs of the mother and fetus, whereas the changes in maternal nitrogen and protein metabolism occur early in pregnancy, before fetal demand" (Blackburn, 2018, pp. 543–544).

Maternal basal metabolic rate increases, which, along with other alterations in maternal metabolism and fetal heat dissipation, increases heat generation during pregnancy by 30% to 40% (Cunningham et al., 2014). As a result, maternal temperature increases by about 0.5°C.

Pregnancy can be divided into two metabolic phases: an initial anabolism dominant phase and a later catabolism predominant phase. During the first part of pregnancy, anabolism is prominent with nutrient uptake, energy stored as fat, and maternal weight gain. Estrogen stimulates pancreatic beta cell hypertrophy and hyperplasia with increased insulin production. During this phase, insulin sensitivity is not significantly affected; insulin responses are enhanced with a normal glucose tolerance. The increased insulin promotes storage of glucose as glycogen, increased fat synthesis, storage of triglycerides and fat, fat cell hypertrophy, and inhibition of lipolysis. Both low-density and high-density lipoproteins increase (Herrera & Lasuncion, 2017). Maternal protein storage increases, with a net retention of 1.3 g/day of nitrogen for use both by the mother and the fetus (Blackburn, 2018).

As pregnancy progresses, the maternal metabolic status becomes more catabolic, and maternal weight gain is due primarily to fetal growth. Adipose tissue lipolytic activity is enhanced, and plasma free fatty acids, glycerol, and ketones increase (Herrera & Lasuncion, 2017). These provide alternate energy sources for maternal needs, conserving glucose for transfer to the fetus. This is important because the fetus is an obligatory glucose user whose enzyme systems promote fat storage and who cannot readily breakdown fat to use for energy. During this phase, maternal urinary nitrogen excretion decreases, conserving protein for fetal transfer. Maternal insulin levels increase as insulin resistance in the peripheral tissues becomes prominent (Blackburn, 2018; Mouzon & Lassance, 2015).

Insulin antagonism is caused by hCS and other placental hormones (i.e., progesterone, estrogen, cortisol, and prolactin) that oppose the action of insulin and promote maternal lipolysis (Moore, Mouzon, & Catalano, 2014). Insulin normally helps to clear glucose from the blood and promotes glycogen and fat storage. Insulin resistance (mean insulin sensitivity decreases 50% to 70%) means that maternal glucose levels remain higher for a longer period after a meal to promote fetal transfer (Herrera & Lasuncion, 2017; Mouzon & Lassance, 2015). Thus, decreased sensitivity to insulin in the liver and peripheral tissues leads to a persistent relative hyperglycemia after meals. This relative hyperinsulinemia and hyperglycemia of pregnancy has been referred to as a diabetogenic state.

Maternal metabolic responses alter responses on glucose tolerance tests so that these tests need to be interpreted using pregnancy-specific norms. These changes, in comparison to a nonpregnant individual, include (1) a lower initial fasting blood glucose value (due to decreased glucose utilization and increased fat utilization enhancing glucose availability for the fetus) and (2) elevated blood glucose for a longer period after ingestion of carbohydrates (due to insulin antagonism and decreased insulin sensitivity) (Moore et al., 2014; Mouzon & Lassance, 2015).

ENDOCRINE SYSTEM

Thyroid Gland

The production, circulation, and disposal of thyroid hormone are altered in pregnancy to support maternal metabolic changes and fetal growth and development. Increased vascularity and hyperplasia of the thyroid gland result in increased hormone production and an increase in thyroid size, although not in the form of a goiter in populations with adequate iodine intake (Nader, 2014b; Patton, Samuels, Trinidad, & Caughey, 2014). Most of the changes in the thyroid gland occur during the first half of pregnancy and lead to a state of "euthyroid hyperthyroxinemia," in which levels of thyroxine (T4) are elevated. These changes are due to estrogen (increasing thyroxine-binding globulin [TBG] production by the liver), hCG, and increased urinary iodide excretion (Nader, 2014b; Patton et al., 2014). hCG, which has mild thyroid-stimulating–like activity, stimulates production of T4 and triiodothyronine (T3).

Total T4 and T3 increase markedly, peaking by 10 to 15 weeks and remain higher to term (Patton et al., 2014). Free T4 and T3 increase during the first trimester but decrease during the second and third trimesters as levels of TBG increase. Thus, more T3 and T4 are produced (increased total), but because much of the extra thyroid hormone is bound to TBG, the amount of free hormone is reduced. Serum protein–bound iodine increases. Increased production of thyroid hormone increases thyroid iodine uptake. At the same time, urinary iodide excretion increases and iodide is sent to the fetus, leading to a smaller iodine pool. These changes are partially compensated for by increased thyroid clearance and recycling of iodide; however, maternal iodide needs increase during pregnancy (Blackburn, 2018).

Maternal thyroid hormone is critical for fetal central nervous system (CNS) development, especially in early pregnancy, when the CNS undergoes critical development prior to the time the fetus is able to produce T4. Untreated maternal hypothyroidism increases the risk of pregnancy loss and altered fetal brain development and later neurocognitive impairment and neurodevelopmental problems (Huang, 2017; Korevaar, Medici, Visser, & Peeters, 2017; Patton et al., 2014). Iodine supplementation has been found to decrease the incidence of these complications in populations with high endemic levels of hypothyroidism (Melse-Boonstra & Jaiswal, 2010).

Subclinical hyperthyroidism occurs in 3.5% to 18% of healthy pregnant women (Korevaar et al., 2017). Screening for symptoms of both hypothyroidism and hyperthyroidism during pregnancy is challenging because pregnancy is commonly associated with heat intolerance, tachycardia, wide pulse pressure, and vomiting (all signs seen with hyperthyroidism, whereas fatigue, constipation, weight gain, and muscle cramps are also seen with hypothyroidism) (Nader, 2014b). Poor control during pregnancy can result in preterm labor, fetal loss, or thyroid crisis in these women. Diagnosis of abnormal thyroid function in the pregnant woman requires an understanding of the normal changes in thyroid function during pregnancy in order to appropriately interpret results of laboratory tests.

Transient postpartum thyroid disorder (PPTD) is seen in 4% to 9% of postpartum women and is thought to have an autoimmune basis. PPTD is usually characterized by a period (average, 2 to 4 months) of mild hyperthyroidism, followed by a period of hypothyroidism, with a return to normal thyroid function in most women by 12 months postpartum. Some women only experience one of these phases. Up to one fourth of these women develop permanent hypothyroidism within 5 to 15 years (De Groot et al., 2012).

Pituitary Gland

The anterior pituitary enlarges, with a 30% increase in weight and twofold increase in volume and becomes more convex and dome shaped (Blackburn, 2018). These changes are primarily due to an increase in the group of cells that produce prolactin. Adrenocorticotropic hormone (ACTH) secretion and serum levels increase, peaking during the intrapartum period (Vrekoussis et al., 2010). This increase is probably due primarily to stimulation by increased placental rather than hypothalamic CRH. Pituitary growth hormone secretion is suppressed by placental growth hormone, which increases from 15 to 20 weeks to term (Nader, 2014a). FSH (stimulates ovum follicle growth) and LH (needed for ovulation) are both inhibited during pregnancy.

The posterior pituitary hormones are oxytocin and AVP. Oxytocin influences contractility of the uterus, and after birth, it stimulates milk ejection from the breasts. Secretion increases during the intrapartum and postpartum periods. AVP, also called antidiuretic hormone, causes vasoconstriction when released in large amounts, which increases BP. The major role of AVP is its antidiuretic action in the regulation of water balance. Secretion of AVP is controlled by changes in plasma osmolarity and blood volume. Plasma levels of AVP do not change during pregnancy, despite the changes in blood volume, indicating that AVP is secreted at a lower plasma osmolality in pregnancy (Blackburn, 2018).

Adrenal Glands

The elevated ACTH stimulates increased cortisol production by the adrenal glands during pregnancy. The adrenal gland undergoes hypertrophy with increases in the zona fasciculata (the portion of the adrenal that produces glucocorticoids such as cortisol) (Nader, 2014a). Plasma levels of CRH progressively increase during the second and third trimesters of pregnancy. Circulating cortisol levels regulate carbohydrate and protein metabolism. Total and free cortisol increase two- to eightfold leading to a transient hypercortisolemia (Nader, 2014a). Normally increased cortisol would turn off ACTH release. Therefore, the increased ACTH with increased cortisol during pregnancy suggests changes in the set point for cortisol release. Thus, in spite of the elevated cortisol and ACTH, physiologic responses to stress (such as BP, heart rate, and cortisol reactivity) are maintained during pregnancy, although they may be somewhat blunted, with wide individual differences reported (Blackburn, 2018).

Other adrenal cortex hormones, aldosterone (see "Fluid and Electrolyte Balance" under "Renal System" section), and steroid hormones also increase. Total testosterone levels also increase in pregnancy because of an increase in sex hormone–binding globulin. Free testosterone levels are low normal before 28 weeks' gestation.

Parathyroid Glands

Parathyroid hormone (PTH) decreases during the first trimester and then increases to term. The early decrease is due to increased 1,25-dihydroxyvitamin D in response to PTHrP production by the fetus and placenta (Nader, 2014a). Regulation of calcium is closely related to magnesium, phosphate, PTH, vitamin D, and calcitonin levels. Any alteration in one may alter the others. Increases in serum-ionized calcium or magnesium suppress PTH levels, whereas decreases in serum-ionized calcium or magnesium stimulate the release of PTH.

Maternal calcium homeostasis changes during pregnancy. Total serum calcium decreases, primarily related to the fall in albumin, reaching its lowest at 28 to 32 weeks, and then plateaus or increases slightly to term (Blackburn, 2018). There is no significant change in mean serum-ionized calcium. Daily maternal intestinal calcium absorption increases and doubles by the third trimester due to increased calciferol (active form of vitamin D) and its binding proteins (Nader, 2014a). This change begins in the first trimester, before fetal demand, so that maternal bone stores of calcium are increased during early pregnancy. These stores are used to meet the increased fetal demand in late pregnancy. Overall significant maternal bone mass is not lost during pregnancy.

IMMUNE SYSTEM

During pregnancy, the mother's immune system remains tolerant of the foreign paternal antigens on fetal tissues and yet maintains adequate immune competence against most microorganisms. Protection of the fetus from rejection is a multifactorial, complex process that seems to be predominately a localized uterine response, although there are also systemic responses mediated primarily by endocrine factors. The maternal microbiome is altered during pregnancy with changes in gut, vaginal tract, oral and placenta microbiota, and increase in anti-inflammatory species (Neuman & Koren, 2017). These changes are thought to enhance development of the fetal immune and other systems (Hsu & Nanan, 2014).

Adaptations in the maternal immune system protect both the mother and fetus during pregnancy. "Within adaptive responses, the cell-mediated (T helper 1, or Th1) response is reduced, the antibody-mediated (T helper 2, or Th2) response is enhanced, and the relation between the two is dysregulated. These alterations, which help prevent the mother's immune system from rejecting the semiallogenic fetus, may increase her risk of developing certain infections and influence the course of chronic disorders such as autoimmune diseases" (Blackburn, 2018, p. 435). The major changes in the immune system during pregnancy are seen at the maternal–fetal interface where maternal and fetal–placental immune systems work together to provide support and protection for the fetus (Blackburn, 2018). "The uniqueness of the immune system during pregnancy is the interaction between the maternal immune system (characterized by a reinforced network of recognition, communication, trafficking, and repair) and the presence of a developing active fetal immune system that can modify maternal response to the environment" (Shynloya, Lee, Srikhajon, & Lye, 2013, p. 156).

Immunologic adaptation during pregnancy has been characterized by four stages: (1) initiation (during implantation, placentation, and the first and early second trimesters), (2) tolerance (second and third trimesters), (3) activation (late third trimester and parturition), and (4) restoration (postpartum period) (Mor & Abrahams, 2014; Shynloya et al., 2013). During the initial stages, the mother recognizes and protects the fetus. These responses are mediated by Th2 cytokines (interleukins) and growth factors. Factors that enhance

maternal tolerance at the maternal–fetal interface include (1) progesterone; (2) blocking factors induced by progesterone; (3) placental histocompatibility antigen, class 1, G; (4) altered natural killer (NK) cell function; (5) changes in the Th1 to Th2 cytokine balance; (6) decidual macrophages; and (7) toll-like receptor (Blackburn, 2018; Mor & Abrahams, 2014; Munoz-Suano, Hamilton, & Betz, 2011). Cytokines, prostaglandin E2, steroid hormones, estrogen, hCG, and various pregnancy-specific proteins exert immunosuppressive effects during pregnancy.

Immune responses include innate responses and adaptive responses. Both types of responses are altered during pregnancy with enhancement of innate and antibody-mediated responses in the systemic circulation of the pregnant woman. Innate responses include initial actions to the entry of pathogens and inflammatory reactions. Circulating WBCs (especially neutrophils and monocytes) are increased. However, decreased neutrophil chemotaxis (organized movement of neutrophils toward the site of pathogen entry) may delay initial responses to infection (Mor & Abrahams, 2014). Systemic NK cell cytotoxic activity is down-regulated by progesterone especially in the second and third trimesters and immediately postpartum. Decidual NK cells support implantation, placental development, and remodeling of maternal spiral arteries. Enhanced monocyte and neutrophil activity may enhance phagocytosis. Complement levels and activity are normal to increased but may be delayed (Blackburn, 2018).

Adaptive responses include antibody-mediated (B lymphocyte) and cell-mediated (T lymphocyte) responses. Pregnancy is characterized by a switch in the balance of Th1 to Th2 cytokines (Cappelletti, Della Bella, Ferrazzi, Mavilio, & Divanovic, 2016). Th1 and Th2 are subsets of T-lymphocyte helper cells that facilitate different components of the immune response. During pregnancy, Th2 anti-inflammatory cytokines are increased (most prominent in second trimester), enhancing antibody-mediated immunity, whereas Th1 proinflammatory cytokines are decreased (most prominent in first and third trimesters), reducing cell-mediated responses (associated with tissue rejection). B-lymphocyte function (antibody-mediated immunity) is not significantly altered and may be enhanced by the increase in Th2 cytokines. The slight decrease in immunoglobulin G may increase the risk of bacterial colonization. Cell-mediated (T lymphocyte) immunity is somewhat suppressed during pregnancy, which may help prevent maternal rejection of the fetus. This suppression is mediated by cortisol, hCG, progesterone, and alpha-fetoprotein (Blackburn, 2018). T-cell total numbers are probably unchanged and systemic T-cell function maintained. However, selective localized (reproductive) immunosuppression may occur that may increase the risk of viral and mycotic infections.

NEUROMUSCULAR AND SENSORY SYSTEMS

In general, there are no major CNS changes during pregnancy, although changes occur in cerebral circulation with a shift in the cerebral autoregulation to compensate for changes in fluid and electrolyte balance and for cardiovascular changes (Johnson & Cipolla, 2015). Several discomforts reported by pregnant women are associated with the nervous system. Mild frontal headaches may occur in the first and second trimesters and may be caused by tension or related to hormonal changes (Nappi et al., 2011). Severe headache, especially after 20 weeks' gestation, may be associated with preeclampsia. This type of headache is a result of cerebral edema from vasoconstriction. Dizziness may result from vasomotor instability, postural hypotension, or hypoglycemia, especially after prolonged periods of sitting or standing. Paresthesia of the lower extremities can occur because of pressure from the gravid uterus, interfering with circulation. Excessive hyperventilation, resulting in lower P_aCO_2 levels, creates a tingling sensation in the hands (Blackburn, 2018).

Musculoskeletal alterations during pregnancy include changes in posture, gait, and ligament laxity (Thabah & Ravindran, 2015). Early in pregnancy, the ligaments of the pregnant woman soften from the effects of progesterone and relaxin. This softening, especially evident in the sacroiliac, sacrococcygeal, and pubic joints of the pelvis, facilitates birth. The center of gravity changes with advancing pregnancy because of the increase in weight gain, fluid retention, lordosis, and mobilization of ligaments. To accommodate the increased weight of the uterus, the lumbodorsal spinal curve is accentuated, and the woman's posture changes. The rectus abdominis muscle may separate because of the pressure exerted by the growing uterus, producing diastasis recti. The risks of ligament injury, muscle cramps, back and joint pain, and falls are increased during pregnancy (Cakmak, Ribeiro, & Inanir, 2016; Casagrande, Gugala, Clark, & Lindsey, 2015). Approximately 15% to 26% of pregnant women develop restless legs syndrome (RLS), also called Willis-Ekbom disease, which is a rate 2 to 3 times higher than in the general population. RLS is a transient disorder that usually develops in the third trimester and may interfere with sleep. The exact cause of RLS is unknown; it usually disappears by 1 month postpartum but may recur (Picchietti et al., 2015).

Sleep patterns change during pregnancy, mediated by hormonal changes and mechanical forces. Changes include increases in total sleep time, insomnia, night awakenings, and daytime sleepiness and decreased stage 3 and 4 non–rapid eye movement sleep (Blackburn, 2018; Santiago, Nolledo, Kinzler, & Santiago, 2001). Night awakenings are often related to nocturia, fetal activity, backache, dyspnea, and heartburn. Sleep is also altered in the postpartum period, especially in the first few weeks.

The pregnant woman may experience ocular and otolaryngeal changes. Intraocular pressure tends to drop during the second half of gestation. The cornea becomes thicker, and mild corneal edema may be present. These changes can slightly alter refractory power and may lead to mild discomforts in women who wear contact lenses. Otolaryngeal changes are due to altered fluid dynamics, increased vascular permeability, vasomotor changes, increased vascularization, and the effects of estrogen. These changes can lead to an increase in ear and nasal stuffiness, hoarseness, and snoring (Blackburn, 2018; Sarberg et al., 2014).

INTEGUMENTARY SYSTEM

Skin changes induced by pregnancy include vascular alterations, variations in nail and hair growth, connective tissue changes, and altered pigmentation (Blackburn, 2018; Rapini, 2014; Tyler, 2015). Blood flow to the skin increases 3 to 4 times above prepregnancy levels. Vascular spider nevi appear on the face, neck, chest, arms, and legs. These are small, bright red elevations of the skin radiating from a central body. Spider nevi are related to increased subcutaneous blood flow and potentially to increased estrogen levels in the tissue. Palmar erythema is a normal vascular change during pregnancy, but it has also been associated with liver and collagen vascular diseases.

Hair growth is altered during pregnancy. During early pregnancy, the number of hairs in the growth phase remains stable. In the later stages of pregnancy, however, hormonal levels apparently increase the number of hairs in the growth phase and decrease the number of hairs in the resting phase. After birth, the proportion of hairs that enters the resting phase doubles, and women may experience an increase in hair loss 2 to 4 months postpartum (Camacho-Martínez, 2009). Occasionally, nail growth may be affected, and nail changes include transverse grooving, softening, and increased brittleness.

Striae gravidarum (i.e., stretch marks) may occur on the skin of the breasts, hips, and upper thighs and are usually most pronounced on the abdomen. Striae, which result from the normal stretching of the skin and softening and relaxing of the dermal collagenous and elastic tissues during the last months of pregnancy, occur in about 50% of pregnant women (Blackburn, 2018).

Increases in estrogen and progesterone may cause an increase in melanocyte-stimulating hormone, causing hyperpigmentation in the integumentary system. Darkening of the nipples, areolae, and perianal and genital areas occurs. The linea alba becomes the linea nigra and divides the abdomen longitudinally from the sternum to the symphysis. Melasma (i.e., the "mask of pregnancy," previously referred to as chloasma) appears as irregularly shaped brown blotches on the face, with a masklike distribution on the cheekbones and forehead and around the eyes. Melasma is thought to result from elevated serum levels of estrogen and progesterone, which also stimulate melanin deposits. Melasma disappears after pregnancy but may reappear with excessive sun exposure or with oral contraceptive use (Rapini, 2014; Tyler, 2015).

REPRODUCTIVE ORGANS

Uterus

Before pregnancy, the uterus is a small, semisolid, pear-shaped organ that weighs 40 to 50 g. During pregnancy, the uterus becomes globular and increases in length. At term, the uterus weighs approximately 1,100 to 1,200 g due to hypertrophy of the myometrial cells (Norwitz et al., 2014). Ten percent to 20% of the maternal cardiac output flows through the vascular system of the uterus (Monga & Mastrobattista, 2014). During the first few months of pregnancy, the wall of the uterus thickens due to myometrial hyperplasia and hypertrophy in response to elevated estrogen and progesterone levels. After this time, the muscle wall thins, allowing easier palpation of the fetus. The size and number of blood and lymphatic vessels increase.

The uterus remains relatively quiescent during most of pregnancy, although even in nonpregnant women, the myometrium has periodic low-frequency, low-amplitude activity. This baseline activity increases during pregnancy and becomes more apparent to the women as gestation progresses. Near the end of pregnancy, the myometrium goes through a preparatory stage for labor involving activation of uterine contractility, cervical ripening, and activation of fetal membranes. Activation is thought to be stimulated by uterotrophins such as estrogen and by increased formation of gap junctions (needed for transmission of the action potential between muscle cells), oxytocin receptors, PG receptor activation, and ion channels to enhance movement of calcium (essential for muscle contraction) into the myocytes (Norwitz et al., 2014).

Uteroplacental blood flow is essential for adequate fetal growth and survival. By term, the blood flow from the uterine and ovarian arteries to the uterus is approximately 500 to 800 mL/min, 80% of which is directed to the placental bed (Monga & Mastrobattista, 2014).

Maternal position, maternal arterial pressure, and uterine contractility influence uterine blood flow. The uterine spiral arteries are altered by the fetal trophoblast cells, which migrate out of the placenta and remodel the elastic and muscle elements of the maternal spiral arteries underlying the site of placental implantation. As a result of these changes, the spiral arteries (often called uteroplacental arteries during pregnancy) are greatly increased in diameter and can accommodate the vast supply of blood needed to supply the placenta.

Cervix

The cervix undergoes changes characterized by increased vascularity and water content, softening, and dilation (Myers et al., 2015). Estrogen stimulates glandular tissue of the cervix, which increases the number of cells. Early in pregnancy, increased vascularity causes a softening and a bluish discoloration of the cervix known as Chadwick sign. Endocervical glands, which occupy one half of the mass of the cervix at term, secrete a thick, tenacious mucus that forms the mucous plug and prevents bacteria and other substances from entering the uterus. This mucous plug is expelled before the onset of labor and may be associated with a bloody show. Hyperactive glandular tissue also causes an increase in the normal mucus production during pregnancy.

Ovaries

Ovulation ceases during pregnancy. Cells that line the follicles, known as thecal cells, become active in hormone production and serve as the interstitial glands of pregnancy. The corpus luteum persists and secretes progesterone until the 10th to 12th week, which maintains the endometrium until adequate progesterone is secreted by the placenta.

Vagina

Vaginal epithelium and muscle layers undergo hypertrophy, increased vascularization, and hyperplasia during pregnancy in response to estrogen levels. Loosening of the connective tissue and thickening of the mucosa increase vaginal secretions. These secretions are thick, white, and acidic and play a role in preventing infection. By the end of pregnancy, the vaginal wall and perineal body become relaxed enough to permit stretching of the tissues to accommodate the birth of the infant.

Breasts

Breasts increase in size and nodularity to prepare for lactation. Nipples become more easily erectile, and veins are more prominent. Areolar pigmentation increases. Montgomery glands or tubercles, the sebaceous glands located in the areola, hypertrophy. Striae may develop as the breasts enlarge. Colostrum, a yellow secretion rich in antibodies, may leak from the nipples during the last trimester of pregnancy. Feelings of fullness, tingling, and increased sensitivity begin in the first few weeks of gestation.

SUMMARY

Significant physical, metabolic, and structural changes occur from conception until weeks into the postpartum period. A thorough understanding of these changes facilitates assessment of normal pregnancy progression. Recognition of variations from normal may result in early identification of risk factors and potential complications. Prompt management can be initiated to help ensure optimal outcomes for both mother and fetus.

REFERENCES

Abbassi-Ghanavati, M., Greer, L. G., & Cunningham, F. G. (2009). Pregnancy and laboratory studies: A reference table for clinicians. *Obstetrics and Gynecology, 114*(6), 1326–1331. doi:10.1097/AOG.0b013e3181c2bde8

Anthony, K. M., Racusin, D. A., Aagaard, K., & Dildy, G. A. (2017). Maternal physiology. In S. G. Gabbe, J. R. Niebyl, J. L. Simpson, M. B. Landon, H. L. Galan, E. R. M. Jauniaux, . . . W. A. Grobman (Eds.), *Normal and problems pregnancies* (7th ed., pp. 38–63). Philadelphia, PA: Elsevier.

Blackburn, S. T. (2018). *Maternal, fetal, and neonatal physiology: A clinical perspective* (5th ed.). Philadelphia, PA: Elsevier.

Bobrowski, R. A. (2010). Pulmonary physiology in pregnancy. *Clinical Obstetrics and Gynecology, 53*(2), 285–300. doi:10/1097/GRF.ob013e3181e04776

Bustos, M., Venkataramanan, R., & Caritis, S. (2017). Nausea and vomiting of pregnancy—What's new? *Autonomic Neuroscience, 202*, 62–72. doi:10.1016/j.autneu.2016.05.002

Cakmak, B., Ribeiro, A. P., & Inanir, A. (2016). Postural balance and the risk of falling during pregnancy. *Journal of Maternal Fetal and Neonatal Medicine, 29*(10), 1623–1625. doi:10.3109/14767058.2015.1057490

Camacho-Martínez, F. M. (2009). Hair loss in women. *Seminars in Cutaneous Medicine and Surgery, 28*(1), 19–32. doi:10.1016/j.sder.2009.01.001

Caparroz, F. A., Gregorio, L. L., Bongiovanni, G., Izu, S. C., & Kosugi, E. M. (2016). Rhinitis and pregnancy: Literature review. *Brazilian Journal of Otorhinolaryngology, 82*(1), 105–111. doi:10.1016/j.bjorl.2015.04.011

Cappelletti, M., Della Bella, S., Ferrazzi, E., Mavilio, D., & Divanovic, S. (2016). Inflammation and preterm birth. *Journal of Leukocyte Biology, 99*(1), 67–78. doi:10.1189/jlb.3MR0615-272RR

Carlson, L. M., & Vora, N. L. (2017). Prenatal diagnosis: Screening and diagnostic tools. *Obstetric and Gynecologic Clinics of North America, 44*(2), 245–256. doi:10.1016/j.ogc.2017.02.004

Casagrande, D., Gugala, Z., Clark, S. M., & Lindsey, R. W. (2015). Low back pain and pelvic girdle pain in pregnancy. *The Journal of the American Academy of Orthopaedic Surgeons, 23*(9), 539–549. doi:10.5435/JAAOS-D-14-00248

Chen, A., Xu, F., Xie, C., Wu, T., Vuong, A. M., Miao, M., . . . DeFranco, E. A. (2015). Gestational weight gain trend and population attributable risks of adverse fetal growth outcomes in Ohio. *Paediatric and Perinatal Epidemiology, 29*(4), 346–350. doi:10.1111/ppe.12197

Cheung, K. L., & Lafayette, R. A. (2013). Renal physiology of pregnancy. *Advances in Chronic Kidney Disease, 20*(3), 209–214. doi:10.1053/j.ackd.2013.01.012

Cole, L. A. (2010). Hyperglycosylated hCG, a review. *Placenta, 31*(8), 653–664. doi:10.1016/j.placenta.2010.06.005

Cunningham, F. G., Leveno, K. J., Bloom, S. L., Spong, C. Y., Dashe, J. S., Hoffman, B. L., . . . Sheffield, J. S. (Eds.). (2014). *Williams obstetrics* (24th ed.). New York, NY: McGraw-Hill.

De Groot, L., Abalovich, M., Alexander, E. K., Amino, N., Barbour, L., Cobin, R. H., . . . Sullivan, S. (2012). Management of thyroid dysfunction during pregnancy and postpartum: An Endocrine Society clinical practice guideline. *The Journal of Clinical Endocrinology and Metabolism, 97*(8), 2543–2565. doi:10.1210/jc.2011-2803

Fiadjoe, P., Kannan, K., & Rane, A. (2010). Maternal urological problems in pregnancy. *European Journal of Obstetrics, Gynecology, and Reproductive Biology, 152*(1), 13–17. doi:10.1016/j.ejogrb.2010.04.013

Fournier, T., Guibourdenche, J., & Evain-Brion, D. (2015). Review: hCGs: Different sources of production, different glycoforms and functions. *Placenta, 36*(1 Suppl.), S60–S65. doi:10.1016/j.placenta.2015.02.002

Gandhi, M., & Martin, S. R. (2015). Cardiac disease in pregnancy. *Obstetrics and Gynecology Clinics of North America, 42*(2), 315–333. doi:10.1016/j.ogc.2015.01.012

Harris, I. S. (2011). Management of pregnancy in patients with congenital heart disease. *Progress in Cardiovascular Diseases, 53*(4), 305–311. doi:10.1016/j.pcad.2010.08.001

Hegewald, M. J., & Crapo, R. O. (2011). Respiratory physiology in pregnancy. *Clinics in Chest Medicine, 32*(1), 1–13. doi:10.1016/j.ccm.2010.11.001

Herrera, E., & Lasuncion, M. A. (2017). Maternal-fetal transfer of lipid metabolites. In R. A. Polin, S. H. Abman, D. H. Rowitch, W. E. Benitz, & W. W. Fox (Eds.), *Fetal and neonatal physiology* (4th ed., pp. 342–353). Philadelphia, PA: Saunders Elsevier.

Hsu, P., & Nanan, R. (2014). Foetal immune programming: Hormones, cytokines, microbes and regulatory T cells. *Journal of Reproductive Immunology, 104–105*, 2–7. doi:10.1016/j.jri.2014.02.005

Huang, S. A. (2017). Fetal and neonatal thyroid physiology. In R. A. Polin, S. H. Abman, D. H. Rowitch, W. E. Benitz, & W. W. Fox (Eds.), *Fetal and neonatal physiology* (4th ed., pp. 1503–1509). Philadelphia, PA: Saunders Elsevier.

Johnson, A. C., & Cipolla, M. J. (2015). The cerebral circulation during pregnancy: Adapting to preserve normalcy. *Physiology (Bethesda), 30*(2), 139–147. doi:10.1152/physiol.00048.2014

Katz, D., & Beilin, Y. (2015). Disorders of coagulation in pregnancy. *British Journal of Anaesthesia, 115*(2 Suppl.), ii75–ii88. doi:10.1093/bja/aev374

Kelly, T. F., & Savides, T. J. (2014). Gastrointestinal disease in pregnancy. In R. K. Creasy, R. Resnik, J. D. Iams, C. J. Lockwood, T. Moore, & M. F. Greene (Eds.), *Creasy & Resnik's maternal-fetal medicine: Principles and practice* (7th ed., pp. 1059–1074). Philadelphia, PA: Saunders Elsevier.

Kilpatrick, S. J. (2014). Anemia and pregnancy. In R. K. Creasy, R. Resnik, J. D. Iams, C. J. Lockwood, T. Moore, & M. F. Greene (Eds.), *Creasy & Resnik's maternal-fetal medicine: Principles and practice* (7th ed., pp. 918–931). Philadelphia, PA: Saunders Elsevier.

Korevaar, T. I. M., Medici, M., Visser, T. J., & Peeters, R. P. (2017). Thyroid disease in pregnancy: New insights and clinical management. *Nature Reviews: Endocrinology, 13*(10), 610–622. doi:10.1038/nrendo.2017.93

Lindheimer, M. D., Conrad, K. P., & Ananth Karumanchi, S. (2013). Renal physiology and disease in pregnancy. In R. J. Alpern, M. J. Caplan, & O. W. Moe (Eds.), *Seldin and Giebisch's the kidney: Physiology and pathophysiology* (5th ed., pp. 2689–2762). San Diego, CA: Academic Press.

Liu, J. H. (2014). Endocrinology of pregnancy. In R. K. Creasy, R. Resnik, J. D. Iams, C. J. Lockwood, T. Moore, & M. F. Greene (Eds.), *Creasy & Resnik's maternal-fetal medicine: Principles and practice* (7th ed., pp. 100–111). Philadelphia, PA: Saunders Elsevier.

Lumbers, E. R., & Pringle, K. G. (2014). Roles of the circulating renin-angiotensin-aldosterone system in human pregnancy. *American Journal of Physiology, Regulatory, Integrative and Comparative Physiology, 306*(2), R91–101. doi:10.1152/ajpregu.00034.2013

Melse-Boonstra, A., & Jaiswal, N. (2010). Iodine deficiency in pregnancy, infancy and childhood and its consequences for brain development. Best Practice & Research. *Clinical Endocrinology & Metabolism, 24*(1), 29–38. doi:10.1016/j.beem.2009.09.002

Monga, M., & Mastrobattista, J. (2014). Maternal cardiovascular, respiratory and renal adaptation to pregnancy. In R. K. Creasy, R. Resnik, J. D. Iams, C. J. Lockwood, T. Moore, & M. F. Greene (Eds.), *Creasy & Resnik's maternal-fetal medicine: Principles and practice* (7th ed., pp. 93–99). Philadelphia, PA: Saunders Elsevier.

Moore, K. L., Persaud, T. V. N., & Torchia, M. G. (2015). *The developing human: Clinically oriented embryology* (10th ed.). Philadelphia, PA: Saunders Elsevier.

Moore, T. R., Mouzon, S. H., & Catalano, P. (2014). Diabetes and pregnancy. In R. K. Creasy, R. Resnik, J. D. Iams, C. J. Lockwood, T. Moore, & M. F. Greene (Eds.), *Creasy & Resnik's maternal-fetal medicine: Principles and practice* (7th ed., pp. 988–1021). Philadelphia, PA: Saunders Elsevier.

Mor, G., & Abrahams, V. M. (2014). Immunology of pregnancy. In R. K. Creasy, R. Resnik, J. D. Iams, C. J. Lockwood, T. Moore, & M. F. Greene (Eds.), *Creasy & Resnik's maternal-fetal medicine: Principles and practice* (7th ed., pp. 80–92). Philadelphia, PA: Saunders Elsevier.

Mouzon, S. H., & Lassance, L. (2015). Endocrine and metabolic adaptations to pregnancy; impact of obesity. *Hormone Molecular Biology and Clinical Investigation, 24*(1), 65–72. doi:10.1515/hmbci-2015-0042

Munoz-Suano, A., Hamilton, A. B., & Betz, A. G. (2011). Gimme shelter: The immune system during pregnancy. *Immunological Reviews, 241*(1), 20–38. doi:10.1111/j.1600-065X.2011.01002

Myers, K. M., Feltovich, H., Mazza, E., Vink, J., Bajka, M., Wapner, R. J., . . . House, M. (2015). The mechanical role of the cervix in pregnancy. *Journal of Biomechanics, 48*(9), 1511–1523. doi:10.1016/j.jbiomech.2015.02.065

Nader, S. (2014a). Other endocrine disorders of pregnancy. In R. K. Creasy, R. Resnik, J. D. Iams, C. J. Lockwood, T. Moore, & M. F. Greene (Eds.), *Maternal-fetal medicine: Principles and practice* (7th ed., pp. 1038–1058). Philadelphia, PA: Saunders.

Nader, S. (2014b). Thyroid disease and pregnancy. In R. K. Creasy, R. Resnik, J. D. Iams, C. J. Lockwood, T. Moore, & M. F. Greene (Eds.), *Maternal-fetal medicine: Principles and practice* (7th ed., pp. 1022–1037). Philadelphia, PA: Saunders Elsevier.

Nappi, R. E., Albani, F., Sances, G., Terreno, E., Brambilla, E., & Polatti, F. (2011). Headaches during pregnancy. *Current Pain and Headache Reports, 15*(4), 289–294. doi:10.1007/s11916-011-0200-8

Neuman, H., & Koren, O. (2017). The pregnancy microbiome. *Nestle Nutrition Institute Workshop Series, 88*, 1–9. doi:10.1159/000455207

Norwitz, E. R., Mahendroo, M., & Lye, S. J. (2014). Biology of parturition. In R. K. Creasy, R. Resnik, J. D. Iams, C. J. Lockwood, T. Moore, & M. F. Greene (Eds.), *Creasy & Resnik's maternal-fetal medicine: Principles and practice* (7th ed., pp. 66–79). Philadelphia, PA: Saunders Elsevier.

Patton, P. E., Samuels, M. H., Trinidad, R., & Caughey, A. B. (2014). Controversies in the management of hypothyroidism during pregnancy. *Obstetric & Gynecological Survey, 69*(6), 346–358. doi:10.1097/OGX.0000000000000075

Penn, A. K. (2017). Endocrine and paracrine function of the human placenta. In R. A. Polin, S. H. Abman, D. H. Rowitch, W. E. Benitz, & W. W. Fox (Eds.), *Fetal and neonatal physiology* (4th ed., pp. 134–143). Philadelphia, PA: Saunders Elsevier.

Peña-Rosas, J. P., De-Regil, L. M., Garcia-Casal, M. N., & Dowswell, T. (2015). Daily oral iron or iron supplementation during pregnancy. *Cochrane Database of Systematic Reviews,* (7), CD004736. doi:10.1002/14651858.CD004736.pub5

Picchietti, D. L., Hensley, J. G., Bainbridge, J. L., Lee, K. A., Manconi, M., McGregor, J. A., . . . Walters, A. S. (2015). Consensus clinical practice guidelines for the diagnosis and treatment of restless legs syndrome/Willis-Ekbom disease during pregnancy and lactation. *Sleep Medicine Reviews, 22*, 64–77. doi:10.1016/j.smrv.2014.10.009

Podymow, T., August, P., & Akbari, A. (2010). Management of renal disease in pregnancy. *Obstetrics and Gynecology Clinics of North America, 37*(2), 195–210. doi:10.1016/j.ogc.2010.02.012

Rapini, R. P. (2014). The skin and pregnancy. In R. K. Creasy, R. Resnik, J. D. Iams, C. J. Lockwood, T. Moore, & M. F. Greene (Eds.), *Creasy & Resnik's maternal-fetal medicine: Principles and practice* (7th ed., pp. 1146–1145). Philadelphia, PA: Saunders Elsevier.

Rasmussen, K. M., Abrams, B., Bodnar, L. M., Butte, N. F., Catalano, P. M., & Maria Siega-Riz, A. (2010). Recommendations for weight gain during pregnancy in the context of the obesity epidemic. *Obstetrics and Gynecology, 116*(5), 1191–1195. doi:10.1097/AOG.0b013e3181f60da7

Sanghavi, M., & Rutherford, J. D. (2014). Cardiovascular physiology of pregnancy. *Circulation, 130*(12), 1003–1008. doi:10.1161/CIRCULATIONAHA.114.009029

Santiago, J. R., Nolledo, M. S., Kinzler, W., & Santiago, T. V. (2001). Sleep and sleep disorders in pregnancy. *Annals of Internal Medicine, 134*(5), 396–408.

Sarberg, M., Svanborg, E., Wiréhn, A. B., & Josefsson, A. (2014). Snoring during pregnancy and its relation to sleepiness and pregnancy outcomes—A prospective study. *BMC Pregnancy Childbirth, 14*, 15. doi:10.1186/1471-2393-14-15

Shynloya, O., Lee, Y. H., Srikhajon, K., & Lye, S. J. (2013). Physiologic uterine inflammation and labor onset: Integration of endocrine and mechanical signals. *Reproductive Sciences, 20*(2), 154–167. doi:10.1177/1933719112446084

Siu, A. L. (2015). Screening for iron deficiency anemia and iron supplementation in pregnant women to improve maternal health and birth outcomes: U.S. Preventive Services Task Force recommendation statement. *Annals of Internal Medicine, 163*(7), 529–536. doi:10.7326/M15-1707

Stotland, N. E., Bodnar, L. M., & Abrams, B. (2014). Maternal nutrition. In R. K. Creasy, R. Resnik, J. D. Iams, C. J. Lockwood, T. Moore, & M. F. Greene (Eds.), *Creasy & Resnik's maternal-fetal medicine: Principles and practice* (7th ed., pp. 131–138). Philadelphia, PA: Saunders Elsevier.

Thabah, M., & Ravindran, V. (2015). Musculoskeletal problems in pregnancy. *Rheumatology International, 35*(4), 581–587. doi:10.1007/s00296-014-3135-7

Thomas, J., Fairclough, A., Kavanagh, J., & Kelly, A. J. (2014). Vaginal prostaglandin (PGE2 and PGF2a) for induction of labour at term. *Cochrane Database of Systematic Reviews,* (6), CD003101. doi:10.1002/14651858.CD003101.pub3

Tyler, K. H. (2015). Physiological skin changes during pregnancy. *Clinical Obstetrics and Gynecology, 58*(1), 119–124. doi:10.1097/GRF.0000000000000077

Vrekoussis, T., Kalantaridou, S. N., Mastorakos, G., Zoumakis, E., Makrigiannakis, A., Syrrou, M., . . . Chrousos, G. P. (2010). The role of stress in female reproduction and pregnancy: An update. *Annals of the New York Academy of Science, 1205*, 69–75. doi:10.1111/j.1749-6632.2010.05686.x

Whitty, J. E., & Dombrowski, M. P. (2014). Respiratory diseases in pregnancy. In R. K. Creasy, R. Resnik, J. D. Iams, C. J. Lockwood, T. Moore, & M. F. Greene (Eds.), *Creasy & Resnik's maternal-fetal medicine: Principles and practice* (7th ed., pp. 965–987). Philadelphia, PA: Saunders Elsevier.

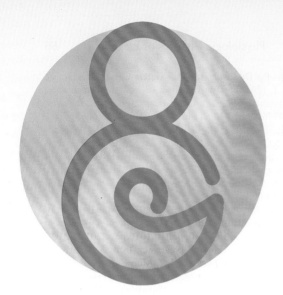

CHAPTER 4

Antenatal Care

Ellise D. Adams

INTRODUCTION

Care of the pregnant woman in the antenatal setting is multifaceted, requiring knowledge of the normal and abnormal pregnancy, risk factors affecting pregnancy outcome, screening tests, common pregnancy discomforts and treatments, and psychosocial tasks and issues surrounding the childbearing continuum and appropriate nursing interventions. The purpose of this chapter is to present an overview of essential aspects of preconception and prenatal care for perinatal nurses caring for women during the childbearing process. Complications that may result in a high-risk pregnancy and require additional medical and nursing intervention are discussed in detail in Chapters 5 to 12.

PRECONCEPTION CARE

Prenatal care begins with preconception healthcare. The purpose of preconception care is to deliver risk screening, health promotion, and effective interventions as a part of routine healthcare. The behaviors and exposures that occur before prenatal care is initiated may affect fetal development and subsequent maternal and perinatal outcomes; therefore, preconception healthcare is critical. The Centers for Disease and Prevention (CDC) (Johnson et al., 2006) developed 10 recommendations for improving preconception and interconception care as part of a strategic plan to improve the health of women, their children, and their families (Display 4–1). These recommendations, based on existing knowledge and evidence-based practice, were developed for improving preconception health through changes in consumer knowledge, clinical practice, public health programs, healthcare financing, and data and

research activities. Each recommendation has specific action steps toward the continuing goal of achieving the *Healthy People 2020* objectives to improve maternal and child health outcomes. The recommendations are aimed at achieving four goals, based on personal health outcomes.

Goal 1. Improve the knowledge and attitudes and behaviors of men and women related to preconception health.

Goal 2. Ensure that all women of childbearing age in the United States receive preconception care services (i.e., evidence-based risk screening, health promotion, and interventions) that will enable them to enter pregnancy in optimal health.

Goal 3. Reduce risks indicated by a previous adverse pregnancy outcome through interventions during the interconception period.

Goal 4. Reduce the disparities in adverse pregnancy outcomes.

Preconception care should be tailored to meet the needs of the individual woman. Because preconception care needs to be provided across the life span and not during only one visit, certain recommendations will be more relevant to women at different life stages and with varying levels of risk. Intuitively, it makes sense to provide preconception care in the context of primary care. All women attempting a pregnancy should follow the same behavioral recommendations for a healthy pregnancy: avoiding smoking and alcohol and avoiding medications known to be unsafe in pregnancy. Use of a health screening tool such as Health Screening for Women of Reproductive Age (American Academy of Pediatrics [AAP] & American College of Obstetricians and Gynecologists [ACOG], 2017) can be useful.

DISPLAY 4–1

Recommendations to Improve Preconception Health

Recommendation 1. Individual responsibility across the life span. Each woman, man, and couple should be encouraged to have a reproductive life plan.

Recommendation 2. Consumer awareness. Increase public awareness of the importance of preconception health behaviors and preconception care services by using information and tools appropriate across various ages; literacy, including health literacy; and cultural/linguistic contexts.

Recommendation 3. Preventive visits. As a part of primary care visits, provide risk assessment and educational and health promotion counseling to all women of childbearing age to reduce reproductive risks and improve pregnancy outcomes.

Recommendation 4. Interventions for identified risks. Increase the proportion of women who receive interventions as follow-up to preconception risk screening, focusing on high-priority interventions (i.e., those with evidence of effectiveness and greatest potential impact).

Recommendation 5. Interconception care. Use the interconception period to provide additional intensive interventions to women who have had a previous pregnancy that ended in an adverse outcome (e.g., infant death, fetal loss, birth defects, low birth weight, or preterm birth).

Recommendation 6. Prepregnancy checkup. Offer, as a component of maternity care, one prepregnancy visit for couples and persons planning pregnancy.

Recommendation 7. Health insurance coverage for women with low incomes. Increase public and private health insurance coverage for women with low incomes to improve access to preventive women's health and preconception and interconception care.

Recommendation 8. Public health programs and strategies. Integrate components of preconception health into existing local public health and related programs, including emphasis on interconception interventions for women with previous adverse outcomes.

Recommendation 9. Research. Increase the evidence base and promote the use of the evidence to improve preconception health.

Recommendation 10. Monitoring improvements. Maximize public health surveillance and related research mechanisms to monitor preconception health.

From Johnson, K., Posner, S. F., Biermann, J., Cordero, J. F., Atrash, H. K., Parker, C. S., . . . Curtis, M. G. (2006). Recommendations to improve preconception health and health care—United States: A report of the CDC/ATSDR Preconception Care Work Group and the select panel on preconception care. *MMWR. Recommendations and Reports, 55*(RR-6), 1–23.

It is vital that women who present for preconception care have a thorough medication review to allow efforts make medication adjustments reducing risk in early pregnancy. Of concern are antihypertensive and antiseizure medications, some of which are considered safe in pregnancy and some of which are contraindicated (Brown & Garovic, 2014). Women who are not counseled before pregnancy regarding their medications often stop taking their prescriptions when they have a positive home pregnancy test, putting their health at risk. All women of childbearing age should take 0.4 mg (400 mcg) folic acid daily, regardless of their pregnancy intention. As many as half of pregnancies are unplanned, and adequate folic acid is most vital in preventing neural tube defects (NTDs) (ACOG, 2017a; U.S. Preventive Services Task Force [USPSTF], 2009b). Beginning pregnancy with nondepleted iron stores is beneficial for the maternal iron status during pregnancy and for infant birth weight (Ribot et al., 2012). The importance of preconception advice to ensure that women have adequate iron stores prior to, or early in, pregnancy when supplemented with moderate daily iron doses should not be underestimated.

Health promotion, risk screening, and interventions are different for a young woman who has never experienced pregnancy than for women who are older or have had multiple pregnancies. Women who present with chronic diseases, previous pregnancy complications, or behavioral risk factors might need more intensive interventions. Social determinants of women's health also play a role in birth outcome. Low socioeconomic status is a long-known risk factor for preterm birth. Identified modifiable risk factors include isotretinoins (Accutane) use, alcohol misuse, antiepileptic drug use, diabetes (preconception), folic acid deficiency, hepatitis B, HIV/AIDS, hypothyroidism, maternal phenylketonuria, rubella seronegativity, obesity, oral anticoagulant use, sexually transmitted disease, and smoking (Johnson et al., 2006). The ACOG (2005), reaffirmed in 2017, identified the following as core preconception care factors:

- Undiagnosed, untreated, or poorly controlled medical conditions
- Immunization history
- Medication and radiation exposure in early pregnancy
- Nutritional issues
- Family history and genetic risk
- Tobacco and substance abuse and other high-risk behaviors
- Occupational and environmental exposures
- Social issues
- Mental health issues

Implementation of the CDC (Johnson et al., 2006) recommendations is targeted to (1) women and men of childbearing age having high reproductive awareness (i.e., they understand risk factors related to childbearing), (2) women and men who have a reproductive life plan, (3) pregnancies that are intended and planned, (4) women and men of childbearing age who have healthcare coverage, (5) women of childbearing age who are screened before pregnancy for risks that could affect the pregnancy, and (6) women with previous adverse pregnancy outcomes (e.g., infant death, very low birth weight, or preterm birth) who have access to interconception care aimed at reducing their risks.

PRENATAL CARE

As per AAP and ACOG (2017), prenatal care is a comprehensive antepartum care program that involves a coordinated approach to medical care and psychosocial support that ideally begins before conception and extends throughout pregnancy. This comprehensive program includes (1) preconception care, (2) prompt diagnosis of pregnancy, (3) initial prenatal evaluation, and (4) follow-up prenatal visits. Quality prenatal care includes education and support for the pregnant woman, ongoing maternal–fetal assessment, preparation for parenting, and promotion of a positive physical and emotional family experience. Comprehensive services include health education; nutrition education; the Women, Infants, and Children's (WIC) program; social services assessment; assessment for intimate partner violence, depression screening, and medical risk assessment; and referral as appropriate. To provide optimal, individualized care, nurses must recognize the effect of pregnancy on a woman's life span. Although a woman's preconception health has an impact on pregnancy, it is also true that childbearing is an event that may affect her long-term health. It is important to consider pregnancy within the larger context of women's health and primary care.

Continued contact with the pregnant woman through comprehensive prenatal care provides an ideal opportunity for the healthcare provider to assess for and identify potential problems that may place the woman and fetus at risk. AAP and ACOG (2017) recommend prenatal visits at 4 weeks in the first 28 weeks of pregnancy, every 2 weeks until 36 weeks, and once weekly until birth. Dowswell et al. (2010) reported that in settings with limited resources, reduced visit programs are associated with higher perinatal mortality when compared to standard prenatal care. Women in all settings were less satisfied with the reduced visits schedule and perceived the gap between visits as too long. Although reduced visits may be associated with lower costs, visits should not be reduced without close monitoring on fetal and neonatal outcomes. If a reduced visit schedule is used,

specific guidelines for low-risk pregnancies should be used and must include adequate education for the women regarding risk factors and recommendations for contacting their healthcare providers in between visits. See Display 4–2 for guidelines for routine prenatal care visits.

Another model of prenatal care, CenteringPregnancy, was developed in 1998 and integrates group support with prenatal care. CenteringPregnancy uses the essential components of prenatal care: risk assessment, health promotion, medical and psychosocial interventions, and follow-up. Group prenatal care intuitively seems to be an efficient method of simultaneously communicating the same message to multiple patients as well as promoting the development of an instant support group for women and families. This model involves ten 90- to 120-minute sessions that begin at 16 weeks' gestation and conclude with a postpartum meeting (Rising, 1998; Rising, Kennedy, & Klima, 2004). The initial prenatal visit is an individual appointment. Each woman is invited to join a group of 8 to 12 other women with similar estimated dates of birth. Sessions allow for individual time with the care provider and group sharing and education. Groups are led by advanced practice nurses or other healthcare professionals with expertise in group process. Group prenatal care results in equal or improved perinatal outcomes without added cost and provider satisfaction (Ickovics et al., 2016; Kania-Richmond, et al., 2017; Kennedy et al., 2011). Other group prenatal care models have been developed by individual healthcare providers and facilities to enhance their prenatal care structures. Nurses must be familiar with these prenatal care models to offer the highest quality evidence-based care to pregnant women. Guidelines for prenatal care visits and screening is established through the practice of evidenced-based care and clinical guidelines provided by professional organizations. Display 4–2 is a summary of the content, timing, counseling, and education that should be delivered in prenatal care.

Because early initiation of prenatal care is important to the health of the mother and to try to optimize pregnancy outcomes, a goal of increasing the proportion of pregnant women who initiate prenatal care in the first trimester to 77.9% was established as one of the *Healthy People 2020* objectives (U.S. Department of Health and Human Services [USDHHS], 2010). Achieving this goal will be a challenge with significant barriers to overcome such as access to care and issues of health disparity of women achieving a live birth to receive prenatal care in the first trimester. Some of the factors that might affect this trend include lack of education in recognizing the early signs of pregnancy, lack of insurance coverage for prenatal care, and difficulty accessing prenatal care providers. Promotion of early pregnancy

Guidelines for Preconception and Prenatal Care Visits

Event	Preconception Visit	Visit 1* 6 to 8 weeks	Visit 2 10 to 12 weeks	Visit 3 16 to 18 weeks	Visit 4 22 weeks	Visit 5 28 weeks	Visit 6 32 weeks	Visit 7 36 weeks	Visit 8 to 11 38 to 41 weeks
Health Screening	Height and weight/BMI Blood pressure History (personal and family) and Physical Exam Consider genetic screening, if applicable. Risk profiles (sexually transmitted diseases, substance abuse, environmental and occupational exposures) STI, Hepatitis A and B screening, if necessary Rubella/rubeola Varicella Intimate partner violence Depression Social support Personal resources	Height and weight/BMI Blood pressure History (personal and family) and Physical Exam† Estimated due date evaluation Rubella Varicella Intimate partner violence Depression CBC ABO/Rh/Ab Syphilis Urine culture Hepatitis B HIV GC/chlamydia TB, if high risk [Blood lead screening] [VBAC] Risk profiles (sexually transmitted diseases, substance abuse, environmental and occupational exposures)	Weight Blood pressure Estimated due date evaluation Fetal aneuploidy screening Fetal heart tones	Weight Blood pressure Estimated due date evaluation Urine (albumin/glucose) Depression Fetal aneuploidy screening Fetal heart tones OB ultrasound (optional) Fundal height	Weight Blood pressure Urine (albumin/glucose) Fetal heart tones Fundal height	Preterm labor risk Weight Blood pressure Urine (albumin/glucose) Depression Fetal heart tones Fundal height GDM Domestic abuse [Rh antibody status] [Hepatitis B surface Ag] [GC/Chlamydia]	Weight Blood pressure Urine (albumin/glucose) Fetal heart tones Fundal height	Weight Blood pressure Urine (albumin/glucose) Fetal heart tones Fundal height Cervix exam Confirm fetal position Culture for group B streptococcus	Weight Blood pressure Urine (albumin/glucose) Fetal heart tones Fundal height Cervix exam

(continued)

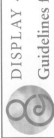

DISPLAY 4–2
Guidelines for Preconception and Prenatal Care Visits

Event	Preconception Visit	Visit 1* 6 to 8 weeks	Visit 2 10 to 12 weeks	Visit 3 16 to 18 weeks	Visit 4 22 weeks	Visit 5 28 weeks	Visit 6 32 weeks	Visit 7 36 weeks	Visit 8 to 11 38 to 41 weeks
Counseling Education Intervention	Nutrition and weight; Preterm labor education and prevention; Prenatal and life-style education; Substance use; Intimate partner violence; List of medications, herbal supplements, vitamins; Accurate recording of menstrual dates; Family planning/pregnancy spacing	Preterm labor education and prevention; Prenatal and life-style education • Physical activity • Nutrition • Follow-up of modifiable risk factors • Nausea and vomiting • Warning signs • Course of care • Physiology of pregnancy; Discuss fetal aneuploidy screening	Preterm labor education and prevention; Prenatal and life-style education • Fetal growth • Review lab results from visit 1. • Breastfeeding • Nausea and vomiting • Physiology of pregnancy • Follow-up of modifiable risk factors	Preterm labor education and prevention; Prenatal and lifestyle education • Follow-up of modifiable risk factors • Physiology of pregnancy • Second trimester growth • Quickening	Preterm labor education and prevention; Prenatal and lifestyle education • Follow-up of modifiable risk factors • Classes • Family issues • Length of stay • GDM • [RhoGAM]	Psychosocial risk factors; Preterm labor education and prevention; Prenatal and life-style education • Follow-up modifiable risk factors • Work • Physiology of pregnancy • Preregistration • Fetal growth • Awareness of fetal movement	Preterm labor education and prevention; Prenatal and lifestyle education • Follow-up of modifiable risk factors • Travel • Sexuality • Infant feeding choices • Pediatric care • Episiotomy • Awareness of fetal movement • Labor and delivery issues • Warning signs/pregnancy-induced hypertension [VBAC]	Prenatal and postpartum lifestyle education • Follow-up of modifiable risk factors • Management of late pregnancy symptoms • When to call provider • Postpartum care • Postpartum contraception • Discussion of postpartum depression Awareness of fetal movement	Prenatal and postpartum lifestyle education • Follow-up of modifiable risk factors • Postpartum vaccinations • Infant CPR • Post-term management Awareness of fetal movement Labor and delivery update
Immunization and Chemoprophylaxis	Tetanus booster; Rubella/MMR; [Varicella/VZIG]; Hepatitis B vaccine; HPV vaccine (until age 27); Folic acid supplement	Nutritional supplements; Influenza; [Varicella/VZIG]†		[Progesterone]		Tdap [ABO/Rh/Ab] [RhoGAM]			

Bracketed items refer to high-risk groups only. Ab, antibody; ABO, blood group system; Ag, antigen; BMI, body mass index; CBC, complete blood count; CPR, cardiopulmonary resuscitation; GC, gonococci; GDM, gestational diabetes mellitus; MMR, measles/mumps/rubella; OB, obstetrics; Rh, Rhesus; RhoGAM, Rho(D) immune globulin; STI, sexually transmitted infection; TB, tuberculosis; Tdap, tetanus, diphtheria, and pertussis; VBAC, vaginal birth after cesarean; VZIG, varicella zoster immune globulin.

*Should also include all subjects listed for the preconception visit if none occurred.

†It is acceptable for the history and physical and laboratory tests listed under visit 1 to be deferred to visit 2 with the agreement of both the patient and the provider.

*Administration of the varicella vaccine during pregnancy is contraindicated.

From American Academy of Pediatrics & American College of Obstetricians and Gynecologists. (2017). *Guidelines for perinatal care* (8th ed.). Washington, DC: Author.

recognition could be a means of improving birth outcomes because early pregnancy recognition is associated with improved timing and number of prenatal care visits (Ayoola, Nettleman, Stommel, & Canady, 2010). Nurses can encourage and empower women to access prenatal care at a critical point in fetal development.

PRENATAL RISK ASSESSMENT

The goal of risk assessment is to identify women and fetuses at risk for developing antepartum, intrapartum, postpartum, or neonatal complications and to promote risk-appropriate care that will enhance the perinatal outcome. The underlying causes of preterm labor and intrauterine growth restriction (IUGR) are not fully understood. However, a large body of knowledge on risk factors associated with prematurity and low birth weight has developed. These factors include demographic, medical, obstetric, sociocultural, lifestyle, and environmental risks. It is important to note that many risk factors have been identified in studies of women who develop complications of pregnancy or deliver preterm; however, no firm cause-and-effect relationship between some of the commonly associated risk factors and poor outcome has been established. Risk assessment tools may be helpful in distinguishing between women at high and low risk (Display 4–3). Unfortunately, the predictive value of these tools is limited. Enthusiasm for risk assessment must be tempered with reality. Identification of real or potential problems should be a shared process in which the nurse assesses the woman's individual perception of risk. Risk presented as a calculation of odds may not resonate with the pregnant woman; most women use a set of values that is rooted in their lives, personal philosophies, family, and health histories to make sense of risk (Carolan, 2009). Approximately one third of the potential complications of pregnancy occur during the intrapartum period and are not predictable by current risk-assessment systems (AAP & ACOG, 2017). However, risk assessment directs the provider toward areas in which intervention can have a positive impact on perinatal outcomes. The nurse's knowledge of prenatal risk assessment allows for anticipatory planning, individualized education, and appropriate referral. Outcomes of risk assessment provide guidelines by which the effectiveness of the care can be evaluated. The nurse's role in prenatal care is discussed within these parameters.

Initial Prenatal Visit

Antepartum assessment begins with the first prenatal visit. Generally, a woman with an uncomplicated pregnancy is examined approximately every 4 weeks for the first 28 weeks of pregnancy, every 2 to 3 weeks until 36 weeks' gestation, and weekly thereafter.

Women with medical or obstetric problems may require closer surveillance. Intervals between visits are determined by the nature and severity of the problem (AAP & ACOG, 2017).

The initial prenatal visit is of vital importance and requires careful attention to detail. The nurse is obligated to practice within the framework of professional standards, such as the Association of Women's Health, Obstetric and Neonatal Nurses' (AWHONN) *Standards and Guidelines* (2019) and *Guidelines for Perinatal Care* (AAP & ACOG, 2017), which provide guidelines for practice in the ambulatory care setting. During the first prenatal visit, baseline health data are obtained and assessed, a patient-centered relationship is established, and the plan of care is initiated. Risk assessment during the initial prenatal visit should include the following:

- Careful family medical history, individual medical history, reproductive health history, psychosocial history, and genetic history
- Comprehensive physical examination designed to evaluate potential risk factors
- Appropriate prenatal laboratory screening
- Individualized, risk-appropriate laboratory and genetic screening or diagnostic testing if desired
- Fetal assessment, as developmentally appropriate (e.g., fetal heart rate [FHR], fetal activity, kick counts), and individualized fetal surveillance, as indicated (e.g., ultrasonography, biophysical profile [BPP])

Maternal Age

The association between Down syndrome and advanced maternal age has been long documented (Hook, 1981). Maternal age of 35 years and older is associated with an increased risk of poor fetal outcomes, obstetrical complications, and perinatal morbidity and mortality (Khalil, Syngelaki, Maiz, Zinevich, & Nicolaides, 2013; McCall, Nair, & Knight, 2017; Silver, 2007). Children born to mothers younger than 19 or older than 35 years of age have an increased risk of prematurity, congenital anomalies, and risks from other complications of pregnancy (March of Dimes, 2010). However, researchers report that pregnancy outcomes previously linked to maternal age are mitigated by poverty (Cunningham et al., 2014; Markovitz, Cook, Flick, & Leet, 2005). With poor socioeconomic status, the risk of perinatal morbidity increases after the age of 35 years, but with adequate income and healthcare, women in that age group experienced only a slight increase in gestational diabetes, pregnancy-induced hypertension, placenta previa or abruption, and cesarean birth (Markovitz et al., 2005).

Complications common in pregnant adolescents include low birth weight, preeclampsia and pregnancy-induced hypertension, IUGR, and preterm labor.

DISPLAY 4-3
Risk Assessment

Obstetric History

History of infertility

Grand multiparity

Previous stillborn/neonatal death

Incompetent cervix

Previous multiple gestation

Uterine or cervical anomaly

Previous prolonged labor

Previous preterm labor or preterm birth

Previous low-birth-weight infant

Previous cesarean birth

Previous midforceps delivery

Previous macrosomic infant

Previous pregnancy loss (spontaneous or induced)

Last delivery <1 year before present conception

Previous hydatidiform mole or choriocarcinoma

Previous infant with neurologic deficit, birth injury, or congenital anomaly

Medical History

Cardiac disease	History of abnormal Pap smear
Metabolic disease	Previous surgeries, particularly
Gastrointestinal disorders	involving the reproductive
Seizure disorders	organs
Malignancy	Pulmonary disease
Reproductive tract anomalies	Chronic hypertension
Renal disease, repeat urinary	Endocrine disorders
tract infections, bacteriuria	Hemoglobinopathies
Emotional disorders, mental	Sexually transmitted diseases
retardation	Surgery during pregnancy
Family history of severe	
inherited disorders	

Current Obstetric Status

Inadequate prenatal care	Rh sensitization
Intrauterine growth–restricted	Preterm labor
fetus	Overweight or underweight
Polyhydramnios	Immunization status

Large-for-gestational-age fetus	Fetal or placental malformations
Placenta previa	Abnormal fetal surveillance tests
Abnormal presentation	Abruptio placentae
Maternal anemia	Multiple gestation
Weight gain <10 lb	Postdatism
Weight loss >5 lb	Fibroids
Sexually transmitted diseases	Fetal manipulation
Pregnancy-induced hyperten-	Cervical cerclage
sion, preeclampsia	Maternal infection
Premature rupture of	
membranes	

Psychosocial Factors

Inadequate finances

Poor housing

Social problems

Unwed, father of baby uninvolved or unsupportive

Adolescent

Minority status

Poor nutrition

Parental occupation

More than two children at home, no help

Inadequate support systems

Unacceptance of pregnancy

Dysfunctional grieving

Psychiatric history

Attempt or ideation of suicide

Intimate partner violence

Demographic factors

    Maternal age <16 years or >35 years

    Education <11 years

Lifestyle

    Smokes >10 cigarettes per day

    Alcohol intake

    Substance abuse

    Heavy lifting, long periods of standing

    Long commute

    Unusual stress

In younger mothers, socioeconomic factors largely explain increased neonatal mortality risk (Markovitz et al., 2005). Although much of the literature links advanced maternal age to adverse perinatal outcomes, there is a paucity of data linking advanced maternal age with outcomes of preterm newborns. Kanungo and colleagues (2011) reported that among preterm newborns, the odds of survival without major morbidity improved by 5% and mortality (8%), necrotizing enterocolitis (11%), and sepsis (9%) reduced as maternal age group increased by 5 years. Knowledge of these risks and outcomes serves as a guide for counseling women for whom age is a risk factor.

Medical and Obstetric History

Assessment of health factors that may influence pregnancy outcome includes careful evaluation of the woman's individual medical, gynecologic, obstetric, psychosocial, and environmental history. Pertinent family history of the woman and her partner is necessary for complete evaluation. Maternal–family reproductive health history (e.g., preeclampsia, hypertension, diabetes, preterm birth) may be particularly significant. The additional physiologic stress of pregnancy affects chronic conditions (e.g., asthma, diabetes, hypertension, or cardiac disease). Likewise, factors such as a recent history of sexually transmitted infections (STIs) or chemical dependency may be indicative of lifestyle behaviors that threaten maternal–fetal well-being.

Obstetric history, such as length of previous labors, cesarean birth, birth weight, gestational age, history of preterm labor or preterm birth, grand multiparity, elective or spontaneous abortion, instrument-assisted birth, previous stillbirth, or uterine or cervical anomaly, may indicate potential risks for the current pregnancy. Apply these risk factors within the context of the gestational age. For example, a history of preterm birth would be a pertinent risk to a woman who is presently at 20 weeks' gestation but is not relevant when the woman is at 37 weeks' gestation. Note familial history, including cardiac disease, diabetes, and bleeding disorders. The woman's risk profile may also be affected by her mother's obstetric history. There is a familial predisposition to develop preeclampsia. The medical and genetic history of the birth parents serves to guide counseling and testing for predisposed genetic complications. The family history is the most important source of genetic information. While the ideal time for genetic screening is before attempting pregnancy, genetic screening is still recommended during early pregnancy.

The most common indications for genetic counseling and prenatal diagnosis are maternal age and abnormal maternal serum screening. If the initial prenatal risk assessment reveals factors that carry risk for the baby (e.g., Tay-Sachs disease, sickle cell disease/trait, thalassemia, and cystic fibrosis), the woman (and her partner) should be offered genetic counseling and additional testing if the woman so desires.

Genetic counseling has grown into a well-recognized specialty. Our understanding of genetics and genomics in healthcare has changed in recent years, however. Genetic conditions inherited in families are caused by gene mutations present on one or both chromosomes of a pair. The three main patterns of Mendelian inheritance are autosomal dominant, autosomal recessive, and X-linked (Fig. 4–1). The term *genomics* refers to the study of all the genes in the human genome together, including their interactions with each other and the environment (Feetham, Thomson, & Hinshaw, 2005). Genes can cause diseases, and they also may affect disease susceptibility and resistance, prognosis and progression, and responses to illnesses and their treatments. This range of responsiveness results in variable testing sensitivity, specificity, and predictive value of the genetic test (Feetham et al., 2005).

As knowledge of the behavioral, environmental, and genetic mechanisms of disease increases, individuals and families may need to consider methods of prevention or seek diagnosis and treatment of genetic disorders if applicable (Feetham et al., 2005). Therefore, individualized education, planning, and support are vital to the process of genetic counseling. Genetic counseling and fetal surveillance techniques allow a woman (and her partner) to consider (1) the amount and kind of information desired, (2) subsequent decisions related to that information, and (3) how those decisions may reflect about their self-image and personal values. Genetic screening options are changing and multiplying rapidly, and all women should be offered the opportunity to receive information on those options, to have an opportunity to explore insurance coverage for genetic screening, and to discuss their concerns with their healthcare providers and/or a genetic counselor before and after testing is performed. Nurses are knowledgeable, nonthreatening confidants as the woman and her partner sort

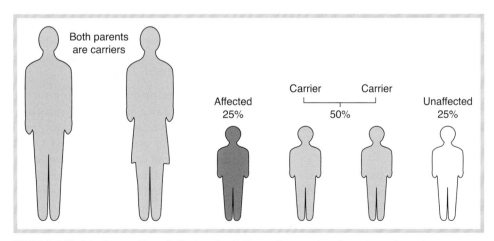

FIGURE 4–1. The inheritance pattern of offspring when both parents are carriers of an autosomal recessive gene.

through the information and decision making. Nurses, therefore, need to be cognizant of the benefits, limitations, and social implications of the genetic counseling and testing process.

Lifestyle Factors

Lifestyle or behavioral factors significantly affect women's health in general and perinatal health specifically. Living conditions; marital status; occupation; nutrition; and use of tobacco, alcohol, and illicit substances can all affect pregnancy outcome. Socioeconomic factors may influence gestational age at entry to prenatal care, nutritional status, and availability of support systems. Number of years of completed maternal education has been correlated with birth weight, perinatal mortality and morbidity, and neonatal neurologic sequelae. In general, as years of maternal education increase, incidence of perinatal mortality and morbidity decreases. Not surprising, adolescents are more likely to begin prenatal care later than adults (March of Dimes, 2019). Pregnant women who have more education are more likely to start prenatal care early and have more visits. Women in lower socioeconomic groups tend to initiate prenatal care later than their middle socioeconomic group counterparts. Late entry to prenatal care has been found to be associated with maternal age, race, economic status, education level, and drug or alcohol use (Baer et al., 2018).

The marital status of the mother and the presence of the father as related to perinatal outcome is a complex social phenomenon. Marital status may be a marker for the presence or absence of social, emotional, and financial resources. Infants of mothers who are not married have been shown to be at higher risk for poor outcomes. In 2013, infants of unmarried mothers had an infant mortality rate of 7.96 per 1,000, 73% higher than the rate for infants of married mothers (Matthews, MacDorman, & Thoma, 2015).

Births to women who live in an intimate relationship with a partner but without legal marriage have become increasingly common and widely accepted in many Western societies. However, pregnancy outcomes are worse among mothers in common-law unions versus traditional marriage relationships. One study found an overall 20% increase of adverse outcomes in unmarried, cohabiting mothers and that free maternity care did not overcome the difference (Raatikainen, Heiskanen, & Heinonen, 2005).

When employment status of the Finnish parents in 24,939 pregnancies was examined, unemployment was associated with adolescent maternal age, unmarried status, excessive body weight, anemia, smoking, alcohol consumption, and prior pregnancy terminations. Although antenatal care is free in Finland, this did not affect the adverse pregnancy outcomes associated with unemployment. Small-for-gestational-age risk was highest when both parents were unemployed (Raatikainen, Heiskanen, Verkasalo, & Heinonen, 2006).

Teratogen Exposure

The cause of congenital malformations can be divided into three categories: unknown, genetic, and environmental. The cause of a majority of human malformations is unknown. Both maternal and paternal environmental exposures can produce human developmental disease including preterm birth, growth restriction, functional or structural abnormalities, or death. "Whereas single genes and individual chemical exposures are responsible for some instances of adverse pregnancy outcome or developmental disease, gene–environment interactions are responsible for the majority. These gene–environment interactions may occur in the father, mother, placenta or fetus" (Mattison, 2010, p. 210).

More than 50 teratogenic environmental drugs, chemicals, and physical agents have been described using modern epidemiologic tools and clinical dysmorphology. Major birth defects occur in 2-3 percent of the population (AAP & ACOG, 2017). According to the CDC, the leading congenital anomalies are hypospadias, cyanotic congenital heart disease, Down syndrome, cleft lip with or without cleft palate, unsuspected chromosomal disorder, cleft palate alone, gastroschisis, menigomyelocele, omphalocele, limb reduction defect and anencephaly (Martin, Hamilton, Osterman, Driscoll, & Drake, 2018). In 2017, 14,389 congenital anomalies were reported in the US (Martin et al., 2018). Our understanding of this process is evolving:

"Whereas single genes and individual chemical exposures are responsible for some instances of adverse pregnancy outcome or developmental disease, gene–environment interactions are responsible for the majority. These gene–environment interactions may occur in the father, mother, placenta or fetus, suggesting that critical attention be given to maternal and paternal exposures and gene expression as they relate to the mode of action of the putative developmental toxicant both prior to and during pregnancy." (Mattison, 2010, p. 208)

Counseling on possible teratogenic influences should be performed in a factual yet sympathetic and supportive way so that the woman is not unduly alarmed or burdened with guilt (AAP & ACOG, 2017). Nurses should also be cognizant of the common potential teratogens in the population for which they provide care. For example, if the majority of the women come from an urban setting in which it is known that lead exposure is problematic, the history should include special attention to the risk. Maternal blood lead levels of approximately 10 mcg/dL have been linked to increased risks of pregnancy hypertension, spontaneous abortion, and reduced neurobehavioral development in the child (Bellinger, 2005).

Teratogen exposure may be associated with an occupation (e.g., X-rays, chemicals, viruses) or a lifestyle. The most common substances used by pregnant women include tobacco, alcohol, and marijuana. Alcohol is a potent teratogen in humans, and prenatal alcohol exposure is a leading preventable cause of birth defects and developmental disabilities. The harm from substance use and abuse is well known and may have disastrous effects in pregnancy, affecting all body systems and causing cardiac, pulmonary, gastrointestinal, and psychiatric complications. "Although the prevalence of substance abuse is significantly lower in pregnant women compared to nonpregnant women, some groups remain vulnerable to continued use, including those who did not intend to get pregnant and those who are less educated, unemployed, unmarried, and exposed to violence" (Massey et al., 2011, p. 143). Effects of tobacco use in pregnancy are well documented. No amount of alcohol is safe in pregnancy. Marijuana is the most commonly used illicit substance taken during pregnancy, especially in the first trimester, when women may use marijuana to combat nausea and increase appetite. The impact on the child is not clear. While prenatal marijuana use does not increase the risk of preterm birth, birth defects, or mortality in the first 2 years of life in exposed infants, emerging evidence indicates effects on later functioning. These effects include cognitive deficits, especially in visuospatial function, impulsivity, inattention and hyperactivity, depressive symptoms and substance use disorders, and cancer (Singer et al., 2018; Huizink & Mulder, 2006). Methamphetamine abuse is becoming more common among women of reproductive age. "Meth," also known as speed or chalk, or as ice, crystal, and glass when smoked, is a powerfully addictive stimulant and a known neurotoxic agent, which damages the endings of brain cells containing dopamine. Definitive information on the impact of exposure to methamphetamine in utero is lacking. There is fair to good evidence that amphetamines do not cause congenital anomalies. Amphetamine exposure during pregnancy is associated with an increased risk of preterm birth, low birth weight, and birth of small-for-gestational-age infants, but most of these studies have not adjusted for confounding factors, such as tobacco use, polydrug exposure, nutrition, and access to prenatal care (Chang, 2019). Screening for alcohol and substance use and abuse is discussed in more detail later in this chapter.

Approximately 90% of pregnant women use medications during pregnancy, including over-the-counter and prescription medications (Schonfeld, Schmid, Brown, Amora, & Gordon, 2013). Approximately half of pregnant women take at least 4 medication at some point while they are pregnant (Schonfeld et al., 2013). Some medications can increase risk to the pregnant woman and her fetus, with 10% of all birth defects directly linked to medications taken during pregnancy (Stanley, Durham, Sterrett, & Wallace, 2019).

Assessing the use of prescription or over-the-counter medications and use of complementary and alternative therapies such as herbs, homeopathy, and folk remedies is crucial. This provides nurses with a more complete picture of the woman's approach to healthcare and allows them to identify potentially harmful practices. Commonly, pregnant women are counseled that using acetaminophen is safe, whereas using a nonsteroidal anti-inflammatory drug such as ibuprofen is not. Both medications cross the placenta, however nonsteroidal anti-inflammatory drugs have potentially more side effects (Stanley et al., 2019).

Over the last three decades, first trimester use of prescription medications increased by more than 60% and the use of four or more medications more than tripled; approximately half of women of childbearing age use at least one medication (Mitchell et al., 2011). As more women delay childbearing and as the population has grown more obese, there are more likely to be women of childbearing age using medications for chronic diseases such as diabetes, hypertension, and hyperlipidemia. Medications to treat the later disorders include angiotensin-converting enzyme (ACE) inhibitor, angiotensin receptor blocker (ARB), or HMG-coenzyme A reductase inhibitor (statin). Use of ACE inhibitors and ARBs is associated with well-established risks: oligohydramnios, fetal renal dysplasia, IUGR, and fetal death (Morrical-Kline, Walton, & Guildenbecher, 2011). Statin use during pregnancy is contraindicated with case reports demonstrating vertebral, anal, cardiac, tracheal, esophageal, renal, and limb anomalies (Patel, Edgerton, Flake, & Smits, 2006). Consequently, it is important for providers in primary care as well in women's health to be cognizant of this growing shift in the population of childbearing women about medication use and to counsel women appropriately.

Nutrition

The impact of nutrition on maternal and fetal well-being cannot be underestimated. The unique physiology of a woman creates variable nutrient requirements during different stages of the life cycle. Nutritional practices influence every pregnancy as well as a woman's risk for anemia, diabetes mellitus, cardiovascular disease, osteoporosis, and several types of cancer. Specific complications of pregnancy, such as preeclampsia, preterm birth, intrauterine growth retardation, and low-birth-weight infants with associated detrimental outcomes, can be correlated to nutritional status.

A healthy, well-nourished woman has a surplus of all nutrients. The key components of a health-promoting lifestyle during pregnancy include appropriate weight gain; appropriate physical activity; consumption of a variety of foods in accordance with the *Dietary Guidelines for Americans 2015–2020* (https://health.gov/dietaryguidelines/2015/resources/2015-2020_Dietary_Guidelines.pdf); appropriate and timely vitamin and mineral supplementation; avoidance of alcohol, tobacco, and other harmful substances; and safe food handling.

Approximately 60% of American women do not gain the appropriate amount of weight during pregnancy, with more gaining too much, especially those with a high prepregnancy body mass index (Olson, 2008). Current weight gain guidelines are described in Table 4–1. In 2011, the U.S. Department of Agriculture created an interactive Web-based MyPlate. The Web site provides food intake and physical activity recommendations for persons aged 2 years and older, replacing healthy foods for unhealthful, diet tracking, menu planning, nutrition information, and personalized advice. The strategies are easy to understand for the lay public. The information should be used to complement and not substitute for prenatal education (Shieh & Carter, 2011). The nurse is encouraged to explore the Web site for use with preconception, prenatal, and lactating women: http://choosemyplate.gov.

The nutrition assessment includes diet intake information (3-day recall), monitoring weight gain, and hematologic assessment. Assessment of usual dietary patterns provides a basis for understanding nutritional health. Variations from the normal dietary routine, such as eating disorders, food avoidance or special diets, food resources, and metabolic disorders such as diabetes, warrant additional interventions. Women who have eating disorders may be reticent to reveal this information. The nutritional assessment may require several prenatal visits and a trusting relationship between the nurse and the woman. After an eating disorder is revealed, the nurse should ask the woman how she manages eating food and meals as well as what her attitude is toward eating (e.g., preoccupation with food, feeling guilty after eating, engaging in dieting, enjoyment of food).

The current dietary recommendations include (1) increased intake of protein from 60 to 80 g/day (1.1 g/kg/day), (2) 340 additional calories per day in the second trimester and 452 calories per day in the third trimester, (3) increased iron intake from 15 to 30 g/day, and (4) increased folate consumption from 400 to 800 mcg/day. The recommended amount of calcium for women ages 19 to 50 years, pregnant or not, is 1,000 mg/day; for adolescents up to age 18 years, it is 1,300 mg daily. There are certain special circumstances that may affect these recommendations. For example, if there is a history of a child with an NTD, the folic acid recommendation is increased to 4 mg rather than 0.4 to 0.8 mg/day. Nurses should encourage women to consume a variety of foods, eat at regular intervals (three meals a day and healthy snacks), drink milk two to three times per day, reduce caffeine, and avoid alcohol. Common discomforts (e.g., nausea and vomiting of pregnancy, heartburn, and varied reactions to taste or smell of food) can prove challenging to the woman who is trying to follow pregnancy dietary recommendations. Knowledge of safe remedies is the basis for advice when helping women with these discomforts. For example, acupressure wristbands and small, frequent meals with adequate protein can be of help to some women to decrease nausea.

Another aspect of the nutritional assessment is the use of vitamins and herbs. Because herbs and vitamins are considered dietary supplements, these products are not regulated in the same manner as prescription and over-the-counter medications. Often, the products are labeled as "natural," and the woman may conclude that the product is therefore not harmful. Excesses of one nutrient can alter the need for, absorption of, or use of other nutrients. Supernutrient regimens or megadoses of vitamins (especially those that are fat soluble) may be harmful during pregnancy.

Vitamin D deficiency is the most common nutritional deficiency worldwide in both children and adults. It has also been observed that vitamin D deficiency is linked to preeclampsia during pregnancy and an increased risk of cesarean (Achkar et al., 2015; Scholl, Chen, & Stein, 2012). However, it is not necessary to screen vitamin D levels in the general population of pregnant women. Instead, a dietary supplement of 400 IU (10 mcg) daily is recommended and can be found in most prenatal

TABLE 4–1. Recommendations for Weight Gain during Pregnancy

Prepregnant status	BMI	Recommended Range of Total Weight Gain (Pounds)
Underweight	<18.5	28 to 40 lb
Normal weight	18.5 to 24.9	25 to 35 lb
Overweight	25.0 to 29.9	15 to 25 lb
Obese (includes all classes)	≥30	11 to 20 lb

BMI, body mass index.
From Institute of Medicine. (2009). *Weight gain during pregnancy: Reexamining the guidelines.* Washington, DC: National Academies Press. American Academy of Pediatrics & American College of Obstetricians and Gynecologists. (2017). *Guidelines for perinatal care* (8th ed.). Washington DC: Author; American College of Obstetricians and Gynecologists. (2013b, reaffirmed 2018). *Weight gain during pregnancy* (Committee Opinion No. 548). Washington, DC: Author.

vitamins. There is insufficient evidence to recommend more than what is contained in prenatal vitamins. Women at risk of vitamin D deficiency (low dietary intake as in vegetarians, inadequate sunlight exposure, and ethnic minorities especially those with darker skin) can be screened and treated (1,000 to 2,000 IU per day) if low levels are found (ACOG, 2011).

Many women have concerns about consuming fish during pregnancy and will need appropriate education regarding safe fish consumption. Fish is an excellent source of protein, is low in saturated fats, and contains omega-3 fatty acids and is therefore a healthy source of nutrients for the pregnant woman. Nearly all fish and shellfish contain trace amounts of mercury. Pregnant and lactating women are advised to avoid fish with potentially high methylmercury levels such as shark, swordfish, king mackerel, and tile fish. Pregnant women are advised to ingest no more than 12 oz or two servings of canned tuna per week and no more than 6 oz of albacore or "white" tuna (U.S. Food and Drug Administration, 2019). If the mercury content of locally caught fish is unknown, then overall fish consumption should be limited to 6 oz per week.

Avoidance of foodborne illnesses (e.g., norovirus causing acute gastroenteritis, salmonella, listeriosis, *Escherichia coli*, hepatitis A), which cause maternal disease, congenital defects, preterm labor, miscarriage, and fetal death, is also important for the nurse to assess and to teach the woman. To reduce the risk of foodborne illness, it is important for the woman to do the following:

- Practice good personal hygiene (handwashing and care of kitchen utensils, cookware, and surfaces).
- Consume meats, fish, poultry, eggs that are fully cooked.
- Avoid unpasteurized dairy, fruit/vegetable products.
- Wash fresh fruits and vegetables prior to eating.
- Avoid raw sprouts (alfalfa, clover, radish, and mung bean).
- Avoid listeriosis by refraining from processed/deli meats, hot dogs, soft cheeses, smoked seafood, meat spreads, and pâté. Processed meats must be heated to 165°F (or "steaming hot") in order to destroy bacteria prior to consumption.

The U.S. Food and Drug Administration provides advice on food safety for women at https://www.fda .gov/media/83740/download.

Many pregnant women experience pica (craving and eating nonfood substances) during pregnancy. Some women are embarrassed to tell the nurse about these cravings, yet they may significantly interfere with dietary intake of proper nutrients during pregnancy. Pica cravings are not limited to any educational level, race, ethnic group, income level, or religious belief but rather are universal; however, the type of substance ingested does seem to be culturally influenced (Young, 2010). In the United States, the practice of pica during pregnancy is linked to lower income women, African American heritage, family or personal history of pica during childhood or before pregnancy, strong cravings during pregnancy, and cultural groups that endorse pica during pregnancy as important for fertility and femininity (Corbett, Ryan, & Weinrich, 2003). As a part of nutrition assessment, nurses should question (in a nonjudgmental style) patients at each prenatal visit regarding pica practice. Pica may be practiced for cultural or other reasons unknown to nurses. Some common nonfood substances that may be ingested include ice, starch, laundry powder, paper, clay, and dirt. Working with patients to discover what they are eating, and helping them to substitute foods with nutritional value, can be a part of a nursing care plan that results in a positive pregnancy outcome (Corbett et al., 2003).

Occupation

Women employed prior to pregnancy should be able to continue employment unless the pregnancy becomes complicated or the nature of the employment puts an undue physical stress on the pregnancy. Concerns during pregnancy would be activities that cause excessive fatigue, such as heavy work, job-related stress, or psychosocial stress. Because of a relationship between preterm birth, small-for-gestational-age infants, and occupations that are physically demanding (AAP & ACOG, 2017), it is important for the nurse to inquire about the woman's type of job. Question to include are whether she sits or stands continuously, lifts heavy objects, perceives problems with ventilation, or is exposed to toxic chemicals or radiation. Hobbies and the home environment should be assessed also. Household tasks may be a source of fatigue equal to or greater than job-related fatigue. It should be considered that decreasing or eliminating work during pregnancy may place the woman at greater socioeconomic risk by threatening her livelihood.

Psychosocial Screening

Psychosocial screening of every woman presenting for prenatal care is an important step toward improving the woman's health and birth outcomes. Psychosocial screening allows the nurse to identify areas of concern, validate major issues, and make suggestions for possible changes. Depending on the nature of the identified problem, a referral may be made to an appropriate member of the healthcare team. A woman may be reluctant to share information until a trusting relationship has been formed. Questions asked at the first prenatal visit bear repeating with ongoing prenatal care. The woman may need reassurance that information shared will be confidential. For example, if she reveals she uses cocaine, would she be turned over to the judicial system and possibly jailed? Nurses are obligated to know how to answer the woman when these issues arise.

Pregnancy affects the entire family, and, therefore, assessment and intervention must be considered in a family-centered perspective. Stress has been suggested as a potential contributor to preterm birth and physical complications during pregnancy and birth, including prolonged labor, increased use of intrapartum analgesics and barbiturates, and other complications. Unusual stressful events, such as the death of a significant family member or friend, job loss, or a problematic relationship with the newborn's father, may increase risk of poor pregnancy outcomes. Home conditions (e.g., private or government housing), quality of comfort (e.g., heat, water), housekeeping burden, and the number and age of previous children influence stress levels. Nurses should be aware that many women continue to work under hazardous or stressful conditions out of economic necessity but may attempt to minimize known risk factors. Nurses should assess how the woman appraises her situation (e.g., what one woman finds stressful, another may not). Nurses should identify resources available to the pregnant woman (e.g., support groups, social worker, counselor).

Symptoms of dysfunctional family relationships, such as violence toward the pregnant woman, child abuse, or psychosomatic illnesses, are also indicative of risk and warrant investigation. One in 3 American women has experienced intimate partner violence, and greater than 300,000 of these women were pregnant when the violence occurred (ACOG, 2012; Bianchi, Cesario, & McFarlane, 2016). Victims are found among women of all ages, socioeconomic classes, and ethnicities. Intimate partner violence against women covers a broad spectrum of behaviors, including actual or threatened physical, sexual, or psychological abuse between family members or intimate partners. Exposure to intimate partner violence is associated with a range of negative psychobehavioral risks and health outcomes including increased risk of late entry to prenatal care, high blood pressure, increased urinary tract infections, vaginal bleeding, nausea, vomiting and dehydration, physical disability, posttraumatic stress disorder, depression, decreased ability to bond with the baby, and heightened substance use including alcohol and illicit drugs (Bianchi, Cesario, et al., 2016; Kiely, El-Mohandes, El-Khorazaty, Blake, & Gantz, 2010). Risks to the newborn include preterm birth, low birth weight, intrauterine growth retardation, fetal death, increased newborn intensive care unit admissions, poor infant weight gain, and behavioral difficulties up to 42 months of age (Bianchi, Cesario, et al., 2016; Bianchi, McFarlane, Cesario, Symes, & Maddoux, 2016; Vu, Jouriles, McDonald, & Rosenfield, 2016).

Yost, Bloom, McIntire, and Leveno (2005) surveyed 16,041 women presenting to a labor and delivery unit.

They found that when compared with women denying intimate partner violence, women ($n = 949$) reporting verbal abuse had an increased rate of low-birth-weight infants, and neonatal deaths were significantly increased in women experiencing physical abuse. Second, women who declined to participate ($n = 94$) in their survey were found to have significantly increased rates of a variety of pregnancy complications that adversely affected their infants' outcomes (Yost et al., 2005).

The National Violence Against Women Survey report demonstrated that women had an increased risk of injury if the perpetrator was an intimate partner (vs. a nonintimate partner) (Tjaden & Thoennes, 2000). There is an increased risk of intimate partner violence if the couple was cohabitating rather than married. Married women living apart from their husbands were more likely to be victims of rape, physical assault, and/or stalking (Tjaden & Thoennes, 2000).

AWHONN (2004) has a history of urging nurses to routinely assess all pregnant women for intimate partner violence. ACOG (2012) recommends screening at the initial prenatal visit, once per trimester, and in the postpartum follow-up visit. Initiating this screening for women experiencing intimate partner violence may be difficult because this population typically accesses prenatal care later in pregnancy. Screening for intimate partner violence during pregnancy should be sensitive, demonstrate caring, and be done in a nonjudgmental manner for the woman to be most likely to tell her story (Bianchi, 2016). Nurses must be prepared to assess the woman's safety, physical injuries, and then make proper referrals immediately after disclosure of any violence she has experienced. Integrating a standardized screening protocol into routine history-taking procedures increases identification, documentation, and referral for intimate partner violence (AAP & ACOG, 2017; ACOG, 2012).

Nurses should document the frequency and severity of present and past abuse (using patient quotes as much as possible), location and extent of injuries, treatments, interventions, escape plan, and educational materials (including phone numbers to a shelter and the police). Discuss a plan of escape and document whether shelter assistance was declined or accepted by the woman. Counseling and intervention can reduce intimate partner violence and improve pregnancy outcome (Kiely et al., 2010).

Addressing psychosocial issues during pregnancy has the potential to reduce costs to the individual and to society (AWHONN, 2004; Lancaster et al., 2010). A simple screening system was developed by the Healthy Start program of the Florida Department of Health and has been refined and in use since 1992. This tool is a concise (nine questions) way to open the questioning about perinatal psychosocial risk factors

DISPLAY 4–4
Psychosocial Screening Tool

1. Yes   No   Do you have any problems (job, transportation, etc.) that prevent you from keeping your healthcare appointments?

2. Yes   No   Do you feel unsafe where you live?

3. Yes   No   In the past 2 months, have you used any form of tobacco?

4. Yes   No   In the past 2 months, have you used drugs or alcohol (including beer, wine, or mixed drinks)?

5. Yes   No   In the past year, have you been threatened, hit, slapped, or kicked by anyone you know?

6. Yes   No   Has anyone forced you to perform any sexual act that you did not want to do?

7. On a 1 to 5 scale, how do you rate your current stress level?

1	2	3	4	5
Low				High

8. How many times have you moved in the past 12 months?

———————————

9. If you could change the timing of this pregnancy, would you want it
earlier
later
not at all
no change

———————————

From American College of Obstetricians and Gynecologists. (2006). *Psychosocial risk factors: Perinatal screening and intervention* (Committee Opinion No. 343). Washington, DC: Author.

(Display 4–4). If the patient answers in a way indicative of risk to any of the questions, the nurse can further explore the topic with the woman.

Major depression is one of the most frequently encountered medical complications in pregnancy, and the risk for depression increases even more during the postpartum period. As many as 1 in 7 women are treated for depression sometime 1 year prior to pregnancy and 1 year following pregnancy (AAP & ACOG, 2017). These numbers represent both high patient volume and high healthcare costs. Depression in pregnancy is associated with greater maternal lifestyle risks, increased incidence of postpartum depression, suicide, and adverse birth outcomes (Beck, 2008; Pereira et al., 2011). The impact of depression during pregnancy is significant for the mother and to her baby. Rahman, Bunn, Lovel, and Creed (2007) and Van den Bergh, Mulder, Mennes, and Glover (2005) have identified that untreated maternal depression that extends into the postpartum period has a negative effect on the emotional, cognitive, and developmental growth

of young infants. While it is unclear why pregnancy and childbirth represent a time of increased vulnerability for the onset or exacerbation of depression, it may be that it is the combination of hormonal shifts, neuroendocrine changes, and psychosocial adjustments (Pereira et al., 2011).

Recognition, diagnosis, and treatment of depression in pregnancy are vital. Brief screens for symptoms of depression in pregnancy during the initial interview assist clinicians in identifying pregnant women who have symptoms of depression. Effective identification of depression in obstetrical practice meets *Healthy People 2020's* (USDHHS, 2010) recommendation for additional research to discover health indicators that place women at risk in pregnancy. The U.S. Preventive Services Task Force (Pignone et al., 2002) recommended that the following two questions be part of the basic repertoire of every adult patient visit:

- "Over the past 2 weeks have you felt down, depressed, or hopeless?"
- "Over the past 2 weeks, have you felt little interest in doing things?"

Jesse and Graham (2005) validated the use of these two questions in pregnancy; sensitivity was 91%, and specificity was 52%. If the responses are positive, nurses must assess the patient's safety (i.e., risk of suicide). These questions can be the first step in determining which women should be referred for a clinical diagnostic evaluation by a psychiatric nurse practitioner, social worker, psychologist, or a psychiatrist. A pregnancy support group may be helpful. Women who are diagnosed with depression during pregnancy should be followed carefully for postpartum depression. Predisposing risk factors for the development of postpartum depression have been identified (Display 4–5).

It is possible to identify prenatally women who are at risk for experiencing parenting difficulties. Asking the woman how she thinks her pregnancy is progressing and questions about her preparations for the care of the baby provides opportunities for discussion that may provide insight into positive or negative reactions to the experience of pregnancy and preparation for parenthood. Women should be given the opportunity to verbalize thoughts about changes she is experiencing, fantasies about the baby, acceptance of pregnancy, and, after birth, acceptance of the child by the family.

Substance Use

Alcohol use has long been identified as a preventable cause of birth defects. Drinking while pregnant is still a problem; 1 in 8 pregnant women drink alcohol (Denny, Tsai, Floyd, & Green, 2009). Fetal alcohol spectrum disorder (FASD) is associated with

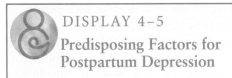

DISPLAY 4–5

Predisposing Factors for Postpartum Depression

Anxiety or depression during pregnancy

History of depression

Not being married or cohabiting with partner; poor marital relationship

Poor social support

Low socioeconomic status; Medicaid insurance

Intimate partner violence

Unintended pregnancy

Smoking

Stressful life event during pregnancy and/or puerperium
- Loss of loved one (fetus, newborn, partner, or other child)
- Illness of partner, parent, or child
- Financial difficulties
- Job loss
- Move of household

Adapted from Beck, C. T. (2008). State of the science on postpartum depression: What nurse researchers have contributed—Part 1. *MCN: The American Journal of Maternal Child Nursing, 33*(2), 121–126; Lancaster, C., Gold, K., Flynn, H., Yoo, H., Marcus, S., & Davis, M. (2010). Risk factors for depressive symptoms during pregnancy: A systematic review. *American Journal of Obstetrics & Gynecology, 202,* 5–14. doi:10.1016/j.ajog.2009.09.007

four characteristics: (1) maternal drinking during pregnancy, (2) a characteristic pattern of facial abnormalities, (3) growth restriction, and (4) central nervous system dysfunction (often manifested by intellectual difficulties or behavioral problems) (AAP & ACOG, 2017). As surveillance and research have progressed, it has become clear that FAS is a rare example of a wide array of defects that can occur from fetal exposure to alcohol.

Substance abuse or chemical dependency affects all body systems and can cause cardiac, pulmonary, gastrointestinal, and psychiatric complications. The relationships between substance abuse, stress, psychiatric comorbidities, intimate partner violence, and the lack of healthcare are striking. Simmons, Havens, Whiting, and Bada (2009) note the connections:

- General health status declines with use of illicit drugs, including cocaine, opiates, and amphetamines, even after controlling for other psychosocial and biologic covariates.
- Stress is strongly associated with substance use. Stress has been associated with abnormal functioning of the hypothalamic–pituitary–adrenal axis.
- Psychiatric comorbidity is also common in individuals with substance use disorders. Individuals with mental and substance use comorbidities are less likely to receive mental health treatment.

- Research demonstrates women who use drugs or drink alcohol are more likely to be battered and injured.
- Women who experience intimate partner violence are more likely to be frequent substance users and have a greater number of substance disorder symptoms than women who do not experience intimate partner violence.
- Previous research has demonstrated a link between receipt of welfare benefits and increased risk of illicit drug use, but Medicaid policies make it difficult for clients to obtain substance abuse treatment services.

Chasnoff, Wells, McGourty, and Bailey (2007) validated a four-item brief screening instrument, 4Ps Plus©, to identify pregnant women at highest risk for substance use receiving prenatal care. The questions are easily integrated into prenatal care. The four screening questions are the following:

1. Did either of your parents ever have a problem with alcohol or drugs?
2. Does your partner have a problem with alcohol or drugs?
3. Have you ever drunk beer, wine, or liquor?
4. In the month before you knew you were pregnant, how many cigarettes did you smoke? In the month before you knew you were pregnant, how many beers/how much wine/how much liquor did you drink?

The women fall into low-, average-, and high-risk categories based on these questions. High risk are those women who used any alcohol or smoked three or more cigarettes in the month before pregnancy. Because substance abuse or chemical dependency can adversely affect the health of the woman and the fetus, it is essential to include drug use assessment and education strategies in prenatal and women's healthcare encounters.

Cigarette Smoking

Cigarette smoking has been linked to an increased incidence of low birth weight and prematurity (ACOG, 2017b) and remains a problem. In the United States, combined data for 2000 to 2005 indicated that 22.5% of those surveyed reported smoking before or during pregnancy or after delivery. Compared with nonsmokers, women who smoked were significantly more likely to be younger (aged <25 years), be non-Hispanic White, have <12 years of education, be unmarried, have an annual income of <$15,000, be underweight, have an unintended pregnancy, be first-time mothers, have initiated prenatal care later, be Medicaid enrolled, and be enrolled in WIC during pregnancy (Tong, Jones, Dietz, D'Angelo, & Bombard, 2009).

From a preventive perspective, it is not enough to discourage smoking in pregnant women. The focus must be on discouraging smoking in any woman of childbearing age who may potentially become pregnant. Smoking during pregnancy presents major, avoidable health risks to the fetus. Smoking has been linked to increased risk of miscarriage, IUGR, low birth weight and very low birth weight, preterm labor and premature birth, placenta previa, placental abruption, perinatal loss, and sudden infant death syndrome. Infants and young children are affected by environmental tobacco smoke, which has been linked with an increased risk of lower respiratory infections in children, acute and chronic otitis media, reduced lung function, and neurobehavioral disorders (AWHONN, 2017).

The risk of fetal death is typically 1.5-fold over nonsmokers; the risk decreases to that of nonsmokers in women who stop smoking after the first trimester (Silver, 2007). Infants who live with a smoker face an increased risk of sudden infant death syndrome. During pregnancy, many women are more highly motivated to stop or decrease their smoking; however, simply providing information may not be enough for the pregnant woman with a long history of smoking. The USPSTF (2009a) recommends that clinicians ask all pregnant women about tobacco use and provide augmented, pregnancy-tailored counseling for those who smoke. In pregnant women, the USPSTF found convincing evidence that smoking cessation counseling sessions, augmented with messages and self-help materials tailored for pregnant smokers, increases abstinence rates during pregnancy compared with brief, generic counseling interventions alone. Tobacco cessation at any point during pregnancy yields substantial health benefits for the expectant mother and baby. Some insurance companies will cover smoking cessation aids such as behavioral interventions, which may increase a woman's ability to obtain assistance in her efforts to quit using tobacco. Nicotine replacement however is not recommended during pregnancy.

Methods of achieving smoking cessation during pregnancy include adequate screening, counseling, feedback, and incentives (AWHONN, 2017; Chamberlain et al., 2017). In practices that have used the 5 A's approach, quit rates among pregnant women have risen by 30% or more (Martin et al., 2006). One evidence-based approach is the "5 A's." This approach to smoking cessation is easily integrated into prenatal care.

- *Ask*: Ask the patient to choose a statement that best describes her smoking status.
- *Advise*: Ask permission to share the health message about smoking during pregnancy.
- *Assess*: Assess readiness to change.
- *Assist*: Briefly explore problem-solving methods and skills for smoking cessation.
- *Arrange*: Let the woman know that you will be following up on each visit; assess smoking status at subsequent prenatal visits; affirm efforts to quit (ACOG, 2017b).

Physical Activity

Even though pregnancy is associated with profound anatomic and physiologic changes, there are confirmed benefits of exercise with minimal risks for most women. A woman's overall health, including obstetric and medical risks, should be assessed before initiating an exercise program (Display 4–6). Generally, participation in a wide range of recreational activities is safe during pregnancy; however, each sport should be reviewed individually for its potential risk. Activities with a high risk of falling or those with a high risk of abdominal trauma should be avoided during pregnancy. Scuba diving should be avoided throughout pregnancy because the fetus is at an increased risk for decompression sickness during this activity. In the absence of either medical or obstetric complications, 30 minutes or more of moderate exercise a day on most, if not all, days of the week is recommended for pregnant women (AAP & ACOG, 2017).

Exercise benefits the woman psychologically and physically. Recreational and competitive athletes with uncomplicated pregnancies may remain active during pregnancy and modify their usual exercise routines to refrain from contact sports or other activities that might possibly cause abdominal trauma. It is important for the pregnant woman to maintain proper hydration during exercise sessions. Pregnant women with diabetes, morbid obesity, or chronic hypertension should have an individualized exercise prescription. Women with medical or obstetric complications should be carefully evaluated before recommendations on physical activity participation during pregnancy are made. Because of increased relaxation of ligaments during pregnancy, flexibility exercise should be individualized. It is important to advise women to avoid lying flat on the back after 26 weeks' gestation due to vascular compression, which could lead to reduced perfusion for mother and baby. Exercise positions where the head is below the level of the heart can increase the risk of dizziness and fainting and should also be avoided after 26 weeks' gestation. A typical exercise prescription should promote musculoskeletal fitness and address type, intensity and progression, quantity and duration, and frequency. A typical session includes the following:

- Warm-ups and stretching (5 to 10 minutes)
- Exercise program (30 to 45 minutes)
- Cool down (5 to 10 minutes)

Maternal Infections

Maternal infections are recognized as risk factors for adverse pregnancy outcomes. Infections have been reported to account for 10% to 25% of fetal deaths in developed countries (Cunningham et al., 2014). Factors such as maternal serologic status, timing of infection during pregnancy, mode of acquisition,

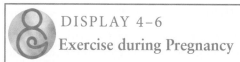

DISPLAY 4-6

Exercise during Pregnancy

Absolute Contraindications to Aerobic Exercise during Pregnancy
- Hemodynamically significant heart disease
- Restrictive lung disease
- Incompetent cervix/cerclage
- Multiple gestation at risk for premature labor
- Persistent second- or third-trimester bleeding
- Placenta previa after 26 weeks' gestation
- Premature labor during the current pregnancy
- Ruptured membranes
- Preeclampsia/pregnancy-induced hypertension
- Severe anemia

Relative Contraindications to Aerobic Exercise during Pregnancy
- Anemia
- Unevaluated maternal cardiac arrhythmia
- Chronic bronchitis
- Poorly controlled type 1 diabetes

- Extreme morbid obesity
- Extreme underweight (BMI <12)
- History of extremely sedentary lifestyle
- Intrauterine growth restriction in current pregnancy
- Poorly controlled hypertension
- Orthopedic limitations
- Poorly controlled seizure disorder
- Poorly controlled hyperthyroidism
- Heavy smoker

Warning Signs to Terminate Exercise while Pregnant
- Vaginal bleeding
- Dyspnea prior to exertion
- Dizziness
- Headache
- Chest pain
- Muscle weakness affecting balance
- Calf pain or swelling
- Regular painful contractions
- Amniotic fluid leakage

BMI, body mass index.
From American College of Obstetricians and Gynecologists. (2015). *Physical activity and exercise during pregnancy and the postpartum period* (Committee Opinion No. 650; Reaffirmed 2019). Washington, DC: Author.

and immunologic status influence both the course of the disease and pregnancy outcomes (Cunningham et al., 2014). There is epidemiologic, microbiologic, and clinical evidence of an association between infection and preterm birth. Spontaneous preterm birth epidemiologic studies reveal that births at less than 34 weeks' gestation are much more frequently accompanied by clinical or subclinical infection than those at more than 34 weeks. Both maternal and neonatal infections are more common after preterm than term birth. The proportion of fetal deaths due to viral infections is uncertain because there is no of systematic evaluation. Prevention of infection is key to preventing the complications associated with infections (see Appendix 4–A for information on vaccination in pregnancy).

Parvovirus B19 (B19V) is perhaps the most common viral infection to cause pregnancy loss (Dijkmans et al., 2012). The infection caused by B19V, erythema infectiosum, also known as fifth disease, is a relatively benign disease affecting mainly children and young adults. Infection with B19V usually occurs through respiratory droplets but can be transmitted vertically from mother to fetus via the placenta (Dijkmans et al., 2012). Approximately half of pregnant women are already immune to B19V and are not at risk of transmitting an infection to the fetus. Maternal infection can occur without symptoms, and the fetus is at little risk of being affected by the infection. When the fetus is affected, there is risk of severe fetal anemia and miscarriage related to hydrops. In the childbearing

population, 50% to 65% of women are seropositive for B19V (AAP & ACOG, 2017). No vertical transmission has been described if the mother has immunoglobulin G antibodies against B19V at the time of exposure. When maternal infection occurs, maternal viremia peaks at approximately 1 week and the risk of vertical transmission has been estimated to be approximately 25% (de Jong, Walther, Kroes, & Oepkes, 2011).

Another common viral infection is cytomegalovirus (CMV). The rate of infection in pregnant women in the United States is reported to be 2.3% (Hyde, Schmid, & Cannon, 2010). Day care providers, who are exposed to common childhood illnesses on a regular basis, have an annual infection rate of 8.5% (Hyde et al., 2010). Transmission usually occurs by contact with infected nasopharyngeal secretions or other body fluids. Maternal transmission to the fetus or newborn is most common following primary maternal infection. Routine screening is not recommended because of the following:

- No vaccine is available.
- In seropositive pregnant women, it is difficult to distinguish between primary and nonprimary infection.
- There is no evidence that antiviral drug treatment of primary infection in pregnant women changes the outcome in the neonate.
- When fetal infection occurs, there is no way to accurately predict whether the fetus will develop significant sequelae.

Coxsackie virus, along with other sporadically occurring viruses (e.g., echoviruses, enteroviruses, chickenpox, measles, mumps, and rubella), has also been reported to cause fetal death. Genital herpes simplex virus (HSV) is one of the most common STIs but is rarely transmitted in utero. National HSV-2 prevalence rates remain high (16.2%), and the disease continues to disproportionately burden African Americans (39.2% prevalence), particularly Black women (48.0% prevalence). Because HSV-2 is asymptomatic in most persons, many carry the virus yet have *not* received a diagnosis and therefore treatment (AAP & ACOG, 2017).

Currently, AAP & ACOG (2017) do not recommend routine HSV screening of pregnant women. There is controversy over the cost/benefit ratio of universal screening and the number of neonatal deaths prevented from this type of screening. Most primary and first-episode infections in early pregnancy are not associated with spontaneous abortion or stillbirth but a late pregnancy primary infection may be associated with preterm labor. Neonatal transmission occurs through three routes: (1) intrauterine, 5%; (2) peripartum, 85%; or (3) postnatal, 10% (Cunningham et al., 2014). The fetus becomes infected by virus shed from the cervix and/or lower genital tract. The virus either invades the uterus following membrane rupture or is transmitted by contact with the fetus at birth. Rate of transmission is 1 in 3,200 to 1 in 30,000 births depending on the population studied (Cunningham et al., 2014). Antiviral therapy with acyclovir or valacyclovir has been used for treatment and will decrease the duration of symptoms and viral shedding in women with a primary outbreak in pregnancy. Acyclovir and valacyclovir appear safe for pregnant women and may reduce the risk of outbreaks at the time of labor that would lead to a cesarean section delivery in efforts to prevent transmission of HSV to the baby. AAP & ACOG (2017) recommend antiviral therapy at or beyond 36 weeks for women who have any recurrence during pregnancy. Whether suppression is needed for women with outbreaks before but not during pregnancy has not been determined (Cunningham et al., 2014).

HIV attacks the CD4 cells of the immune system. Infection with HIV occurs primarily through sexual contact, contaminated blood or blood products, through exposure to contaminated needles and syringes, and mother-to-child transmission. High-risk factors include injection of nonmedical drugs, prostitution, a suspected or known HIV-infected sexual partner, multiple sexual partners, or a diagnosis of another STI. HIV is transmitted during pregnancy via the placenta, during vaginal birth, and through the breast milk of an HIV-infected woman.

According to the CDC (2017) HIV surveillance report, the number of women with HIV who give birth annually in the United States is unknown. An estimate for 2006 suggested that approximately 8,500 women with HIV gave birth each year. More recent evidence suggests that the number is less than 5,000. At the end of 2016, 1,814 children were living with diagnosed perinatal HIV in the United States and dependent areas. Of these approximately 63% were Black, 15% were Hispanic, and 11% were White (CDC, 2017). The decrease in perinatally acquired HIV is predominantly due to the implementation of prenatal HIV testing with antiretroviral therapy given to the pregnant woman and then to her neonate. Testing for HIV infection during prenatal care, with patient notification, should be a routine part of prenatal lab work unless the woman declines the test (AAP & ACOG, 2017). If the woman declines HIV testing (i.e., the opt-out approach), as permitted by local and state regulations, her refusal should be documented in the medical record (AAP & ACOG, 2017). When a pregnant woman with unknown HIV status presents to the hospital for care, rapid HIV testing is recommended (AAP & ACOG, 2017).

In addition to the standard prenatal assessment for all pregnant women, the initial laboratory evaluation of an HIV-infected woman should include the following:

- History of use (prior and current) of antiretroviral medications
- Renal and liver function
- HIV-1 RNA viral level
- CD4$^+$ lymphocyte count, CD4$^+$ percentage
- Complete blood count (CBC) with differential
- Platelet count
- Screen for other STIs, including gonorrhea and chlamydia
- Screen for hepatitis B and C
- Screen for CMV and toxoplasmosis
- Cervical cancer screening
- Purified protein derivative for tuberculosis
- Assessment of supportive care needs

During pregnancy, most women with HIV are advised to take combination antiretroviral regimens to reduce perinatal transmission treatment and treatment of maternal HIV (National Institutes of Health, 2018). This regimen may need adjustment in the woman who was already taking a regimen of medications. When possible, zidovudine is included because it has been shown to significantly reduce the risk of passing HIV to the infant and is thought to be safe to take during pregnancy. A combination regimen is more effective in reducing HIV transmission than a single-drug regimen (AAP & ACOG, 2017).

Medical and nursing care of HIV-infected pregnant women requires coordination and communication between HIV specialists and obstetrical healthcare providers. General counseling should include current knowledge about risk factors for perinatal transmission. Risk of perinatal transmission of HIV has been associated with potentially modifiable factors including cigarette smoking, illicit drug use, genital tract infections, and unprotected sexual intercourse with multiple partners during pregnancy. Besides improving maternal health, cessation of cigarette smoking and drug use, treatment of genital tract infections, and use of condoms with sexual intercourse during pregnancy may reduce risk of perinatal transmission (NIH, 2018). A resource available to nurses is the Perinatal HIV Consultation line (1-888-448-8765), a federally funded service providing free clinical consultation to providers caring for HIV-infected women and their infants.

Maternal genitourinary and reproductive tract infections have been implicated as a main risk factor in 15% to 25% of preterm deliveries (Denney & Culhane, 2009). Bacterial vaginosis is a maldistribution of normal vaginal flora occurring in up to 20% of all pregnancies (Boggess, 2005). Numbers of lactobacilli are decreased, and overrepresented species are anaerobic bacteria, including *Gardnerella vaginalis*, *Mobiluncus*, and some *Bacteroides* species. Treatment is reserved for symptomatic women who usually complain of a fishy-smelling discharge or burning and itching. However, treatment does not reduce preterm birth, and routine screening is not recommended (ACOG, 2016a).

As a routine part of prenatal practice, nurses can assess maternal dentition and advise on proper brushing and flossing techniques and encourage women to seek dental care. Continuing or acquiring dental care during pregnancy should be a routine recommendation to pregnant women because there has been evidence to support an association between gingivitis and preterm birth, low birth weight, and preeclampsia (Xiong, Buekens, Fraser, Beck, & Offenbacher, 2006). Gingivitis occurs in 60% to 75% of pregnant women, and it surfaces most frequently during the second trimester (Khader & Ta'ani, 2005). Symptoms include swollen red gums and bleeding with brushing. Elevated levels of estrogen and progesterone cause the gums to react differently to the bacteria found in plaque.

Although multiple studies have shown an association between periodontal infection and adverse pregnancy outcomes, treatment of periodontal disease during pregnancy has not been shown to improve birth outcomes. Recently, Jeffcoat et al. (2011) demonstrated that successful routine periodontal treatment (scaling and root planing plus oral hygiene instruction) is associated with a decreased incidence of spontaneous preterm birth.

Culture

Cultural assessment is an important part of prenatal care. A comprehensive discussion of culture as it relates to pregnancy and childbirth practices is presented in Chapter 2. Cultural beliefs and practices can affect the health status of the woman by influencing her use of healthcare services; confidence in and acceptance of recommended prevention and treatment strategies; and global beliefs regarding her body, illness, religion, and so forth (Seidel et al., 2010). Principal beliefs, values, and behaviors that relate to pregnancy and childbirth should be identified, taking care to avoid sweeping generalizations about cultural characteristics or cultural values. Not every individual in a culture may display certain characteristics because there are variations among cultures and within cultures. Planning culturally specific care requires information about ethnicity, degree of affiliation with the ethnic group, religion, patterns of decision making, language, style of communication, norms of etiquette, and expectations about the healthcare system (Seidel et al., 2010). Nutritional practices and beliefs about medication are particularly significant during pregnancy. Certain behavioral differences can be expected if a culture views pregnancy as an illness, as opposed to a natural occurrence; for example, seeking prenatal care may or may not be important if pregnancy is viewed as a natural occurrence. Healthcare practices during pregnancy are influenced by numerous factors, such as the prevalence of folk remedies, the prevalence of indigenous healers, and the influence of professional healthcare workers. Socioeconomic status and living in an urban or rural setting affect patterns of use of home remedies and use of the healthcare system.

Without cultural awareness, nurses and other healthcare providers tend to project their own cultural responses onto women and families from different socioeconomic, religious, or educational groups. This leads caregivers to assume patients are demonstrating a certain type of behavior for the same reason that they themselves would. Additionally, some nurses may fail to recognize that healthcare has its own culture, which has been dominated historically by traditional middle-class values and beliefs. In an ethnocentric approach, caregivers sometimes believe that if members of other cultures do not share Western values, they should adopt them. An example of this is a nurse who values equality of the sexes dealing with an Asian woman who defers to the husband to make the decisions. Encouraging women to defy cultural values and beliefs can prove stressful for the woman and significantly interfere with a therapeutic relationship.

When a language barrier exists, the woman may be reluctant to provide information if the interpreter is male, a relative, or a child of the pregnant woman. Reviewing the goals and purposes of the interview with the interpreter in advance generally enhances the interaction with the woman. Efforts should be made to have a medical interpreter available for the interview in order to ensure the woman's privacy is protected and that the information shared between patient and provider is translated correctly. Gender is an important factor in health beliefs. In many cultures, a male provider would not be allowed to examine a woman, much less deliver her baby. In these cases, a female provider should be made available if possible. Nurses cannot expect to be culturally competent for every woman they care for. However, culturally responsive behaviors can enhance prenatal care. If a particular ethnic group dominates the local population, it is a professional responsibility to learn as much about that culture so as to provide optimal care.

Current Pregnancy Status

Assessment of current pregnancy status includes an analysis of current pregnancy history, psychosocial factors, nutritional status, and laboratory data; a review of symptoms guided by the gestational age and that may reflect medical or pregnancy complications; an assessment of the pregnant woman's concerns; and a complete physical examination. Symptom review includes questions about nausea and vomiting, headache, abdominal or epigastric pain, visual changes, fever, viral illness, vaginal bleeding, dysuria, cramping, and other concerns. This screening process incorporates assessment of historical and social factors with current health status. Evaluation of current pregnancy status provides baseline data that guide planning for future evaluation and health promotion activities.

The physical examination is comprehensive and covers a review of the cardiovascular, respiratory, neurologic, endocrine, gastrointestinal, reproductive, and genitourinary systems. An anthropometric assessment, including the woman's height, weight, and pelvimetry data may positively influence the course of pregnancy and birth (Cunningham et al., 2014). Pelvic examination includes measurement of cervical length, a Pap smear, and assessment for STIs. The abdominal examination compares data from the woman's report of her last menstrual period with physical findings. Depending on weeks of gestation, the FHR may be auscultated with a handheld Doppler.

Selected laboratory data are valuable to the assessment process. Biochemical information provides information about current prenatal health as well as general wellness status. Evaluation of specific laboratory data is discussed later in this chapter.

ONGOING PRENATAL CARE

Nurses who interact with the childbearing family in the prenatal period assess the well-being of the woman and the growth and well-being of the fetus. Nursing intervention is directed by the data obtained from ongoing comprehensive maternal–fetal assessments.

Evaluation of the growth and development of the fetus can be shared with the parents to promote prenatal parent–infant attachment.

Risk status in pregnancy is a dynamic process that affects clinical and nonclinical parameters. Psychosocial factors, socioeconomic factors, and lifestyle patterns also require ongoing evaluation. Employment status, family economic status, and relationship status could change from visit to visit. These changes affect the woman's psychosocial stress level, potentiating existing risk factors. In general, factors with potential to affect the pregnancy are in a constant state of fluctuation and require continued surveillance.

Subsequent prenatal visits should be structured to promote continuous, rather than episodic, risk assessment. Each prenatal visit should include a maternal–fetal physical assessment, including vital signs, weight, fundal height, FHR, and fetal movement as well as a review of pertinent laboratory data, dating data, the problem list, and the woman's response to recommended interventions (e.g., smoking cessation). At return prenatal visits, risk factors must be analyzed to evaluate their relevance to the gestational age. For example, if a woman has a history of preterm labor and is at 37 weeks' gestation in the current pregnancy, this risk factor would no longer be relevant. Conversely, new risk factors may develop during the pregnancy, such as preeclampsia or gestational diabetes. Ongoing prenatal care is a dynamic process in which risk factors may change from month to month. Achieving healthy pregnancy outcomes is a multifaceted and sometimes complex process. Nurses can be credible sources of information, offering support as the woman and her partner or family sort through information and decision making during pregnancy.

Evaluation of maternal blood pressure trends is a critical nursing intervention (see Chapter 5 for a complete discussion of hypertensive disease during pregnancy). During pregnancy, blood pressure values decrease slightly during the second trimester but return to early pregnancy values by the third trimester. Ideally, during preconception care or early prenatal care, a baseline blood pressure is noted. It is important to evaluate and document blood pressure measurements in the same arm with the woman in the same position (e.g., sitting or semi-Fowler) with the blood pressure cuff at the level of the heart. Use of the same device for assessing blood pressure is also critical to accuracy. Consistency in blood pressure monitoring allows for more accurate assessment and comparison across prenatal visits.

A blood pressure reading of >140 mm Hg systolic, 90 mm Hg diastolic, or both is considered elevated (AAP & ACOG, 2017). Other clinical data are important to assess because blood pressure change is not usually a lone sign of complications. When there is a change in blood pressure, the woman should be assessed for the concurrent development of proteinuria, headaches, dizziness, visual disturbances, epigastric pain, or edema. Gestational hypertension is defined as systolic blood pressure ≥140 mm Hg and/or diastolic blood pressure ≥90 mm Hg in a previously normotensive pregnant woman who is ≥20 weeks of gestation and has no proteinuria (ACOG, 2013a). The blood pressure readings should be documented on at least two occasions at least 6 hours apart. It is considered severe when sustained elevations in systolic blood pressure ≥160 mm Hg and/or diastolic blood pressure ≥110 mm Hg are present for at least 6 hours (ACOG, 2013c). Gestational hypertension is a temporary diagnosis for hypertensive pregnant women who do not meet criteria for preeclampsia (both hypertension and proteinuria) or chronic hypertension (hypertension first detected before the 20th week of pregnancy). The diagnosis is changed to the following:

- Preeclampsia, if proteinuria develops
- Chronic hypertension, if blood pressure elevation persists ≥12 weeks postpartum
- Transient hypertension of pregnancy, if blood pressure returns to normal by 12 weeks postpartum

Basic fetal surveillance includes assessment of fundal height, FHR, and fetal activity. Fundal height is the measurement of the uterus from the symphysis pubis to the top of the fundus. The measurement of the fundal height in centimeters (±2 cm) should correlate with gestational age between 22 and 34 weeks. Fundal height less than gestational age may be indicative of IUGR. Fundal height greater than gestational age may indicate multiple gestation, polyhydramnios, macrosomia, fibroids, or other conditions that cause uterine distension. Fetal activity is an indirect measure of central nervous system function and is predictive of fetal well-being. Fetal movement counting (i.e., "kick counts") is discussed later in this chapter.

Preterm Labor and Birth

Preterm and low-birth-weight births are considered by many to be the most urgent problems in the care of pregnant women. In the United States, preterm birth rates declined from 10.4% to 9.5% of all live births from 2007 to 2014 (Ferré, Callaghan, Olson, Sharma, & Barfield, 2016). This decline was due in part to effective teen pregnancy prevention programs and fewer unintended pregnancies. However, the implications of preterm birth are great and the reader is referred to Chapter 7 for an in-depth discussion of this topic.

Biochemical Screening and Laboratory Assessment

Selected biochemical screens may be repeated at specific intervals during pregnancy. Subsequent prenatal visits usually include urinalysis by dipstick for evidence of proteinuria, glucosuria, and ketonuria. Although it is common practice, there is little evidence to suggest routine urinalysis by means of dipstick provides useful clinical information or is predictive of women who will develop complications of pregnancy (AAP & ACOG, 2017). Dipstick urinalysis does not detect proteinuria reliably in patients with early preeclampsia; measurement of 24-hour urinary protein excretion is the gold standard but is not always practical. Trace glycosuria also is unreliable, although higher concentrations may be useful (Kirkham, Harris, & Grzybowski, 2005).

After a baseline CBC is obtained, periodic assessment of hematocrit and hemoglobin values may be indicated for certain at-risk populations. Additionally, laboratory data such as urinalysis, urine culture, blood type and Rhesus (Rh) factor, antibody screen, rubella titer, rapid plasma reagin test, hepatitis B surface antigen, gonorrhea and chlamydia testing, and cervical cytology should be obtained from all pregnant women. Additional laboratory tests (e.g., STI screens, group B streptococci, fetal fibronectin [fFN], TORCH titers, tuberculin testing, toxicology screens, and genetic screens) should be performed as indicated based on historical indicators or clinical findings (AAP & ACOG, 2017).

Chlamydia testing is recommended for all pregnant women (AAP & ACOG, 2017). A nucleic acid amplification test of the cervix is the most sensitive test available with excellent specificity (CDC, 2002). Universal HIV testing of pregnant women is recommended (AAP & ACOG, 2017) early in the pregnancy using an "opt-out" approach, that is, the test is offered to all and the woman may opt-out if she desires to decline testing. In this way, appropriate medical management can be initiated early to reduce the possibility of perinatal transmission. Appropriate counseling and referral services should be available for women with positive test results.

Screening for gestational diabetes mellitus (GDM) occurs at 24 to 28 weeks' gestation using a 1-hour, 50-g glucose challenge test (AAP & ACOG, 2017). Serum glucose evaluation before 24 to 28 weeks' gestation (i.e., at the first visit) may be indicated based on family history or maternal factors such as glucosuria, advanced maternal age, marked obesity, family history of diabetes mellitus, personal history of GDM, previous macrosomic infant, or previous unexplained fetal loss. The woman does not need to be fasting for the screening test. One hour after ingesting a glucose load (Glucola), the serum glucose level should be less than 140 mg/dL. The American Diabetes Association (ADA) recommends a cutoff value after 1 hour of either 140 mg/dL (7.8 mmol/L), which is said to identify 80% of women with GDM, or 130 mg/dL (7.2 mmol/L), which should identify 90%. Problems have also been reported for the glucose challenge test: There are many false positives, and sensitivity is only 86% at best (Menato et al., 2008) Nonfasting plasma glucose over 200 mg/dL on screening or a fasting greater than 105 mg/dL is indicative of diabetes mellitus and no oral glucose tolerance test (OGTT) is necessary for diagnosis.

If the screening result is greater than or equal to 140 mg/dL, a diagnostic test using a 3-hour, 100-g OGTT is recommended. The diagnostic test for GDM is administered after a fast of at least 8 hours, but with the patient consuming her usual unrestricted daily diet in the days preceding the test. On the day of the test, only water may be consumed, and cigarette smoking should be avoided.

The diagnosis of gestational diabetes is made when two or more of the values at the 3-hour OGTT are elevated above the following values (in plasma mg/dL):

Fasting: 105
1 hour: 190
2 hour: 165
3 hour: 145

If only one level is elevated, repeat testing at a later gestation may be ordered or dietary restriction recommended. Women diagnosed with GDM require education about appropriate nutrition, self-management, and self-glucose monitoring and referral for appropriate medical care and counseling. Approximately 15% to 20% of those with GDM will develop overt diabetes mellitus.

Genetic screening should be offered to all pregnant women during the first trimester and no later than between 15 and 20 weeks' gestation (AAP & ACOG, 2017). The goal of commonly used genetic screening tests is to identify women who have an increased risk of NTD, Down syndrome, or trisomy 21. Screening should be voluntary, and the woman should be counseled about its limitations and benefits (ACOG, 2016b).

One part of genetic screening is maternal serum alpha-fetoprotein (MSAFP). Alpha-fetoprotein (AFP) is a protein that is produced in the fetal yolk sac during the first trimester and in the fetal liver during later gestation. The concentration of AFP in maternal serum is altered by factors that include inaccurate dating of gestational age, maternal weight and race, multiple gestation, and maternal diabetes. Most screening programs establish a cutoff of 2 to 2.5 times the median values (2 to 2.5 MoM) to be designated as a positive result for NTD (AAP & ACOG, 2017). There is a direct relationship between the age of the patient and the chance of her result being designated as positive.

Abnormally elevated MSAFP levels have been associated with birth defects and chromosomal anomalies, such as open NTDs, open abdominal defects, and congenital nephrosis (AAP & ACOG, 2017). High MSAFP levels also may result from multiple gestations.

Low MSAFP levels have been associated with Down syndrome and other chromosomal anomalies (AAP & ACOG, 2017). Double-marker screening (i.e., AFP and human chorionic gonadotropin [hCG]), triple-marker screening (i.e., AFP, hCG, and estriol), and quadruple-marker screening (AFP, hCG, estriol, and inhibin A) are also available to screen for trisomy 18, trisomy 21, and NTDs. In pregnancies with Down syndrome, average hCG levels are higher and unconjugated estriol levels are lower than normal. In pregnancies with trisomy 18, the hCG and estriol levels are lower than normal. When more parameters are evaluated, there is an increased accuracy in diagnosis. Although maternal serum screening with the use of double and triple markers is superior to the use of MSAFP alone when screening for fetal Down syndrome, this method still fails to detect Down syndrome in women less than 35 years of age (AAP & ACOG, 2017). The quadruple is the most effective multiple-marker screening test for Down syndrome in the second trimester. This approach yields an 81% detection rate and a false-positive rate of 5% (ACOG, 2016b).

Women should be counseled that maternal serum screening tests are optional, that the screening tests have limited sensitivity and specificity, and that there may be psychological implications of a positive test prior to the performance of the tests. Any abnormal finding warrants additional testing; however, screening protocols vary. If the initial ultrasound examination does not provide an explanation for the MSAFP elevation (such as inaccurate dating, multiple gestation, or fetal demise), a comprehensive (level II) ultrasound examination is performed to evaluate the fetus for malformations.

Nuchal Translucency

An ultrasound scan is carried out to assess the amount of fluid behind the neck of the fetus—known as nuchal translucency (NT). Fetuses at risk for Down syndrome tend to have a higher amount of fluid around the neck. The nuchal scan is most accurate between 11 and 14 weeks. The scan is obtained with the fetus in sagittal section and a neutral position of the fetal head (neither hyperflexed nor extended, either of which can influence the NT thickness). The fetal image is enlarged to fill 75% of the screen, and the maximum thickness is measured, from leading edge to leading edge. When combined with serum markers, such as those included in the quad screen earlier, NT measurement detects 79% to 87% of Down syndrome fetuses (ACOG, 2016b).

Noninvasive Prenatal Testing

In addition to the long-used screening mentioned earlier, newer screening is becoming more commonly used in certain high-risk populations, including women >35 years old, women with previous pregnancies affected by genetic conditions, and women with abnormal results on initial genetic screening. Noninvasive prenatal testing, or NIPT, involves a blood draw from the women, thereby limiting the risk to the fetus. The blood is then sent to a specialty laboratory where fetal fraction DNA is separated from maternal DNA and chromosomal defects can be identified, including trisomy 21, trisomy 13, trisomy 18, and sex chromosome disorders. When abnormal results are received, follow-up ultrasound imaging is usually performed; amniocentesis is not as commonly used now due to the excellent sensitivity and specificity of the newer NIPT. Genetic counseling should be offered before and after testing to ensure that women are aware of the risks and benefits of such testing.

Hemoglobinopathies

Hemoglobin electrophoresis is used to detect genetic hemoglobin disorders, including sickle cell anemia, sickle cell disease, and thalassemia. These recessive inherited conditions occur in the United States primarily in families of African descent but can also be found in families of Asian, Middle Eastern, or Mediterranean descent (Larrabee & Cowan, 1995). Women of African descent are routinely screened for these disorders. Although prevalence of sickle cell trait is common among African Americans (8% to 12%), information related to inheritance patterns is not well known to those at risk. Figure 4–1 and Display 4–7 provide teaching tools that may be helpful in explaining the genetic transfer of sickle cell trait and sickle cell disease to women and their partners.

Prenatal Diagnosis

Prenatal diagnostic evaluation should be offered to families with any of the following: maternal age of 35 years or more, maternal age of 32 years or more and pregnant with twins, women carrying a fetus with a sonographically identified structural anomaly, women with ultrasound markers of aneuploidy (including increased nuchal thickness), women with a known positive serum screen, a family history of chromosomal anomalies, parental balanced translocation carrier, the mother with a known or at-risk carrier for X-linked disorder, parents who are carriers of an autosomal recessive disorder detectable in utero, a parent affected with an autosomal dominant disorder detectable in utero, a family history of NTDs (Kirkham et al., 2005).

Ultrasonography

Ultrasonography (i.e., fetal imaging by intermittent, high-frequency sound waves) is the most commonly

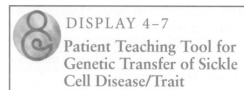

DISPLAY 4–7
Patient Teaching Tool for Genetic Transfer of Sickle Cell Disease/Trait

1. Two parents affected with sickle cell trait:
   SA + SA = 25% of children will have sickle cell disease.
   50% of children will have sickle cell trait.
   25% of children will not be affected by the trait or disease.
2. One parent affected with sickle cell trait, one parent affected with sickle cell disease:
   SA + SS = 50% of children will have sickle cell disease.
   50% of children will have sickle cell trait.
   0 children will not be affected by the trait or disease.
3. Two parents affected by sickle cell disease:
   SS + SS = 100% of children will have sickle cell disease.
   0 children will have sickle cell trait.
   0 children will not be affected by the disease.
4. One parent affected by sickle cell disease, one parent unaffected:
   SS + AA = 100% of children will have sickle cell trait.
   0 children will have sickle cell disease.
   0 children will not be affected by trait.
5. One parent affected by sickle cell trait, one parent unaffected:
   SA + AA = 50% of children will have sickle cell trait.
   50% of children will not be affected by the trait.
   0 children will not be affected by sickle cell disease.

AA = unaffected; SA = sickle cell trait; SS = sickle cell disease.
From Larrabee, K., & Cowan, M. (1995). Clinical nursing management of sickle cell disease and trait during pregnancy. *The Journal of Perinatal & Neonatal Nursing, 9*(2), 29–41.

used prenatal diagnostic procedure. Indications vary widely and depend on gestational age and type of diagnostic information sought. During early pregnancy, ultrasound is frequently used to determine presence of an intrauterine gestational sac, fetal number, and cardiac activity and to measure crown-rump length. Early ultrasonography (i.e., before 14 weeks' gestation) accurately determines gestational age (±1 week), decreases the need for labor induction after 41 weeks' gestation, and detects multiple pregnancies (ACOG, 2016c). Components of the basic ultrasound examination include the following:

- Presence of gestational sac and an evaluation of uterus and adnexa when performed during the first trimester
- Estimated gestational age
- Number of fetuses
- Viability
- Location of placenta
- Volume of amniotic fluid
- Fetal presentation and anatomic survey when performed during the second and third trimesters

Ultrasound during the second and third trimesters can be useful when there is a discrepancy between the woman's last menstrual period and uterine size, to detect fetal anatomic defects or abnormal fetal growth, and for placental localization and amniotic fluid volume estimates. When maternal or fetal complications are suspected or identified, ultrasonography serves as a valuable tool to confirm the diagnosis and follow-up on fetal status. Ultrasonography is also used to guide the obstetrician during other diagnostic procedures, such as chorionic villus sampling (CVS), amniocentesis, and fetal blood sampling. In women for whom preterm birth is a concern, cervical length can be measured via ultrasound. However, the value of doing this test lies in its negative predictive value. That is, the test is more useful for those women who have normal results and are not likely to experience preterm labor than for predicting preterm labor in women with abnormal results (ACOG, 2016a).

Controversy exists over the benefits of routine ultrasound examination for all pregnant women. Advocates suggest routine screening can decrease incidence of labor induction for suspected postdate pregnancies and avoid undiagnosed fetal anomalies and twin gestations. However, no evidence directly links improved fetal outcomes with routine ultrasound screening (Kirkham et al., 2005).

Chorionic Villus Sampling

CVS involves the removal of a small sample of chorionic (placental) tissue through a catheter inserted through the cervix. The villi are harvested and cultured for chromosomal analysis and processed for DNA and enzymatic analysis as indicated. Results are available in 4 days. CVS is ideally performed between 10 and 11.5 weeks' gestation. The risk of fetal loss is approximately 1%. As with amniocentesis, information about benefits and risks must be provided before the procedure (Cunningham et al., 2014).

Amniocentesis

Amniocentesis is the collection of a sample of amniotic fluid from the amniotic sac for identification of genetic diseases, selected birth defects, and fetal lung maturity; therapy for polyhydramnios; and progressive evaluation of isoimmunized pregnancies. Amniocentesis for genetic evaluation may be performed between 15 and 20 weeks' gestation. Genetic amniocentesis allows for detection of chromosomal anomalies, biochemical disorders, NTDs, some ventral wall defects, and DNA analysis for many single-gene disorders. Early amniocentesis, between 11 and 14 weeks' gestation, is offered at some centers with outcomes like midtrimester amniocentesis (Cunningham et al., 2014). Before testing, families should be given information about indications for amniocentesis, how the procedure is done, risks involved, and ramifications of findings.

Fetal Blood Sampling

Fetal blood sampling, also known as percutaneous umbilical cord blood sampling or cordocentesis, allows direct evaluation of fetal blood obtained from the umbilical cord. The procedure is not often performed and only done in centers that have the expertise. Using ultrasonography to guide placement, a needle is inserted into one of the umbilical vessels (usually the vein), and a small amount of blood is withdrawn. Valuable information can be gained from analysis of fetal blood, including prenatal diagnosis of fetal blood disorders, isoimmunization, metabolic disorders, infections, and karyotyping (Cunningham et al., 2014). Cordocentesis can also be used for fetal therapies such as red blood cell and platelet transfusions.

Biochemical Markers

fFN, a protein secreted by the trophoblast, can be detected by use of a monoclonal antibody: FDC-6. The exact function is unknown, but this protein is thought to play a role in mediating placental–uterine attachment. fFN is normally present in the cervical or vaginal fluid before 20 weeks' gestation. However, after 20 weeks, the presence of fFN may indicate a disruption of the attachment of the fetal membranes, and therefore, it has been investigated as an early marker for preterm birth.

Predicting women truly at risk for preterm birth as opposed to those destined to deliver at term may aid in the ability to initiate interventions to prolong pregnancy and avoid preterm birth (see Chapter 7). fFN is a glycoprotein found in high concentrations in the amniotic fluid. It is normally found in the cervical and vaginal secretions before 16 to 20 weeks' gestation, but its presence in the cervicovaginal secretion after 20 weeks' gestation is abnormal, except as a marker of the imminent onset of labor at term (Cunningham et al., 2014). Elevation of fFN levels is hypothesized to reflect mechanical or inflammatory damage to the membranes or placenta. The fFN cutoff for a positive test is ≥ 50 ng/mL (Cunningham et al., 2014). The cervicovaginal fFN assay has limited accuracy in predicting preterm within 7 days of sampling in symptomatic pregnant women (Sanchez-Ramos, Delke, Zamora, & Kaunitz, 2009).

The fFN test is best used in the evaluation of women with preterm contractions in whom the diagnosis of preterm labor is uncertain. A negative test together with other reassuring factors (e.g., no signs of intrauterine infection or active abruption and no progressive cervical change or increase in uterine contraction intensity) can be used to avoid interventions (e.g., admission to the hospital, tocolysis, glucocorticoid administration). The high negative predictive value has proved most useful. Unfortunately, the positive predictive value is not as high, and women with a positive fFN may or may not actually experience preterm labor and birth.

To collect a specimen for fFN testing, a Dacron swab is placed in the posterior fornix of the vagina and rotated for 10 seconds. Sexual activity within 24 hours of sample collection, recent cervical examination, and vaginal bleeding may result in false-positive tests (Adeza Biomedical, 2005). For this reason, a specimen should not be collected if the patient has had intercourse within 24 hours, and the specimen should be collected before performance of a digital cervical exam, measurement of transvaginal cervical length, or cervical cultures. fFN testing should be limited to women with intact amniotic membranes and cervical dilatation <3 cm. This provides the nurse with the opportunity to review signs and symptoms of preterm labor and to address any fears or anxieties the woman or family may have regarding preterm birth.

FETAL SURVEILLANCE

Fetal assessment is an integral component of prenatal care. Careful assessment of fetal well-being enhances perinatal outcome through early identification and intervention for fetal compromise. The goal of antepartum fetal surveillance is to prevent fetal death. Display 4–8 provides the indications for antepartum fetal surveillance. Techniques based on FHR patterns have been in use since the 1970s. Ultrasonography may be used as indicated throughout the pregnancy to assess fetal growth and development. See Chapter 15 for more details about fetal assessment.

Assessment of Fetal Activity

Fetal movement counting (i.e., "kick counts") has been proposed as a primary method of fetal surveillance for all pregnancies. Cessation of fetal movement is correlated with fetal death. The mother's observation of fetal movement has been validated through an 80% to 90% correlation of maternal perception of movement with movement detected on real-time ultrasonography (AAP & ACOG, 2017).

Several methods of fetal movement counting have been proposed. Perception of 10 distinct movements in a period of up to 2 hours is considered reassuring. After 10 movements have been perceived, the count may be discontinued. Another approach is to instruct women to count fetal movements for 1 hour three times per week. The count is considered reassuring if it equals or exceeds the woman's established baseline count (AAP & ACOG, 2017). Monitoring of fetal movement is recommended for pregnant women at high risk for antepartum fetal death beginning as early as 26 to

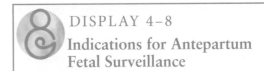

DISPLAY 4–8

Indications for Antepartum Fetal Surveillance

Maternal Conditions
- Pregestational diabetes mellitus
- Hypertension
- Antiphospholipid syndrome
- Hyperthyroidism (poorly controlled)
- Hemoglobinopathies (hemoglobin SS, SC, or S-thalassemia)
- Cyanotic heart disease
- Systemic lupus erythematosus
- Chronic renal disease

Pregnancy-Related Conditions
- Gestational hypertension
- Preeclampsia
- Decreased fetal movement
- Gestational diabetes (poorly controlled or medically treated)
- Oligohydramnios
- Fetal growth restriction
- Late term or postterm pregnancy
- Isoimmunization
- Previous fetal demise (unexplained or recurrent risk)
- Monochorionic multiple gestation (with significant growth discrepancy)

From American College of Obstetricians and Gynecologists. (2014). *Antepartum fetal surveillance* (Practice Bulletin No. 145). Washington, DC: Author.

28 weeks' gestation. Because fetal movement counting is inexpensive, reassuring, and a relatively easily taught skill, all women could benefit from instruction on fetal activity assessment.

Although fetal activity is a reassuring sign, decreased fetal movement is not necessarily ominous. A healthy fetus usually has perceptible movements within 10 to 60 minutes (Cunningham et al., 2014). However, perception of fetal movement can be influenced by many factors, including time of day, gestational age, placental location, glucose loading, maternal smoking, maternal medications, and decreased uterine space as gestation increases. Decreased fetal movement may also reflect the fetal sleep state. Early identification of conditions that can affect pregnancy outcome can minimize perinatal morbidity by allowing for the establishment of an appropriate treatment plan and referrals (AAP & ACOG, 2017). Report of decreased fetal movement is an indication for further assessment. The woman should be instructed to have something to eat and drink, rest, and focus on fetal movement for 1 hour. Four movements in 1 hour are considered reassuring. If fewer than four movements are perceived in 2 hours, the woman should call her primary healthcare provider immediately.

Nonstress Test

The nonstress test (NST) is one of the most common methods of prenatal screening and involves electronic FHR monitoring for approximately 20 minutes. The NST is based on the premise that the normal fetus moves at various intervals and that the central nervous system and myocardium respond to movement with acceleration of the FHR. Acceleration of the FHR during fetal activity is a sign of fetal well-being (ACOG, 2014). Various definitions of reactivity have been used. Using the most common definition, the NST is reactive when two or more FHR accelerations of 15 beats per minute above baseline and lasting at least 15 seconds occur within a 20-minute time frame with or without perception of fetal movement by the woman (ACOG, 2014). These accelerations should occur within 40 minutes of testing. An NST that does not meet these criteria is nonreactive. A reactive NST is reassuring, indicating less than a 1% chance of fetal death within 1 week of a reactive NST. Most deaths within 1 week of a reactive NST fall into nonpreventable categories, such as abruptio placentae, sepsis, and cord accidents. However, a nonreactive NST is not necessarily an ominous sign. Rather, the nonreactive NST indicates a need for further testing and should be followed by a contraction stress test or a BPP (Cunningham et al., 2014). The NST of the uncompromised preterm fetus (24 to 28 weeks' gestation) is frequently nonreactive, and up to 50% of NSTs may not be reactive from 28 to 32 weeks' gestation (ACOG, 2014). Prior to 32 weeks, some practitioners consider that the test is reactive if FHR increases 10 beats for 10 seconds twice in a 20-minute period.

Biophysical Profile

The BPP combines electronic FHR monitoring with ultrasonography to evaluate fetal well-being based on multiple biophysical variables. Five parameters are assessed: fetal muscle tone, fetal movement, fetal breathing movements, amniotic fluid volume, and FHR reactivity as demonstrated by NST. Each item has a maximum score of 2, with a summed score of 8 to 10 indicating fetal well-being (i.e., reassuring). A score of 6 is considered "equivocal," and the test should be repeated the next day in a preterm fetus. A term fetus should be delivered if the score is less than 8. A score of 4 usually indicates that birth is warranted, although for extremely premature pregnancies, management is individualized. Scores of 0 or 2 are "abnormal," with expeditious birth considered (ACOG, 2014). Indications for BPP are those listed for antepartum fetal surveillance with weekly testing usually recommended.

Modified Biophysical Profile

The modified BPP combines two of the components of the regular BPP: the use of an NST as a short-term indicator of fetal well-being and the assessment of amniotic fluid index (AFI) as an indicator of long-term placental function. The AFI is the sum of the measurements of the deepest cord-free amniotic fluid pocket in each of the four abdominal quadrants. An AFI value greater than 5 cm generally is considered adequate. A modified BPP is considered reassuring if the NST is reactive and the AFI is greater than 5 cm but abnormal if the NST is nonreactive or the AFI is 5 cm or less (ACOG, 2014). The modified BPP is less cumbersome and may be as predictive of fetal status as other approaches of biophysical fetal surveillance (AAP & ACOG, 2017).

NURSING ASSESSMENT AND INTERVENTIONS

Nursing interventions are based on a collaborative approach. These interventions are based on a woman's strengths and any conditions with potential to increase risk of complications. Together, the nurse and woman set goals and strategize ways to implement a plan of care to meet these goals. During the antepartum period, nursing care typically includes comfort promotion (i.e., measures to relieve discomforts caused by the physiologic changes of pregnancy), counseling for family adaptation in planning the addition of a new member, and encouraging behaviors to enhance maternal and fetal well-being. Providing education, especially for the woman experiencing a first-time pregnancy, is an important aspect of antepartum care. The nurse has the opportunity and the responsibility to teach the woman and her family about beneficial and detrimental lifestyle practices, potential risks, and care required to promote maternal and fetal well-being. The nurse in ambulatory care provides anticipatory planning, assesses all available data, and structures education and nursing interventions accordingly. Inherent in competent antenatal nursing practice is the ability to differentiate between normal pregnancy variations and high-risk complications and the initiation of appropriate nursing interventions.

Total care management of the childbearing family requires cooperation, collaboration, and communication across disciplines. Risk factors must be evaluated in terms of individual risk versus benefit to be effective. Healthcare providers are charged with the task of finding the goodness of fit between the recommended healthcare regimen and the individual's reality to optimize outcome. Case management allows for a single healthcare professional to coordinate healthcare management in collaboration with the pregnant woman.

Case Management

The childbearing woman and her family are the core of the perinatal healthcare team. Family-centered perinatal care is a model of care based on the philosophy that the physical, social, spiritual, and economic needs of the total family unit should be integrated and considered collectively. The nurse's role as case manager, advocate, and educator is of primary importance in facilitating a family-friendly system that validates the woman's own knowledge and promotes empowered healthcare decision making.

Nutrition

Nutrition assessment and counseling is a vital component of prenatal care. The woman may benefit from regularly scheduled appointments with the nutritionist during an early prenatal visit and again at 28 weeks' gestation. Additional visits with the nutritionist should be scheduled as indicated (e.g., for inadequate or excessive weight gain, anemia, metabolic disorders such as GDM). Weight-gain charts; 24-hour diet recall; or simple, self-report dietary assessment tools are valuable education resources.

Nutritional status may change because of availability of appropriate foods and financial resources for groceries. The most significant food shortages for low-income women occur at the end of the month, when federal and local resources are depleted or when food is shared among a disproportionate number of household members. Likewise, religious practices may dictate fasting during specific times of the year (e.g., Lent or Ramadan), limiting the woman's food intake. Awareness and ongoing assessment of these factors allow for timely interventions and appropriate referral to nutrition counseling, social work, and community support services. Referrals to food and nutrition supplement programs may be warranted. Women in the United States should be referred to the Special Supplemental Nutrition Program. Other supplemental food and nutrition programs are available to childbearing families on a regional or local basis. The prenatal healthcare team must be knowledgeable about such resources in their area.

Social Services

The emphasis on individualized, holistic prenatal care, encompassing physiologic and psychosocial needs, promotes a prevention-oriented model of care. Today's families may face unemployment, homelessness, chemical dependency, increased family and neighborhood violence, and lack of support systems precipitating crises and affecting perinatal outcomes. Early recognition of potential risk allows for prompt intervention and referral. The role of the perinatal social worker is critical in providing interventions that relieve stress, providing for woman's basic needs, following crisis situations, and facilitating healthcare decision making. Social work referrals are appropriate for pregnant women experiencing medical, psychological, or socioeconomic crises. Psychosocial and socioeconomic factors are

evaluated on a continuing basis, with referral to social services as needed.

From a practical point of view, pregnant women have much to benefit from a team approach. The woman has access to health professionals offering expertise in a specific area, and the perinatal team may be more likely to thoroughly assess and plan for a woman's individual needs. A pregnant woman may communicate about some concern to a nutritionist or social worker regarding a problem area that she did not reveal to the physician or nurse. With professional collaboration and communication among team members, problems can be better identified and addressed.

Education and Counseling

Educational and health promotional activities that include the father (depending on his relationship with the pregnant woman) can be integrated into prenatal care. Prenatal education should focus not only on a positive labor and birth experience but also on a successful pregnancy outcome. Education regarding nutrition, sexuality, stress reduction, lifestyle behaviors, and hazards in the work place is appropriate to include in prenatal education (Display 4–9).

Early identification of conditions that can affect pregnancy outcome can minimize perinatal morbidity by allowing for the establishment of an appropriate treatment plan and referrals (AAP & ACOG, 2017). Women must receive information regarding risk factors, warning signs, and criteria for provider notification. Routine prenatal care should include education to enhance recognition of warning signs of preterm labor and preeclampsia, fever, rupture of membranes or leaking of fluid, decreased fetal movement, vaginal bleeding, persistent nausea and vomiting, and signs and symptoms of viral or bacterial infection.

With current postpartum lengths of stay, it is increasingly difficult to teach the woman and family all they need to know about maternal–newborn care during hospitalization. The last trimester of pregnancy may be a potentially effective time to introduce maternal–newborn care content, including parenting issues and family planning information. Because there is no accurate way to predict which women will develop postpartum emotional disorders, all childbearing women and family members should be provided information about postpartum depression and where to seek help.

Confidence-building strategies that promote breastfeeding are an important component of prenatal nutrition education. Providing information about breastfeeding convenience, infant benefits, and potential formula cost savings can enhance maternal motivation. Acknowledging that some women may feel embarrassed or uncomfortable about breastfeeding and providing tips for discreet breastfeeding techniques are also helpful approaches.

DISPLAY 4-9
Prenatal Education Topics

First Trimester

What to expect during prenatal care; scope of services offered in the practice which the patient is attending; anticipated schedule of visits

Healthy lifestyle

Nutrition

Dental care

Smoking cessation

Teratogen avoidance including medication use, hot tub exposure

Alcohol avoidance

Illicit drug avoidance

Seat belt use

Sexuality

Work and rest patterns

Physiologic changes of pregnancy

Emotional changes of pregnancy

Discomforts of pregnancy

Screening, diagnostic tests

Nipple assessment, breastfeeding promotion

Warning signs of pregnancy complications

Criteria and mechanism for notification of healthcare provider

(Information may be given at individual prenatal care visit or early pregnancy class.)

Second Trimester

Nutrition

Smoking cessation

Teratogen avoidance

Alcohol avoidance

Illicit drug avoidance

Prenatal laboratory tests

Physiologic changes of pregnancy

Emotional changes of pregnancy

Healthy lifestyle

Discomforts of pregnancy

Sexuality

Family roles

Fetal growth and development

Breastfeeding promotion

Childbirth education

Travel

Perineal exercises

Clothing choices/shoes

Body mechanics

Preterm birth prevention

Preeclampsia precautions/warning signs of pregnancy complications

Third Trimester

Reproductive health; family planning

Discomforts of pregnancy

When to stop working

Where to go/whom to call; physician coverage in labor and delivery

Warning signs of pregnancy complications

Fetal growth and development

Cord blood banking

Newborn care

Infant car seat use

Discussion of planned infant feeding

Childbirth education

Postpartum self-care choices

Postpartum emotional changes

Preparation for childbirth

Maternal breastfeeding self-efficacy is a significant predictor of breastfeeding duration and level. Breastfeeding duration is significantly associated with psychological factors including dispositional optimism, breastfeeding self-efficacy, faith in breast milk, breastfeeding expectations, anxiety, planned duration of breastfeeding, and the time of the infant feeding decision (O'Brien, Buikstra, & Hegney, 2008). Self-efficacy enhancing strategies to increase a new mother's confidence in her ability to breastfeed can easily be integrated into prenatal nursing care. Breastfeeding promotion interventions increase duration of breastfeeding (Chung, Raman, Trikalinos, Lau, & Ip, 2008). However, combining both pre- and postnatal interventions are more effective than either pre- or postnatal alone. Group education (peer support) is a more effective strategy to extend the duration of breastfeeding than usual prenatal care. Class information commonly given to pregnant mothers includes benefits of breastfeeding, early initiation, how breast milk is produced, hazards of bottle feeding, breastfeeding on demand, prolonged breastfeeding, family planning, and the lactational amenorrhea method. A session with the nutritionist, focusing on nutrition during lactation, may be helpful in encouraging initiation of breastfeeding and a successful breastfeeding experience. Chapter 20 provides an in-depth discussion about breastfeeding.

The childbearing continuum is a transition involving each family member. Childbirth education provides the opportunity for enhancement of family systems and facilitation of empowered behaviors that may last a lifetime. Over 40 years ago, the first childbirth education classes began to provide information for women wishing to be awake, active participants in the birth of their child. Since then, childbirth education focusing on coping strategies for labor has been shown to decrease use of anesthesia in labor and enhance maternal confidence and satisfaction. Today, childbirth education goes well beyond basics to include information about birth as a natural process, environments that enhance the woman's ability to give birth, care options, and, most important, the tools necessary to make informed healthcare decisions that are appropriate for individual families. Childbirth education has expanded in some centers to meet consumers' need for information concerning preconception wellness, care provider and birthing options, and maternal–newborn care during the postpartum period. Current, accurate information; effective coping skills; and intact support systems fostered by childbirth education provide families with the skills to explore alternatives and make informed decisions that are congruent with their personal goals. It is important that childbirth education is available to all women. Perinatal nurses are challenged to move childbirth education from traditional services to time frames and locations that meet consumer needs or increase availability through social media and distance learning avenues.

Health Promotion

Preconception health promotion is increasingly recognized as an important factor influencing perinatal outcome. The addition of a prepregnancy visit and the recommended prenatal and postpartum visits has been identified as an essential step toward improving pregnancy outcomes, particularly for those planning pregnancy (Johnson et al., 2006). If women have not been exposed to this information before pregnancy, healthcare professionals should seize the opportunity to provide information and experiences that promote these activities during prenatal care. Awareness of reproductive risk, healthy lifestyle behaviors, and reproductive options is essential in improving pregnancy outcome. Additionally, use the interconception period to provide additional intensive interventions to women who have had a previous pregnancy that ended in an adverse outcome (e.g., infant death, fetal loss, birth defects, low birth weight, or preterm birth). Experiencing an adverse outcome in a previous pregnancy is an important predictor of future reproductive risk. However, many women with adverse pregnancy outcomes do not receive targeted interventions to reduce risks during future pregnancies (Johnson et al., 2006). Whereas a preterm birth is identified on birth certificates and a woman's primary care provider typically knows this information, professional guidelines do not include systematic follow-up and intervention for women with this critical predictor of risk.

SUMMARY

Prenatal care provides numerous opportunities for increasing reproductive awareness from a woman's health perspective. Aside from providing valuable information about the current pregnancy, laboratory evaluation also provides indicators of general health status and opportunities for health promotion. Screening tests that allow for health promotion are also offered during pregnancy. Nursing care during the prenatal period is multifaceted, requiring knowledge of the psychosocial tasks and issues surrounding the childbearing continuum as well as knowledge of normal physiologic processes and potential risks. Anticipatory guidance during the prenatal period can have a significant impact on perinatal outcome. Education based on individual assessment empowers women and underscores their partnership in healthcare decision making. The goal of prenatal care must go a step farther than targeting a positive physical outcome. Rather, we must work toward providing care and education that facilitate holistic family wellness and the best possible outcomes for mothers and babies.

REFERENCES

Achkar, M., Dodds, L., Giguère, Y., Forrest, J. C., Armson, B. A., Woolcott, C., . . . Weiler, H. A. (2015). Vitamin D status in early pregnancy and risk of preeclampsia. *American Journal of Obstetrics & Gynecology*, 212(4), 1–7. doi:10.1016/j.ajog.2014.11.009

Adeza Biomedical. (2005). *Fetal fibronectin enzyme immunoassay and rapid fFN for the TLi™ system: Information for health care providers*. Sunnyvale, CA: Author.

American Academy of Pediatrics & American College of Obstetricians and Gynecologists. (2017). *Guidelines for perinatal care* (8th ed.). Washington, DC: Author.

American College of Obstetricians and Gynecologists. (2005). *The importance of preconception care in the continuum of women's health care* (Committee Opinion No. 313). Washington, DC: Author.

American College of Obstetricians and Gynecologists. (2011). *Vitamin D: Screening and supplementation during pregnancy* (Committee Opinion No. 495). Washington, DC: Author.

American College of Obstetricians and Gynecologists. (2012). *Intimate partner violence* (Committee Opinion No. 518). Washington, DC: Author.

American College of Obstetricians and Gynecologists. (2013a). *Hypertension in pregnancy*. Washington, DC: Author.

American College of Obstetricians and Gynecologists. (2013b). *Weight gain during pregnancy* (Committee Opinion No. 548; Reaffirmed, 2018). Washington, DC: Author.

American College of Obstetricians and Gynecologists. (2014). *Antepartum fetal surveillance* (Practice Bulletin No. 145 Reaffirmed, 2019). Washington, DC: Author. doi:10.1097/01. AOG.0000451759.90082.7b

American College of Obstetricians and Gynecologists. (2015). *Exercise during pregnancy and the postpartum period* (Committee Opinion No. 650; Reaffirmed, 2019). Washington, DC: Author.

American College of Obstetricians and Gynecologists. (2016a). *Management of preterm labor* (Practice Bulletin No. 171). Washington, DC: Author.

American College of Obstetricians and Gynecologists. (2016b). *Prenatal diagnostic testing for genetic disorders* (Practice Bulletin No. 162). Washington, DC: Author.

American College of Obstetricians and Gynecologists. (2016c). *Ultrasound in pregnancy* (Practice Bulletin No. 175). Washington, DC: Author. doi:10.1097/AOG.0000000000001815

American College of Obstetricians and Gynecologists. (2017a). *Neural tube defects* (Practice Bulletin No. 187). Washington, DC: Author.

American College of Obstetricians and Gynecologists. (2017b). *Smoking cessation during pregnancy* (Committee Opinion No. 721). Washington, DC: Author.

Association of Women's Health, Obstetric and Neonatal Nurses. (2004). *Response to the U.S. Preventive Services Task Force Report on Screening for Family and Intimate Partner Violence published in the March 2 Annals of Internal Medicine*. Washington, DC: Author.

Association of Women's Health, Obstetric and Neonatal Nurses. (2017). Tobacco use and women's health (Clinical Position Statement). *Journal of Obstetric, Gynecologic, and Neonatal Nursing, 46*(5), 794–796. doi:10.1016/j.jogn.2017.07.002

Association of Women's Health, Obstetric and Neonatal Nurses. (2019). *Standards and guidelines for professional nursing practice in the care of women and newborns* (8th ed.). Washington, DC: Author.

Ayoola, A. B., Nettleman, M., Stommel, M., & Canady, R. B. (2010). Time of pregnancy recognition and prenatal care use: A population-based study in the United States. *Birth, 37*(1), 37–43. doi:10.1111/j.1523-536X.2009.00376.x

Baer, R., Altman, M., Oltman, S., Ryckman, K., Chamber, C., Rand, L., & Jelliffe-Pawlowski, L. (2018). Maternal factors influencing late entry into prenatal care: A stratified analysis by race or ethnicity and insurance status. *The Journal of Maternal-Fetal & Neonatal Medicine, 32*(20), 3336–3342. doi:10.1080/14767058.2018.1463366

Beck, C. T. (2008). State of the science on postpartum depression: What nurse researchers have contributed—Part 1. *MCN. The American Journal of Maternal Child Nursing, 33*(2), 121–126. doi:10.1097/01.NMC.0000313421.97236.cf

Bellinger, D. C. (2005). Teratogen update: Lead and pregnancy. *Birth Defects Research, 73*(6), 409–420. doi:10.1002/bdra.20127

Bianchi, A. (2016). Intimate partner violence during the childbearing years. *Journal of Obstetric, Gynecologic, and Neonatal Nursing, 45*, 577–578.

Bianchi, A., Cesario, S., & McFarlane, J. (2016). Interrupting intimate partner violence during pregnancy with an effective screening and assessment program. *Journal of Obstetric, Gynecologic, and Neonatal Nursing, 45*, 579–591.

Bianchi, A., McFarlane, J., Cesario, S., Symes, L., & Maddoux, J. (2016). Continued intimate partner violence during pregnancy and after birth and its effect on child functioning. *Journal of Obstetric, Gynecologic, and Neonatal Nursing, 45*, 601–609.

Boggess, K. A. (2005). Pathophysiology of preterm birth: Emerging concepts of maternal infection. *Clinics in Perinatology, 32*(3), 561–569. doi:10.1016/j.clp.2005.05.002

Brown, C., & Garovic, V. (2014). Drug treatment of hypertension in pregnancy. *Drugs, 74*(3), 283–296.

Carolan, M. (2009). Towards understanding the concept of risk for pregnant women: Some nursing and midwifery implications. *Journal of Clinical Nursing, 18*(5), 652–658. doi:10.1111/j.1365-2702.2008.02480.x

Centers for Disease Control and Prevention. (2002). Screening tests to detect chlamydia trachomatis and Neisseria gonorrhoeae infections—2002. *MMWR Morbidity and Mortality Weekly Report, 51*(RR-15), 1.

Centers for Disease Control and Prevention. (2016). *Guidelines for vaccinating pregnant women*. Atlanta, GA: Author. Retrieved from https://www.cdc.gov/vaccines/pregnancy/hcp-toolkit/guidelines.html

Centers for Disease Control and Prevention. (2017). *Diagnosis of HIV infection in the United States and dependent areas, 2016*. HIV Surveillance Report, 28, 1–125. Retrieved from http://www.cdc.gov/hiv/library/reports/hiv-surveillance.html.

Chamberlain, C., O'Mara-Eves, A., Porter, J., Coleman, T., Perlen, S. M., Thomas, J., & McKenzie, J. E. (2017). Psychosocial interventions for supporting women to stop smoking in pregnancy. *Cochrane Database of Systematic Reviews*, (2), CD001055. doi:10.1002/14651858.CD001055.pub5

Chang, G. (2019). *Substance use by pregnant women*. http://www.uptodate.com/contents/substance-use-in-pregnancy

Chasnoff, I. J., Wells, A. M., McGourty, R. F., & Bailey, L. K. (2007). Validation of the 4P's Plus screen for substance use in pregnancy validation of the 4P's Plus. *Journal of Perinatology, 27*(12), 744–748. doi:10.1038/sj.jp.7211823

Chung, M., Raman, G., Trikalinos, T., Lau, J., & Ip, S. (2008). Interventions in primary care to promote breastfeeding: An evidence review for the U.S. Preventive Services Task Force. *Annals of Internal Medicine, 149*, 565–582.

Corbett, R. W., Ryan, C., & Weinrich, S. P. (2003). Pica in pregnancy: Does it affect pregnancy outcomes? *MCN. The American Journal of Maternal Child Nursing, 28*(3), 183–191.

Cunningham, F. G., Leveno, K. J., Bloom, S. L., Spong, C. Y., Dashe, J. S., Hoffman, B. L., . . . Sheffield, J. S. (2014). *William's obstetrics* (4th ed.). New York, NY: McGraw-Hill.

de Jong, E. P., Walther, F. J., Kroes, A. C., & Oepkes, D. (2011). Parvovirus B19 infection in pregnancy: New insights and management. *Prenatal Diagnosis, 31*(5), 419–425. doi:10.1002/pd.2714

Denney, J., & Culhane, J. (2009). Bacterial vaginosis: A problematic infection from both a perinatal and neonatal perspective. *Seminars in Fetal & Neonatal Medicine, 14*(4), 200–203. doi:10.1016/j.siny.2009.01.008

Denny, C. H., Tsai, J., Floyd, R. L., & Green, P. P. (2009). Alcohol use among pregnant and nonpregnant women of childbearing age—United States, 1991–2005. *MMWR Morbidity and Mortality Weekly Report, 58*, 529–532.

Dijkmans, A. C., de Jong, E. P., Dijkmans, B. A., Lopriore, E., Vossen, A., Walther, F. J., & Oepkes, D. (2012). Parvovirus B19 in pregnancy: Prenatal diagnosis and management of fetal complications. *Current Opinion in Obstetrics & Gynecology, 24*(2), 95–101. doi:10.1097/GCO.0b013e3283505a9d

Dowswell, T., Carroli, G., Duley, L., Gates, S., Gülmezoglu, A. M., Khan-Neelofur, D., & Piaggio, G. G. (2010). Alternative versus standard packages of antenatal care for low-risk pregnancy. *Cochrane Database of Systematic Reviews*, (10), CD000934.

Feetham, S., Thomson, E. J., & Hinshaw, A. S. (2005). Nursing leadership in genomics for health and society. *Journal of Nursing Scholarship, 37*(2), 102–110. doi:10.1111/j.1547-5069.2005.00021.x

Ferré, C., Callaghan, W., Olson, C., Sharma, A., & Barfield, W. (2016). Effects of maternal age and age-specific preterm birth rates on overall preterm birth rates—United States, 2007 and 2014. *MMWR Morbidity and Mortality Weekly Report, 65*(43), 1181–1184. doi:10.15585/mmwr.mm6543a1

Hook, E. B. (1981). Rates of chromosome abnormalities at different maternal ages. *Obstetrics & Gynecology, 58*, 282–285.

Huizink, A. C., & Mulder, E. J. (2006). Maternal smoking, drinking or cannabis use during pregnancy and neurobehavioral and cognitive functioning in human offspring. *Neuroscience and Biobehavioral Reviews, 30*(1), 24–41. doi:10.1016/j.neubiorev.2005.04.005

Hyde, T. B., Schmid, D. S., & Cannon, M. J. (2010). Cytomegalovirus seroconversion rates and risk factors: Implications for congenital CMV. *Reviews in Medical Virology, 20*(5), 311–326. doi:10.1002/rmv.659

Ickovics, J., Earnshaw, V., Lewis, J., Kershaw, R., Magriples, U., Stasko, E., . . . Tobin, J. (2016). Cluster randomized controlled trial of group prenatal care: Perinatal outcomes among adolescents in

New York City health centers. *American Journal of Public Health*, *106*(2), 359–365. doi:10.2105/AJPH.2015.302960

Institute of Medicine. (2009). *Weight gain during pregnancy: Reexamining the guidelines* (Report Brief). Washington, DC: National Academy Press.

Jeffcoat, M., Parry, S., Sammel, M., Clothier, B., Catlin, A., & Macones, G. (2011). Periodontal infection and preterm birth: Successful periodontal therapy reduces the risk of preterm birth. *BJOG*, *118*, 250–256. doi:10.1111/j.1471-0528.2010.02713.x

Jesse, D. E., & Graham, M. (2005). Are you often sad and depressed? Brief measures to identify women at risk for depression in pregnancy. *MCN: The American Journal of Maternal Child Nursing*, *30*(1), 40–45.

Johnson, K., Posner, S. F., Biermann, J., Cordero, J. F., Atrash, H. K., Parker, C. S., . . . Curtis, M. G. (2006). Recommendations to improve preconception health and health care—United States: A report of the CDC/ATSDR Preconception Care Work Group and the select panel on preconception care. *MMWR. Recommendations and Reports*, *55*(RR-6), 1–23.

Kania-Richmond, A., Hetherington, E., McNeil, D., Bayrampour, H., Tough, S., & Metcalfe, A. (2017). The impact of introducing Centering Pregnancy in a community health setting: A qualitative study of experiences and perspectives of health center clinical and support staff. *Maternal and Child Health Journal*, *21*, 1327–1335. doi:10.1007/s10995-016-2236-1

Kanungo, J., James, A., McMillan, D., Lodha, A., Faucher, D., Lee, S., & Shah, P. (2011). Advanced maternal age and the outcomes of preterm neonates: A social paradox? *Obstetrics & Gynecology*, *118*(4), 872–877. doi:10.1097/AOG.0b013e31822add60

Kennedy, H., Farrell, T., Paden, R., Hill, S., Jolivet, R., Cooper, B., & Rising, S. (2011). A randomized clinical trial of group prenatal care in two military settings. *Military Medicine*, *176*, 1169–1177.

Khader, Y. S., & Ta'ani, Q. (2005). Periodontal diseases and the risk of preterm birth and low birth weight: A meta-analysis. *Journal of Periodontology*, *76*(2), 161–165. doi:10.1902/jop.2005.76.2.161

Khalil, A., Syngelaki, A., Maiz, N., Zinevich, Y., & Nicolaides, H. (2013). Maternal age and adverse pregnancy outcome: A cohort study. *Ultrasound in Obstetrics & Gynecology*, *42*, 634–643. doi:10.1002/uog.12494

Kiely, M., El-Mohandes, A. A., El-Khorazaty, M. N., Blake, S. M., & Gantz, M. G. (2010). An integrated intervention to reduce intimate partner violence in pregnancy: A randomized controlled trial. *Obstetrics & Gynecology*, *115*(2 Pt 1), 273–283. doi:10.1097/AOG.0b013e3181cbd482

Kirkham, C., Harris, S., & Grzybowski, S. (2005). Evidence-based prenatal care: Part I. General prenatal care and counseling issues. *American Family Physician*, *71*(7), 1307–1316.

Lancaster, C., Gold, K., Flynn, H., Yoo, H., Marcus, S., & Davis, M. (2010). Risk factors for depressive symptoms during pregnancy: A systematic review. *American Journal of Obstetrics & Gynecology*, *202*(1), 5–14. doi:10.1016/j.ajog.2009.09.007

Larrabee, K., & Cowan, M. (1995). Clinical nursing management of sickle cell disease and trait during pregnancy. *The Journal of Perinatal & Neonatal Nursing*, *9*(2), 29–41.

March of Dimes. (2010). *Toward improving the outcome of pregnancy III*. White Plains, NY: Author.

March of Dimes. (2019). *Peristats*. White Plains, NY: Author. Retrieved from https://www.marchofdimes.org/peristats/Peristats.aspx

Markovitz, B. P., Cook, R., Flick, L. H., & Leet, T. L. (2005). Socioeconomic factors and adolescent pregnancy outcomes: Distinctions between neonatal and post-neonatal deaths? *BMC Public Health*, *5*, 79. doi:10.1186/1471-2458-5-79

Martin, J. A., Hamilton, B. E., Osterman, M. J. K., Driscoll, A. K., & Drake, P. (2018). Births: Final data for 2017. *National Vital Statistics Reports*, *67*(8), 1–50.

Martin, J. A., Hamilton, B. E., Sutton, P. D., Ventura, S. J., Menacker, F., & Kirmeyer, S. (2006). Births: Final data for 2004. *National Vital Statistics Reports*, *55*(1), 1–101.

Massey, S. H., Lieberman, D. Z., Reiss, D., Leve, L. D., Shaw, D. S., & Neiderhiser, J. M. (2011). Association of clinical characteristics and cessation of tobacco, alcohol, and illicit drug use during pregnancy. *The American Journal on Addictions*, *20*, 143–150. doi:10.1111/j.1521-0391.2010.00110.x

Matthews, T. J., MacDorman, M. F., & Thoma, M. E. (2015). Infant mortality statistics from the 2013 period linked birth/infant death data set. *National Vital Statistics Reports*, *64*(9), 1–30.

Mattison, D. R. (2010). Environmental exposures and development. *Current Opinion in Pediatrics*, *22*(2), 208–218. doi:10.1097/MOP.0b013e32833779bf

McCall, S., Nair, M., & Knight, M. (2017). Factors associated with maternal mortality at advanced maternal age: A population-based case-control study. *BJOG*, *124*, 1225–1233. doi:10.1111/1471-0528.14216

Menato, G., Bo, S., Signorile, A., Gallo, M., Cotrino, I., Poala, C. B., . . . Massobrio, M. (2008). Current management of gestational diabetes mellitus. *Expert Review of Obstetrics & Gynecology*, *3*(1), 73–91. doi:10.1586/17474108.3.1.73

Mitchell, A. A., Gilboa, S. M., Werler, M. M., Kelley, K. E., Louik, C., & Hernàndez-Díaz, S. (2011). Medication use during pregnancy, with particular focus on prescription drugs: 1976-2008. *American Journal of Obstetrics & Gynecology*, *205*(1), 51.e1–51.e8. doi:10.1016/j.ajog.2011.02.029

Morrical-Kline, K. A., Walton, A. M., & Guildenbecher, T. M. (2011). Teratogen use in women of childbearing potential: An intervention study. *Journal of the American Board of Family Medicine*, *24*(3), 262–271. doi:10.3122/jabfm.2011.03.100198

National Institutes of Health. (2018). *Recommendations for the use of antiretroviral drugs in pregnant women with HIV infection and interventions to reduce perinatal HIV transmission in the United States*. Retrieved from https://aidsinfo.nih.gov/guidelines/html/3/perinatal/180/intrapartum-antiretroviral-therapy-prophylaxis

O'Brien, M., Buikstra, E., & Hegney, D. (2008). The influence of psychological factors on breastfeeding duration. *Journal of Advanced Nursing*, *63*(4), 397–408. doi:10.1111/j.1365-2648.2008.04722.x

Olson, C. M. (2008). Achieving a healthy weight gain during pregnancy. *Annual Review of Nutrition*, *28*, 411–423.

Patel, C., Edgerton, L., Flake, D., & Smits, A. (2006). Clinical inquiries. What precautions should we use with statins for women of childbearing age? *The Journal of Family Practice*, *55*(1), 75–77.

Pereira, A., Bos, S., Marques, M., Maia, B., Soares, M., Valente, J., . . . Azevedo, M. (2011). The Postpartum Depression Screening Scale: Is it valid to screen for antenatal depression? *Archives of Women's Mental Health*, *14*, 227–238.

Pignone, M. P., Gaynes, B. N., Rushton, J. L., Burchell, C. M., Orleans, C. T., Mulrow, C. D., . . . Lohr, K. N. (2002). Screening for depression in adults: A summary of the evidence for the U.S. Preventive Services Task Force. *Annals of Internal Medicine*, *136*(10), 765–776.

Raatikainen, K., Heiskanen, N., & Heinonen, S. (2005). Marriage still protects pregnancy. *BJOG*, *112*(10), 1411–1416. doi:10.1111/j.1471-0528.2005.00667.x

Raatikainen, K., Heiskanen, N., Verkasalo, P., & Heinonen, S. (2006). Good outcome of teenage pregnancies in high-quality maternity care. *European Journal of Public Health*, *16*(2), 157–161. doi:10.1093/eurpub/cki158

Rahman, A., Bunn, J., Lovel, H., & Creed, F. (2007). Association between antenatal depression and low birthweight in a developing country. *Acta Psychiatrica Scandinavica*, *115*, 481–486. doi:10.1111/j.1600-0447.2006.00950.x

Ribot, B., Aranda, F., Viteri, F., Hernández-Martínez, C., Canals, J., & Arija, V. (2012). Depleted iron stores without anaemia early in pregnancy carries increased risk of lower birthweight even when supplemented daily with moderate iron. *Human Reproduction*, 27(5), 1260–1266. doi:10.1093/humrep/des026

Rising, S. S. (1998). Centering Pregnancy. An interdisciplinary model of empowerment. *Journal of Nurse-Midwifery*, 43(1), 46–54. doi:10.1016/S0091-2182(97)00117-1

Rising, S., Kennedy, H., & Klima, C. (2004). Redesigning prenatal care through CenteringPregnancy. *Journal of Midwifery & Women's Health*, 49(5), 398–404. doi:10.1111/j.1542-2011.2004.tb04433.x

Sanchez-Ramos, L., Delke, I., Zamora, J., & Kaunitz, A. M. (2009). Fetal fibronectin as a short-term predictor of preterm birth in symptomatic patients: A meta-analysis. *Obstetrics & Gynecology*, 114(3), 631–640. doi:10.1097/AOG.0b013e3181b47217

Scholl, T., Chen, X., & Stein, P. (2012). Maternal vitamin D status and delivery by cesarean. *Nutrients*, 4(4), 319–330. doi:10.3390/nu4040319

Schonfeld, T., Schmid, K. K., Brown, J. S., Amoura, N. J., & Gordon, B. (2013). A pregnancy testing policy for women enrolled in clinical trials. *IRB*, 35(6), 9–15.

Seidel, H. M., Ball, J. W., Dains, J. E., Flynn, J. A., Solomon, B. S., & Stewart, R. W. (2010). *Mosby's guide to physical examination* (6th ed.). Philadelphia, PA: Mosby.

Shieh, C., & Carter, A. (2011). Online prenatal nutrition education: Helping pregnant women eat healthfully using MyPyramid.gov. *Nursing for Women's Health*, 15(1), 26–35. doi:10.1111/j.1751-486X.2011.01608.x

Silver, R. M. (2007). Fetal death. *Obstetrics & Gynecology*, 109(1), 153–167. doi:10.1097/01.AOG.0000248537.89739.96

Simmons, L. A., Havens, J. R., Whiting, J. B., Holz, J. L., & Bada, H. (2009). Illicit drug use among women with children in the United States: 2002–2003. *Annals of Epidemiology*, 19, 187–193. doi:10.1016/j.annepidem.2008.12.007

Singer, L., Min, M., Minnes, S., Short, E., Lewis, B., Lang, A., & Wu, M. (2018). Prenatal and concurrent cocaine, alcohol, marijuana and tobacco effects on adolescent cognition and attention. *Drug and Alcohol Dependence*, 191, 37–44. doi:10.1016/j.drugalcdep.2018.06.022

Stanley, A. Y., Durham, C. O., Sterrett, J. J., & Wallace, J. B. (2019). Safety of over-the-counter medications in pregnancy. *MCN: The American Journal of Maternal/Child Nursing*, 44(4), 196–205. doi:10.1097/NMC.0000000000000537

Tjaden, P., & Thoennes, T. (2000). *Extent, nature, and consequences of intimate partner violence*. Washington, DC: National Institute of Justice.

Tong, V. T., Jones, J. R., Dietz, P. M., D'Angelo, D., & Bombard, J. M. (2009). Trends in smoking before, during, and after pregnancy—Pregnancy Risk Assessment Monitoring System (PRAMS), United States, 31 sites, 2000-2005. *MMWR Morbidity and Mortality Weekly Report*, 58, 1–29.

U.S. Department of Health and Human Services. (2010). *Healthy People 2020: Understanding and improving health* (2nd ed.). Washington, DC: U.S. Government Printing Office.

U.S. Food and Drug Administration. (2019). Advice about eating fish: For women who are or might become pregnant, breastfeeding mothers, and young children. Retrieved from https://www.fda.gov/media/129959/download

U.S. Preventive Services Task Force. (2009a). Counseling and interventions to prevent tobacco use and tobacco-caused disease in adults and pregnant women: U.S. Preventive Services Task Force reaffirmation recommendation statement. *Annals of Internal Medicine*, 150, 551–555.

U.S. Preventive Services Task Force. (2009b). Folic acid for the prevention of neural tube defects: U.S. Preventive Services Task Force recommendation statement. *Annals of Internal Medicine*, 150, 626–631.

Van den Bergh, B. R., Mulder, E. J., Mennes, M., & Glover, V. (2005). Antenatal maternal anxiety and stress and the neurobehavioural development of the fetus and child: Links and possible mechanisms. A review. *Neuroscience and Biobehavioral Reviews*, 29(2), 237–258. doi:10.1016/j.neubiorev.2004.10.007

Vu, N., Jouriles, E., McDonald, R., & Rosenfield, D. (2016). Children's exposure to intimate partner violence: A meta-analysis of longitudinal associations with child adjustment problems. *Clinical Psychology Review*, 46, 25–33.

Xiong, X., Buekens, P., Fraser, W. D., Beck, J., & Offenbacher, S. (2006). Periodontal disease and adverse pregnancy outcomes: A systematic review. *BJOG*, 113(2), 135–143. doi:10.1111/j.1471-0528.2005.00827.x

Yost, N. P., Bloom, S. L., McIntire, D. D., & Leveno, K. J. (2005). A prospective observational study of domestic violence during pregnancy. *Obstetrics & Gynecology*, 106(1), 61–65. doi:10.1097/01.AOG.0000164468.06070.2a

Young, S. L. (2010). Pica in pregnancy: New ideas about an old condition. *Annual Review of Nutrition*, 30, 403–422. doi:10.1146/annurev.nutr.012809.104713

APPENDIX 4–A. Guidelines For Vaccinating Pregnant Women

	Vaccine	General Recommendation for Use in Pregnant Women
Routine	Hepatitis A	Base decision on risk vs. benefit.
	Hepatitis B	Recommended in some circumstances.
	Human Papillomavirus (HPV)	Not recommended.
	Influenza (Inactivated)	Recommended.
	Influenza (LAIV)	Contraindicated.
	MMR	Contraindicated.
	Meningococcal (ACWY)	May be used if otherwise indicated.
	Meningococcal (B)	Base decision on risk vs. benefit.
	PCV13	No recommendation.
	PPSV23	Inadequate data for specific recommendation.
	Polio	May be used if needed.
	Td	Should be used if otherwise indicated (Tdap preferred).
	Tdap	Recommended.
	Varicella	Contraindicated.
	Zoster	Contraindicated.
Travel & Other	Anthrax	Low risk of exposure — not recommended. High risk of exposure — may be used.
	BCG	Contraindicated.
	Japanese Encephalitis	Inadequate data for specific recommendation.
	Rabies	May be used if otherwise indicated.
	Typhoid	Inadequate data. Give Vi polysaccharide if needed.
	Smallpox	Pre-exposure — contraindicated. Post-exposure — recommended.
	Yellow Fever	May be used if benefit outweighs risk.

BCG, bacille Calmette-Guerin; LAIV, live attenuated influenza vaccine; PCV13, pneumococcal conjugate; PPSV23, pneumococcal polysaccharide; Td, tetanus and diphtheria; Tdap, tetanus, diphtheria, and pertussis.
From Centers for Disease Control and Prevention. (2016). *Guidelines for vaccinating pregnant women*. Atlanta, GA: Author. Retrieved from https://www.cdc.gov/vaccines/pregnancy/hcp-toolkit/guidelines.html

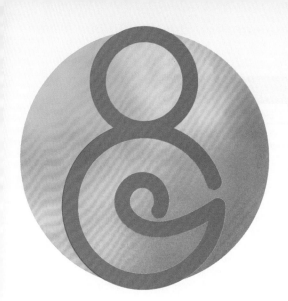

CHAPTER 5

Hypertensive Disorders of Pregnancy

Adriane Burgess

HYPERTENSIVE DISORDERS

Hypertensive disorders of pregnancy affect 5% to 8% of pregnancies globally and are a leading cause of maternal and infant morbidity and mortality (Umesawa & Kobashi, 2017). Women may present with hypertension that predates pregnancy or be diagnosed in pregnancy or during the postpartum period. Regardless of when the diagnosis is made, it is important for healthcare providers to recognize that hypertensive disorders of pregnancy are part of a spectrum of diagnoses. This spectrum of diagnoses is often associated with the gestational age at onset of hypertension as well the presence or absence of other symptomology. This chapter discusses diagnostic criteria associated with each hypertensive disorder of pregnancy, common risk factors, pathophysiology, management, and health promotion strategies. Assessment of maternal–fetal status and implications for the perinatal nurse are included.

CURRENT CLASSIFICATION AND DEFINITIONS

Terminology used to describe hypertensive disorders of pregnancy has included imprecise usage, resulting in confusion among healthcare providers and subsequently has resulted in difficulty in synthesizing research on the topic. The International Society for the Study of Hypertension in Pregnancy (ISSHP) (Tranquilli et al., 2014) as well as the American College of Obstetricians and Gynecologists (ACOG, 2013) have issued revised guidelines regarding the classification, diagnosis, and management of the hypertensive disorders

of pregnancy. See Table 5–1 for the current classifications of hypertension in pregnancy.

Clinically, ACOG (2013) states that there are four basic types of hypertension, which can occur during pregnancy or in the postpartum period: chronic hypertension, gestational hypertension, preeclampsia or eclampsia, and chronic hypertension with superimposed preeclampsia. Diagnosis is based on the gestational age at onset of hypertension and the presence or absence of other symptomology, which can include proteinuria, thrombocytopenia, cerebral or visual disturbances, impaired liver function, renal insufficiency, or pulmonary edema.

Chronic Hypertension

Hypertension is defined as a systolic blood pressure greater than or equal to 140 mm Hg or a diastolic blood pressure greater than or equal to 90 mm Hg (ACOG, 2019b; Society for Maternal-Fetal Medicine [SMFM], 2015). Hypertension is diagnosed when either value is elevated; elevation of both systolic and diastolic pressures is not required for the diagnosis. Chronic hypertension is defined as hypertension present and observable before pregnancy or diagnosed before 20 weeks' gestation (ACOG, 2019b). It is important to monitor maternal trends in blood pressure. If blood pressure is normal in the first trimester then begins to increase as the woman nears 20 weeks' gestation, gestational hypertension or early preeclampsia should be considered (ACOG, 2019b; SMFM, 2015). Due to the pathophysiologic effects of pregnancy on blood pressure, it is important to determine a baseline blood pressure early in pregnancy or have a recent prepregnancy blood pressure documented in the woman's health record (Tranquilli et al., 2014).

TABLE 5–1. Classification of Hypertensive Disorders of Pregnancy

Type of hypertension	Diagnostic criteria	Significance

Gestational hypertension	• New onset of hypertension, generally after 20 weeks of gestation
	• Hypertension defined as
	  • SBP ≥140 mm Hg *or*
	  • DBP ≥90 mm Hg
	• Absence of proteinuria
		• Replaces PIH
		• BP normalizes to prepregnancy values by 12 weeks' postpartum.

Preeclampsia	• Hypertension in a previously normotensive woman after 20 weeks of gestation
	• Proteinuria defined as
	  • >300 mg on 24-hr urine
	  • ≥1+ on dipstick
		• In absence of proteinuria, diagnosed if any of the following are present:
		  • Headache
		  • Blurred vision, scotomata
		  • Abnormal laboratory tests (↓ platelet, ↑ serum creatinine or liver transaminase)

Preeclampsia with severe features	• Diagnosis of preeclampsia plus at least one of the following:
	  • SBP ≥160 mm Hg
	  • DBP ≥110 mm Hg
	  • Serum creatinine >1.1 mg/dL or doubling of serum creatinine in the absence of renal disease
	  • Platelets <100,000/μL
	  • Elevated serum liver enzymes to twice normal
	  • New-onset cerebral/visual disturbances
	  • Persistent epigastric pain
		• At increased risk for complications
		• Treat with magnesium and antihypertensive quickly.

HELLP syndrome	• Diagnosis based on presence of
	  • Hemolysis
	    • Abnormal peripheral smear
	    • LDH >600 U/L
	    • Total bilirubin ≥1.2 mg/dL
	  • Elevated liver enzymes
	    • Serum AST ≥70 U/L
	    • LDH >600 U/L
	  • Low platelets <100,000/μL
		• Severe form/complication of preeclampsia
		• Severity associated with platelet count
		• Laboratory diagnosis
		• Impairs oxygenation and perfusion
		• Common complications included abruptio placentae, DIC, and subsequent severe postpartum bleeding.

Eclampsia	• Diagnosis of preeclampsia • Occurrence of grand mal seizures • No other possible etiology for seizure	• Critically ill patient • Timely treatment of preeclampsia with severe features with magnesium sulfate is necessary to prevent eclampsia. • At risk for cerebral hemorrhage, aspiration, and death

Chronic hypertension	• Hypertension defined as
	  • SBP ≥140 mm Hg *or*
	  • DBP ≥90 mm Hg
	• Hypertension
	  • Present and observable before pregnancy
	  • Diagnosed before 20 weeks' gestation
	  • Persists beyond 12 weeks postpartum
		• Diagnosis may not be known prior to pregnancy.
		• Increased risk for preeclampsia
		• Places pregnancy at increased risk for abruption

Superimposed preeclampsia	• Diagnosis based on presence of one or more of the following in the woman with chronic hypertension:
	  • New onset of proteinuria or sudden ↑ in proteinuria
	  • Headache
	  • Blurred vision, scotomata
	  • Abnormal laboratory tests (↓ platelet, ↑ serum creatinine or liver transaminase)
	• Pulmonary edema
		• Prognosis worse for woman and fetus
		• Timing of birth indicated by overall assessment of maternal–fetal well-being rather than fixed end point

AST, aspartate aminotransferase; BP, blood pressure; DBP, diastolic blood pressure; DIC, disseminated intravascular coagulation; LDH, lactate dehydrogenase; PIH, pregnancy-induced hypertension; SBP, systolic blood pressure.
Adapted from American College of Obstetricians and Gynecologists (2013). *Hypertension in Pregnancy.* Washington, DC; Author.
Haram, K., Svendsen, E., & Abildgaard, U. (2009). The HELLP syndrome: Clinical issues and management. A review. *BMC Pregnancy and Childbirth, 9*(1), 8–22. doi:10.1186/1471-2393-9-8

Gestational Hypertension

Gestational hypertension is the onset of hypertension, generally after the 20th week of gestation, in a previously normotensive woman. If hypertension is first diagnosed during pregnancy, does not progress into preeclampsia, and is normotensive by 12 weeks postpartum, a diagnosis of gestational hypertension is made; if the blood pressure elevation persists past 12 weeks postpartum, then the diagnosis is chronic hypertension (ACOG, 2019b; Tranquilli et al., 2014). Gestational hypertension progresses to preeclampsia in 25% of cases; therefore, increased maternal–fetal surveillance is required (ACOG, 2019b; Tranquilli et al., 2014).

Preeclampsia

Preeclampsia is characterized by ACOG (2013) and the ISSHP (Tranquilli et al., 2014) as the new onset of hypertension with blood pressure greater than or equal to 140 mm Hg systolic or greater than or equal to 90 mm Hg diastolic on two occasions at least 4 hours apart after 20 weeks 0 days' gestation in a previously normotensive women and proteinuria ($\geq$300 mg in a 24-hour urine collection). However, proteinuria is not required to be present for the diagnosis to be made. In the absence of proteinuria, the client must meet blood pressure parameters as well as have any one or more of the following in order to meet preeclampsia diagnostic criteria:

- "Platelets <100,000 μL
- Serum creatinine >1.1 or doubling of serum creatinine in the absence of renal disease
- Elevated concentrations of blood liver transaminases to at least twice normal
- Pulmonary edema
- New onset of cerebral or visual disturbances" (ACOG, 2019b, p. 4)

According to ACOG (2013), preeclampsia is defined as with *severe features* or *without severe features*. Preeclampsia *with severe features* is documented when patients meet diagnostic criteria and reach severe blood pressure (systolic blood pressure $\geq$160 mm Hg and/or diastolic blood pressure $\geq$10 mm Hg) or any one of the other diagnostic criteria aside from proteinuria.

Preeclampsia is heterogeneous in nature, and there seem to be several subtypes of the disease. Most commonly, these subtypes are associated with their timing of onset within pregnancy or in the postpartum. *Early-onset preeclampsia* occurs prior to 34 weeks' gestation (Tranquilli et al., 2014). *Late-onset preeclampsia* occurs on or after 34 weeks' gestation (Tranquilli et al., 2014). *Postpartum preeclampsia* can occur up to 6 weeks postpartum.

If signs and symptoms of preeclampsia or eclampsia occur in women with chronic hypertension, the diagnosis of *chronic hypertension with superimposed preeclampsia* or *eclampsia* is made.

HELLP Syndrome

HELLP syndrome is a clinical and laboratory diagnosis characterized by hepatic involvement as evidenced by *h*emolysis, *e*levated *l*iver enzymes, and *l*ow *p*latelet count. HELLP syndrome is a complication of preeclampsia or eclampsia. Due to the severity of this complication, women with this condition often require immediate treatment, urgent delivery, and transport to a tertiary care facility (ACOG, 2019b; Tranquilli et al., 2014).

Eclampsia

Eclampsia is characterized by the onset of grand mal seizures in the woman diagnosed with preeclampsia with no history of preexisting neurologic pathology or other identifiable cause (ACOG, 2019b).

SIGNIFICANCE AND INCIDENCE

Hypertensive disorders of pregnancy are some of the most common medical complications during pregnancy, labor, birth, and the postpartum period. Increasing numbers of women enter into pregnancy with chronic health conditions such as hypertension, diabetes, and chronic heart disease (Centers for Disease Control and Prevention [CDC], 2018a). In the United States, rates of chronic hypertension in pregnancy have increased from 65.1 per 10,000 birth hospitalizations in 1993 to 166.9 per 10,000 birth hospitalizations in 2014 (CDC, 2018a).

A diagnosis of hypertension complicating pregnancy challenges the care provider, who must weigh the risk, benefits, and alternatives of treatment related to maternal, fetal, and neonatal well-being. Everyone caring for the woman during her pregnancy must be aware of the significance of the disease process, current diagnostic criteria, and management recommendations. Prompt recognition of the disease process and monitoring for potential complications decrease the risk of significant morbidity for the woman and her baby.

In the United States, rates of hypertensive disorders of pregnancy have increased from 528.9 per 10,000 birth hospitalizations in 1993 to 912.4 per 10,000 birth hospitalizations in 2014 (CDC, 2018a). Specifically, preeclampsia is a significant contributor to maternal, fetal, and neonatal morbidity and mortality, complicating approximately 5% to 8% of all pregnancies, with an increase in incidence with gestational age (Umesawa & Kobashi, 2017).

Maternal race influences the rate of gestational hypertension complicating pregnancy, with the highest rates seen for non-Hispanic Black women (50.2 per 1,000 live births). The rate for non-Hispanic White women is 46.1 per 1,000 live births, and for Hispanic women, the rate is 28.9 per 1,000 live births. Non-Hispanic Black women also have higher rates for chronic hypertension (25.7 per 1,000) when compared to non-Hispanic White (12.3 per 1,000) and Hispanic (6.8 per 1,000) women. Maternal age distributions demonstrate women older than 30 years of age have the highest rates of hypertension for all reported races (Martin et al., 2011).

MORBIDITY AND MORTALITY

The CDC (2018b) reports that in 2014, there were 18.0 all-cause pregnancy-related deaths per 100,000 live births. The overall maternal death rate for African American women was 26.5 per 100,000 live births in 2007, compared with 10.0 per 100,000 for White women and 21.7 per 100,000 for all other races. From 2011 to 2014 in the United States, hypertensive disorders of pregnancy accounted for 6.8% of pregnancy related deaths (CDC, 2018b). There is a large disparity among rates of maternal death by race. Specifically, African American women are more likely to die of preeclampsia. Of those maternal deaths from preeclampsia or eclampsia, the maternal mortality rate was 6.6% for whites, 17.3% for African Americans, and 14.6% for all other races (Xu, Kochanek, Murphy, Tejada-Vera, 2010). Nurses and healthcare providers must address the role implicit bias plays in the disparities noted in these outcomes.

The U.S. Department of Health and Human Services and the CDC published data from the Pregnancy Mortality Surveillance System reporting pregnancy-related mortality from 2011 to 2013 (Creanga, Syverson, Seed, & Callaghan, 2017). There has been a decline in pregnancy related mortality associated with hypertensive disorders in pregnancy. In 2006, hypertensive disorders of pregnancy accounted for 9.4% of mortality in pregnancy as compared with 6.8% of deaths from 2011-2014 (CDC, 2018a). This reduction may be related to improved treatment with magnesium sulfate and antihypertensive medications. Yet, deaths from hypertensive disorders of pregnancy continue to account for a significant portion of all pregnancy-related mortality. For women who had a hypertensive disorder of pregnancy as the cause of death, 10.1% gave birth to a living infant and 12.2% had a stillbirth; for 5.5%, the pregnancy outcome was unknown (Creanga et al., 2017). Almost all (96.8%) of pregnancy-related deaths attributed to hypertensive disorders of pregnancy occurred by 42 days postpartum (Creanga et al., 2017). Maternal intracranial hemorrhage remains a leading cause of death in preeclampsia (Martin et al., 2005) and subsequently supports immediate treatment of hypertensive crisis aimed to improve outcomes and prevent severe morbidity or death.

As many as 60% of maternal deaths from preeclampsia may be preventable (Main, McCain, Morton, Holtby, & Lawton, 2015). Delay in seeking medical care, diagnosis, or treatment can result in increased morbidity or mortality associated with preeclampsia. Early recognition of signs and symptoms of preeclampsia and timely treatment of hypertension are key components to improving maternal, fetal, and neonatal outcomes. Historically, major emphasis has been placed on the delivery of the fetus and placenta as well as maternal treatment with magnesium sulfate for seizure prophylaxis and less emphasis placed on pharmacologic treatment of hypertension. More recently, the *National Partnership for Maternal Safety* created Maternal Early Warning Criteria to outline vital signs and abnormal parameters to facilitate urgent bedside evaluation and escalation in care for pregnant women (Mhyre et al., 2014). Perinatal units may consider using the Preeclampsia Early Recognition Tool (Display 5–1), which outlines assessment findings that trigger follow-up assessments, consultation, and treatments.

The *Council on Patient Safety in Women's Health Care* created a safety bundle to improve readiness and standardize recognition and response in the care of women with severe hypertension. In addition to improving provider response, maternal awareness of signs and symptoms is integral to improving outcomes. Using protocols and toolkits, such those created by the California Maternal Quality Care Collaborative (CMQCC, 2014) or the Northern New England Perinatal Quality Improvement Network (2019), may continue to reduce preventable maternal death from hypertensive disorders of pregnancy.

Hypertension during pregnancy predisposes the woman to potentially lethal complications such as abruptio placentae, disseminated intravascular coagulation (DIC), cerebral hemorrhage, cerebral vascular accident, hepatic failure, and acute renal failure. Leading causes of maternal death from hypertension complicating pregnancy include complications from abruptio placentae, hepatic rupture, and eclampsia (Roberts, 2004). The risk of stroke is disproportionately high among women diagnosed with either preeclampsia or eclampsia. Although rare, there is a fourfold increased risk of stroke in this population either during the pregnancy or later in life (Bushnell & Chireau, 2011).

Maternal hypertension is associated with increased risk of fetal and neonatal death. There is a twofold risk of neonatal death in infants born to women diagnosed with preeclampsia and significant associated neonatal morbidity, such as lower Apgar scores, seizures, and neonatal encephalopathy (Lisonkova & Joseph, 2013).

DISPLAY 5–1
Preeclampsia Early Recognition Tool

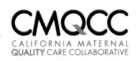

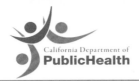
California Department of
PublicHealth

CMQCC PREECLAMPSIA TOOLKIT
PREECLAMPSIA CARE GUIDELINES
CDPH-MCAH Approved: 12/20/13

PREECLAMPSIA EARLY RECOGNITION TOOL (PERT)

Preeclampsia Early Recognition Tool (PERT)

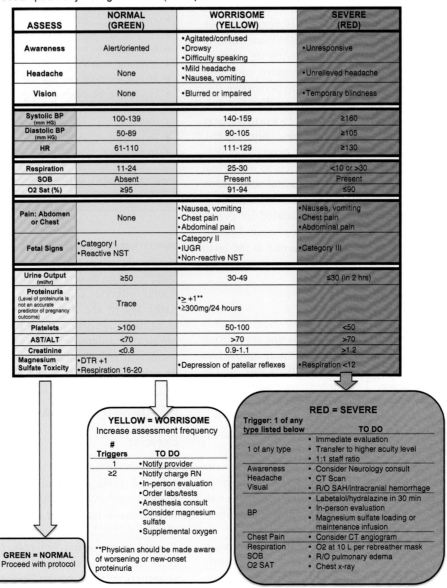

ASSESS	NORMAL (GREEN)	WORRISOME (YELLOW)	SEVERE (RED)
Awareness	Alert/oriented	•Agitated/confused •Drowsy •Difficulty speaking	•Unresponsive
Headache	None	•Mild headache •Nausea, vomiting	•Unrelieved headache
Vision	None	•Blurred or impaired	•Temporary blindness
Systolic BP (mm HG)	100-139	140-159	≥160
Diastolic BP (mm HG)	50-89	90-105	≥105
HR	61-110	111-129	≥130
Respiration	11-24	25-30	<10 or >30
SOB	Absent	Present	Present
O2 Sat (%)	≥95	91-94	≤90
Pain: Abdomen or Chest	None	•Nausea, vomiting •Chest pain •Abdominal pain	•Nausea, vomiting •Chest pain •Abdominal pain
Fetal Signs	•Category I •Reactive NST	•Category II •IUGR •Non-reactive NST	•Category III
Urine Output (ml/hr)	≥50	30-49	≤30 (in 2 hrs)
Proteinuria (Level of proteinuria is not an accurate predictor of pregnancy outcome)	Trace	•≥ +1** •≥300mg/24 hours	
Platelets	>100	50-100	<50
AST/ALT	<70	>70	>70
Creatinine	<0.8	0.9-1.1	>1.2
Magnesium Sulfate Toxicity	•DTR +1 •Respiration 16-20	•Depression of patellar reflexes	•Respiration <12

GREEN = NORMAL
Proceed with protocol

YELLOW = WORRISOME
Increase assessment frequency

# Triggers	TO DO
1	•Notify provider
≥2	•Notify charge RN •In-person evaluation •Order labs/tests •Anesthesia consult •Consider magnesium sulfate •Supplemental oxygen

**Physician should be made aware of worsening or new-onset proteinuria

RED = SEVERE
Trigger: 1 of any type listed below

	TO DO
1 of any type	• Immediate evaluation • Transfer to higher acuity level • 1:1 staff ratio
Awareness Headache Visual	• Consider Neurology consult • CT Scan • R/O SAH/intracranial hemorrhage
BP	• Labetalol/hydralazine in 30 min • In-person evaluation • Magnesium sulfate loading or maintenance infusion
Chest Pain	• Consider CT angiogram
Respiration SOB O2 SAT	• O2 at 10 L per rebreather mask • R/O pulmonary edema • Chest x-ray

11.8.13.v1

Eclampsia/preeclampsia is listed as the primary obstetrical cause for one of four perinatal deaths (Hodgins, 2015). Of pregnancies that end in stillbirth, approximately 16% occur in pregnancies effected by a gestational hypertensive disorder, specifically, 11% from chronic hypertension and 5% from preeclampsia (Lawn et al., 2016). Ten percent of early neonatal deaths occur in newborns who were born to a mother with a hypertensive disorder of pregnancy (Vogel, Souza, & Mori, 2014). Poor placentation occurs early in pregnancy in pregnancies effected by preeclampsia. Abnormal vascular remodeling limits oxygenation, nutrition, and the removal of waste products of the fetus. This can result in fetal growth restriction (Hodgins, 2015). The main causes of neonatal death in newborns effected by preeclampsia during gestation are placental insufficiency and abruptio placentae (Roberts, 2004). Intrauterine growth restriction (IUGR) is common in babies of women with preeclampsia. Among preterm infants admitted to the neonatal intensive care unit (NICU), those born to mothers with hypertensive disorders of pregnancy are more often smaller for gestational age compared to those born to normotensive women (Avorgbedor, Silva, Merwin, Blumenthal, & Holditch-Davis, 2019). Fetal and neonatal consequences of preeclampsia may be related to abnormal vascular remodeling of the uteroplacental unit; however, the exact cause is unknown. Histologic findings of placentas from pregnancies complicated by preeclampsia are consistent with poor uteroplacental perfusion, which can lead to chronic hypoxemia in the fetus (Roberts, 2004).

RISK FACTORS

Preeclampsia is a subtle and dangerous disease process unique to human pregnancy. Signs and symptoms of preeclampsia become apparent relatively late in the course of the disease. The highest morbidity occurs in women who present in second trimester and give birth to extremely preterm infants <28 weeks' gestation. The underlying pathophysiology may be present as early as 8 weeks of gestation. Historically, several well-defined risk factors have been identified for the development of preeclampsia (Display 5–2). Although risk factors are identified, the individual predictive values of the risk factors for screening and risk identification purposes have not been verified.

Of interest today is the identification of physiologic or biochemical markers that would allow early identification of the woman at risk for the development of preeclampsia. Theoretically, such markers would permit healthcare providers the opportunity to target close surveillance and timely interventions to the subpopulation of hypertensive women that would best benefit from the interventions. There are many

DISPLAY 5–2
Risk Factors for the Development of Preeclampsia

- First pregnancy (nulliparity) or pregnancy of a new genetic makeup
- Pregnancy achieved through artificial reproductive technology
- Use of barrier contraceptives that prevent exposure to sperm
- Multiple pregnancy
- Gestational diabetes
- Preexisting diabetes
- Preexisting collagen vascular disease (systemic lupus erythematosus)
- Preexisting chronic hypertension
- Preexisting renal disease
- Antiphospholipid antibody syndrome
- Hydatidiform mole
- Fetal hydrops
- Older maternal age
- African American race (racism)
- Socioeconomic status
- Personal or family history of preeclampsia
- Obesity
- Periodontal disease
- Thrombophilic disorders, including hyperhomocysteinemia

Adapted from Saito, S. (2018). *Preeclampsia: Basic, genomic, and clinical.* Singapore: Springer.

biomarkers under investigation. Pregnancy-associated placental protein A, placental protein 13, uterine Doppler flow and placental growth factor are of particular interest. Due to the variation of physiologic pathways of the disease, a predictive algorithm will most likely need to include biomarkers as well as biophysical characteristics in order to accurately identify women at risk (Eastabrook, Aksoy, Bedell, Penava, & de Vrijer, 2018).

PREVENTION STRATEGIES
Exercise

In healthy pregnancy, there is significant cardiovascular adaptation to include increased blood volume, blood vessel remodeling, and arterial compliance as well as vasodilation and enhanced endothelial function (Boeldt & Bird, 2017). Theoretically, regular physical activity may further enhance the positive cardiovascular adaptation that occurs in healthy pregnancy. A systematic review of the literature was performed in 2017, which included 17 randomized control trials and 5,075 women, to evaluate the effect of exercise during pregnancy on the risk of gestational hypertensive disorders (Magro-Malosso, Saccone, Di Mascio, Di Tommaso, & Berghella, 2017). Findings from this review were mixed. Several studies in the review found that women who performed regular (30 to 60 minutes two to seven times per week) prenatal exercise of moderate intensity (e.g., 140 minutes per week of brisk walking) had significantly lower incidence of gestational hypertensive disorders (Davenport et al., 2018; Magro-Malosso et al., 2017). Conversely, other authors did not report an association between exercise and risk of gestational hypertension or preeclampsia (Du, Ouyang, Nie, Huang, & Redding, 2019; Syngelaki, Sequeira Campos, Roberge, Andrade, & Nicolaides, 2018). Once diagnosed with preeclampsia, exercise is contraindicated. However, additional research needs to be done to determine the impact prepregnancy and prenatal exercise has on the risk of developing gestational hypertensive disorders. Regardless, there are many other maternal benefits of regular prenatal exercise, which in turn, further support the need for prenatal education on the importance of exercise during pregnancy in healthy women.

Low-Dose Aspirin Therapy

The ACOG Task Force on Hypertension in Pregnancy initially recommended the use of low-dose aspirin for the prevention of preeclampsia in 2013, and the U.S. Preventive Services Task Force (Henderson et al., 2014) expanded the recommendation to include administration of low-dose aspirin (81 mg/day) prophylaxis for women at high risk for preeclampsia. Aspirin prophylaxis should be initiated early in gestation between 12–16 weeks gestation and should be continued daily until birth (ACOG, 2018). Research supports low-dose aspirin therapy started earlier in pregnancy (<16 weeks) is more effective particularly in reducing fetal growth restriction and preeclampsia with severe features (Roberge et al., 2017). The use of low-dose aspirin during pregnancy is considered safe. Research has not shown an increase in risk of maternal hemorrhagic complications, such as placental abruption or postpartum hemorrhage (ACOG, 2018) in women taking low-dose aspirin during pregnancy, nor was there an increased risk of intracranial hemorrhage in neonates born to these women (Henderson et al., 2014). In 2018, ACOG published *Committee Opinion No. 743: Low-Dose Aspirin Use during Pregnancy*, which further supports the USPSTF guideline. Specifically, ACOG (2018) states that in women with a history of early-onset preeclampsia or preeclampsia in more than one pregnancy, low-dose aspirin should be initiated in the first trimester. Theoretically, poor placental perfusion leads to ischemia, which results in systemic inflammation and oxidative stress. The therapeutic properties of low-dose aspirin may reduce inflammation, promote normal blood vessel formation, and inhibit blood clot formation that promotes normal fetal growth (ACOG, 2019b; Henderson et al., 2014).

Dietary Supplementation

Calcium supplementation may be effective in reducing risk of preeclampsia because of its ability to decrease smooth muscle contractility and increase vasodilation (Villar, Repke, & Belizan, 1989). For women with low dietary calcium intake, supplementation may decrease the severity of the disease ACOG (2013). In the United States, calcium supplementation is not universally recommended to women at risk for preeclampsia (Khaing et al., 2017). However, due to the significant gap in calcium intake during pregnancy between women in low- and high-income countries, calcium supplementation may be beneficial in the prevention of preeclampsia for women in low-income countries (Cormick et al., 2019). Currently, there are no data to support the use of antioxidants (e.g., vitamin C, vitamin E, selenium, lycopene) to reduce the risk of preeclampsia and are not universally recommended (Rumbold, Duley, Crowther, & Haslam, 2008).

PATHOPHYSIOLOGY OF PREECLAMPSIA

Preeclampsia has been called the "disease of theories." The disease is heterogeneous, and thus, each subtype of preeclampsia may have varying pathophysiology (Founds et al., 2011; Myatt et al., 2014). Research is ongoing to identify the pathophysiology and genetic, immunologic, biologic, and pathophysiologic causes (Founds et al., 2011; Ilekis, Reddy, & Roberts, 2007). Although the exact mechanism is unknown, preeclampsia is thought to occur due to a complex interplay between maternal and fetal factors (Hermes et al., 2013). Historically, preeclampsia had been modeled in two stages—the first stage encompassing poor placentation and the second the new onset of hypertension and proteinuria (Roberts & Hubel, 2009). More recently, alternations to this model have been proposed, specifically suggesting that factors (immune, genetic, and biologic) prior to pregnancy may influence onset of the disease very early after conception.

Normal physiologic adaptations to pregnancy include an increase in plasma volume, vasodilation of the vascular bed, decreased systemic vascular resistance, elevation of cardiac output, and increased prostacyclin production. Physical assessment findings consistent with these changes are dilutional anemia, lower systemic blood pressures and mean arterial pressure, a slight increase in heart rate, and peripheral edema. In preeclampsia, these normal adaptations are altered. Instead of plasma volume expansion and hemodilution, there is a decrease in circulating plasma volume, resulting in hemoconcentration. Women with preeclampsia have inadequate plasma volume expansion, with an average plasma volume 9% below expected values for disease and up to 40% below normal with severe disease.

Further intravascular volume depletion may occur from endothelial injury and increased capillary permeability. The volume depletion may result in increased blood viscosity, leading to a decrease in maternal organ perfusion, including the uteroplacental unit.

The reduction in plasma volume may be more closely related to IUGR than hypertension. The vascular bed demonstrates increased sensitivity to vasoactive substances, resulting in vasoconstriction and increased vascular tone. Vasoconstriction results in increased systemic vascular resistance and hypertension. Maternal hypertension is further aggravated by vasospasms of the arterial bed. Decreased intravascular volume and vasoconstriction lead to a decreased organ perfusion. As the process worsens, red blood cell hemolysis may further impair tissue oxygenation.

During normal pregnancy adaptation, cardiac output increases. Vasoconstriction, arterial vasospasms, endothelial damage, and prostacyclin and thromboxane imbalances impair organ perfusion and blood clot formation. Tables 5–2 and 5–3 provide highlights of the pathophysiology of disease progression and multiple organ system involvement.

Of interest is ongoing research examining the relationship of endothelial dysfunction and alterations in the immune response with the development of preeclampsia (Chaiworapongsa et al., 2004; Dechend et al., 2005; González-Quintero et al., 2004; Mignini et al., 2005; National High Blood Pressure Education Program [NHBPEP] Working Group on High Blood Pressure in Pregnancy, 2000; Waite, Louie, & Taylor, 2005; Wang, Gu, Zhang, & Lewis, 2004; Yamamoto, Suzuki, Kojima, & Suzumori, 2005). Vascular endothelial cells play a role in the modulation of vascular smooth muscle contractile activity and the coagulation and regulation of blood flow. Receptors within the endothelial cells respond to vasodilators and vasoconstrictors, while producing vasoactive substances such as hormones and cytokines, including prostaglandin I2, nitric oxide, and endothelin. The underlying processes are not fully understood, but women diagnosed with preeclampsia exhibit histologic evidence of increased circulating markers of endothelial activation. Endothelial dysfunction and subsequent increased capillary permeability in turn leads to the pathway of reduced organ perfusion.

TABLE 5–2. Physiologic and Pathophysiologic Changes Associated with Preeclampsia

Feature	Normal pregnancy	Preeclampsia alterations
Blood volume	50% ↑	Smaller ↑
Plasma volume	50% ↑	Little or no change
Red cell mass	20% ↑	Hemoconcentration
Cardiac output	40%–50% ↑	Variable
	Widening pulse pressure	↓ Vascular compliance
Blood pressure	↓ Initially with return to prepregnant values by third trimester	Hypertension
Peripheral vascular resistance	↓ Total peripheral resistance	↑ Resistance
		↑ Vascular reactivity
Renal function	↑ Venous capacitance	Vasospasms
RPF	↑	↓
GFR	75% ↑	↓
BUN	50% ↑	↓
Creatinine clearance	↓	↑
Serum creatinine	↑	↓
Uric acid	↓	↑
Renin–angiotensin–aldosterone system	Markedly activated and responds appropriately to posture and salt intake	Plasma renin concentration and activity suppressed
		Loss of antagonists (vasodilators) to AII
		Increased sensitivity to vasoactive substances
Coagulation system		
Fibrinogen	↑	Normal with disease
Factors VII, VIII, IX, X	All ↑	Normal initially, then ↓
		Increase in ratio of von Willebrand factor to factor VII, coagulant activity increased leading to consumption of factor VI
Fibrinolytic activity	↓	↑
Platelet count	Normal	↓
Bleeding time	Normal	Prolonged

AII, angiotensin II; BUN, blood urea nitrogen; GFR, glomerular filtration rate; RPF, renal plasma flow.
Adapted from Roberts, J. (1994). Current perspectives on preeclampsia. *Journal of Nurse-Midwifery, 39*(2), 70–90. doi:10.1016/0091-2182(94)90015-9

TABLE 5–3. Preeclampsia Pathophysiology as a Multiorgan System Disease

System	Effect of preeclampsia	Clinical implications
Vascular bed 1. Endothelial dysfunction 2. Altered coagulation 3. Altered response to vasoactive substances	• Increased release of cellular fibronectin, growth factors, VCAM-1, factor VIII antigen, and peptides • Endothelial cell injury initiates coagulation by either intrinsic pathway (contact adhesion) or extrinsic pathway (tissue factor). • Decreased production of prostacyclin and alteration in prostacyclin/thromboxane ratio	Endothelial dysfunction present before clinical signs of disease Increased thrombus formation, including pulmonary and cerebral emboli Vasoconstriction and vasospasm Increased sensitivity to vasoactive substance Capillary permeability, which contributes to edema formation
Cardiovascular and pulmonary 1. ↑ Vascular resistance 2. ↑ Cardiac output and stroke volume 3. ↓ Colloid osmotic pressure	• Arteriolar narrowing • ↑ Sympathetic activity • ↑ Levels of endothelin-1, a vasoconstrictor • ↑ Sensitivity to endogenous pressors, including vasopressin, epinephrine, and norepinephrine • ↑ Capillary permeability • Further depletion of intravascular colloids through capillary permeability and renal excretion of proteins	Increased blood pressure Hyperdynamic cardiac activity Epidurals can be used safely but must be cautious if ephedrine is used to correct hypotension. Subendocardial hemorrhages are present in >50% of women who die of eclampsia. At risk for pulmonary edema, myocardial ischemia, left ventricular dysfunction
Renal 1. Proteinuria 2. Altered function	• Slight decrease in glomerular size • Diameter of glomerular capillary lumen decreased • Glomerular endothelial cells are greatly enlarged and may occlude the capillary lumen. • Glomerular capillary endotheliosis • Thickening of renal arterioles	Proteinuria plus hypertension is the most reliable indicator of fetal jeopardy; indicative of glomerular dysfunction ↑ Serum uric acid secondary to a ↓ urate clearance (uric acid better predictor of outcome than blood pressure) ↓ Creatinine clearance with an elevation of serum creatinine levels ↑ BUN mirrors changes in creatinine clearance and also a function of protein intake and liver function Urine sediment analysis may not be beneficial. At risk for oliguria, ATN, renal failure
Hepatic 1. Hepatic dysfunction 2. Hepatic rupture	• Changes consistent with hemorrhage into hepatic tissue • Later changes consistent with hepatic infarction • ↑ Hepatic artery resistance • Fibrin deposition • Hepatocellular necrosis	Elevations of liver function tests; the association of microangiopathic anemia and elevations of AST/ALT carries ominous prognosis for mother and fetus. HELLP syndrome Possible elevations in bilirubin Signs of liver failure: malaise, nausea, epigastric pain, hypoglycemia, hemolysis, anemia
Hematologic 1. Thrombocytopenia 2. Altered platelet function 3. Hemolysis	• ↑ Platelet destruction • ↑ Platelet aggregation • ↓ Platelet life span • Hemolytic anemia • Destruction of RBCs in microvasculature	Platelets <100,000 increased risk of coagulopathy Platelets <50,000 increased risk of hemorrhage Platelets <20,000 increased risk for spontaneous bleeding Decreased oxygen-carrying capacity and organ oxygenation
CNS 1. Hyperreflexia	• May indicate increasing CNS involvement but not diagnostic of disease • Alteration of cerebral autoregulation with seizures • ↑ Intracranial pressures	Cerebral edema with severe disease Signs of CNS alterations: headache, dizziness, changes in vital signs, diplopia, scotomata, blurred vision, amaurosis, tachycardia, alteration in level of consciousness
Fetal/neonatal 1. Fetal intolerance to labor 2. Preterm birth 3. Oligohydramnios 4. IUGR 5. IUFD 6. Abruptio placentae	• Alteration in placental function • At risk for indicated preterm birth secondary to maternal disease process	Must monitor for signs of fetal compromise Monitoring for IUGR and IUFD At risk for abruptio placentae, oligohydramnios, indeterminate or abnormal fetal heart rate patterns
Uteroplacental 1. Spiral arteries 2. Changes consistent with hypoxia	• Abnormal invasion • Retain nonpregnant characteristics • Limited vasodilatation • Vessel necrosis	Decreases in uteroplacental perfusion Increased risk for fetal compromise and IUGR

ALT, alanine aminotransferase; AST, aspartate aminotransferase; ATN, acute tubular necrosis; BUN, blood urea nitrogen; CNS, central nervous system; IUFD, intrauterine fetal demise; IUGR, intrauterine growth restriction; RBCs, red blood cells; VCAM-1, vascular cell adhesion molecule 1.

CLINICAL MANIFESTATIONS OF PREECLAMPSIA–ECLAMPSIA

The clinical manifestations of preeclampsia are directly related to the presence of vascular vasospasms. Vasospasm results in endothelial injury, red blood cell destruction, platelet aggregation, increased capillary permeability, increased systemic vascular resistance, renal and hepatic dysfunction, and other systemic changes. Hypertension and proteinuria are the most significant clinical manifestations of preeclampsia. Edema is significant when hypertension, proteinuria, or signs of multisystem organ involvement are present. Fetal growth restriction is not diagnostic and, however, requires close assessment and monitoring for the development of preeclampsia.

Hypertension

In 2013, ACOG defined gestational hypertension as a sustained blood pressure elevation of 140 mm Hg or more systolic or 90 mm Hg or more diastolic after the 20th week of gestation that is recorded on two or more measurements. Although blood pressure elevations above baseline, specifically a 30-mm Hg increase in systolic blood pressure or a 15-mm Hg increase in diastolic blood pressure, are not diagnostic of preeclampsia, these increases in baseline values should warrant close observation for impending preeclampsia (ACOG, 2019b; NHBPEP, 2000; NHBPEP Working Group on High Blood Pressure in Pregnancy, 2000).

Appropriate Measurement of Blood Pressure

Measurement of blood pressure is important in the evaluation, diagnosis, and management of hypertension. It is important to ensure that the appropriate size blood pressure cuff has been chosen because considerable overestimation can occur when the cuff used is too small.

To obtain the most accurate reading, allow the patient to sit quietly for 5–10 minutes before obtaining the reading. Patient position will influence blood pressure readings. Historically, blood pressure determinations were obtained in a left lateral position with the blood pressure cuff placed on the upper right arm superior to the heart. However, this position will falsely lower systolic, diastolic, and mean pressures. Current recommendations are to evaluate the blood pressure with the woman in a sitting position, legs uncrossed, and feet flat on the floor, with placement of the cuff on a bare upper arm with the arm positioned at heart level. The patient should not have had alcohol or tobacco in the previous 30 minutes and should not be talking during the reading. If a patient must remain in bed, blood pressure can either be taken in the sitting position or in the left lateral recumbent position with the patient's arm at the level of the heart (ACOG, 2019b).

The diagnosis of hypertension is not made solely on one blood pressure measurement. The degree of hypertension and clinical condition will determine the frequency of nursing reassessment. If the patient has hypertension, reevaluation is required within 15 minutes. If blood pressure remains greater than or equal to 140/90 mm Hg, immediate bedside evaluation by an obstetric provider is warranted. If blood pressure remains greater than 160/110 mm Hg, antihypertensive medication should be administered as soon as reasonably possible, within 30 to 60 minutes (ACOG, 2019b).

Proteinuria

Protein in the urine may increase up to 300 mg in 24 hours during normal pregnancy. Proteinuria is defined as urinary excretion of 0.3 g of protein/L (300 mg/L) in a 24-hour urine specimen or a protein/creatinine ratio of at least 0.3 mg/dL (ACOG, 2019b). The level of protein in the urine fluctuates throughout the day and may miss detection at a given time. Urine dipstick analysis is only moderately reliable and may lead to false-negative analysis and is no longer recommended for diagnostic purposes unless no other methods are available. The stated threshold of 0.3 g/L correlates with 30 mg/dL or "1+" or greater on dipstick analysis (NHBPEP, 2000) and is diagnostic for preeclampsia. Studies comparing traditional urine dipstick analysis to 24-hour urine protein quantitation to determine proteinuria found that in routine clinical practice, a finding of "negative" or "trace" proteinuria misses significant proteinuria in up to 40% of hypertensive women (NHBPEP, 2000; NHBPEP Working Group on High Blood Pressure in Pregnancy, 2000). It is important to remember that proteinuria is not required to make a diagnosis of preeclampsia. Preeclampsia without proteinuria is atypical and, however, may occur in 10% to 25% of patients with preeclampsia (Dong et al., 2017; Tranquilli et al., 2014). Diagnosis and treatment of preeclampsia should not be delayed while waiting for results of a 24-hour urine, and amounts of proteinuria should not be used to inform decisions regarding delivery.

In 2013, ACOG removed massive proteinuria (>5 g in 24 hours) from criteria that classifies severe features of preeclampsia because it was not correlated with adverse outcomes. Urinary protein concentration is influenced by factors such as contamination of the specimen with vaginal secretions, blood, or bacteria; urine specific gravity and pH; exercise; and posture.

Edema

Dependent edema is a common finding in the third trimester of pregnancy and is not diagnostic of preeclampsia (ACOG, 2019b). In the absence of hypertension or proteinuria, dependent edema is generally related to changes in interstitial and intravascular hydrostatic and osmotic pressures that facilitate movement of intravascular fluid into the tissues. Compression of the iliac vein increases venous hydrostatic pressure; this promotes fluid shifting into the interstitial space. Increased plasma volume reduces serum albumin levels; this lowers the colloid osmotic pressure causing additional fluid shift into the intravascular space. Together, these two physiologic adaptations of pregnancy result in benign dependent edema.

With preeclampsia, edema becomes pathologic when accompanied by hypertension, proteinuria, or signs of organ dysfunction. Clinically, rapid weight gain or the development of significant edema should raise suspicion of preeclampsia (ACOG, 2019b). Intracellular and extracellular edema represents a generalized and excessive accumulation of fluid in tissue. As vasospasms worsen, capillary endothelial damage results in increased systemic capillary permeability (i.e., leakage), which leads to hemoconcentration and increases the risk of pulmonary or cerebral edema (Yogev & Sheiner, 2014).

Hyperreflexia

Hyperreflexia is not considered diagnostic but may be a nervous system manifestation in preeclampsia. In healthy young women, hyperreflexia can be a common finding. Deep tendon reflexes (DTRs) should be evaluated prior to magnesium sulfate therapy to establish a baseline and reassessed every 15 minutes during a bolus dose and hourly until otherwise ordered during continuous intravenous (IV) magnesium administration. Absent DTRs, respiratory rate less than 12 breaths per minute, and decreased level of consciousness are signs of magnesium toxicity.

PREECLAMPSIA WITHOUT SEVERE FEATURES VERSUS PREECLAMPSIA WITH SEVERE FEATURES

Preeclampsia is no longer classified as mild or severe but rather with severe features or without severe features (ACOG, 2019b). The diagnosis of preeclampsia has significant implications for both maternal and fetal/neonatal well-being. Because other conditions can mimic preeclampsia, it is important to look for systemic manifestations of disease progression such as cerebral and visual disturbances, epigastric pain, and pulmonary edema. To identify increasing progression in the severity of preeclampsia, or to increase the certainty of the diagnosis, nursing management requires accurate and thorough observation and assessments as well as possible preparation for birth of the baby.

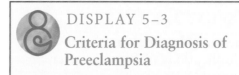

DISPLAY 5–3

Criteria for Diagnosis of Preeclampsia

In previously normotensive women >20 weeks' gestation

- Blood pressure ≥140 mm Hg systolic *or* ≥90 mm Hg diastolic on two occasions at least 4 hr or more apart
- Proteinuria of ≥300 mg in 24-urine collection or a protein/creatinine ratio of ≥0.3 mg/dL or dipstick reading of 1+

In the absence of proteinuria, a woman meeting the hypertension criteria and any of the following can be diagnosed with preeclampsia.

- Serum creatinine >1.1 mg/dL or a doubling of serum creatinine in women without preexisting renal disease
- Platelet count <100,000 cells/mm³
- Elevated serum liver transaminases to twice normal concentrations (alanine aminotransferase or aspartate aminotransferase)
- Persistent headache or other cerebral or visual disturbances
- Pulmonary edema

A classification of preeclampsia with severe features is made if the woman has any of the above bulleted features and/or a systolic blood pressure of ≥160 mm Hg and/or a diastolic blood pressure of ≥110 mm Hg on two occasions at least 4 hours or more apart. If severe hypertension is present, immediate bedside evaluation should occur by an obstetric provider, and antihypertensive therapy should be provided as soon as possible and not wait for follow-up blood pressure to establish diagnosis.

From American College of Obstetricians and Gynecologists. (2013). *Hypertension in pregnancy.* Washington, DC: Author.

Display 5–3 lists criteria for confirming the diagnosis of preeclampsia and progression to preeclampsia with severe features. Display 5–4 lists the potential maternal and fetal complications of preeclampsia with severe features.

While caring for women with hypertensive disorders of pregnancy, nursing assessments focus on identification of severe features and disease progression. Preeclampsia is a systemic disease with multiorgan involve. The wide range of symptomatology and multiple organ system involvement can sometimes result in misdiagnosis and delay in treatment. Cocaine intoxication, lupus nephritis, chronic renal failure, and acute fatty liver of pregnancy are examples of conditions that may mimic preeclampsia and eclampsia. Women with chronic hypertension or any preexisting medical condition that predisposes to the development of hypertension are at increased risk for superimposed preeclampsia and eclampsia. Care of the woman with preeclampsia with severe features at less than 34 weeks or HELLP syndrome is best referred to a tertiary perinatal center if stable for transfer (ACOG & SMFM, 2019).

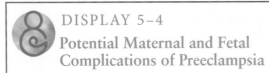

DISPLAY 5–4
Potential Maternal and Fetal Complications of Preeclampsia

- Cardiovascular
  - Hypoperfusion
  - Severe hypertension
  - Hypertensive crisis
  - Pulmonary edema
  - Congestive heart failure
  - Future cardiac dysfunction
- Pulmonary
  - Pulmonary edema
  - Hypoxemia/acidemia
- Renal
  - Oliguria
  - Acute renal failure
  - Impaired drug metabolism and excretion
- Hematologic
  - Hemolysis
  - Decreased oxygen-carrying capacity
  - Thrombocytopenia
  - Coagulation defects, including disseminated intravascular coagulation
  - Anemia
- Neurologic
  - Eclampsia
  - Cerebral edema
  - Cerebral hemorrhage
  - Stroke
  - Amaurosis (cortical blindness)
- Hepatic
  - Hepatocellular dysfunction
  - Hepatic rupture
  - Hypoglycemia
  - Coagulation defects
  - Impaired drug metabolism and excretion
- Uteroplacental
  - Abruptio placentae
  - Decreased uteroplacental perfusion
- Fetal
  - Intrauterine growth restriction
  - Intrauterine fetal demise
  - Fetal intolerance to labor
  - Preterm birth
  - Low birth weight
  - Decreased oxygenation

Early- versus Late-Onset Preeclampsia

Early and late onset are two subtypes of preeclampsia and are classified according to gestational age at onset. Early-onset preeclampsia that occurs at <34 weeks gestation is often associated with poor placentation; there may be a significant genetic component associated with this subtype (Boyd, Tahir, Wohlfahrt, & Melbye, 2013; Lisonkova & Joseph, 2013; Myatt et al., 2014;

Steegers, Von Dadelszen, Duvekot, & Pijnenborg, 2010). The early-onset subtype is often more severe and is associated with adverse maternal and neonatal outcomes such as fetal growth restriction and HELLP, and eclampsia in women effected by the disease (Kucukgoz Gulec et al., 2013). It is important to note that severe features of the disease can occur at any time, and severity is not determined by gestational age at onset (ACOG, 2019b; Kucukgoz Gulec et al., 2013).

NURSING ASSESSMENT AND INTERVENTIONS FOR PREECLAMPSIA

Delivery of the fetus remains the definitive treatment; however, it is important to note this is not a "cure." The decision to initiate birth versus expectant management must be individualized and is determined by maternal and fetal status and gestational age. In women with gestational hypertension and preeclampsia without severe features less than 37 weeks 0 days' gestation and with no other indications for delivery, expectant management may be appropriate until the women reaches 37 weeks 0 days' gestation or the disease increases in severity. In women with preeclampsia without severe features or gestational hypertension, induction of labor at 37 weeks 0 days' gestation is recommended and is associated with lower rates of maternal and fetal complications (ACOG, 2019b; Sibai, 2011). If being expectantly managed at less than 37 weeks' gestation, steroid administration is recommended; however, this should not delay delivery if required due to increasing severity of the disease (ACOG, 2019b).

Home Care Management

Women at less than 37 weeks' gestation with preeclampsia without severe features may be managed at home, unless there are other complications such as fetal growth restriction, which may warrant in-hospital surveillance. However, if managed at home, these women require frequent maternal/fetal follow-up care including biweekly blood pressure monitoring, weekly weight assessment, maternal symptom assessment, twice weekly fetal nonstress testing, daily maternal observation of fetal kick counts, and weekly laboratory assessment to include complete blood count, liver enzymes, serum creatinine, and urine protein/creatinine ratio. Fetal growth should be evaluated every 3 weeks and amniotic fluid volume weekly. Frequency of follow-up surveillance may be increased based on maternal/fetal clinical findings. Criteria for home management vary among primary perinatal healthcare providers and home care agencies. The woman must be in a stable condition with no evidence of worsening maternal or fetal status. Remote blood pressure monitoring could be used to ensure timely recognition of changes in the severity of blood pressure readings and allow for close monitoring of blood pressure trends. Nurses should provide patients with education on how to properly self-measure blood pressure. Consider observing patients demonstrate self-monitoring of blood pressure in order to ensure reliable results. It is also important to educate women to immediately report any signs and symptoms of preeclampsia, severe hypertension, or decrease in fetal movement to their provider.

Inpatient Management

Women with preeclampsia without severe features may be evaluated in the inpatient setting and remain hospitalized. Women with preeclampsia with severe features or eclampsia are managed in the hospital. Nursing care involves accurate and astute observations and assessments. Comprehensive knowledge regarding pharmacologic therapies, management regimens, and possible complications is required.

An important aspect of care for women with hypertension in pregnancy is recognition of the abilities of the facility and the obstetric and neonatal staff to handle potential emergencies. The decision to transfer a patient to a higher level of care should be made based on the increasing severity of the disease and/or because the fetus is preterm and will require neonatal support. It is optimal for expectant management of patients with preeclampsia with severe features at <34 weeks to be cared for in a tertiary care center. Providers of obstetric care, regardless of the level of care, must be able to stabilize the woman before transport to a higher level of care.

Fluid Management

Endothelial damage that occurs in preeclampsia results in the leakage of fluid from the intravascular space. Shifting of fluid to the interstitial space results in peripheral edema and/or central edema (pulmonary or cerebral edema). This shift in fluid to the interstitial space may be associated with a decrease in plasma volume, leading to hemoconcentration and hypovolemia. Careful administration of IV fluid (less than 125 mL/hr) and intake and output measurement is warranted. Lactated Ringer's is typically used for maintenance IV fluid therapy (Archer & Champagne, 2014). Prior to epidural administration, thoughtful consideration should be given prior to the provision of an IV fluid bolus because the administration of excess fluids may increase risk of pulmonary edema (Archer & Champagne, 2014).

The CMQCC Preeclampsia Toolkit Care Guidelines on Fluid Management (Archer & Champagne, 2014) suggest that in the context of oliguria (<30 mL/hr or <500 mL/24 hr), a 250 to 500 mL IV bolus of normal saline or lactated Ringer's may be considered. If total IV fluid administration reaches 1,000 mL, and oliguria has not improved, other modalities such as the use of colloids or diuretics may be used depending on the suspected cause of the oliguria. The use of a fluid bolus, colloids, and diuretics, even in the context of oliguria, needs to be used with caution due to the increased risk of pulmonary edema. Oxygen saturation (SaO_2) levels less than 95% are abnormal and requires prompt notification to the obstetric provider. Nursing care includes a heightened surveillance for pulmonary edema: complaints of chest pain, SaO_2 <96%, cough, shortness of breath, dyspnea, tachypnea, tachycardia, and adventitious breath sounds (Archer & Champagne, 2014; Huwe et al., 2019).

Antepartum Management

Antepartum management of the woman diagnosed with preeclampsia without severe features may occur at home or in the hospital. However, in the face of severe features, the woman should be hospitalized with the timing of birth dictated by maternal/fetal status and gestational age. Historically, women diagnosed with preeclampsia without severe features were admitted to the hospital for two reasons: to prevent eclampsia and to improve perinatal outcome. However, researchers have questioned the practice of routine hospitalization of women diagnosed with preeclampsia without severe features. Outpatient management for women with preeclampsia without severe features is a viable option for those who agree to follow established protocols, can have frequent office or home visits, and can perform blood pressure monitoring.

The use of antihypertensive medication in the expectant management of women with preeclampsia without severe features is not recommended. Antihypertensive regimens reported in prospective and retrospective studies include hydralazine, methyldopa, nifedipine, prazosin, diuretics, and beta-blockers. Although these studies examined the effect of different antihypertensive agents, none reported a better perinatal outcome compared with management without antihypertensives. There are insufficient data to support prophylactic use of antihypertensive therapy in the management of preeclampsia without severe features.

Women diagnosed with preeclampsia with severe features remote from term are delivered expeditiously. The use of expectant management of preeclampsia with severe features remote from term suggests that pregnancy may be prolonged to gain fetal maturity without increased risk to the woman (Coppage & Sibai, 2004; Haddad et al., 2004). Antihypertensives are indicated and may include labetalol, hydralazine, and/or nifedipine (calcium channel blockers) (ACOG, 2019b). With strict criteria for patient selection and intensive maternal and fetal surveillance, pregnancy may be prolonged. Assessments are aimed at early identification of worsening maternal or fetal status or evidence of end-organ dysfunction because immediate birth may be required.

Activity Restriction

Activity restriction, varying from frequent rest periods with legs elevated to complete bed rest in the full lateral position, is frequently prescribed for women with preeclampsia. There is not enough evidence to support that strict bed rest reduces risk of preeclampsia (ACOG, 2019b; Meher, Abalos, & Carroli, 2005). Women with preeclampsia may require hospitalization for maternal and fetal surveillance, and reduced physical activity is recommended.

Ongoing Assessment

Preeclampsia can occur without warning or be recognized with the gradual development of symptoms. A review of the major organ systems adds to the database for detecting changes from baseline in blood pressure, weight gain and patterns of weight gain, increasing edema, and presence of proteinuria. The nurse should note whether the woman complains of unusual, frequent, or severe headaches; visual disturbances; or epigastric pain. Presence of edema, in addition to hypertension, warrants additional investigation, although it is not diagnostic. Edema, assessed by distribution and degree, is described as dependent or pitting. If periorbital or facial edema is not obvious, the pregnant woman should be asked if it was present when she awoke. DTRs are evaluated if preeclampsia is suspected. The biceps and patellar reflexes and ankle clonus should be assessed and documented.

A 24-hour urine collection for protein and creatinine clearance is most reflective of true renal status because proteinuria is a later sign in the course of preeclampsia. A protein/creatinine ratio of at least 0.3 mg/dL can also be diagnostic of proteinuria. Dipstick testing of a clean-catch or catheter urine specimen may be used to initially determine proteinuria; however, this method should not be diagnostic when other methods are available. Urine output should also be assessed for a volume of at least 30 mL/hr or $\geq$500 mL/24 hr. Placement of an indwelling Foley catheter with an urometer facilitates accurate assessment of urine output and may assist with the detection of early signs of renal compromise. This is especially important in those patients receiving magnesium sulfate because any decrease in urine output could result in decreased clearance of magnesium sulfate, which increases the risk for magnesium toxicity.

An important ongoing assessment is determination of fetal status. Uteroplacental perfusion decreases in women with preeclampsia, thereby placing the fetus at risk of intrauterine fetal growth restriction or death. The uterine spiral arteries of the placental bed are subject to vasospasm. When this occurs, perfusion between maternal circulation and intervillous space is compromised, decreasing blood flow and oxygenation to the fetus. Oligohydramnios, IUGR, fetal compromise, and intrauterine fetal death all are associated with preeclampsia. The fetal heart rate (FHR) should be assessed for baseline rate, variability, and normal versus indeterminate or abnormal patterns. The presence of abnormal baseline rate, minimal or absent variability, or late decelerations may indicate fetal intolerance to the intrauterine environment. Because of the poor positive predictive value of indeterminate or abnormal fetal findings to detect fetal acidemia at birth, maternal and fetal status is evaluated to determine when birth should occur. The presence of variable decelerations, antepartum or intrapartum, may suggest decreased amniotic fluid volume (i.e., oligohydramnios), increasing the risk of umbilical cord compression, and possible fetal compromise. Biophysical or biometric monitoring for fetal well-being may be ordered. These tests include fetal movement counting, nonstress testing, contraction stress test, biophysical profile, and serial ultrasonography to include Doppler flow velocimetry (ACOG, 2019b; Sotiriadis et al., 2019). As long as the fetus continues to grow in an appropriate manner and biophysical findings are reassuring, it can be inferred that the placenta and uterine blood flow are appropriate.

If labor is suspected, a vaginal examination for cervical changes is indicated. Uterine tonicity is evaluated for signs of labor and abruptio placentae. Preterm contractions or a tense, tender uterus may be early indications of an abruptio placentae.

Assessments target signs of deterioration from preeclampsia without severe features to preeclampsia with severe features or eclampsia. Signs of liver involvement (e.g., epigastric pain, elevated liver function test, and thrombocytopenia), renal failure, worsening hypertension, cerebral involvement (e.g., headache, blurry vision, spots before eyes), and developing coagulopathies must be assessed and documented. Lung sounds are assessed for rales (i.e., crackles) or diminished breath sounds, which may indicate pulmonary edema. Noninvasive assessment parameters to assess maternal status include level of consciousness, blood pressure, hemoglobin SaO_2 (i.e., pulse oximetry), electrocardiogram (ECG) findings, and urine output. Invasive hemodynamic monitoring with a flow-directed pulmonary artery catheter (Swan-Ganz) may be indicated in selected patients, particularly in those with oliguria and pulmonary edema. Invasive monitoring may require that the patient be transferred to an intensive care unit.

Laboratory Tests

The nurse assists in obtaining a number of blood and urine specimens to aid in the diagnosis of preeclampsia, HELLP syndrome, or chronic hypertension.

No known laboratory tests predict the development of preeclampsia. Laboratory abnormalities are nonspecific in preeclampsia, but changes can reflect underlying multiorgan system dysfunctions. Thrombocytopenia is the most common hematologic abnormality, and routine assessment of other coagulation factors is not recommended until the platelet concentration is less than 100,000/mm^3. Unless a preexisting coagulopathy is present, the woman is not at an increased risk for developing a coagulopathy until the platelet level falls below 100,000/mm^3. Elevated liver transaminases and creatinine are also diagnostic of preeclampsia and should be assessed. Baseline laboratory test information is useful in the early diagnosis of preeclampsia and for comparison with results obtained to evaluate progression and severity of disease. Display 5–5 provides the common laboratory assessments for a woman with hypertension during pregnancy.

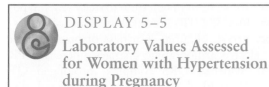

DISPLAY 5–5
Laboratory Values Assessed for Women with Hypertension during Pregnancy

Complete blood count
- Hemoglobin
- Hematocrit
- Platelet count

Chemistry
- Electrolytes
- Blood urea nitrogen
- Serum creatinine
- Serum albumin
- Uric acid
- Serum calcium
- Serum sodium
- Serum magnesium
- Serum glucose
- Liver function tests: lactate dehydrogenase, aspartate aminotransferase, alanine aminotransferase
- May consider serum amylase and lipase
- May consider cardiac enzymes

Urine
- Urinalysis for protein
- The 24-hr creatinine clearance may be measured in patients with chronic hypertension or renal disease.
- 24-hr urine for sodium excretion
- Specific gravity

Coagulation profile
- Platelet count and function
- Prothrombin and partial thromboplastin times
- Fibrinogen
- Fibrin split or fibrin degradation products
- Bleeding time
- D-dimer

Pharmacologic Therapies

Pharmacologic therapies are instituted for two purposes: seizure prophylaxis and antihypertensive management.

Magnesium Sulfate

Magnesium sulfate is the drug of choice in the management of preeclampsia to prevent seizure activity and should be used in all patients with preeclampsia with severe features or with HELLP syndrome (ACOG, 2019b). (Magnesium sulfate safety is also presented in Chapter 7, Preterm Labor and Birth.) The Institute for Safe Medication Practices (2018) lists magnesium sulfate as a high-alert medication and often requires one to one nursing care. When used for seizure prophylaxis, magnesium sulfate is administered as a secondary infusion by an infusion-controlled device to achieve serum levels of approximately 4.8 to 8.4 mg/dL (4 to 7 mEq/dL). The loading dose is a 4- to 6-g IV bolus over 15 to 20 minutes. This should be administered via a separate admixture bag from the maintenance dose. The IV bag and tubing should be clearly labeled as magnesium sulfate. The loading dose is followed by a maintenance infusion of 1 to 2 g/hr. An independent double check by two nurses should be done when magnesium sulfate is initiated, when the dose changes, and at change of shift (Berg, Lee, & Chagolla, 2014). After initiation, magnesium sulfate should continue to be administered until 24 to 48 hours after birth or after the last seizure.

Magnesium is a calcium antagonist. The action of magnesium sulfate as an anticonvulsant is controversial, but it is thought to block neuromuscular transmission and decrease acetylcholine excretion at the end plate, depressing the vasomotor center and thereby depressing central nervous system (CNS) irritability. Magnesium circulates largely unbound to protein and is almost exclusively excreted in the urine. In patients with normal renal function, the half time for excretion of magnesium is approximately 4 hours. In women with decreased glomerular filtration and renal hypoperfusion, such as seen in preeclampsia, the half time for excretion is delayed, increasing the risk for slowed clearance and resulting toxicity.

Signs and symptoms of hypermagnesemia are assessed for the duration of the infusion. Women receiving magnesium for preeclampsia/eclampsia most often require one to one nursing care. Clinically significant findings of hypermagnesemia are related primarily to magnesium's cellular effects. IV magnesium, more so than oral, slows or blocks neuromuscular and cardiac conducting system transmission, decreases smooth muscle contractility, and depresses CNS irritability. Although the desired anticonvulsant effect can be achieved easily with current dosing regimens, the nurse must be aware of the potential for untoward effects, including decreased uterine and myocardial contractility, depressed respirations, and interference with cardiac conduction that places the woman at risk for cardiac dysrhythmias or cardiac arrest. Subsequently, if magnesium toxicity is suspected, calcium gluconate should be administered. Magnesium sulfate has little effect on maternal blood pressure when administered appropriately.

The effect of magnesium sulfate on fetal heart baseline variability is controversial. Fetal serum levels for magnesium will approximate maternal levels so fetal sedation is possible, particularly following the loading dose. Minimal to absent baseline variability should not be seen as a side effect of maternal magnesium sulfate therapy until fetal hypoxemia has been ruled out.

Nursing responsibilities and assessments for women receiving magnesium sulfate include the following:

- Obtain patient history, including drug history and any known allergies; note renal function or history of heart block, myocardial damage, and myasthenia gravis or concurrent use of CNS depressants, digoxin, or neuromuscular blocking agents. Magnesium sulfate may be contraindicated in some of these conditions.
- Make sure anesthesia personnel are aware of infusion.
- Assess maternal baseline vital signs, DTRs, neurologic status, and urinary output before initiation of therapy and reassess per institution protocol.
- Administer magnesium sulfate according to protocol; all infusions should be prepared by the facility pharmacy, or the facility should use commercially prepared solutions.
- Establish the primary IV line and intravenously administer magnesium sulfate piggyback by means of a controlled infusion device; infuse via a separate line and do not mix with other IV drugs unless compatibility has been established.
- Perform an independent double check with two nurses to confirm dose at initiation, when the dose changes, and at change of shift.
- Avoid administration of any solution of magnesium sulfate if particulate matter, cloudiness, or discoloration is noted.
- Document magnesium sulfate infusion in grams per hour.
- Continue fetal assessment.
- Keep calcium gluconate (1 g of a 10% solution) immediately available in a secure medication area on the unit (e.g., drug dispenser system or locked emergency medication area).
- Be cautious with concurrent administration of narcotics, CNS depressants, calcium channel blockers, and beta-blockers. Magnesium sulfate dose may need to be adjusted or discontinued. Notify the physician if signs of toxicity occur.

TABLE 5–4. Serum Magnesium Levels and Associated Effects

Effect	Serum level (mg/dL)
Anticonvulsant prophylaxis	5–8
Electrocardiographic changes	5–10
Loss of deep tendon reflexes	8–12
Somnolence	10–12
Slurred speech	10–12
Muscular paralysis	15–17
Respiratory difficulty	15–17
Cardiac arrest	20–35

Adapted from Coppage, K. H., & Sibai, B. M. (2004). Hypertensive emergencies. In M. R. Foley, T. H. Strong, Jr., & T. J. Garite (Eds.), *Obstetric intensive care manual* (2nd ed., pp. 51–65). New York, NY: McGraw-Hill; Roberts, J. M. (2004). Pregnancy-related hypertension. In R. K. Creasy, R. Resnik, & J. D. Iams (Eds.), *Maternal-fetal medicine: Principles and practice* (5th ed., pp. 859–900). Philadelphia, PA: Saunders.

- Monitor for signs of magnesium toxicity (e.g., hypotension, loss of DTRs, respiratory depression, respiratory arrest, oliguria, shortness of breath, chest pains, electrocardiographic changes [increased PR interval, widened QRS complex, prolonged QT interval, heart block]); if toxicity is suspected, discontinue infusion and notify provider.
- Monitor serum magnesium levels as indicated based on maternal status or if toxicity suspected; routine serum magnesium levels are not required in the absence of comorbidities. Depression of DTRs occurs at serum concentrations lower than those associated with adverse cardiopulmonary effects, and the presence of DTRs indicates magnesium levels that are not too high. See Table 5–4 for effects associated with various serum magnesium levels.
- Maintain strict intake and output and keep patient hydrated; many recommend that total hourly intake be ≤125 mL/hr (range 60 to ≤125 mL/hr); urine output should be at least 30 mL/hr (≥500 mL/24 hr) while administering parenteral magnesium; magnesium sulfate may cause a transient osmotic diuresis.
- Common side effects of magnesium sulfate include flushing, sweating, weakness, and drowsiness. Educate patient regarding the side effects, provide cool environment, offer cold packs, and cool wash rags for comfort.
- Maintain seizure precautions and neurologic evaluations.
- Prepare for neonatal resuscitation.

Anticonvulsant Therapy

Magnesium sulfate is the first-line therapy for seizure prophylaxis. If recurrent seizures occur in women already on magnesium sulfate, the CMQCC Preeclampsia Toolkit guidelines recommend another loading dose of magnesium sulfate, 2 g IV over 5 minutes

(Berg et al., 2014). Use of other anticonvulsants should be considered if seizure reoccurs after the second loading dose. Other anticonvulsants suggested for use in the management of seizures in this population include lorazepam (Ativan), midazolam (Versed), phenytoin (Dilantin), and levetiracetam (Keppra). A 2010 Cochrane review supports that the use of magnesium sulfate is better in the prevention of seizure and reducing risk of maternal death in women with preeclampsia/eclampsia than in phenytoin (Duley, Henderson-Smart, & Chou, 2010). Because of a lack of experience with phenytoin and the significant maternal side effects, magnesium sulfate remains the first-line drug in the United States. However, anticonvulsants, such as phenytoin, may be considered when the use of magnesium sulfate is associated with increased risk of maternal complications, such as with myasthenia gravis or markedly reduced renal function or if seizures are recurrent after second loading dose of magnesium (Berg et al., 2014). If other anticonvulsants are used, extreme care must be taken and staff must be familiar with the expected side effects and potential complications. Phenytoin in particular may cause QRS or QT prolongation, and resuscitation equipment must be immediately available (Berg et al., 2014).

Antihypertensive Therapy

Pharmacologic therapies directed at the control of severe hypertension include a variety of agents. Several general precautions should be considered when antihypertensive agents are ordered: During pregnancy, antihypertensive therapy is initiated when diastolic blood pressure is sustained at greater than or equal to 105 to 110 mm Hg or systolic blood pressure is sustained at greater than or equal to 160 mm Hg to prevent maternal cerebral vascular accident (ACOG, 2018). The effect of the antihypertensive agent may depend on intravascular volume status and hypovolemia resulting from increased capillary permeability, and hemoconcentration may need correction before the initiation of therapy. Treatment of hypertension may be especially challenging in women with chronic cocaine/amphetamine abuse and may result in significant hypotension. Antihypertensive therapy is not suggested for use in women with gestational hypertension or preeclampsia without severe features. Careful monitoring of blood pressure after antihypertensive therapy is essential in order to maintain uteroplacental perfusion. The aim of antihypertensive treatment is not to return blood pressures to normal but rather to maintain blood pressure between 140 to 150 mm Hg systolic and 90 to 100 mg Hg diastolic to prevent repeated prolonged exposure to severe systolic hypertension, with subsequent loss of cerebral vasculature autoregulation (ACOG, 2019a). See Display 5–6 for indications for antihypertensive therapy. See Table 5–5

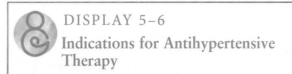

for dosing, mechanism of action, and considerations for commonly used antihypertensive agents. First-line antihypertensive agents include IV hydralazine and labetalol. If no IV access is readily available, oral immediate release nifedipine should be considered. In rare cases that blood pressure is resistant to these agents, in consultation with anesthesiologists, maternal–fetal medicine, or critical care specialists, a second-line antihypertensive such as esmolol, sodium nitroprusside, or nicardipine may be used. Providers should be especially cautious with sodium nitroprusside due to the risk of cyanide and thiocyanate toxicity in the mother, fetus, and newborn (ACOG, 2019a). The use of these second-line medications often requires invasive hemodynamic monitoring.

Hydralazine Hydrochloride

Hydralazine hydrochloride (Apresoline) is a first-line agent in the treatment of hypertension in women requiring urgent blood pressure control. The recommended dosage regimens calls for intermittent IV boluses every 20 to 40 minutes (ACOG, 2019b) (see Table 5–5). Because the response cannot be predicted, it is recommended that 5 to 10 mg IV or IM be the initial dose administered (ACOG, 2019a,b). Side effects of hydralazine include flushing, headache, maternal and fetal tachycardia, palpitations, and uteroplacental insufficiency with subsequent fetal tachycardia and late decelerations. Because hydralazine increases maternal cardiac output and heart rate, if hypertension is more of a force issue (i.e., elevated cardiac output, hypervolemia, or tachycardia), the clinical state may worsen with blood pressure either not lowering or possibly increasing.

TABLE 5-5. Antihypertensive Therapy for Urgent Blood Pressure Control in Pregnancy

Generic name	Trade name	Mechanism of action	Dosage	Considerations
Hydralazine	Apresoline	• Direct-acting dilator of smooth muscle • Primary effect is arterial dilation, with minor venodilator effects. • ↓ Systemic, pulmonary, and renal resistance • Systemic vasodilation results in ↓ systemic vascular resistance, ↓ arterial pressure, ↑ SV, ↑ rate of ventricular pressure rise • Reflex tachycardia may occur secondary to vasodilation. • Onset of action in 10 to 20 min; peak action in 15–30 min • Duration of effect is approximately 2–6 hr. • Metabolized by liver	• 5 mg IV for more than 2 min • If either BP threshold is still exceeded after 20 min, administer 5 to 10 mg IV for more than 2 min to a maximum cumulative dosage of 20 mg or constant infusion of 0.5 to 10 mg/hr. • If either threshold is still exceeded, administer labetalol.	• Must wait 20 min for response between IV doses • After dosing, if either threshold is exceeded, repeat dose and continue to monitor blood pressure closely. • After second dose, if either threshold is exceeded, change to labetalol. • Rebound hypotension • Reflex ↑ in CO and HR (Hyperdynamic circulatory changes also include ↑ LV pressure rise, and SV may be dangerous in patients with certain cardiovascular disorders.) • Monitor BP and HR. Cardiac monitoring is not required. • Maximal BP ↓ within 10 min • ↓ Dose with hepatic dysfunction, low cardiac output, and severe renal dysfunction • Use with caution in patients with coronary artery disease (reflex tachycardia can produce anginal attacks or AMI). • Contraindicated in patients with rheumatic mitral valve disease (↑ PAP) • Not recommended for blood pressure control in patients with dissecting aortic aneurysm (↑ rate of LV pressure rise stresses dissecting aortic segment and worsens aortic injury and propagates dissection.) • Because of postural hypotension, give with caution in patients with cerebrovascular disease. • Excessive dosing may result in too rapid and too profound a reduction in BP causing ↓ uteroplacental blood flow and ↓ oxygen delivery to the fetus. • May ↓ hemoglobin, neutrophil, WBC, granulocyte, platelet, and RBC counts
Labetalol	Normodyne Trandate	• Selective (alpha-adrenergic and nonselective beta-adrenergic) blocking agent • Induces a controlled rapid decrease in BP • ↓ in catecholamine–induced cardiac stimulation and direct vasodilation • ↓ SVR and arterial pressure without reflex tachycardia • Beta-blocking effects also blunt rate of LV pressure rise usually associated with vasodilator drugs, ↓ stress on aortic wall • Onset of action in 1 to 2 min. Hypotensive effect usually seen within 2 to 5 min, peaks at 5 min, and persists for 2 to 6 hr after IV administration • Metabolized by liver and excreted in urine and bile	• Initial dose 10 to 20 mg IV for more than 2 min • If either threshold is exceeded after 10 min, repeat with 40 mg IV for more than 2 min. • If either threshold is exceeded after 10 min, repeat with 80 mg. • If either threshold is exceeded after 10 min, move to hydralazine protocol (10 mg IV for more than 2 min).	• Must wait 10 min between doses for response • Monitor HR and BP. Cardiac monitoring is not required. • Hold IV labetalol if maternal pulse <60 beats per minute. • Monitor blood glucose levels. • ↓ Amplitude and frequency of FHR accelerations; may lower FHR baseline • Monitor newborn for hypoglycemia, hypotension, and bradycardia. • Avoid in women with asthma, heart disease, and congestive heart failure. • A 200-mg oral dose can be administered if no IV access is available nor is immediate release nifedipine.

- Not a titratable drug; effect of increases in IV infusion rate may not be noted for approximately 10 min; diminution of the drug effect may not be noted for several hours following reduction of dose or discontinuation of drug.
- Valuable in managing hypertensive crisis as a result of dissecting aortic aneurysm or traumatic dissection of aorta
- Effectively ↓ cerebral perfusion pressures without ↓ cerebral perfusion
- ↓ Dose with hepatic dysfunction or hepatic hypoperfusion
- ↓ Dosage necessary in patients with creatinine clearances <10 mL/min
- Adverse reactions related to alpha-blockade include orthostatic hypotension.
- Potential beta-blockade reactions include bronchospasm, ↓ myocardial contractility and SV, and bradycardia (dose related).
- Patient should not be quickly raised to a sitting position during therapy and for at least 2 hr after last dose.
- ↑ Uteroplacental perfusion and ↓ uterine vascular resistance
- May exert a positive effect on early fetal lung maturation in patients remote from term
- May ↑ transaminase and urea levels

Drug	Mechanism	Dosing	Considerations
Nifedipine (immediate release) Procardia Adalat	Calcium channel blocker. Thought to inhibit calcium ion influx across cardiac and smooth muscle cells, decreasing contractility and oxygen demand. May dilate coronary arteries and arterioles. Onset of action in 5 to 10 min. Effect seen within 5 to 20 min, with peak action within 30 to 60 min with duration of 4 to 8 hr	10 to 20 mg immediate-release capsules PO, may be repeated after 20 min. If not effective after 2 to 3 doses, consider IV administration of labetalol or hydralazine.	Oral route only; should not be given sublingually due to excessive hypotension, acute myocardial ischemia, and death. Monitor HR and BP. Cardiac monitoring is not required. Good option for treatment in patients with severe hypertension and no immediate IV access. Possible exaggerated effect if used with MgSO₄, including severe hypotension with resulting ↓ uteroplacental perfusion and maternal neuromuscular blockade (muscle weakness, jerky movements of extremities, difficulty in swallowing, paradoxical respirations, and inability to lift head from pillow). Principal side effects include headache and cutaneous flushing. May ↑ ALT, AST, alkaline phosphatase, and LDH levels

ALT, alanine aminotransferase; AMI, acute myocardial infarction; AST, aspartate aminotransferase; BP, blood pressure; CO, cardiac output; ECG, electrocardiogram; FHR, fetal heart rate; HR, heart rate; IV, intravenous; LDH, lactate dehydrogenase; LV, left ventricular; MgSO₄, magnesium sulfate; PAP, pulmonary artery pressure; PO, by mouth; RBC, red blood cell; SV, stroke volume; SVR, systemic vascular resistance; WBC, white blood cell.

From American College of Obstetricians and Gynecologists. (2019a). *Emergent therapy for acute-onset, severe hypertension during pregnancy and the postpartum period* (Committee Opinion No. 767). Washington, DC: Author. American College of Obstetricians and Gynecologists. (2019b). *Gestational hypertension and preeclampsia* (Practice Bulletin No. 202). Washington, DC: Author. Please note, these two ACOG resources suggest slightly different doses. Provider orders, institutional protocols, and patient condition should guide care.

Labetalol Hydrochloride

Labetalol hydrochloride (Normodyne or Trandate) is also a first-line medication for the management of hypertension (ACOG, 2019b). Labetalol seems to have less side effects than hydralazine (see Table 5–5). Labetalol hydrochloride is contraindicated in women with asthma, those with greater than first-degree heart block, and congestive heart failure. Because of labetalol's alpha- and beta-adrenergic blockage, transient fetal and neonatal hypotension, bradycardia, and hypoglycemia are possible. The combined alpha- and beta-adrenergic blockades decrease the incidence of rebound maternal tachycardia, making it an attractive alternative to hydralazine, especially in women with cardiac disease who cannot tolerate tachycardia.

Nifedipine

Nifedipine, a calcium channel blocker, is considered a second-line drug used to control blood pressure in women requiring treatment (ACOG, 2019b) (see Table 5–5). An oral dose of 10 to 20 mg should be given and can be repeated in 20 minutes if necessary. Because nifedipine is an immediate release capsule, the capsule should not be broken or should it be given sublingually. Nifedipine should be considered as a first-line agent in the event that acute blood pressure treatment is needed in a patient without IV access (Archer, Druzin, Shields, & Peterson, 2014).

Postpartum Management

Most women are clinically stable within 48 hours after birth. However, because of the risk of eclampsia during the first 24 to 48 hours postpartum, careful monitoring is essential and should include frequent assessments of vital signs, level of consciousness, DTRs, urinary output, and laboratory data. IV magnesium sulfate is usually continued for 24 to 48 hours postpartum. Due to the tocolytic effect of magnesium, it is important for the nurse to remain vigilant for uterine atony as well as for early signs and symptoms of complications of preeclampsia such as postpartum hemorrhage, DIC, pulmonary edema, HELLP syndrome, increased intracranial pressure, and intracranial hemorrhage. Intensity of monitoring and progression of activity are based on the patient's condition. After vital signs and mental status are stable, laboratory data indicate condition is improving, urinary output is reassuring, and IV magnesium sulfate is discontinued, the frequency of maternal assessments can be decreased from 1 to 2 hours to 4 to 8 hours, the Foley catheter is removed, and the patient is encouraged to ambulate. It is important to provide assistance and assess stability during initial ambulation, after bed rest, and after IV administration of magnesium sulfate. Efforts should be made to initiate maternal–newborn attachment by bringing the newborn, if stable, to visit the mother or facilitating a maternal visit to the NICU. Photographs can be provided or a video feed of the newborn set up to support maternal newborn bonding if the maternal or newborn condition prevents visitation. Breastfeeding should be initiated soon after delivery. Due to the increased lifetime cardiovascular risk associated with preeclampsia, and the cardioprotective effect of lactation, human milk feeding should be encouraged and supported (Anderson, 2018; Nguyen, Jin, & Ding, 2017). If mother and newborn are separated, research shows that initiating pumping within 1 hour after birth results in improved milk supply. Subsequently, labor and delivery nurses should work to support early initiation of pumping, particularly due to the benefits human milk feeding offers to critically ill newborns (Spatz et al., 2015). Magnesium sulfate and most antihypertensive medications used after preeclampsia are compatible with breastfeeding; any concerns may be addressed with a lactation consultant.

ACOG (2018) recommends that women with gestational hypertension, preeclampsia, or superimposed preeclampsia be monitored in the hospital for 72 hours or receive the equivalent monitoring outpatient. Nurses should ensure that discharge education clearly outlines signs and symptoms of preeclampsia and includes information on when to call their healthcare provider. Encourage patients to remind all providers of their delivery date when reporting any signs and symptoms. If blood pressure is persistently elevated—≥150 mm Hg systolic or ≥100 mm Hg diastolic—on two occasions 4 to 6 hours apart, antihypertensive treatment should be initiated (ACOG, 2018). Women with preeclampsia should follow up with their healthcare provider within 7 to 14 days postpartum (Council on Patient Safety in Women's Health Care, 2015).

HELLP SYNDROME

It is estimated that approximately 5% to 10% of women who develop preeclampsia will develop HELLP syndrome (Berry & Iqbal, 2014). HELLP syndrome, a multisystem disease, is a severe complication of preeclampsia in which the woman presents with a variety of complaints and exhibits common laboratory markers to include hemolysis (H), elevated liver enzymes (EL), and low platelets (LP). This subset of women often rapidly progress from preeclampsia to the development of multiple-organ involvement and damage. The complaints range from malaise, epigastric pain, nausea, and vomiting to nonspecific viral syndrome–like symptoms. Patients may present in the antepartum or postpartum period; due to the significant associated maternal and fetal morbidity and mortality, immediate delivery is often required, particularly if after 34 weeks of gestation or if symptoms are severe (ACOG, 2019b).

On presentation, these patients are generally in the second or early third trimester and initially may show few signs of preeclampsia. Because of the presenting symptoms, these patients may receive a nonobstetric diagnosis, delaying treatment and increasing maternal and perinatal morbidity and mortality. Maternal morbidity and mortality are often associated with DIC, pulmonary edema, renal failure, and stroke. Some authors suggest considering corticosteroid therapy to decrease maternal morbidity (Martin et al., 2012). Early diagnosis and treatment are key to improved outcomes. Assessments and management of the woman diagnosed with HELLP syndrome are the same as those for the woman with preeclampsia with severe features.

ECLAMPSIA

Eclampsia is the development of grand mal seizures or coma or both in a woman with signs and symptoms of preeclampsia (ACOG, 2019b). Other causes of seizures must be excluded. Eclampsia can occur antepartum, intrapartum, or postpartum. The prevalence of eclampsia has declined due to improved medical management in preeclampsia with magnesium sulfate. The nurse should be alert for the following signs and symptoms that are often seen in women prior to seizing: headache, blurry vision, photophobia, altered mental status, and epigastric pain and/or right upper quadrant pain (Cooray, Edmonds, Tong, Samarasekera, & Whitehead, 2011). Neurologic deficits and aspiration pneumonia are the leading causes of maternal morbidity after an eclamptic seizure. Placental abruption occurs in 10% of cases (Taylor et al., 2015).

If a seizure occurs, call all emergency team members immediately. Turn the patient to a lateral recumbent position to improve perfusion, which also allows for the patient's tongue to fall to the side. Ensure a patent airway and work to protect the patient from injury. Laryngoscopy can result in an acute increase in blood pressure, so this should be carefully considered and done with anesthesia present. The provision of supplemental oxygen via non-rebreather should be used once stabilized to decrease risk of aspiration. Magnesium sulfate should be given according to institutional protocol, and in the case of recurrent seizure, midazolam, lorazepam, and phenytoin may also be given. After initial stabilization and airway management, the nurse should carefully monitor blood pressure, respirations, and pulse oximetry and anticipate orders for a chest radiograph and possibly arterial blood gas (ABG) determinations to exclude the possibility of aspiration (Berg et al., 2014). Rapid assessments of uterine activity, cervical status, and fetal status are performed. During the seizure, membranes may rupture and the cervix may dilate because the uterus becomes hypercontractile and hypertonic. Often, after a seizure, fetal bradycardia is noted but typically recovers within 3 to 5 minutes, and often, baseline variability does not return to normal until approximately an hour after the seizure occurred (Taylor et al., 2015). In women with eclampsia, if cesarean delivery is required, it should only occur after maternal stabilization. If birth is not imminent, the timing and route of delivery and the induction of labor versus cesarean birth depend on maternal and fetal status.

Many cases of eclampsia occur greater than 48 hours postpartum; it is important for women and their families to be educated on the signs and symptoms of preeclampsia, so they can remain vigilant and seek medical attention as appropriate (Sibai, 2005). Nurses should consider using Association of Women's Health, Obstetric and Neonatal Nurses POST-BIRTH Warning Signs tool in order to provide women and their families with clear, concise instructions at discharge on when to follow up postpartum if preeclampsia is suspected. Clinical drills can improve recognition and response in the care of women with eclamptic seizures. Healthcare providers caring for this population should consider the use of simulation to improve their readiness for this obstetrical emergency. The CMQCC has a variety of simulations on the care of women with preeclampsia and eclampsia that could help address this educational need.

CARDIOVASCULAR IMPLICATIONS OF PREECLAMPSIA

A history of preeclampsia has been linked to increased lifetime risk of cardiovascular disease (CVD), and the American Heart Association (Mosca et al., 2011) lists preeclampsia as a major risk factor for CVD. Specifically, women with early-onset preeclampsia are at approximately 7 to 9 times the risk of CVD than women who had a normotensive pregnancy, and women with late-onset preeclampsia have approximately 2 times the increased risk of CVD (Mongraw-Chaffin, Cirillo, & Cohn, 2010; van Rijn et al., 2013). Bushnell and colleagues (2014) reported that 18.2% of women with a history of preeclampsia had a cardiovascular event in the 10 years following the delivery of the effected pregnancy compared to 1.7% of women with uncomplicated pregnancies. Education on the association between preeclampsia and cardiovascular risk should be provided to women soon after delivery so that cardiovascular risk reduction behaviors can be instituted early in the life course. Specifically, women with a history of preeclampsia should receive education on the importance of smoking cessation; weight management; physical activity; a healthy diet; and annual assessment of blood pressure, lipids, cholesterol, and glucose (Bushnell et al., 2014). Nurses are uniquely situated to provide targeted patient education, create creative programs in order to engage women with history of preeclampsia in heart healthy behaviors, encourage adherence, and follow up with primary care provider within 6 months to 1 year postpartum (Burgess & Founds, 2016).

Emotional Support after Preeclampsia

Due to the life-threatening and stressful nature of preeclampsia, eclampsia, and HELLP syndrome, in addition to the physical effects, these disorders can increase risk for posttraumatic stress disorder (Modarres, Afrasiabi, Rahnama, & Montazeri, 2012). It is important for nurses in the postpartum to assess emotional status, provide emotional support, and educate women and families on supportive resources available after a pregnancy effected by a hypertensive disorder of pregnancy.

QUALITY CARE OF WOMEN WITH PREECLAMPSIA

Education on the signs and symptoms of preeclampsia, early recognition, and treatment as well as ensuring appropriate follow-up are essential to improving outcomes in women with preeclampsia. There are a variety of resources available to nurses and healthcare providers in order to improve the care provided to women with preeclampsia. The CMQCC offers a *preeclampsia toolkit* with a variety of resources for standardizing the care provided to women with preeclampsia. The Council on Patient Safety in Women's Health Care offers a patient safety bundle on *severe hypertension in pregnancy* and provides guidelines for care, recognition and response. Finally, the Preeclampsia Foundation offers a variety of educational materials that can be used to standardize education provided to patients on signs and symptoms of preeclampsia antenatally and in the postpartum and on cardiovascular risk after preeclampsia.

SUMMARY

Perinatal nurses may be challenged by complications of pregnancy, especially when they occur unexpectedly in the low-risk setting. Nurses in the outpatient setting should provide education on the signs and symptoms of preeclampsia starting early in pregnancy. In the antepartum and intrapartum setting, a thorough knowledge of the nursing care of women with hypertensive disorders of pregnancy, including timely identification and appropriate interventions, is required to ensure optimal outcomes for mothers and babies. In postpartum, nurses should ensure that women are aware of their continued risk of preeclampsia and of the associated signs and symptoms. Maternal newborn nurses

should educate women with a history of preeclampsia on the cardiovascular risk associated with preeclampsia as well as on cardiovascular risk reduction strategies so that women receive the appropriate follow-up and have an opportunity to initiate cardiopreventive strategies earlier in their life course.

REFERENCES

American College of Obstetricians and Gynecologists. (2013). *Hypertension in pregnancy*. Washington, DC: Author.

American College of Obstetricians and Gynecologists. (2018). *Low-dose aspirin use during pregnancy* (Committee Opinion No. 743). Washington, DC: Author.

American College of Obstetricians and Gynecologists. (2019a). *Emergent therapy for acute-onset, severe hypertension during pregnancy and the postpartum period* (Committee Opinion No. 767). Washington, DC: Author.

American College of Obstetricians and Gynecologists. (2019b). *Gestational hypertension and preeclampsia* (Practice Bulletin No. 202). Washington, DC: Author.

American College of Obstetricians and Gynecologists & Society for Maternal–Fetal Medicine. (2019). Levels of maternal care (Obstetric Care Consensus No. 9). *American Journal of Obstetrics & Gynecology, 221*(2), B1–B12. doi:10.1016/j.ajog.2019.05.046

Anderson, P. O. (2018). Treating hypertension during breastfeeding. *Breastfeeding Medicine, 13*(2), 95–96. doi:10.1089/bfm.2017.0236

Archer, T., & Champagne, H. (2014). Fluid management in preeclampsia. In Preeclampsia Task Force (Ed.), *Preeclampsia toolkit: Improving health care response to preeclampsia*. Stanford, CA: California Maternal Quality Care Collaborative.

Archer, T., Druzin, M., Shields, L., & Peterson, N. (2014). Antihypertensive agents in preeclampsia. In Preeclampsia Task Force (Ed.), *Preeclampsia toolkit: Improving health care response to preeclampsia*. Stanford, CA: California Maternal Quality Care Collaborative.

Avorgbedor, F., Silva, S., Merwin, E., Blumenthal, J., & Holditch-Davis, D. (2019). Health, physical growth, and neurodevelopmental outcomes in preterm infants of women with hypertensive disorders of pregnancy. *Journal of Obstetric, Gynecologic & Neonatal Nursing, 48*(1), 69–77. doi:10.1016/j.jogn.2018.10.003

Berg, O., Lee, R., & Chagolla, B. (2014). Magnesium sulfate. In Preeclampsia Task Force (Ed.), *Preeclampsia toolkit: Improving health care response to preeclampsia*. Stanford, CA: California Maternal Quality Care Collaborative.

Berry, E. L., & Iqbal, S. N. (2014). HELLP syndrome at 17 weeks gestation: A rare and catastrophic phenomenon. *Journal of Clinical Gynecology and Obstetrics, 3*(4), 147–150. doi:10.14740/jcgo297w

Boeldt, D. S., & Bird, I. M. (2017). Vascular adaptation in pregnancy and endothelial dysfunction in preeclampsia. *Journal of Endocrinology, 232*(1), R27–R44. doi:10.1530/JOE-16-0340

Boyd, H. A., Tahir, H., Wohlfahrt, J., & Melbye, M. (2013). Associations of personal and family preeclampsia history with the risk of early-, intermediate- and late-onset preeclampsia. *American Journal of Epidemiology, 178*(11), 1611–1619. doi:10.1093/aje/kwt189

Burgess, A., & Founds, S. (2016). Cardiovascular implications of preeclampsia. *MCN: The American Journal of Maternal Child Nursing, 41*(1), 8–15. doi:10.1097/NMC.0000000000000204

Bushnell, C., & Chireau, M. (2011). Preeclampsia and stroke: Risks during and after pregnancy. *Stroke Research and Treatment, 2011*, 858134. doi:10.4061/2011/858134

Bushnell, C., McCullough, L., Awad, I., Chireau, M., Fedder, W., Furie, K., . . . Walters, M. (2014). Guidelines for the prevention of stroke in women: A statement for healthcare professionals from the American Heart Association/American Stroke Association. *Stroke, 45*(5), 1545–1588. doi:10.1161/01.str.0000442009.06663.48

California Maternal Quality Care Collaborative. (2014). Eclampsia algorithm. In Preeclampsia Task Force (Ed.), *Preeclampsia toolkit: Improving health care response to preeclampsia.* Stanford, CA: Author.

Centers for Disease Control and Prevention. (2018a). *Data on selected pregnancy complications in the United States.* Retrieved from https://www.cdc.gov/reproductivehealth/maternalinfanthealth/pregnancy-complications-data.htm

Centers for Disease Control and Prevention. (2018b). *Pregnancy mortality surveillance system.* Retrieved from http://www.cdc.gov/reproductivehealth/maternalinfanthealth/pregnancy-mortality-surveillance-system.htm

Chaiworapongsa, T., Romero, R., Espinoza, J., Bujold, E., Mee Kim, Y., Gonçalves, L. F., . . . Edwin, S. (2004). Evidence supporting a role for blockade of the vascular endothelial growth factor system in the pathophysiology of preeclampsia. *American Journal of Obstetrics & Gynecology, 190*(6), 1541–1550. doi:10.1016/j.ajog.2004.03.043

Cooray, S., Edmonds, S., Tong, S., Samarasekera, S., & Whitehead, C. (2011). Characterization of symptoms immediately preceding eclampsia. *Obstetrics & Gynecology, 118*(5), 995–999. doi:10.1097/AOG.0b013e3182324570

Coppage, K. H., & Sibai, B. M. (2004). Hypertensive emergencies. In M. R. Foley, T. H. Strong Jr., & T. J. Garite (Eds.), *Obstetric intensive care manual* (2nd ed., pp. 51–65). New York, NY: McGraw-Hill.

Cormick, G., Betrán, A. P., Romero, I. B., Lombardo, C. F., Gülmezoglu, A. M., Ciapponi, A., & Belizán, J. M. (2019). Global inequities in dietary calcium intake during pregnancy: A systematic review and meta-analysis. *BJOG, 126*(4), 444–456. doi:10.1111/1471-0528.15512

Council on Patient Safety in Women's Health Care. (2015). *Severe hypertension in pregnancy* Washington, DC: Author.

Creanga, A. A., Syverson, C., Seed, K., & Callaghan, W. M. (2017). Pregnancy-related mortality in the United States, 2011–2013. *Obstetrics & Gynecology, 130*(2), 366–373. doi:10.1097/AOG.0000000000002114

Davenport, M. H., Ruchat, S. M., Poitras, V. J., Jaramillo Garcia, A., Gray, C. E., Barrowman, N., . . . Mottola, M. F. (2018). Prenatal exercise for the prevention of gestational diabetes mellitus and hypertensive disorders of pregnancy: A systematic review and meta-analysis. *British Journal of Sports Medicine, 52*(21), 1367–1375. doi:10.1136/bjsports-2018-099355

Dechend, R., Gratze, P., Wallukat, G., Shagdarsuren, E., Plehm, R., Bräsen, J. H., . . . Müller, D. N. (2005). Agonistic autoantibodies to the AT1 receptor in a transgenic rat model of preeclampsia. *Hypertension, 45*(4), 742–746. doi:10.1161/01.HYP.0000154785.50570.63

Dong, X., Gou, W., Li, C., Wu, M., Han, Z., Li, X., & Chen, Q. (2017). Proteinuria in preeclampsia: Not essential to diagnosis but related to disease severity and fetal outcomes. *Pregnancy Hypertension, 8*, 60–64. doi:10.1016/j.preghy.2017.03.005

Du, M., Ouyang, Y., Nie, X., Huang, Y., & Redding, S. R. (2019). Effects of physical exercise during pregnancy on maternal and infant outcomes in overweight and obese pregnant women: A meta-analysis. *Birth, 46*, 211–221. doi:10.1111/birt.12396

Duley, L., Henderson-Smart, D. J., & Chou, D. (2010). Magnesium sulphate versus phenytoin for eclampsia. *Cochrane Database of Systematic Reviews,* (10), CD000128. doi:10.1002/14651858.CD000128.pub2

Eastabrook, G., Aksoy, T., Bedell, S., Penava, D., & de Vrijer, B. (2018). Preeclampsia biomarkers: An assessment of maternal cardiometabolic health. *Pregnancy Hypertension, 13*, 204–213. doi:10.1016/j.preghy.2018.06.005

Founds, S., Catov, J., Gallaher, M., Harger, G., Markovic, N., & Roberts, J. (2011). Is there evidence of separate inflammatory or metabolic forms of preeclampsia? *Hypertension in Pregnancy, 30*, 1–10. doi:10.3109/10641950903322907

González-Quintero, V. H., Smarkusky, L. P., Jiménez, J. J., Mauro, L. M., Jy, W., Hortsman, L. L., . . . Ahn, Y. S. (2004). Elevated plasma endothelial microparticles: Preeclampsia versus gestational hypertension. *American Journal of Obstetrics & Gynecology, 191*(4), 1418–1424. doi:10.1016/j.ajog.2004.06.044

Haddad, B., Deis, S., Goffinet, F., Paniel, B. J., Cabrol, D., & Siba, B. M. (2004). Maternal and perinatal outcomes during expectant management of 239 severe preeclamptic women between 24 and 33 weeks' gestation. *American Journal of Obstetrics & Gynecology, 190*(6), 1590–1597. doi:10.1016/j.ajog.2004.03.050

Haram, K., Svendsen, E., & Abildgaard, U. (2009). The HELLP syndrome: Clinical issues and management. A review. *BMC Pregnancy and Childbirth, 9*(1), 8–22. doi:10.1186/1471-2393-9-8

Henderson, J. T., Whitlock, E. P., O'Conner, E., Senger, C. A., Thompson, J. H., & Rowland, M. G. (2014). *Low-dose aspirin for the prevention of morbidity and mortality from preeclampsia: A systematic evidence review for the U.S. Preventive Services Task Force* (Evidence Syntheses, No. 112). Rockville, MD: Agency for Healthcare Research and Quality.

Hermes, W., Tamsma, J. T., Grootendorst, D. C., Franx, A., van der Post, J., van Pampus, M., . . . de Groot, C. J. (2013). Cardiovascular risk estimation in women with a history of hypertensive pregnancy disorders at term: A longitudinal follow-up study. *BMC Pregnancy and Childbirth, 13*, 126. doi:10.1186/1471-2393-13-126

Hodgins, S. (2015). Pre-eclampsia as underlying cause for perinatal deaths: Time for action. *Global Health, Science and Practice, 3*(4), 525–527. doi:10.9745/GHSP-D-15-00350

Huwe, V. Y., Puck, A. L., Vasher, J., Baird, S. M., Witcher, P. M., & Troiano, N. H. (2019). Guidelines for the care of the patient with hypertension during pregnancy. In N. H. Troiano, P. M. Witcher, & S. M. Baird (Eds.), *AWHONN's high-risk and critical care obstetrics* (4th ed., pp. 371–375). Philadelphia, PA: Wolters Kluwer.

Ilekis, J., Reddy, U., & Roberts, J. (2007). Preeclampsia—A pressing problem: An executive summary of a National Institute of Child Health and Human Development workshop. *Reproductive Sciences, 14*(6), 508–523. doi:10.1177/1933719107306232

Institute for Safe Medication Practices. (2018). *High-alert medications in acute care settings.* Horsham, PA: Author.

Khaing, W., Vallibhakara, S. A., Tantrakul, V., Vallibhakara, O., Rattanasiri, S., McEvoy, M., . . . Thakkinstian, A. (2017). Calcium and vitamin D supplementation for prevention of preeclampsia: A systematic review and network meta-analysis. *Nutrients, 9*(10), E1141. doi:10.3390/nu9101141

Kucukgoz Gulec, U., Ozgunen, F. T., Buyukkurt, S., Guzel, A. B., Urunsak, I. F., Demir, S. C., & Evruke, I. C. (2013). Comparison of clinical and laboratory findings in early- and late-onset preeclampsia. *Journal of Maternal-Fetal and Neonatal Medicine, 26*(12), 1228–1233. doi:10.3109/14767058.2013.776533

Lawn, J. E., Blencowe, H., Waiswa, P., Amouzou, A., Mathers, C., Hogan, D., . . . Cousens, S. (2016). Stillbirths: Rates, risk factors, and acceleration towards 2030. *Lancet, 387*(10018), 587–603. doi:10.1016/S0140-6736(15)00837-5

Lisonkova, S., & Joseph, K. (2013). Incidence of preeclampsia: Risk factors and outcomes associated with early—Versus late-onset disease. *American Journal of Obstetrics & Gynecology, 209*(6), 544.e1–544.e12. doi:10.1016/j.ajog.2013.08.019

Magro-Malosso, E., Saccone, G., Di Mascio, Di Tommaso, M., & Berghella, V. (2017). Exercise during pregnancy and risk of preterm birth in overweight and obese women: A systematic review and meta-analysis of randomized controlled trials. *Acta Obstetricia et Gynecologica Scandinavica, 96*, 263–273. doi:10.1111/aogs.13087

Main, E., McCain, C., Morton, C., Holtby, S., & Lawton, E. S. (2015). Pregnancy-related mortality in California: Causes, characteristics, and improvement opportunities. *Obstetrics & Gynecology*, *125*(4), 938–947. doi:10.1097/AOG.0000000000000746

Martin, J. A., Hamilton, B. E., Ventura, S. J., Osterman, M. J. K., Kirmeyer, S., Mathews, T. J., & Wilson, E. C. (2011). Births: Final data for 2009. *National Vital Statistics Reports*, *60*(1), 1–70.

Martin, J. A., Owens, M., Keiser, S., Parrish, M., Tam Tam, K., Brewer, J. . . . May, W. L. (2012). Standardized Mississippi Protocol treatment of 190 patients with HELLP syndrome: Slowing disease progression and preventing new major maternal morbidity. *Hypertension in Pregnancy*, *31*(1), 79–90. doi:10.3109/10641955.2010.525277

Martin, J. A., Thigpen, B., Moore, R., Rose, C., Cushman, J., & May, W. (2005). Stroke and severe preeclampsia and eclampsia: A paradigm shift focusing on systolic blood pressure. *Obstetrics & Gynecology*, *105*(2), 246–254. doi:10.1097/01.AOG.0000151116.84113.56

Meher, S., Abalos, E., & Carroli, G. (2005). Bed rest with or without hospitalisation for hypertension during pregnancy. *Cochrane Database of Systematic Reviews*, (4), CD003514. doi:10.1002/14651858.CD003514.pub2

Mhyre, S., D'Oria, R., Hameed, A., Lappen, J., Holley, S., Hunter, S., . . . D'Alton, M. (2014). The Maternal Early Warning Criteria: A proposal from the National Partnership for Maternal Safety. *Obstetrics & Gynecology*, *124*(4), 782–786. doi:10.1097/AOG.0000000000000480

Mignini, L. E., Latthe, P. M., Villar, J., Kilby, M. D., Carroli, G., & Khan, K. S. (2005). Mapping the theories of preeclampsia: The role of homocysteine. *Obstetrics & Gynecology*, *105*(2), 411–425. doi:10.1097/01.AOG.0000151117.52952

Modarres, M., Afrasiabi, S., Rahnama, P., & Montazeri, A. (2012). Prevalence and risk factors of childbirth-related post-traumatic stress symptoms. *BMC Pregnancy and Childbirth*, *12*, 88. doi:10.1186/1471-2393-12-88

Mongraw-Chaffin, M. L., Cirillo, P. M., & Cohn, B. A. (2010). Preeclampsia and cardiovascular disease death: Prospective evidence from the child health and development studies cohort. *Hypertension*, *56*(1), 166–171.

Mosca, L., Benjamin, E. J., Berra, K., Bezanson, J. L., Dolor, R. J., Lloyd-Jones, D. M., . . . Wenger, N. K. (2011). Effectiveness-based guidelines for the prevention of cardiovascular disease in women—2011 Update: A guideline from the American Heart Association. *Circulation*, *123*, 1243–1262. doi:10.1161/CIR.0b013e31820faaf8

Myatt, L., Redman, C., Staff, A., Hansson, S., Wilson, M., Laivuori, H., . . . Roberts, J. (2014). Strategy for standardization of preeclampsia research study design. *Hypertension*, *63*(6), 1293–1301. doi:10.1161/HYPERTENSIONAHA.113.02664

National High Blood Pressure Education Program. (2000). *National High Blood Pressure Education Program Working group report on high blood pressure in pregnancy* (NIH Publication No. 00-3029). Bethesda, MD: National High Blood Pressure Education Program, National Heart, Lung, and Blood Institute, National Institutes of Health. Retrieved from http://www.nhlbi.nih.gov/files/docs/guidelines/hbp_preg_archive.pdf

National High Blood Pressure Education Program Working Group on High Blood Pressure in Pregnancy. (2000). Report of the National High Blood Pressure Education Program Working Group on high blood pressure in pregnancy. *American Journal of Obstetrics & Gynecology*, *183*(1), S1–S22. doi:10.1067/mob.2000.107928

Nguyen, B., Jin, K., & Ding, D. (2017). Breastfeeding and maternal cardiovascular risk factors and outcomes: A systematic review. *PLoS One*, *12*(11), e0187923. doi:10.1371/journal.pone.0187923

Northern New England Perinatal Quality Improvement Network. (2019). *NNEPQIN guideline for the management of hypertensive disorders of pregnancy*. Lebanon, NH.

Roberge, S., Nicolaides, K., Demers, S., Hyett, J., Chaillet, N., & Bujold, E. (2017). The role of aspirin dose on the prevention of preeclampsia and fetal growth restriction: Systematic review and meta-analysis. *American Journal of Obstetrics & Gynecology*, *216*(2), 110.e6–120.e6. doi:10.1016/j.ajog.2016.09.076

Roberts, J. (1994). Current perspectives on preeclampsia. *Journal of Nurse-Midwifery*, *39*(2), 70–90. doi:10.1016/0091-2182(94)90015-9

Roberts, J. M. (2004). Pregnancy-related hypertension. In R. K. Creasy, R. Resnik, & J. D. Iams (Eds.), *Maternal-fetal medicine: Principles & practice* (5th ed., pp. 859–900). Philadelphia, PA: Saunders.

Roberts, J., & Hubel, C. (2009). The two stage model of preeclampsia: Variations on the theme. *Placenta*, *30*(Suppl. A), S32–S37. doi:10.1016/j.placenta.2008.11.009

Rumbold, A., Duley, L., Crowther, C. A., & Haslam, R. R. (2008). Antioxidants for preventing pre-eclampsia. *Cochrane Database of Systematic Reviews*, (1), CD004227. doi:10.1002/14651858.CD004227.pub3

Saito, S. (2018). *Preeclampsia: basic, genomic, and clinical*. Singapore: Springer.

Sibai, B. M. (2005). Diagnosis, prevention, and management of eclampsia. *Obstetrics & Gynecology*, *105*(2), 402–410. doi:10.1097/01.AOG.0000152351.13671.99

Sibai, B. M. (2011). Management of late preterm and early-term pregnancies complicated by mild gestational hypertension/pre-eclampsia. *Seminars in Perinatology*, *35*(5), 292–296. doi:10.1053/j.semperi.2011.05.010

Society for Maternal Fetal Medicine Publications Committee. (2015). *SMFM statement: Benefit of antihypertensive therapy for mild-to-moderate chronic hypertension during pregnancy remains uncertain*. Washington, DC: Author.

Sotiriadis, A., Hernandez-Andrade, E., da Silva Costa, F., Ghi, T., Glanc, P., Khalil, A., . . . Thilaganathan, B. (2019). ISUOG practice guidelines: Role of ultrasound in screening for and follow-up of pre-eclampsia. *Ultrasound in Obstetrics and Gynecology*, *53*(1), 7–22. doi:10.1002/uog.20105

Spatz, D. L., Froh, E. B., Schwarz, J., Houng, K., Brewster, I., Myers, C., . . . Olkkola, M. (2015). Pump early, pump often: A continuous quality improvement project. *The Journal of Perinatal Education*, *24*(3), 160–170. doi:10.1891/1058-1243.24.3.160

Steegers, E., von Dadelszen, P., Duvekot, J. J., & Pijnenborg, R. (2010). Pre-eclampsia. *Lancet*, *376*(9741), 631–644.

Syngelaki, A., Sequeira Campos, M., Roberge, S., Andrade, W., & Nicolaides, K. H. (2018). Diet and exercise for preeclampsia prevention in overweight and obese pregnant women: Systematic review and meta-analysis. *Journal of Maternal-Fetal and Neonatal Medicine*, 1–7. doi:10.1080/14767058.2018.1481037

Taylor, R., Roberts, J., Cunningham, F., & Lindheimer, M. (2015). *Chesley's hypertensive disorders in pregnancy* (4th ed.). Amsterdam, Netherlands: Elsevier. doi:10.1016/C2012-0-02662-2

Tranquilli, A. L., Dekker, G., Magee, L., Roberts, J., Sibai, B. M., Steyn, W., . . . Brown, M. A. (2014).The classification, diagnosis and management of the hypertensive disorders of pregnancy: A revised statement from the ISSHP. *Pregnancy Hypertension*, *4*(2), 97–104. doi:10.1016/j.preghy.2014.02.001

Umesawa, M., & Kobashi, G. (2017). Epidemiology of hypertensive disorders in pregnancy: Prevalence, risk factors, predictors and prognosis. *Hypertension Research*, *40*(3), 213–220. doi:10.1038/hr.2016.126

van Rijn, B., Nijdam, M., Bruinse, H., Roest, M., Uiterwaal, C., Grobbee, D., . . . Franx, A. (2013). Cardiovascular disease risk factors in women with a history of early-onset preeclampsia. *Obstetrics & Gynecology*, *121*(5), 1040–1048. doi:10.1097/AOG.0b013e31828ea3b5

Villar, J., Repke, J., & Belizan, J. (1989). Relationship of blood pressure, calcium intake, and parathyroid hormone. *American Journal of Clinical Nutrition, 49,* 183–184. doi:10.1093/ajcn/49.1.183a

Vogel, J. P., Souza, J. P., & Mori, R. (2014). Maternal complications and perinatal mortality: Findings of the World Health Organization multicountry survey on maternal and newborn health. *BJOG, 121*(Suppl. 1), 76–88. doi:10.1111/1471-0528.12633

Waite, L. L., Louie, R. E., & Taylor, R. N. (2005). Circulating activators of peroxisome proliferator-activated receptors are reduced in preeclamptic pregnancy. *Journal of Clinical Endocrinology and Metabolism, 90*(2), 620–626. doi:10.1210/jc.2004-0849

Wang, Y., Gu, Y., Zhang, Y., & Lewis, D. F. (2004). Evidence of endothelial dysfunction in preeclampsia: Decreased endothelial nitric oxide synthase expression is associated with increased cell permeability in endothelial cells from preeclampsia. *American Journal of Obstetrics & Gynecology, 190*(3), 817–824. doi:10.1016/j.ajog.2003.09.049

Xu, J. Q., Kochanek, K. D., Murphy, S. L., & Tejada-Vera, B. (2010). Deaths: Final data for 2007. *National Vital Statistics Reports, 58*(19), 1–19. Retrieved from http://www.cdc.gov/nchs/data/nvsr/nvsr58/nvsr58_19.pdf

Yamamoto, T., Suzuki, Y., Kojima, K., & Suzumori, K. (2005). Reduced flow-mediated vasodilation is not due to a decrease in production of nitric oxide in preeclampsia. *American Journal of Obstetrics & Gynecology, 192*(2), 558–563. doi:10.1016/j.ajog.2004.08.031

Yogev, Y., & Sheiner, E. (2014). *Controversies in preeclampsia.* New York, NY: Nova Science.

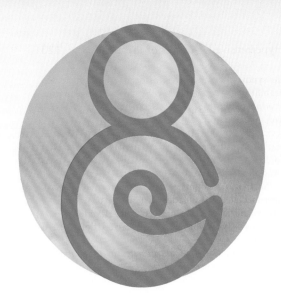

CHAPTER 6

Bleeding in Pregnancy

Jean Salera-Vieira

SIGNIFICANCE AND INCIDENCE

Hemorrhagic complications during pregnancy are a significant causative factor of adverse maternal–fetal outcomes. Major blood loss predisposes the woman to an increased risk of hypovolemia, anemia, infection, preterm labor/birth, and maternal death. Although bleeding can cause considerable problems for the mother, the fetus is especially in jeopardy because significant maternal blood loss can result in negative alterations in maternal hemodynamic status and decreased oxygen-carrying capacity. When bleeding decreases blood flow to the placenta, maternal–fetal gas exchange is reduced and the fetus is at risk for progressive physiologic deterioration (e.g., hypoxemia, hypoxia, asphyxia, and death). This risk is directly related to the amount and duration of blood loss.

Hemorrhage during pregnancy is one of the leading causes of maternal mortality in the United States, along with cardiovascular disease, infection/sepsis, and hypertensive disorders (Berg, Callaghan, Syverson, & Henderson, 2010; Centers for Disease Control and Prevention [CDC], 2017; Main et al., 2015; Paxton & Wardlaw, 2011; The Joint Commission, 2010). The pregnancy-related mortality ratio continues to show an upward trend with a rate of 17.3 deaths per 100,000 live births in 2013 (CDC, 2017). Racial disparities exist in pregnancy-related mortality. Between 2011 and 2013, pregnancy-related deaths for black women were 43.5 deaths per 100,000 live births as compared to 12.7 deaths per 100,000 live births for white women and 14.4 deaths per 100,000 live births for women of other races (CDC, 2017). The proportion of deaths attributable to hemorrhage and hypertensive disorders declined from previous years, whereas the proportion from medical conditions, particularly cardiovascular,

increased (Berg et al., 2010; CDC, 2017). Hemorrhage related to pregnancy still remains a significant issue in the United States and globally. Postpartum hemorrhage remains one of the leading causes of maternal death worldwide (Burke, 2010; Callaghan, Kuklina, & Berg, 2010; Oyelese & Ananth, 2010).

The concern over the maternal morbidity and mortality in the United States has recently come to the forefront. The American College of Obstetricians and Gynecologists (ACOG) and the Society for Maternal-Fetal Medicine (SMFM) have developed an Obstetric Care Consensus statement on *Severe Maternal Mortality: Screening and Review* (ACOG, 2016) to provide guidance on screening women at risk for severe maternal mortality and conducting quality reviews of the same. Maternal mortality review boards do not exist in every state, so it is difficult to assess the actual rates and preventability of pregnancy-related deaths.

Obstetric hemorrhage is viewed as a preventable cause of maternal mortality (Main et al., 2015). When the outcome of pregnancy was live birth, maternal deaths were caused by a number of factors including uterine rupture, placental abruption, placenta previa, placenta accreta, retained placental fragments, coagulopathies, and uterine atony (Berg et al., 2010). Significant causes of death in women whose pregnancy ends in stillbirth are hemorrhage from placental abruption and uterine rupture (Berg et al., 2010; Chang et al., 2003). Placental abruption and uterine dehiscence or rupture also are significant causes of fetal death (ACOG, 2017a; Silver, 2007).

Vaginal bleeding in pregnancy may occur during each trimester. Up to 20% of maternal cardiac output (500 to 1,000 mL/min) flows through the placental bed at term; unresolved bleeding can result in maternal exsanguination in 8 to 10 minutes (Blackburn, 2018; Poole & White, 2005; Rajan & Wing, 2010). Most bleeding occurring in the first trimester of pregnancy is nontraumatic, is related to spontaneous abortion, and is generally not life-threatening. Ectopic pregnancy is a cause of maternal morbidity and mortality, with a prevalence rate up to 2% of all pregnancies (Jurkovic & Wilkinson, 2011). Hemorrhage during the antepartum period usually results from disruption of the placental implantation site (involving a normally implanted placenta or placenta previa) (Hull & Resnik, 2014). Symptomatic placenta previa is identified in approximately 0.3% to 0.5% of pregnancies (Harper, Obido, Macones, Crane, & Cahill, 2010; Oyelese & Smulian, 2006). Low implantation of the placenta is much more common during early pregnancy; however, most of these cases resolve or are not found to be clinically significant as pregnancy progresses (Harper et al., 2010; Oyelese & Smulian, 2006). Placentas may be classified as low lying during the second trimester by routine abdominal ultrasonography because it is difficult to determine placental lie during ultrasonographic examination in early pregnancy. Transvaginal ultrasound remains a more accurate way to diagnose placenta previa and to measure the distance from the placental edge to the cervical os (Oyelese & Smulian, 2006; Vergani et al., 2009). The incidence of placenta previa is increasing, most likely secondary to the increasing cesarean birth rate (Hull & Resnik, 2014).

Placenta accreta is an uncommon abnormality of placental implantation in which the placenta attaches abnormally to the myometrium. Placenta accreta is one of the most serious complications of placenta previa. In addition to placenta previa, prior uterine surgery significantly increases the risk of placenta accreta (ACOG, 2012b; Comstock, 2011). Silver et al. (2006) found that when placenta previa is present, the risk of placenta accreta was 3%, 11%, 40%, 61%, and 67% for the first, second, third, fourth, and fifth or greater repeat cesarean deliveries, respectively. The incidence of placenta accreta is rising secondary to an increase in the cesarean birth rate (ACOG, 2012b; Eller et al., 2011; Mahlmeister, 2010).

The incidence of placental abruption varies in the literature according to the population studied and diagnostic criteria. In the United States, the reported incidence of placental abruption is approximately 0.5% to 1% of all pregnancies (Hull & Resnik, 2014; SMFM & Gyamfi-Bannerman, 2018). Risk of recurrence in subsequent pregnancies has been reported to be as high as 5.8% compared to women without a previous abruption (0.06%) (adjusted odds ratio = 93) (Ruiter, Ravelli, de Graaf, Mol, & Pajkrt, 2015). The strongest risk factor for abruption is a history of placental abruption in a previous pregnancy (Hull & Resnik, 2014). The risk of recurrence for women

with a history of two placental abruptions increases to approximately 25% (Hull & Resnik, 2014).

Vasa previa is a condition in which umbilical arteries and veins abnormally implanted throughout the amnion traverse the cervical os in front of the presenting part of the fetus. Vasa previa is a rare but life-threatening complication for the fetus at the time of rupture of membranes (Oyelese & Smulian, 2006; Robinson & Grobman, 2011). The reported incidence of vasa previa is approximately 1 in 2,500 births (Robinson & Grobman, 2011). Rupture of the vessels during spontaneous or artificial rupture of membranes usually leads to fetal exsanguination or severe neurologic fetal injury secondary to fetal hemorrhage before the cause of bleeding is recognized and before an emergent cesarean birth can be accomplished (Silver, 2007). Fetal death occurs in 60% to 75% of cases of ruptured vasa previa (Oyelese & Smulian, 2006). Prenatal diagnosis of vasa previa increases the survival rate (SMFM & Gyamfi-Bannerman, 2018).

Uterine rupture is another significant cause of maternal hemorrhage. The risk of uterine rupture for women attempting a trial of labor after cesarean delivery (TOLAC) is less than 1% for spontaneous labor; however, the consequences can be catastrophic for the mother and baby (ACOG, 2017b; Spong & Queenan, 2011; Tillett, 2010). The risk of uterine rupture depends on the number, type, and location of the previous incisions (ACOG, 2017b; Lang & Landon, 2010). A large multicenter study did not find a difference in rupture rates in patient having one versus more than one previous cesarean deliveries (Tahseen & Griffiths, 2010). Women with a previous low-vertical uterine incision have a similar success rate for having a vaginal birth after cesarean birth (VBAC) as those women with a previous low transverse incision (ACOG, 2010; Cahill & Macones, 2007). The risk of uterine rupture is increased for women with a T-shaped incision (ACOG, 2010).

Waiting for spontaneous labor, thus avoiding pharmacologic cervical ripening agents, appears to significantly decrease the risk of uterine rupture for women attempting TOLAC (ACOG, 2010, 2017b; Landon et al., 2005; Lang & Landon, 2010). The rate of uterine rupture with spontaneous labor is lower than the rate with labor induced with oxytocin alone (ACOG, 2017b). Spontaneous labor when attempting a TOLAC leads to higher VBAC success rate (ACOG, 2017b). There are enough data to suggest that prostaglandins and high rates of oxytocin infusion increase the risk for rupture (ACOG, 2017b; Lang & Landon, 2010). Uterine ruptures at the scar site and remote from the previous scar site have been reported with high doses of oxytocin (Lang & Landon, 2010). It has been theorized that prostaglandins induce local biochemical modifications that weaken the prior uterine scar, thus predisposing it to rupture (Lang & Landon, 2010). Due to the risk of uterine rupture with the use of misoprostol or any prostaglandin agent for cervical ripening or induction, ACOG (2017b) does not recommend prostaglandins for women attempting a TOLAC. If labor needs to be induced in a patient with a previous scar for a clear and compelling clinical indication, the potential increased risk of uterine rupture with the use of prostaglandins should be discussed with the patient and documented in the medical record (ACOG, 2017b).

The incidence of uterine inversion is approximately 1 case in 2,500 births, although the range varies among studies (You & Zahn, 2006). It is difficult to ascertain the true incidence because uterine inversion is not often reported in the literature. Improper management of the third stage of labor increases the likelihood of iatrogenic uterine inversion (Oyelese & Ananth, 2010).

DEFINITIONS AND CLINICAL MANIFESTATIONS

The definitions, cause, pathophysiology, and clinical manifestations of the most frequently occurring causes of bleeding and bleeding disorders in pregnancy are described in the following sections. A diagnosis-specific summary of expected management is included. A more detailed summary of nursing interventions for bleeding during pregnancy concludes this section.

Placenta Previa

Placenta previa is the abnormal implantation of the placenta extending over or abutting the internal cervical os (SMFM & Gyamfi-Bannerman, 2018). Asymptomatic placenta previa is often diagnosed during routine ultrasound performed in the second trimester; most cases of placenta previa are detected before the third trimester (Oyelese & Smulian, 2006) and is more accurately diagnosed with transvaginal ultrasound (SMFM & Gyamfi-Bannerman, 2018). These women are at increased risk for other obstetric complications, such as placental abruption, intrauterine growth restriction (IUGR), and hemorrhage. It has been theorized that the placental tissue that surrounds the cervical os does not develop as well as the placental tissue that is in the myometrium (Hull & Resnik, 2014; Oyelese & Smulian, 2006). By the end of 40 weeks of pregnancy, the incidence of placenta previa is approximately 0.3% to 0.05% (SMFM & Gyamfi-Bannerman, 2018). The most significant risk factors include prior uterine surgery resulting in uterine scarring and history of a prior placenta previa (Hull & Resnik, 2014; Oyelese & Smulian, 2006). Late development and implantation of the ovum, more frequently occurring in older women, may also play a role in placenta previa. Display 6–1 lists the risk factors associated with placenta previa.

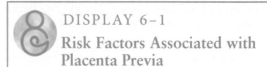

DISPLAY 6–1

Risk Factors Associated with Placenta Previa

- Previous placenta previa
- Previous cesarean birth
- Induced or spontaneous abortions involving suction curettage
- Multiparity
- Advanced maternal age (>35 years)
- Cigarette smoking
- Nonwhite race (all)

Adapted from Hull, A. D., & Resnik, R. (2014). Placenta previa, placenta accreta, abruptio placentae, and vasa previa. In R. K. Creasy, R. Resnik, J. D. Iams, C. J. Lockwood, T. R. Moore, & M. F. Greene (Eds.), *Creasy and Resnik's maternal–fetal medicine: Principles and practice* (7th ed., p. 733). Philadelphia, PA: Saunders Elsevier. Copyright 2014 by Saunders Elsevier.

Placental implantation has traditionally been classified as normal, low-lying, partial placenta previa, and total placenta previa (Fig. 6–1). Clark (1999) proposed a new classification system: placenta previa, in which the placenta covers the internal os in the third trimester, and marginal placenta previa, in which the placenta is within 2 to 3 cm of the internal os but does not cover the os. The rationale for this classification system is the ambiguity and lack of clinical utility of the term *low-lying placenta*. Until recently, there had been no accepted definition of how close the placenta must be to mandate cesarean birth or double setup examination. There is no increased risk of intrapartum hemorrhage if the distance from the lower margin of the placenta to the internal os is at least 2 to 3 cm (Vergani et al., 2009). The term *placental migration* (a misnomer) has been used to describe the apparent movement of the placenta away from the cervical os. The placenta does not move; it remains in place as the uterus expands away from the os.

Clinical Manifestations

Painless uterine bleeding during the second or third trimester characterizes placenta previa. The first significant bleeding episode may occur before 30 weeks' gestation; some women never exhibit bleeding as a symptom until labor develops (Hull & Resnik, 2014). Rarely is the first bleeding episode life-threatening or a cause of hypovolemic shock due to the increased blood volume in pregnancy. The bright red bleeding may be intermittent or continuous. After the initial bleeding episode, women may demonstrate "spotting" of bright red or dark brown blood on the peripad. Second or third episodes of bleeding can be sudden and have significant consequences for the oxygenation of the mother and fetus.

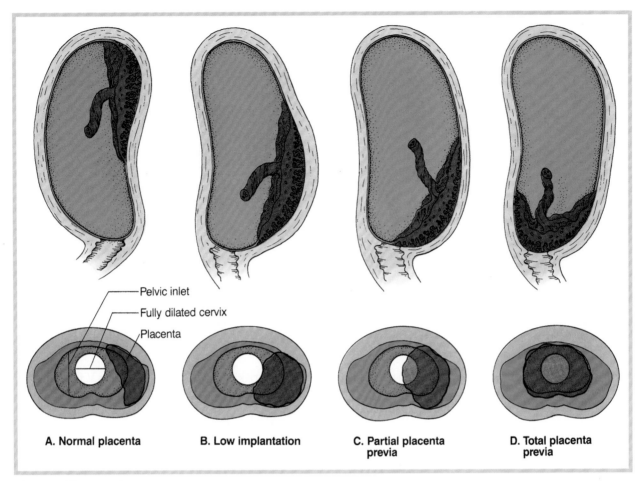

- Pelvic inlet
- Fully dilated cervix
- Placenta

A. Normal placenta   **B. Low implantation**   **C. Partial placenta previa**   **D. Total placenta previa**

FIGURE 6–1. Placenta previa.

Diagnosis

The standard for the diagnosis of placenta previa is an ultrasound examination. Transvaginal ultrasound provides precise information regarding the placement of the placenta in relation to the cervical os (Hull & Resnik, 2014; Oyelese & Smulian, 2006; SMFM & Gyamfi-Bannerman, 2018). If ultrasound reveals a normally implanted placenta, a speculum examination is performed to exclude local causes of bleeding (e.g., cervicitis, polyps, carcinoma of the cervix), and a coagulation profile is obtained to exclude other causes of bleeding. Diagnosis of placenta previa increased dramatically with the advent of transabdominal ultrasound; the rate has decreased with the use of transvaginal or translabial ultrasound (Oyelese & Smulian, 2006). Placenta previa is most often diagnosed before the onset of bleeding when an ultrasound examination is performed for other indications.

Management

Conservative management is usually possible when the fetus is not mature and maternal status is stable. For women with placenta previa who are stable and without bleeding or complications, delivery is recommended at 36 to 36 6/7 weeks (SMFM & Gyamfi-Bannerman, 2018).

Most births are by cesarean section, although vaginal birth may be achieved if the placental edge does not completely cover the cervical os. This type of vaginal birth should occur in the operating room with personnel and equipment available for a cesarean birth if needed (i.e., a double setup).

Patients are frequently hospitalized with the initial bleeding episode. Those with recurrent bleeding episodes, recurrent uterine activity associated with bleeding, or evidence of fetal or maternal compromise usually remain hospitalized until the birth. Some women will have a life-threatening bleeding event. For women who are unstable, blood should be cross-matched and intravenous (IV) access maintained. For stable patients with occasional spotting, a saline lock may be used to maintain an IV access site. In the event of sudden-onset hemorrhage, a second IV line should be initiated with a large-bore catheter because it is very difficult to obtain IV access when the woman is in shock. Recommended management for women who experience an initial mild bleeding episode at 34 to 35 weeks that resolves, are hemodynamically stable, demonstrate fetal well-being, and have emergency services readily available to them is less clear (Hull & Resnik, 2014; Oyelese & Smulian, 2006; SMFM & Gyamfi-Bannerman, 2018). Cervical

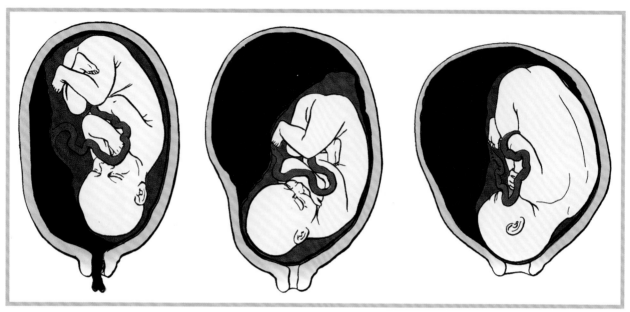

FIGURE 6–2. Abruptio placentae at various separation sites: external hemorrhage (*left*), internal or concealed hemorrhage (*center*), and complete separation (*right*).

length screening is not recommended as a method to assess which women are more or less likely to have another bleed (SMFM & Gyamfi-Bannerman, 2018).

Placental Abruption

Placental abruption is the detachment of a part or all of the placenta from its implantation site before delivery, typically occurring after the 20th week of pregnancy (Fig. 6–2). Recent studies have shown an increase in adverse outcomes with severe abruption, including Apgar scores of less than 7 at 1 and 5 minutes, neonatal and maternal complications (Ananth et al., 2016; Pariente et al., 2011). Risk factors associated with placental abruption are listed in Display 6–2. Despite these reported risk factors, the exact cause of placental abruption is unknown. There may be some type of disease or damage to the blood vessels; this may be of long duration. The risk of recurrence in subsequent pregnancies has been reported as high as 5% to 16% (Hull & Resnik, 2014). Women with two previous placental abruptions have a risk of recurrence of 25% (Hull & Resnik, 2014). Women with severe preeclampsia and eclampsia are at high risk for placental abruption. This high-risk status includes women with mild pregnancy-induced or chronic hypertension. A placental abruption significant enough to cause fetal death is less common (1 in 420 births), but as use of cocaine has increased, fetal death associated with abruptio placentae has risen in selected populations (Hull & Resnik, 2014). Thrombophilias, such as factor V Leiden or the antiphospholipid antibody syndrome (APS), were thought to be associated with an increased risk of abruption (Sibai, 2005); however, studies have shown that there is no increased risk of abruption with factor V Leiden mutation (Hull & Resnik, 2014).

Clinical Manifestations

Placental abruption is suspected in the woman presenting with sudden-onset, intense, often localized, uterine pain or tenderness with or without vaginal bleeding. The woman may also present with preterm contractions with vaginal bleeding or with an occult abruption in the absence of abdominal pain. The pain from abruption may be difficult to distinguish from the pain of labor contractions. Pain may be localized to the area

---

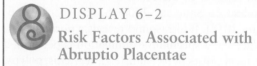

DISPLAY 6–2
Risk Factors Associated with Abruptio Placentae

- Partial abruption of current pregnancy
- Prior abruptio placentae
- Hypertension, chronic
- Gestational hypertension or preeclampsia
- Cigarette smoking (dose-related risk)
- Thrombophilias (not factor V Leiden or MTFHR)
- Blunt abdominal trauma, motor vehicle accidents
- Preterm premature rupture of membranes <34 weeks' gestation
- Early pregnancy bleeding with subchorionic hemorrhage
- Cocaine use

Adapted from Hull, A. D., & Resnik, R. (2014). Placenta previa, placenta accreta, abruptio placentae, and vasa previa. In R. K. Creasy, R. Resnik, J. D. Iams, C. J. Lockwood, T. R. Moore, & M. F. Greene (Eds.), *Creasy and Resnik's maternal–fetal medicine: Principles and practice* (7th ed., p. 739). Philadelphia, PA: Saunders Elsevier. Copyright 2014 by Saunders Elsevier.

of the abruption. When placental implantation is posterior, lower back pain may be more prominent than uterine tenderness. Occasionally, nausea and vomiting may occur. Vaginal bleeding from a placental abruption is not usually proportional to the degree of placental detachment because blood may become trapped behind the placenta. Approximately 10% of women present with concealed hemorrhage when the abruption is located centrally, and no vaginal bleeding is visualized initially (Hull & Resnik, 2014). Marginal separations and large abruptions are associated with bright red bleeding and are almost always accompanied by contractions that are usually of low amplitude and high frequency (Hull & Resnik, 2014; Oyelese & Ananth, 2010; Oyelese & Smulian, 2006). Contractions may be difficult to record if there is an increase in uterine resting tone and for women at earlier gestations. Palpation for uterine contractions or hypertonus is necessary. The contraction pattern of women with an evolving placental abruption often will show frequent contractions of short duration. Fetal assessment by electronic fetal monitoring (EFM) should be accomplished before obtaining a full uterine ultrasound because ultrasound cannot accurately identify a placental abruption in up to 50% of cases (SMFM & Gyamfi-Bannerman, 2018).

The fetal response to placental abruption depends on the volume of blood loss and the extent of uteroplacental insufficiency. Anticipatory nursing care includes being alert to the possibility of an abruption in the presence of any or all of the following: fetal tachycardia, bradycardia, loss of variability, presence of late decelerations, decreasing baseline (especially from tachycardia to a normal or near-normal baseline with minimal or absent variability), a sinusoidal fetal heart rate (FHR) pattern, uterine irritability, uterine hypertonus, or abdominal pain.

The Kleihauer–Betke (KB) test may be performed on the mother's serum or vaginal blood to test for the presence of fetal red blood cells (RBCs). Fetal–maternal transfer of blood is documented by a positive KB, indicating the presence of fetal RBCs in maternal serum (Silver, 2007). Cesarean birth is not always indicated. The decision to proceed with cesarean birth is usually based on fetal status. In the setting of a category I FHR tracing, expectant management may be appropriate for those women who are preterm and not in labor, providing the abruption is small and the mother and fetus are stable. Vaginal or cesarean birth, whichever mode presents the fewest risks to the woman and/or fetus, is indicated for significant bleeding or coagulopathy. Some women with an abruption may demonstrate very rapid labor progress (Hull & Resnik, 2014). Chronic placental abruption may develop, with the woman experiencing episodic bleeding, subjecting the fetus to prolonged stress and increased risk of IUGR (Hull & Resnik, 2014; Oyelese & Ananth, 2010). Risk of developing

disseminated intravascular coagulation (DIC) exists during placental abruption because of release of thromboplastin from the site into the maternal bloodstream.

Diagnosis

The diagnosis of placental abruption is based on the woman's history, clinical presentation, physical examination, and laboratory studies. Examination of the placenta at birth or by a pathologist confirms the diagnosis. Ultrasonography is used to exclude placenta previa; however, it is not diagnostic for abruption (Hull & Resnik, 2014). Abruptions are classified as partial, marginal (i.e., only the margin of the placenta is involved), or total (i.e., complete).

Management

Treatment depends on maternal and fetal status. In the presence of fetal compromise, severe hemorrhage, coagulopathy, poor labor progress, or increasing uterine resting tone, an emergent cesarean birth is performed once efforts to stabilize the woman have been initiated. A vaginal birth may be attempted if the mother is hemodynamically stable and the fetus is alive with a normal FHR tracing, vaginal birth is imminent, or if mother is stable and the fetus is demised. If the mother is hemodynamically unstable, attempts are first directed at maternal stabilization.

IV access is established; if possible, two lines are placed. Blood replacement products and lactated Ringer's solution are infused in quantities necessary to maintain urine output of 30 to 60 mL/hr and a minimal hematocrit of approximately 21% to 24% (Lyndon et al., 2015). Blood loss is almost always underestimated, leading to the current recommendations of quantifying blood loss (Lyndon et al., 2015). Replacement of blood products resuscitation is aggressive in the presence of hemorrhage. Obstetric safety bundles and massive transfusion protocols include a recommended ratio of blood replacement products, such as a ratio of 4 to 6 units of packed red blood cells (PRBCs) to 4 units of fresh frozen plasma (FFP) to 1 unit of apheresis platelets, possibly including 10 units of cryoprecipitate (Lyndon et al., 2015; Roth, Parfitt, Hering, & Dent, 2014). With rapid volume IV infusions, the nurse anticipates the possibility of pulmonary edema due to lower colloid osmotic pressure in pregnancy. DIC may develop, placing the mother at significant risk for maternal morbidity and mortality.

Abnormal Placental Implantation

Abnormal adherence of the placenta is thought to be the result of blastocyst implantation in an area of defective decidua basalis where there is a uterine scar or damage to the area where the endometrium–myometrium join

(Jauniaux, Collins, & Burton, 2018). The rising rate of cesarean births has contributed to the increased rate of abnormal implantation (ACOG, 2017b; Eller et al., 2011; You & Zahn, 2006). The risk of placenta accreta is increased with the number of previous cesarean births; the odds ratio increases from 1.3 for a second cesarean birth to 29.8 for the sixth or greater cesarean births (ACOG, 2017b; Comstock, 2011; Wright et al., 2011). Artificial reproductive technology, dilation and curettage, and minor surgical procedures may also lead to abnormal placental adherence (Jauniaux et al., 2018). When pregnancy is complicated by placenta previa, the risk of accreta is much greater, increasing to 67% for women with four or more cesarean births presenting with anterior or central placenta previa (Lyndon et al., 2015; Wright et al., 2011). Patients with one prior cesarean birth who present with anterior or central placenta previa in the subsequent pregnancy have a 24% risk of placenta accreta (ACOG, 2012b). Placenta accreta and uterine atony are the two most common causes of postpartum hysterectomy (ACOG, 2017a; Eller et al., 2011). Other risk factors include advanced maternal age, smoking, and a short interconception period.

Clinical Manifestations

Placenta accreta spectrum (PAS) is a term encompassing abnormal placental adherence and abnormal invasion (Jauniaux et al., 2018). Previously, PAS was described as placenta accreta, placenta increta, or placenta percreta. All grades of adherence abnormalities may occur in the same placental bed (Jauniaux et al., 2018). Placenta accreta occurs when there is a lack of decidua basalis so that the placenta is implanted directly into the myometrium. Complete accreta occurs when the entire placenta is adherent, partial accreta occurs with one or more cotyledons adherent, and focal accreta occurs with one piece of a cotyledon adherent. Placenta increta is the abnormal invasion of the trophoblastic cells into the uterine wall and myometrium circulation. Placenta percreta occurs when the trophoblast cells penetrate the uterine musculature, and the placenta develops on organs in the vicinity of the percreta. Placenta percreta can adhere to the bladder and other pelvic organs and vessels. Placenta percreta accounts for only 5% to 7% of cases of abnormal adherence. Placenta increta occurs in 15% to 18% of cases, and accreta is the most common form accounting for 75% to 80% of PAS cases (Comstock, 2011; You & Zahn, 2006). Figure 6–3 demonstrates abnormal adherence of the placenta.

Diagnosis

PAS is most often diagnosed in late in the second trimester or early in the third trimester with transabdominal ultrasound (Jauniaux et al., 2018). Second trimester elevated maternal serum alpha-fetoprotein levels were

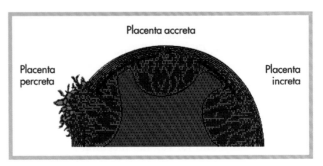

FIGURE 6–3. Abnormal adherence of the placenta.

noted in studies to be elevated in women with placenta previa and accreta (Lyndon et al., 2015). The diagnosis of an abnormally adherent placenta was made historically when manual separation of a retained placenta was attempted. If the placenta does not separate readily, rapid surgical intervention may be indicated. The woman with an abnormally attached placenta is at increased risk for hemorrhage; 90% of women lose more than 3,000 mL of blood intraoperatively, and the maternal mortality rate has been reported as high as 7% to 10% (Wright et al., 2011; You & Zahn, 2006).

Management

It is recommended that women with a history of prior cesarean birth have an ultrasound to determine if there is a placenta previa. If so, further screening for an accreta via ultrasound and/or magnetic resonance imaging (MRI) is recommended (Lyndon et al., 2015). However, use of MRI is not recommended for women who are acutely bleeding between 34 and 36 weeks' gestation (SMFM & Gyamfi-Bannerman, 2018). Planning for the potential of significant maternal blood loss and its sequelae is critical. If there is a diagnosis or strong suspicion of placenta accreta prior to birth, ACOG (2012b) recommends the following measures: The woman should be counseled about the likelihood of hysterectomy and blood transfusion; blood products and clotting factors should be available, and cell saver technology should be considered if available; the appropriate location and timing of birth should be considered to allow access to adequate surgical personnel and equipment; and preoperative anesthesia assessment should be obtained. These anticipatory steps improve the potential for the best possible outcome.

Women who are diagnosed with placental attachment disorders at the time of delivery are at higher risk for developing shock, thrombosis, infection, ureteral injury, and acute respiratory distress syndrome (ARDS) as well as for an increased risk of death. Management includes late preterm delivery for women diagnosed with placenta previa with PAS (ACOG, 2019). Mobilization of a multidisciplinary team including nursing and medical staff, anesthesia, blood bank, surgery, and radiology is necessary immediately to perform the cesarean hysterectomy if necessary (Shamshirsaz et al., 2018;

Snegovskikh, Clebone, & Norwitz, 2011). An interventional radiologist may be needed if selective embolization of the hypogastric arteries with an absorbable gel is needed to reduce blood loss (Eller et al., 2011; You & Zahn, 2006). In hospitals where specialized services may not be immediately available, the nurse can anticipate the need for calling in extra staff, alerting on-call physicians, obtaining uncrossed O-negative blood, and proceeding to hysterectomy. Patients may receive erythropoietin before the surgery, with thrombosis prevention, antibiotics, and fluid resuscitation during the surgery. Invasive hemodynamic monitoring is continuous. It is recommended that 8 to 10 units of PRBCs be available in the operating room, with the blood bank maintaining the same amount (Eller et al., 2011).

Vasa Previa

Clinical Manifestations/Diagnosis

Vasa previa is the result of a velamentous insertion of the umbilical cord. With vasa previa, the umbilical cord is implanted into the membranes rather than into the placenta. The vessels then traverse within the membrane, crossing the cervical os before reaching the placenta. The umbilical vein and arteries are not surrounded by Wharton's jelly, so they have no supportive tissue, which predisposes the umbilical blood vessels to laceration; this condition occurs most often during either spontaneous or artificial rupture of the membranes (Oyelese & Smulian, 2006; Robinson & Grobman, 2011). The sudden appearance of bright red blood at the time of spontaneous or artificial rupture of the membranes, coupled with the sudden onset of an indeterminate or abnormal FHR pattern, should immediately alert the nurse to the possibility of vasa previa. Bleeding that is fetal in origin is always significant because of the small volume of fetal blood. Total blood volume in the fetus is approximately 80 to 100 mL/kg, and rapid exsanguination can result in severe neurologic injury or fetal death (Silver, 2007).

Management

Immediate cesarean birth is indicated in the presence of vasa previa. Vasa previa rupture may also occur before or after rupture of the membranes; the diagnosis is considered for women with limited antenatal bleeding and indeterminate or abnormal FHR patterns. Risk factors associated with vasa previa are listed in Display 6–3.

Although it rarely occurs (approximately 1 in 2,500 births or 1 in 50 cases in which there is a velamentous insertion of the cord), vasa previa is associated with high incidence of fetal morbidity and mortality because fetal bleeding rapidly leads to shock and exsanguination (Oyelese et al., 2004; Robinson & Grobman, 2011; SMFM & Gyamfi-Bannerman, 2018). Diagnosis before birth may be made with color Doppler ultrasound. Transvaginal ultrasound is indicated if placental

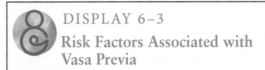

DISPLAY 6–3

Risk Factors Associated with Vasa Previa

- Succenturiate-lobed placenta
- Bilobed placenta
- Velamentous cord insertion
- Low-lying placenta observed in the second trimester
- In vitro fertilization
- Multiple gestation

Adapted from Hull, A. D., & Resnik, R. (2014). Placenta previa, placenta accreta, abruptio placentae, and vasa previa. In R. K. Creasy, R. Resnik, J. D. Iams, C. J. Lockwood, T. R. Moore, & M. F. Greene (Eds.), *Creasy and Resnik's maternal–fetal medicine: Principles and practice* (7th ed., p. 737). Philadelphia, PA: Saunders Elsevier. Copyright 2014 by Saunders Elsevier.

cord insertion cannot be determined transabdominally (Hull & Resnik, 2014; Oyelese & Smulian, 2006). If noted, planned cesarean birth is accomplished at 34 to 35 weeks' gestation (Robinson & Grobman, 2011). The survival rate in one retrospective study was 56% without a prenatal diagnosis versus 97% with a prenatal diagnosis (Oyelese et al., 2004).

In the case of an antenatal bleeding event, some practitioners suggest obtaining a KB test, an Apt test, a rosette test, or a flow cytometry to determine if the blood is fetal in origin. These tests have limited clinical utility during labor because of the short time required from rupture to birth to save the fetus; complete exsanguination can occur in less than 10 minutes as all of the fetal cardiac output moves through the umbilical cord (Hull & Resnik, 2014).

Uterine Rupture

Uterine rupture may be a catastrophic event for the woman and fetus, whether related to rupture of a uterine scar from prior uterine surgery, tachysystole, trauma, or, rarely, spontaneous rupture of the uterus. The terms *uterine rupture* and *uterine dehiscence* are sometimes used interchangeably in the literature. Uterine rupture refers to the actual separation of the uterine myometrium or previous uterine scar, with rupture of the membranes and possible extrusion of the fetus or fetal parts into the peritoneal cavity. Dehiscence refers to a separation of the old scar with the uterine serosa remaining intact; the fetus remains inside the uterus (Lang & Landon, 2010). Excessive bleeding usually occurs with uterine rupture, whereas bleeding is generally minimal with dehiscence.

Uterine rupture occurs most frequently in women with a previous uterine incision through the myometrium and usually occurs during labor, although it can occur in the antepartum period. Hyperstimulation or hypertonus of the uterus by oxytocin or prostaglandin administration can cause uterine rupture even in the

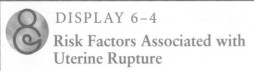

DISPLAY 6–4

Risk Factors Associated with Uterine Rupture

- Sequential labor induction with prostaglandins and oxytocin
- Previous uterine surgery
- Labor augmentation with oxytocin
- Antepartum fetal death
- Previous first trimester miscarriages
- <16-month interdelivery interval
- Previous cesarean delivery with severe postpartum hemorrhage

Adapted from Al-Zirqi, I., Daltveit, A. K., Forsén, L., Stray-Pedersen, B., & Vangen, S. (2017). Risk factors for complete uterine rupture. *American Journal of Obstetrics & Gynecology, 216*(2), 165.

unscarred uterus (Catanzarite, Cousins, Dowling, & Daneshmand, 2006; Lang & Landon, 2010; Mazzone & Woolever, 2006). The use of misoprostol is contraindicated for third trimester use in patients with a previously scarred uterus from cesarean section, myomectomy, or other uterine surgeries (ACOG, 2017b; Scott, 2011). Invasive or blunt trauma, seen in women after a motor vehicle accident, battery, fall, or with knife or gunshot wound, is an additional cause of uterine rupture. Uterine rupture may also occur spontaneously with no history of uterine surgery or terminations of pregnancy. Display 6–4 describes the risk factors associated with uterine rupture.

Clinical Manifestations

The clinical presentation of the woman experiencing a uterine rupture depends on the specific type of rupture and may develop over several hours or may be sudden. Impending rupture may be preceded by increasing uterine hypertonus or tachysystole (Lang & Landon, 2010; Sheiner et al., 2004). Contrary to earlier reports, there is usually no decrease in uterine tone or cessation of contractions prior to or during uterine rupture (ACOG, 2010; Lang & Landon, 2010), although this finding has been reported by some researchers (Sheiner et al., 2004). Indeterminate or abnormal changes in the FHR pattern are early signs of impending or evolving uterine rupture and are seen in up to 70% of cases of uterine rupture (ACOG, 2010, 2017b; Cahill & Macones, 2007; Lang & Landon, 2010; Sheiner et al., 2004). The FHR pattern prior to rupture or as the rupture is evolving may be characterized by a decrease in variability, recurrent variables, prolonged or late decelerations followed by bradycardia, or sudden onset of fetal bradycardia (Ayres, Johnson, & Hayashi, 2001; Lang & Landon, 2010; Menihan, 1999; Ridgeway, Weyrich, & Benedetti, 2004). The most consistent FHR patterns noted with uterine rupture are recurrent variable or late decelerations and fetal bradycardia (ACOG, 2010,

2017b; Ayres et al., 2001; Lang & Landon, 2010; Ridgeway et al., 2004). If the uterine rupture is preceded by late decelerations, the fetus will tolerate a shorter period of prolonged decelerations. Significant neonatal morbidity has been reported when the time between onset of prolonged decelerations and birth is equal to or greater than 17 minutes (Scott, 2011). Jauregui, Kirkendall, Ahn, and Phelan (2000) reported a significant risk of brain damage, intrapartum death, and death within 1 year of life for infants who were partially or completely extruded into the maternal abdomen during uterine rupture.

The woman with a uterine rupture may complain of abdominal pain and tenderness and/or have vomiting, syncope, vaginal bleeding, tachycardia, or pallor. If unrecognized, bleeding can quickly cause maternal hypotension and shock. A traumatic rupture may be apparent almost immediately in the woman who complains of sharp, tearing pain. There may be an inability on the part of the practitioner to reach the presenting part on vaginal examination, demonstrating loss of fetal station. Uterine contractions may decrease in frequency and intensity or demonstrate tachysystole (Lang & Landon, 2010; Scott, 2011). The fetus may be palpated through the abdominal wall. Bleeding may be vaginal or into the abdominal cavity or both. Intraabdominal bleeding is suspected if the woman has a tense, acute abdomen with shoulder pain. Signs of shock appear soon after a catastrophic rupture, and complete cardiovascular collapse rapidly follows without prompt intervention.

Dehiscence of a prior lower segment cesarean scar is usually initially asymptomatic. The woman may continue to have contractions without further dilation of the cervix. If an intrauterine pressure catheter is in place for labor assessments, there may be little or no change in intrauterine pressure or resting tone pressures. If the dehiscence extends past the scar tissue, the woman may begin to complain of pain in the lower abdomen that is unrelieved with analgesia or epidural anesthesia.

Common sequelae associated with uterine rupture include excessive hemorrhage requiring surgical exploration; need for hysterectomy; need for blood product transfusion; hypovolemia; hypovolemic shock; injury to the bladder or ureters; bowel laceration; extrusion of any part of the fetus, umbilical cord, or placenta through the disruption; emergent cesarean birth for suspected rupture; emergent cesarean birth for indeterminate or abnormal fetal status; and general anesthesia (ACOG, 2010; Landon et al., 2004; Paré, Quiñones, & Macones, 2006; Scott, 2011).

Diagnosis

The key to diagnosis is suspicion that uterine rupture has occurred. The nurse immediately should inform the primary healthcare provider at the first suspicion of a uterine rupture based on characteristics of the FHR pattern and maternal condition. Diagnosis is confirmed at birth.

Management

Treatment includes maternal hemodynamic stabilization and immediate cesarean birth. If possible, the uterine defect is repaired, or hysterectomy is performed. Uterine rupture is discussed further in Chapter 14.

NURSING ASSESSMENT

A medical history may be available in the prenatal record and can be assessed for previous bleeding or bleeding disorders in order to assist the nurse in identifying risk factors for obstetrical precursors to hemorrhage. Assessment of the woman who is bleeding begins with careful evaluation of amount and color of blood loss, character of uterine activity, presence of abdominal pain, stability of maternal vital signs, and fetal status. Bright red vaginal bleeding suggests active bleeding, and dark or brown blood may indicate past blood loss. Skin and mucous membrane color is noted. Inspection also includes looking for oozing at the sites of incisions or injections and detecting petechiae or ecchymosis in areas not associated with surgery or trauma. Display 6–5 presents nursing assessments and interventions for abnormal bleeding and/or hemorrhage.

Maternal or fetal tachycardia and maternal hypotension suggest hypovolemia; however, hypotension is a late sign. Historically, the frequency of vital signs depends on patient stability. Vital signs are usually repeated every 15 minutes until the bleeding is controlled and the vital signs remain or return to normal. Vital signs are performed more frequently (every 1 to 5 minutes) when there is evidence of instability, including systolic blood pressure less than 90 mm Hg, maternal tachycardia, decreasing level of consciousness, and oliguria.

Many automatic blood pressure monitors calculate mean arterial pressure (MAP = systolic blood pressure + 2 × diastolic blood pressure / 3), which provides a quick number for reference and is a more stable parameter of hemodynamic function. The normal value for mean arterial pressure in the second trimester of pregnancy is approximately 80 mm Hg (Page & Christianson, 1976) and is 90 mm Hg at term. When the blood pressure cannot be assessed with a blood pressure cuff, systolic blood pressure may be estimated by the presence of a radial, femoral, or brachial pulse. The presence of a radial pulse is associated with a systolic blood pressure of approximately 80 mm Hg, a femoral pulse with a blood pressure of 70 mm Hg, and a carotid pulse with a blood pressure of 60 mm Hg (Ruth & Mighty, 2019). Placement of an arterial line in the woman who is hemorrhaging allows

DISPLAY 6–5
Nursing Assessments and Interventions for Abnormal Bleeding/Hemorrhage

Initial Nursing Interventions
- Notify physician and/or nurse midwife and anesthesia providers.
- Secure airway; start oxygen via nonrebreather mask at 10 L/min.
- Establish intravenous (IV) access if there is not an existing IV line: Infuse lactated Ringer's solution (or normal saline) wide open, start another IV with a 16-gauge catheter. (Do not infuse IV solutions containing glucose.)
- Perform uterine massage.
- Obtain complete blood count (CBC), fibrinogen, prothrombin time (PT), partial thromboplastin time (PTT), and other laboratory tests as ordered.
- Draw 5 mL of the patient's blood in a red-top tube and observe frequently. If no clot forms within 5 to 10 minutes, suspect coagulopathy.
- Type and cross-match 4 units of packed red blood cells (PRBCs).
- Administer oxytocin, methylergonovine, prostaglandin $F_{2\alpha}$, misoprostol, tranexamic acid, or factor VII as ordered.
- Administer blood products as ordered. Institute massive transfusion protocol if available.

Secondary Nursing Interventions
- Insert Foley catheter with urometer; assess for output of at least 30 mL/hr.
- Apply oxygen saturation monitor.
- Assess maternal vital signs per hospital policy.
- Call for additional nursing help so that one nurse can be responsible for patient care and another nurse is available for obtaining necessary medications, administering IV fluids, and monitoring intake and output if possible.
- Obtain CBC, PT, PTT, fibrinogen, ionized calcium, and potassium after 5 to 7 units of PRBCs.
- Anticipate surgical intervention such as exploratory laparotomy, Bakri balloon, uterine artery embolization, bilateral uterine artery ligation, B-lynch suture, hypogastric artery ligation, and hysterectomy. Notify members of the surgical team and ensure that a surgical suite is readied.

for continuous, accurate blood pressure monitoring and provides a means for drawing blood for arterial blood gas analysis and other laboratory values. Invasive hemodynamic monitoring with a flow-directed pulmonary artery catheter (Swan-Ganz) may be indicated in selected patients, especially in patients who remain oliguric after fluid resuscitation (Clark, Greenspoon, Aldahl, & Phelan, 1986) or who have other complications such as sepsis, cardiac or pulmonary disease, or severe hypertension related to preeclampsia.

Antenatally, FHR is continuously assessed, and the uterus is palpated for contractions, especially in early gestations. In an emergent situation, use of electronic FHR and uterine monitoring provides continuous data about the fetus and uterus, allowing the nurse time to

DISPLAY 6–6

Laboratory Values Assessed in Pregnant Women Who Are Bleeding

- Complete blood count
- Fibrinogen concentration
- Prothrombin time
- Activated partial thromboplastin time
- Fibrin degradation products or fibrin split products
- Platelet count
- Blood type, Rh, and antibody screen
- Whole blood clotting time

Possibly Indicated

- Kleihauer-Betke test
- Apt test
- Bleeding time
- D-dimer
- Serum creatinine
- Blood urea nitrogen
- Urine creatinine clearance
- Urine sodium excretion
- Liver function test, including serum glucose
- Antithrombin III
- Arterial blood gases
- Urine or serum drug screen

by nonrebreather facemask at 10 L/min to maintain maternal–fetal oxygen saturation. Mentation is assessed frequently and provides additional indication of maternal blood volume and oxygen saturation.

Blood is drawn to assess maternal hemoglobin, hematocrit, platelet count, and coagulation profile. Display 6–6 lists the blood tests commonly ordered for the woman who is bleeding. In an emergent situation, blood may be drawn into a red-top (plain) tube, the tube taped to a wall and then visually evaluated for clot formation. Treatment for a significant coagulopathy should be initiated if no sign of clotting is evident within 5 to 10 minutes (Lyndon et al., 2015; Rajan & Wing, 2010; SMFM & Gyamfi-Bannerman, 2018). Massive hemorrhage protocols offer guidance for volume replacement. The California Maternal Quality Care Collaborative (CMQCC) recommends a ratio of 4 to 6 units PRBCs, 4 units FFP, and 1 unit apheresis platelets (Lyndon et al., 2015). Cryoprecipitate should be considered for patients who have a fibrinogen <80 or a specific clotting disorder needing such factors (Lyndon et al., 2015). Table 6–1 lists blood replacement products, factors present, and the expected effect per unit administered.

Circulating volume is usually restored with IV crystalloid solution administration. Two large-bore IV lines are needed for fluid replacement and administration of drug therapies. Blood and blood products are administered as needed or as soon as they are available. Breath sounds are auscultated before fluid volume replacement, if possible, to provide a baseline for future assessment. Massive fluid replacement during pregnancy or the immediate postpartum period for the woman who is hemorrhaging increases the potential for development of pulmonary edema. However, fluid replacement is necessary to restore circulatory volume, and the nurse anticipates and assesses for the development of peripheral or pulmonary edema and treatment

simultaneously initiate other needed treatments. The pregnant woman is positioned in the lateral or modified Trendelenburg position, if possible. If the patient is in Trendelenburg or supine position, a wedge is placed under one hip to alleviate compression of the vena cava and aorta by the gravid uterus. Caution must be used in placing a pregnant woman in Trendelenburg because the pressure of the gravid uterus may interfere with optimal cardiopulmonary functioning. If the mother is hemodynamically unstable, oxygen is administered

TABLE 6–1. Blood Replacement Products

| | | Blood component therapy | |
Product	Volume (mL)*	Contents	Effect (per unit)
Fresh whole blood	500	Red blood cells, all procoagulants	Increase hematocrit by 3 percentage points, hemoglobin by 1 g/dL
Packed red blood cells	240	Red blood cells, white blood cells, plasma	Increase hematocrit by 3 percentage points, hemoglobin by 1 g/dL
Platelets	50	Platelets, red blood cells, plasma; small amounts of fibrinogen, factors V and VIII	Increase platelet count 5,000 to 10,000/mm^3 per unit
Fresh frozen plasma	250	Fibrinogen, antithrombin III, factors V and VIII	Increase fibrinogen by 10 mg/dL to 25 mg/dL
Cryoprecipitate	40	Fibrinogen, factors VIII and XIII, von Willebrand factor	Increase fibrinogen by 10 mg/dL to 25 mg/dL

*Volume depends on individual blood bank.
Adapted from American College of Obstetricians and Gynecologists. (2017a). *Postpartum hemorrhage* (Practice Bulletin No. 183). Washington, DC: Author; Rajan, P. V., & Wing, D. A. (2010). Postpartum hemorrhage: Evidence-based medical interventions for prevention and treatment. *Clinical Obstetrics and Gynecology, 53*(1), 165–181. doi:10.1097/GRF.0b013e3181ce0965

with furosemide as ordered. Hemoglobin arterial oxygen saturation is monitored with a pulse oximeter. Pulse oximeters are an adjunct to assessment; they are not always accurate, especially in a patient in hypovolemic shock. In the hemorrhagic patient, blood flow to the extremities is decreased, and the oxygen saturation displayed may not accurately reflect tissue oxygenation status or the pulse oximeter may not be able to display a value at all. Arterial blood gas analysis may therefore be necessary to determine oxygen status. A maternal oxygen saturation of at least 95% and a partial pressure of oxygen (P_aO_2) of at least 65 mm Hg are necessary for the fetus to maintain adequate oxygenation.

Continuous electrocardiogram monitoring is indicated for the woman who is hypotensive or tachycardic, continuing to bleed profusely, or in shock. Maternal hypovolemia leading to hypoxia and acidosis may result in maternal heart rate dysrhythmias, including premature ventricular contractions, sinus or atrial tachycardia, and atrial or ventricular fibrillation.

A Foley catheter with a urometer is inserted to allow for hourly assessment of urine output. The most objective and least invasive assessment of adequate organ perfusion and oxygenation is urinary output of at least 30 mL/hr (Ruth & Kennedy, 2011). In addition to volume, urine is assessed for the presence of blood and protein and for specific gravity.

NURSING INTERVENTIONS

Evaluation and management of acute episodes of bleeding during pregnancy usually occur in the inpatient setting. An exception is spotting during early gestation. After stabilization and a period of hospitalization, women may be managed at home or in the hospital.

Inpatient Management

When the woman is admitted to the hospital, the nurse begins assessment of the bleeding. The woman with acute bleeding requires continuous, ongoing nursing assessments and interventions. Maternal vital signs are assessed frequently, according to individual clinical situations. Vital signs and noninvasive assessments of cardiac output (e.g., skin color, skin temperature, pulse oximetry, mentation, urinary output) are obtained frequently to observe for signs of declining hemodynamic status.

Because an indeterminate or abnormal FHR pattern may be the first sign of maternal or fetal hemodynamic compromise, electronic FHR and uterine activity monitoring should be continuous. It is important to appreciate how rapidly maternal–fetal status can deteriorate as a result of maternal hemorrhage. Blood is shunted away from the uterus when the mother experiences hypotension or hypovolemic shock. Because of

the potential for maternal–fetal mortality, it is essential to be prepared for an emergent birth at all times when caring for a pregnant woman who is bleeding. Supportive staff necessary for an emergency cesarean birth (i.e., anesthesia personnel, surgical team, and neonatal resuscitation team) should be notified and on standby (if possible, in the hospital). Hemorrhage from placenta previa, abruptio placentae, or uterine rupture requires expeditious birth. The need to replace fluids and blood is determined by a number of parameters, including vital signs, amount of blood loss, mental status, laboratory values, and fetal condition.

Communication with the blood bank is essential. Significant hemorrhage resulting in syncope or hypovolemic shock generally necessitates transfusion. Two large-bore IV catheters (at least 18 gauge) are placed if the woman is experiencing heavy bleeding. If consistent with institution policy, a 14- or 16-gauge IV catheter may be considered. Fluid replacement consists of administering lactated Ringer's or normal saline solution, PRBC, FFP, cryoprecipitate, and, possibly, platelets.

Blood type, Rhesus (Rh), and antibody screen should be obtained on admission; cross-matching is ordered as necessary. The use of blood components in conjunction with crystalloid solutions, rather than with whole blood, is usually a better treatment option because it provides only the specific components needed (Fuller & Bucklin, 2010; Ruth & Kennedy, 2011). By using only the specific products required for the emergency, blood resources are conserved, and there is a decreased risk of blood replacement complications. Transfusion reactions may be demonstrated by chills, fever, tachycardia, hypotension, shortness of breath, muscle cramps, itching, convulsions, and, ultimately, cardiac arrest. The woman is assessed throughout the procedure. In the event of a reaction, the transfusion is immediately discontinued, and the IV line is flushed with normal saline. Treatment is then based on clinical symptoms. The development of anaphylaxis should be considered and appropriate treatment made available.

Careful fetal surveillance is critical to ensure fetal well-being during transfusion of multiple blood products. The increased incidence of uteroplacental insufficiency is related to complications of coagulation factor replacement therapy (Simpson, Luppi, & O'Brien-Abel, 1998) and the amount and duration of blood loss (Ruth & Kennedy, 2011). Administration of multiple replacement blood products leads to increased intravascular fibrin formation. Deposition of fibrin in the decidual vasculature of the chorionic villi may cause fetal compromise.

Because of the normal hemodynamic changes that occur, pregnant women may lose more than one fourth of their fluid volume before displaying signs of shock (Clark, 2004). Women who are bleeding should be monitored carefully for the actual amount of blood loss, although this is sometimes difficult to assess in an emergent situation and is usually underestimated (Ruth & Kennedy, 2011). Quantified blood loss should be followed closely in order to accurately assess blood loss. Accurate intake and output measurement and documentation are critical. Ideally, one nurse is assigned to monitor intake and output during a period of massive fluid and blood replacement. In an emergent situation in which the obstetrician and anesthesiologist may be ordering or adding replacement fluid to multiple IV lines, it becomes essential that nurses record and maintain a running total of intake and output in addition to signing for blood products and overseeing administration.

The woman may develop a coagulopathy. Display 6–7 lists the risk factors for DIC. Pulmonary edema and renal failure, as evidenced by oliguria proceeding to anuria, must be anticipated. Systolic blood pressures of less than 60 mm Hg are associated with acute renal failure. The woman is at risk for development of acute tubular necrosis from lack of perfusion to the kidneys (i.e., prerenal failure). Prolonged periods of severe hypotension may result in renal cortical necrosis. Urine output of less than 30 mL/hr should be reported to the primary care provider immediately.

In the case of severe hemorrhage, control of abdominal bleeding may be achieved by the placement of medical antishock trousers (MAST) suit, which are used in prehospital settings and in emergency and trauma units to control bleeding. Consensus does not exist about the benefits of using MAST suits; however, MAST suits are used in many institutions. Care must be taken not to put any pressure on the pregnant abdomen past midgestation, but MAST suits can be used for postpartum hemorrhage (Brown, 2009). A nonpneumatic antishock garment is also available, and there is some data to support its use during a hemorrhagic situation (Lyndon et al., 2015).

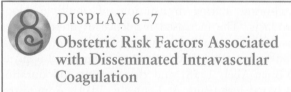

DISPLAY 6–7
Obstetric Risk Factors Associated with Disseminated Intravascular Coagulation

- Abruptio placentae
- Hemorrhage
- Preeclampsia or eclampsia
- Amniotic fluid embolism
- Saline termination of pregnancy
- Sepsis
- Dead fetus syndrome
- Cardiopulmonary arrest
- Massive transfusion therapy

HEMORRHAGIC AND HYPOVOLEMIC SHOCK

Hemorrhagic and hypovolemic shock is an emergent situation in which the perfusion of body organs may become severely compromised and death may ensue. Aggressive treatment is necessary to prevent adverse sequelae (e.g., cellular death, fluid overload, ARDS, or oxygen toxicity). Common clinical symptoms of inadequate intravascular volume (i.e., hypovolemia) that necessitates blood replacement include evidence of hemorrhage (i.e., loss of a large amount of blood externally or internally in a short period of time), evidence of hypovolemic shock (i.e., increasing pulse; cool, clammy skin; rapid breathing; restlessness; and reduced urine output), or a decrease in hemoglobin and hematocrit below acceptable levels for trimester of pregnancy or the nonpregnant state.

Aggressive fluid and blood replacement is not without risk. The 24 hours after the shock period are critical. Observe for fluid overload, ARDS, and oxygen toxicity. Transfusion reactions may follow administration of blood or blood components. Even in an emergency, each unit should be checked per hospital protocol. Rapid transfusion with cold blood can chill the woman and cause vasoconstriction, arrhythmia, or cardiac arrest. Banked blood may be calcium deficient, increasing the risk for arrhythmias and further bleeding. Potassium levels may increase to dangerous levels. Laboratory values for other parameters are usually checked at least every 4 to 6 hours or as indicated by the woman's condition. Display 6–8 suggests a management plan for hypovolemic shock (Fuller & Bucklin, 2010; Ruth & Kennedy, 2011). Most hospitals have developed massive transfusion guidelines or policies for patients who are anticipated to or who need blood product replacement. Infection is another complication of hemorrhage. Causes of infection may include surgical procedures, multiple pelvic examinations, anemia, and loss of the white blood cell component of the blood. It is anticipated that the patient may receive prophylactic antibiotics or treatment for signs of infection.

Hemorrhage is a nursing and medical emergency requiring rapid and efficient teamwork from all members of the healthcare team. Perinatal nurses play an important role in the initial assessments, early interventions, and stabilization of the woman. Recognition that blood loss is out of proportion to the patient's clinical presentation is important because initial vital signs may remain within normal range in the presence of a significant hemorrhage. Anticipating that a woman who is bleeding may rapidly proceed to hypovolemic shock can prevent complications and decrease maternal and fetal morbidity and mortality.

DISPLAY 6–8

Management Plan for Obstetric Hypovolemic Shock

Goals

- Maintain systolic blood pressure ≥90 mm Hg, urine output ≥30 mL/hr, and normal mental status.
- Identify and eliminate source of hemorrhage.
- Avoid overzealous volume replacement that may contribute to pulmonary edema.

Management

- Establish two large-bore intravenous lines.
- Place woman in Trendelenburg position (wedge under hip if undelivered).
- Rapidly infuse 5% dextrose in lactated Ringer's solution while blood products are obtained.
- Infuse fresh whole blood or packed red blood cells, as available.
- Infuse platelets and fresh frozen plasma only as indicated by documented deficiencies in platelets (<30,000/mL) or clotting parameters (fibrinogen, prothrombin time [PT], partial thromboplastin time [PTT]).
- Search for and eliminate the source of hemorrhage.
- Use invasive hemodynamic monitoring if the woman fails to respond to clinically adequate volume replacement.
- Critical laboratory tests include complete blood count, platelet count, fibrinogen, PT, PTT, and arterial blood gas determinations.

THROMBOPHILIAS IN PREGNANCY

Acquired and/or inherited thrombophilias in pregnancy are associated with a myriad of maternal and fetal complications, including maternal thrombosis/embolism. The evidence is insufficient as to if and how strong an association there is with adverse outcomes, including early-onset severe preeclampsia, abruption, fetal growth restriction, fetal loss, and recurrent miscarriage for most thrombophilias (ACOG, 2013; Silver, 2007). The most common acquired thrombophilia during pregnancy is APS (Blackburn, 2018; Sibai, 2005). There is compelling evidence to support an association between APS and adverse outcomes such as fetal loss during pregnancy, preeclampsia, and IUGR (ACOG, 2012a). Of the antiphospholipid antibodies, lupus anticoagulant (a misnomer because it causes thrombosis), anticardiolipin antibody, and anti–beta-2 glycoprotein have the highest association with pregnancy complications. The antibodies are the result of antigenic changes in endothelial and platelet cell membranes, which promote thrombosis (ACOG, 2012a).

Inherited thrombophilias vary in prevalence and ability to cause thrombosis. The most common inherited thrombophilias most likely to cause thrombosis in pregnancy are mutations in factor V Leiden, antithrombin deficiency, prothrombin gene G20210A mutation, tetrahydrofolate reductase, deficiencies in proteins C and S, and platelet collagen receptor alpha-2-beta-1 (ACOG, 2013; Sibai, 2005). Other factors that contribute to thrombosis formation in pregnancy include the normal hypercoagulable state and venous stasis.

Management

Women who have been identified as having a thrombophilia need to be counseled as to current recommendations regarding anticoagulation during pregnancy. Surveillance alone versus prophylaxis/anticoagulation therapy is individualized by history and current clinical indicators. Anticoagulation is not recommended if the woman has no history of venous thromboembolism (VTE) or poor pregnancy outcome. Full- or adjusted-dose anticoagulation with low molecular weight heparin (LMWH) is recommended antenatally and 6 weeks postpartum for women who have antithrombin deficiency, homozygosity for the factor V Leiden mutation, the prothrombin gene G20210A mutation, compound heterozygosity for both mutations, or a current VTE. The same is recommended antenatally and long term for women receiving vitamin K antagonist therapy (ACOG, 2013; James, Abel, & Brancazio, 2006). Women with a history of APS with a previous thrombosis (history of two or more early pregnancy losses, one or more late loss, IUGR, abruption, or preeclampsia) are offered during antepartum a low dose of aspirin, an intermediate dose of unfractionated heparin (UFH), or prophylactic LMWH. Women who have a history of a single episode of VTE and thrombophilia or a strong family history of thrombosis may receive intermediate dose LMWH or UFH antepartum followed with postpartum anticoagulants (ACOG, 2012a).

LMWH has fewer side effects and a longer half-life than UFH. Because of the longer half-life of LMWH, women may not be able to receive regional anesthesia; many women are switched to UFH at 36 weeks (ACOG, 2013). Heparin may be discontinued 24 to 36 hours before a schedule cesarean delivery or induction of labor (ACOG, 2013). Controversy exists regarding which women should be screened for thrombophilias. Individual screening is done based on the woman's history and current pregnancy status. Screening for thrombophilias is considered for women with a history of a VTE with nonrecurrent condition or women with a first-degree relative with a history of high risk for VTE or a VTE prior to the age of 50 years with no known risk factors. Thrombophilia screening is no longer recommended for women with a history of recurrent fetal loss, IUGR, preeclampsia, or abruption (ACOG, 2013). As the current pregnancy progresses, the woman can be tested for thrombophilias if she develops signs and symptoms of VTE.

UFH is associated with the development of osteoporosis and a 2% risk of vertebral fracture as well as heparin-induced thrombocytopenia (HIT). LMWHs are actually fragments of UFHs, which have more activity against factor Xa. There is a lower risk of developing osteoporosis and HIT (James et al., 2006). However, LMWH is costlier, and the longer half-life increases the risk of bleeding in the intrapartum period. Neither UFH nor LMWH crosses the placenta.

Fetal surveillance may be beneficial. Serial ultrasounds for growth and twice-weekly nonstress tests or biophysical profiles can be instituted at 24 to 25 weeks' gestation. The mother can be monitored closely for the development of preeclampsia.

MATERNAL TRAUMA

The perinatal nurse may encounter pregnant women who have experienced trauma as they may be admitted to the labor and delivery unit, the obstetric triage unit, or the obstetric emergency department. In most institutions, women with major trauma are stabilized in the emergency department with the assistance of perinatal healthcare providers who are called to the department for consultation and assessment of fetal well-being, whereas women with minor trauma may be sent directly to the labor and delivery unit. It is important for the obstetric nurse to understand the importance of a thorough assessment of all trauma patients, as approximately 5% to 25% of women who experience minor trauma have an adverse maternal or fetal outcome (Curet, Schermer, Demarest, Bieneik, & Curet, 2000; El Kady et al., 2004). A thorough knowledge of the normal physiologic changes during pregnancy, complications of bleeding and preterm labor, and maternal–fetal assessment is necessary to provide optimum care for pregnant women after trauma.

Approximately 5% to 8% of women experience trauma during pregnancy (Barraco et al., 2010; Brown, 2010). Of women who present to the hospital for treatment, approximately 6% of maternal trauma patients have significant orthopedic injuries, which often are associated with additional adverse outcomes such as increased risk of preterm birth, placental abruption, and perinatal mortality, when compared to pregnant women with trauma excluding orthopedic injuries (Cannada et al., 2010). Therefore, traumatized pregnant women with orthopedic injuries are high-risk obstetrical patients and may benefit from referral to a medical center capable of handling both the primary injury and the potential preterm birth associated with the injury (Cannada et al., 2010). Approximately two thirds of all trauma events during pregnancy are the result of motor vehicle accidents (which may or may not include an orthopedic injury). Motor vehicle accidents are the most significant cause of fetal death due to trauma (Barraco et al., 2010; Brown, 2010). The incidence and severity of injuries can be reduced by appropriate use of automobile safety restraints, education for use of safety restraints while driving, or riding as a passenger in a car should be included in prenatal teaching.

Other significant causes of trauma during pregnancy are falls and direct assaults to the abdomen. During pregnancy, falls are of the most common cause of minor injury and are estimated to cause 17% to 39% of trauma that results in emergency department visits and hospital admissions, second only to motor vehicle accidents (Dunning, LeMasters, & Bhattacharya, 2010). In a study of 3,997 women who had given birth within the previous 2-month period, 27% reported falling at least once during their pregnancy and 10% indicated they fell at least twice (Dunning et al., 2010). Of those who fell, 20% sought medical care and 21% had 2 or more days of restricted activity. Women aged 20 to 24 years had an almost twofold risk of falling more than those over 35 years. Approximately 56% of falls occurred indoors, 39% on stairs, and 9% reported falling from a height greater than 3 ft (Dunning et al., 2010). Injuries associated with falls during pregnancy include fractures, sprains/strains, head injury, rupture of internal organs, placental abruption, uterine rupture, rupture of membranes, and occasionally maternal or fetal death (Dunning et al., 2010).

Intimate partner violence is an increasing source of trauma during pregnancy. Data about incidence of intimate partner violence have been difficult to accumulate because of reporting issues and the frequency of inaccurate description of the causative factors for injury given by the woman. It is estimated that up to 1 out of every 4 women in the United States are victims of intimate partner violence each year (Shay-Zapien & Bullock, 2010). Fetal loss resulting from abdominal trauma may occur because of abruptio placentae or other placenta injury, direct fetal injury, uterine rupture, maternal shock, maternal death, or a combination of these events (Barraco et al., 2010; Oxford & Ludmir, 2009).

Nursing assessment and interventions for the pregnant woman who has experienced trauma are based on the clinical situation and maternal–fetal status. A thorough history is essential and should include the nature of the trauma event, condition and symptoms at time of injury, and current clinical symptoms. The principles of management of preterm labor and complications of bleeding are applied based on the clinical situation. Ongoing maternal–fetal assessments and accurate reporting of findings to the primary healthcare provider are important.

Fortunately, most women who experience trauma suffer only minor injuries that do not require inpatient evaluation for the nonpregnant population. Careful evaluation of maternal–fetal status is warranted when pregnant women present with reports of any type of trauma (Cannada et al., 2010). Reliability of methods to predict which women are at risk for adverse outcomes remains low. The usual signs of complications, including bleeding, uterine tenderness, contractions, and loss of amniotic fluid, are valuable, but they may not be present in all cases (Curet et al., 2000; Muench et al., 2004). Use of ultrasound to exclude placental abruption has the potential to miss 20% to 50% of cases (SMFM & Gyamfi-Bannerman, 2018). Continuous EFM is useful for ongoing evaluation of fetal status and uterine activity. Recommended duration of continuous EFM after trauma ranges from 6 to 24 hours based on clinical signs and symptoms and the mechanism of injury (Curet et al., 2000; Mattox & Goetzl, 2005). Monitoring should be continued, and further evaluation is warranted if uterine contractions, an indeterminate or abnormal FHR pattern, vaginal bleeding, significant uterine tenderness or irritability, serious maternal injury, or rupture of the membranes occurs (Mattox & Goetzl, 2005). Women with a positive KB test may benefit greatly from continuous EFM and assessment of serial KB testing every 6 to 12 hours to determine if the KB value is falling. If the KB value decreases and EFM is normal, the woman may be evaluated for discharge. Rh immune globulin may need to be administered for the Rh-negative woman (Muench et al., 2004). The decision to continue inpatient evaluation, discharge to home, or transfer to another facility is made in collaboration with the primary healthcare provider, consistent with maternal–fetal status, and as outlined in the federal Emergency Medical Treatment and Active Labor Act (EMTALA). See Chapter 13 for maternal transport and discussion of EMTALA.

SUMMARY

When bleeding complicates pregnancy, there is significant risk for adverse outcomes. A thorough knowledge of the nursing care for bleeding complications, including timely identification and appropriate interventions, is required to ensure optimal outcomes for mothers and babies. Postpartum hemorrhage is covered in Chapter 17.

REFERENCES

Al-Zirqi, I., Daltveit, A. K., Forsén, L., Stray-Pedersen, B., & Vangen, S. (2017). Risk factors for complete uterine rupture. *American Journal of Obstetrics & Gynecology, 216*(2), 165.e1–165.e8. doi:10.1016/j.ajog.2016.10.017

American College of Obstetricians and Gynecologists. (2010). *Vaginal birth after previous cesarean delivery* (Practice Bulletin No. 115). Washington, DC: Author.

American College of Obstetricians and Gynecologists. (2012a). *Antiphospholipid syndrome* (Practice Bulletin No. 132; Reaffirmed, 2017). Washington, DC: Author.

American College of Obstetricians and Gynecologists. (2012b). *Placenta accreta* (Committee Opinion No. 529; Reaffirmed, 2017). Washington, DC: Author.

American College of Obstetricians and Gynecologists. (2013). *Inherited thrombophilias in pregnancy* (Practice Bulletin No. 138; Reaffirmed, 2017). Washington, DC: Author.

American College of Obstetricians and Gynecologists. (2016). *Severe maternal morbidity: Screening and review* (Obstetric Care Consensus No. 5). Washington, DC: Author.

American College of Obstetricians and Gynecologists. (2017a). *Postpartum hemorrhage* (Practice Bulletin No. 183). Washington, DC: Author.

American College of Obstetricians and Gynecologists. (2017b). *Vaginal birth after previous cesarean delivery* (Practice Bulletin No. 184). Washington, DC: Author.

American College of Obstetricians and Gynecologists. (2019). *Medical indicated late-preterm and early-term deliveries* (Committee Opinion No. 764). Washington, DC: Author.

Ananth, C. V., Lavery, J. A., Vintzileos, A. M., Skupski, D. W., Varner, M., Saade, G., . . . Wright, J. D. (2016). Severe placental abruption: Clinical definition and associations with maternal complications. *American Journal of Obstetrics & Gynecology, 214*, 272.e1–272.e9. doi:10.1016/j.ajog.2015.09.069

Ayres, A. W., Johnson, T. R., & Hayashi, R. (2001). Characteristics of fetal heart rate tracings prior to uterine rupture. *International Journal of Gynaecology and Obstetrics, 74*(3), 235–240.

Barraco, R. D., Chiu, W. C., Clancy, T. V., Como, J. J., Ebert, J. B., Hess, L. W., . . . Weiss, P. M. (2010). Practice management guidelines for the diagnosis and management of injury in the pregnant patient: The EAST Practice Management Guidelines Work Group. *The Journal of Trauma, 69*(1), 211–214. doi:10.1097/TA.0b013e3181dbe1ea

Berg, C. J., Callaghan, W. M., Syverson, C., & Henderson, Z. (2010). Pregnancy-related mortality in the United States, 1998 to 2005. *Obstetrics & Gynecology, 116*(6), 1302–1309. doi:10.1097/AOG.0b013e3181fdfb11

Blackburn, S. T. (2018). *Maternal, fetal, & neonatal physiology* (5th ed.). Maryland Heights, MO: Elsevier Saunders.

Brown, H. L. (2009). Trauma in pregnancy. *Obstetrics & Gynecology, 114*(1), 147–160. doi:10.1097/AOG.0b013e3181ab6014

Brown, H. L. (2010). Trauma in pregnancy. *Obstetric Anesthesia Digest, 30*(3), 144–145. doi:10.1097/01.aoa.0000386814.84816.cd

Burke, C. (2010). Active versus expectant management of the third stage of labor and implementation of a protocol. *The Journal of Perinatal & Neonatal Nursing, 24*(3), 215–228. doi:10.1097/JPN.0b013e3181e8ce90

Cahill, A. G., & Macones, G. A. (2007). Vaginal birth after cesarean delivery: Evidence-based practice. *Clinical Obstetrics and Gynecology, 50*(2), 518–525. doi:10.1097/GRF.0b013e31804bde7b

Callaghan, W. M., Kuklina, E. V., & Berg, C. J. (2010). Trends in postpartum hemorrhage: United States, 1994–2006. *American Journal of Obstetrics & Gynecology, 202*(4), 353.e1–353.e6. doi:10.1016/j.ajog.2010.01.011

Cannada, L. K., Pan, P., Casey, B. M., McIntire, D. D., Shafi, S., & Leveno, K. J. (2010). Pregnancy outcomes after orthopedic trauma. *The Journal of Trauma, 69*(3), 694–698. doi:10.1097/TA.0b013e3181e97ed8

Catanzarite, V., Cousins, L., Dowling, D., & Daneshmand, S. (2006). Oxytocin-associated rupture of an unscarred uterus in a primigravida. *Obstetrics & Gynecology, 108*(3, Pt. 2), 723–725. doi:10.1097/01.AOG.0000215559.21051.dc

Centers for Disease Control and Prevention. (2017). *Pregnancy Mortality Surveillance System*. Atlanta, GA: Author.

Chang, J., Elam-Evans, L. D., Berg, C. J., Herndon, J., Flowers, L., Seed, K., & Syversen, C. J. (2003). Pregnancy-related mortality surveillance—United States, 1991–1999. *Morbidity and Mortality Weekly Report, 52*(2), 1–8.

Clark, S. L. (1999). Placenta previa and abruptio placenta. In R. K. Creasy, R. Resnik, & J. Iams (Eds.), *Maternal–fetal medicine* (4th ed., pp. 616–631). Philadelphia, PA: Saunders.

Clark, S. L. (2004). Placenta previa and abruptio placenta. In R. K. Creasy, R. Resnik, & J. Iams (Eds.), *Maternal–fetal medicine* (5th ed., pp. 707–722). Philadelphia, PA: Saunders.

Clark, S. L., Greenspoon, J. S., Aldahl, D., & Phelan, J. P. (1986). Severe preeclampsia with persistent oliguria: Management of hemodynamic subsets. *American Journal of Obstetrics & Gynecology, 154*(3), 490–494.

Comstock, C. (2011). The antenatal diagnosis of placental attachment disorders. *Current Opinion in Obstetrics & Gynecology, 23*(2), 117–122. doi:10.1097/GCO.0b013e328342b730

Curet, M. J., Schermer, C. R., Demarest, G. B., Bieneik, E. J., III, & Curet, L. B. (2000). Predictors of outcome in trauma during pregnancy: Identification of patients who can be monitored for less than 6 hours. *Journal of Trauma, 49*(1), 18–25.

Dunning, K., LeMasters, G., & Bhattacharya, A. (2010). A major public health issue: The high incidence of falls during pregnancy. *Maternal Child Health Journal, 14*(5), 720–725. doi:10.1007/s10995-009-0511-0

El Kady, D., Gilbert, W. M., Anderson, J., Danielsen, B., Towner, D., & Smith, L. H. (2004). Trauma during pregnancy: An analysis of maternal and fetal outcomes in a large population. *American Journal of Obstetrics & Gynecology, 190*(6), 1661–1668. doi:10.1016/j.ajog.2004.02.051

Eller, A. G., Bennett, M. A., Sharshiner, M., Masheter, C., Soisson, A. P., Dodson, M., & Silver, R. M. (2011). Maternal morbidity in cases of placenta accreta managed by a multidisciplinary care team compared with standard obstetric care. *Obstetrics & Gynecology, 117*(2, Pt. 1), 331–337. doi:10.1097/AOG.0b013e3182051db2

Fuller, A. J., & Bucklin, B. A. (2010). Blood product replacement for postpartum hemorrhage. *Clinical Obstetrics and Gynecology, 53*(1), 196–208. doi:10.1097/GRF.0b013e3181cc42a0

Harper, L. M., Obido, A. O., Macones, G. A., Crane, J. P., & Cahill, A. G. (2010). Effect of placenta previa on fetal growth. *American Journal of Obstetrics & Gynecology, 203*(4), 330.e1–330.e5. doi:10.1016/j.ajog.2010.05.014

Hull, A. D., & Resnik, R. (2014). Placenta previa, placenta accreta, abruptio placentae, and vasa previa. In R. K. Creasy, R. Resnik, J. D. Iams, C. J. Lockwood, T. R. Moore, & M. F. Greene (Eds.), *Creasy and Resnik's maternal–fetal medicine: Principles and practice* (7th ed., pp. 732–742). Philadelphia, PA: Saunders Elsevier.

James, A. H., Abel, D. E., & Brancazio, L. R. (2006). Anticoagulants in pregnancy. *Obstetrical & Gynecological Survey, 61*(1), 59–69.

Jauniaux, E., Collins, S., & Burton, G. J. (2018). Placenta accreta spectrum: Pathophysiology and evidence-based anatomy for prenatal ultrasound imaging. *American Journal of Obstetrics & Gynecology, 218*(1), 75–87. doi:10.1016/j.ajog.2017.05.067

Jauregui, I., Kirkendall, C., Ahn, M. O., & Phelan, J. (2000). Uterine rupture: A placentally mediated event? *Obstetrics & Gynecology, 95*(4, Suppl. 1), S75. doi:10.1016/S0029-7844(00)00754-7

Jurkovic, D., & Wilkinson, H. (2011). Diagnosis and management of ectopic pregnancy. *BMJ, 342*, d3397. doi:10.1136/bmj.d3397

Landon, M. B., Hauth, J. C., Leveno, K. J., Spong, C. Y., Leindecker, S., Varner, M. W., . . . Gabbe, S. G. (2004). Maternal and perinatal outcomes associated with a trial of labor after prior cesarean delivery. *The New England Journal of Medicine, 351*(25), 2581–2589. doi:10.1056/NEJMoa040405

Landon, M. B., Leindecker, S., Spong, C. Y., Hauth, J. C., Bloom, S., Varner, M. W., . . . Gabbe, S. G. (2005). The MFMU Cesarean Registry: Factors affecting the success of trial of labor after previous cesarean delivery. *American Journal of Obstetrics & Gynecology, 193*(3, Pt. 2), 1016–1023. doi:10.1016/j.ajog.2005.05.066

Lang, C., & Landon, M. (2010). Uterine rupture as a source of obstetrical hemorrhage. *Clinical Obstetrics and Gynecology, 53*(1), 237–251. doi:10.1097/GRF.0b013e3181cc4538

Lyndon, A., Lagrew, D., Shields, L., Melsop, K., Main, E., & Cape, V. (Eds.). (2015). *Improving health care response to obstetric hemorrhage version 2.0.* Retrieved from http://www.cmqcc.org/ob_hemorrhage

Mahlmeister, L. R. (2010). Best practices in perinatal care: Strategies for reducing the maternal death rate in the United States. *The Journal of Perinatal & Neonatal Nursing, 24*(4), 297–301. doi:10.1097/JPN.0b013e3181f918bb

Main, E. K., Goffman, D., Scavone, B. M., Low, L. K., Bingham, D., Fontaine, P. L., . . . Levy, B. S. (2015). National partnership for maternal safety: Consensus bundle on obstetric hemorrhage. *Anesthesia and Analgesia, 121*(1), 142–148.

Mattox, K. L., & Goetzl, L. (2005). Trauma in pregnancy. *Critical Care Medicine, 33*(10), S385–S389.

Mazzone, M. E., & Woolever, J. (2006). Uterine rupture in a patient with an unscarred uterus: A case study. *WMJ, 105*(2), 64–66.

Menihan, C. A. (1999). The effect of uterine rupture on fetal heart rate patterns. *Journal of Nurse-Midwifery, 44*(1), 40–46. doi:10.1016/S0091-2182(98)00076-7

Muench, M. V., Baschat, A. A., Reddy, U. M., Mighty, H. E., Weiner, C. P., Scalea, T. M., & Harman, C. R. (2004). Kleihauer-Betke testing is important in all cases of maternal trauma. *The Journal of Trauma, 57*(5), 1094–1098.

Oxford, C. M., & Ludmir, J. (2009). Trauma in pregnancy. *Clinical Obstetrics and Gynecology, 52*(4), 611–629. doi:10.1097/GRF.0b013e3181c11edf

Oyelese, Y., & Ananth, C. V. (2010). Postpartum hemorrhage: Epidemiology, risk factors, and causes. *Clinical Obstetrics and Gynecology, 53*(1), 147–156. doi:10.1097/GRF.0b013e3181cc406d

Oyelese, Y., Catanzarite, V., Prefumo, F., Lashley, S., Schachter, M., Tovbin, Y., . . . Smulian, J. C. (2004). Vasa previa: The impact of prenatal diagnosis on outcomes. *Obstetrics & Gynecology, 103*(5, Pt 1), 937–942. doi:10.1097/01.AOG.0000123245.48645.98

Oyelese, Y., & Smulian, J. C. (2006). Placenta previa, placenta accreta, and vasa previa. *Obstetrics & Gynecology, 107*(4), 927–941. doi:10.1097/01.AOG.0000207559.15715.98

Page, E. W., & Christianson, R. (1976). The impact of mean arterial pressure in the middle trimester upon the outcome of pregnancy. *American Journal of Obstetrics & Gynecology, 125*(6), 740–746.

Paré, E., Quiñones, J. N., & Macones, G. A. (2006). Vaginal birth after caesarean section versus elective repeat caesarean section: Assessment of maternal downstream health outcomes. *BJOG, 113*(1), 75–85. doi:10.1111/j.1471-0528.2005.00793.x

Pariente, G., Wiznitzer, A., Sergienko, R., Mazor, M., Holcberg, G., & Sheiner, E. (2011). Placental abruption: Critical analysis of risk factors and perinatal outcomes. *The Journal of Maternal-Fetal & Neonatal Medicine, 24*(5), 698–702. doi:10.3109/14767058.2010.511346

Paxton, A., & Wardlaw, T. (2011). Are we making progress in maternal mortality? *The New England Journal of Medicine, 364*(21), 1990–1993. doi:10.1056/NEJMp1012860

Poole, J. H., & White, D. (2005). *Obstetrical emergencies for the perinatal nurse* (2nd ed.). White Plains, NY: March of Dimes Birth Defects Foundation.

Rajan, P. V., & Wing, D. A. (2010). Postpartum hemorrhage: Evidence-based medical interventions for prevention and treatment. *Clinical Obstetrics and Gynecology, 53*(1), 165–181. doi:10.1097/GRF.0b013e3181ce0965

Ridgeway, J. J., Weyrich, D. L., & Benedetti, T. J. (2004). Fetal heart rate changes associated with uterine rupture. *Obstetrics & Gynecology, 103*(3), 506–512.

Robinson, B. K., & Grobman, W. A. (2011). Effectiveness of timing strategies for delivery of individuals with vasa previa. *Obstetrics & Gynecology, 117*(3), 542–549. doi:10.1097/AOG.0b013e31820b0ace

Roth, C. K., Parfitt, S. E., Hering, S. L., & Dent, S. A. (2014). Developing protocols for obstetric emergencies. *Nursing for Women's Health, 18*(5), 378–390. doi:10.1111/1751-486X.12146

Ruiter, L., Ravelli, A. C., de Graaf, I. M., Mol, B. W., & Pajkrt, E. (2015). Incidence and recurrence rate of placental abruption: A longitudinal linked national cohort study in the Netherlands. *American Journal of Obstetrics & Gynecology, 213*(4), 573.e1–573.e8. doi:10.1016/j.ajog.2015.06.019

Ruth, D., & Kennedy, B. B. (2011). Acute volume resuscitation following obstetric hemorrhage. *The Journal of Perinatal & Neonatal Nursing, 25*(3), 253–260. doi:10.1097/JPN.0b013e31822539e3

Ruth, D., & Mighty, H. E. (2019). Trauma in pregnancy. In N. H. Troiano, P. M. Witcher, & S. M. Baird (Eds.), *High-risk & critical care obstetrics* (4th ed., pp. 331–343). Philadelphia, PA: Wolters Kluwer.

Scott, J. R. (2011). Vaginal birth after cesarean delivery: A common-sense approach. *Obstetrics & Gynecology, 118*(2, Pt. 1), 342–350. doi:10.1097/AOG.0b013e3182245b39

Shamshirsaz, A. A., Fox, K. A., Erfani, H., Clark, S. L., Shamshirsaz, A. A., Nassr, A. A., . . . Belfort, M. A. (2018). Outcomes of planned compared with urgent deliveries using a multidisciplinary team approach for morbidly adherent placenta. *Obstetrics & Gynecology, 131*(2), 234–241. doi:10.1097/AOG.0000000000002442

Shay-Zapien, G., & Bullock, L. (2010). Impact of intimate partner violence on maternal child health. *MCN: The American Journal of Maternal/Child Nursing, 35*(4), 206–212. doi:10.1097/NMC.0b013e3181dd9d6e

Sheiner, E., Levy, A., Ofir, K., Hadar, A., Shoham-Vardi, I., Hallak, M., . . . Mazor, M. (2004). Changes in fetal heart rate and uterine patterns associated with uterine rupture. *The Journal of Reproductive Medicine, 49*(5), 373–378.

Sibai, B. M. (2005). Thrombophilia and severe preeclampsia: Time to screen and treat in future pregnancies? *Hypertension, 46*(6), 1252–1253. doi:10.1161/01.HYP.0000188904.47575.7e

Silver, R. M. (2007). Fetal death. *Obstetrics & Gynecology, 109*(1), 153–167. doi:10.1097/01.AOG.0000248537.89739.96

Silver, R. M., Landon, M. B., Rouse, D., Leveno, K. J., Spong, C. Y., Thom, E. A., . . . Mercer, B. M. (2006). Maternal morbidity associated with multiple repeat cesarean deliveries. *Obstetrics & Gynecology, 107*(6), 1226–1232. doi:10.1097/01.AOG.0000219750.79480.84

Simpson, K. R., Luppi, C. J., & O'Brien-Abel, N. (1998). Acute fatty liver of pregnancy. *The Journal of Perinatal & Neonatal Nursing, 11*(4), 35–44.

Snegovskikh, D., Clebone, A., & Norwitz, E. (2011). Anesthetic management of patients with placenta accreta and resuscitation strategies for associated massive hemorrhage. *Current Opinion in Anaesthesiology, 24*(3), 274–281. doi:10.1097/ACO.0b013e328345d8b7

Society for Maternal-Fetal Medicine & Gyamfi-Bannerman, C. (2018). Society for Maternal-Fetal Medicine (SMFM) Consult Series #44: Management of bleeding in the late preterm period. *American Journal of Obstetrics & Gynecology, 218*(1), B2–B8. doi:10/1016/j.ajog.2017.10.019

Spong, C. Y., & Queenan, J. T. (2011). Uterine scar assessment: How should it be done before trial of labor after cesarean delivery? *Obstetrics & Gynecology, 117*(3), 521–522. doi:10.1097/AOG.0b013e31820ce593

Tahseen, S., & Griffiths, M. (2010). Vaginal birth after two caesarean sections (VBAC-2)—A systematic review with meta-analysis of success rate and adverse outcomes of VBAC-2 versus VBAC-1 and repeat (third) caesarean sections. *BJOG, 117*(1), 5–19. doi:10.1111/j.1471-0528.2009.02351.x

The Joint Commission. (2010). *Preventing maternal death* (Sentinel Event Alert No. 44). Oak Brook Terrace, IL: Author.

Tillett, J. (2010). Understanding and explaining risk. *The Journal of Perinatal & Neonatal Nursing, 24*(3), 196–198. doi:10.1097/JPN.0b013e3181e7c6f9

Vergani, P., Ornaghi, S., Pozzi, I., Beretta, P., Russo, F. M., Follesa, I., & Ghidini, A. (2009). Placenta previa: Distance to internal os and mode of delivery. *American Journal of Obstetrics & Gynecology, 201*(3), 266.e1–266.e5. doi:10.1016/j.ajog.2009.06.009

Wright, J. D., Pri-Paz, S., Herzog, T. J., Shah, M., Bonanno, C., Lewin, S. N., . . . Devine, P. (2011). Predictors of massive blood loss in women with placenta accreta. *American Journal of Obstetrics & Gynecology, 205*(1), 38.e1–38.e6. doi:10.1016/j.ajog.2011.01.040

You, W. B., & Zahn, C. M. (2006). Postpartum hemorrhage: Abnormally adherent placenta, uterine inversion, and puerperal hematomas. *Clinical Obstetrics and Gynecology, 49*(1), 184–197.

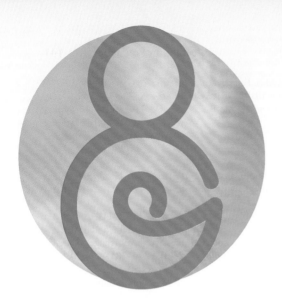

CHAPTER 7

Preterm Labor and Birth

Sheryl E. Parfitt

SIGNIFICANCE AND INCIDENCE

Preterm labor and birth are critical conditions that threaten the health of children and stability of families. Worldwide, approximately 15 million babies are born preterm (World Health Organization [WHO], 2018). In the United States, 9.6% of pregnancies are complicated by preterm birth (PTB), which results in about 1 in 10 infants being born prematurely (Centers for Disease Control and Prevention [CDC], 2019). There was a decline in the PTB rate between 2006 (12.8%) and 2014 (9.57%), but research from the CDC demonstrated a concerning rise in both 2015 and 2016 (CDC, 2019). Causes of this increase are multifactorial and not completely understood (Frey & Klebanoff, 2016).

According to the March of Dimes (MOD, 2017) *2017 Premature Birth Report Cards*, the United States received a "C" grade due to significant disparities in prematurity rates when comparing different races and ethnicities. Rates of PTB among non-Hispanic blacks rose from 13.2% in 2014 to 13.4% in 2015, placing them at a 48% higher risk over women in other racial groups (MOD, 2019b). Whereas other ethnicities have lower rates, all remain unacceptably high. The rate of PTB for American Indians/Alaska natives is 10.5%; for Hispanics, 9.1%; for non-Hispanic whites, 9.0%; and for Asian/Pacific Islanders, 8.5% (MOD, 2019b).

The rising rates of PTB in the United States contrast with the decrease in rates of infant mortality since the 1950s. In 2013, the rate of infant mortality for the United States was 5.96 per 1,000 live births; in 1950, by comparison, it was 29.2 per 1,000 live births (Matthews, MacDorman, & Thoma, 2015; National Center for Health Statistics, 2005). This dramatic change occurred because of the emergence of the science of neonatal care, with more babies now living past their first birthdays despite being born at earlier gestational ages. Sophisticated neonatal care has also allowed more preterm babies to survive, although for many of the smallest preterm babies survival is liable to come with significant morbidity, which can last throughout their lifetime.

PTB is defined as birth occurring before 37 completed weeks of gestation. It can be further subdivided into categories of late preterm (34 to 36 weeks and 6 days), moderately preterm (32 to 33 weeks and 6 days), very preterm (28 to 31 weeks and 6 days), and extremely preterm (<28 weeks) (MOD, Partnership for Maternal, Newborn & Child Health, Save the Children, & WHO, 2012; Rundell & Panchal, 2017). "Spontaneous" and "medically indicated" are additional classifications of PTB (Purisch & Gyamfi-Bannerman, 2017). Spontaneous preterm delivery is responsible for approximately 75% of all PTBs and is one of the leading reasons for hospitalization during pregnancy as well as neonatal morbidity (Purisch & Gyamfi-Bannerman, 2017; Rundell & Panchal, 2017). Causes include "spontaneous preterm labor, preterm premature rupture of membranes, and second trimester spontaneous pregnancy loss" (Purisch & Gyamfi-Bannerman, 2017, p. 388). Women with a history of prior spontaneous PTB, shortened cervix, non-Hispanic black race, multiple gestations, uterine anomalies, multiples, and short interval between pregnancies are at highest risk of PTB. The principal risk factor is prior spontaneous PTB with a 15% to 50% recurrence rate depending on the number of preterm births and gestational age of the mother's previous PTBs (Goldenberg, Culhane, Iams, & Romero, 2008). It should be noted that spontaneous PTBs can also occur in primigravida women without any known risk factors (Purisch & Gyamfi-Bannerman, 2017).

Approximately 25% of all preterm births fall into the medically indicated category. Maternal and fetal complications such as preeclampsia, uncontrolled diabetes, abnormalities of the placenta, and intrauterine growth restriction may necessitate a medically indicated PTB (Purisch & Gyamfi-Bannerman, 2017). In 2017, the majority of preterm births in the United States were late PTBs, comprising 7.17% of all births. The rate of early preterm births comprise 2.76% of all births (Martin, Hamilton, Osterman, Driscoll, & Drake, 2018).

It is important when discussing PTB that everyone uses the same definitions. Although they are different entities, often with separate etiologies, the terms *PTB* and *low birth weight* (LBW) are commonly used interchangeably. Most of the long-term follow-up studies of children and adults quoted in the literature are of very LBW (VLBW) or extremely LBW (ELBW) children because assessment of gestational age was not common in perinatal care until recent decades. Birth weight has been, and continues to be, a simple and definitive assessment, thus easier to access. PTB refers only to gestational age at birth, no matter the birth weight. In 2014, the National Center for Health Statistics moved away from using the mother's last menstrual period for determination of gestational age and recommends use of the obstetric estimate of gestation at delivery as the new measurement (Martin, Osterman, Kirmeyer, & Gregory, 2015). Although many preterm infants are LBW, maternal conditions such as gestational diabetes may lead to a normal birth weight in a preterm baby. The prematurity would then dictate the health problems of the baby, as lung, central nervous system, or gastrointestinal immaturity would pose health risks.

LBW refers only to weight at birth, no matter the gestational age. A baby is considered LBW if it is born with a weight less than 2,500 g (5.5 lb). Moderately LBW (MLBW) infants weigh 1,500 g to less than 2,500 g, VLBW is less than 1,500 g (3.5 lb), and ELBW is less than 1,000 g (less than 2.2 lb) (Tchamo, Prista, & Leandro, 2016). LBW babies may be born before 37 weeks but can also be born at term (e.g., a baby at 41 weeks gestational age could weigh 1,800 g because of intrauterine growth restriction). Risk factors, causes, and outcomes for LBW, growth restriction, and PTB are interrelated. It has been noted that approximately one third of infants born in an LBW category are also preterm (Yang, Chen, Yen, & Chen, 2015). This close correlation can cause some confusion when reviewing the literature. The rates of LBW and PTB in the United States are different. The LBW rate increased more than 20% from the mid-1980s to 2006 with a peak of 8.26% but then trended down slightly until 2014. In 2017, the percentage of LBW infants rose for the third year in a row, to 8.28% (Martin et al., 2018). Percentages for MLBW infants increased from

6.77% in 2016 to 6.87% in 2017, whereas the rate of VLBW remained unchanged at 1.40% during the same time period (Martin et al., 2018).

Research has been conducted on the sequelae of LBW, MLBW, VLBW, and ELBW infants. Babies born in these categories have greater risk factors related to death or severe neurosensory impairment. According to a study on ELBW infants, those who received cardiopulmonary resuscitation (CPR) in the delivery room had a greater risk of mortality and neurodevelopmental abnormalities than those who did not receive CPR (Wyckoff et al., 2012). Other risk factors for LBW and ELBW infants include bronchopulmonary dysplasia, brain injury, severe retinopathy of prematurity, and infections (Bassler et al., 2009; Schmidt et al., 2015). Low gestational age is also a corresponding risk factor for neonatal morbidity. Babies born at less than or equal to 25 weeks' gestation have about a 50% mortality rate and are at greatest risk for morbidities. Mortality rates associated with preterm babies demonstrate that survival rates worsen as gestational age and birth weight decrease. As a result, infants presenting with the lowest gestational age and birth weight have the greatest effect on infant mortality rates due to their higher risk of death (Matthews et al., 2015).

VLBW children followed through adulthood have exhibited lower educational achievements, higher blood pressures, and generally lower physical abilities than their peers who were born at normal birth weight (Davies, Smith, May, & Ben-Shlomo, 2006; Yang et al., 2015). A meta-analysis of studies of overall brain growth revealed a reduction in size of all major brain structures in 818 children and adolescents born at less than 32 weeks or less than 1,500 g when compared with 450 peers born at term (de Kieviet, Zoetebier, van Elburg, Vermeulen, & Oosterlaan, 2012). An analysis of adolescent children born preterm with VLBW demonstrated a higher risk of neurodevelopmental disorders: 26.2% of the adolescents required educational plans individualized to meet their needs; 52.5% were diagnosed with at least one neuropsychiatric disorder such as cerebral palsy, intellectual disabilities, or attention deficit/hyperactivity disorder; and 32.8% were disabled (Yang et al., 2015). Research findings that followed infants born with ELBW noted that poor growth continued into school age. These children were lighter, shorter, and had smaller head circumferences and body mass index (Bocca-Tjeertes, Kerstjens, Reijneveld, de Winter, & Bos, 2011). It has also been shown that there are racial and gender differences in the viability of LBW and preterm infants. Male infants have more adverse neurologic outcomes and higher mortality rates than female infants, while the leading cause of infant death in black babies is PTB and LBW (Kent, Wright, & Abdel-Latif, 2012; Martin et al., 2018).

Consequences of PTB continue to devastate families, communities, and healthcare in general, especially related to financial costs associated with patient care. It is estimated that PTBs are responsible for approximately 70% of neonatal deaths and 36% of infant deaths as well as 25% to 50% of cases of long-term neurologic impairment in children within the United States (American College of Obstetricians and Gynecologists [ACOG], 2016b; MacDorman, Callaghan, Mathews, Hoyert, & Kochanek, 2007; Mathews & MacDorman, 2010; Volpe, 1997). Costs to society in the United States alone for prematurity complications were estimated to be $26.2 billion in 2007 (MOD, 2015a). According to the MOD, premature births cost society $16.9 billion in medical and healthcare costs associated with the baby, $1.9 billion for labor and delivery costs for the mother, $611 million for programs to assist children with disabilities and developmental delays from birth to age 3, $1.1 billion for special educations services, and $5.7 billion for lost work and pay in individuals born prematurely (MOD, 2015a). Furthermore, there is an impact on businesses from prematurity. An analysis prepared by Truven Health Analytics, Inc. for MOD (2015b) reported that approximately 11% of babies covered by employee health plans were born prematurely. Employers were billed an excess of $12 billion annually for costs associated with lost productivity of employees and excess healthcare costs related to this condition. They also paid 12 times more in healthcare costs for premature/LBW babies compared to those without this complication. When costs for the mother are added, employees pay $58,917 more for a premature infant. Studies show that employers spend more on one premature infant than on eight babies who are born at term (MOD, 2015b). There is great need for more research about this costly public health problem to find successful methods of prevention.

LATE PRETERM BIRTHS

Late preterm infants may not present with the most severe morbidities. They do have their own set of physiologic, metabolic, and developmental problems and demonstrate a 6 to 7 times greater rate of complications than babies born at term (Shapiro-Mendoza et al., 2008). In the past, these issues were not recognized because of concentration on the dramatically severe difficulties encountered by infants less than 32 weeks' gestation. But with newer evidence, late preterm infants are now the focus of much research and intervention (Machado, Passini, Rosa, & Carvalho, 2014).

In July 2005, the National Institute of Child Health and Human Development (NICHD, 2005) convened a panel of experts to discuss the definition and terminology, epidemiology, etiology, biology or maturation,

clinical care, surveillance, and public health aspects of "near-term" PTB and "near-term" infants (Raju, Higgins, Stark, & Leveno, 2006). However, the panel came to the consensus that "late PTB" and "late preterm infants" were better descriptors because they highlight the physiologic vulnerability of this group of preterm infants. Along with the MOD, ACOG, and the American Academy of Pediatrics (AAP), the Association of Women's Health, Obstetric and Neonatal Nurses (AWHONN) was an invited participant and has been one of the professional organizations leading the way to increase awareness among healthcare providers and the public to promote better outcomes. Before the NICHD expert panel meeting, AWHONN established its "Late Preterm Infant Initiative," a conceptual framework for optimizing the health of these babies (Medoff-Cooper, Bakewell-Sachs, Buus-Frank, & Santa-Donato, 2005; Santa-Donato, 2005). This ongoing program is focused on developing evidence-based practices when caring for subsets of preterm babies born between 34 weeks and 0 days and 36 weeks and 6 days (Raju et al., 2006).

It is believed that the practice of elective inductions may be a contributor to the rise in late PTBs (Baker, 2015; Newnham et al., 2014). Other possible causes for the increase in late PTBs include maternal complications resulting in medically indicated births, inaccurate dating of the pregnancy, increasing proportions of pregnant women over 35 years of age, multiple births, and rising rates of maternal obesity (Engle & Kominiarek, 2008; Goldenberg et al., 2008; Martin et al., 2018; Spong et al., 2011).

In 2012, AWHONN initiated its "Go the Full 40" program to further educate consumers and healthcare providers on the importance of delivery at 40 weeks' gestation and avoidance of elective inductions before term (Bingham, Ruhl, & Cockey, 2013). Since that time, organizations such as the MOD (2019d), ACOG and the Society for Maternal-Fetal Medicine (SMFM) (2017a), AWHONN (2017), and The Joint Commission (TJC, 2017) have developed guidelines to assist in the development of quality improvement programs aimed at reducing elective births before 39 weeks' gestation. TJC published the *Perinatal Care PC-01: Elective Delivery* (TJC, 2017) in an effort to increase awareness of this issue. This measure requires institutions accredited by TJC to submit data on all inductions that are performed before 39 weeks' gestation. Other professional entities that have added their support include the National Quality Forum, the Centers for Medicare & Medicaid Services, and Leapfrog, a public reporting agency (Baker, 2015). Evaluation of the issue of late preterm infants by AWHONN (Baker, 2015) found that these infants were often overlooked in research because they did not appear dramatically sick. They are, however, immature at birth and have

DISPLAY 7–1

Adverse Outcomes Significantly Increased in Late Preterm Infants

- Respiratory distress syndrome
- Transient tachypnea of the newborn
- Pulmonary infection
- Unspecified respiratory failure
- Recurrent apnea
- Temperature instability
- Jaundice as a cause for discharge delay
- Bilirubin-induced brain injury
- Clinical problems with one or more diagnoses
- Rehospitalization for all causes
- Rehospitalization for neonatal dehydration
- Feeding difficulties
- Long-term neurodevelopmental delay
- Periventricular leukomalacia

missed 4 to 6 weeks of the third trimester of gestation, putting them at risk for many health problems. There is a growing body of evidence that compared to term babies, late preterm babies have more problems with temperature stability, feeding, hypoglycemia, respiratory distress, apnea/bradycardia, symptoms suggesting the need for sepsis evaluation, and clinical jaundice. They also are at greater risk for neurodevelopmental disorders such as cerebral palsy and mental retardation as well as longer hospitalization stays and rehospitalization (Engle, Tomashek, Wallman, & the Committee on Fetus and Newborn, 2007; Leone et al., 2012; Machado et al., 2014; Medoff-Cooper et al., 2012). It is estimated that the brain size of a baby born at approximately 35 weeks' gestation is only 65% of that of a baby born at term, reducing the amount of external surface sulci accordingly, putting them at risk for neurologic compromise (Billiards, Pierson, Haynes, Folkerth, & Kinney, 2006; Kinney, 2006). Display 7–1 lists adverse outcomes that are significantly increased in late preterm infants. Because late preterm babies reflect such a large proportion of all preterm babies, even a modest increase in the PTB rate can have a significant impact on human and healthcare costs. Late preterm infants are discussed in detail in Chapter 21.

EARLY TERM BIRTHS

In the past, infants born between 37 and 41 weeks' gestation were considered to be term births (Fleischman, Oinuma, & Clark, 2010). But research demonstrates that babies born between 37 weeks' and 38 completed weeks' gestation have higher rates of morbidity and mortality compared with infants born at 39 weeks or

greater (ACOG & SMFM, 2017b; Parikh et al., 2014). As this issue became more apparent, NICHD, ACOG, the AAP, SMFM, MOD, and the WHO assembled in 2012 to redefine and expand the definition of term *birth* (Spong, 2013). They recommended that the period of time from 37 weeks and 0 days to 38 weeks and 6 days be categorized as early term. Full term would encompass 39 weeks and 0 days to 40 weeks and 6 days, and 41 weeks and 0 days to 41 weeks and 6 days would be considered late term (Raju et al., 2006).

The Consortium on Safe Labor performed a retrospective cohort study of 233,844 infants born at 37 weeks' gestation. These babies were shown to have higher rates of respiratory failure, ventilator use, respiratory distress syndrome, transient tachypnea, pneumonia, and surfactant and oscillator use when compared with infants born at 39 weeks (Hibbard et al., 2010). Other morbidities associated with early term births include hypoglycemia, 5-minute Apgar score less than 7, neonatal mortality, and higher neonatal intensive care unit (NICU) admission rates (Hibbard et al., 2010). NICU admission rates for deliveries not initiated by induction of labor or rupture of membranes were examined for 3 months within 27 hospitals in the United States. Infants born at 37 to 38 completed weeks were compared with those born at 39 weeks' gestation. Of these births, neonates born in the early term period were shown to have higher NICU admission rates, feeding challenges, and learning difficulties requiring special educational interventions than those born at 39 weeks' gestation or beyond (Clark et al., 2009).

Lung maturity has been used historically as a determining factor in predicting risks of neonatal morbidity and mortality related to PTB; however, lung maturity is not necessarily an indicator of maturation of other organ systems (ACOG & SMFM, 2017a). For example, the brain continues to develop throughout pregnancy, including rapid growth in the last month (Bouyssi-Kobar et al., 2016). Being born at term, but earlier than 39 weeks' gestation, can have significant negative neurologic effects as children develop. A population-based prospective study performed in England of children born at early term compared to those born after 39 weeks' gestation showed statistically worse performance scores for all five subject domains except writing (Chan & Quigley, 2014).

Although it is well documented that significant excess costs are associated with elective births before 37 completed weeks of gestation (MOD, 2015b), electively born early term babies also generate appreciable costs, including admission to the NICU due to iatrogenic morbidity and educational interventions related to being born too soon (Craighead, 2012). Elective labor inductions and cesarean births are preventable factors contributing to the increase in late preterm and early term births and associated costs (ACOG & SMFM, 2017a; Bingham et al., 2013; Craighead, 2012). Evidence supports induction of labor for post-term gestation, premature rupture of membranes, and Intrauterine Inflammation, Infection, or both (Triple I) (Peng, Chang, Lin, Cheng, & Su, 2018) as well as significant maternal compromise such as Hemolysis, Elevated Liver Enzymes, and Low Platelets (HELLP) syndrome or nonremedial fetal compromise such as fetal hydrops (ACOG, 2009; Mozurkewich, Chilimigras, Koepke, Keeton, & King, 2009). Other medical indications for induction before 39 completed weeks' gestation suggested by ACOG and SMFM (2017a) include prior myomectomy, prior classical cesarean, placenta previa, multiple gestation, preterm premature rupture of membranes (PPROM), Triple I, fetal demise, gestational hypertension, preeclampsia, eclampsia, maternal medical conditions (e.g., diabetes mellitus, renal disease, chronic pulmonary disease, chronic hypertension, and antiphospholipid syndrome), and fetal compromise (e.g., severe fetal growth restriction, isoimmunization, and oligohydramnios) (ACOG & SMFM, 2017a). See Table 7–1 for ACOG and SMFM recommendations for timing of medically indicated births before 39 completed weeks of gestation.

Because late preterm and early term births without medical indications have potential to result in preventable neonatal morbidities, professional organizations have promulgated recommendations to avoid their occurrence. Estimations of the "due date" can often be miscalculated by up to 2 weeks; therefore, ACOG and SMFM (2017a) recommend that gestational age of 39 completed weeks of gestation be confirmed by at least one method before elective labor induction, repeat cesarean birth, or nonmedically indicated cesarean birth to avoid iatrogenic PTB (AAP & ACOG, 2017; ACOG, 2009; ACOG & SMFM, 2017a). These methods include an ultrasound measurement in the first trimester (up to 13 weeks and 6 days' gestation) and determination of the last menstrual period to calculate the most accurate estimated due date (ACOG, American Institute of Ultrasound in Medicine, & SMFM, 2017). In 2016, ACOG reinvented the Pregnancy Wheel by developing a new Estimated Due Date Calculator app that includes ACOG guidelines that are built into the logic. This app is unique because it has the ability to reconcile differences in due dates between the first ultrasound and date of the last menstrual period. It can also be used to recalculate due dates based on ultrasound or assisted reproductive technologies (ART) (ACOG, 2016a). Testing for fetal lung maturity should not be performed and is contraindicated when birth is required for fetal or maternal indications (ACOG & SMFM, 2017a). Conversely, a mature fetal lung maturity test result before 39 weeks of gestation, in the absence of appropriate clinical circumstances, is not an indication for birth (ACOG & SMFM, 2017a).

The American College of Nurse-Midwives (ACNM, 2016) and AWHONN (AWHONN, 2019; Bingham et al., 2013) recommend awaiting spontaneous onset of labor unless there are evidence-based medical indications that outweigh the risks of induction. New research linking potential long-term effects from induction of labor are being studied. While the information is still evolving with an unknown extent, there is developing concern regarding outcomes associated with fetal brain development near term and the potential for autism spectrum disorder (ACNM, 2016). Adoption and consistent use of guidelines for medically indicated births before 39 weeks should have a positive influence on avoidance of preventable adverse neonatal morbidity related to elective early term births (ACOG & SMFM, 2017a).

WHY HAS THE RATE OF PRETERM BIRTH INCREASED?

Some of the contributing factors to the rise in PTBs over the last three decades include the following (Georgiou, Di Quinzio, Permezel, & Brennecke, 2015; Goldenberg et al., 2008; Spong et al., 2011):

- Increasing use of infertility treatments producing twins and higher order multiples
- More births to women at older ages (greater than 35 years of age)
- More medically induced prematurity (including early labor inductions)
- Early repeat cesarean births
- Primary cesarean births without a medical indication
- Advances in maternal and fetal medicine and neonatal care (which leads both providers and patients to believe that birth at earlier gestations is not an insurmountable health hazard)
- More pregnancies in very-high-risk women who then require early birth
- An increase in fetal complications, such as intrauterine growth restriction, leading to early birth

The issue of PTB of multiples and higher order multiples is particularly problematic, although the rate of twin births declined by an average of 1% a year from 2014 (33.9) through 2018 (32.6) for a total decrease of 4% (Martin & Osterman, 2019). For the first time in more than three decades, from 2014 through 2018, the twin birth rate for the United States trended downward. Of the 3,855,500 U.S. live births in 2017, there were 133,155 twin births, 3,675 triplet births, 193 quadruplet births, and 49 quintuplet and higher-order multiple births (Martin et al., 2018). The rate of

TABLE 7–1. Guidance Regarding Timing of Delivery When Conditions Complicate Pregnancy at or After 34 Weeks of Gestation

Condition	Gestational age* at delivery	Grade of recommendation[†]
Placental and uterine issues		
Placenta previa[†]	36–37 wk	B
Suspected placenta accreta, increta, or percreta with placenta previa[†]	34–35 wk	B
Prior classical cesarean (upper segment uterine incision)[†]	36–37 wk	B
Prior myomectomy necessitating cesarean delivery[†]	37–38 wk (may require earlier delivery, similar to prior classical cesarean, in situations with more extensive or complicated myomectomy)	B
Fetal issues		
Fetal growth restriction-singleton	**38–39 wk:**	
	• Otherwise uncomplicated, no concurrent findings	B
	34–37 wk:	
	• Concurrent conditions (oligohydramnios, abnormal Doppler studies, maternal risk factors, co-morbidity)	B
	Expeditious delivery regardless of gestational age:	
	• Persistent abnormal fetal surveillance suggesting imminent fetal jeopardy	
Fetal growth restriction-twin gestation	**36–37 wk:**	
	• Dichorionic-diamniotic twins with isolated fetal growth restriction	B
	32–34 wk:	
	• Monochorionic-diamniotic twins with isolated fetal growth restriction	B
	• Concurrent conditions (oligohydramnios, abnormal Doppler studies, maternal risk factors, co-morbidity)	
	Expeditious delivery regardless of gestational age:	
	• Persistent abnormal fetal surveillance suggesting imminent fetal jeopardy	
Fetal congenital malformations[†]	**34–39 wk:**	B
	• Suspected worsening of fetal organ damage	
	• Potential for fetal intracranial hemorrhage (eg, vein of Galen aneurysm, neonatal alloimmune thrombocytopenia)	
	• When delivery prior to labor is preferred (eg, EXIT procedure)	
	• Previous fetal intervention	
	• Concurrent maternal disease (eg, preeclampsia, chronic hypertension)	
	• Potential for adverse maternal effect from fetal condition	
	Expeditious delivery regardless of gestational age:	B
	• When intervention is expected to be beneficial	
	• Fetal complications develop (abnormal fetal surveillance, new-onset hydrops fetalis, progressive or new-onset organ injury)	
	• Maternal complications develop (mirror syndrome)	
Multiple gestations: dichorionic-diamniotic[†]	38 wk	B
Multiple gestations: monochorionic-diamniotic[†]	34–37 wk	B
Multiple gestations: dichorionic-diamniotic or monochorionic-diamniotic with single fetal death[†]	If occurs at or after 34 wk, consider delivery (recommendation limited to pregnancies at or after 34 wk; if occurs before 34 wk, individualize based on concurrent maternal or fetal conditions)	B
Multiple gestations: monochorionic-monoamniotic[†]	32–34 wk	B
Multiple gestations: Monochorionic-monoamniotic with single fetal death[†]	Consider delivery; individualized according to gestational age and concurrent complications	B
Oligohydramnios—isolated and persistent[†]	36–37 wk	B
Maternal issues		
Chronic hypertension—no medications[†]	38–39 wk	B
Chronic hypertension—controlled on medication[†]	37–39 wk	B
Chronic hypertension—difficult to control (requiring frequent medication adjustments)[†]	36–37 wk	B
Gestational hypertension[§]	37–38 wk	B
Preeclampsia—severe[†]	At diagnosis (recommendation limited to pregnancies at or after 34 wk)	C
Preeclampsia—mild[†]	37 wk	B
Diabetes—pregestational well controlled[†]	LPTB or ETB not recommended	B
Diabetes—pregestational with vascular disease[†]	37–39 wk	B

(continued)

TABLE 7–1. Guidance Regarding Timing of Delivery When Conditions Complicate Pregnancy at or After 34 Weeks of Gestation *(Continued)*

Condition	Gestational age* at delivery	Grade of recommendation[†]
Diabetes—pregestational, poorly controlled[†]	**34–39 wk** (individualized to situation)	B
Diabetes—gestational well controlled on diet[†]	LPTB or ETB not recommended	B
Diabetes—gestational well controlled on medication[†]	LPTB or ETB not recommended	B
Diabetes—gestational poorly controlled on medication[†]	**34–39 wk** (individualized to situation)	B
Obstetric issues		
Prior stillbirth-unexplained[†]	LPTB or ETB not recommended	B
	Consider amniocentesis for fetal pulmonary maturity if delivery planned at less than 39 wk	C
Spontaneous preterm birth: preterm premature rupture of membranes[†]	**34 wk** (recommendation limited to pregnancies at or after 34 wk)	B
Spontaneous preterm birth: active preterm labor[†]	Delivery if progressive labor or additional maternal or fetal indication	B

LPTB, late-preterm birth at 34 weeks 0 days through 36 weeks and 6 days; ETB, early-term birth at 37 weeks and 0 days through 38 weeks and 6 days.

*Gestational age is in completed weeks; thus, 34 weeks includes 34 weeks and 0 days through 34 weeks and 6 days.

[†]Grade of recommendations are based on the following: recommendations or conclusions or both are based on good and consistent scientific evidence (A); limited or inconsistent scientific evidence (B); primarily consensus and expert opinion (C). The recommendations regarding expeditious delivery for imminent fetal jeopardy were not given a grade. The recommendation regarding severe preeclampsia is based largely on expert opinion; however, higher-level evidence is not likely to be forthcoming because this condition is believed to carry significant maternal risk with limited potential fetal benefit from expectant management after 34 weeks.

[†]Uncomplicated, thus no fetal growth restriction, superimposed preeclampsia, etc. If these are present, then the complicating conditions take precedence and earlier delivery may be indicated.

[§]Maintenance antihypertensive therapy should not be used to treat gestational hypertension.

Reprinted with permission from Spong, C. Y., Mercer, B. M., D'Alton, M., Kilpatrick, S., Blackwell, S., & Saade, G. (2011). Timing of indicated late-preterm and early-term birth. *Obstetrics & Gynecology, 118*(2, Pt. 1), 323–333. doi:10.1097/AOG.0b013e3182255999

triplet and other higher order multiple births in 2017 was 101.6 per 100,000 births. The triplet/+ birth rate (number of triplets, quadruplets, and quintuplets and other higher-order multiples per 100,000 births), rose more than 400% from 1980 to 1998, but it has fallen 47% since the 1998 peak of 193.5 per 100,000 births (Martin et al., 2018). The current rates of triplet and higher-order multiple are the lowest reported in more than 2 decades. This reduction is thought to be due to changes in artificial reproductive therapies. In 2017, 59.43% of twins and >98% of triplets were born at less than 37 weeks' gestation (Martin et al., 2018).

WHAT IS PRETERM LABOR?

The diagnosis of preterm labor is generally based on clinical criteria of regular uterine contractions accompanied by a change in cervical dilation, effacement, or both, or initial presentation with regular contractions and cervical dilation of at least 2 cm (ACOG, 2016b). Display 7–2 lists diagnostic criteria for preterm labor. Less than 10% of women with a clinical diagnosis of preterm labor actually give birth within 7 days of presentation (ACOG, 2016b). It is estimated that approximately 30% of preterm labor resolves spontaneously, and 50% of women hospitalized for preterm labor

actually give birth at term (ACOG, 2016b). It is important, though, to educate and reinforce the significance of careful assessment and follow-up to women who present with irregular contractions that do not meet diagnostic criteria (ACOG, 2016b) in order to decrease the risk of potentially progressing to active preterm labor.

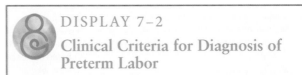

DISPLAY 7–2

Clinical Criteria for Diagnosis of Preterm Labor

- 20 to 36 weeks' gestation
  and
- Regular uterine contractions
  and
- Change in cervical dilation
  and/or
- Change in cervical effacement by digital examination or transvaginal assessment of cervical length
  or
- Initial presentation with regular contractions and cervical dilation ≥2 cm

Adapted from American College of Obstetricians. (2016b). *Management of preterm labor* (Practice Bulletin No. 171). Washington, DC: Author.

PATHOPHYSIOLOGY OF PRETERM LABOR AND BIRTH

In nearly 50% of spontaneous PTBs, the cause is unknown (MOD, 2019a). Based on what has been learned from research over the past few decades, it is doubtful that one causative factor for preterm labor will be discovered. All indications are that preterm labor has multiple causes, including social, physiologic, medical history, and illness factors. Recent research is finding that genetics may also play a role. Studies are currently being performed on different genomes in an attempt to find variant genes that may trigger labor (Hirbo, Eidem, Rokas, & Abbot, 2015; Manuck, 2016; MOD, 2019a; Monangi, Brockway, House, Zhang, & Muglia, 2015; Nan & Li, 2015). Whatever the cause, there appears to be a common pathway that ultimately ends in a process that promotes rupture of the membranes, cervical change, and uterine activity that ends in PTB (Monangi et al., 2015) (see Fig. 7–1 for potential determinants of preterm labor).

An inflammatory response is associated with approximately 50% of spontaneous PTBs (Tambor et al., 2015). It is known that the hormone progesterone is necessary for the formation and preservation of a pregnancy. Current research suggests that stimuli from an inflammatory response causes a withdrawal of functional progesterone leading to preterm labor and birth (Talati, Hackney, & Mesiano, 2017). Potential triggers of inflammation include microbial invasion into the amniotic cavity (Goldenberg, Hauth, & Andrews, 2000), maternal obesity which is associated with higher rates of low-grade prolonged inflammation

that can result in Triple I (Hadley et al., 2017), and uterine overdistention from multiples or polyhydramnios, which in turn can cause an inflammatory response associated with preterm labor (Adams Waldorf et al., 2015).

The external environment can also play a role in the development of preterm labor and delivery. Personal behaviors (e.g., smoking and drug use); psychosocial factors such as depression, post-traumatic stress disorder, and use of antidepressant agents (Cantarutti, Merlino, Monzani, Giaquinto, & Corrao, 2016; Huybrechts, Sanghani, Avorn, & Urato, 2014; Shaw et al., 2014; Staneva, Bogossian, Pritchard, & Wittkowski, 2015); sleep disorders (Felder, Baer, Rand, Jelliffe-Pawlowski, & Prather, 2017; Kajeepeta et al., 2014); and nutritional factors including emesis in the first trimester, underweight and overweight conditions, and low levels of vitamin D have been implicated in the development of preterm labor (Hu et al., 2017; MOD, 2018; McDonnell et al., 2017).

Maternal immune status, medical conditions, and medical interventions interact with genetics and family history through pathways that include inflammation and infection, maternal/fetal stress, abnormal uterine distention, cesarean section at full dilation (Cong, de Vries, & Ludlow, 2018), bleeding/thrombophilia, and other possible pathways including hormones and toxins that when combined with racial and ethnic disparities, fetal growth, and PPROM can also result in spontaneous preterm labor/birth (Goldenberg et al., 2008; Institute of Medicine [IOM], 2007; MOD, 2018, 2019a; Menon, 2008; Romero, Dey, & Fisher, 2014). When thought of in this manner, it is clear that there is no

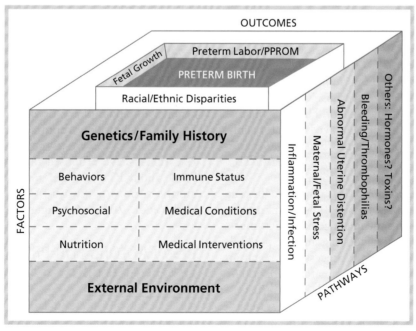

FIGURE 7–1. Determinants of preterm labor.

one "cause" of preterm labor and birth and, therefore, no one single "cure." Multiple causes require research into many cures and preventive measures. One of the significant barriers in studying the causative factors of preterm labor and birth is the lack of knowledge regarding the exact physiologic mechanism responsible for initiation of term labor and birth. As with preterm labor, multiple theories have been proposed concerning which factors are responsible for spontaneous term labor, but none has proven conclusive yet. New research in the roles of maternal metabolism, genetics, maternal microbiomes, and inflammation is showing promise in potentially identifying causative factors of preterm labor and birth. These include the following:

1. *Association between lipid levels and spontaneous preterm delivery*: A case-controlled study of lipid levels (cholesterol, triglycerides, high-density lipoprotein, and low-density cholesterol) in maternal blood and in cord blood revealed that abnormal lipid metabolism may occur in women and preterm infants experiencing spontaneous preterm delivery (Li, Hua, Jian-Ping, & Yan, 2015).

2. *Genetic contributions*: Scientists are finding that certain genomes are associated with the duration of pregnancy as well as spontaneous PTB. Ongoing studies of genetic variants and loci associated with PTB are currently being performed (Zhang et al., 2017).

3. *Maternal microbiomes*: Microbiomes are basically normal bacteria that inhabit the body and assist with normal functions and health. Researchers are hypothesizing that with the physiologic changes of pregnancy that occur, immunologic changes may also transpire in the gut, placenta, and reproductive tract, leading to adverse outcomes like PTB (Parnell, Briggs, & Mysorekar, 2017). Current research suggests that women with PPROM who will develop preterm labor have different microbiomes in the second trimester than those who will reach term gestation. Studies of non-Hispanic black women indicate they may have less lactobacillus in their vaginal microbiome than non-Hispanic white women, leading to a higher rate of PTB (Fettweis et al., 2014; Manuck, 2017).

4. *Infections/inflammation*: It is now thought that at least half of spontaneous PTBs of unknown origin are due to subclinical genital tract infections. Researchers are looking into the possibility that the inflammatory process may result in repression of the anti-inflammatory function of progesterone (Di Renzo, Pacella, Di Fabrizio, & Giardina, 2017); B lymphocytes have been known to help the body fight off infection by producing antibodies. A recent study found that B lymphocytes are present in the uterine lining during late pregnancy and have the ability to not only detect inflammation and uterine stress but also produce molecules that can then suppress the inflammatory process that leads to PTB (Huang et al., 2017).

5. *Prenatal stress*: Studies on the effects of hormones related to prenatal stress show that maternal production of glucocorticoids, prostaglandins, and circulating inflammatory markers may contribute to the development of preterm labor. Furthermore, recent research proposes that the fetus may also play an important role in stress-induced PTB with production of adrenal hormones (Boateng, 2011; Rood & Buhimschi, 2017).

6. *Cervical remodeling*: In order for any birth to occur, the cervix must dilate enough for the fetus to be delivered. Because of this fact, researchers are now taking a new in-depth look at the structure and function of the cervix in relationship to spontaneous PTB. They have rediscovered a large amount of smooth muscle that borders the periphery of the internal os. These findings suggest the possibility that this smooth muscle is actually a form of a specialized sphincter, and when cervical funneling or dilation of the internal os is present, it is in fact related to "sphincter failure." Additional multidisciplinary studies are recommended to further research in this area (Vink & Mourad, 2017; Vink et al., 2016). Proteins potentially involved in the regulation of cervical remodeling that leads to PPROM were identified in a recent study suggesting that causes of premature labor are multifactorial with potential different pathways for PPROM and preterm labor (Makieva et al., 2017).

Not all PTBs can or should be prevented. About 25% of PTBs are intentional and occur because of health problems of the mother or the fetus (e.g., intrauterine growth restriction, preeclampsia, abruptio placentae, and pulmonary or cardiac disease); another 25% of PTBs follow rupture of membranes (a cause not currently known to be preventable). Recently, researchers have proposed reconceptualizing how we think about PTB in order to more clearly differentiate the various pathways (ACOG & SMFM, 2017a; Hirbo et al., 2015; Monangi et al., 2015).

RISK FACTORS FOR PRETERM LABOR AND BIRTH

Risk factors for preterm labor and birth have been published and refined since the early 1980s (IOM, 1985). Historically, risk factors and gestational age have defined the conversation about preterm labor and birth. However, recent discussions are showing that many risk factors are interrelated making it difficult to pinpoint a single etiology for preterm labor and birth (Manuck, 2017).

In addressing prevention of PTB, the MOD suggested that there are three important known risk factors for preterm labor and birth (current multifetal pregnancy, history of a PTB, and uterine/cervical abnormalities), along with multiple categories of risk for subgroups of women (MOD, 2018). Additional risk factors include medical conditions predating the pregnancy, demographic factors, behavioral and environmental factors, illnesses occurring during the pregnancy, and genetics. These factors are listed in Displays 7–3 and 7–4. One of the risk factors that has received attention in the literature is periodontal disease. Follow-up studies of interventions in periodontal disease have attempted to identify an association between adverse pregnancy outcomes, including spontaneous PTB. Research has been unable to provide conclusive evidence that treatment of periodontal disease does indeed improve rates of PTB and LBW. Instead, it is hypothesized that any association between periodontal disease and PTB may be due to an exaggerated inflammatory response to the bacteria, which in turn leads to both conditions. Consequently, it is thought that there may be an epidemiologic link but not a causally related link between periodontal disease and PTB (Sanz & Kornman, 2013).

Some of the risks of preterm labor and birth have been known for decades, and some are new to the list (IOM, 1985, 2007). Knowledge of the genetics of PTB (see next section) is clearly a new and evolving phenomenon. The risk of preterm labor after the use of ART is another concern that is currently being studied. Qin and colleagues (2015) performed a meta-analysis of 39 studies, examining the outcomes of 146,008 multiple births. They found significantly higher odds ratios for PTB and other adverse perinatal outcomes in the multiples conceived through ART. Further risks of ART include PPROM, pregnancy-induced hypertension, gestational diabetes mellitus, LBW and VLBW, and congenital malformations (Qin et al., 2015). Of live births from pregnancies conceived in ART cycles using fresh nondonor eggs or embryos in 2015, 77.2% were singletons, 22.1% were twins, and 0.6% were

higher order multiples (Sunderam et al., 2018). Among ART births in 2015, 58.2% of twins, 96.3% of higher order multiples were born preterm, and 55.9% of twins and 93.5% of higher order multiples were LBW (Sunderam et al., 2018).

Genetic Influences

In the late 1970s when the topic of preterm labor and birth became prominent as an important entity for research and prevention, no thought was given to the possibility that preterm labor could have a genetic component. For decades, researchers in medicine, epidemiology, public health, and nursing focused on physical symptoms, biologic pathways, and social

DISPLAY 7–4

Other Possible Risk Factors for Preterm Labor

Chronic health problems
- Hypertension
- Diabetes mellitus
- Clotting disorders/thrombophilia
- Low prepregnancy weight
- Obesity
- Abnormal lipid metabolism

Behavioral and environmental risks
- Late or no prenatal care
- Smoking
- Alcohol abuse
- Use of illicit drugs
- Diethylstilbestrol exposure
- Intimate partner violence
- Lack of social support
- High levels of stress
- Long working hours
- Long periods of standing

Demographic risks
- Non-Hispanic black race
- Age <17 years old
- Age >35 years old
- Low socioeconomic status

Genetics

Cervical remodeling

Assisted reproductive technologies

Medical risks in current pregnancy
- Infection (especially genitourinary infections)
- Changes in the maternal microbiome
- Short interpregnancy interval
- Fetal anomalies
- Preterm premature rupture of membranes
- Vaginal bleeding (especially in the second trimester or in more than one trimester)
- Periodontal disease with potential epidemiologic link
- Being underweight prior to the pregnancy

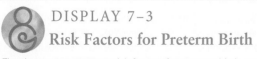

DISPLAY 7–3

Risk Factors for Preterm Birth

The three most common risk factors for preterm birth are
- Current multifetal pregnancy
- History of a preterm birth
- Uterine/cervical abnormalities

interventions in their efforts to prevent this costly and dangerous complication of pregnancy. It was not until 2003 that the director of the National Human Genome Research Institute at the National Institutes of Health announced that sequencing of the human genome had been completed (National Human Genome Research Institute, 2003). This event ushered in the genomic era of health research and has impacted the study of PTB in extraordinary ways. What we once thought of as strictly a social phenomenon or a biologic accident is now showing that 30% to 40% of PTBs may be related to genetics (Bezold, Karjalainen, Hallman, Teramo, & Muglia, 2013; Boyd et al., 2009; Plunkett et al., 2009; York et al., 2013). The possibility that preterm labor and birth has a genetic component provides us with new targets for prevention.

Because almost 50% of preterm births are associated with an inflammatory response, a considerable amount of research in genetics and protein fingerprints have concentrated on this pathway (Tambor et al., 2015). One study identified proteins in amniotic fluid that were associated with an infectious inflammatory complication related to spontaneous PTB (Tambor et al., 2015). Other areas of new research are looking at causes of PTB when infection and inflammation are not present. Ongoing studies on twin births and preterm labor demonstrate the potential role of maternal genetic factors. Using this information, researchers were able to identify 33 genes, including 217 variants from five modules that differed profoundly between study cases with preterm labor and controls without preterm labor. Furthermore, the study indicated that there is a 36% to 40% increased chance that future generations will also experience a PTB (Uzun et al., 2016); a thorough review of studies on single nucleotide gene polymorphisms identified 119 genes potentially associated with PTB (Sheikh et al., 2016);

another study on more than 44,000 women of European and Nordic descent identified six genes associated with PTB. Researchers also found that one of the implicated genes found in the cellular lining of the uterus appears to affect the length of pregnancy. Last of all, they identified a gene that is involved in the body's use of selenium and preterm labor (Rayman, Wijnen, Vader, Kooistra, & Pop, 2011; Zhang et al., 2017). In this patient population, treatment for preterm labor could potentially be found by simply adding selenium supplements in expectant mothers' diets. This sort of tailored intervention is an example of how advances in our understanding of genetics and biomarkers could transform the way we look at PTB prevention and presents a new avenue for future studies on PTB (Rayman et al., 2011).

Currently, the number of mothers and infants that have been phenotyped and genotyped for preterm labor risk is small (Monangi et al., 2015). Data gleaned from this information is providing insights into new areas of genetic research related to preterm labor and birth. Scientists are hopeful that as the number of participants grows, new gene-related targets for therapy and prevention will be discovered. (See Tables 7–2 to 7–4 for genes that control pro-inflammatory cytokines involved in possible infection and PPROM, the labor cascade genes [being studied for their role in the initiation of labor], and vasculopathic genes [involved in vascular problems such as preeclampsia and thrombophilias]).

PRETERM BIRTH RISK IN THE CONTEXT OF THE LIFE COURSE

Several investigators have observed that PTB is characterized by complex interactions between genes, environment, and socioeconomic factors. It is presently

TABLE 7–2. Pro-inflammatory Cytokines

Candidate genes	Symbol	Polymorphisms	Role of candidate gene in preterm labor and birth	Speculated impact of the polymorphism
Interleukin 6	IL-6	G-174C Other SNPs: C/C G/G G/C	Critical in the cascade of host response; activates the acute phase response, stimulates T lymphocytes, induces differentiation of B lymphocytes; increases seen in gestational tissues in PTL	Women with C/C variation produce less IL-6 and are less likely to manifest the inflammatory cascade leading to PTL. C/C variation lacking in African American women in PTB cases <34 weeks.
Interleukin 1 beta	IL-1β	IL-1β+3953*1 IL 1RN*2	A key pro-inflammatory cytokine correlated to prostaglandin production and increased uterine activity; found in membranes in PTL	Fetal carriage of these variations possibly increases the IL-1β cytokine production and risk for PTB.
Tumor necrosis factor-α promotor gene	TNF-α	G-308A (TNFA2 or Allele 2)	Pro-inflammatory cytokine; elevated in the amniotic fluid of women experiencing preterm labor, PPROM, and positive amniotic fluid cultures	TNFA2 allele causes elevated levels of TNF-α protein, leading to immune hyperresponsiveness to environmental factors, such as bacterial vaginosis, causing chorioamnionitis

PPROM, preterm premature rupture of membranes; PTB, preterm birth; PTL, preterm labor; SNPs, single nucleotide polymorphisms.
Adapted from Giarratano, G. (2006). Genetic influences on preterm birth. *MCN: The American Journal of Maternal/Child Nursing, 31*(3), 169–175.

TABLE 7–3. Labor Cascade Pathways

Candidate genes	Symbol	Polymorphisms	Role of candidate gene in preterm labor and birth	Speculated impact of the polymorphism
Oxytocin receptors	OTRs	No association found with OTRs rs2254298, rs53576, rs2228485, rs237911	In normal labor onset, OTRs are thought to increase myometrial sensitivity to oxytocin before labor onset. The binding of oxytocin to the myometrial receptor promotes the influx of calcium from the intracellular stores, as one pathway to activate contractions.	Findings on study of 100 women with preterm labor. No association between the presence of four common OTR gene polymorphisms and preterm labor noted. But the combination of three haplotype genes were found to be significantly associated with PTB.
Combination of haplotype OTRs	OTRs	Association found: rs2254298 A allele OTR rs2228485 C allele OTR rs237911 G allele		
Corticotropin-releasing hormone	CRH	T255G Other SNPs: T/T T/G G/G CRF CRH1	CRH is synthesized in the hypothalamus in response to stress, and in the placenta and membranes in pregnancy. CRH metabolic pathway promotes production of prostaglandins and PTL onset.	A rapid increase of CRH occurs at high levels of stress as well as the onset of labor. Studies suggest that this stress may be a trigger for preterm labor/birth; in an obesity study, T/G variation in combination with a glucocorticoid polymorphism increased cortisol levels.

PTB, preterm birth; PTL, preterm labor; SNPs, single nucleotide polymorphisms.
Adapted from Giarratano, G. (2006). Genetic influences on preterm birth. *MCN: The American Journal of Maternal/Child Nursing, 31*(3), 169–175; Kuessel, L., Grimm, C., Knöfler, M., Haslinger, P., Leipold, H., Heinze, G., . . . Schmid, M. (2013). Common oxytocin receptor gene polymorphisms and the risk for preterm birth. *Disease Markers, 34*(1), 51–56. doi:10.3233/DMA-2012-00936; National Center for Biotechnology Information. (2019). *CRH corticotropin releasing hormone receptor 1 [Homo sapiens (human)]*. Retrieved from https://www.ncbi.nlm.nih.gov/gene/1392

believed that preconception stress and/or cumulative activation of stressors, such as racism and economic stress across the life course may contribute to the observed racial disparity in PTB in the United States. Although the exact mechanisms of these effects are unclear, it does appear as though stress-induced production of biologically active glucocorticoids, prostaglandins, and corticotropin-releasing hormone may be related to stress-associated PTBs, especially if they occur during the second half of the pregnancy (Frey & Klebanoff, 2016; Wadhwa, Entringer, Buss, & Lu, 2011). Better understanding of social inequities, including local environmental exposures, in conjunction with genetic responses, gene-environment interaction, and microbiomes may

TABLE 7–4. Vasculopathic Pathways

Candidate genes	Symbol	Polymorphisms	Role of candidate gene in preterm labor and birth	Speculated impact of the polymorphism
Vascular endothelial growth factor	VEGF	C936T Other SNPs: T/T	VEGF is a major angiogenic factor and regulates endothelial cell proliferation. Threshold levels are required for fetal and placental vascular development and inhibition of cell death in the placenta.	C936T is associated with lower VEGF production; an association was found between this variation and an increased risk of spontaneous PTB. VEGF/inflammatory markers in midtrimester amniotic fluid may be predictive values in determining risk for spontaneous PTB.
		C677T A1298C	An abnormal vascular network is hypothesized to predispose to spontaneous abortion or to early labor and birth.	
		IL-6 MMP-8		
Methylenetra-hydrofolate reductase (enzyme)	MTHFR	Risks results from a vitamin B_{12} deficiency, plus mutation	Elevates homocysteine, a risk factor associated with many vascular disorders in adults. In pregnancy, associated with uteroplacental vasculopathy, such as thrombosis and placental infarcts, seen with PTB.	Both mutations associated with decreased MTHFR activity, which increases homocysteine concentrations, particularly with low folate. Association of this mutation with PTB is unknown.

PTB, preterm birth; SNPs, single nucleotide polymorphisms.
From Giarratano, G. (2006). Genetic influences on preterm birth. *MCN: The American Journal of Maternal/Child Nursing, 31*(3), 169–175; Kim, A., Lee, E. S., Shin, J. C., & Kim, H. Y. (2013). Identification of biomarkers for preterm delivery in mid-trimester amniotic fluid. *Placenta, 34*(10), 873–878. doi:10.1016/j.placenta.2013.06.306

ultimately explain disparities in U.S. birth outcomes and contribute to the development of more effective prevention strategies (Frey & Klebanoff, 2016; MOD, 2018; McPherson & Manuck, 2016; Parnell et al., 2017).

Risk Factors as Screening Methods to Predict Preterm Labor and Birth

Because there is, as yet, no known single causative factor for preterm labor and about 50% of all PTBs occur in women with no known risk factors (Sheikh et al., 2016), it must be concluded that all pregnant women are at some risk for preterm labor and birth. Therefore, risk screening for PTB (as well as other obstetric or medical complications of pregnancy) should be conducted during the prenatal period as part of a comprehensive assessment process. Women with a history of PTB or second trimester miscarriages are at greatest risk of PTB. Furthermore, the risk appears to increase with the numbers of abortions a patient has had in the past (Di Renzo, Pacella, et al., 2017). This knowledge, along with other known risk factors, can assist healthcare providers in hopefully identifying early signs of impending preterm labor. A problem as pervasive as preterm labor and birth must be explained to all pregnant women during routine prenatal care, with instructions to report any symptoms of early labor to their healthcare providers immediately.

CAN PRETERM LABOR AND BIRTH BE PREVENTED?

The search for prevention of PTB has been ongoing for decades. It would be comforting to think that simple strategies such as prenatal care could prevent PTB, but studies have not shown that to be true (Rundell & Panchal, 2017). Current thinking in this field proposes that preconception, prenatal, and postpartum care provide opportunities to educate women regarding their ability to reduce or eliminate modifiable risk factors for PTB (Johnson et al., 2006; O'Connor & Gennaro, 2017). Ongoing education can potentially ameliorate some preexisting factors such as smoking cessation, substance abuse, interpersonal violence, tight regulation of preexisting diabetes, hypertension, obesity, optimal interpregnancy intervals, nutritional status, or optimal control of chronic diseases prior to and during pregnancy (Johnson et al., 2006; MOD, 2018; O'Connor & Gennaro, 2017; van Zijl, Koullali, Mol, Pajkrt, & Oudijk, 2016).

Mental health can be an important factor in predicting a healthy pregnancy outcome. Studies involving maternal depression and use of selective serotonin reuptake inhibitors during pregnancy demonstrate an increased risk of spontaneous PTB, although higher rates of risky behaviors such as smoking, poor nutrition,

alcohol use, and irregular attendance at prenatal visits may be confounding factors that also increase the risk (Cantarutti et al., 2016; Huybrechts et al., 2014; Staneva et al., 2015). Those involved in mental healthcare, as well as obstetric healthcare providers, can assist in possible prevention of preterm labor and birth with early identification of maternal psychological needs. Planning strategies that help patients manage mental health issues during pregnancy may reduce the potential for prematurity. More research into perinatal mood disorders and standardized treatment plans is needed in this area (Staneva et al., 2015).

In an attempt to assist with prevention and reduction of PTB, the MOD Prematurity Campaign instituted goals to reduce PTBs to 8.1% by 2020 and 5.5% by 2030 (MOD, 2016). Plans to accomplish these goals include reduction of elective deliveries, progesterone therapy for women with a history of prior PTB, reduction or cessation of smoking when pregnant, encouraging birth spacing of at least 18 months apart, use of low-dose aspirin for women at risk for preeclampsia, universal screening for short cervix, and reduction of multiple births using ART (MOD, 2016).

Biochemical Markers

The search for early predictive factors for preterm labor and birth has included the use of biochemical markers, most notably fetal fibronectin. The U.S. Food and Drug Administration (FDA) approved fetal fibronectin testing for preterm labor in 1995. Fetal fibronectin is an extracellular matrix glycoprotein produced in the decidual cells of the uterus and is thought to be the trophoblastic "glue" in the formation of the uteroplacental junction. Lockwood et al. (1991) first published a study suggesting that fetal fibronectin found in vaginal secretions between 24 and 34 weeks at a level greater than 50 ng/mL is a predictor of preterm labor.

Fetal fibronectin is present in the cervical–vaginal secretions between 16 and 19 weeks of gestation and then disappears until around term gestation. It can become detectable approximately 1 week prior to the onset of preterm labor (Di Renzo, Pacella, et al., 2017). It has been theorized that preterm labor breaks the bonds between the placenta and the amniotic membranes, causing release of fetal fibronectin into the vaginal secretions. Several factors may affect the accuracy of the results of fetal fibronectin testing, including sexual activity within 24 hours of sample collection, cervical examination within 24 hours of sample collection, vaginal probe ultrasound, vaginal bleeding, intraamniotic and vaginal infections, and use of douches or vaginal lubricants. When a woman presents with signs and symptoms of preterm labor that is a potential candidate for fetal fibronectin testing, it is important to delay digital examination of the cervix until the test has been completed.

The potential value of the test is in deciding who is at immediate risk for preterm labor and who is not. The negative predictive value (NPV) of the fetal fibronectin test is high (up to 95%), whereas the positive predictive value (PPV) is low (25% to 40%). Therefore, the test is most effective in predicting who will not experience preterm labor rather than who will experience it. Studies combining the use of the fetal fibronectin test and cervical length measurement have shown some limited value in determining risk for PTB (Son & Miller, 2017).

Another biochemical marker test using placental alpha microglobulin-1 (PAMG-1) in cervical–vaginal secretions was studied in the United States (Wing et al., 2017). PAMG-1 is a glycoprotein released from the decidual cells and is found in high concentrations only in the amniotic fluid. The presence of PAMG-1 in cervical–vaginal fluid when labor and delivery is imminent is likely due to a hydrostatic or osmotic pressure gradient that allows passage of the protein (PAMG-1) through preexisting pores in the chorioamniotic membranes during uterine contractions and, potentially, degradation of the extracellular matrix of fetal membranes due to an inflammatory process of labor or infection (Bolotskikh & Borisova, 2017). Two recent large-scale studies have directly compared the predictive ability of both fetal fibronectin and PAMG-1 tests for the prediction of spontaneous preterm delivery among singletons within 7 days of testing. A prospective observational clinical trial was conducted at 15 academic and community hospital centers across the United States. Wing and colleagues (2017) reported the presence of PAMG-1 in vaginal secretions at a level greater than 1 ng/mL, between 24 and 34 weeks and 6 days to be a predictor of imminent spontaneous preterm delivery in women with intact membranes and cervical dilation less than 3 cm who presented with signs or symptoms of preterm labor (Wing et al., 2017). Of the 711 women included in the study, the PPV for fetal fibronectin was only 4.3%, whereas the PAMG-1 PPV was 23.1%. The study concluded that although PAMG-1 and fetal fibronectin NPVs were similar (PAMG-1 99.5%; fetal fibronectin 99.6%), PAMG-1 demonstrated statistical superiority in predicting spontaneous preterm labor (Wing et al., 2017). Another study conducted in Spain included women with singleton gestations between 24 and 34 weeks and 6 days gestation with symptoms of early preterm labor, intact membranes, and cervical dilation less than 3 cm. Results demonstrated a fetal fibronectin PPV of 7.9% and NPV of 97.9% compared to a PPV of 35.3% and NPV of 98.3% using PAMG-1. Over the course of separate 1-year periods, the study found that researchers were more than 2 times more likely to have a positive fetal fibronectin test than a PAMG-1 test. Yet, the rate of women who ended up delivering within 14 days of testing was not affected. They also found that a positive PAMG-1 test was more than 4 times more reliable than a positive fetal fibronectin test in predicting impending spontaneous preterm delivery (Melchor et al., 2017). Given the location of PAMG-1 inside the amniotic cavity, collections of a PAMG-1 specimen following a recent vaginal examination or intercourse are not expected to lead to false-positive test results and can be collected without the use of a speculum (Melchor et al., 2017).

The potential value of biochemical tests is in their ability to correctly determine patients at immediate risk for preterm labor versus those who are not. Researchers continue to be challenged to develop sensitive and specific tests that can detect markers of preterm labor and delivery before they become irreversible. Benefits of biochemical testing can assist in reducing unnecessary hospital admissions, transfers of patients to a higher level of care, and decreased NICU admissions. These benefits can result in decreased medical interventions and in cost savings to patients and hospitals (Di Renzo, Pacella, et al., 2017).

Cervical Length Measurements

Measuring cervical length has been thought to be predictive of PTB because, in some populations, it has been shown that a short cervical length can be a precursor to preterm labor. Women who experience significant cervical shortening in the second trimester have been shown to be at increased risk for spontaneous PTB (Berghella, Roman, Daskalakis, Ness, & Baxter 2007; SMFM, McIntosh, Feltovich, Berghella, & Manuck, 2016). Under normal circumstances, cervical length does not undergo changes between 14 and 28 weeks of gestation. Median cervical lengths at 22 weeks should be around 40 mm and approximately 35 mm at 22 to 32 weeks' gestation. After 28 to 32 weeks, the cervical length will slowly shorten and reach an average of 30 mm. Short cervix is diagnosed when the cervical length is less than or equal to 25 mm at 16 to 24 weeks' gestation (Romero et al., 2012). SMFM guidelines recommend cervical length measurements in the second trimester for women with a singleton pregnancy and a history of previous spontaneous PTB. At this time, there is insufficient evidence to mandate universal cervical length screening for all pregnant women (SMFM et al., 2016).

Transvaginal ultrasound is the gold standard for cervical length measurement and has been shown to be more sensitive than transabdominal ultrasound. This technology does require significant skill and training, though, to assure consistency and accuracy of results (SMFM et al., 2016; Wax, Cartin, & Pinette, 2016). Studies are also showing that use of transabdominal ultrasound in conjunction with biochemical screening tests can be beneficial in identifying patients at risk for spontaneous PTB (Bolotskikh & Borisova, 2017).

If ultrasound is not available or easily accessible, use of a nonsonographic cervical length measurement using a measuring probe (Cervilenz) may be valuable as a screening tool. This can be a cost-saving method to identify women who truly need sonographic evaluation (Möller, Henderson, Nathan, & Pennell, 2013).

Cervical Cerclage

Cervical cerclage is a surgical procedure that involves stitching a piece of suture around the neck of the cervix to give additional support in an attempt to reduce the risk of PTB or second trimester miscarriage (Alfirevic, Stampalija, & Medley, 2017). Most cervical cerclages performed to reduce rates of preterm birth are placed transvaginal, although on rare occasions, the transabdominal route may be used if there is extreme shortening of the cervix, scarring, or lacerations. The transabdominal cerclage is placed by laparotomy, and the patient is then delivered by cesarean section (Burger, Brölmann, Einarsson, Langebrekke, & Huirne, 2011). Use of a cerclage is indicated in women with a history of spontaneous PTB at 17 to 33 weeks and 6 days gestation and a cervical length less than 25 mm before 23 weeks gestation (Owen et al., 2009; SMFM, 2015).

A Cochrane review analyzed 15 trials that assessed cerclage use in singleton pregnancies with history of pregnancy loss and/or shortened cervix. The authors concluded that use of a cervical cerclage in women at high risk for preterm delivery decreased the risks of PTB and potentially decreased the risk of perinatal deaths. But they were unable to state whether other treatments for preterm delivery would be just as effective (Alfirevic et al., 2017). Studies of progesterone use with cerclage are limited at this time, but SMFM does include administration of 17-alpha hydroxyprogesterone caproate (17OHP-C) in its management strategies for cervical cerclage (SMFM, 2015). Utilization of cervical cerclage with multiples has been found to increase the risk of preterm birth twofold (Berghella, Odibo, To, Rust, & Althuisius, 2005; Di Renzo, Roura, et al., 2017). Because of this, use of cervical cerclage in multiple gestations is not recommended (Di Renzo, Roura, et al., 2017).

Cervical cerclage placement is usually performed as an outpatient procedure with discharge once the woman is able to void and ambulate. Patients should be educated to report any leaking of vaginal fluid, bleeding, or uterine contractions to their provider.

Pessary

Use of a silicone pessary to decrease rates of spontaneous preterm birth is a noninvasive intervention that has been studied recently. The pessary is flexible and is thought to actually change cervical position away from the internal cervical os and toward the sacrum. This action redistributes the weight of the uterus to the vaginal floor and surrounding areas (Di Renzo, Roura, et al., 2017; Saccone, Maruotti, Giudicepietro, & Martinelli, 2017; SMFM, 2017b). The pessary may also form a barrier between the chorion and vaginal flora that can potentially cause spontaneous preterm labor and birth (Jones, Clark, & Bewley, 1998).

Two randomized controlled trials using cervical pessaries were performed in multiple institutions with almost 2,000 twin pregnancies. Results did not demonstrate a significant drop in the rate of PTBs (Liem et al., 2013; Nicolaides et al., 2016). Trials in women with a singleton pregnancy and short cervix has shown contradictory data. In one trial, a cervical pessary decreased PTBs from 27% to 6%, whereas another study group increased the PTB rate from 5.5% to 9.4% (Goya et al., 2012; Hui, Chor, Lau, Lao, & Leung, 2013). More recently, Saccone and colleagues (2017) found that women presenting with a short transvaginal cervical length, without a prior history of PTB and a singleton pregnancy without contractions, demonstrated lower rates of spontaneous PTB before 34 weeks' gestation with use of a pessary, compared to those who did not have a pessary (Saccone et al., 2017). Further studies need to be performed to assess whether this device can provide an additional noninvasive method of decreasing rates of PTB.

Progesterone

Progesterone appears to play an important role in keeping uterine activity at a minimum, especially during the latter portion of the pregnancy. With the onset of both term and preterm labor, scientists have noted that progesterone levels in pregnant women appear to drop, leading to increased uterine activity (Lockwood et al., 2010; Mesiano, Wang, & Norwitz, 2011). Although the mechanism of how this occurs is unknown, progesterone supplementation has been shown to decrease PTB rates in women with a singleton pregnancy and a history of PTB by approximately 30% (Dodd, Jones, Flenady, Cincotta, & Crowther, 2013). Progesterone administration in this patient population also resulted in lower rates of neonatal morbidities including death, use of assisted ventilation, necrotizing enterocolitis, and decreased NICU admissions (Dodd et al., 2013).

According to the SMFM (2012), there is inadequate evidence recommending progesterone therapy for singleton pregnancies with no history of PTB and an unknown cervical length. For women who present with a cervical length less than 20 mm at less than 24 weeks' gestation, vaginal progesterone has been shown to decrease the rate of PTB and perinatal morbidity and mortality and may be considered as a treatment option. Women who have previously experienced a spontaneous PTB (20 to 36 weeks and 6 days) with a singleton pregnancy are recommended weekly intramuscular 17OHP-C therapy in subsequent singleton pregnancies, starting at 16 to 20 weeks' gestation until 36 weeks' gestation (SMFM, 2012, 2017a). Administration of progesterone to women with multiple gestations and preterm labor or PPROM has not been associated with the prevention of preterm delivery. Although some experts have offered 17OHP-C to this patient population who have previously experienced a spontaneous PTB, there is insufficient information to adequately assess risks and benefits associated with the intervention (SMFM, 2012). See Figure 7–2 for

SMFM (2012) algorithm for use of progesterone in prevention of PTB in clinical care.

Studies to determine if progesterone administration could be used for maintenance tocolysis after preterm labor was arrested in women with intact membranes have concluded that it is not effective and should not be used routinely (Eke, Chalaan, Shukr, Eleje, & Okafor, 2016; Wood, Rabi, Tang, Brant, & Ross, 2017). Administration of 17OHP-C to women who had undergone placement of a transvaginal cerclage showed a 73% reduction in delivery at less than 24 weeks' gestation compared to women with cerclage surgery only, demonstrating that the addition of progesterone increases the

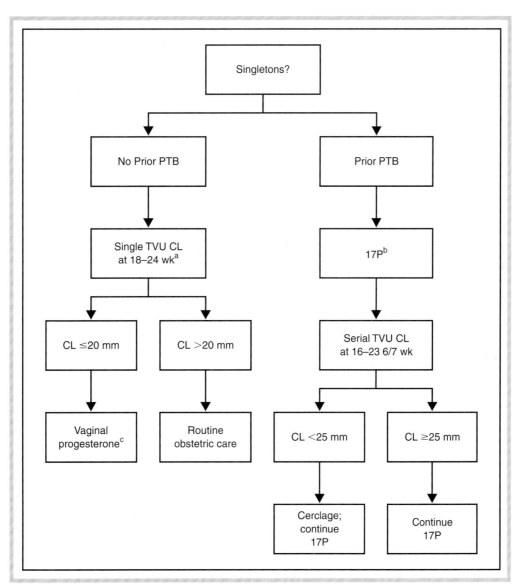

FIGURE 7–2. Algorithm for use of progestogens in prevention of PTB in clinical care. [a]If TVU CL screening is performed. [b]17P 250 mg intramuscularly every week from 16 to 20 weeks to 36 weeks. [c]For example, daily 200-mg suppository or 90-mg gel from time of diagnosis of short CL to 36 weeks. CL, cervical length; PTB, preterm birth; 17P, 17-alpha-hydroxy-progesterone caproate; TVU, transvaginal ultrasound. (From Society for Maternal-Fetal Medicine. [2012]. Progesterone and preterm birth prevention: Translating clinical trials data into clinical practice. *American Journal of Obstetrics & Gynecology, 206*[5], 376–386.)

chance of delivering a viable neonate (Stetson, Hibbard, Wilkins, & Leftwich, 2016).

Findings on safety, side effects, and adverse reactions associated with progesterone administration as a means to prevent PTB, do not show an increase risk of major complications for women or their infants 2 years after they received the medication (Norman et al., 2016).

Bed Rest

Although bed rest, either in the hospital setting or at home, for treatment of spontaneous PTB is occasionally still recommended by some practitioners, evidence for or against it is lacking. A Cochrane review revealed two studies that met inclusion criteria for bed rest. One study combined singleton and multiple pregnancies and showed no differences in perinatal outcomes using bed rest (Sosa, Althabe, Belizán, & Bergel, 2015). The other study reviewed results of bed rest for 432 women compared to 834 women who either received a placebo or had no intervention. Outcomes showed similar rates of PTB before 37 weeks' gestation in both groups (Sosa et al., 2015). An analysis performed by Grobman and colleagues (2013) in conjunction with the NICHD and Maternal-Fetal Medicine Units Network determined that restriction of activity did not lessen the rate of PTB in nulliparous women receiving 17OHP-C therapy who presented with a short cervix and no symptoms of preterm labor (Grobman et al., 2013). On the other hand, risks of thromboembolic events in pregnancy related to bed rest and hospitalization have been noted (Sultan et al., 2013). Sultan et al. (2013) found that 3 or more days in the hospital led to the highest rate of developing venous thromboembolism. They also discovered a fourfold increase in the risk of developing a thrombosis in women admitted to the hospital for less than 3 days. The rate of venous thromboembolism was also high in the 28 days following discharge. They concluded that pregnant women admitted to the hospital, not related to delivery, should receive thromboprophylaxis therapy (Sultan et al., 2013). Bed rest has also demonstrated negative psychological effects, loss of muscle mass, poorer nutrition, orthostatic hypotension, as well as other symptoms related to a deconditioned state (Convertino, Bloomfield, Greenleaf, 1997; Murray & McKinney, 2014). Display 7–5 describes nursing care measures for women who are prescribed bed rest during pregnancy. At this time, ACOG (2016b) recommends that bed rest not be used routinely, as studies have not demonstrated this intervention to be effective in preventing spontaneous PTB.

Intravenous Hydration

One common strategy used in inpatient settings to reduce preterm contractions is intravenous (IV) hydration. Significant amounts of IV fluids are usually administered to increase vascular volume and because,

DISPLAY 7–5
Nursing Care for Women Prescribed Bed Rest as Therapy

- Assist the family in becoming involved in the nursing care plan.
- Assist the woman and healthcare team in clarifying what is meant by "bed rest" (e.g., Allowed to sit up? Shower? Make dinner? Use the stairs __ times per day?).
- If the family is not available, suggest that the woman ask friends for help during this time.
- Maintaining hydration while on bed rest is important; suggest that a cooler be kept beside the bed.
- Bed rest can lead to muscle wasting; teach passive limb exercises.
- Anxiety and depression are common during bed rest; teach the family to expect this and talk about their feelings.
- The woman should be in a place where she can interact with her family rather than in a bedroom alone.
- Instruct the woman not to do any nipple preparation for breastfeeding; nipple stimulation can cause uterine contractions.
- Some women find that keeping a journal helps them deal with the isolation and boredom of bed rest.
- Household jobs that can be done while in bed (e.g., paying bills, mending, folding laundry) help the woman feel more a part of the family.
- This is a good time to provide short educational videos about all aspects of pregnancy, labor, birth, and parenting.
- A laptop computer or tablet with Internet access can help the woman keep in touch with friends and access support and information.
- Provide referral information for online support groups to women with computer and Internet access.
- Encourage the woman to develop a support system of people with whom she can talk and vent her feelings.
- Educate the family about the emotional and behavioral responses they can expect from other children, according to the ages and developmental stages of other children in the family.

anecdotally, it is thought that uterine contractions are quieted by hydration. There has been no evidence found that hydration indeed can avert PTBs (ACOG, 2016b; Stan, Boulvain, Pfister, & Hirsbrunner-Almagbaly, 2013). Similar to bed rest therapy, however, IV fluid therapy is a traditional treatment that continues to be used despite recommendations to the contrary (ACOG, 2016b). This therapy is not without side effects. Nurses should be cautious when administering IV fluids for this purpose. If uterine activity continues, the next treatment could be administration of tocolytic agents, which carry a possible side effect of pulmonary edema. Careful attention to intake and output and auscultation of the lungs are essential to monitor for the development of pulmonary edema.

According to a review in the *Cochrane Database of Systematic Reviews*, available data does not demonstrate any advantage of hydration as a treatment for women who present in preterm labor, although hydration may be beneficial for women with evidence of dehydration (Stan et al., 2013). Based on the preponderance of the evidence that bed rest, hydration, and pelvic rest do not appear to improve rates of PTB, ACOG (2016b) does not recommend routine use of these measures.

Prophylactic Antibiotics

Prophylactic antibiotics to prevent PTB have been studied, and no evidence exists that they can prevent PTB or improve newborn outcomes in women experiencing preterm labor without rupture of membranes. Furthermore, studies indicate that prophylactic antibiotic therapy may cause lasting harm (ACOG, 2018b). This may be due in part to an active inflammatory cascade from a subclinical infection that is too advanced for antibiotic treatment to be effective (Acosta et al., 2014). ACOG (2018b, 2019) supports CDC-recommended antibiotic therapy protocols for prevention of early-onset perinatal group B *Streptococcus* (GBS) (Verani, McGee, & Schrag, 2010) in women with preterm labor because it can prevent infections in newborns (ACOG, 2018b). ACOG (2016b, 2018b) also recommends antibiotics to prolong latency (the period between rupture of membranes and onset of labor) in women with PPROM. Figure 7–3 presents the ACOG (2019) and CDC (Verani et al., 2010)

algorithm for screening for GBS colonization and use of intrapartum prophylaxis for women with preterm labor. Table 7–5 depicts the ACOG (2019) and CDC-recommended (Verani et al., 2010) regimens for intrapartum antimicrobial prophylaxis for perinatal GBS disease prevention. Figure 7–4 portrays the ACOG (2019) and CDC (Verani et al., 2010) algorithm for screening for GBS colonization and use of intrapartum prophylaxis for women with PPROM. Figure 7–5 presents the ACOG (2019) and CDC-recommended (Verani et al., 2010) regimens for intrapartum antibiotic prophylaxis for prevention of early-onset GBS disease. Care of the baby exposed to GBS is presented in Chapter 21.

Tocolytics

Although once thought of as the "magic bullet" for prevention of PTB, tocolytic drugs used to inhibit uterine contractions are now more commonly thought to be most useful in delaying birth up to 48 hours in women at 23 to 33 weeks and 6 days gestation who are diagnosed with true spontaneous preterm labor (Navathe & Berghella, 2016). This time frame allows for interventions that have been shown to improve neonatal outcomes, such as administration of antenatal glucocorticoids to help mature fetal lungs, administration of magnesium sulfate for fetal neuroprotection, and transport of the mother to a regional care center (Navathe & Berghella, 2016). Evidence does not

TABLE 7–5. Indications for Intrapartum Antibiotic Prophylaxis to Prevent Neonatal Group B Streptococcal Early-Onset Disease*

Intrapartum GBS Prophylaxis Indicated	Intrapartum GBS Prophylaxis Not Indicated

Maternal history
  Previous neonate with invasive GBS disease
Current pregnancy
  Positive GBS culture obtained at 36 weeks and 0 days of gestation or more during current pregnancy (unless a cesarean birth is performed before onset of labor for a woman with intact amniotic membranes)
  GBS bacteriuria during any trimester of the current pregnancy
Intrapartum
  Unknown GBS status at the onset of labor (culture not done or results unknown) and any of the following:
    Birth at less than 37 weeks and 0 days of gestation
    Amniotic membrane rupture 18 hours or more
    Intrapartum temperature 100.4°F (38.0°C) or higher*
    Intrapartum NAAT result positive for GBS
    Intrapartum NAAT result negative but risk factors develop (i.e., less than 37 weeks and 0 days of gestation, amniotic membrane rupture 18 hours or more, or maternal temperature 100.4°F (38.0°C) or higher)
    Known GBS-positive status in a previous pregnancy
	Colonization with GBS during a previous pregnancy (unless colonization status in current pregnancy is unknown at onset of labor at term)
	Negative vaginal–rectal GBS culture obtained at 36 weeks and 0 days of gestation or more during the current pregnancy
	Cesarean birth performed before onset of labor on a woman with intact amniotic membranes, regardless of GBS colonization status or gestational age
	
	Negative vaginal–rectal GBS culture obtained at 36 weeks and 0 days of gestation or more during the current pregnancy, regardless of intrapartum risk factors
	Unknown GBS status at onset of labor, NAAT result negative and no intrapartum risk factors present (i.e., less than 37 weeks and 0 days of gestation, amniotic membrane rupture 18 hours or more, or maternal temperature 100.4°F [38°C] or higher)

GBS, group B *Streptococcus*; NAAT, nucleic acid amplification test.
*If intraamniotic infection is suspected, broad-spectrum antibiotic therapy that includes an agent known to be active against GBS should replace GBS prophylaxis.
From American College of Obstetricians and Gynecologists. (2019). *Prevention of group B streptococcal early-onset disease in newborns* (Committee Opinion No. 782). Washington, DC: Author. Modified from Verani, J. R., McGee, L., & Schrag, S. J. (2010). Prevention of perinatal group B streptococcal disease: Revised guidelines from CDC, 2010. *Morbidity and Mortality Weekly Report Recommendations and Reports, 59*(RR-10), 1–32.

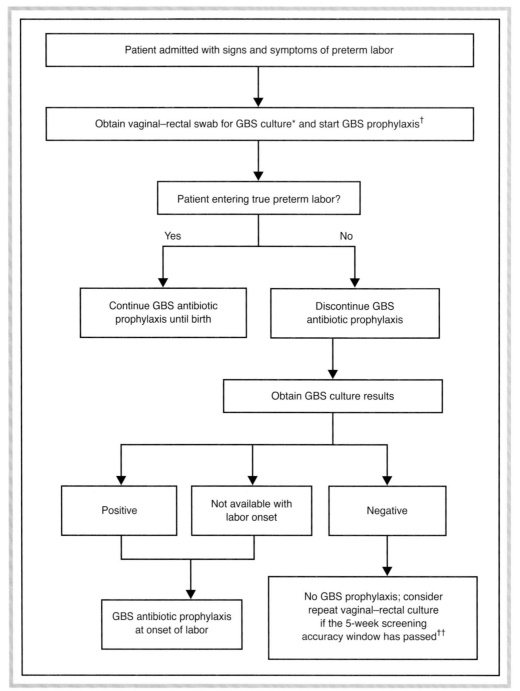

FIGURE 7–3. Management of women with preterm labor <37 weeks and 0 days of gestation. *If the patient has undergone vaginal–rectal group B *Streptococcus* (GBS) screening culture within the preceding 5 weeks, the results of that culture should guide management. Women colonized with GBS should receive intrapartum antibiotic prophylaxis. Although a negative GBS culture is considered valid for 5 weeks, the number of weeks is based on early-term screening and data in preterm gestations is lacking. †See Figure 7–5 for recommended antibiotic regimens. ††A negative GBS culture is considered valid for 5 weeks. However, the number of weeks is based on early-term screening, and data in preterm gestations is lacking. If a patient with preterm labor is entering true labor and had a negative GBS culture more than 5 weeks previously, she should be rescreened and treated according to this algorithm at that time. (American College of Obstetricians and Gynecologists. [2019]. *Prevention of group B streptococcal early-onset disease in newborns* [Committee Opinion No. 782]. Washington, DC: Author. Modified from Verani, J. R., McGee, L., & Schrag, S. J. [2010]. Prevention of perinatal group B streptococcal disease: Revised guidelines from CDC, 2010. *Morbidity and Mortality Weekly Report Recommendations and Reports, 59*[RR-10], 1–32.)

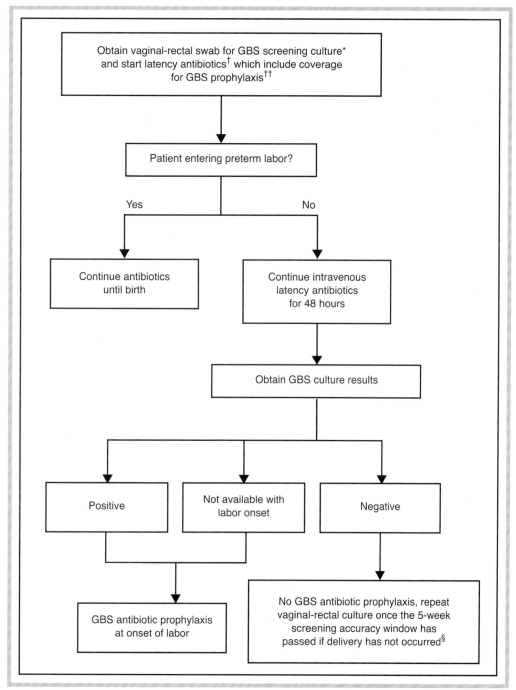

FIGURE 7–4. Management of women with preterm prelabor rupture of membranes. *If a woman has undergone vaginal–rectal group B *Streptococcus* (GBS) culture within the preceding 5 weeks, the results of that culture should guide management. Women colonized with GBS should receive intrapartum antibiotic prophylaxis. Although a negative GBS culture is considered valid for 5 weeks, the number of weeks is based on early-term screening and data in preterm gestations is lacking. †Latency antibiotics that include ampicillin given in the setting of preterm prelabor rupture of membranes are adequate for GBS prophylaxis. The optimal latency antibiotic regimen is unclear, but one of the established protocols should be used. (See ACOG [2018a] Prelabor Rupture of Membranes [Practice Bulletin No. 188].) If other regimens are used that do not provide adequate GBS coverage, GBS prophylaxis should be initiated in addition. ††See Figure 7–5 for recommended antibiotic regimens. A negative GBS culture is considered valid for 5 weeks. However, the number of weeks is based on early-term screening, and data in preterm gestations is lacking. §If a patient with preterm prelabor rupture of membranes is entering labor and had a negative GBS culture more than 5 weeks previously, she should be rescreened and managed according to this algorithm at that time. (American College of Obstetricians and Gynecologists. [2019]. *Prevention of group B streptococcal early-onset disease in newborns* [Committee Opinion No. 782]. Washington, DC: Author. Modified from Verani, J. R., McGee, L., & Schrag, S. J. [2010]. Prevention of perinatal group B streptococcal disease: Revised guidelines from CDC, 2010. *Morbidity and Mortality Weekly Report Recommendations and Reports, 59*[RR-10], 1–32.)

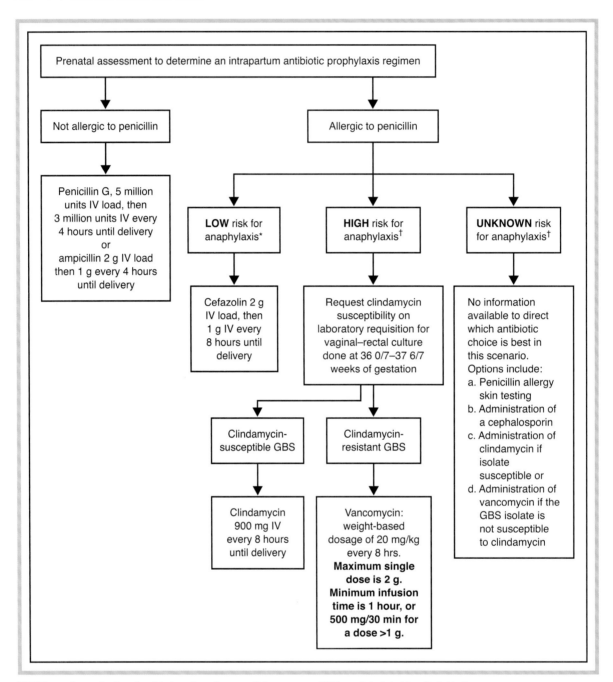

FIGURE 7–5. Determination of antibiotic regimen for group B *Streptococcus* (GBS) prophylaxis in labor. *Individuals with a history of any of the following: nonurticarial maculopapular (morbilliform) rash without systemic symptoms; family history of penicillin allergy but no personal history; nonspecific symptoms such as nausea, diarrhea, yeast vaginitis; patient reports history but has no recollection of symptoms or treatment. †Individuals with a history of any of the following after administration of a penicillin; urticarial rash (hives), intense pruritus, anaphylaxis, angioedema, laryngeal edema, respiratory distress, hypotension, immediate flushing or rare delayed reactions, such as eosin necrolysis. Individuals with recurrent reactions, reactions to multiple beta-lactam antibiotics, or those with positive skin testing also are considered high risk. (American College of Obstetricians and Gynecologists. [2019]. Prevention of group B streptococcal early-onset disease in newborns [Committee Opinion No. 782]. Washington, DC: Author. Modified from Verani, J. R., McGee, L., & Schrag, S. J. [2010]. Prevention of perinatal group B streptococcal disease: Revised guidelines from CDC, 2010. *Morbidity and Mortality Weekly Report Recommendations and Reports, 59*[RR-10], 1–32.)

support the use of tocolytic maintenance therapy, nor is there sufficient evidence to support a clear choice for the first-line agent to use for short-term therapy (ACOG, 2016b). All drugs used for tocolysis are used "off-label" (i.e., used for a purpose other than that approved by the FDA [2017a]).

Gestational age limits for administration of tocolytics remain controversial. Suggested lower limits are dependent on the situation surrounding the need for intervention. For instance, tocolytics may be given to a patient undergoing an appendectomy to inhibit uterine contractions as long as sepsis is not present. On the other hand, tocolytic therapy after 34 weeks' gestation is not justified given the potential for increased costs of care and potential fetal and maternal complications that may occur (ACOG, 2016b). Given the possibility of serious adverse effect from all tocolytic agents, neither maintenance treatment nor repeated acute tocolysis should be undertaken as a general practice (ACOG, 2016b). Furthermore, careful expert nursing care is essential for all women who receive tocolytic therapy to reduce potential harm.

If a tocolytic drug is used to stop preterm contractions, the choice of that drug can only be made based on the individual woman and her health status at the time. All drugs used for tocolysis have major side effects for the mother or fetus and should be used with extreme care. Generally, tocolysis should not be administered in cases where fetal distress, infection, or maternal instability is present (Haas et al., 2009). Available data does not support the role of tocolytic agents in reducing the incidence of preterm labor, increasing the interval from onset to birth, or reducing the incidence of PTB (ACOG, 2016b), but they are still frequently used as a secondary intervention in the United States. Displays 7–6, 7–7, and 7–8 describe contraindications to tocolytic therapy, complications that can arise when tocolytics are used, and nursing care for women undergoing tocolytic therapy, respectively.

Beta-mimetics

Beta-mimetics (also called beta-adrenergic receptor agonists) stimulate beta-receptor cells located in smooth muscle. Theoretically, beta-agonist agents work by relaxing the smooth muscle, which decreases or stops uterine contractions. The beta-receptors are also located in smooth muscle in the cardiovascular, pulmonary, and gastrointestinal systems. Effects of beta-mimetic agents are related directly to dosage and route of administration. Maternal side effects are

---

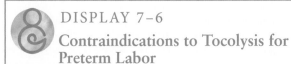

DISPLAY 7–6

Contraindications to Tocolysis for Preterm Labor

General Contraindications*
- Acute fetal compromise (except for intrauterine resuscitation)
- Intraamniotic infection/Triple I
- Eclampsia or severe preeclampsia
- Intrauterine fetal demise
- Lethal fetal anomaly
- Fetal maturity
- Placental abruption
- Maternal bleeding with hemodynamic instability
- Intolerance to tocolytics
- Pulmonary hypertension
- Preterm premature rupture of membranes (except for the purpose of maternal transport, steroid administration, or both)

Contraindications for Specific Tocolytic Agents
Beta-mimetic Agents
- Tachycardia-sensitive maternal cardiac disease
- Poorly controlled maternal diabetes mellitus
- Maternal hyperthyroidism
- Maternal seizure disorders

Magnesium Sulfate
- Maternal hypocalcemia
- Maternal myasthenia gravis
- Maternal renal failure

Indomethacin
- Gestation ≥32 weeks
- Maternal asthma
- Coronary artery disease
- Maternal gastrointestinal bleeding (current or past)
- Platelet dysfunction or bleeding disorder
- Oligohydramnios
- Renal failure
- Suspected fetal cardiac or renal anomaly
- Maternal liver disease
- Allergy to aspirin or other nonsteroidal anti-inflammatory drug
- Presence of fetal growth restriction

Calcium Channel Blockers
- Maternal cardiovascular disease
- Maternal preload-dependent cardiac lesions such as aortic insufficiency
- Maternal hemodynamic instability
- Maternal hypotension
- Avoid combination with beta-sympathomimetic drugs

*Relative and absolute contraindications to tocolysis are based on the clinical circumstances and should take into account the risks of continuing the pregnancy versus those of birth.
From American College of Obstetricians and Gynecologists. (2016c). *Management of preterm labor* (Practice Bulletin No. 171). Washington, DC; Author; Lowe, N. K., Openshaw, M., & King, T. L. (2017). Treatments for women in preterm labor. In M. C. Brucker & T. L. King (Eds.), *Pharmacology for women's health* (2nd ed., pp. 1069–1073). Burlington, MA: Jones & Bartlett.

DISPLAY 7–7

Potential Complications and/or Side Effects of Tocolytic Agents

Beta-adrenergic Agents

Maternal

- Hyperglycemia
- Hypokalemia
- Hypotension
- Flushing
- Pulmonary edema
- Cardiac insufficiency
- Tachycardia
- Arrhythmias
- Palpitations
- Nausea and vomiting
- Shortness of breath
- Chest discomfort
- Maternal death

Fetal/Neonatal

- Fetal cardiac effects such as tachycardia
- Alterations in fetal glucose metabolism/hyperglycemia/hyperinsulinemia
- Neonatal hypoglycemia, hypocalcemia, hypotension

Magnesium Sulfate

Maternal

- Maternal lethargy
- Flushing
- Drowsiness
- Double vision
- Nausea
- Vomiting
- Diaphoresis
- Headache
- Pulmonary edema
- Loss of deep tendon reflexes
- Respiratory depression*
- Cardiac arrest*
- Maternal tetany*
- Profound muscular paralysis*

- Profound hypotension*
- When used with calcium channel blockers: suppresses heart rate, contractility and left ventricular systolic pressure; produces neuromuscular blockade

Fetal/Neonatal

- Hypotonia
- Lethargy
- Bone demineralization
- Neonatal depression

Indomethacin

Maternal

- Nausea and vomiting
- Esophageal reflux
- Gastritis
- Hepatitis[†]
- Renal failure[†]
- Gastrointestinal bleeding[†]

Fetal/Neonatal

- Oligohydramnios
- Transient hypotension
- Premature closure of fetal ductus arteriosus
- Necrotizing enterocolitis in preterm newborn
- Intraventricular hemorrhage in newborn

Calcium Channel Blockers

Maternal

- Dizziness
- Flushing
- Transient hypotension
- Headache
- Nausea
- Palpitations
- Edema
- Elevation of hepatic transaminases
- When used with magnesium sulfate: suppression of heart rate, contractility, and left ventricular systolic pressure

Fetal/Neonatal

- No known adverse effects

*Effect is rare and seen with toxic levels.
[†]Effect is rare and associated with chronic use.
From American College of Obstetricians and Gynecologists. (2016c). *Management of preterm labor* (Practice Bulletin No. 171). Washington, DC: Author.; Lowe, N. K., Openshaw, M., & King, T. L. (2017). Treatments for women in preterm labor. In M. C. Brucker & T. L. King (Eds.), *Pharmacology for women's health* (2nd ed., pp. 1069–1073). Burlington, MA: Jones & Bartlett.

common and uncomfortable. Fetal side effects are thought to be the same as those in the mother because beta-mimetics rapidly cross the placenta. Beta-mimetic agents are contraindicated in patients with known cardiac disease.

Terbutaline (Brethine) is a beta-agonist commonly administered for asthma and is sometimes used off-label for tocolysis. In 1997 and 1998, the FDA issued warnings to healthcare providers about the potential risks of using terbutaline pumps to prevent PTBs

(Nightingale, 1998). More recently, the FDA issued a warning to the public and healthcare providers that injectable terbutaline should also not be administered to pregnant women (FDA, 2017b). They cited data on serious side effects, including maternal cardiac issues and death. They did acknowledge potential use of the drug for 48 to 72 hours but condemned usage on an outpatient basis or beyond 72 hours. Moreover, the FDA has warned against using oral terbutaline in pregnancy, citing the same dangers and no evidence of efficacy (FDA, 2017b). Taking into consideration these warnings, terbutaline may be given by injection in an inpatient setting for 24 to 72 hours only. Terbutaline pumps and oral terbutaline for tocolysis are strongly cautioned against and not recommended.

Conscientious nursing care for the woman receiving beta-mimetic therapy is essential and includes ongoing assessment and monitoring of side effects. Maternal pulse rate must be monitored for any patient who is administered a beta-mimetic agent. A heart rate of 120 beats per minute or greater may warrant continuous electrocardiogram monitoring and discontinuation of tocolytic therapy. A heart rate greater than 120 beats per minute is associated with a decreased ventricular filling time and, therefore, with decreased cardiac output. Over time, if the left ventricular filling time is decreased, less blood is pumped to the myocardium, resulting in decreased perfusion. This is reflected by the patient's complaints of chest heaviness, shortness of breath, or chest pain. Myocardial infarction may result if the agent is not discontinued. Mothers may also experience hypotension, cardiac arrhythmias, pulmonary edema, and alterations in metabolism. Fetal effects can include tachycardia, hyperglycemia, and hyperinsulinemia (Lowe, Openshaw, & King, 2017; Neilson, West, & Dowswell, 2014).

Oxytocin Receptor Antagonists

Atosiban, an oxytocin receptor antagonist, was tested in the United States as a tocolytic agent during the 1990s. It was felt that this tocolytic could be effective in stopping preterm labor and also demonstrated fewer side effects in the mother and baby. A systematic review and meta-analysis of randomized trials using Atosiban was performed in 2014. Use of the drug versus a placebo did not demonstrate a reduction in the rate of spontaneous PTB within 48 hours of administration (Flenady, Reinebrant, Liley, Tambimuttu, & Papatsonis, 2014). Approval for use of Atosiban within the United States has not been approved, although this medication is widely used throughout Europe and other countries.

Magnesium Sulfate

IV magnesium sulfate is a pharmacologic agent commonly used to stop preterm contractions in intrapartum settings. Despite its widespread use in the United States, the effectiveness of magnesium sulfate therapy for tocolysis remains controversial because studies and meta-analyses have shown conflicting results. A systematic review comparing magnesium sulfate with a placebo concluded that magnesium was ineffective as a tocolytic agent and did not improve maternal or neonatal outcomes (Crowther, Brown, McKinlay, & Middleton, 2014). Magnesium sulfate was also examined in 33 comparative trials. Although it was found to be comparable to other tocolytics, reviews cautioned that the studies were not designed as equivalence trials; thus, results may not be accurate (Crowther et al., 2014). At this time, ACOG and SMFM maintain that magnesium sulfate may be used for up to 48 hours to prolong pregnancy in women who may experience preterm delivery within 7 days (ACOG & SMFM, 2016b).

The exact mechanism of action of magnesium sulfate is unknown. Theoretically, magnesium interferes with calcium uptake in the cells of the myometrium. Because myometrial cells are thought to need calcium to contract, decreasing the amount of calcium lessens or stops contractions. Magnesium sulfate relaxes smooth muscle throughout the body, and a decrease in blood pressure may be observed with the administration of a loading dose or at high infusion rates. Maternal side effects include flushing, headache, nausea and vomiting, loss of deep tendon reflexes, shortness of breath, respiratory depression, chest pain, pulmonary edema, and death (Bain, Middleton, & Crowther, 2013). Many practitioners feel comfortable using this agent because they have experience in its administration for the prevention of eclamptic seizures. Institutional protocols may differ for how this drug is used in women with preterm labor.

Magnesium sulfate should be administered by nurses who are skilled in resuscitation and knowledgeable regarding dosing regimens and side effects of the medication. If using this medication for preterm labor, the patient's uterine activity and fetal heart rate should be monitored. During administration of the bolus dose, the nurse should remain at the patient's bedside and vital signs, including oxygen saturation and patella reflexes, should be obtained at a minimum of every 15 minutes for the first hour, every 30 minutes for the second hour, and hourly thereafter (Grissinger, 2009).

If at any time the patient's respiratory rate drops to less than 12 breaths per minute, or if her respirations are 4 breaths per minute below the initial assessment, or the pulse oximeter reading is less than 95%, infusion of the magnesium sulfate should be discontinued. Likewise, a drop in blood pressure 15 mm Hg below the initial reading should also warrant discontinuation of the drug and physician notification. Continuous monitoring of the fetal heart rate and contraction pattern is recommended (Murray & McKinney, 2014; Simpson & Knox, 2004).

Women in preterm labor often receive magnesium sulfate after significant amounts of IV fluids have been infused in an effort to inhibit contractions. This practice increases the risk for pulmonary edema. Therefore, careful assessment of respiratory status, including rate and clarity of breath sounds, is required as well as accurate recording of fluid intake and output (Simpson & Knox, 2004). Signs and symptoms of pulmonary edema include shortness of breath, chest tightening or discomfort, cough, oxygen saturation below 95%, increased respiratory and heart rates, and adventitious breath sounds. Changes in behavior such as apprehension, anxiety, or restlessness may be additional signs of pulmonary edema or hypoxemia and should be closely monitored, documented, and reported (Simpson & Knox, 2004). The provider should be notified if a woman experiences any of the following symptoms (Simpson & Knox, 2004):

- Significant changes in blood pressure from baseline values
- Double (or blurring of) vision
- Tachycardia or bradycardia
- Respiratory rate below 12 or above 24
- Oxygen saturation below 95%
- Changes in breath sounds suggestive of pulmonary edema
- Changes in level of consciousness or neurologic status
- Absent deep tendon reflexes
- Sweating or flushing
- Serum magnesium level above therapeutic range of 4 to 8 mg/dL
- Urinary output less than 30 mL/hr
- Indeterminate or abnormal fetal heart rate pattern

Maternal respiratory rate, oxygen saturation, deep tendon reflexes, and state of consciousness should be monitored closely to detect progressive magnesium toxicity (Display 7–9). Magnesium toxicity results in loss of deep tendon reflexes and progressive muscle weakness, including the diaphragm and other respiratory muscles, leading to acute respiratory failure. In addition, an overdose of magnesium sulfate depresses the respiratory center in the brain, further inhibiting respirations. Hypotension, complete heart block, and cardiac arrest can occur. One ampule of calcium gluconate, 1 g (10 mL of a 10% solution), should be clearly labeled with directions for administration and kept in the nearest locked drug cabinet (Murray & McKinney, 2014). If respiratory depression occurs, the magnesium sulfate infusion must be discontinued immediately and 1 g calcium gluconate (10 mL of 10% solution) should be administered intravenously over 1 to 2 minutes while respiratory support is provided (Murray & McKinney, 2014; Simpson et al., 2018). Although significantly high values are frequently reported as being necessary to cause cardiac arrest, it is important to remember that an untreated respiratory arrest will lead to cardiac arrest as the heart muscle becomes hypoxic and ischemic. Thus, cardiac arrest can occur at magnesium levels consistent with respiratory failure if the respiratory failure is not identified and treated immediately. Magnesium levels causing cardiotoxicity are not required to cause cardiac arrest.

In October 2005 and June 2006, the Institute for Safe Medication Practices (ISMP) issued Medication Safety Alerts Preventing Magnesium Toxicity in Obstetrics (ISMP, 2006). Numerous cases of magnesium overdoses resulting in maternal respiratory arrest, as well as some maternal deaths, have been reported to ISMP in past years (ISMP, 2010). Although errors with magnesium sulfate infusions may not be more common than those with other medications, consequences are more devastating (ISMP, 2006). Essential components of safe nursing care for women receiving IV magnesium sulfate have been described (ISMP, 2006; Murray & McKinney, 2014; Simpson & Knox, 2004). See Display 7–9 for safe care practices when using magnesium sulfate in obstetrics. Because accidents and adverse outcomes continue to occur with magnesium sulfate in obstetrics, it is important to review important safety procedures that can minimize risk.

Magnesium Sulfate for Neuroprotection. In 2016, ACOG and SMFM reaffirmed use of magnesium sulfate as a potential benefit to preterm newborns when given to women at high risk for birth before 32 weeks' gestation (ACOG & SMFM, 2016b). However, the potential neuroprotective effects of magnesium sulfate should not be the basis for decision making about which agent to use for tocolysis. Hospitals that elect to use magnesium sulfate for fetal neuroprotection should develop uniform and specific guidelines for their departments regarding inclusion criteria, treatment regimens, concurrent tocolysis, and monitoring in accordance with one of the larger clinical trials that showed effectiveness (ACOG & SMFM, 2016b). Suggestions for dosing of IV magnesium sulfate for neuroprotection were based on one of three previous clinical trials (Crowther, Hiller, Doyle, & Haslam, 2003; Marret et al., 2007; Rouse et al., 2008). Therefore, three different dosing regimens are listed as appropriate (ACOG & SMFM, 2016a). Although the duration of magnesium sulfate administration for neuroprotection is not known, current recommendations are less than 24 hours (ACOG &

DISPLAY 7–9

Safe Care Practices for the Use of Intravenous Magnesium Sulfate in Obstetrics

Intravenous (IV) magnesium sulfate may be administered to pregnant women for preterm labor prophylaxis, neuroprotection of the preterm fetus, or seizure prophylaxis for women with preeclampsia.

- The pharmacy should supply high-risk IV medications such as magnesium sulfate in prepackaged–premixed solutions.
- Magnesium sulfate only should be administered via controlled infusion pump.
- The infusion pump should not be preprogrammed to change the dose in the absence of direct bedside attendance of the nurse.
- A second nurse should double-check all doses and pump settings.
- Use a 100 mL (4 g)/150 mL (6 g) IV piggyback solution for the initial bolus instead of bolusing from the main bag with a rate change on the pump.
- Use 500-mL IV bags with 20 g of magnesium sulfate versus 1,000-mL IV bags with 40 g of magnesium sulfate for the maintenance fluids.
- Use color-coded tags on the lines as they go into the pumps and into the IV ports.
- Maternal–fetal status should be assessed and documented before the medication is administered. Assessments include maternal vital signs, oxygen saturation, level of consciousness, characteristics of the fetal heart rate, and uterine activity.
- All maternal–fetal status parameters, including how the woman is tolerating magnesium sulfate, should be documented in the medical record every 15 minutes during the first hour, every 30 minutes during the second hour, and at least every hour while the maintenance dose is infusing (even for those patients who are considered to be stable).
- Signs and symptoms of magnesium toxicity should be evaluated and ruled out during each assessment. Deep tendon reflexes

should be assessed prior to administration of the medication, at least every 2 hours thereafter, and as needed based on maternal signs and symptoms. Oxygen saturation should be assessed once per hour. Continuous pulse oximetry is not recommended. Breath sounds should be auscultated before the initial administration of magnesium sulfate and then every 2 hours thereafter.

- Provide one nurse to one woman continuous nursing care at the bedside during the first hour of administration.
- Provide one nurse to one woman ratio during labor and until at least 2 hours postpartum.
- Patient assignment should be no more than one additional couplet or woman for a nurse caring for a woman receiving IV magnesium sulfate in a maintenance dose.
- Provide nursing care during the maintenance dose in a clinical setting where the patient is close to the nurses' station rather than on the general antepartum or postpartum nursing unit where there is less intensive nursing care.
- Consider that a woman receiving magnesium sulfate remains high risk even when symptoms of preeclampsia or preterm labor are stable.
- When care is transferred to another nurse, have both nurses together at the bedside assess patient status, review dosage and pump settings, and review written physician medication orders.
- After the medication therapy is completed, discontinue the medication by removing the line from the IV port to prevent accidental infusion and potential magnesium sulfate overdose.
- Conduct periodic magnesium overdose drills with airway management and calcium administration with physician and nurse team members participating together.
- Maintain calcium antidote in an easily accessible locked medication kit with the dosage and administration (1 g of calcium gluconate should be given intravenously over 3 minutes) clearly printed on the kit.

Adapted from Murray, S. S., & McKinney, E. S. (2014). Intrapartum complications. In *Foundations of maternal-newborn and women's health nursing* (6th ed., pp. 568–597). St. Louis, MO: Elsevier; Simpson, K. R. (2006). Minimizing risk of magnesium sulfate overdose in obstetrics. *MCN: The American Journal of Maternal/Child Nursing, 31*(5), 340; Simpson, K. R., & Knox, G. E. (2004). Obstetrical accidents involving intravenous magnesium sulfate: Recommendations to promote patient safety. *MCN: The American Journal of Maternal/Child Nursing, 29*(3), 170–171.

SMFM, 2016a). The clinical leadership team at each site can determine which regimen will work best for their perinatal service. For medication safety reasons, ideally one regimen should be chosen for each perinatal service. There remains many unanswered questions about the use of magnesium sulfate for neuroprotection, including which women and fetuses are the best candidates and optimal dosing regimens. More research is needed for answers on safety and benefit for preterm newborns.

Calcium Channel Blockers

Calcium channel blockers (CCB) are another class of drugs that have been used to suppress contractions. They cause myometrial muscles to relax by interfering with the movement of extracellular calcium into the calcium channels of the cells. This action prevents the electrical system from generating a current through the

cells, thus preventing contractions (Lowe et al., 2017). Studies comparing CCBs and beta-agonists demonstrated comparable effectiveness, but CCBs resulted in fewer negative side effects making them a more desirable drug choice (Di Renzo, Roura, et al., 2017). Another analysis comparing CCBs with beta-mimetics, oxytocin receptor antagonists, and magnesium sulfate indicated that CCBs were superior in decreasing rates of PTB, respiratory distress syndrome in the neonate, NICU admissions, as well as adverse outcomes for the mother (Flenady et al., 2014; Naik Gaunekar, Raman, Bain, & Crowther, 2013). Research looking at pharmacogenomics of PTB treatment drugs found that CCBs are metabolized by a family of metabolic enzymes (CYP3A) found in the liver. Investigators noted that when women had a higher expressor genotype of these enzymes, they metabolized CCBs at a higher rate leading to decreased levels of the CCB and increased uterine activity (Manuck, 2016). More studies are needed in this area to better understand why the same medication can act differently within a similar patient population.

CCBs are peripheral vasodilators so maternal side effects will reflect physiologic processes associated with this condition. These include nausea, headache, dizziness, flushing, tachycardia, hypotension, and slight increase in blood glucose (Murray & McKinney, 2014).

Prostaglandin or Cyclooxygenase Inhibitors

Prostaglandin is a naturally produced agent that is thought to cause uterine contractions and cervical ripening in term pregnancies. The enzymes cyclooxygenase (COX)-1 and COX-2 are essential to the biosynthesis of prostaglandin that is necessary for labor and/or birth (Lowe et al., 2017). Because little prostaglandin has been found in women who are not in labor, the use of drugs that inhibit the production of prostaglandin has been hypothesized as a possible treatment for preterm labor. Several types of prostaglandins affect uterine contractions and cervical ripening. The most well-known and well-studied prostaglandin inhibitor for use as a tocolytic agent is indomethacin. It competes with other factors in a long-term process whereby prostacyclin is the end product blocking the production of prostaglandin (Lowe et al., 2017). Indomethacin is not without side effects. Patients may experience nausea and/or vomiting, gastrointestinal–esophageal reflux, or generalized irritation of the intestinal system. There are concerns regarding side effects for the fetus with indomethacin administration. Oligohydramnios can occur secondary to reduced fetal urine output. Premature closure of the ductus arteriosus can also ensue causing pulmonary hypertension as well as tricuspid regurgitation. This condition appears to be dependent on the gestational age of the fetus and the length of drug use. Studies have shown effects as early as 24 weeks, although they are most commonly seen after 31 to 32 weeks' gestation (Vermillion, Scardo, Lashus, & Wiles, 1997). Because of this, use of indomethacin is not recommended for longer than 48 to 72 hours or after 32 weeks' gestation (Murry & McKinney, 2014).

IS THERE ANY GOOD NEWS?

Antenatal Corticosteroids

Antenatal corticosteroid use for prevention of respiratory distress syndrome in premature infants is endorsed by ACOG, SMFM, WHO, and other organizations (ACOG, 2017a; SMFM, 2016; WHO, 2015). This class of medication does not prevent PTB; rather, it prevents major complications in the neonate, which is the best outcome possible at this time. Because PTB cannot effectively be prevented currently, ACOG (2017a) has recommended either of the following antenatal corticosteroid courses:

Betamethasone
- 12 mg given intramuscularly (IM) 24 hours apart for two doses

Dexamethasone
- 6 mg given IM every 12 hours for four doses

Either medication should be given to any woman at 24 to 33 weeks and 6 days' gestation at risk for PTB within 7 days. Recent updates from ACOG (2017a) also state that based on family input and considerations regarding resuscitation, antenatal corticosteroid therapy can be considered for women at 23 weeks and 0 days or during the periviable period who may deliver within 7 days, despite fetal numbers (ACOG, 2017a). Administration of a single dose of betamethasone in women who have not previously had a course of corticosteroids, are between 34 weeks and 0 days and 36 weeks and 6 days, and likely to delivery within 7 days is now recommended (ACOG, 2017a). Based on a Cochrane review, ACOG (2017a) supports a single course of antenatal corticosteroids in patients with multiples, between 24 weeks and 0 days and 33 weeks and 6 days, and at risk for delivery within 7 days regardless of fetal number.

The greatest benefit of treatment occurs between 24 hours and 7 days of administration; however, the medication can still benefit the newborn before 24 hours, so it should be given unless birth is imminent (ACOG, 2017a). An additional rescue dose may be considered 2 weeks following the initial dose of corticosteroids in women who are less than 34 weeks and 0 days and likely to give birth within the next 7 days. Depending on the clinical picture, ACOG (2017a) also states that a single rescue dose may be given 7 days following the first course, if needed. Multiple courses of corticosteroids (more than two) have not shown benefit, and several studies have found decreased birth weight, decreased head circumference, and the potential development of cerebral palsy (ACOG, 2017a). In women presenting with PPROM, repeat or rescue treatment of corticosteroids remains controversial and is not currently recommended (ACOG, 2017a). Research continues in this area, especially with long-term outcomes in children whose mothers received antenatal corticosteroid therapy. Another area of study is in maternal critical care. At this time, ACOG continues to recommend this course of treatment even when sepsis is present (ACOG, 2017a).

NURSING CARE FOR THE PREVENTION OF PRETERM BIRTH

Education About Signs and Symptoms of Preterm Labor

Educating women about signs and symptoms of preterm labor has been a hallmark of PTB prevention programs since the early 1980s (Herron, Katz, & Creasy, 1982). Patient education is one of nursing's core areas of practice; therefore, nurses are well qualified to teach women about signs and symptoms of preterm labor. If possible, education for prevention of PTB should begin within the community before a woman becomes pregnant. Nurses working in clinics are in unique positions to provide this information to their patients of childbearing age. Topics should include the importance of prenatal and dental care, activities that can increase risks associated with PTB, and outcomes for the entire family when PTB occurs (Murray & McKinney, 2014). Once a woman is pregnant, education for her and her partner on preventive measures to decrease rates of PTB should continue to be provided.

Because all pregnant women should be considered at risk for preterm labor, ongoing education regarding subtle signs and symptoms of preterm labor and how they differ from those of true labor should be provided by healthcare workers in clinics as well as hospital settings. Specific instructions regarding contractions or cramping between 20 and 36 weeks' gestation should include telling patients that these symptoms are not normal discomforts in pregnancy and that contractions or cramping that do not go away should prompt them to contact their healthcare providers immediately so interventions can be instituted in a timely manner (Ladewig, London, & Davidson, 2017; Murray & McKinney, 2014). Furthermore, antenatal glucocorticoids, which are the most effective therapy for avoiding neonatal health problems such as respiratory distress syndrome, can be administered to hasten fetal lung maturity (ACOG, 2017a; SMFM, 2016; WHO, 2015). In addition to teaching symptoms of preterm labor, it is essential that nurses in the antepartum or intrapartum setting establish a therapeutic relationship with the pregnant woman, so she will feel comfortable reporting vague, nonspecific complaints and will come in or call her primary healthcare provider if she experiences any of the following signs or symptoms of preterm labor (Ladewig et al., 2017; Murray & McKinney, 2014):

- Uterine cramping (menstrual-like cramps, intermittent or constant)
- Uterine contractions (four in 20 minutes/eight in 1 hour) that may or may not be painful (Ladewig et al., 2017, p. 408)
- Low abdominal pressure (pelvic pressure)
- Dull low backache (intermittent or constant)
- Increase or change in vaginal discharge
- Feeling that the baby is "pushing down"
- Abdominal cramping with or without diarrhea
- A sense of "coming down with something" or "just feeling bad" (Murray & McKinney, 2014, p. 580)

Once the patient comes in, she should be assessed for cervical effacement or dilation as well as uterine contractions. If she is sent home, encourage her to call the provider or come back to the hospital if symptoms reappear. It is also important to be sensitive to women who have been identified as at risk for PTB because they may have difficulty balancing concern about bodily symptoms versus overreaction. They may become confused when symptoms that were previously identified as alarming turn out to be "nothing" when they present to the office or hospital for evaluation (Murray & McKinney, 2014). If healthcare providers minimize women's symptoms, they may not return early enough for needed interventions.

Although many nurses teach their patients in a one-on-one manner, the use of electronic educational methods for education regarding preterm symptoms may also be effective. The MOD *PTB PSA/Causes of Premature Birth and Preterm Labor* YouTube video and Sidelines National High-Risk Pregnancy Support Web site are just two examples of online patient education. No matter which method of instruction is used, patient education on preterm labor should be reviewed at each visit, along with an assessment of any symptoms that may have been experienced since the last visit (Murray & McKinney, 2014).

Education About Timing of Elective Birth

Perinatal nurses can offer patient education to prevent elective, early term births. Pregnant women are receiving mixed messages as to the ideal time for their babies to be born when they are healthy and their pregnancy has been uncomplicated. Many women interpret 9 months to mean 36 weeks of pregnancy as full term. For some time, messages from healthcare providers have conveyed that term pregnancy is between 37 and 42 weeks' gestation and that preterm babies are those born before 37 weeks' gestation. This wide time frame is confusing for women who are considering their options in the last weeks of pregnancy. Recently, there has been education from multiple sources encouraging pregnant women to wait until at least 39 completed weeks before asking their primary care provider for elective labor induction. However well intended, this message implies that 39 weeks is an ideal time for birth. Benefits to the mother and baby of awaiting the onset of spontaneous labor and risks of elective labor induction, especially for nulliparous women with an unfavorable cervix, have been overlooked in some patient education materials. Patient education materials from AWHONN (Bingham et al., 2013) focuses on 40 weeks of pregnancy as normal and ideal: *40 Reasons to Go the Full 40*. This messaging is clear that at least 40 weeks, rather than 39 weeks, is best for healthy mothers and babies. The emphasis is on finishing pregnancy, labor, and birth healthy and well; managing risks; and enjoying the final weeks of pregnancy (Bingham et al., 2013). Although the main points of patient education are serious and targeted to risks of asking to be induced early, there are also lighthearted reasons included for awaiting spontaneous labor. This innovative patient education pamphlet published by AWHONN can be used as part of prenatal visits, prepared childbirth classes, and other patient interactions during the last weeks of pregnancy.

Lifestyle Modification

Evidence exists that some women experience more preterm symptoms when engaged in certain activities. We have known for many years through research that when women are able to modify those lifestyle factors, they have fewer PTBs (Murray & McKinney, 2014). Patients should be encouraged to rest frequently throughout the day, drink plenty of fluids, avoid caffeine, keep their bladder emptied, and avoid lifting objects (Ladewig et al., 2017).

Smoking Cessation

Smoking is a modifiable lifestyle factor strongly associated with PTB and LBW. It is associated with impaired lung development and chromosomal abnormalities in the fetus, small-for-gestational-age and LBW infants, preterm infants, and infant deaths. Cigarette smoking before conception can cause reduced fertility and conception delay among women (American Society for Reproductive Medicine, 2012). Maternal cigarette smoking during pregnancy increases the risk for pregnancy complications (e.g., placental previa, placental abruption, premature rupture of membranes, and preeclampsia) and poor pregnancy outcomes (e.g., preterm delivery, restricted fetal growth, stillbirth, and sudden infant death syndrome) (MOD, 2019c; Pineles, Hsu, Park, & Samet, 2016; American Society for Reproductive Medicine, 2012). It is estimated that there would be a 10% reduction in perinatal mortality and an 11% reduction in LBW if smoking during pregnancy were eliminated. The risk of fetal death for pregnant women who smoke is generally 1.5-fold over that for pregnant nonsmokers (Silver, 2007).

Pregnant women are also at risk for secondhand and thirdhand smoke in their homes or public areas (MOD, 2019c). Secondhand smoke is associated with similar complications seen in women who do smoke. These include PTB, placental abruption and previa, PPROM, and adverse neonatal outcome, including intrauterine growth restriction, increased respiratory problems (e.g., bronchitis and pneumonia), ear infections, dying from sudden infant death syndrome, and NICU admission (Crane, Keough, Murphy, Burrage, & Hutchens, 2011; Leonardi-Bee, Britton, & Venn, 2011; MOD, 2019c). Thirdhand smoke is the residue from any tobacco product that is left on clothing, furniture, walls, carpet, and so forth. It is what can be smelled when entering a room. Because of its saturation levels, simply opening the window in a room with thirdhand smoke will not help the patient or newborn baby from being exposed. Thirdhand smoke can cause asthma, breathing problems, learning disabilities, as well as cancer in those who are exposed to it (MOD, 2019c).

According to the 2011 Pregnancy Risk Assessment Monitoring System data from 24 states (CDC, 2017), around 10% of pregnant women admitted to smoking during the last 3 months of their pregnancy (Cheng, Salimi, Terplan, & Chisolm, 2015). Approximately 55% of women who smoked 3 months before getting pregnant were able to quit at some point during the pregnancy (CDC, 2017). It can be difficult, though, to know if the statistics truly reflect the amount pregnant women actually smoke because self-reported behaviors are often understated.

The physiologic effects of smoking occur as a result of transient intrauterine hypoxemia. When a pregnant woman smokes, carbon monoxide crosses the placenta and binds with maternal and fetal hemoglobin, producing carboxyhemoglobin. Carboxyhemoglobin interferes with the normal binding process of oxygen to the hemoglobin molecule, reducing the ability of the blood to carry adequate levels of oxygen to the fetus (Stone, Bailey, & Khraisha, 2014). Smoking also causes physical changes to the placenta. These changes include less blood flow within the capillary system and thickening of the villous membrane which makes oxygen exchange more difficult (Larsen, Clausen, & Jønsson, 2002).

Studies involving genetic susceptibility and smoking have reported that certain maternal genotypes may increase both maternal and fetal adverse responses to smoking and its residual components. Infants born to smoking mothers and those exposed to tobacco in the surrounding environment demonstrated significantly lower birth weights and length of gestation compared to infants not exposed to any tobacco during gestation. Additional studies in genotypes need to be completed to assist in identifying patient populations that are at greatest risk (Aagaard-Tillery et al., 2010; Huang et al., 2018).

An opportunity to reduce the risk of PTB and LBW exists if education for pregnant women about the effects of smoking on the fetus begins early in pregnancy. Identification of risk factors associated with cigarette smoking is an important step in knowing which smoking cessation programs can be most effective. Choosing programs that are tailored to meet the demographics of the patient may be more valuable and successful (Newnham et al., 2014). One intervention to reduce smoking during pregnancy is to encourage women to institute a no-smoking policy at home (Mullen, Richardson, Quinn, & Ershoff, 1997).

As more employers and cities institute no smoking policies, restaurants, work environments, and public places are becoming off-limits for smokers; a no-smoking policy at home can be even more helpful in eliminating opportunities to smoke. Another effective measure is including partners in the smoking cessation process because one of the primary barriers to smoking cessation among pregnant women who smoke is having a partner who smokes (Duckworth & Chertok, 2012). It can be extremely challenging to quit smoking without partner support and with the partner continuing to smoke in front of the pregnant woman (Duckworth & Chertok, 2012). Partners influence health behaviors of pregnant women, so nurses should try to include partners whenever possible in all efforts to assist the pregnant woman and postpartum woman to stop smoking.

Another useful incentive for smoking cessation is biochemically verified abstinence with a conditional incentive. Testing for urinary cotinine levels can detect tobacco use 5 days following exposure (Raja, Garg, Yadav, Jha, & Handa, 2016). Analysis of carbon monoxide is an additional method of abstinence testing. In a 2017 systematic review of psychosocial interventions, women who received monetary vouchers with negative carbon monoxide levels demonstrated a higher quit rate. However, when the voucher amount was reduced, the smoking rate increased somewhat. Further studies on how to provide cost-effective incentives need to be performed (Chamberlain et al., 2017). Counseling and feedback cessation programs in conjunction with other strategies such as health education and social support have also shown a decrease in smoking. Studies involving women who were provided information on risks associated with smoking in the form of a handout, self-help manual, and video tapes from their physicians have shown significant reductions in smoking rates. In spite of these encouraging statistics, it is thought that only 49% of obstetricians actually provide routine as assessments and follow-up with their patients who smoke, and only 28% will provide actual education and tactics for successful smoking cessation (Orleans, Barker, Kaufman, & Marx, 2000).

Use of pharmacologic interventions have been tested for smoking cessation in pregnancy. Studies associated with this intervention have been conflicting. A review of six trials was unable to validate the advantage of nicotine replacement therapy (Coleman, Chamberlain, Davey, Cooper, & Leonardi-Bee, 2012). If physicians are going to prescribe nicotine replacement therapy, interventions for behavior changes, as well as counseling, should be offered on an ongoing basis throughout the pregnancy and postpartum period. ACOG (2017c) reported that use of varenicline and bupropion appears to be safe for use in pregnancy. There is limited data available, though, and the FDA has added warnings of psychiatric manifestations and suicide related

to their use. Additional studies need to be performed to adequately assess safety in the pregnant population (ACOG, 2017c).

E-cigarettes and vaping have become popular substitutes for smoking. They do contain nicotine, though, which can cause poor outcomes related to the fetal brain and lungs. In a study of nonpregnant patients' use of electronic nicotine delivery systems, researchers found that there was poor evidence that they actually helped aid smoking cessation (ACOG, 2017c). There is a need for evaluation in the pregnant population to assess whether these devices cause harm and whether they are helpful for those wishing to quit smoking completely.

Another area of assistance in decreasing exposure of tobacco to the fetus has come in the form of legislation. In a review of 11 studies that looked at the effects of local and national legislative action banning smoking in public places and its relationship to PTBs, researchers found a 10% reduction in the rate of PTBs compared with areas that did not have the same legislation (Been et al., 2014).

Given the difficulty many pregnant women addicted to tobacco have quitting during pregnancy, ACOG (2017c) has promoted using the 5 As approach to smoking cessation in pregnancy for every pregnant smoker. These include (1) ask about tobacco use, (2) advise to quit, (3) assess willingness to make an attempt, (4) assist in quit attempt, and (5) arrange follow-up. Although cessation of smoking in pregnancy is important, women should also be taught about the hazards of postpartum smoking for their own health and the health of their children.

When women are successful in stopping or reducing smoking during their pregnancy, this does not necessary equal to permanent positive lifestyle changes. Relapse in the postpartum period is a significant problem. Approximately 50% to 60% of women who stop smoking during pregnancy will resume smoking within 1 year postpartum (ACOG, 2017c). According to the most recent data available from the Pregnancy Risk Assessment Monitoring System, 42% of women who quit smoking during the last 3 months of pregnancy relapsed within 6 months after giving birth (Rockhill et al., 2016). A study using focus groups found that some women did not believe that smoking by themselves or family members caused harm to their fetus or newborn or that it was addictive. Some patients were amenable to use of nicotine patches, however, there were others that doubted the safety of the patch and felt that smoking was a better choice (Hotham, Atkinson, & Gilbert, 2002). More research about smoking cessation for childbearing women is greatly needed; this is an opportunity for nurse researchers to make a significant contribution to the health and well-being of women and newborns.

Illicit Drug Use

Pregnancy and neonatal complications have been noted with illicit drug use. Women who are substance abusers may not even realize they are pregnant, thinking instead that signs of pregnancy such as nausea, vomiting, and cramping are actually withdrawal symptoms (Heil et al., 2011). Once they are aware of the pregnancy, they may not pursue prenatal care because of embarrassment, feelings of shame, or fear of legal ramifications. Risk factors associated with substance abuse and pregnancy include unmarried young women, less education, late and/or missed prenatal visits, erratic changes in behavior, and volatile home situations (Klein, Friedman-Campbell, & Tocco, 1993; Unger et al., 2010).

A national survey taken within the United States showed that 57% of women using illicit drugs who became pregnant quit using for the remainder of their pregnancy. Further analysis revealed that many of them unfortunately returned to drug use within the first year after delivery (Ebrahim & Gfroerer, 2003). Opioid use during pregnancy is associated with placental abruption, preeclampsia, PPROM, preterm labor and delivery, postpartum hemorrhage, fetal growth restriction, and fetal death (Maeda, Bateman, Clancy, Creanga, & Leffert, 2014). Use of methadone or buprenorphine as an opioid substitute has been shown to be a safe alternative with improved outcomes for both the mother and the fetus. It is felt as though use of these medications is more advantageous than sending patients for detoxification (Alto & O'Connor, 2011). Patients using opioid substitution therapy also demonstrated lower rates of relapse (Jones, O'Grady, Malfi, & Tuten, 2008). A meta-analysis of 31 studies evaluating maternal cocaine use and adverse perinatal outcomes showed significant risk for PTB, LBW, and small-for-gestation infants (Gouin, Murphy, & Shah, 2011). The placenta and fetal blood–brain barrier allow cocaine to easily pass through resulting in vasoconstriction in the fetus and placenta. Furthermore, cocaine toxicity can occur causing maternal hypertension. Use of beta-blockers such as labetalol is contraindicated as they can cause unopposed coronary vasoconstriction and end-organ damage. Pregnant women using cocaine and presenting with hypertension should be treated with hydralazine (Kuczkowski, 2007). Methamphetamines are neurotoxic agents that destroy the end terminals of brain cells containing dopamine. A two- to fourfold risk of gestational hypertension, preeclampsia, abruption, PTB, fetal demise, and neonatal/infant death has been reported in patients using methamphetamines during pregnancy (Gorman, Orme, Nguyen, Kent, & Caughey, 2014). Although marijuana use in pregnancy does not appear to cause preterm labor, its use was shown by the Stillbirth Collaborative Research Network to be related to a threefold increased risk of morbidity or death in the neonate (Conner et al., 2016). Because of this risk and unknown chemical products found in marijuana that pass through the placental barrier and breast milk, both ACOG and the Academy of Breastfeeding Medicine oppose its use during pregnancy and in the postpartum period (ACOG, 2017b; Reece-Stremtan, Marinelli, & Academy of Breastfeeding Medicine, 2015).

It is important for nurses to know and understand the processes of addiction, how to assess for illicit drug use, and how to intervene to best help the woman and her baby. Research is showing that substance abuse of alcohol, nicotine, and illicit drugs are heritable traits related to certain gene sequences (Gelernter & Kranzler, 2015). These women suffer from an addiction cycle that includes an inability to abstain from illicit drug use. They need understanding, not condemnation, from healthcare personnel. Nurses working in prenatal, intrapartum, or postpartum care are in a unique position to assist in education regarding risks associated with illicit drug use. Use of a screening tool that asks specific questions regarding drug usage appears to be more helpful in obtaining accurate information (WHO, 2014). Mothers who use illicit substances should be told that these drugs can be found in breast milk and have a deleterious effect on newborns. At this time, the AAP does not recommend breastfeeding for women who are currently using any type of amphetamine (AAP & ACOG, 2017). Nurses should also know how to contact social services to ensure that appropriate referrals for drug-using women can be made to local treatment facilities, so they and their infants have the best chance to improve outcomes of the pregnancy. Illicit drug use is generally not an isolated risk behavior; rather, it is often consistent with a life span risk framework for alcohol use, childhood abuse, familial alcoholism, and lifetime major depressive disorder (Flynn & Chermack, 2008).

Intimate Partner Violence

Intimate partner violence (IPV) is one of the most critical, preventable public health problems in the United States. It can happen to any person regardless of age, race, socioeconomic status, or sexual orientation. Even though research has shown that many IPV occurrences are not reported, it is still estimated that 1 in 4 women (27.4%) in the United States have experienced some form of IPV (Smith et al., 2017). There are three main forms of IPV: psychological/emotional, physical, or sexual. A person can experience one or all of these types (WHO, 2012).

Parker, McFarlane, and Soeken (1994) were the first to correlate IPV (domestic violence) with preterm labor and birth. Their work showed that IPV is a health problem, not a social problem, and that women who are battered have more LBW and PTB than women who are not. Donovan, Spracklen, Schweizer, Ryckman, and Saftlas (2016) performed a meta-analysis of 50 studies and found that occurrences of IPV have not declined but continue to be a significant cause of PTB as well as LBW and small for gestational age found in infants. Other factors have also been identified. A national survey of women who experienced vaginal bleeding, PTB, LBW, kidney infections, and other complications during their pregnancy revealed that they had experienced IPV in the year prior to becoming pregnant (Dutton et al., 2006; Silverman, Decker, Reed, & Raj, 2006). Depression is also a known consequence of IPV (Ludermir, Lewis, Valongueiro, de Araújo, & Araya, 2010). This condition has been linked to increased rates of PTB.

Screening for IPV should occur at many different times during a woman's pregnancy. At a minimum, women should be screened at their first prenatal visit, at least once in each trimester, and during the postpartum period, when violence may escalate (ACOG, 2012). In a meta-analysis of qualitative studies on patient expectations during assessment for IPV, it was found that women wanted a nonjudgmental and compassionate healthcare provider who would provide time for discussion, supportive listening, and validation that this was not their fault yet not put pressure on them to leave the relationship or press charges (Feder, Hutson, Ramsay, & Taket, 2006). In a busy obstetrical unit, there may not be time to provide an in-depth screening for IPV, though, but nursing care for these at-risk women should include some type of assessment for family stress and abuse. Screening assessments that range from a single question to three or four questions can help to increase detection and should be included in the initial admission assessment and postpartum period for all patients (Nelson, Bougatsos, & Blazina, 2012). Identification of patients who are at risk and care management that focuses on education and assistance in leaving an unhealthy relationship may be able to help decrease rates of PTB and other bad outcomes associated with domestic violence.

INTRAPARTUM NURSING CARE OF THE WOMAN IN PRETERM LABOR

The goals of intrapartum care for women with a diagnosis of preterm labor are to achieve a reduction in uterine activity that is long enough to allow for administration of antenatal corticosteroids, transfer of the mother to a facility with the appropriate level of neonatal care for current gestational age, administration of antibiotics for GBS prophylaxis, and consideration of magnesium sulfate for neuroprotection. Nursing care is then delivered by nurses competent to care for the high-risk pregnant woman. The recommended nurse-to-patient ratio for women with high-risk obstetric conditions during labor is 1:1 (AAP & ACOG, 2017; AWHONN, 2010). Ladewig and colleagues (2017) have described this care, which includes monitoring of the fetus, uterine contractions, maternal hydration, laboratory testing, and ultrasound. Careful attention to maternal positions that facilitate the transfer of oxygen from the mother to the fetus and maternal intake and output are especially important (Ladewig et al., 2017). See Chapter 15 for a discussion of monitoring the preterm fetus.

Stress reduction for mothers with threatened PTB in antepartum units is an area of care that intrapartum nurses may be able to assist with. One such risk reduction strategy aimed at reducing stress in this patient population is the "Stress Coping App" (Jallo, Thacker, Menzies, Stojanovic, & Svikis, 2017). Researchers found that use of the stress coping interventional application led to a significant drop in the visual analog stress scale scores. All participants reported benefits from its use (Jallo et al., 2017).

Women in preterm labor need emotional support and information about the potential risks to their baby if preterm labor proceeds to PTB. In institutions that provide a special care nursery or neonatal intensive care, a visit from the neonatal nurse practitioner or neonatologist prior to the birth can be helpful in explaining what to expect and how their baby will be cared for in the nursery. This process is preferred over the neonatal resuscitation team rushing in the room at birth without prior introductions and explanations. If the baby's gestational age or condition is such that it is anticipated that an immediate admission to the nursery will be required, every effort should be made to assure that birth occurs in a facility equipped to care for the estimated gestational age of the baby (AAP & ACOG, 2017) and to communicate maternal–fetal status to the neonatal team. See Chapter 13 for details of maternal transfer. Equal effort should be made to allow the mother to see and touch the baby before the neonatal team leaves the birthing room or surgical suite. The father of the baby or other support person should be encouraged to visit the nursery as soon as possible, and the family should be provided visiting policy information. Some nurseries have cameras that can be used to provide the mother with a picture while she is in the post-anesthesia recovery period before she is able to visit the nursery. With the widespread use of cell phones and tablets with cameras, mothers will likely be able to see a picture of the baby quickly. Because premature infants benefit tremendously from receiving human milk, nurses need to ensure they engage parents in early discussion of the medical importance of breast milk and support early initiation of pumping.

AAP & ACOG (2017) consider provision of breast milk a key intervention for preterm infants because of its effects on short- and long-term health outcomes. See Chapter 20 for a full discussion of breastfeeding.

FURTHER RESEARCH

Although extensive research has been dedicated to preterm labor and birth, a definitive cause or cure still alludes the medical profession. The MOD and the International Federation of Gynecology and Obstetrics Working Group on PTB recently reported data from a widespread, cross-country analysis of 4.1 million individual patients (Martin, D'Alton, Jacobsson, & Norman, 2017). They found seven areas of research that need more emphasis if global PTB is effectively going to be reduced in the future. These include the following (Martin, D'Alton, et al., 2017, pp. 716–718):

- Prior PTB and preeclampsia that presents before term are factors that confer the highest risk of PTB when present in an individual.
- On a population basis, nulliparity in the mother and male gender in the fetus have the largest overall association with PTB.
- Individual risk factors for PTB (less than 37 weeks of gestation) and very PTB (less than 32 weeks of gestation) vary somewhat.
- Individual patient and population risks are similar among high-income countries.
- The majority of patients with PTB have no apparent risk factor(s) or identifiable mechanism to explain its occurrence.
- Using population data accrued for this study, it will be possible to estimate the PTB risk for subpopulations of patients.
- A strong emphasis on new basic research is ultimately more likely to mitigate the problem of PTB than either policy or public health actions or more widespread use of currently available clinical interventions and medications.

SUMMARY

PTB remains one of the most pressing problems in perinatal health. Nurses have the ability to participate in PTB prevention research and enhance their clinical knowledge and skills regarding this topic. One of the most important interventions nurses can implement is their ability to effectively teach pregnant women about the symptoms of preterm labor and birth. This can result in women obtaining the essential antenatal steroids at the earliest time possible. Although we may not yet know how to prevent PTBs, nurses can make a difference in how many babies are born with potentially devastating sequelae associated with PTB through patient education, sharing of knowledge, advocating for women and newborns, and participation in ongoing research.

REFERENCES

Aagaard-Tillery, K., Spong, C. Y., Thom, E., Sibai, B., Wendel, G., Jr., Wenstrom, K., . . . Wapner, R. J. (2010). Pharmacogenomics of maternal tobacco use: Metabolic gene polymorphisms and risk of adverse pregnancy outcomes. *Obstetrics & Gynecology*, 115(3), 568–577. doi:10.1097/AOG.0b013e3181d06faf

Acosta, E. P., Grigsby, P. L., Larson, K. B., James, A. M., Long, M. C., Duffy, L. B., . . . Novy, M. J. (2014). Transplacental transfer of azithromycin and its use for eradicating intra-amniotic *Ureaplasma* infection in a primate model. *Journal of Infectious Diseases*, 209(6), 898–904. doi:10.1093/infdis/jit578

Adams Waldorf, K. M., Singh, N., Mohan, A. R., Young, R. C., Ngo, L., Das, A., . . . Johnson, M. R. (2015). Uterine overdistention induces preterm labor mediated by inflammation: Observations in pregnant women and nonhuman primates. *American Journal of Obstetrics & Gynecology*, 213(6), 830.e1–830.e19. doi:10.1016/j.ajog.2015.08.028

Alfirevic, Z., Stampalija, T., & Medley, N. (2017). Cervical stitch (cerclage) for preventing preterm birth in singleton pregnancy. *Cochrane Database of Systematic Reviews*, (6), CD08991. doi:10.1002/14651858.CD008991.pub3

Alto, W. A., & O'Connor, A. B. (2011). Management of women treated with buprenorphine during pregnancy. *American Journal of Obstetrics & Gynecology*, 205(4), 302–308. doi:10.1016/j.ajog.2011.04.001

American Academy of Pediatrics & American College of Obstetricians and Gynecologists. (2017). *Guidelines for perinatal care* (8th ed.). Elk Grove Village, IL: American Academy of Pediatrics.

American College of Nurse-Midwives. (2016). *Induction of labor* [Position statement]. Silver Springs, MD: Author.

American College of Obstetricians and Gynecologists. (2009). *Induction of labor* (Practice Bulletin No. 107). Washington, DC: Author.

American College of Obstetricians and Gynecologists. (2012). *Intimate partner violence* (Committee Opinion No. 518). Washington DC: Author.

American College of Obstetricians and Gynecologists. (2016a). *ACOG reinvents the pregnancy wheel*. Washington, DC: Author.

American College of Obstetricians and Gynecologists. (2016b). *Management of preterm labor* (Practice Bulletin No. 171). Washington, DC: Author.

American College of Obstetricians and Gynecologists. (2017a). *Antenatal corticosteroid therapy for fetal maturation* (Committee Opinion No. 713). Washington, DC: Author.

American College of Obstetricians and Gynecologists. (2017b). *Marijuana use during pregnancy and lactation* (Committee Opinion No. 722). Washington, DC: Author.

American College of Obstetricians and Gynecologists. (2017c). *Smoking cessation during pregnancy* (Committee Opinion No. 721). Washington, DC: Author.

American College of Obstetricians and Gynecologists. (2018a). *Prelabor rupture of membranes* (Practice Bulletin No. 188). Washington, DC: Author.

American College of Obstetricians and Gynecologists. (2018b). *Use of prophylactic antibiotics in labor and delivery* (Practice Bulletin No. 199). Washington, DC: Author.

American College of Obstetricians and Gynecologists. (2019). *Prevention of group B streptococcal early-onset disease in newborns* (Committee Opinion No. 782). Washington, DC: Author.

American College of Obstetricians and Gynecologists, American Institute of Ultrasound in Medicine, & Society for Maternal-Fetal Medicine. (2017). *Methods for estimating the due date* (Practice Bulletin No. 700). Washington, DC: Author.

American College of Obstetricians and Gynecologists & Society for Maternal-Fetal Medicine. (2016a). *Magnesium sulfate before anticipated preterm birth for neuroprotection* (Committee Opinion No. 455). Washington DC: Author.

American College of Obstetricians and Gynecologists & Society for Maternal-Fetal Medicine. (2016b). *Magnesium sulfate use in obstetrics* (Committee Opinion No. 652). Washington, DC; Author.

American College of Obstetricians and Gynecologists & Society for Maternal-Fetal Medicine. (2017a). *Medically indicated late-preterm and early-term deliveries* (Practice Bulletin No. 560). Washington, DC: Author.

American College of Obstetricians and Gynecologists & Society for Maternal-Fetal Medicine. (2017b). *Nonmedically indicated early-term deliveries* (Committee Opinion No. 561). Washington, DC: Author.

American Society for Reproductive Medicine. (2012). Smoking and infertility: A committee opinion. *Fertility and Sterility, 98*(6), 1400–1406. doi:10.1016/j.fertnstert.2012.07.1146

Association of Women's Health, Obstetric and Neonatal Nurses. (2010). *Guidelines for professional registered nurse staffing for perinatal units*. Washington, DC: Author.

Association of Women's Health, Obstetric and Neonatal Nurses. (2017). *Assessment and care of the late preterm infant* (2nd ed.). Washington, DC: Author.

Association of Women's Health, Obstetric and Neonatal Nurses. (2019). Elective induction of labor. *Nursing for Women's Health, 23*(2), 177–179. doi:10.1016/j.nwh.2019.03.001

Bain, E. S., Middleton, P. F., & Crowther, C. A. (2013). Maternal adverse effects of different antenatal magnesium sulphate regimens for improving maternal and infant outcomes: A systematic review. *BMC Pregnancy and Childbirth, 13*, 195. doi:10.1186/1471-2393-13-195

Baker, B. (2015). Improving outcomes for late preterm infants and their mothers. *Journal of Obstetric, Gynecologic, & Neonatal Nursing, 44*(1), 100–101. doi:10.1111/1552-6909.12520

Bassler, D., Stoll, B. J., Schmidt, B., Asztalos, E. V., Roberts, R. S., Robertson, C. M., & Sauve, R. S. (2009). Using a count of neonatal morbidities to predict poor outcome in extremely low birth weight infants: Added role of neonatal infection. *Pediatrics, 123*(1), 313–318. doi:10.1542/peds.2008-0377

Been, J. V., Nurmatov, U. B., Cox, B., Nawrot, T. S., van Schayck, C. P., & Sheikh, A. (2014). Effect of smoke-free legislation on perinatal and child health: A systematic review and meta-analysis. *Lancet, 383*(9928), 1549–1560. doi:10.1016/S0140-6736(14)60082-9

Berghella, V., Odibo, A. O., To, M. S., Rust, O. A., & Althuisius, S. M. (2005). Cerclage for short cervix on ultrasonography: Meta-analysis of trials using individual patient-level data. *Obstetrics & Gynecology, 106*(1), 181–189. doi:10.1097/01.AOG.0000168435.17200.53

Berghella, V., Roman, A., Daskalakis, C., Ness, A., & Baxter, J. K. (2007). Gestational age at cervical length measurement and incidence of preterm birth. *Obstetrics & Gynecology, 110*(2, Pt. 1), 311–317. doi:10.1097/01.AOG.0000270112.05025.1d

Bezold, K. Y., Karjalainen, M. K., Hallman, M., Teramo, K., & Muglia, L. J. (2013). The genomics of preterm birth: From animal models to human studies. *Genome Medicine, 5*(4), 34. doi:10.1186/gm438

Billiards, S. S., Pierson, C. R., Haynes, R. L., Folkerth, R. D., & Kinney, H. C. (2006). Is the late preterm infant more vulnerable to gray matter injury than the term infant? *Clinics in Perinatology, 33*(4), 915–933, abstract x–xi. doi:10.1016/j.clp.2006.10.003

Bingham, D., Ruhl, C., & Cockey, C. D. (2013). Don't rush me . . . go the full 40: AWHONN's public health campaign promotes spontaneous labor and normal birth to reduce overuse of inductions and cesareans. *Journal of Perinatal Education, 22*(4), 189–193. doi:10.1891/1058-1243.22.4.189

Boateng, C. (2011). An examination of maternal stress, inflammatory markers, and preterm labor in pregnant women. *Kaleidoscope, 10*(39), 1–6.

Bocca-Tjeertes, I. F. A., Kerstjens, J. M., Reijneveld, S. A., de Winter, A. F., & Bos, A. F. (2011). Growth and predictors of growth restraint in moderately preterm children aged 0 to 4 years. *Pediatrics, 128*(5), e1187–e1194. doi:10.1542/peds.2010-3781

Bolotskikh, V., & Borisova, V. (2017). Combined value of placental alpha macroglobulin-1 detection and cervical length via transvaginal ultrasound in the diagnosis of preterm labor in symptomatic patients. *The Journal of Obstetrics and Gynaecology Research, 43*(8), 1263–1269. doi:10.1111/jog.13366

Bouyssi-Kobar, M., du Plessis, A. J., McCarter, R., Brossard-Racine, M., Murnick, J., Tinkleman, L., . . . Limperopoulos, C. (2016). Third trimester brain growth in preterm infants compared with in utero healthy fetuses. *Pediatrics, 138*(5), 1–11.

Boyd, H. A., Poulsen, G., Wohlfahrt, J., Murray, J. C., Feenstra, B., & Melbye, M. (2009). Maternal contributions to preterm delivery. *American Journal of Epidemiology, 170*(11):1358–1364. doi:10.1093/aje/kwp324

Burger, N. B., Brölmann, H. A., Einarsson, J. I., Langebrekke, A., & Huirne, J. A. (2011). Effectiveness of abdominal cerclage placed via laparotomy or laparoscopy: Systematic review. *Journal of Minimally Invasive Gynecology, 18*(6), 696–704. doi:10.1016/j.jmig.2011.07.009

Cantarutti, A., Merlino, L., Monzani, E., Giaquinto, C., & Corrao, G. (2016). Is the risk of preterm birth and low birth weight affected by the use of antidepressant agents during pregnancy? A population-based investigation. *PLoS ONE, 11*(12), e0168114, 1–10. doi:10.1371/journal.pone.0168115

Centers for Disease Control and Prevention. (2017). *Substance use during pregnancy*. Atlanta, GA: Author.

Centers for Disease Control and Prevention. (2019). *Premature birth*. Atlanta, GA: Author.

Chamberlain, C., O'Mara-Eves, A., Porter, J., Coleman, T., Perlen, S. M., Thomas, J., & McKenzie, J. E. (2017). Psychosocial interventions for supporting women to stop smoking in pregnancy. *Cochrane Database of Systematic Reviews*, (2), CD001055. doi:10.1002/14651858.CD001055.pub5

Chan, E., & Quigley, M. A. (2014). School performance at age 7 years in late preterm and early term birth: A cohort study. *Archives of Disease in Childhood: Fetal and Neonatal Edition, 99*, F451–F457. doi:10.1136/archdischild-2014-306124

Cheng, D., Salimi, S., Terplan, M., & Chisolm, M. S. (2015). Intimate partner violence and maternal cigarette smoking before and during pregnancy. *Obstetrics & Gynecology, 125*(2), 356–362. doi:10.1097/AOG.0000000000000609

Clark, S. L., Miller, D. D., Belfort, M. A., Dildy, G. A., Frye, D. K., & Meyers, J. A. (2009). Neonatal and maternal outcomes associated with elective term delivery. *American Journal of Obstetrics & Gynecology, 200*(2), 156.e1–156.e4. doi:10.1016/j.ajog.2008.08.068

Coleman, T., Chamberlain, C., Davey, M. A., Cooper, S. E., & Leonardi-Bee, J. (2012). Pharmacological interventions for promoting smoking cessation during pregnancy. *Cochrane Database of Systematic Reviews*, (9), CD010078. doi:10.1002/14651858.CD010078.pub2

Cong, A., de Vries, B., & Ludlow, J. (2018). Does previous caesarean section at full dilatation increase the likelihood of subsequent spontaneous preterm birth? *Australian and New Zealand Journal of Obstetrics and Gynaecology, 58*(3), 267–273. doi:10.1111/ajo.12713

Conner, S. N., Bedell, V., Lipsey, K., Macones, G. A., Cahill, A. G., & Tuuli, M. G. (2016). Maternal marijuana use and adverse neonatal outcomes: A systematic review and meta-analysis. *Obstetrics & Gynecology, 128*(4), 713–723. doi:10.1097/AOG.0000000000001649

Convertino, V. A., Bloomfield, S. A., & Greenleaf, J. E. (1997). An overview of the issues: Physiological effects of bed rest and restricted physical activity. *Medicine & Science in Sports & Exercise, 29*(2), 187–190. doi:10.1097/00005768-199702000-00004

Craighead, D. V. (2012). Early term birth. *Nursing for Women's Health, 16*(2), 136–145. doi:10.1111/j.1751-486X.2012.01719.x

Crane, J. M., Keough, M., Murphy, P., Burrage, L., & Hutchens, D. (2011). Effects of environmental tobacco smoke on perinatal outcomes: A retrospective cohort study. *BJOG, 118*(7), 865–871. doi:10.1111/j.1471-0528.2011.02941.x

Crowther, C. A., Brown, J., McKinlay, C. J., & Middleton, P. (2014). Magnesium sulphate for preventing preterm birth in threatened preterm labour. *Cochrane Database of Systematic Reviews*, (8), CD001060. doi:10.1002/14651858.CD001060.pub2

Crowther, C. A., Hiller, J. E., Doyle, L. W., & Haslam, R. R. (2003). Effect of magnesium sulfate given for neuroprotection before preterm birth: A randomized controlled trial. *JAMA, 290*(20), 2669–2676. doi:10.1001/jama.290.20.2669

Davies, A. A., Smith, G. D., May, M. T., & Ben-Shlomo, Y. (2006). Association between birth weight and blood pressure is robust, amplifies with age, and may be underestimated. *Hypertension, 48*(3), 431–436. doi:10.1161/01.HYP.0000236551.00191.61

de Kieviet, J. F., Zoetebier, L., van Elburg, R. M., Vermeulen, R. J., & Oosterlaan, J. (2012). Brain development of very preterm and very low-birthweight children in childhood and adolescence: A meta-analysis. *Developmental Medicine and Child Neurology, 54*(4), 313–323. doi:10.1111/j.1469-8749.2011.04216.x

Di Renzo, G. C., Pacella, E., Di Fabrizio, L., & Giardina, I. (2017). Preterm birth: Risk factors, identification and management. In A. Malvasi, A. Tineli, & G. C. Di Renzo (Eds.), *Management and therapy of late pregnancy complications third trimester and puerperium* (pp. 81–94). Cham, Switzerland: Springer International.

Di Renzo, G. C., Roura, L. C., Facchinetti, F., Helmer, H., Hubinont, C., Jacobsson, B., . . . Visser, G. H. (2017). Preterm labor and birth management: Recommendations from the European Association of Perinatal Medicine. *The Journal of Maternal-Fetal & Neonatal Medicine, 30*(17), 2011–2030. doi:10.1080/14767058.2017.1323860

Dodd, J. M., Jones, L., Flenady, V., Cincotta, R., & Crowther, C. A. (2013). Prenatal administration of progesterone for preventing preterm birth in women considered to be at risk of preterm birth. *Cochrane Database of Systematic Reviews*, (7), CD004947. doi:10.1002/14651858.CD004947

Donovan, B. M., Spracklen, C. N., Schweizer, M. L., Ryckman, K. K., & Saftlas, A. F. (2016). Intimate partner violence during pregnancy and the risk for adverse infant outcomes: A systematic review and meta-analysis. *BJOG, 123*(8), 1289–1299. doi:10.1111/1471-0528.13928

Duckworth, A. L., & Chertok, I. R. (2012). Review of perinatal partner-focused smoking cessation interventions. *MCN: The American Journal of Maternal/Child Nursing, 37*(3), 174–181. doi:10.1097/NMC.0b013e31824921b4

Dutton, M. A., Green, B. L., Kaltman, S. I., Roesch, D. M., Zeffiro, T. A., & Krause, E. D. (2006). Intimate partner violence, PTSD, and adverse health outcomes. *Journal of Interpersonal Violence, 21*(7), 955–968. doi:10.1177/0886260506289178

Ebrahim, S. H., & Gfroerer, J. (2003). Pregnancy-related substance use in the United States during 1996–1998. *Obstetrics & Gynecology, 101*(2), 374–379. doi:10.1016/S0029-7844(02)02588-7

Eke, A. C., Chalaan, T., Shukr, G., Eleje, G. U., & Okafor, C. I. (2016). A systematic review and meta-analysis of progestogen

use for maintenance tocolysis after preterm labor in women with intact membranes. *International Journal of Gynecology & Obstetrics, 132*, 11–16. doi:10.1016/j.ijgo.2015.06.058

Engle, W. A., & Kominiarek, M. A. (2008). Late preterm infants, early term infants, and timing of elective deliveries. *Clinics in Perinatology, 35*(2), 325–341, vi. doi:10.1016/j.clp.2008.03.003

Engle, W. A., Tomashek, K. M., Wallman, C., & the Committee on Fetus and Newborn. (2007). "Late-preterm" infants: A population at risk (Reaffirmed, 2013). *Pediatrics, 120*(6), 1390–1401. doi:10.1542/peds.2007-2952

Feder, G. S., Hutson, M., Ramsay, J., & Taket, A. R. (2006). Women exposed to intimate partner violence: Expectations and experiences when they encounter health care professionals: A meta-analysis of qualitative studies. *Archives of Internal Medicine, 166*(1), 22–37. doi:10.1001/archinte.166.1.22

Felder, J. N., Baer, R. J., Rand, L., Jelliffe-Pawlowski, L. L., & Prather, A. A. (2017). Sleep disorder diagnosis during pregnancy and risk of preterm birth. *Obstetrics & Gynecology, 130*(3), 573–581. doi:10.1097/AOG.0000000000002132

Fettweis, J. M., Brooks, J. P., Serrano, M. G., Sheth, N. U., Girerd, P. H., Edwards, D. J., . . . Buck, G. A. (2014). Differences in vaginal microbiome in African American women versus women of European ancestry. *Microbiology, 160*(Pt. 10), 2272–2282. doi:10.1099/mic.0.081034-0

Fleischman, A. R., Oinuma, M., & Clark, S. L. (2010). Rethinking the definition of "term pregnancy." *Obstetrics & Gynecology, 116*(1), 136–139. doi:10.1097/AOG.0b013e3181e24f28

Flenady, V., Reinebrant, H. E., Liley, H. G., Tambimuttu, E. G., & Papatsonis, D. N. M. (2014). Oxytocin receptor antagonists for inhibiting preterm labour. *Cochrane Database of Systematic Reviews*, (6), CD004452. doi:10.1002/14651858.CD004452.pub3

Flynn, H. A., & Chermack, S. T. (2008). Prenatal alcohol use: The role of lifetime problems with alcohol, drugs, depression, and violence. *Journal of Studies on Alcohol and Drugs, 69*(4), 500–509. doi:10.15288/jsad.2008.69.500

Frey, H. A., & Klebanoff, M. A. (2016). The epidemiology, etiology, and costs of preterm birth. *Seminars in Fetal & Neonatal Medicine, 21*(2), 68–73. doi:10.1016/j.siny.2015.12.011

Gelernter, J., & Kranzler, H. R. (2015). Genetics of addiction. In M. Galanter, H. D. Kleber, & K. T. Brady (Eds.), *Textbook of substance abuse treatment* (5th ed., pp. 25–46). Washington, DC: American Psychiatric Publishing.

Georgiou, H. M., Di Quinzio, M. K., Permezel, M., & Brennecke, S. P. (2015). Predicting preterm labour: Current status and future prospects. *Disease Markers, 2015*, 1–9. doi:10.1155/2015/435014

Giarratano, G. (2006). Genetic influences on preterm birth. *MCN: The American Journal of Maternal/Child Nursing, 31*(3), 169–175.

Goldenberg, R. L., Culhane, J. F., Iams, J. D., & Romero, R. (2008). Epidemiology and causes of preterm birth. *Lancet, 371*(9606), 75–84. doi:10.1016/S0140-6736(08)60074-4

Goldenberg, R. L., Hauth, J. C., & Andrews, W. W. (2000). Intrauterine infection and preterm delivery. *The New England Journal of Medicine, 342*(20), 1500–1507. doi:10.1056/NEJM200005183422007

Gorman, M. C., Orme, K. S., Nguyen, N. T., Kent, E. J., III, & Caughey, A. B. (2014). Outcomes in pregnancies complicated by methamphetamine use. *American Journal of Obstetrics & Gynecology, 211*(4), 429.e1–429.e7. doi:10.1016/j.ajog.2014.06.005

Gouin, K., Murphy, K., & Shah, P. S. (2011). Effects of cocaine use during pregnancy on low birthweight and preterm birth: Systematic review and metaanalyses. *American Journal of Obstetrics & Gynecology, 204*(4), 340.e1–340.e12. doi:10.1016/j.ajog.2010.11.013

Goya, M., Pratcorona, L., Merced, C., Rodó, C., Valle, L., Romero, A., . . . Carreras, E. (2012). Cervical pessary in pregnant women with a short cervix (PECEP): An open-label randomised controlled trial. *Lancet, 379*(9828), 1800–1806. doi:10.1016/S0140-6736(12)60030-0

Grissinger, M. (2009). Preventing magnesium toxicity in obstetrics. *Pharmacy and Therapeutics, 34*(8), 403.

Grobman, W. A., Gilbert, S. A., Iams, J. D., Spong, C. Y., Saade, G., Mercer, B. M., . . . Van Dorsten, P. (2013). Activity restriction among women with a short cervix. *Obstetrics & Gynecology, 121*(6), 1181–1186. doi:10.1097/AOG.0b013e3182917529

Haas, D. M., Imperiale, T. F., Kirkpatrick, P. R., Klein, R. W., Zollinger, T. W., & Golichowski, A. M. (2009). Tocolytic therapy: A meta-analysis and decision analysis. *Obstetrics & Gynecology, 113*(3):585–594. doi:10.1097/AOG.0b013e318199924a

Hadley, E. E., Discacciati, A., Costantine, M. M., Munn, M. B., Pacheco, L. D., Saade, G. R., & Chiossi, G. (2017). Maternal obesity is associated with chorioamnionitis and earlier indicated preterm delivery among expectantly managed women with preterm premature rupture of membranes. *The Journal of Maternal-Fetal & Neonatal Medicine, 32*(2),271–278. doi: 10.1080/14767058.2017.1378329

Heil, S. H., Jones, H. E., Arria, A., Kaltenbach, K., Coyle, M., Fischer, G., . . . Martin, P. R. (2011). Unintended pregnancy in opioid-abusing women. *Journal of Substance Abuse Treatment, 40*(2), 199–202. doi:10.1016/j.jsat.2010.08.011

Herron, M. A., Katz, M., & Creasy, R. K. (1982). Evaluation of a preterm birth prevention program: Preliminary report. *Obstetrics & Gynecology, 59*(4), 442–446.

Hibbard, J. U., Wilkins, I., Sun, L., Gregory, K., Haberman, S., Hoffman, M., . . . Zhang, J. (2010). Respiratory morbidity in late preterm births. *JAMA, 304*(4), 419–425. doi:10.1001/jama.2010.1015

Hirbo, J., Eidem, H., Rokas, A., & Abbot, P. (2015). Integrating diverse types of genomic data to identify genes that underlie adverse pregnancy phenotypes. *PLoS ONE, 10*(12), e0144155. doi:10.1371/journal.pone.0144155

Hotham, E. D., Atkinson, E. R., & Gilbert, A. L. (2002). Focus groups with pregnant smokers: Barriers to cessation, attitudes to nicotine patch use and perceptions of cessation counselling by care providers. *Drug and Alcohol Review, 21*, 163. doi:10.1080/09595230220139064

Hu, R., Chen, Y., Zhang, Y., Qian, Z., Liu, Y., Vaughn, M. G., . . . Zhang, B. (2017). Association between vomiting in the first trimester and preterm birth: A retrospective birth cohort study in Wuhan, China. *BMJ Open, 7*, e017309, 1–6. doi:10.1136/bmjopen-2017-017309

Huang, B., Faucette, A. N., Pawlitz, M. D., Pei, B., Goyert, J. W., Zhou, J. Z., . . . Chen, K. (2017). Interleukin-33-induced expression of PIBF1 by decidual B cells protects against preterm labor. *Nature Medicine, 23*(1), 128–135. doi:10.1038/nm.4244

Huang, L., Luo, Y., Wen, X., He, Y. H., Ding, P., Xie, C., . . . Chen, W. Q. (2019). Gene–gene-environment interactions of prenatal exposed to environmental tobacco smoke, CYP1A1 and GSTs polymorphisms on full-term low birth weight: relationship of maternal passive smoking, gene polymorphisms, and FT-LBW. *The Journal of Maternal-Fetal & Neonatal Medicine, 32*(13), 2200–2208. doi:10.1080/14767058.2018.1429394

Hui, S. Y., Chor, C. M., Lau, T. K., Lao, T. T., & Leung, T. Y. (2013). Cerclage pessary for preventing preterm birth in women with a singleton pregnancy and a short cervix at 20 to 24 weeks: A randomized controlled trial. *American Journal of Perinatology, 30*(4), 283–288. doi:10.1055/s-0032-1322550

Huybrechts, K. F., Sanghani, R. S., Avorn, J., & Urato, A. C. (2014). Preterm birth and antidepressant medication use during pregnancy: A systematic review and meta-analysis. *PLoS ONE, 9*(3), e92778, 1–13. doi:10.1371/journal.pone.0092778

Institute for Safe Medication Practices. (2006). Preventing magnesium toxicity in obstetrics. *Nurse Advise-ERR: ISMP Medication Safety Alert, 4*(6), 1–2.

Institute for Safe Medication Practices. (2010). Failure to set a volume limit for a magnesium bolus dose leads to harm. *Acute Care: ISMP Medication Safety Alert*, (June 3, 2010 issue), 1–3.

Institute of Medicine. (1985). *Preventing low birthweight*. Washington, DC: National Academy Press.

Institute of Medicine. (2007). *Preterm birth: Causes, consequences, and prevention*. Washington, DC: National Academy Press.

Jallo, N., Thacker, L. R., Menzies, V., Stojanovic, P., & Svikis, D. S. (2017). A stress coping app for hospitalized pregnant women at risk for preterm birth. *MCN: The Journal of Maternal/Child Nursing, 42*(5), 257–262. doi:10.1097/NMC.0000000000000355

Johnson, K., Posner, S. F., Biermann, J., Cordero, J. F., Atrash, H. K., Parker, C. S., . . . Curtis, M. G. (2006). Recommendations to improve preconception health and health care—United States. A report of the CDC/ATSDR Preconception Care Work Group and the Select Panel on Preconception Care. *MMWR. Recommendations and Reports, 55*(RR-6), 1–23.

Jones, G., Clark, T., & Bewley, S. (1998). The weak cervix: Failing to keep the baby in or infection out? *British Journal of Obstetrics and Gynaecology, 105*(11), 1214–1215.

Jones, H. E., O'Grady, K. E., Malfi, D., & Tuten, M. (2008). Methadone maintenance vs. methadone taper during pregnancy: Maternal and neonatal outcomes. *American Journal on Addictions, 17*(5), 372–386. doi:10.1080/10550490802266276

Kajeepeta, S., Sanchez, S. E., Gelaye, B., Qiu, C., Barrios, Y. V., Enquobahrie, D. A., & Williams, M. A. (2014). Sleep duration, vital exhaustion, and odds of spontaneous preterm birth: A case-control study. *BMC Pregnancy & Childbirth, 14*, 337. doi:10.1186/1471-2393-14-337

Kent, A. L., Wright, I. M., & Abdel-Latif, M. E. (2012). Mortality and adverse neurologic outcomes are greater in preterm male infants. *Pediatrics, 129*(1), 124–131. doi:10.1542/peds.2011-1578

Kim, A., Lee, E. S., Shin, J. C., & Kim, H. Y. (2013). Identification of biomarkers for preterm delivery in mid-trimester amniotic fluid. *Placenta, 34*(10), 873–878. doi:10.1016/j.placenta.2013.06.306

Kinney, H. C. (2006). The near-term (late preterm) human brain and risk for periventricular leukomalacia: A review. *Seminars in Perinatology, 30*(2), 81–88. doi:10.1053/j.semperi.2006.02.006

Klein, R. F., Friedman-Campbell, M., & Tocco, R. V. (1993). History taking and substance abuse counseling with the pregnant patient. *Clinical Obstetrics and Gynecology, 36*(2), 338–346. doi:10.1097/00003081-199306000-00012

Kuczkowski, K. M. (2007). The effects of drug abuse on pregnancy. *Current Opinions in Obstetrics and Gynecology, 19*(6), 578–585. doi:10.1097/GCO.0b013e3282f1bf17

Kuessel, L., Grimm, C., Knöfler, M., Haslinger, P., Leipold, H., Heinze, G., . . . Schmid, M. (2013). Common oxytocin receptor gene polymorphisms and the risk for preterm birth. *Disease Markers, 34*(1), 51–56. doi:10.3233/DMA-2012-00936

Ladewig, P. W., London, M. L., & Davidson, M. R. (2017). Care of the woman at risk because of preterm labor. In *Contemporary maternal-newborn nursing care* (9th ed., pp. 407–411). Hoboken, NJ: Pearson Education.

Larsen, L. G., Clausen, H. V., & Jønsson, L. (2002). Stereologic examination of placentas from mothers who smoke during pregnancy. *American Journal of Obstetrics & Gynecology, 186*(3), 531–537. doi:10.1067/mob.2002.120481

Leonardi-Bee, J., Britton, J., & Venn, A. (2011). Secondhand smoke and adverse fetal outcomes in nonsmoking pregnant women: A meta-analysis. *Pediatrics, 127*(4), 734–741. doi:10.1542/peds.2010-3041

Leone, A., Ersfeld, P., Adams, M., Schiffer, P. M., Bucher, H. U., & Arlettaz, R. (2012). Neonatal morbidity in singleton late preterm infants compared with full-term infants. *Acta Paediatrica, 101*(1), e6–e10. doi:10.1111/j.1651-2227.2011.02459.x

Li, J., Hua, J., Jian-Ping, H., & Yan, L. (2015). Association between the lipid levels and single nucleotide polymorphisms of ABCA1,

APOE and HMGCR genes in subjects with spontaneous preterm delivery. *PLoS ONE, 10*(8), e0135785. doi:10.1371/journal .pone.0135785

Liem, S., Schuit, E., Hegeman, M., Bais, J., de Boer, K., Bloemenkamp, K., . . . Bekedam, D. (2013). Cervical pessaries for prevention of preterm birth in women with a multiple pregnancy (ProTWIN): A multicentre, open-label randomised controlled trial. *Lancet, 382*(9901), 1341–1349. doi:10.1016/S0140-6736(13)61408-7

Lockwood, C. J., Senyei, A. E., Dische, M. R., Casal, D., Shah, K. D., Thung, S. N., . . . Garite, T. J. (1991). Fetal fibronectin in cervical and vaginal secretions as a predictor of preterm delivery. *The New England Journal of Medicine, 325*(10), 669–674. doi:10.1056/NEJM199109053251001

Lockwood, C. J., Stocco, C., Murk, W., Kayisli, U. A., Funai, E. F., & Schatz, F. (2010). Human labor is associated with reduced decidual cell expression of progesterone, but not glucocorticoid, receptors. *The Journal of Clinical Endocrinology & Metabolism, 95*(5), 2271–2275. doi:10.1210/jc.2009-2136

Lowe, N. K., Openshaw, M., & King, T. L. (2017). Treatments for women in preterm labor. In M. C. Brucker & T. L. King (Eds.), *Pharmacology for women's health* (2nd ed., pp. 1069–1073). Burlington, MA: Jones & Bartlett.

Ludermir, A. B., Lewis, G., Valongueiro, S. A., de Araújo, T. V., & Araya, R. (2010). Violence against women by their intimate partner during pregnancy and postnatal depression: A prospective cohort study. *Lancet, 376*(9744), 903–910. doi:10.1016/S0140 -6736(10)60887-2

MacDorman, M. F., Callaghan, W. M., Mathews, T. J., Hoyert, D. L., & Kochanek, K. D. (2007). Trends in preterm-related infant mortality by race and ethnicity, United States, 1999–2004. *International Journal of Health Services, 37*(4), 635–641. doi:10.2190/HS.37.4.c

Machado, L. C., Jr., Passini, R., Jr., Rosa, I. R., & Carvalho, H. B. (2014). Neonatal outcomes of late preterm and early term birth. *European Journal of Obstetrics & Gynecology and Reproductive Biology, 179*, 204–208. doi:10.1016/j.ejogrb.2014.04.042

Maeda, A., Bateman, B. T., Clancy, C. R., Creanga, A. A., & Leffert, L. R. (2014). Opioid abuse and dependence during pregnancy: Temporal trends and obstetrical outcomes. *Anesthesiology, 121*(6), 1158–1165. doi:10.1097/ALN.0000000000000472

Makieva, S., Dubicke, A., Rinaldi, S. F., Fransson, E., Ekman-Ordeberg, G., & Norman, J. E. (2017). The preterm cervix reveals a transcriptomic signature in the presence of premature prelabor rupture of membranes. *American Journal of Obstetrics & Gynecology, 216*, 602.e1–602.e21. doi:10.1016/j.ajog.2017.02.009

Manuck, T. A. (2016). Pharmacogenomics of preterm birth prevention and treatment: A review. *BJOG, 123*(3), 368–375. doi:10.1111/1471-0528.13744

Manuck, T. A. (2017). Racial and ethnic differences in preterm birth: A complex, multifactorial problem. *Seminars in Perinatology.* doi:10.1053/j.semperi.2017.08.010

March of Dimes. (2015a). *The impact of premature birth on society.* Retrieved from https://www.marchofdimes.org/mission/the -economic-and-societal-costs.aspx

March of Dimes. (2015b). *The cost to business.* Retrieved from https://www.marchofdimes.org/mission/the-cost-to-business .aspx

March of Dimes. (2016). *March of Dimes foundation data book for policy makers: Maternal, infant, and child health in the United States, 2016.* Retrieved from https://www.marchofdimes.org /materials/March-of-Dimes-2016-Databook.pdf

March of Dimes. (2017). *2017 Premature birth report cards.* Retrieved from https://www.marchofdimes.org/materials/Premature BirthReportCard-United-States-2017.pdf

March of Dimes. (2018). *Preterm labor and premature birth: Are you at risk?* Retrieved from https://www.marchofdimes.org /complications/preterm-labor-and-premature-birth-are-you-at -risk.aspx

March of Dimes. (2019a). *Finding the causes of prematurity.* Retrieved from https://www.marchofdimes.org/research/finding-the -causes-of-prematurity.aspx

March of Dimes. (2019b). *Peristats.* Retrieved from http://www .marchofdimes.org/peristats

March of Dimes. (2019c). *Smoking during pregnancy.* Retrieved from https://www.marchofdimes.org/pregnancy/smoking-during -pregnancy.aspx

March of Dimes. (2019d). *39+ Weeks quality improvement.* Retrieved from https://www.marchofdimes.org/mission/39-weeks -quality-improvement.aspx

March of Dimes, Partnership for Maternal, Newborn & Child Health, Save the Children, & World Health Organization. (2012). *Born too soon: The global action report on preterm birth.* Geneva, Switzerland: World Health Organization.

Marret, S., Marpeau, L., Zupan-Simunek, V., Eurin, D., Lévêque, C., Hellot, M.-F., & Bénichou, J. (2007). Magnesium sulfate given before very-preterm birth to protect infant brain: The randomised controlled PREMAG trial. *BJOG, 114*(3), 310–318. doi:10.1111/j.1471-0528.2006.01162.x

Martin, J. A., Hamilton, B. E., Osterman, M. J. K., Driscoll, A. K., & Drake, P. (2018). Births: Final data for 2017. *National Vital Statistics Reports, 67*(8), 1–50.

Martin, J. A., & Osterman, M. J. K. (2019). *Is twin childbearing on the decline? Twin births in the United States, 2014–2018* (NCHS Data Brief No. 351). Hyattsville, MD: National Center for Health Statistics.

Martin, J. A., Osterman, M. J., Kirmeyer, S. E., & Gregory, E. C. (2015). Measuring gestational age in vital statistics data: Transitioning to the obstetric estimate. *National Vital Statistics Report, 64*(5), 1–20.

Martin, J. N., Jr., D'Alton, M., Jacobsson, B., & Norman, J. E. (2017). In pursuit of progress toward effective preterm birth reduction. *Obstetrics & Gynecology, 129*(4), 715–719. doi:10.1097/AOG.0000000000001923

Mathews, T. J., & MacDorman, M. F. (2010). Infant mortality statistics from the 2006 period linked birth/infant death data set. *National Vital Statistics Report, 58*(17), 1–31.

Matthews, M. S., MacDorman, M. F., & Thoma, M. E. (2015). Infant mortality statistics from the 2013 period linked birth/infant death data set. *National Vital Statistics Report, 64*(9), 1–30.

McDonnell, S. L., Baggerly, K. A., Baggerly, C. A., Aliano, J. L., French, C. B., Baggerly, L. L., . . . Wagner, C. L. (2017). Maternal 25(OH)D concentrations ≥40 ng/mL associated with 60% lower preterm birth risk among general obstetrical patients at an urban medical center. *PLoS ONE, 12*(7), e0180483. doi:10.1371 /journal.pone.0180483

McPherson, J. A., & Manuck, T. A. (2016). Genomics of preterm birth—Evidence of association and evolving investigations. *American Journal of Perinatology, 33*(3), 222–228. doi:10.1055/s-0035-1571144

Medoff-Cooper, B., Bakewell-Sachs, S., Buus-Frank, M. E., & Santa-Donato, A. (2005). The AWHONN Near-Term Initiative: A conceptual framework for optimizing health for near-term infants. *Journal of Obstetric, Gynecologic & Neonatal Nursing, 34*(6), 666–671. doi:10.1177/0884217505281873

Medoff-Cooper, B., Holditch-Davis, D., Verklan, M. T., Fraser-Askin, D., Lamp, J., Santa-Donato, A., . . . Bingham, D. (2012). Newborn clinical outcomes of the AWHONN late preterm infant research-based practice project. *Journal of Obstetric, Gynecologic, and Neonatal Nursing, 41*(6), 774–785. doi:10.1111 /j.1552-6909.2012.01401.x

Melchor, J. C., Navas, H., Marcos, N., Iza, A., de Diego, N., Rando, D., . . . Burgos, J. (2017). Retrospective cohort study of PAMG-1 and fetal fibronectin test performance in assessing spontaneous preterm birth risk in symptomatic women attending an emergency obstetrical unit. *Ultrasound in Obstetrics and Gynecology, 51*(5). doi:10.1002/uog.18892

Menon, R. (2008). Spontaneous preterm birth, a clinical dilemma: Etiologic, pathophysiologic and genetic heterogeneities and racial disparity. *Acta Obstetricia et Gynecologica Scandinavica*, *87*(6), 590–600. doi:10.1080/00016340802005126

Mesiano, S., Wang, Y., & Norwitz, E. R. (2011). Progesterone receptors in the human pregnancy uterus: Do they hold the key to birth timing? *Reproductive Sciences*, *18*(1), 6–19. doi:10.1177/1933719110382922

Möller, M. I., Henderson, J. J., Nathan, E. A., & Pennell, C. E. (2013). Cervilenz™ is an effective tool for screening cervical-length in comparison to transvaginal ultrasound. *Journal of Maternal-Fetal & Neonatal Medicine*, *26*(4), 378–382. doi:10.3109/14767058.2012.712564

Monangi, N. K., Brockway, H. M., House, M., Zhang, G., & Muglia, L. J. (2015). The genetics of preterm birth: Progress and promise. *Seminars in Perinatology*, *39*, 574–583. doi:10.1053/j.semperi.2015.09.005

Mozurkewich, E., Chilimigras, J., Koepke, E., Keeton, K., & King, V. J. (2009). Indications for induction of labour: A best-evidence review. *BJOG*, *116*(5), 626–636. doi:10.1111/j.1471-0528.2008.02065.x

Mullen, P. D., Richardson, M. A., Quinn, V. P., & Ershoff, D. H. (1997). Postpartum return to smoking: Who is at risk and when. *American Journal of Health Promotion*, *11*(5), 323–330. doi:10.4278/0890-1171-11.5.323

Murray, S. S., & McKinney, E. S. (2014). Intrapartum complications. In *Foundations of maternal-newborn and women's health nursing* (6th ed., pp. 568–597). St. Louis, MO: Elsevier.

Naik Gaunekar, N., Raman, P., Bain, E., & Crowther, C. A. (2013). Maintenance therapy with calcium channel blockers for preventing preterm birth after threatened preterm labour. *Cochrane Database of Systematic Reviews*, (10), CD004071. doi:10.1002/14651858.CD004071.pub3

Nan, Y., & Li, H. (2015). MTHFR genetic polymorphism increases the risk of preterm delivery. *International Journal of Clinical and Experimental Pathology*, *8*(6), 7397–7402.

National Center for Biotechnology Information. (2019). *CRHR corticotropin releasing hormone receptor 1 [Homo sapiens (human)]*. Retrieved from https://www.ncbi.nlm.nih.gov/gene/1392

National Center for Health Statistics. (2005). *Chartbook on trends in the health of Americans*. Hyattsville, MD: Authors.

National Human Genome Research Institute. (2003). *International consortium completes human genome project*. Bethesda, MD: Author.

National Institute of Child Health and Human Development. (2005). *Optimizing care and long-term outcomes of near-term pregnancy and near-term newborn infants*. Bethesda, MD: Authors.

Navathe, R., & Berghella, V. (2016). Tocolysis for acute preterm labor: Where have we been, where are we now, and where are we going? *American Journal of Perinatology*, *33*(3), 229–235. doi:10.1055/s-0035-1571147

Neilson, J. P., West, H. M., & Dowswell, T. (2014). Betamimetics for inhibiting preterm labour. *Cochrane Database of Systematic Reviews*, (2), CD004352. doi:10.1002/14651858.CD004352.pub3

Nelson, H. D., Bougatsos, C., & Blazina, I. (2012). Screening women for intimate partner violence: A systematic review to update the U.S. Preventive Services Task Force recommendation. *Annals of Internal Medicine*, *156*(11), 796–808, W-279–W-282. doi:10.7326/0003-4819-156-11-201206050-00447

Newnham, J. P., Dickinson, J. E., Hart, R. J., Pennell, C. E., Arrese, C. A., & Keelan, J. A. (2014). Strategies to prevent preterm birth. *Frontiers in Immunology*, *5*, 584. doi:10.3389/fimmu.2014.00584

Nicolaides, K. H., Syngelaki, A., Poon, L. C., de Paco Matallana, C., Plasencia, W., Molina, F. S., . . . Conturso, R. (2016). Cervical pessary placement for prevention of preterm birth in unselected twin pregnancies: A randomized controlled trial. *American Journal of Obstetrics & Gynecology*, *214*(1), 3.e1–3.e9. doi:10.1016/j.ajog.2015.08.051

Nightingale, S. L. (1998). Warning use of terbutaline sulfate for preterm labor. *JAMA*, *279*(1), 9. doi:10.1001/jama.279.1.9-JFD71011-2-1

Norman, J. E., Marlow, N., Messow, C.-M., Shennan, A., Bennett, P. R., Thornton, S., . . . Norrie, J. (2016). Vaginal progesterone prophylaxis for preterm birth (the OPPTIMUM study): A multicentre, randomised, double-blind trial. *Lancet*, *387*(10033), 2106–2116. doi:10.1016/S0140-6736(16)00350-0

O'Connor, C., & Gennaro, S. (2017). Preventing prematurity: Preconception, prenatal and postpartum nursing care. *March of Dimes*. Retrieved from https://www.marchofdimes.org/nursing/modnemedia/othermedia/articles/art06_preventing_prematurity_text.pdf

Orleans, C. T., Barker, D. C., Kaufman, N. J., & Marx, J. F. (2000). Helping pregnant smokers quit: Meeting the challenge in the next decade. *Tobacco Control*, *9*(Suppl. 3), iii6–iii11. doi:10.1136/tc.9.suppl_3.iii6

Owen, J., Hankins, G., Iams, J. D., Berghella, V., Sheffield, J. S., Perez-Delboy, A., . . . Hauth, J. C. (2009). Multicenter randomized trial of cerclage for preterm delivery prevention in high-risk women with shortened midtrimester cervical length. *American Journal of Obstetric & Gynecology*, *201*(4), 375.e1–375.e8. doi:10.1016/j.ajog.2009.08.015

Parikh, L. I., Reddy, U. M., Männistö, T., Mendola, P., Sjaarda, L., Hinkle, S., & Laughon, K. (2014). Neonatal outcomes in early term birth. *American Journal of Obstetrics & Gynecology*, *211*(3), 265.e1–265.e11. doi:10.1016/j.ajog.2014.03.021

Parker, B., McFarlane, J., & Soeken, K. (1994). Abuse during pregnancy: Effects on maternal complications and birth weight in adult and teenage women. *Obstetrics & Gynecology*, *84*(3), 323–328.

Parnell, L. A., Briggs, C. M., & Mysorekar, I. U. (2017). Maternal microbiomes in preterm birth: Recent progress and analytical pipelines. *Seminars in Perinatology*, *41*, 392–400. doi:10.1053/j.semperi.2017.07.010

Peng, C. C., Chang, J. H., Lin, H. Y., Cheng, P. J., & Su, B. H. (2018). Intrauterine inflammation, infection, or both (Triple I): A new concept for chorioamnionitis. *Pediatric Neonatology*, *59*(3), 231–237. doi: 10.1016/j.pedneo.2017.09.001

Pineles, B. L., Hsu, S., Park, E., & Samet, J. M. (2016). Systematic review and meta-analyses of perinatal death and maternal exposure to tobacco smoke during pregnancy. *American Journal of Epidemiology*, *184*(2), 87–97. doi:https://doi.org/10.1093/aje/kwv301

Plunkett, J., Feitosa, M. F., Trusgnich, M., Wangler, M. F., Palomar, L., Kistka, Z. A., . . . Muglia, L. J. (2009). Mother's genome or maternally-inherited genes acting in the fetus influence gestational age in familial preterm birth. *Human Heredity*, *68*(3), 209–219. doi:10.1159/000224641

Purisch, S. E., & Gyamfi-Bannerman, C. (2017). Epidemiology of preterm birth. *Seminars in Perinatology*, *41*(7), 387–391. doi:10.1053/j.semperi.2017.07.009

Qin, J., Wang, H., Sheng, X., Liang, D., Tan, H., & Xia, J. (2015). Pregnancy-related complications and adverse pregnancy outcomes in multiple pregnancies resulting from assisted reproductive technology: A meta-analysis of cohort studies. *Fertility and Sterility*, *103*(6), 1492–1508. doi:10.1016/j.fertnstert.2015.03.018

Raja, M., Garg, A., Yadav, P., Jha, K., & Handa, S. (2016). Diagnostic methods for detection of cotinine level in tobacco users: A review. *Journal of Clinical and Diagnostic Research*, *10*(3), ZE04–ZE06. doi:10.7860/JCDR/2016/17360.7423

Raju, T. N. K., Higgins, R. D., Stark, A. R., & Leveno, K. J. (2006). Optimizing care and outcome for late-preterm (near-term) infants: A summary of the workshop sponsored by the National Institute of Child Health and Human Development. *Pediatrics*, *118*(3), 1207–1214. doi:10.1542/peds.2006-0018

Rayman, M. P., Wijnen, H., Vader, H., Kooistra, L., & Pop, V. (2011). Maternal selenium status during early gestation and risk for preterm birth. *Canadian Medical Association Journal*, *183*(5), 549–555. doi:10.1503/cmaj.101095

Reece-Stremtan, S., Marinelli, K. A., & Academy of Breastfeeding Medicine. (2015). ABM Clinical Protocol #21: Guidelines for breastfeeding and substance use or substance use disorder, revised 2015. *Breastfeeding Medicine*, *10*(3), 135–141. doi:10.1089/bfm.2015.9992

Rockhill, K. M., Tong, V. T., Farr, S. L., Robbins, C. L., D'Angelo, D. V., & England, L. J. (2016). Postpartum smoking relapse after quitting during pregnancy: Pregnancy risk assessment monitoring system, 2000-2011. *Journal of Women's Health*, *25*(5), 480–488. doi:10.1089/jwh.2015.5244

Romero, R., Dey, S. K., & Fisher, S. J. (2014). Preterm labor: One syndrome, many causes. *Science*, *345*(6198), 760–765. doi:10.1126/science.1251816

Romero, R., Nicolaides, K., Conde-Agudelo, A., Tabor, A., O'Brien, J. M., Cetingoz, E., . . . Hassan, S. S. (2012). Vaginal progesterone in women with an asymptomatic sonographic short cervix in the midtrimester decreases preterm delivery and neonatal morbidity: A systematic review and metaanalysis of individual patient data. *American Journal of Obstetrics & Gynecology*, *206*(2), 124.e1–124.e19. doi:10.1016/j.ajog.2011.12.003

Rood, K. M., & Buhimschi, C. S. (2017). Genetics, hormonal influences, and preterm birth. *Seminars in Perinatology*, *41*, 401–408. doi:10.1053/j.semperi.2017.07.011

Rouse, D. J., Hirtz, D. G., Thom, E., Varner, M. W., Spong, C. Y., Mercer, B. M., . . . Roberts, J. M. (2008). A randomized, controlled trial of magnesium sulfate for the prevention of cerebral palsy. *The New England Journal of Medicine*, *359*(9), 895–905. doi:10.1056/NEJMoa0801187

Rundell, K., & Panchal, B. (2017). Preterm labor: Prevention and management. *American Family Physician*, *95*(6), 366–372.

Saccone, G., Maruotti, G. M., Giudicepietro, A., & Martinelli, P. (2017). Effect of cervical pessary on spontaneous preterm birth in women with singleton pregnancies and short cervical length: A randomized clinical trial. *JAMA*, *318*(23), 2317–2324. doi:10.1001/jama.2017.18956

Santa-Donato, A. (2005). Near-term infants: What experts say health care providers and parents need to know. *AWHONN Lifelines*, *9*(6), 456–462. doi:10.1177/1091592305285274

Sanz, M., & Kornman, K. (2013). Periodontitis and adverse pregnancy outcomes: Consensus report of the Joint EFP/AAP Workshop on Periodontitis and Systemic Diseases. *Journal of Periodontology*, *84*(4 Suppl.), S164–S169. doi:10.1902/jop.2013.1340016

Sunderam, S., Kissin, D. M., Crawford, S. B., Folger, S. G., Boulet, S. L., Warner, L., & Barfield, W. D. (2018). Assisted reproductive technology surveillance—United States, 2015. *Morbidity and Mortality Weekly Report*, *67*(3), 1–20. doi:10.15585/mmwr.ss6703al

Schmidt, B., Roberts, R. S., Davis, P. G., Doyle, L. W., Asztalos, E. V., Opie, G., . . . Sauve, R. S. (2015). Prediction of late death or disability at age 5 years using a count of 3 neonatal morbidities in very low birth weight infants. *Journal of Pediatrics*, *167*(5), 982.e2–986.e2. doi:10.1016/j.jpeds.2015.07.067

Shapiro-Mendoza, C. K., Tomashek, K. M., Kotelchuck, M., Barfield, W., Nannini, A., Weiss, J., & Declercq, E. (2008). Effect of late-preterm birth and maternal medical conditions on newborn morbidity risk. *Pediatrics*, *121*(2), e223–e232. doi:10.1542/peds.2006-3629

Shaw, J. G., Asch, S. M., Kimerling, R., Frayne, S. M., Shaw, K. A., & Phibbs, C. S. (2014). Posttraumatic stress disorder and risk of spontaneous preterm birth. *Obstetrics & Gynecology*, *124*(6), 1111–1119. doi:10.1097/AOG.0000000000000542

Sheikh, I. A., Ahmad, E., Jamal, M. S., Rehan, M., Assidi, M., Tayubi, I. A., . . . Al-Qahtani, M. (2016). Spontaneous preterm birth and single nucleotide gene polymorphisms: A recent update. *BMC Genomics*, *17*(Suppl. 9), 759. doi:10.1186/s12864-016-3089-0

Silver, R. M. (2007). Fetal death. *Obstetrics & Gynecology*, *109*(1), 153–167. doi:10.1097/01.AOG.0000248537.89739.96

Silverman, J. G., Decker, M. R., Reed, E., & Raj, A. (2006). Intimate partner violence victimization prior to and during pregnancy among women residing in 26 U.S. states: Associations with maternal and neonatal health. *American Journal of Obstetrics & Gynecology*, *195*(1), 140–148. doi:10.1016/j.ajog.2005.12.052

Simpson, K. R. (2006). Minimizing risk of magnesium sulfate overdose in obstetrics. *MCN: The American Journal of Maternal/Child Nursing*, *31*(5), 340.

Simpson, K. R., & Knox, G. E. (2004). Obstetrical accidents involving intravenous magnesium sulfate: Recommendations to promote patient safety. *MCN: The American Journal of Maternal/Child Nursing*, *29*(3), 170–171.

Simpson, L. L., Rochelson, B., Ananth, C. V., Bernstein, P. S., D'Alton, M., Chazotte, C., . . . Zielinski K. (2018). Safe motherhood initiative: Early impact of severe hypertension in pregnancy bundle implementation. *AJP Reports*, *8*(4), e212–e218. doi:10.1055/s-0038-1673632

Smith, S. G., Chen, J., Basile, K. C., Gilbert, L. K., Merrick, M. T., Patel, N., . . . Jain, A. (2017). *The National Intimate Partner and Sexual Violence Survey: 2010-2012 State report*. Atlanta, GA: National Center for Injury Prevention and Control, Centers for Disease Control and Prevention.

Society for Maternal-Fetal Medicine. (2012). *Progesterone and preterm birth prevention: Translating clinical trials data into clinical practice*. Washington, DC: Author.

Society for Maternal-Fetal Medicine. (2015). *Cervical cerclage for the woman with prior adverse pregnancy outcome*. Washington, DC: Author.

Society for Maternal-Fetal Medicine. (2016). Implementation of the use of antenatal corticosteroids in the late preterm birth period in women at risk for preterm delivery. *American Journal of Obstetrics & Gynecology*, *215*(2), B13–B15. doi:10.1016/j.ajog.2016.03.013

Society for Maternal-Fetal Medicine. (2017a). The choice of progestogen for the prevention of preterm birth in women with singleton pregnancy and prior preterm birth. *American Journal of Obstetrics & Gynecology*, *216*(3), B11–B13. doi:10.1016/j.ajog.2017.01.022

Society for Maternal-Fetal Medicine. (2017b). *The role of cervical pessary placement to prevent preterm birth in clinical practice*. Washington, DC: Author.

Society for Maternal-Fetal Medicine, McIntosh, J., Feltovich, H., Berghella, V., & Manuck, T. (2016). *The role of routine cervical length screening in selected high- and low-risk women for preterm birth prevention* (Society for Maternal-Fetal Medicine Consult Series #40).

Son, M., & Miller, E. S. (2017). Predicting preterm birth: Cervical length and fetal fibronectin. *Seminars in Perinatology*, *41*(8), 445–451. doi:10.1053/j.semperi.2017.08.002

Sosa, C. G., Althabe, F., Belizán, J. M., & Bergel, E. (2015). Bed rest in singleton pregnancies for preventing preterm birth. *Cochrane Database of Systematic Reviews*, (3), CD003581. doi:10.1002/14651858.CD003581.pub3

Spong, C. Y. (2013). Defining "term" pregnancy: Recommendations from the defining "term" pregnancy workgroup. *JAMA*, *309*(23), 2445–2446. doi:10.1001/jama.2013.6235

Spong, C. Y., Mercer, B. M., D'Alton, M., Kilpatrick, S., Blackwell, S., & Saade, G. (2011). Timing of indicated late-preterm and early-term birth. *Obstetrics & Gynecology*, *118*(2, Pt. 1), 323–333. doi:10.1097/AOG.0b013e3182255999

Stan, C., Boulvain, M., Pfister, R., & Hirsbrunner-Almagbaly, P. (2013). Hydration for treatment of preterm labour. *Cochrane Database of Systematic Reviews*, (11), CD003096. doi:10.1002/14651858.CD003096.pub2

Staneva, A., Bogossian, F., Pritchard, M., & Wittkowski, A. (2015). The effects of maternal depression, anxiety, and perceived stress during pregnancy on preterm birth: A systematic review. *Women and Birth, 28,* 179–193. doi:10.1016/j.wombi.2015.02.003

Stetson, B., Hibbard, J. U., Wilkins, I., & Leftwich, H. (2016). Outcomes with cerclage alone compared with cerclage plus 17α-hydroxyprogesterone caproate. *Obstetrics & Gynecology, 128*(5), 983–988. doi:10.1097/AOG.0000000000001681

Stone, W. L., Bailey, B., & Khraisha, N. (2014). The pathophysiology of smoking during pregnancy: A systems biology approach. *Frontiers in Bioscience (Elite Edition), 6,* 318–328. doi:10.2741/708

Sultan, A. A., West, J., Tata, L. J., Fleming, K. M., Nelson-Piercy, C., & Grainge, M. J. (2013). Risk of first venous thromboembolism in pregnant women in hospital: Population based cohort study from England. *BMJ, 347,* f6099. doi:10.1136/bmj.f6099

Talati, A. N., Hackney, D. H., & Mesiano, S. (2017). Pathophysiology of preterm labor with intact membranes. *Seminars in Perinatology, 41,* 420–426. doi:10.1053/j.semperi.2017.07.013

Tambor, V., Vajrychova, M., Kacerovsky, M., Link, M., Domasinska, P., Menon, R., & Lenco, J. (2015). Potential peripartum markers of infectious-inflammatory complications in spontaneous preterm birth. *Biomed Research International, 2015*(343501), 1–13. doi:10.1155/2015/343501

Tchamo, M. E., Prista, A., & Leandro, C. G. (2016). Low birth weight, very low birth weight and extremely low birth weight in African children aged between 0 and 5 years old: A systematic review. *Journal of Developmental Origins of Health and Disease, 7*(4), 408–415. doi:10.1017/S2040174416000131

The Joint Commission. (2017). *Perinatal care PC-01: Elective delivery.* Oakbrook Terrace, IL: Author.

Unger, A. S., Martin, P. R., Kaltenbach, K., Stine, S. M., Heil, S. H., Jones, H. E., . . . Fischer, G. (2010). Clinical characteristics of Central European and North American samples of pregnant women screened for opioid agonist treatment. *European Addiction Research, 16*(2), 99–107. doi:10.1159/000284683

U.S. Food and Drug Administration. (2017a). *FDA drug safety communication: New warnings against use of terbutaline to treat preterm labor.* Washington, DC: Author.

U.S. Food and Drug Administration. (2017b). *New warnings against use of terbutaline to treat preterm labor* (FDA Drug Safety Communication). Silver Spring, MD: Author.

Uzun, A., Schuster, J., McGonnigal, B., Schorl, C., Dewan, A., & Padbury, J. (2016). Targeted sequencing and meta-analysis of preterm birth. *PLoS ONE, 11*(5), 1–17. doi:10.1371/journal.pone.0155021

van Zijl, M. D., Koullali, B., Mol, B. W., Pajkrt, E., & Oudijk, M. A. (2016). Prevention of preterm delivery: Current challenges and future prospects. *International Journal of Women's Health, 8,* 633–645.

Verani, J. R., McGee, L., & Schrag, S. J. (2010). Prevention of perinatal group B streptococcal disease: Revised guidelines from CDC, 2010. *Morbidity and Mortality Weekly Report Recommendations and Reports, 59*(RR-10), 1–32.

Vermillion, S. T., Scardo, J. A., Lashus, A. G., & Wiles, H. B. (1997). The effect of indomethacin tocolysis on fetal ductus arteriosus constriction with advancing gestational age. *American Journal of Obstetrics & Gynecology, 177*(2), 256–261. doi:10.1016/S0002-9378(97)70184-4

Vink, J., & Mourad, M. (2017). The pathophysiology of human premature cervical remodeling resulting in spontaneous preterm birth: Where are we now? *Seminars in Perinatology, 41,* 427–437. doi:10.1053/j.semperi.2017.07.014

Vink, J. Y., Qin, S., Brock, C. O., Zork, N. M., Feltovich, H. M., Chen, X., . . . Gallos, G. (2016). A new paradigm for the role of smooth muscle cells in the human cervix. *American Journal of Obstetrics & Gynecology, 215*(4), 478.e1–478.e11. doi:10.1016/j.ajog.2016.04.053

Volpe, J. J. (1997). Overview: Perinatal and neonatal brain injury. *Mental Retardation and Developmental Disabilities Reserves, 3,* 1–2. doi:10.1002/(SICI)1098-2779(1997)3:1<1::AID-MRDD1>3.0.CO;2-W

Wadhwa, P. D., Entringer, S., Buss, C., & Lu, M. C. (2011). The contribution of maternal stress to preterm birth: Issues and considerations. *Clinics in Perinatology, 38*(3), 351–384. doi:10.1016/j.clp.2011.06.007

Wax, J. R., Cartin, A., & Pinette, M. G. (2016). Biophysical and biochemical screening for the risk of preterm labor. *Clinics in Laboratory Medicine, 30*(3), 693–707. doi:10.1016/j.cll.2010.04.006

Wing, D. A., Haeri, S., Silber, A. C., Roth, C. K., Weiner, C. P., Echebiri, N. C., . . . Norton, M. E. (2017). Placental alpha macroglobulin-1 compared with fetal fibronectin to predict preterm delivery in symptomatic women. *Obstetrics & Gynecology, 130*(6), 1183–1191. doi:10.1097/AOG.0000000000002367

Wood, S., Rabi, Y., Tang, S., Brant, R., & Ross, S. (2017). Progesterone in women with arrested premature labor, a report of a randomized clinical trial and updated meta-analysis. *BMC Pregnancy and Childbirth, 17,* 258. doi:10.1186/s12884-017-1400-y

World Health Organization. (2012). *Intimate partner violence.* Geneva, Switzerland: Author.

World Health Organization. (2014). *Guidelines for the identification and management of substance use and substance use disorders in pregnancy.* Geneva, Switzerland: Author.

World Health Organization. (2015). *WHO recommendations on interventions to improve preterm birth outcomes.* Geneva, Switzerland: Author.

World Health Organization. (2018). *Preterm birth: Fact sheet 2018.* Geneva, Switzerland: Author.

Wyckoff, M. H., Salhab, W. A., Heyne, R. J., Kendrick, D. E., Stoll, B. J., & Laptook, A. R. (2012). Outcome of extremely low birth weight infants who received delivery room cardiopulmonary resuscitation. *Journal of Pediatrics, 160,* 239.e2–244.e2. doi:10.1016/j.jpeds.2011.07.041

Yang, P., Chen, Y., Yen, C., & Chen, H. (2015). Psychiatric diagnosis, emotional-behavioral symptoms and functional outcomes in adolescents born preterm with very low birth weights. *Child Psychiatry Human Development, 46,* 358–366. doi:10.1007/s10578-014-0475-1

York, T. P., Eaves, L. J., Lichtenstein, P., Neale, M. C., Svensson, A., Latendresse, S., . . . Strauss, J. F. (2013). Fetal and maternal genes' influence on gestational age in a quantitative genetic analysis of 244,000 Swedish births. *American Journal of Epidemiology, 178*(4), 543–550. doi:10.1093/aje/kwt005

Zhang, G., Feenstra, B., Bacelis, J., Liu, X., Muglia, L. M., Juodakis, J., . . . Muglia, L. J. (2017). Genetic associations with gestational duration and spontaneous preterm birth. *The New England Journal of Medicine, 377,* 1156–1167. doi:10.1056/NEJMoa1612665

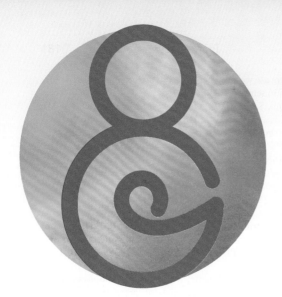

CHAPTER 8
Diabetes in Pregnancy

Cheryl K. Roth

SIGNIFICANCE AND INCIDENCE

Approximately 30.3 million people in the United States, or 9.4% of the nation's population, has diabetes (Centers for Disease Control and Prevention [CDC], 2019). It is estimated that 7.2 million people have diabetes that has not yet been diagnosed (CDC, 2017b). About 4.6 million people aged 18 to 44 years have diagnosed or undiagnosed diabetes. Women older than the age of 18 years who are of minority racial and ethnic groups have a higher prevalence of diagnosed diabetes than Caucasian women (6.8%), including African Americans (13.2%), Hispanics (11.7%), American Indians (15.3%), and Asian/Pacific Islanders (7.3%) (CDC, 2017a). Approximately 6% to 9% of pregnancies in the United States are complicated by gestational diabetes (also known as gestational diabetes mellitus or GDM) and this number has increased in the last decade (Casagrande, Linder, & Cowie, 2018; Deputy, Kim, Conrey, & Bullard, 2018).

Although comprehensive obstetric care and intensive metabolic management have reduced perinatal risk in pregnancies complicated by types 1 and 2 diabetes, morbidity and mortality still remain higher than in the general population. Preconception and early pregnancy glycemic control, as evidenced by a near-normal glycosylated hemoglobin (A1c), during the period of organogenesis greatly reduces the risk of birth defects (Pearson, Kernaghan, Lee, & Penney, 2007; Rezai et al., 2016). Pregnant women with types 1 and 2 diabetes have a 3.21-fold increase in risk of fetal death (Patel, Goodnight, James, & Grotegut, 2015).

Women with GDM are at higher risk of perinatal morbidity, such as obesity, preeclampsia, and cesarean birth (American College of Obstetricians and Gynecologists [ACOG], 2018a; Persson, Pasupathy, Hanson,

Westgren, & Norman, 2012). Approximately 50% of pregnant women in the United States are overweight (25.6%) or obese (24.8%) before starting their pregnancy (Branum, Kirmeyer, & Gregory, 2016). Being overweight or obese further complicates pregnancies with diabetes. The higher the prepregnancy body mass index (BMI) of the woman with diabetes, the more risks of adverse outcomes to the mother and fetus (Persson et al., 2012). Risks for type 2 diabetes, such as obesity and increased age, are similarly associated with GDM (Bouthoorn et al., 2015).

Risks during pregnancy for the woman with type 1 or type 2 diabetes include an increased incidence of hypoglycemia (blood glucose less than 60 mg/dL) as a result of stricter control (Mathiesen, 2016). Hypoglycemia is more common in early pregnancy due to nausea and vomiting and increasing insulin sensitivity to rising estrogen levels (Mathiesen, 2016). Hypoglycemia does not seem to cause problems for the fetus unless blood sugar levels are chronically low, but hypoglycemia does threaten the well-being of the mother. Educational efforts focusing on prevention and appropriate management of hypoglycemia can decrease this risk. Continuous glucose management (CGM) and electronic apps to follow blood sugars may assist the patient in managing her glucose levels.

Diabetic ketoacidosis (DKA) is a rare complication for women with diabetes. Most diabetic patients will present with nausea and vomiting and must be treated aggressively with insulin, intravenous (IV) fluid, and symptomatic support (Bryant, Herrera, Nelson, & Cunningham, 2017). The occurrence of DKA carries serious morbidity and mortality for the mother and the fetus and may occur at lower glucose levels (Mathiesen, 2016; Sibai & Viteri, 2014). Fetal loss may occur through spontaneous abortion in the first and early second trimesters or as an intrauterine fetal death during an episode of DKA in late second and third trimesters.

Women with microvascular complications, poor glycemic control, and a longer duration of diabetes have poorer outcomes. Retinopathy encountered in women of reproductive age may present in pregnancy and may also progress rapidly in patient with a previous diagnosis during pregnancy (Pescosolido, Campagna, & Barbato, 2014). Dilated eye examination should occur in the first trimester with continued surveillance throughout pregnancy. Laser photocoagulation therapy can be performed during pregnancy if indicated (Pescosolido et al., 2014). Nephropathy is a more serious microvascular complication that has been associated with adverse outcomes, including intrauterine growth restriction (IUGR) and preterm birth (Mathiesen, 2015). Excellent control of blood glucose levels and hypertension can reduce perinatal complications and preserve kidney function (Mathiesen, 2015).

Women with all types of diabetes are at increased risk for hypertensive disorders including chronic hypertension, gestational hypertension, and preeclampsia. Women with hypertensive disorders are at higher risk of preterm birth and cesarean birth, with resultant need for neonatal intensive care. Angiotensin-converting enzyme inhibitors and angiotensin receptor blockers are contraindicated during pregnancy and should be stopped prior to conception or as soon as possible after discovery of pregnancy. Renal failure is a potential complication without meticulous control of blood pressure. Hypertensive disorders of pregnancy also increase the risk of chronic hypertension and cardiovascular events (Sullivan, Umans, & Ratner, 2011).

Gastroparesis or gastropathy is a neuropathic complication that causes chronic upper abdominal pain, constipation, and may exacerbate nausea and vomiting. This can result in irregular absorption of nutrients, inadequate nutrition, and poor glycemic control (Fuglsang & Ovesen, 2015). Gastrostimulators may be implanted to improve symptoms, but very little information is available regarding use in pregnancy.

Macrosomia has been defined as a weight greater than the 90th percentile for gestational age and sex or a birth weight of 4,000 g (8 lb, 13 oz) to 4,500 g (9 lb, 15 oz) (ACOG, 2016, 2017a). Other factors such as morbid maternal obesity and postmaturity are also associated with fetal macrosomia and, when combined with insulin-controlled diabetes, lead to an even higher occurrence. Fetal macrosomia predisposes the mother to a higher risk of postpartum hemorrhage and vaginal lacerations, and the newborn to a variety of traumatic injuries such as shoulder dystocia with associated risk for brachial plexus injury and clavicular fracture (ACOG, 2017a; Scifres et al., 2015). Shoulder dystocia is the most common injury related to fetal macrosomia but occurs only in approximately 0.2 to 3% of all vaginal births (ACOG, 2017a). When birth weight exceeds 4,500 g, the risk of brachial plexus injury related to shoulder dystocia has been reported to increase 18- to 21-fold (ACOG, 2016). Fetal macrosomia contributes to an increased risk of cesarean birth, with resultant increased surgical morbidity in the mother (ACOG, 2016).

Epigenetics, including study of the human/fetal genome, is demonstrating that metabolic disturbances during fetal development can permanently alter gene expression throughout the lifetime of the individual. A link has emerged between fetal nutrition, birth weight, and metabolic profile in adulthood. Abnormal "programming" of nutrient management increases risk for developing metabolic diseases such as obesity, hypertension, cardiovascular disease, and type 2 diabetes (Monteiro, Norman, Rice, & Illanes, 2016). Hyperglycemia in pregnancy is associated with a higher risk of childhood obesity (Tam et al., 2017) as well as a higher risk of prediabetes and type 2 diabetes in adult offspring of women with diabetes (Monteiro et al., 2016).

In addition to the risk of fetal macrosomia for all women with diabetes, the other extreme of weight, IUGR, is a risk for infants born to women who have complications of diabetes. Nephropathy associated with poor renal function may contribute to uteroplacental insufficiency that leads to infants who are small for their gestational age (Bramham, 2017). Gestational hypertension, to which women with diabetes (with or without vascular disease) are predisposed, also decreases uterine blood flow, compromising intrauterine fetal growth. Maintaining excellent control of blood glucose levels and blood pressure can help to decrease the risk of IUGR.

Neonatal metabolic abnormalities may occur with a higher frequency in offspring of women with diabetes. Hypoglycemia, whose precise definition may vary by institution, occurs with increased frequency in babies of mothers with uncontrolled diabetes (Ogunyemi et al., 2017). (See Chapter 21 for hypoglycemia in the newborn definitions.) Preterm and large-for-gestational-age infants are at greatest risk for the development of hypoglycemia in the neonatal period. Chronic maternal hyperglycemia leads to excessive insulin production in the fetus (i.e., fetal hyperinsulinemia), which lowers fetal plasma glucose and inhibits glycogen release from the fetal liver as a normal physiologic response to hypoglycemia. This combination contributes to the risk for hypoglycemia development in the first 24 hours of life when cutting the umbilical cord interrupts transplacental glucose delivery. Early detection and prompt treatment prevent the potential severe neurologic sequelae associated with profound hypoglycemia.

Infants of diabetic mothers may exhibit polycythemia, a venous hematocrit of greater than 65%. Chronic hyperglycemia and hyperinsulinemia cause increased oxygen consumption and decreased fetal arterial oxygen content. Erythropoietin production increases, resulting in polycythemia. The elevated red blood cell mass can also result in hyperbilirubinemia (Lloreda-García, Sevilla-Denia, Rodríguez-Sánchez, Muñoz-Martínez, & Díaz-Ruiz, 2016). Hypocalcemia and hypomagnesemia are other metabolic abnormalities occasionally seen in infants of women with types 1 and 2 diabetes, the exact causes of which are unknown.

Strict maternal glycemic control has decreased the incidence of respiratory distress syndrome significantly, but other factors such as iatrogenic prematurity due to early birth as a result of maternal or fetal compromise continue to contribute to the risk. Fetal surfactant production is inhibited by hyperinsulinemia, which occurs more frequently in women with poor diabetes control and is the underlying mechanism for respiratory distress syndrome in this group (Lloreda-García et al., 2016).

DEFINITIONS AND CLASSIFICATION

Women with diabetes during pregnancy can be divided into two groups. The first group consists of women who have pregestational diabetes (type 1 or type 2 diabetes), including women diagnosed with diabetes at the first prenatal visit. The second group consists of women with gestational diabetes or diabetes diagnosed during or after the second trimester.

Pregestational Diabetes (Type 1 or Type 2 Diabetes)

Type 1 diabetes accounts for about 5% of pregestational diabetes in the United States (CDC, 2017a). Type 1 diabetes is hyperglycemia as a result of absolute insulin deficiency. It occurs as a result of genetic autoimmunity directed at the beta cells of the pancreas after an environmental trigger turns on antibodies that attack the islet cells of the pancreas, resulting in a total lack of insulin production. Exogenous insulin administration and medical nutrition therapy are the mainstays of treatment. Type 1 diabetes is more often diagnosed in people younger than 30 years old but can develop at any age. Type 2 diabetes accounts for approximately 95% of pregestational diabetes in the United States (CDC, 2017a). Insulin resistance and relative insulin deficiency characterize type 2 diabetes. Insulin resistance at the cellular level may exist because of genetic defects in insulin binding to receptor sites or in glucose transport within the cell. This condition demands an increase in insulin secretion

from the pancreas to maintain normoglycemia. Eventually, the beta cells exhaust and insulin production is diminished, resulting in hyperglycemia. Type 2 diabetes is the result of either genetic predisposition or environmental factors, such as obesity, or a combination of both. To achieve euglycemia, patients with type 2 diabetes may require not only medical nutrition therapy and exercise but also medication. Oral medications that increase the sensitivity of cells to insulin are first-line therapy, after diet and exercise, for type 2 diabetes, but additional types of medication and/or insulin may be necessary to maintain normoglycemia during pregnancy. Type 2 diabetes is increasingly seen in pregnancy because obesity and inactivity in the general population is increasing.

Gestational Diabetes Mellitus

GDM is currently defined as "glucose intolerance with onset or first recognition during pregnancy. The definition applies whether insulin or only diet modification is used for treatment and whether or not the condition persists after pregnancy" (American Diabetes Association [ADA], 2003, p. S013). GDM has been subdivided further to designate those women whose GDM is diet controlled (GDM A_1) or insulin controlled (GDM A_2) (Gibson, Waters, & Catalano, 2012). It is possible that early diagnosed cases of gestational diabetes may actually represent type 2 diabetes that was first recognized during pregnancy rather than true gestational diabetes. The ADA (2017a) recommends that women who meet screening criteria (Display 8–1) at the first prenatal visit be tested for diabetes. If they screen negative, blood glucose testing should be repeated at 24 to 28 weeks' gestation to rule out GDM.

Pathophysiology of Diabetes in Pregnancy

Profound metabolic changes occur in normal pregnancy to allow for a continuously feeding fetus in an intermittently feeding mother. These alterations must be understood to comprehend the effects that diabetes has on a progressively changing metabolic state. In early pregnancy, beta-cell hyperplasia results in increased insulin production, as a result of progesterone and estrogen increases, which also contributes to increased tissue sensitivity to insulin. This hyperinsulinemic state allows increased lipogenesis and fat deposition in early pregnancy in preparation for the dramatic rise in energy needs of the growing fetus in the latter half of pregnancy. As a result of these changes, along with nausea and vomiting, the mother has an increased risk for hypoglycemia in the first trimester. In women with type 1 diabetes and insulin-controlled type 2 diabetes, exogenous insulin needs may decrease.

The second half of pregnancy is characterized by accelerated growth of the fetus and rapidly increasing

Criteria for Early Screening for
Gestational Diabetes Mellitus

BMI >25 (>23 in Asian Americans) with at least one of
the following:

- Physical inactivity
- First-degree relative with diabetes
- African American, Latino, Native American, Asian American,
  Pacific Islander
- Previous birth of infant ≥4,000 g
- Previous GDM
- BP ≥140/90 mm Hg or on medication for hypertension
- Abnormal cholesterol (HDL <35 mg/dL or triglycerides
  >250 mg/dL)
- Polycystic ovarian syndrome
- Hgb A1c ≥5.7%, impaired glucose fasting or glucose tolerance
- Clinical conditions associated with insulin resistance BMI
  ≥40, acanthosis nigricans
- History of cardiovascular disease

BMI, body mass index; BP, blood pressure; GDM, gestational diabetes mellitus;
HDL, high-density lipoprotein; Hgb A1c, glycosylated hemoglobin.
Adapted from American Diabetes Association. (2017a). Classification and
diagnosis of diabetes. *Diabetes Care, 40*(1), S11–S24.

levels of maternal and placental diabetogenic hormones, which include human placental lactogen, cortisol, estrogen, progesterone, and prolactin. Insulin resistance and increased insulin production result from increased circulating levels of insulin-antagonizing hormones, including soluble prorenin receptor (Bonakdaran, Azami, Tara, & Poorali, 2017; Lain & Catalano, 2007; Parker & Conway, 2007).

The anabolic phase (i.e., fat storage) of the first 20 weeks of pregnancy is followed by a catabolic phase (i.e., fat breakdown or lipolysis) in the latter half of pregnancy (Lain & Catalano, 2007). During the third trimester, women have an exaggerated response to even short periods of fasting (>12 hours), which is referred to as "accelerated starvation." This allows the woman to convert to metabolism of fat more easily, sparing fuels such as glucose and amino acids, which are needed for fetal growth (Sinha, Venkatram, & Diaz-Fuentes, 2014).

In the absence of vascular disease, the pathologic manifestations of diabetes in pregnancy are usually the result of maternal hyperglycemia. Excessive hyperglycemia, as a result of insulin deficiency with a corresponding increase in counterregulatory hormones (e.g., glucagon, epinephrine, growth hormone, and cortisol), may contribute to the development of DKA. Factors in pregnancy that can trigger the release of these hormones leading to the development of DKA are

fasting hyperglycemia, infection, stress, emesis, dehydration, gastroparesis, and beta-cell-sympathomimetic and corticosteroid administration for the treatment of preterm labor (Fuglsang & Ovesen, 2015; Sibai & Viteri, 2014). Continuous subcutaneous insulin infusion (CSII) pump failure and poor patient compliance have also led to the development of DKA during pregnancy.

Excessive hyperglycemia can result from increased hepatic glucose and ketone production and insulin deficiency. Urinary excretion of potassium, sodium, and water occurs as a result of osmotic diuresis due to excessive plasma glucose. Fat metabolism leads to increased circulating levels of free fatty acids and ketonemia, which quickly overwhelm the maternal buffering system, resulting in metabolic acidosis (Mathiesen, 2016). Sustained or intermittent maternal hyperglycemia later in pregnancy stimulates fetal hyperinsulinemia as a normal fetal physiologic response to elevated blood glucose with pathologic consequences such as macrosomia (ACOG, 2017a). Hyperinsulinemia promotes catabolism of the extra fuel, using energy and depleting fetal oxygen stores (Lloreda-García et al., 2016). Fetal hyperinsulinemia also inhibits the release of surfactant that is necessary for pulmonary maturation resulting in respiratory distress syndrome. Prolonged or frequent maternal hyperglycemia may also be associated with other neonatal metabolic abnormalities, including lower IQ scores, and fetal brain injury including a possible link to autism and stroke (Krakowiak et al., 2012; Sibai & Viteri, 2014; Stenerson, Collura, Rose, Lteif, & Carey, 2011). Polyhydramnios, urinary tract infections, pyelonephritis, and monilial vaginitis are other maternal complications of hyperglycemia.

SCREENING AND DIAGNOSIS OF GESTATIONAL DIABETES MELLITUS

Screening for GDM is recommended for all patients between 24 and 28 weeks' gestation, when the diabetogenic hormones are exerting a significant influence on insulin performance. Risk factors identifying women who should undergo early screening for GDM at the first prenatal visit (as soon as risk is identified) are listed in Display 8–1. The ADA (2017a) recommends testing for type 2 diabetes at the first prenatal visit in populations with a high prevalence of type 2 diabetes, such as Latinas, African Americans, Native Americans, Southeast Asians, and Pacific Islanders, with a fasting blood glucose value and an A1c. If the A1c is ≥6.5 mg/dL, the fasting blood glucose is ≥126 mg/dL, a 2-hour postprandial glucose is ≥200 mg/dL after a 75-g load, or a random glucose is ≥200 mg/dL, overt diabetes is diagnosed. If the screening at the first prenatal visit is normal, standard screening is repeated between 24 and 28 weeks of gestation (ADA, 2017a).

Evaluation for GDM in the United States is most often performed in a two-step approach (ACOG, 2018a). The nonfasting screening test consists of ingestion of a 50-g glucose solution, without consideration of time of day or last meal, drawing a plasma or serum glucose level 1 hour after ingestion. The positive thresholds have been described in the literature as 130 to 140 mg/dL. Studies have not shown a clear advantage to either threshold (ACOG, 2018a). The decision for which cutoff to use should be based on cost effectiveness and risk factors in the population to be tested. If the test result is positive, a diagnostic 3-hour 100-g oral glucose tolerance test (OGTT) is administered after an approximately 8-hour fast, preceded by 3 days of unrestricted diet and activity. Women should refrain from smoking or eating before and throughout the test and should remain seated during testing. Plasma glucose determinations are made at fasting and 1-, 2-, and 3-hour intervals after ingestion of the glucose solution. The diagnostic criteria are listed in Table 8–1. One or more thresholds must be met or exceeded to diagnose GDM (ACOG, 2018a).

The Hyperglycemia and Adverse Pregnancy Outcome (HAPO) study was an observational study of 23,325 pregnant women at 15 healthcare centers in 9 countries (HAPO Study Cooperative Research Group, 2008). All women had a 75-g 2-hour OGTT at 28 weeks of gestation, and the results were blinded unless the fasting value exceeded 105 mg/dL and/or the 2-hour value exceeded 200 mg/dL. The goal of the study was to relate the blood glucose levels on the 75-g 2-hour OGTT to pregnancy outcomes. The researchers found that the risk of adverse outcome was a continuum, even at levels that were previously considered normal. As blood glucose levels rose, so did the risk of macrosomia, cesarean birth, and neonatal hypoglycemia. The authors concluded that they could not determine what level of blood glucose is clinically important or what level should be considered abnormal (HAPO Study Cooperative Research Group, 2008).

The International Association of Diabetes and Pregnancy Study Groups (IADPSG), a collection of experts on diabetes and pregnancy and representatives from various organizations who have an interest in diabetes and pregnancy came to a consensus about what criteria should be used to diagnose GDM based on the results of the HAPO study (Metzger, 2010). The IADPSG recommends using *only* the 75-g 2-hour OGTT to diagnose GDM, thus eliminating the two-step process. They do not recommend using an OGTT before 24 weeks of gestation. This approach has been accepted by many internationally (ADA, 2017a) but has not been adopted by the ADA or ACOG as the preferred method (ACOG, 2018a).

The recommended threshold values for the diagnosis of GDM are listed in Table 8–1. These values are based on values in the HAPO study where the odds ratios of birth weight and percentage neonatal body fat greater than the 90th percentile reached 1.75 times the odds of these outcomes at mean glucose values. GDM is diagnosed if only one value exceeds the threshold values (ACOG, 2018a). Using these threshold values, the overall rate of GDM in the HAPO study was 17.8% (Metzger, 2010).

A study done with the Eunice Kennedy Shriver National Institute of Child Health and Human Development compared the two most commonly used criteria to evaluate the results of the 3-hour OGTT in the United States, the Carpenter-Coustan criteria and the National Diabetes Data Group criteria (Harper et al., 2016). They found a favorable treatment effect for preeclampsia, shoulder dystocia, cesarean delivery, and macrosomia for both sets of criteria. They did not find a significant difference in outcomes for either set of criteria.

CLINICAL MANIFESTATIONS

The clinical manifestations of diabetes occur as a result of both hypoglycemia and hyperglycemia. Glycemic goals for pregnancy in women with diabetes reflect the plasma blood glucose values found in pregnant women who do not have diabetes; 60 to 95 mg/dL fasting, 60 to 105 mg/dL before a meal, 140 mg/dL 1 hour after a meal, and 120 mg/dL 2 hours after a meal (ADA, 2017b). Hallmark symptoms of uncontrolled

TABLE 8–1. Diagnostic Criteria for Gestational Diabetes Mellitus

100-g OGTT	Threshold glucose levels (mg/dL)	
	Carpenter and Coustan[a,b]	National diabetes group[c]
Fasting	≥95	≥105
1 hr	≥180	≥190
2 hr	≥155	≥165
3 hr	≥140	≥145

One or more values must be met or exceeded to diagnose gestational diabetes mellitus.

OGTT, oral glucose tolerance test.

[a]Adapted from Carpenter, M. W., & Coustan, D. R. (1982). Criteria for screening tests for gestational diabetes. *American Journal of Obstetrics & Gynecology, 144*(7), 768–773.

[b]Adapted from American College of Obstetricians and Gynecologists. (2017a). Practice Bulletin No. 180: Gestational diabetes mellitus. *Obstetrics & Gynecology, 130*(1), e17–e37. doi:10.1097/AOG.0000000000002159

[c]Adapted from American Diabetes Association. (2017b). Standards of medical care in diabetes–2017. *Diabetes Care, 40*(1 Suppl.), S1–S135. doi:10.2337/dc17-S001

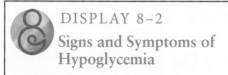

- Mental confusion and irritability
- Somnolence
- Slowed reaction time
- Pallor
- Diaphoresis
- Tachycardia
- Palpitations
- Hunger
- Paresthesias
- Shakiness
- Cold, clammy skin
- Blurred vision
- Extreme fatigue

hyperglycemia include polyuria, polydipsia, blurred vision, and polyphagia. These are usually associated with pregestational diabetes, and women with gestational diabetes rarely experience these symptoms.

Hypoglycemia is defined as a plasma glucose level of 60 mg/dL or below, but patients may feel the symptoms of hypoglycemia at higher levels when the patient's average blood glucose level is higher. Autonomic nervous system stimulation by hypoglycemia results in adrenergic and cholinergic symptoms of pallor, diaphoresis, tachycardia, palpitations, hunger, paresthesias, and shakiness. Moderate hypoglycemia causes glucose deprivation in the central nervous system as evidenced by an inability to concentrate, confusion, slurred speech, irrational behavior, slowed reaction time, blurred vision, numbness, somnolence, or extreme fatigue (Display 8–2). Disorientation, loss of consciousness, seizures, and coma may result from severe hypoglycemia and is primarily seen in type 1 diabetes and not in gestational or type 2 diabetes.

NURSING ASSESSMENTS AND INTERVENTIONS FOR DIABETES MELLITUS

Evaluation and management of women with diabetes, whether pregestational or gestational, generally occur on an outpatient basis. Hospital admission may be advisable for uncontrolled diabetes during the period of organogenesis (prior to 8 weeks) or during an episode of illness, DKA, or other obstetric complication. Nurses can have a profound role in educating and monitoring women with diabetes during pregnancy and are vital members of the multidisciplinary diabetes management team (Association of Women's Health, Obstetric and Neonatal Nurses [AWHONN], 2016). The goal of nursing management focuses on the woman attaining and maintaining self-care behaviors, which result in near-normal blood glucose levels to improve perinatal outcomes. Ideally, a team approach should be used to achieve this goal, which includes a physician with expertise in diabetes; medical nutrition therapy by a registered dietitian; exercise; education about self-monitoring of blood glucose and taking medication (as needed) by a registered nurse, preferably a certified diabetes educator; and stress reduction and management by a social worker or behavioral health specialist, as needed.

AMBULATORY AND HOME CARE MANAGEMENT

Ideally, intensive management of diabetes should begin prior to conception in women with pregestational diabetes. Attaining an A1c <6.5 g/dL and the pregnancy targets for blood glucose levels before pregnancy will decrease the risk of congenital malformations and spontaneous abortion to that of the general population (ADA, 2017b). The ADA also recommends that all women with diabetes of childbearing potential should receive preconception counseling due to the risk of malformations associated with unplanned pregnancies and poor glycemic control. In the absence of preconception care, prenatal care should begin immediately on discovery of the pregnancy and continue throughout the perinatal period. The assessment of women with pregestational diabetes should include a thorough history of diabetes type, duration of disease, self-care practices, acute and chronic complication assessment (may include 24-hour urine for kidney function, baseline electrocardiogram, and eye exam), a review of current glucose values, an A1c, and a food history of at least 3 days. Knowledge deficits should be identified and an individualized teaching plan outlined during this initial assessment. Psychosocial issues should be explored and evaluated periodically, and appropriate referrals made. Display 8–3 lists information that should be discussed with women who have pregestational diabetes.

When women who have type 1 or type 2 diabetes become pregnant, an educational session should be scheduled as soon as possible with a diabetes educator and registered dietitian before, or in conjunction with, the initial prenatal visit. The session should include all aspects of medical nutrition therapy, self-monitoring of blood glucose levels, and insulin therapy, including a demonstration by the woman of the correct method for drawing up and self-injection of insulin or use of an insulin pump. Injection sites should be observed for correct regional rotation as well as for identifying evidence of lipohypertrophy or lipoatrophy, bruising, and signs and symptoms of infection.

DISPLAY 8–3

Educational Guidelines for Women with Pregestational Diabetes Mellitus

- **Healthy Eating**
  - Medical nutrition therapy
- **Being Active**
  - 30 to 60 min/day of activity such as brisk walking
- **Monitoring**
  - Self-monitoring of blood glucose levels, four to eight times per day
  - Glycemic goals for pregnancy
  - Guidelines for ketone testing
- **Taking Medications**
  - Insulin/oral agent therapy
  - Prenatal vitamins with folic acid
  - Medications for other medical conditions
- **Problem Solving**
  - Sick-day management
  - Appropriate treatment of hypoglycemia (correct amount and composition of snack, use of glucagon by family member)
  - Signs and symptoms of diabetic ketoacidosis and contributing factors
  - When and why to call the healthcare provider
- **Healthy Coping**
  - Psychosocial assessment
  - Barriers to optimal care
- **Reducing Risks**
  - Effect pregnancy has on diabetes
  - Potential for fetal or neonatal complications: intrauterine growth restriction, macrosomia, intrauterine fetal demise, birth trauma, prematurity, respiratory distress syndrome, neonatal metabolic disturbances
  - Potential for maternal complications: preterm birth, hypertensive disorders, cesarean birth
  - Association of glycosylated hemoglobin to risk for congenital anomalies or spontaneous abortion
  - Schedule of antenatal visits and testing

Adapted from American Association of Diabetes Educators. (2012). *AADE7 Self-Care Behaviors®*. Retrieved from http://www.diabeteseducator.org /ProfessionalResources/AADE7

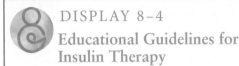

DISPLAY 8–4

Educational Guidelines for Insulin Therapy

- Glycemic goals for treatment
- Onset, peak, and duration of action of insulins to be administered
- Inspection, storage, and traveling with insulin
- Timing of injections, injection technique, site selection, and regional rotation
- Glucagon use and appropriate administration by family or significant other
- Appropriate sick-day management
- Prevention strategies and appropriate management of hypoglycemia
- Syringe disposal guidelines

Women with type 2 diabetes who have been using oral medications for glucose control may be converted to insulin, before conception or after pregnancy diagnosis. Because glycemic control is so important to prevent malformations in the first trimester, the level of control needed may not be achievable on oral medications, and women on oral hypoglycemic agents should not stop those agents until insulin is instituted. These women require more extensive education regarding insulin and additional support with this new aspect of their diabetes management. Display 8–4 lists issues to be reviewed in the educational session about insulin.

Treatment of Hypoglycemia

Glycemic thresholds may shift during pregnancy, causing management of hypoglycemia to be challenging. Generally, patients should be alert to a blood glucose ≤70 mg/dL (Seaquist et al., 2013), although some women are not symptomatic and may be unaware. Appropriate management of hypoglycemia should be reviewed with women with pregestational diabetes. Patients need an explanation that the occurrence of hypoglycemic events may increase with intensive management goals during pregnancy. The level at which symptoms occur may vary. If women have hypoglycemia unawareness (the inability to tell their blood sugar is too low), the risk for a potentially fatal nocturnal episode must be avoided. General guidelines for treatment of hypoglycemia during pregnancy include treatment with 15 g of carbohydrates for a blood glucose of 60 to 70 mg/dL and treatment with 30 g of carbohydrates (divided as half liquid and half solid, preferably) at a level of 40 to 60 mg/ dL. Blood glucose should be tested again 15 minutes after treatment of hypoglycemia. Retreatment should occur if the blood glucose level has not risen. Including protein with the carbohydrate decreases the risk for rebound hypoglycemia and provides a more consistent and stable blood glucose level after treatment. Women with evidence of gastroparesis should use liquids for initial treatment of hypoglycemia because of their slower digestion. Carbohydrates ingested for treatment of hypoglycemia should not count toward the daily carbohydrate goals of the prescribed diet to allow glucagon stores to be replenished. Family members and significant others should be instructed on the use of injectable glucagon, and two kits should be readily available at all times. CGM monitors may help with control, especially in patients who are unaware of hypoglycemic symptoms.

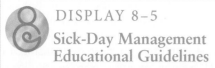

DISPLAY 8–5

Sick-Day Management
Educational Guidelines

- Insulin should be given even with vomiting.
- Urine ketones should be checked every 4 to 6 hr and the healthcare provider notified of ≥ moderate results.
- Blood glucose levels should be checked every 1 to 2 hr.
- Healthcare provider should be notified of blood glucose levels ≥200 mg/dL.
- Liquids or soft foods should be consumed equal to the carbohydrate value of the prescribed diet (sugar-free for blood glucose levels of >120 mg/dL).
- A sipping diet of 15 to 30 g of carbohydrates per hour may be consumed during periods of vomiting.
- Call the healthcare provider if liquids are not tolerated.
- Review signs and symptoms of ketoacidosis to report: abdominal pain, nausea and vomiting, polyuria, polydipsia, fruity breath, leg cramps, altered mental status, and rapid respirations.

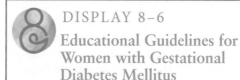

DISPLAY 8–6

Educational Guidelines for Women with Gestational Diabetes Mellitus

- **Healthy Eating**
  - Medical nutrition therapy
- **Being Active**
  - 30 to 60 min/day of activity such as brisk walking
- **Monitoring**
  - Technique of meter use
  - Self-monitoring of blood glucose levels, four times per day
  - Glycemic goals for pregnancy
- **Taking Medications**
  - Insulin/oral agent therapy, as needed
  - Prenatal vitamins
  - Medications for other conditions
- **Problem Solving**
  - Appropriate treatment of hypoglycemia (correct amount and composition of snack)
  - When and why to call the healthcare provider
- **Healthy Coping**
  - Psychosocial assessment
  - Barriers to optimal care
- **Reducing Risks**
  - Explanation of abnormal results from prenatal glucose test
  - Role of glucose and insulin transport and effect of placental hormones
  - Potential for fetal or neonatal complications: intrauterine fetal demise, macrosomia, birth trauma, respiratory distress syndrome, neonatal metabolic disturbances
  - Potential for maternal complications: polyhydramnios, hypertensive disorders, cesarean birth
  - Schedule of antenatal visits and testing

Adapted from American Association of Diabetes Educators. (2012). *AADE7 Self-Care Behaviors®.* Retrieved from http://www.diabeteseducator.org/ProfessionalResources/AADE7

Sick-Day Management

Nurses should also review sick-day management and provide written guidelines (AWHONN, 2016). Understanding appropriate self-care strategies during episodes of nausea and vomiting of early pregnancy is vital to prevent the development of ketoacidosis. Display 8–5 contains specific information that nurses should review with women about sick-day management.

Gestational Diabetes Mellitus

Women who have been diagnosed with GDM need immediate counseling and education. Display 8–6 includes topics that nurses should discuss in the educational session. The diagnosis alone may bring excessive anxiety and fear. Appropriate education and support from the nurse educator should allay the woman's concerns and empower her with the resources she needs to adapt to the diabetic regimen, reducing the risks for perinatal complications (AWHONN, 2016). Including family and significant others in the education and care of women with GDM provides another source of support.

Medical Nutrition Therapy

Medical nutrition therapy is an integral and vital component in the care of women with diabetes, especially during pregnancy, and is best provided by a registered dietitian whenever possible. Therapeutic goals for nutritional intervention are control of postprandial hyperglycemia and appropriate nourishment of mother and fetus while avoiding excessive weight gain or ketosis. Creating a personalized nutrition plan based on the woman's prepregnant BMI is recommended

(ADA, 2017b). An individualized plan will be based on total caloric daily intake, carbohydrate intake, and distribution of calories throughout the day with three meals and three snacks. Carbohydrates should comprise 33% to 40% of the calories, protein should be around 20%, and fats the remaining 40%. No certain type of diet has been proven to be better than another, thus the individualized plan should be created based on the needs and resources of the patient and her family.

A 25- to 35-lb weight gain is encouraged for women with normal prepregnancy weight (prepregnancy BMI 18.5 to 24.9), 28- to 40-lb weight gain for underweight women (BMI <18.5), 15- to 25-lb weight gain for overweight women (BMI 25 to 29.9), and 11- to 20-lb weight gain for obese women (BMI ≥30) (ACOG, 2018c). Nonnutritive sweeteners, including aspartame, saccharin, acesulfame-K, and sucralose, should be used with caution during pregnancy because there are reports that they may be linked to obesity and metabolic syndromes in the infant in later life (Araújo, Martel, & Keating, 2014). More research needs to be done in this area to give clear direction. Women with a positive family history for neural tube defects should take a prenatal vitamin supplement with 400 mcg (4 mg) of folic acid, additional iron if anemic, and supplemental calcium for those women who do not consume enough dietary calcium.

Nutritional counseling should be individualized and culturally sensitive. Significant others and family members should be included in educational sessions to provide support. The person who prepares the meals must be a part of nutrition counseling, and financial constraints determined. The registered dietitian should meet with the woman regularly to assess any dietary problems and to reevaluate nutritional needs after the initial session. More frequent visits are required for women with excessive or low weight gain.

Exercise Therapy

Exercise should be used adjunctively with dietary management of diabetes (ACOG, 2018a). The glucose-lowering mechanism of exercise is unknown but may be related to increased insulin sensitivity, improved first-phase insulin release, and increased caloric expenditure (Halse, Wallman, Newnham, & Guelfi, 2014). Activity can be divided into 10- to 15-minute sessions after each meal. General guidelines for exercise during pregnancy should be followed, with contraindications similar to the nondiabetic pregnant patient. Display 8–7 lists general guidelines for education of diabetic women who plan to exercise during their pregnancy. Women should be counseled to discontinue exercise if uterine activity occurs. Women should be encouraged to record time, duration, and type of exercise on her log and the nurse should review the glucose log to evaluate the effect of exercise on blood sugar values and make appropriate food or insulin adjustment recommendations. Especially in the pregestational diabetic patient, the feet and lower extremities should be inspected for blisters, bruising, or other evidence of trauma because exercise modifications may be required or a change in footwear needed.

Blood Glucose Monitoring

Blood glucose monitoring during pregnancy is directed at detecting hyperglycemia and hypoglycemia and making pharmacologic, dietary, or activity adjustments to maintain euglycemia. Rather than preprandial values, postprandial blood glucose determinations appear to be the most influential in the development of fetal hyperinsulinemia (ACOG, 2018a). Daily self-monitoring allows the woman to know immediately the effect of food intake or activity on her blood sugar. In women with GDM, blood sugar levels should be checked at least four times daily: fasting and 1 or 2 hours after the first bite of each meal. There is insufficient data to indicate if 1- or 2-hour postprandial blood glucose testing is preferable. One method should be chosen and used consistently (ACOG, 2018a). Table 8–2 lists the target glycemic values for pregnancy. These values are usually attainable in women with GDM and type 2 diabetes but may be unrealistic in women with type 1 diabetes who have hypoglycemia unawareness and are generally more difficult to achieve control in. Women with pregestational diabetes should check their blood sugar levels five to eight times daily, depending on their level of control. These determinations may be obtained fasting, preprandial, postprandial, bedtime, and at 2:00 am to 3:00 am for women with a history of nocturnal hypoglycemia or fasting hyperglycemia. Titration of insulin is smoother when based on multiple blood glucose determinations.

All women with diabetes are asked to keep a log of all blood sugars (including the standard prescribed times and any additional measurements for abnormal values, high or low), insulin doses, exercise or activity level, and food intake. These logs allow the nurse

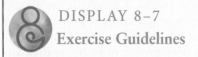

DISPLAY 8–7
Exercise Guidelines

- Proper footwear with silica gel or air midsoles
- Polyester or polyester–cotton-blend socks to promote dryness and prevent blisters
- Wear a visible diabetes identification.
- Carbohydrate (CHO) consumption when blood glucose <100 mg/dL and have CHO snack readily available
- Blood glucose before and after exercise (type 1 diabetes)
- Adequate hydration during and after exercise
- Consult healthcare provider to assist with insulin adjustments.

TABLE 8–2. Recommended Blood Glucose Targets for Women with Gestational Diabetes Mellitus	
Fasting	<95 mg/dL
Postprandial 1 hr	<140 mg/dL
Or	
Postprandial 2 hr	<120 mg/dL
(either 1 or 2 hr may be chosen, should be used consistently)	

Adapted from American College of Obstetricians and Gynecologists. (2018a). *Practice Bulletin No. 1890: Gestational diabetes mellitus.* Washington, DC: Author.

and healthcare provider to accurately evaluate and make necessary adjustments at office visits. These visits should occur weekly for women having insulin adjustments or for women with identified problems. Telephone contact may be necessary to supplement visits. Visits should occur every other week for women with well-controlled diabetes, whether pregestational or gestational, until the latter half of the third trimester, when they are increased to weekly.

The care and use of a blood glucose meter should be reviewed with the woman. Nurses need to know the limits of the meters their patients are using. For women who are newly diagnosed with GDM, a more intensive instructional session should be provided. Meters that have memory capability with date and time are important so that the nurse can correlate the values in the meter to those recorded by the woman. Patients have been reported to falsify blood glucose log entries, perhaps due to a lack of testing or blood glucose outside of target range, and this can lead to poor perinatal outcomes if not detected and managed. If false blood glucose readings are noted, fears or contributory psychosocial issues should be explored. Sometimes, an underlying fear of insulin by women with GDM contributes to this phenomenon. These women need additional support and education and possibly referral for counseling. There are now cell phone and web-based technologies available that can improve compliance and patient satisfaction with monitoring (Bartholomew et al., 2015) including remote sharing of blood glucose logs with their healthcare providers.

Continuous glucose monitoring (CGM) is currently in use by many patients with diabetes. A sensor is placed in subcutaneous tissue, and glucose levels are read from interstitial fluid every 1 to 5 minutes and sent to a screen on a device. Trends in glucose values can be used to adjust insulin therapy. Use of CGM has become more prevalent since publication of a multi-center trial, the CONCEPTT study, which was done to determine the effectiveness of the use of an insulin pump on type 1 diabetic pregnant patients (Feig et al., 2017). The trial found that patients using the insulin pump had improved neonatal outcomes, including lower incidence of large-for-gestation infants, fewer neonatal intensive care unit admissions, fewer incidences of neonatal hypoglycemia, and a 1-day shorter length of stay.

Pharmacologic Therapy

Insulin

Insulin is the preferred pharmacologic agent used in conjunction with nutrition therapy in women with pregestational or gestational diabetes (ADA, 2017b). Insulin requirements during pregnancy increase dramatically from the first to third trimester as the anti-insulin hormones rise and peripheral resistance increases. Requirements in the first trimester may be slightly reduced because of the nausea and vomiting of pregnancy. Initial insulin therapy is generally started at 0.7 to 0.8 U/kg in divided doses. A calculator for dosing is available at http://www.perinatology.com /calculators/GDM.htm. Titration of insulin dosing is dependent on monitored blood glucose values and typically requires increases throughout the pregnancy until the late third trimester when a slight decrease is often required, possibly related to the aging placenta.

Glucose control during pregnancy requires intensive insulin management in women with type 1 diabetes, usually at least three to four injections per day or use of an insulin pump. Women with type 2 diabetes or GDM may require less frequent injections. For example, many women with GDM require only bedtime intermediate-acting insulin to control fasting hyperglycemia. During the day, they may be able to use diet and exercise to manage postmeal excursions of glucose. Women with a prepregnancy BMI of >40 with GDM or type 2 diabetes may require more than 1 U/kg to achieve euglycemia. Long-acting insulins may be more effective in split doses rather than once daily dosing.

Several rapid-acting insulin analogs (e.g., lispro, aspart, and glulisine) are available for postmeal control. They have a quicker onset of action (10 to 15 minutes) and peak effect (60 minutes) than regular insulin and may help prevent hypoglycemia between meals. Regular insulin (U-100 and U-500), insulin aspart, insulin lispro (U-100 and U-200), neutral protamine Hagedorn (NPH), and insulin detemir are pregnancy category B medications and are considered safe to use during pregnancy. Intermediate-acting human NPH insulin is used for basal insulin needs. Insulin glargine no longer is recommended in pregnancy due to lack of clinical trials to establish safety.

For women with GDM who fail to achieve euglycemia (see Table 8–2) with diet and exercise, oral medication or insulin therapy should be initiated. Medication is initiated when fasting blood sugar values are consistently >95 mg/dL, a 1-hour postprandial blood glucose consistently >140 mg/dL, or a 2-hour postprandial consistently >120 mg/dL (ACOG, 2018a). The insulin regimen should be individualized depending on what time of day blood glucose levels are elevated. Use of corticosteroids may drive up the blood glucose levels for up to a week and may require temporary use of insulin therapy.

The educational sessions for women with new onset therapy should follow the guidelines for insulin therapy in women with pregestational diabetes (see Display 8–3). Women who are injecting insulin for the first time may be very fearful and require much support and encouragement from the nurse and family members. They need to be reassured that the inability to control glucose values is not a failure on their part, but a common progression of GDM for many women. Occasionally, a woman may not be able to correctly draw up her insulin. In these situations, a home health referral can be made, another family member can be taught, or the nurse can draw the appropriate insulin to be refrigerated before use. Prefilled syringes may be safely refrigerated for up to 30 days. Prefilled insulin pens may be an option for women who have difficulty mixing insulins in one syringe or seeing the line markings on syringes. For women with needle phobias, self-injectors may be used. Women should be educated that insulin requirements normally increase as the pregnancy progresses for all women, even those without diabetes, and reassured that rising insulin needs do not represent a failure in the woman's ability to follow such a complex medical regimen.

Continuous Subcutaneous Insulin Infusion

An insulin pump is an electronic device that is programmed to deliver rapid-acting insulin subcutaneously through an implanted catheter. Lispro and aspart insulins are most commonly used in pumps. A continuous low-dose amount of basal insulin is infused, which can be set at differing rates throughout the day based on insulin requirements, and boluses are given for hyperglycemia corrections, meals, and snacks based on carbohydrate intake, blood glucose, and the preprogrammed insulin to carbohydrate ratios, insulin sensitivity, and target glucose levels (which can also differ throughout the day). The catheter is changed every 2 to 3 days but may need to be changed daily in pregnancy related to a higher risk of infection. The use of CSII in pregnancy requires careful patient selection, and patients who are already using the device prepregnancy or are very motivated and capable of using the device should be chosen. The risk for pump use during pregnancy is pump malfunction that can lead to the rapid development of DKA. This risk can be reduced by educating the woman to self-inject rapid-acting insulin and check the pump for blood glucose levels of >200 mg/dL. Many insulin pumps also "communicate" with CGMs, and newer models offer a closed-loop system where the insulin pump automatically changes rates to correct blood glucoses out of the target range.

Switching from conventional insulin therapy to pump therapy can be done on an inpatient or outpatient basis, individualizing the decision according to the level of family support and needs of the woman. The total daily insulin dose is divided between basal insulin and meal boluses; 50% to 60% is given as basal insulin, and the remaining 40% to 50% is given as boluses. Boluses may be given, calculated using an insulin-to-carbohydrate ratio. Another method for determining the insulin dose for CSII is based on patient weight and gestational age. Dosing is based on 0.9 U/kg in the first trimester, 1.0 U/kg in the second trimester, and 1.2 U/kg in the third trimester and then reduced by 20% postpartum (Gabbe, Carpenter, & Garrison, 2007). A lower basal rate may be needed during the early nighttime hours to reduce the risk of nocturnal hypoglycemia. However, because of the strong "dawn phenomenon" associated with pregnancy, an increased basal rate may be needed after 3:00 am. Online tools are available to help the provider calculate dosages at http://perinatology.com/calculators/SweetSuccesspumpO.htm, and CGMs may also provide assistance in making insulin adjustments, although it should be noted that their use in pregnancy has not been validated.

Oral Antidiabetes Agents

Treatment methodologies for diabetes in pregnancy are the subject of debate in the literature. Use of oral antidiabetes medications is increasingly being used among women with GDM, although they are not approved for such use by the U.S. Food and Drug Administration. The use of metformin, an oral antidiabetes medication, in pregnant women with type 2 diabetes is currently being studied in a multicenter randomized control trial (MiTy) (Feig et al., 2016). Earlier studies with first-generation sulfonylureas, which crossed the placenta, showed profound hypoglycemia in newborns because these drugs caused the fetal pancreas to secrete more insulin (Kemball et al., 1970). A Cochrane review of short- and long-term outcomes of metformin compared to insulin alone in pregnancy (Butalia et al., 2017) found metformin had no short-term adverse effects on pregnancy, lowered the risk of neonatal hypoglycemia, large-for-gestation babies, pregnancy-induced hypertension, and maternal pregnancy weight gain. Patients who do not have adequate control on metformin may need to convert to insulin therapy. It also recommended that further studies be done on long-term outcomes prior to routine use.

Glyburide is an alternative oral medication used in pregnancy. It is a sulfonylurea and thus should not be used in patients with a sulfa allergy. A systematic review by Balsells et al. (2015) reviewed 15 articles evaluating glyburide as compared to metformin or insulin, including 2,509 subjects. The researchers found that glyburide alone is clearly inferior to metformin and/or insulin and recommended it not be used as first-line therapy.

Fetal Assessment

The best method and the appropriate time to begin antepartum fetal assessment for pregnant women with diabetes have yet to be determined. Most recommend beginning some form of fetal assessment in the third trimester for women with pregestational diabetes (ACOG, 2018b). There is no consensus on when antenatal testing of women with GDM controlled by diet should begin, and testing may be delayed until near term (ACOG, 2018a). Women with poorly controlled GDM or GDM controlled by insulin or oral agents should begin testing at 32 weeks of gestation (ACOG, 2018a). Fetal movement counting is a simple, inexpensive, and appropriate test to begin in all pregnant women with diabetes in the beginning of the third trimester. Women with comorbidities may need more intensive fetal and maternal surveillance. Display 8–8 is a summary of home care management for women with diabetes.

TIMING AND MODE OF BIRTH

The optimal time for birth for a woman with diabetes involves balancing the risk of intrauterine fetal demise with the risks of preterm birth. When glucose control is good, antenatal testing remains reassuring, and no other complications exist, evidence supports awaiting spontaneous labor and birth at 39 weeks of gestation (ACOG, 2018a). ACOG no longer recommends elective induction of labor before 39 weeks, unless it is for fetal or maternal indications. Patients with poorly controlled pre-gestational diabetes may need to be delivered earlier than 39 weeks based on the individualized patient plan of care.

Many women with diabetes are able to have a vaginal birth. An estimated fetal weight of >4,500 g in women with diabetes may be an indication for cesarean birth without a trial of labor (ACOG, 2017b). Cesarean birth increases maternal risks of morbidity and mortality but decreases risks of shoulder dystocia and brachial plexus injury to the fetus.

INPATIENT MANAGEMENT

Women with diabetes require hospitalization during periods of poor control for intensive insulin adjustment, particularly if they are in the critical time of organogenesis (6 to 8 weeks' gestation). Hospitalization may also be required during periods of illness for women with dehydration and is always required for those in DKA. Women who develop complications of pregnancy, such as preterm labor or preeclampsia, may require hospitalization during the third trimester for more intensive maternal and fetal surveillance.

Diabetic Ketoacidosis

DKA is characterized by severe hyperglycemia, ketosis, acidosis, dehydration, hypovolemia, and electrolyte imbalance (Sibai & Viteri, 2014). Kussmaul respirations develop in an effort to correct the ensuing metabolic acidosis. Acetone breath develops as ketone bodies are converted to acetone and excreted by

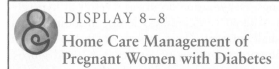

DISPLAY 8–8
Home Care Management of Pregnant Women with Diabetes

The following diagnostic criteria and considerations are suggested for home care management of women with diabetes:

- Patient and family willingness and ability to learn and follow diet, perform blood glucose monitoring, and perform insulin adjustment and administration if needed
- Family member knowledge of signs and symptoms of severe hypoglycemia and ability to administer glucagon (0.5 to 1.0 mg) subcutaneously if this should occur
- Family member knowledge of how and when to call for emergency assistance
- A safe and clean storage place for insulin and other supplies
- Absence of abnormal laboratory values. Glycemic control can be assessed over time (previous 4 to 6 weeks) using measurements of glycosylated hemoglobin (A1c). Fasting and random blood glucose levels provide information about blood glucose levels at the time of testing.

The following parameters should be assessed based on the individual clinical situation. Protocols or physician orders are used to determine threshold for each parameter:

- Diabetes care should be reviewed with the woman and family, including blood glucose monitoring, urine testing for ketones, diet, and insulin administration.
- Assessment for skill in blood glucose monitoring as ordered, including troubleshooting equipment problems
- Review of record of daily dietary intake, blood glucose levels, daily weights, and medications
- Assessment for insulin self-injection
- Home or office visit for comprehensive maternal–fetal assessment, including fundal height, review of daily fetal movement counting log (after 24 weeks' gestation), auscultation fetal heart rate or nonstress test one to two times weekly after 26 to 28 weeks
- Sick-day care management guidelines should be reviewed with the woman and family to ensure knowledge of how to make adjustments in insulin dosages if needed to offset altered food
- Assessment for development of complications such as preterm labor, gestational hypertension, bleeding, or infection
- Review of warning signs to report to primary healthcare provider: hyperglycemia (blood glucose level >200 mg/dL), decreased fetal movement, illness (especially if dietary intake is altered), skin breakdown, visual or neurologic symptoms, and signs of renal involvement

Medications
- Insulin (as prescribed) or oral agents
- Prenatal vitamins and iron

Diet
- Individualized meal plan as recommended by healthcare provider. Current recommendations for dietary management suggest that calories should be consumed in three meals and three snacks, comprising 33% to 40% carbohydrates, 20% protein, and 40% fats.

Activity
- Activities of daily living
- Exercise within parameters recommended by the healthcare provider

the lungs. Dehydration occurs as a result of hyperglycemia. Altered consciousness levels, including coma, are usually present. The diagnosis of DKA is based on the laboratory findings of an elevated blood glucose level, a bicarbonate level below 15 mEq/L, and an arterial pH of less than 7.2. In pregnant women, DKA may occur with only mild elevations in blood glucose values (Sibai & Viteri, 2014).

Care of women in DKA should occur in a tertiary care facility with the support services that can provide intensive care. Nurses in community hospitals should be capable of stabilizing the woman in preparation for, and during transport to, an appropriate facility.

Table 8–3 lists specific interventions nurses use in the care of women experiencing DKA. Initial treatment measures focus on rehydration, which improves tissue perfusion, insulin delivery, and a physiologic lowering of blood glucose by hemodilution. After IV access is established, insulin is administered as ordered to lower blood glucose. Caution should be exercised in lowering the blood glucose because too rapid a fall may result in the serious complication of cerebral edema. With improvement of the intravascular status, fluid shifts result in a potassium deficit that requires replacement. Nurses should continually assess the woman for signs and symptoms of hypokalemia and monitor electrolyte levels in preparation for replacement. Adequate urinary output must also be maintained with potassium replacement to avoid hyperkalemia. In addition to monitoring laboratory electrolyte status, the complete blood cell count and differential also should be monitored as well as the clinical status for signs and symptoms of

TABLE 8–3. Nursing Management of Diabetic Ketoacidosis

Treatment	Nursing intervention
Fluid resuscitation	1. Obtain large-bore peripheral access. 2. Anticipate need for hemodynamic monitoring. 3. Administer fluids as ordered, usually 1,000 to 2,000 mL of normal saline over 1 hr and then 200 to 250 to 500 mL/hr. 4. Assess for signs and symptoms of pulmonary edema—dyspnea, tachypnea, wheezing, cough. 5. Assess for hypovolemia; check vital signs every 15 min; report decrease in blood pressure, increased pulse rate, decrease in central venous and pulmonary capillary wedge pressure, and slow capillary refill. 6. Insert Foley catheter for oliguria or anuria and send specimen for urinalysis, culture, and sensitivity. 7. Hourly intake and output—report output <30 mL/hr. 8. Administer 5% dextrose solution or D5/0.45% normal saline at blood glucose level of 200 mg/dL to prevent hypoglycemia.
Insulin therapy	1. Administer intravenous insulin as ordered—0.1 to 0.2 U/kg of regular insulin as bolus and then 0.1 U/kg/hr. Follow hospital insulin/dextrose drip algorithm if established. 2. Hourly capillary blood glucose determinations (lab correlation with each draw) 3. Monitor urine and blood for ketones. 4. Notify physician when blood glucose level of 250 mg/dL is reached, anticipating a decrease in insulin infusion rate to 0.1 U/kg/hr. 5. Monitor for hypoglycemia. 6. Monitor for cerebral edema—headache, vomiting, deteriorating mental status, bradycardia, sluggish pupillary light reflex, widened pulse pressure.
Electrolyte replacement	1. Obtain electrocardiogram and report ST segment depression, inverted T waves, and appearance of U waves after T waves. 2. Obtain laboratory electrolyte levels every 2 to 4 hr. 3. Anticipate potassium replacement within 2 to 4 hr.
Oxygenation	1. Establish the airway. 2. Anticipate placement of the peripheral arterial catheter. 3. Obtain initial arterial blood gases and then hourly until pH of 7.20 is maintained. 4. Administer oxygen at 10 L/min by a nonrebreather facemask or as ordered to maintain oxygen saturations of 95% per pulse oximeter. 5. Anticipate the need for intubation/mechanical ventilation. 6. Use continuous pulse oximetry. 7. Administer bicarbonate if ordered for pH of 7.10.
Electronic fetal or uterine monitoring	1. Lateral recumbent position 2. Apply external fetal or uterine monitoring (EFM). 3. Observe EFM for evidence of fetal compromise. 4. Observe for uterine activity. 5. Administer tocolytics as ordered (magnesium sulfate or drug of choice). 6. Avoid beta-adrenergic agonists and steroids.

Adapted from Sibai, B. M., & Viteri, O. A. (2014). Diabetic ketoacidosis in pregnancy. *Obstetrics & Gynecology, 123*(1), 167–178. doi:10.1097 /AOG.0000000000000060 infection. Evidence of infection requires prompt and aggressive treatment for DKA treatment to be effective.

Fetal monitoring, even in previable gestations, provides an indication of hydration and perfusion status and should be instituted upon admission. Treatment should, however, not be delayed until monitoring can be instituted in settings where fetal monitoring is not available. Indeterminate fetal status is expected but resolves as the mother is stabilized and should not be an indication for emergent cesarean birth, which could further compromise the mother (Sibai & Viteri, 2014). Maternal oxygenation status should be monitored continually and oxygen administered based on blood gas determinations, bedside oxygen saturation levels, and fetal status. Uterine activity also is associated with severe dehydration but resolves in most cases with improved perfusion. Magnesium sulfate is the drug of choice for treatment of preterm labor because it does not interfere with the action of insulin.

After DKA has been corrected, the underlying cause—whether infection or poor self-care practices—should be discussed with the mother and family, outlining early detection and prevention strategies. For mothers whose infants did not survive, intensive grief support and follow-up should be provided.

Intrapartum Management: Pregestational and Gestational Diabetes Mellitus

Intrapartum management of women with diabetes requires skilled nursing care to prevent maternal and neonatal complications. Hyperglycemia in labor contributes to the development of neonatal hypoglycemia. Blood glucose should be assessed on the first laboratory blood draw and then checked at the bedside every 1 to 2 hours for all women who have previously been controlled by medication. Women with GDM who have been controlled by diet may have their blood glucose levels checked every 2 to 4 hours.

Patients with an insulin pump may continue their pump therapy during labor. Generally, basal rates may be continued while the patient is taking nothing by mouth (NPO), with bolus doses titrated to the patient's hourly blood sugars. Refer to the provider's orders for a specific individualized plan of care.

IV access should be established early so that hydration can be maintained, and insulin should be administered when necessary. Women with GDM and type 2 diabetes may not require insulin during labor. Laboring women with type 1 diabetes will usually require glucose and insulin at some point. If, on hospital admission, the blood glucose level of a woman with type 1 diabetes is 70 mg/dL or below, an infusion with 5% dextrose should be initiated at a rate of 100 to 125 mL/hr. A main line is required, usually of normal saline, at least to keep open. All glucose-containing solutions and insulin-containing solutions should be piggybacked to the main line at ports closest to the hub of IV insertion. These are basic safety measures. Insulin administration should be initiated according to institutional protocol. Women who present in spontaneous labor and who have taken their intermediate- or long-acting insulin may not require insulin during labor but may need a glucose infusion on admission to avoid hypoglycemia.

A standardized solution of 100 units of regular human insulin to 100 mL of normal saline should be used—again, for safety purposes. When a woman is NPO, a rate of 1 unit (1 mL) per hour is often all that is necessary. Most insulin algorithms require IV insulin adjustments according to (at least) hourly blood glucose levels. Polyvinyl tubing should be flushed thoroughly (at least 20 mL) to allow saturation of the insulin to the tubing, allowing the prescribed dose to be infused consistently. Glucose and insulin should be maintained on infusion pumps to enable exact dosing of both solutions.

Insulin is partially catabolized in the kidneys, and in women with nephropathy, the action is unpredictable, requiring closer surveillance of blood sugar levels. Prehydration for conduction anesthesia or IV boluses should use non–glucose-containing solutions and be administered more slowly in the presence of vascular disease. Women with diabetes may have a scheduled induction or cesarean birth. Prior evening or early morning hospital admissions are preferred, withholding the morning insulin dose, with IV glucose and insulin initiated, or insulin pump settings revised as ordered. Cervical ripening and induction procedures should follow institutional protocols and physician orders. Fetal monitoring should be used and assessed for signs of fetal compromise. Continuous electronic fetal monitoring during labor is recommended by ACOG (2009) for women with type 1 diabetes. Women in labor who have diabetes are designated as high-risk by the American Academy of Pediatrics and ACOG (2017) in the *Guidelines for Perinatal Care* and thus require more frequent assessment than low-risk women. See Chapters 14 and 15 for a detailed discussion of maternal and fetal assessment during labor based on risk status. AWHONN (2010) recommends 1 to 1 nursing care during labor for woman who have diabetes. Labor abnormalities that would indicate potential cephalopelvic disproportion should be monitored closely. Nurses caring for laboring women with diabetes should prepare for assisted birth and the possibility of shoulder dystocia. The birth of a potentially high-risk newborn should also be anticipated and preparation made for full resuscitation. A neonatal team should be present at the birth or immediately available. Hypoglycemia during labor is usually avoided with close monitoring but should be recognized and treated aggressively. Observation for signs and symptoms of hypoglycemia should be a continuous nursing assessment. Display 8–2 lists typical signs and symptoms of mild and moderate hypoglycemia.

Concentrated dextrose solutions (10% and 50%) should be immediately available. Treatment should be based on the protocol at the hospital in which the patient is being treated. A common example of a treatment protocol for hypoglycemia in pregnancy may include treatment initiated at a blood glucose level of 70 mg/dL by discontinuing insulin and running only dextrose in the IV to raise the blood glucose level to 80 mg/dL. The insulin drip can then be restarted at an adjusted algorithm or when the blood glucose is 100 to 110 mg/dL. The blood sugar should be rechecked more frequently (every 15 to 30 minutes until resolved) and then every 1 to 2 hours for the duration of the insulin infusion, and further treatment should be administered if the blood glucose remains low. If the woman becomes unconscious, the physician should be notified immediately, and 50% dextrose should be infused intravenously. Vital signs should be assessed every 5 to 10 minutes during episodes of hypoglycemia, including blood glucose checks, until a threshold of 80 mg/dL is reached. Insulin should be resumed when the blood glucose level reaches 120 mg/dL according to a laboratory assessment or 110 mg/dL for a capillary blood glucose determination.

POSTPARTUM MANAGEMENT

Pregestational Diabetes Mellitus

Insulin requirements decrease in the immediate postpartum period when the levels of circulating anti-insulin placental hormones drop. For GDM patients, insulin and glucose infusions are usually stopped completely after delivery as insulin sensitivity returns to normal soon after delivery of the placenta (Kitzmiller, Dang-Kilduff, & Taslimi, 2007; Taylor & Davison, 2007). With oral intake, subcutaneous insulin can be resumed at the prepregnancy dosage or at one half to one third the pregnancy dose for women with types 1 and 2 diabetes. Strict glycemic control can be relaxed somewhat in the postpartum period.

Women with diabetes have a higher incidence of postpartum infections (e.g., mastitis, endometritis, and wound infection). Therefore, nurses should observe for, and teach patients about, signs and symptoms and notify the physician if they occur. Women who have given birth to a macrosomic infant or have had prolonged or induced labors should be closely monitored for hemorrhage.

Contraceptive options should be explored with the woman and her partner, and pregnancy planning should be encouraged to allow for preconception care to decrease the risks for spontaneous abortion and congenital defects in future pregnancies. Counseling and education should be provided regarding long-term consequences of diabetes and the need for glycemic control to decrease adverse sequelae.

Breastfeeding

Breastfeeding is highly recommended for at least 6 months after birth and ideally for 12 months after birth. Mounting evidence indicates that breastfeeding reduces the incidence of childhood obesity and diabetes later in life (Badillo-Suárez, Rodríguez-Crus, & Nieves-Morales, 2017). Evidence also suggests that breastfeeding reduces or delays the onset of type 2 diabetes in women with GDM (Aune, Norat, Romundstad, & Vatten, 2014).

Insulin may be used for women with type 2 diabetes who choose to breastfeed their babies and who cannot achieve normoglycemia by treatment with medical nutrition therapy and exercise alone. Some oral hypoglycemic agents (e.g., glyburide and metformin) may be safe for use while breastfeeding (Balsells et al., 2015; Butalia et al., 2017). The options for medication therapy should be discussed with the provider to optimize patient compliance and blood glucose management.

Caloric needs mandate recalculation based on postpartum body weight and on possible lactation requirements. For those women with BMI >35, a program for exercise and dietary management for weight loss should be outlined. Breastfeeding should be encouraged with adequate support from the nursing staff. Lactating mothers need assistance and education to prevent hypoglycemia while nursing. Most breastfeeding mothers require less insulin due to extra calories expended with nursing and the use of maternal glucose to produce the lactase in their milk. Women with type 1 diabetes should especially be advised regarding the risk of hypoglycemia during breastfeeding and an increase in blood glucose monitoring and/or eating snacks (potentially without insulin coverage) prior to feeds may be warranted, and having fast-acting glucose available nearby is also important.

Gestational Diabetes Mellitus

Most women revert to normal glucose tolerance in the postpartum period. Reclassification of glycemic status should be obtained at the 6- to 12-week postpartum visit for all women with GDM, because up to one third of affected women will have impaired glucose tolerance (Bellamy, Casas, Hingorani, & Williams, 2009). A fasting plasma glucose and a 75-g 2-hour oral OGTT will most accurately identify women with impaired glucose tolerance (ACOG, 2018a). If the glucose tolerance test is normal, repeat testing should occur every 1 to 3 years from the birth of the baby and when pregnancy is being considered (ACOG, 2018a; ADA, 2017b). The risk for development of overt diabetes after GDM increases with time.

Counseling should be provided to women with a history of GDM in the postpartum period for risk-reducing strategies such as weight reduction by diet and exercise. The Diabetes Prevention Program Research Group (2017) showed that a lifestyle modification program could decrease the incidence of type 2 diabetes by 58%. Women also need to know the signs and symptoms of hyperglycemia that would warrant testing for diabetes such as polyuria, polydipsia, polyphagia, persistent vaginal candidiasis, frequent urinary tract infections, excessive fatigue and hunger, or sudden weight loss. Women also should be informed that they have a high risk for development of GDM in subsequent pregnancies. Testing for diabetes is encouraged before conception or at the first prenatal visit, with early prenatal care to allow screening for and intensive management of overt diabetes, which carries a higher perinatal risk than for GDM.

SUMMARY

Diabetes is one of the common medical complications encountered when caring for pregnant women. Diabetes may exist prepregnancy or develop during the pregnancy. Each type of diabetes has specific clinical challenges and the potential for adverse outcomes for the mother and baby. Perinatal nurses should be aware of the required aspects of nursing care for women with diabetes during pregnancy, labor, birth, and postpartum.

REFERENCES

American Academy of Pediatrics & American College of Obstetricians and Gynecologists. (2017). *Guidelines for perinatal care* (8th ed.). Elk Grove Village, IL: American Academy of Pediatrics.

American Association of Diabetes Educators. (2012). *AADE7 Self-Care Behaviors®*. Retrieved from http://www.diabeteseducator.org/ProfessionalResources/AADE7

American College of Obstetricians and Gynecologists. (2009). *Intrapartum fetal heart rate monitoring: Nomenclature, interpretation, and general management principles* (Practice Bulletin No. 106, Reaffirmed 2017). Washington, DC: Author.

American College of Obstetricians and Gynecologists. (2016, Reaffirmed 2018). *Fetal macrosomia* (Practice Bulletin No. 173) Washington, DC: Author.

American College of Obstetricians and Gynecologists. (2017a). *Shoulder dystocia* (Practice Bulletin No. 178). Washington, DC: Author.

American College of Obstetricians and Gynecologists. (2017b). *Vaginal birth after cesarean delivery* (Practice Bulletin No. 184). Washington, DC: Author.

American College of Obstetricians and Gynecologists. (2018a). *Gestational diabetes mellitus* (Practice Bulletin No. 190). Washington, DC: Author.

American College of Obstetricians and Gynecologists. (2018b). *Pregestational diabetes mellitus* (Practice Bulletin No. 201). Washington, DC: Author.

American College of Obstetricians and Gynecologists. (2018c). *Weight gain during pregnancy* (Committee Opinion No. 548, Reaffirmed 2018). Washington, DC: Author.

American Diabetes Association. (2003). Gestational diabetes mellitus. *Diabetes Care, 26*(1 Suppl.), S103–S105. doi:10.2337/diacare.26.2007.S103

American Diabetes Association. (2017a). Classification and diagnosis of diabetes. *Diabetes Care, 40*(1 Suppl.), S11–S24.

American Diabetes Association. (2017b). Standards of medical care in diabetes—2017. *Diabetes Care, 40*(1 Suppl.), S1–S135. doi:10.2337/dc17-S001

Araújo, J. R., Martel, F., & Keating, E. (2014). Exposure to nonnutritive sweeteners during pregnancy and lactation: Impact in programming of metabolic diseases in the progeny later in life. *Reproductive Toxicology, 49*, 196–201. doi:10.1016/j.reprotox.2014.09.007

Association of Women's Health, Obstetric and Neonatal Nurses. (2010). *Guidelines for professional registered nurse staffing for perinatal units*. Washington, DC: Author.

Association of Women's Health, Obstetric and Neonatal Nurses. (2016). *Nursing care of the woman with diabetes in pregnancy: evidence-based clinical practice guideline*. Washington, DC: Author.

Aune, D., Norat, R., Romundstad, P., & Vatten, L. J. (2014). Breastfeeding and the maternal risk of type 2 diabetes: A systematic review and dose-response meta-analysis of cohort studies. *Nutrition, Metabolism, and Cardiovascular Diseases, 24*(2), 107–115. doi:10.1016/j.numecd.2013.10.028

Badillo-Suárez, P. A., Rodríguez-Cruz, M., & Nieves-Morales, X. (2017). Impact of metabolic hormones secreted in human breast milk on nutritional programming in childhood obesity. *Journal of Mammary Gland Biology and Neoplasia, 22*(3), 171–191. doi:10.1007/s1091

Balsells, M., García-Patterson, A., Solà, I., Roqué, M., Gich, I., & Corcoy, R. (2015). Glibenclamide, metformin, and insulin for the treatment of gestational diabetes: A systematic review and meta-analysis. *British Medical Journal, 350*, h102. doi:10.1136/bmj.h102

Bartholomew, M. L., Soules, K., Church, K., Shaha, S., Burlingame, J., Graham, G., . . . Zalud, I. (2015). Managing diabetes in pregnancy using cell phone/internet technology. *Clinical Diabetes, 33*(4), 169–174. doi:10.2337/diaclin.33.4.169

Bellamy, L., Casas, J. P., Hingorani, A. D., & Williams, D. (2009). Type 2 diabetes mellitus after gestational diabetes: A systematic review and meta-analysis. *Lancet, 373*(9677), 1773–1779. doi:10.1016/S0140-6736909060731-5

Bonakdaran, S., Azami, G., Tara, F., & Poorali, L. (2017). Soluble (pro) renin receptor is a predictor of gestational diabetes mellitus. *Current Diabetes Reviews, 13*(6), 555–559. doi:10.2174/1573399812666160919100253

Bouthoorn, S. H., Silva, L. M., Murray, S. E., Steegers, E. A., Jaddoe, V. S, Moll, H., . . . Raat, H. (2015). Low-educated women have an increased risk of gestational diabetes mellitus: The Generation R Study. *Acta Diabetologica, 52*(3), 445–452. doi:10.1007/s00592-014-0668-x

Bramham, K. (2017). Diabetic nephropathy and pregnancy. *Seminars in Nephrology, 37*(4), 362–369. doi:10.1016/j.semnephrol.2017.05.008

Branum, A., Kirmeyer, S. E., & Gregory, E. C. (2016). Prepregnancy body mass index by maternal characteristics and state: Data from the birth certificate, 2014. *National Vital Statistics Reports, 65*(6), 1–11.

Bryant, S. N., Herrera, C. L., Nelson, D. B., & Cunningham, F. G. (2017). Diabetic ketoacidosis complicating pregnancy. *Journal of Neonatal-Perinatal Medicine, 10*(1), 17–23. doi:10.3233/NPM-1663

Butalia, S., Donovan, L., Gutierrez, L., Lodha, A., Aitken, E., Zakariasen, A., & Donovan, L. (2017). Short- and long-term outcomes of metformin compared with insulin alone in pregnancy: A systematic review and meta-analysis. *Diabetic Medicine, 34*(1), 27–36.

Carpenter, M. W., & Coustan, D. R. (1982). Criteria for screening tests for gestational diabetes. *American Journal of Obstetrics & Gynecology, 144*(7), 768–773.

Casagrande, S. S., Linder, B., & Cowie, C. C. (2018). Prevalence of gestational diabetes and subsequent type 2 diabetes among U.S. women. *Diabetes Research and Clinical Practice, 141*(7), 200–208. doi:10.1016/j.diabres.2018.05.010

Centers for Disease Control and Prevention. (2017a). *About diabetes.* Atlanta, GA: Author.

Centers for Disease Control and Prevention. (2017b). *National diabetes statistics report, 2017. Estimates of diabetes and its burden in the United States.* Atlanta, GA: Author.

Centers for Disease Control and Prevention. (2019). *Diabetes and prediabetes.* Atlanta, GA: Author.

Deputy, N. P., Kim, S. Y., Conrey, E. J., & Bullard, K. M. (2018). Prevalence and changes in preexisting diabetes and gestational diabetes among women who had a live birth—United States, 2012–2016. *MMWR. Morbidity and Mortality Weekly Report, 67*(43), 1201–1207.

Diabetes Prevention Program Research Group. (2017). *Diabetes Prevention Program (DPP).* Retrieved from https://niddk.nih .gov/about-niddk/research-areas/diabetes/diabetes-prevention -program-dpp

Feig, D. S., Donovan, L. E., Corcoy, R., Murphy, K. E., Amiel, S. A., Hunt, K. F., . . . Murphy, H. R. (2017). Continuous glucose monitoring in pregnant women with type 1 diabetes (CONCEPTT): A multicenter international randomised controlled trial. *Lancet, 390*(10110), 2347–2359.

Feig, D. S., Murphy, K., Asztalos, E., Tomlinson, G., Sanchez, J., Zinman, B., . . . Barrett, J. F. (2016). Metformin in women with type 2 diabetes in pregnancy (MiTy): A multi-center randomized controlled trial. *BMC Pregnancy and Childbirth, 16*(1), 173. doi:10.1186/s12884-016-0954-4

Fuglsang, J., & Ovesen, P. R. (2015). Pregnancy and delivery in a woman with type 1 diabetes, gastroparesis, and a gastric neurostimulator. *Diabetes Care, 38*(5), e75. doi:10.2337 /dc14-2959

Gabbe, S. G., Carpenter, L. B., & Garrison, E. A. (2007). New strategies for glucose control in patients with type 1 and type 2 diabetes mellitus in pregnancy. *Clinical Obstetrics and Gynecology, 50*(4), 1014–1024. doi:10.1097/GRF.0b013e31815a6435

Gibson, K. S., Waters, T. P., & Catalano, P. M. (2012). Maternal weight gain in women who develop gestational diabetes mellitus. *Obstetrics & Gynecology, 119*(3), 560–565. doi:10.1097/AOG .0b013e31824758e0

Halse, R. E., Wallman, K. E., Newnham, J. P., & Guelfi, K. J. (2014). Home-based exercise training improves capillary glucose profile in women with gestational diabetes. *Medicine and Science in Sports and Exercise, 46*(9),1702–1709. doi:10.1249 /MSS.0000000000000302

HAPO Study Cooperative Research Group. (2008). Hyperglycemia and adverse pregnancy outcomes. *New England Journal of Medicine, 358*(19), 1991–2002.

Harper, L. M., Mele, L., Landon, M. B., Carpenter, M. W., Ramin, S. M., Reddy, U. M., . . . Tolosa, J. E. (2016). Carpenter-Coustan compared with National Diabetes Data Group criteria for diagnosing gestational diabetes. *Obstetrics & Gynecology, 127*(5), 893–898. doi:10.1097/AOG.0000000000001383

Kemball, M. L., McIver, C., Milner, R. D., Nourse, C. H., Schiff, D., & Tiernan, J. R. (1970). Neonatal hypoglycaemia in infants of diabetic mothers given sulphonylurea drugs in pregnancy. *Archives of Disease in Childhood, 45*(243), 696–701.

Kitzmiller, J. L., Dang-Kilduff, L., & Taslimi, M. M. (2007). Gestational diabetes after delivery. *Diabetes Care, 30*(2), S225–S235. doi:10.2337/dc07-s221

Krakowiak, P., Walker, C., Bremer, A., Baker. A. S., Ozonoff, S., Hansen, R. L., Hertz-Picciotto, I. (2012). Maternal metabolic conditions and risk for autism and other neurodevelopmental disorders. *Pediatrics, 129*(5), e1121–e1128.

Lain, K. Y., & Catalano, P. M. (2007). Metabolic changes in pregnancy. *Clinical Obstetrics and Gynecology, 50*(4), 938–948. doi:10.1097/GRF.0b013e31815a5494

Lloreda-García, J. M., Sevilla-Denia, S., Rodríguez-Sánchez, A., Muñoz-Martínez, P., & Díaz-Ruiz, M. (2016). Perinatal outcome of macrosomic infants born to diabetic versus non-diabetic mothers. *Endocrinologia Y Nutricion, 63*(8), 409–413. doi:10 .1016/j.endonu.2016.04.010

Mathiesen, E. R. (2015). Diabetic nephropathy in pregnancy: New insights from a retrospective cohort study. *Diabetologia, 58*(4), 649–650. doi:10.1007/s00125-015-3530-y

Mathiesen, E. R. (2016). Pregnancy outcomes in women with diabetes-lessons learned from clinical research: The 2015 Norbert Freinkel Award lecture. *Diabetes Care, 39*(12), 2111–2117.

Metzger, B. E., Gabbe, S. G., Persson, B., Buchanan, T. A., Catalano, P. A., Damm, P., . . . Schmidt, M. I. (2010). International Association of Diabetes and Pregnancy Study Groups recommendations on the diagnosis and classification of hyperglycemia in pregnancy. *Diabetes Care, 33*(3), 676–682. doi:10.2337/dc09-1848

Monteiro, L. J., Norman, J. E., Rice, G. E., & Illanes, S. E. (2016). Fetal programming and gestational diabetes mellitus. *Placenta, 48*(1 Suppl.), S54–S60. doi:10.1016/j.placenta.2015.11.015

Ogunyemi, D., Friedman, P., Betcher, K., Whitten, A., Sugiyama, N., Qu, L., . . . Paul, H. (2017). Obstetrical correlates and perinatal consequences of neonatal hypoglycemia in term infants. *Journal of Maternal-Fetal & Neonatal Medicine, 30*(11), 1372–1377. doi:10.1080/14767058.2016.1214127

Parker, J. A., & Conway, D. L. (2007). Diabetic ketoacidosis in pregnancy. *Obstetrics and Gynecology Clinics of North America, 34*(3), 533–543. doi:10.1016/j.ogc.2007.08.001

Patel, E. M., Goodnight, W. H., James, A. H., & Grotegut, C. A. (2015). Temporal trends in maternal medical conditions and stillbirth. *American Journal of Obstetrics & Gynecology, 212*, 673.e1–673.e11. doi:10.1016/j.ajog.2014.12.021

Pearson, D. W., Kernaghan, D., Lee, A., & Penney, G. C. (2007). The relationship between pre-pregnancy care and early pregnancy loss, major congenital anomaly or perinatal death in type I diabetes mellitus. *BJOG, 114*(1), 104–107. doi:10.1111/j.1471 -0528.2006.01145.x

Persson, M., Pasupathy, D., Hanson, U., Westgren, M., & Norman, M. (2012). Pre-pregnancy body mass index and the risk of adverse outcome in type 1 diabetic pregnancies: A population-based cohort study. *BMJ Open, 2*(1), e000601. doi:10.1136 /bmjopen-2011-000601

Pescosolido, N., Campagna, O., & Barbato, A. (2014). Diabetic retinopathy and pregnancy. *International Ophthalmology, 34*(4), 989–997. doi:10.1007/s10792-014-9906-z

Rezai, S., Withers Cokes, C., Gottimukkala, S., Penas, R. P., Chadee, A., Chadwick, E., & Henderson, C. (2016). Review of stillbirths among antepartum women with gestational and pregestational diabetes. *Obstetrics & Gynecology International Journal, 4*(4), 00118. doi:10.15406/ogij.2016.04.00118

Scifres, C. M., Feghali, M., Dumont, T., Althouse, A. D., Speer, P., Caritis, S. N., & Catov, J. M. (2015). Large-for-gestational-age ultrasound diagnosis and risk for cesarean delivery in women with gestational diabetes mellitus. *Obstetrics & Gynecology, 126*(5), 978–986. doi:10.1097/AOG.0000000000001097

Seaquist, E. R., Anderson, J., Childs, B., Cryer, P., Dagogo-Jack, S., Fish, L., . . . Vigersky, R. (2013). Hypoglycemia and diabetes: A report of a workgroup of the American Diabetes Association and the Endocrine Society. *The Journal of Clinical Endocrinology & Metabolism, 98*(5), 1845–1859. doi:10.1210/jc.2012-4127

Sibai, B. M., & Viteri, O. A. (2014). Diabetic ketoacidosis in pregnancy. *Obstetrics & Gynecology, 123*(1), 167–178. doi:10.1097/AOG.0000000000000060

Sinha, N., Venkatram, S., & Diaz-Fuentes, G. (2014). Starvation ketoacidosis: A cause of severe anion gap metabolic acidosis in pregnancy. *Case Reports in Critical Care, 2014,* 906283. doi:10.1155/2014/906283

Stenerson, M. B., Collura, C. A., Rose, C. H., Lteif, A. N., & Carey, W. A. (2011). Bilateral basal ganglia infarctions in a neonate born during maternal ketoacidosis. *Pediatrics, 128*(3), e707–e710. doi:10.1542/peds.2010-3597

Sullivan, S. D., Umans, J. G., & Ratner, R. (2011). Hypertension complicating diabetic pregnancies: Pathophysiology, management, and controversies. *Journal of Clinical Hypertension, 13*(4), 275–284. doi:10.1111/j.1751-7176.2011.00440.x

Tam, W. H., Ma, R. C. W., Ozaki, R., Li, A. M., Chan, M. M., Yuen, L. Y., . . . Chan, J. C. N. (2017). In utero exposure to maternal hyperglycemia increases childhood cardiometabolic risk in offspring. *Diabetes Care, 40*(5), 679–686. doi:10.2337/dc16-2397

Taylor, R., & Davison, J. M. (2007). Type 1 diabetes and pregnancy. *BMJ, 334*(7596), 742–745. doi:10.1136/bmj.39154.700417.BE

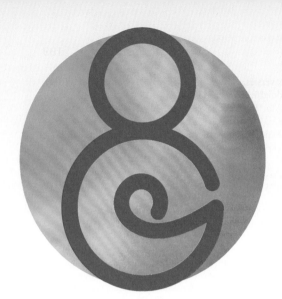

CHAPTER 9

Cardiac Disease in Pregnancy

Julie Arafeh

SIGNIFICANCE AND INCIDENCE

Cardiac disease is present in a relatively small number of pregnancies (Lima, Yang, Xu, & Stergiopoulos, 2017). However, during the years of 2011 to 2013, cardiovascular (CV) disease accounted for 15.5% and cardiomyopathy accounted for 11% of pregnancy-related deaths in the United States making it the leading cause of indirect pregnancy-related mortality (Centers for Disease Control and Prevention, 2017). Indirect pregnancy-related mortality is defined as deaths from preexisting disease influenced by physiologic changes of pregnancy. This trend has been detected in other developed countries, notably the United Kingdom (Knight et al., 2016). The prominence of cardiac disease in maternal mortality and morbidity is attributed to several factors. More women with congenital heart disease (CHD) are reaching childbearing age. Lifestyle trends such as delaying pregnancy until later in life, sedentary routine, obesity, and opioid and tobacco use all play a contributory role. The presence of other chronic medical conditions such as diabetes and hypertension or obstetric conditions such as multiparity also increases the risk of complications during pregnancy (Emmanuel & Thorne, 2015; Rezk, Elkilani, Shaheen, Gamal, & Badr, 2017; Salihu et al., 2017). These conditions and complications, individually or in combination, place an additional burden on the cardiac muscle during pregnancy, labor, and birth, leading to increased risk.

From the years 1995 to 2006, the incidence of women with cardiac disease in the United States had not changed significantly, although the morbidity of pregnant women hospitalized with cardiac disease appeared to be increasing (Kuklina & Callaghan, 2011). In a review of the National Inpatient Sample (NIS) for hospital admission of women with cardiac disease admitted for birth from the years 2003 to 2012, a 24.7% increase was noted. The NIS is the largest database of inpatient care (all payers) in the United States and is useful in analysis of rare patient conditions and special populations. The main objective of the review was to determine overall incidence, types of cardiac disease, and occurrence of adverse cardiac events. In a comparison of 81,295 admissions with cardiac disease and 39,894,032 without, CHD was found to be the most common. Admissions for CHD, pulmonary hypertension and cardiomyopathy all increased, while valvular disease admissions were unchanged. As expected, adverse cardiac events, mortality and severe morbidity were higher in women with cardiac disease when compared to women without. Arrhythmias and heart failure were the most common cardiac events reported and women with pulmonary hypertension and cardiomyopathy had the highest mortality rate. Women with cardiac disease had longer length of stay and higher total cost of care (Lima et al., 2017).

The risks maternal cardiac disease confers on the fetus and neonate can include spontaneous abortion, transference of heart disease in cases of maternal CHD, premature birth, size small for gestational age, respiratory distress syndrome, intraventricular hemorrhage, and death (Canobbio et al., 2017; Ghandi & Shamshirsaz, 2016; Pillutla et al., 2016). Any maternal cardiac disease that significantly impacts cardiac output increases the risk of fetal and neonatal mortality and morbidity. In a study about the effect of maternal cardiac disease on fetal growth and neonatal outcomes, 331 women with cardiac disease were compared to 662 women without cardiac disease (Gelson et al., 2011). Both groups had similar incidence of maternal hypertension and illicit drug and tobacco use. Perinatal complications in the group with cardiac disease were 50% higher than the control group. The most common complications were small-for-gestational-age neonates and preterm birth. No difference in preterm premature rupture of membranes was seen between the two groups. Maternal characteristics most associated with fetal and neonatal adverse outcomes were decreased cardiac output and cyanosis or combination of the two (Gelson et al., 2011).

Earlier studies have also demonstrated the effect reduced maternal cardiac function has on fetal growth. Twenty cases of singleton pregnancies with severe fetal growth restriction were compared to 107 normal singleton pregnancies (Bamfo, Kametas, Turan, Khaw, & Nicolaides, 2006). Two-dimensional and M-mode echocardiography was used to evaluate maternal cardiac function in both groups. Reduction in cardiac output and stroke volume was seen along with an increase in systemic vascular resistance (SVR) in the group with severe fetal growth restriction as compared to pregnancies with normal fetal growth (Bamfo et al., 2006). Another study compared 302 pregnancies with cardiac disease to 572 pregnancies without cardiac disease for neonatal complications (Siu et al., 2002). Neonatal complications included small for gestational age, preterm birth, respiratory distress, intraventricular hemorrhage, and fetal or neonatal death. Neonatal complications occurred over 50% more often in the group with cardiac disease. The subgroup with the highest neonatal complication rate included women with cardiac disease who had the following characteristics: younger than 20 years or older than 35 years, obstetric risk factors, multiple gestation, smoker, anticoagulant therapy, and at least one cardiac risk factor present (Siu et al., 2002).

Despite the significantly increased risk of adverse outcomes, most pregnant women with cardiac disease do well. Careful planning and monitoring prior to, during, and after the pregnancy by an interdisciplinary healthcare team increases the likelihood that the best possible outcome will occur for the mother and baby (Arafeh & Baird, 2006; Deen, Chandrasekaran, Stout, & Easterling, 2017; Hameed, Morton, & Moore, 2017). All members of the team need to possess a thorough understanding of normal cardiac anatomy and physiology, knowledge of how the physiologic changes of pregnancy will influence cardiac function and the mother's cardiac disease, and the ability to estimate the risk pregnancy poses to the mother and her baby and use the most recent and best knowledge to plan comprehensive care for the duration of the pregnancy including follow-up in the postpartum period until the effects of pregnancy have resolved (Deen et al., 2017).

THE CARDIOVASCULAR SYSTEM

The purpose of the CV system is to deliver nutrient-rich oxygenated blood and remove waste products in response to the metabolic needs of the body.

The components of the CV system, the heart, blood, and vascular circulation, all work in a coordinated fashion to achieve this goal (Darovic, 2002a). For example, under normal conditions, the CV system adapts to the need for more oxygen in uterine muscles during labor by increasing the amount of blood flow through the heart and by dilating some vessels while constricting others to direct flow (and oxygen) to the uterus.

The heart has four muscular chambers: two atria or upper chambers and the lower chambers or ventricles. Chamber walls have three layers: the pericardium or sac that surrounds the heart, the myocardium or the muscular layer, and the endocardium or inner lining of the chambers that forms the valves of the heart (Darovic, 2002a). The area between the pericardium and the heart is a potential space, which allows for smooth unrestricted movement of the heart when beating. Accumulation of excessive fluid or inflammation in the pericardial area can interfere with cardiac function. Damage to the heart muscle from overstretching or lack of adequate blood flow can also impact function (Darovic, 2002a). Exposure of the inner lining of the chambers and the valves to bacteria can result in scarring and dysfunction that also impacts flow. In certain situations, prophylactic antibiotics are administered when high levels of bacteria are anticipated in the blood to prevent infection in susceptible women (American College of Obstetricians and Gynecologists [ACOG], 2018b; Nishimura et al., 2014).

Although considered one organ, the heart functions as two pumps. The right side of the heart receives unoxygenated blood from the body in the right atrium. Blood flows through the tricuspid valve to the right ventricle until systole when blood is forced through the pulmonary valve into the pulmonary vasculature primarily for exchange of carbon dioxide for oxygen. Returning from the pulmonary vasculature, blood flows into the left atrium through the mitral valve to the left ventricle where it is pumped through the aortic valve and the systemic circulation during systole. Due to the greater area of circulation and resistance the left side of the heart pumps to, pressure in the left side of the heart is higher than the pressure in the right heart (Darovic, 2002a).

Pressure and functional valves play a key role in blood flow through the heart. As the pressure builds in the atrium during diastole or relaxation, the valve between the atrium and ventricle opens allowing blood to fill the lower chamber. With atrial contraction, more blood is forced into the ventricle. This is called the atrial kick and ensures the ventricle is adequately filled. The difference in pressure between the atria (higher as it is filling) and the ventricles (lower after the majority of blood is ejected during systole) facilitates blood flow. Integrity of the valve connecting the chambers is critical at this point. Healthy valves allow flow in one direction only. Therefore, as pressure

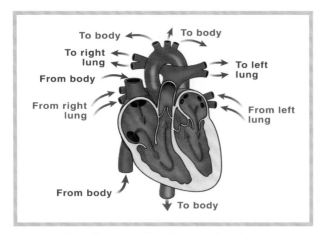

FIGURE 9–1. Linear illustration of blood flow through the heart. (With permission from Association of Women's Health, Obstetric and Neonatal Nurses.)

builds in the ventricle and certainly during ventricular systole, the valve shuts and prevents blood from moving back into the atrium forcing the flow into either the pulmonary (on the right) or systemic (on the left) circulation. The coordination of atrial and ventricular contractions with one way valves is necessary for maximal flow of blood through the heart (Darovic, 2002a). Lack of either can impact cardiac output severely in women with cardiac disease. For this reason, early detection and management of arrhythmias is a key part of the plan of care for women with cardiac disease (Lima et al., 2017). Figure 9–1 offers a conceptualization of the conduit of flow through the heart.

Once blood enters the systemic circulation, a fine meshwork of arteries and veins transport blood through the body. Arteries are muscular vessels that regulate blood flow based on cellular metabolic requirements. Veins return blood back to the heart and serve as a reservoir for as much as 70% of the circulating blood volume. Dilation or constriction of the venous bed occurs to accommodate the needs of the circulatory system. For example, in circumstances of low circulating blood volume, constriction of the veins can redistribute volume to augment circulation (Darovic, 2002a).

The conduction system in the cardiac muscle induces regular coordinated contractions between the upper and lower chambers of the heart to help optimize forward flow of blood. The sinoatrial (SA) node is in the right atrium and is established as the primary pacemaker of the heart, initiating and setting the pulse (Darovic, 2002a). The atrioventricular node offers backup if conduction through the SA node is impaired or damaged. The heart is innervated or stimulated by the autonomic nervous system (i.e., sympathetic and parasympathetic nervous systems). Nerve receptors in the heart are stimulated by the release of epinephrine

and norepinephrine from the sympathetic nervous system. Stimulation of beta-adrenergic receptors results in an increase in discharge from the SA node, augments the automaticity of cells in the heart, and improves contractility of the atria and ventricles (Darovic, 2002a). During pregnancy, the occurrence of arrhythmias is more frequent regardless of the presence of heart disease. Although the exact mechanism is not known, the physiologic CV changes of pregnancy are likely responsible (Deen et al., 2017). Premature atrial contractions, premature ventricular contractions, supraventricular tachycardia, and more rarely ventricular arrhythmias have been reported during pregnancy (Antony, Racusin, Aagaard, & Dildy, 2017; Canobbio et al., 2017).

The CV system undergoes tremendous physiologic change during pregnancy to support the growing fetus and prepare the woman for birth. The tissues of the heart go through a remodeling process during pregnancy that results in enlargement or hypertrophy and expansion of the capillary bed to supply adequate oxygenation for the increased workload. For this reason, a chest X-ray is not used to diagnose cardiac disease during pregnancy as an enlarged heart is a common finding (Antony et al., 2017; Deen et al., 2017). See Table 9–1 for a review of physiologic changes during pregnancy that impact CV disease.

Hemodynamics and Cardiac Output

The movement of blood through the body is essential for life. A major component of the movement of blood or hemodynamics is cardiac output. Cardiac output can be defined as the amount of blood pumped through the heart and is measured in liters per minute (Darovic, Graham, & Pranulis, 2002). Cardiac output is determined by four variables: preload, afterload, contractility, and heart rate. Normal hemodynamic values in pregnancy are listed in Table 9–2. Preload is the volume of blood in the ventricle or tension placed on the myocardial fibers as contraction begins at end diastole. Preload is primarily influenced by circulating blood volume available to fill the ventricle (Darovic, 2002b). If the volume of blood returning to the heart is diminished, as in hypotension, the subsequent decrease in preload reduces cardiac output. The cardiac muscle has the intrinsic ability to respond to variances in filling pressures, which allows for healthy adaptation to stress. This adaptation is challenged by the rise in cardiac output during pregnancy, which usually peaks between the midportion of the second and third trimesters (Antony et al., 2017). Preload is reported as central venous pressure (CVP) in the right side of the heart and as pulmonary capillary wedge pressure in the left side of the heart (Darovic, 2002b; Darovic & Kumar, 2002).

TABLE 9–1. Selected Physiologic Changes of Pregnancy that Impact Cardiac Disease

System	Change
Cardiovascular System	
Total blood volume	Increased 40% to 50%
Plasma volume	Increased 50%
Red cell volume	Increased 18% to 25%
Heart rate	Increased 17% (15 to 20 bpm)
Ejection fraction	Unchanged
Uterine blood flow	Receives 17% of carbon dioxide at term gestation
Coagulation System	
Platelets	Decreased in number, increase in function
Factors I, VII, VIII, IX, X	Greatly increased
Factors II, V, XII	Slightly increased or unchanged
Factors XI, XIII	Decreased
Plasminogen activator	Decreased
Plasminogen activator inhibitor-1	Decreased
Plasminogen activator inhibitor-2	Greatly decreased
Protein S (total and free levels)	Greatly decreased by term
Protein C	Unchanged
Antithrombin III	Unchanged

From Antony, K. M., Racusin, D. A., Aagaard, K., & Dildy, G. A. (2017). Maternal physiology. In S. G. Gabbe, J. R. Niebyl, J. L. Simpson, M. B. Landon, H. L. Galan, E. R. M. Jauniaux, ... W. A. Grobman (Eds.), *Obstetrics: Normal and problem pregnancies* (7th ed., pp. 38–63). Philadelphia, PA: Elsevier; Deen, J., Chandrasekaran, S., Stout, K., & Easterling, T. (2017). Heart disease in pregnancy. In S. G. Gabbe, J. R. Niebyl, J. L. Simpson, M. B. Landon, H. L. Galan, E. R. M. Jauniaux, ... W. A. Grobman (Eds.), *Obstetrics: Normal and problem pregnancies* (7th ed., pp. 803–827). Philadelphia, PA: Elsevier.

Afterload is defined as the resistance the ventricle has to overcome to eject blood during systole (Darovic, 2002b). Afterload the right ventricle pumps against is expressed by pulmonary artery pressure or pulmonary vascular resistance. SVR or the patient's blood pressure provides afterload to the left ventricle. During pregnancy, the influence of progesterone is thought to decrease peripheral vascular resistance, thereby decreasing afterload. As a result, a drop in blood pressure during the second trimester is a common finding (Antony et al., 2017).

TABLE 9–2. Normal Hemodynamic Values in Late Pregnancy

Parameter	Value and standard deviation
Cardiac output (L/min)	6.2 ± 1.0
Systemic vascular resistance (dynes/sec/cm^{-5})	1,210 ± 266
Pulmonary vascular resistance (dynes/sec/cm^{-5})	78 ± 22
Mean arterial pressure (mm Hg)	90 ± 6
Pulmonary capillary wedge pressure (mm Hg)	8 ± 2
Central venous pressure (mm Hg)	4 ± 3
Left ventricular stroke work index (g/min/m^{-2})	48 ± 6

Adapted from Clark, S. L., Cotton, D. B., Lee, W., Bishop, C., Hill, T., Southwick, J., ... Tolley, D. T. (1989). Central hemodynamic assessment of normal term pregnancy. *American Journal of Obstetrics & Gynecology, 161*(6, Pt. 1), 1439–1442. doi:10.1016/0002-9378(89)90900-9

Contractility is an independent intrinsic ability of the cardiac muscle to shorten aside from influences by preload and afterload (Darovic, 2002b). Contractility is measured indirectly by the left ventricular stroke work index. Heart rate is the final component of cardiac output. The speed at which the cardiac muscle pumps can influence output either positively or negatively. Excessively high heart rates lead to a decrease in filling time of the ventricles and reduction in output. During trauma, dysfunction, or disease, the human heart will alter heart rate (i.e., pulse) prior to detectable influences on any of the other remaining parameters (Darovic, 2002a). In cases of severe hypovolemia, the heart rate may rise appreciably before changes in the peripheral vascular resistance (i.e., blood pressure) are evident. Therefore, blood pressure and pulse are two vital signs reflective of cardiac output and cardiac disease. As a result, accuracy of assessment for both parameters and careful evaluation of trends is a key part of thorough patient assessment.

CARDIAC ADAPTATIONS OF PREGNANCY

Normal pregnancy may precipitate signs and symptoms of dyspnea upon exertion, peripheral edema (mild), elevated heart rate (increase of 10 to 20 beats above normal), jugular vein distention (maximum of +2 cm), systolic murmurs, palpitations, and cardiomegaly (Deen et al., 2017; Emmanuel & Thorne, 2015). For this reason, it can be difficult to determine if symptoms experienced by the woman are normal changes found in

TABLE 9–3. Normal Pregnancy Symptoms versus Symptoms of Cardiac Disease

Pregnancy: May be present	Cardiac disease from any cause: May be present
• Fatigue • Exertional dyspnea (usually limited to third trimester) • Irregular or infrequent syncope • Palpations (brief, irregular, and asymptomatic) • Jugular venous distention • Mild tachycardia <15% rise • Grade II/VI systolic murmur • Peripheral edema (mild) • Cardiomegaly	• Decreased ability to perform activities of daily living • Severe breathlessness, orthopnea, paroxysmal nocturnal dyspnea, or cough • Chest pain (not normal in pregnancy) • Cyanosis, clubbing • Jugular venous distention <2 cm • Loud, harsh systolic murmurs • Sustained arrhythmias • Ventricular murmurs • Pleural effusion • Pulmonary edema

From Arif, S., & Thorne, S. A. (2014). Heart disease in pregnancy. *Medicine, 42*(11), 644–649. doi:10.1016/j.mpmed.2014.08.011; Deen, J., Chandrasekaran, S., Stout, K., & Easterling, T. (2017). Heart disease in pregnancy. In S. G. Gabbe, J. R. Niebyl, J. L. Simpson, M. B. Landon, H. L. Galan, E. R. M. Jauniaux, . . . W. A. Grobman (Eds.), *Obstetrics: Normal and problem pregnancies* (7th ed., pp. 803–827). Philadelphia, PA: Elsevier; and Emmanuel, Y., & Thorne, S. A. (2015). Heart disease in pregnancy. *Best Practice & Research. Clinical Obstetrics & Gynaecology, 29*(5), 579–597. doi:10.1016/j.bpobgyn.2015.04.002

pregnancy or an indication of cardiac disease. Table 9–3 outlines normal cardiac changes during pregnancy compared to abnormal signs and symptoms of cardiac disease. Symptoms indicative of heart disease include severe dyspnea, pleural effusion, hemoptysis, paroxysmal nocturnal dyspnea, crackles in the lungs, cyanosis, clubbing, diastolic murmurs, sustained cardiac arrhythmias, loud harsh systolic murmurs, venous jugular distention <2 cm, and chest pain with exertion (Arif & Thorne, 2014; Deen et al., 2017; Emmanuel & Thorne, 2015). Prompt intervention is warranted if signs or symptoms abnormal for pregnancy are present.

The physiologic changes of pregnancy that tend to be problematic for women with cardiac disease include the increase in blood volume, decrease in SVR, the hypercoagulable state of pregnancy, and fluctuations in cardiac output (Deen et al., 2017; Ghandi & Shamshirsaz, 2016). The increase in blood volume may be problematic for women with stenotic heart valves, impaired ventricular function, or congenital artery disease. The inability of the heart to handle the extra volume can lead to failure or an ischemic event. In diseases associated with weakened arterial vessels such as Marfan syndrome (MFS) or coarctation, the pressure from extra blood volume may cause an aneurysm or dissection (Deen et al., 2017; Ghandi & Shamshirsaz, 2016).

Decrease in SVR is problematic for women with abnormal connections between the right and left heart or shunts. Because the left side of the heart is under higher pressure than the right side, oxygenated blood will shunt through defects between the two sides of the heart from the left side to the right side. In the short term, this can be tolerated by the heart and the body as oxygenated blood is being recirculated through the lungs. When the SVR drops in pregnancy, this dynamic can change with potential for blood to shunt from the right side of the heart to the left. In this case, deoxygenated blood is contributing

to cardiac output ultimately resulting in decreased oxygen content in arterial blood (Deen et al., 2017; Ghandi & Shamshirsaz, 2016).

The hypercoagulable state of pregnancy increases the risk of clot formation for women with artificial heart valves and some forms of arrhythmia. Particularly in atrial fibrillation, blood can collect and clots form in the atria due to ineffective emptying from the lack of coordinated atrial and ventricular contractions. The need to achieve anticoagulation can increase the risk of postpartum hemorrhage following birth (Ghandi & Shamshirsaz, 2016). Finally, the dynamic changes in cardiac output throughout pregnancy can precipitate a crisis when disease is present that requires a constant amount of blood volume to maintain output, as in pulmonary hypertension, or when the cardiac output is fixed, as in mitral stenosis. Maternal position has a significant impact on cardiac output. For the majority of women with cardiac disease, the lateral recumbent position is the most desirable and the supine position is avoided, even during birth. The lateral recumbent position supports venous return to the heart, while supine hypotension can result in a precipitous drop in venous return and therefore cardiac output (Arafeh & Baird, 2006; Canobbio et al., 2017).

During pregnancy, cardiac output steadily increases until it is nearly double. An increase of approximately 12% and 51% occurs in the first stage and second stage of labor, respectively (Antony et al., 2017). Uterine contractions may enhance cardiac output by as much as 30% due to the increased blood volume that is displaced back into the systemic circulation (Ghandi & Shamshirsaz, 2016). Uterine contractions also result in marked increases in both systolic and diastolic blood pressure (Antony et al., 2017). The first 30 minutes following birth yields the highest cardiac output during pregnancy, an increase of 60% to 80% over prepregnancy cardiac output. Therefore, the immediate postpartum period is one of the most stressful times (from the standpoint of the CV system) of all pregnancy, labor, and birth (Antony et al., 2017; Canobbio et al., 2017). See Table 9–8.

OBSTETRIC OUTCOMES AND ASSESSMENT OF RISK

When the woman with cardiac disease presents prenatally or ideally for preconception counseling, estimating the risk pregnancy and birth poses to her and her baby is an important part of counseling and developing a plan of care. Risk may occur from cardiac disease as well as other factors such as obesity, tobacco use, and presence of other chronic disease states. Women with congenital heart defects may have increased risk of passing the defect to the baby. The importance of preconception counseling for women with cardiac disease cannot be overstated. Evaluation of the cardiac condition prior to pregnancy will allow the woman to make an informed decision about pursuing pregnancy, and in some situations, correction of a lesion or condition can increase the likelihood of successful pregnancy (ACOG, 2019; Safi & Tsiaras, 2017; Yucel & DeFaria Yeh, 2017).

Assessment of the risk that cardiac disease presents can be evaluated by different methods and testing. For example, women can undergo exercise stress testing before pregnancy to simulate her cardiac response to the physiologic changes of pregnancy (Canobbio et al., 2017; Nishimura et al., 2014; Safi & Tsiaras, 2017; Yucel & DeFaria Yeh, 2017). At a minimum, the following are required for initial evaluation: thorough history with emphasis on cardiac disease, current medication regimen, arterial blood gas measurement, laboratory tests to evaluate blood levels (blood cell counts and electrolyte levels) and basic organ function, electrocardiogram (ECG), echocardiogram, consideration of an exercise stress test, and genetic consult (Canobbio et al., 2017). As stated earlier, chest X-ray is not helpful for evaluation of cardiac disease due to normal physiologic enlargement of the heart during pregnancy. Other imaging tests such as magnetic resonance imaging, computed tomography, and cardiac catheterization are done based on the need for information from the test and risk to the fetus (Canobbio et al., 2017).

Methods of risk assessment are composed of categories that are based on the features of an individual's heart disease or the woman's ability to function without symptoms of heart failure or both. The methods may be used independently but are most often used in a combination of several methods. While it may seem redundant to routinely use several methods, given the relative rarity of cardiac disease in pregnancy and lack of established guidelines to manage cardiac disease in pregnancy, it may be worthwhile to examine risk to the woman from the perspective of each method.

TABLE 9–4. New York Heart Association Functional Classification System

Class	Description
I	Asymptomatic No limitation of physical activity
II	Asymptomatic at rest; symptomatic with heavy physical activity and exertion Slight limitation of physical activity
III	Asymptomatic at rest; symptomatic with minimal or normal physical activity Considerable limitation of physical activity
IV	Symptomatic at rest; symptomatic with any physical activity Severe limitation of physical activity

From Criteria Committee of the New York Heart Association. (1979). *Nomenclature and criteria for diagnosis of diseases of the heart and great vessels* (8th ed.). Boston, MA: Little, Brown.

The first risk assessment method is the New York Heart Association (NYHA) functional classification (Table 9–4). This is the oldest of the methods and is based on the functional ability of the person with cardiac disease regardless of what that disease may be. The patient is assessed either by questioning or by direct observation of symptoms in response to activity. Symptoms of interest include dyspnea, chest pain, and shortness of breath. This risk assessment is particularly helpful in pregnancy to document changes in functional status that are expected in response to the physiologic changes of pregnancy. Progression to a higher NYHA classification should prompt further evaluation due to the association with higher maternal morbidity and mortality. Determining functional classification on a regular basis such as during prenatal visits, frequently during labor, and with each postpartum assessment can uncover a trend that may indicate a decline in status.

Mortality risk can be estimated based on the type of lesion or disease present. In Display 9–1, cardiac disease is divided into groups based on a modification of the World Health Organization (WHO) categorization of heart disease and use of contraceptives. Due to the prominence of cardiac disease in maternal mortality and findings of inadequate care of women with cardiac disease, an expert panel was assembled to develop a category system to guide use of contraception and referral during pregnancy to a knowledgeable health care team. The goals for development were to assist with proper contraception to avoid pregnancy when desirable, alert care providers of the risk pregnancy may entail with specific cardiac disease in hopes of encouraging preconception planning and finally to recommend the proper level of care during pregnancy based on the woman's cardiac disease (Thorne, MacGregor, & Nelson-Piercy, 2006). Group I consists of lesions that generally have a mortality rate that is

DISPLAY 9-1

Maternal Cardiovascular Risk Classification (Modified World Health Organization [WHO] Classification)

Group I

Mortality and morbidity: not detectably greater risk than the general population

- Effectively repaired: atrial septal defect, ventricular septal defect, patent ductus arteriosus, total anomalous pulmonary venous drainage
- Isolated atrial and ventricular ectopic beats
- Uncomplicated or small patent ductus arteriosus, ventricular septal defect, pulmonary stenosis, mitral valve prolapse with insignificant regurgitation

Group II

Mortality and morbidity: slight increase risk

- Woman is well with no other complications:
  - Majority of arrhythmias
  - Tetralogy of Fallot, repaired
  - Unrepaired atrial septal defect

Groups II to III

Mortality and morbidity: encompasses risk of group II to III dependent on the status of the woman

- Aortic dilation <45 mm in bicuspid aortic valve aortopathy
- Bicuspid aortic valve aortopathy (aorta dilated <45 mm)
- Cardiomyopathy (hypertrophic)

- Coarctation (repaired)
- Heart transplant
- Left ventricular dysfunction (mild)
- Native or tissue valvular heart disease that is not in group IV (modified WHO classification)
- Marfan syndrome (no aortic dilation)

Group III

Mortality and morbidity: significant risk requiring care by providers with expertise in cardiac disease during pregnancy (cardiologist, maternal–fetal medicine specialist) from preconception throughout entire pregnancy including postpartum

- Complex congenital heart disease
- Cyanotic heart disease
- Fontan repair
- Mechanical heart valve
- Systemic right ventricle (repaired transposition of great vessels)

Group IV

Mortality and morbidity: very high risk of severe morbidity and of mortality, pregnancy contraindicated. Termination recommended if pregnancy occurs. Ongoing pregnancies require same level of care as group III.

- Left ventricular dysfunction with high New York Heart Association class or ejection fraction <30%
- Marfan syndrome (aortic dilation >40 mm)
- Previous peripartum cardiomyopathy with any residual left ventricular dysfunction
- Pulmonary arterial hypertension
- Severe obstruction in left heart (severe aortic or mitral stenosis)

Adapted from Balci, A., Sollie-Szarynska, K. M., van der Bijl, A. G. L., Ruys, T. P., Mulder, B. J., Roos-Hesselink, J. W., . . . Pieper, P. G. (2014). Prospective validation and assessment of cardiovascular and offspring risk models for pregnant women with congenital heart disease. *Heart (British Cardiac Society)*, *100*(17), 1373–1381. doi:10.1136/heartjnl-2014-305597; Canobbio, M. M., Warnes, C. A., Aboulhosn, J., Connolly, H. M., Khanna, A., Koos, B. J., . . . Stout, K. (2017). Management of pregnancy in patients with complex congenital heart disease: A scientific statement for healthcare professionals from the American Heart Association. *Circulation*, *135*(8), e50–e87. doi:10.1161/CIR.0000000000000458; and Thorne, S., MacGregor, A., & Nelson-Piercy, C. (2006). Risks of contraception and pregnancy in heart disease. *Heart*, *92*(10), 1520–1525. doi:10.1136/hrt.2006.095240

not distinguishable from the general risk of pregnancy. Group II have moderate risk of an adverse event during pregnancy and a slightly higher mortality rate. The risk of complications is considerable in group III with a significant increase of mortality. Women who are in group IV are counseled that the risk of achieving or continuing pregnancy is too great to consider. If pregnancy is continued with group IV disease, care is similar to that recommended for group III disease with a higher risk of mortality and morbidity (Canobbio et al., 2017; Thorne et al., 2006).

In Display 9–2, Siu and colleagues (2001) offer additional guidance regarding potential risk of a cardiac event during pregnancy; 562 women with cardiac disease were followed during pregnancy to determine occurrence of cardiac events. Cardiac events were divided into two groups, primary or secondary. A primary cardiac event was defined as pulmonary edema, persistent symptomatic tachycardia or bradycardia necessitating treatment, stroke, cardiac arrest, or cardiac death. Secondary cardiac events included decrease in functional ability as defined by the NYHA classification and the need for emergent invasive cardiac procedures during pregnancy through 6 months postpartum (Siu et al., 2001). Four predictors of events were identified: previous cardiac complication or arrhythmia, presence of cyanosis or NYHA class II or greater at the beginning of pregnancy, left heart obstruction, and decreased left ventricle function. As the number of predictors that are present increase, so does the risk of a cardiac event. If the woman's cardiac history has all four predictors, then a healthcare provider should counsel her to reconsider attempting pregnancy. It should also be noted that even with no predictors present, risk of having an event is assessed at 5% (Siu et al., 2001).

DISPLAY 9–2
Predictors of Cardiac Events

Prior cardiac event before pregnancy
  Heart failure
  Stroke or transient ischemic attack
Arrhythmia
New York Heart Association > class II
Cyanosis
Obstruction left heart
  Gradient >30 mm Hg peak
  Aortic valve <1.5 cm^2
  Mitral valve prolapse <2 cm^2
Ejection fraction <40%
Number of predictors equals risk of cardiac events during
  pregnancy: 0 = 5%, 1 = 27%, >1 = 75%

Adapted from Siu, S. C., Sermer, M., Colman, J. M., Alvarez, A. N., Mercier, L. A., Morton, B. C., . . . Sorensen, S. (2001). Prospective multicenter study of pregnancy outcomes in women with heart disease. *Circulation, 104*(5), 515–521. doi:10.1161/hc3001.093437

Drenthen et al. (2010) used the risk assessment tool just described in 1,302 pregnancies complicated with CHD. Arrhythmias and heart failure were the most common cardiac events noted in this cohort. When comparing the risk assessment tool prediction to outcomes, it was found that risk was overestimated. The authors caution that use of a risk assessment tool be merely one part of a comprehensive evaluation of the woman and her specific cardiac disease (Drenthen et al., 2010).

Comparison of outcomes from the tools developed by Sui and colleagues (referred to as the CARPREG tool) and the modified WHO classification are of importance when determining risk during pregnancy. An interdisciplinary care team in a university setting followed 164 women who had 179 pregnancies over a 5-year period (January 2007 to 2012) using all of the risk category tools. No maternal deaths occurred and the complication rate was reported at 13.4%. The modified WHO classification was the most accurate tool for predicting cardiac events; however, the findings are limited by the scarce number of women in the higher risk categories prompting a recommendation for further study of all risk assessment tools and classification (Pijuan-Domènech et al., 2015).

Another study used the modified WHO risk scoring classification in 2,742 women globally using the Registry of Pregnancy and Cardiac Disease (ROPAC). The aim of this study was to further validate the modified WHO risk classification and determine if there was a difference in performance in advanced versus emerging countries. The majority of women in the study (1,827) were from advanced countries. The overall rate of cardiac complications was 20.6%, and of this percentage, 12.8% occurred in advanced countries. As expected, over half of the cardiac complications occurred in group IV women, but actually, more cardiac events were reported in group I (9.9%) than group II (7.7%), emphasizing that although risk is low in group I, it does exist. The modified WHO classification was found to be helpful in predicting cardiac complications but was more accurate in advanced than emerging countries. The study also found that adding two qualifiers present prior to pregnancy, atrial fibrillation and signs of heart failure, improved predictive ability (van Hagen et al., 2016). The ROPAC data was used again to determine if the modified WHO classification was predictive of obstetric (such as preeclampsia or hemorrhage) and fetal complications. It was not found be an accurate predictor of either (van Hagen et al., 2017).

Other types of parameters may be used to determine risk. Serum B-type natriuretic peptide (BNP) and N-terminal pro-B-type natriuretic peptide (NT-proBNP) are examples of such parameters. These levels increase in response to stretching of the myocytes in the atria and ventricles as volume in the heart increases with cardiac dysfunction. In nonpregnant adults, BNP and NT-proBNP are used to aid in diagnosis and management of heart failure (Januzzi & Mann, 2015). These levels can be used in a similar way during pregnancy but with different values as both are increased (approximately doubled) even during uncomplicated pregnancies (Canobbio et al., 2017). A study of 78 pregnant women was conducted, 66 with heart disease and 12 without, that followed BNP levels throughout pregnancy to determine if elevated BNP levels correlated with a cardiac event during the pregnancy. BNP levels were lower throughout pregnancy in the group without heart disease. Elevations in BNP were not conclusively predictive of a cardiac event, but a level of less than 100 pg/mL in women with cardiac disease was found to have a negative predictive value of 100% (Tanous et al., 2010). The ability of NT-proBNP to predict a cardiac event was studied in a group of 203 pregnant women with CHD with a total of 213 pregnancies over a 3.5-year period (March 2008 to August 2011). NT-proBNP level was measured at 20 weeks' gestation. Twenty-two women experienced a cardiac complication, and of those, 82.4% had an NT-proBNP level of 128 pg/mL or higher. Similar to findings with BNP, NT-proBNP levels below 128 pg/mL at 20 weeks' gestation successfully predicted no cardiac event later in pregnancy (Kampman et al., 2014). Deen et al. (2017) report using BNP and NT-proBNP as one method of guiding volume replacement during pregnancy. The values used are BNP of 100 pg/mL or less and NT-proBNP of 125 pg/mL or less (Deen et al., 2017).

The risk of cardiac events late after birth can also be predicted. Balint et al. (2010) reviewed 405 pregnancies to determine characteristics predictive of cardiac events that occur greater than 6 months after birth. Late events included cardiac arrest/death, pulmonary edema, arrhythmia, and stroke. Characteristics associated with late events were NYHA class II or higher, presence of cyanosis, subaortic ventricular dysfunction, subpulmonary ventricular dysfunction, pulmonary regurgitation, left heart obstruction, and cardiac complications before pregnancy (Balint et al., 2010). Evaluation for these characteristics can assist in determining how long to carefully assess and hospitalize the woman after birth as well as direct home instructions and guide frequency of follow-up after discharge.

CONGENITAL HEART DISEASE IN PREGNANCY

CHD occurs in approximately 0.8% of live births (Deen et al., 2017). Advances in neonatal care and pediatric cardiac surgery have resulted in a significant improvement in survival rates for babies born with CHD (Canobbio et al., 2017; Emmanuel & Thorne, 2015; Yucel & DeFaria Yeh, 2017). As these infants are reaching reproductive age, more women are beginning pregnancy with medical histories of significant cardiac surgical repairs from CHD (Canobbio et al., 2017; Yucel & DeFaria Yeh, 2017). Even with minor CHD, a woman may be at increased risk during pregnancy if other medical conditions are present such as hypertension. Conditions associated with heart failure in women with complex CHD include development of tachyarrhythmias, obstetric complications, history of heart failure prior to pregnancy, ejection fraction <40%, NYHA class III or greater, and WHO risk group III or greater (Canobbio et al., 2017). When sexual maturity is achieved in girls with CHD, counseling suitable to their age is necessary to review the importance of planning pregnancy in the future due to the impact it will have on their cardiac condition. For all women with CHD, the risk of transference of CHD to the fetus is a critical part of preconception counselling (Canobbio et al., 2017). For ease of discussion, congenital lesions are categorized as acyanotic, cyanotic, or aortic.

Acyanotic Congenital Heart Disease

Acyanotic lesions that involve an abnormal opening in the septum between the right and left side of the heart include atrial septal defect and ventricular septal defect (VSD). Because pressures are typically higher on the left side of the heart, blood flows from left to right, as described earlier. Long-term shunting of extra blood volume to the right side of the heart can cause right ventricular hypertrophy. Extension of that enlargement into the right atrium increases the risk of atrial arrhythmias (Deen et al., 2017). Large septal defects, particularly VSD, can result in hypertension in the pulmonary circulation. Development of pulmonary hypertension can create bidirectional flow or a reverse of the shunt where blood flows from the right to the left side of the heart due to the resistance or afterload exerted by the pulmonary vasculature. This change in shunt flow results in Eisenmenger syndrome and is associated with cyanosis due to unoxygenated blood contributing to cardiac output leading to poor outcomes during pregnancy (Deen et al., 2017). For this reason, large septal defects are usually repaired in childhood. Septal defects also create portals for emboli movement and increase the risk of thromboembolytic injury to the arterial circulation (Deen et al., 2017; Yucel & DeFaria Yeh, 2017). Other acyanotic lesions include pulmonic and aortic stenosis. The degree of stenosis or narrowing of the valve determines the impact on blood flow and cardiac output (Yucel & DeFaria Yeh, 2017).

Cyanotic Congenital Heart Disease

Cyanotic cardiac lesions include tetralogy of Fallot (TOF), transposition of the great vessels, and those with a single functioning ventricle. TOF consists of four defects: (1) VSD, (2) overriding aorta (dextroposition of the aorta so that the aortic orifice sits astride the VSD and overrides the right ventricle), (3) right ventricular hypertrophy, and (4) pulmonary stenosis (Yucel & DeFaria Yeh, 2017). The majority of patients with TOF will have correction of the VSD during childhood (Deen et al., 2017). Although closure of the VSD will decrease risk during pregnancy, a moderate risk of morbidity and small increase in mortality remains. Uncorrected TOF is associated with a higher rate of maternal morbidity and mortality with a poorer prognosis for the fetus (Canobbio et al., 2017; Thorne et al., 2006).

Transposition of the great vessels occurs in two varieties: levo-transposition (L-TGA) and dextro-transposition (D-TGA) (Canobbio et al., 2017; Yucel & DeFaria Yeh, 2017). In L-TGA, the vessels along with the atria and ventricles are switched. This type of TGA is described as congenitally corrected. L-TGA may not be detected until later in life, while D-TGA results in cyanosis soon after birth. In D-TGA, only the great vessels are reversed. D-TGA requires surgical intervention to restore delivery of oxygenated blood to the systemic circulation. The original surgical reversal procedure involved an atrial switch, while more recent procedures perform an arterial switch. Prognosis for the mother and fetus depends on the type of TGA, the type of corrective surgery that was performed, and functional cardiac status (Deen et al., 2017; Yucel & DeFaria Yeh, 2017). Close collaboration between cardiology and obstetric care providers is required to determine current cardiac function and prognosis.

Congenital defects that result in a single ventricle such as hypoplastic left heart or tricuspid atresia require palliative surgery known as the Fontan procedure. Fontan circulation diverts blood from the venous circulation into the pulmonary circulation and utilizes the single ventricle as the "left" ventricle for systemic circulation. The surgical procedure may vary due to the underlying lesion that requires correction. Due to the altered cardiac circulation and hemodynamics, care of the pregnant woman who has undergone a Fontan procedure should occur in a facility with comprehensive experience in cardiac disease in pregnancy (Canobbio et al., 2017; Yucel & DeFaria Yeh, 2017).

Aortic Congenital Heart Disease

Disease of the aorta includes MFS and coarctation. Coarctation of the aorta is an area of narrowing and is usually associated with hypertension of the upper extremities (Ghandi & Shamshirsaz, 2016). Treatment can be challenging when trying to control upper extremity hypertension and still maintain adequate perfusion to the uterus and fetus (Yucel & DeFaria Yeh, 2017). It is important to determine if other defects exist in conjunction with the coarctation and, if so, to utilize risk scoring to assess the risk of pregnancy (Thorne et al., 2006; Yucel & DeFaria Yeh, 2017). The main complications associated with coarctation include aortic dissection, aneurysm, and rupture. If indicated, corrective surgery should precede pregnancy; otherwise, blood pressure titration can be attempted (Yucel & DeFaria Yeh, 2017).

MFS is a connective tissue disorder that is inherited as an autosomal dominant trait. Effect of the disorder on the CV system is the leading cause of death, although connective tissue from other organ systems may also be affected (Yucel & DeFaria Yeh, 2017). In MFS, connective tissue is weakened and, in the case of the aorta, can expand under the constant pressure of blood being pumped from the left ventricle. The expansion further weakens the aorta, making it vulnerable to dissection or rupture. The alterations in hemodynamics during pregnancy can exacerbate the effect. However, aortic involvement such as aortic root dilation, dissection, and rupture are the most significant complications for any person with MFS (Lim et al., 2017). The risk of aortic dissection is based on the amount of dilation that has occurred. Risk is higher when the aorta is 40 mm or greater; however, it should be noted that dissection has occurred with a normal size aortic root (Lim et al., 2017; Yucel & DeFaria Yeh, 2017).

Ideally, the woman with MFS should undergo careful evaluation by a multidisciplinary team prior to pregnancy. The size of the ascending aorta is a key assessment. Usual medical treatment for a patient with a normal size aorta is the use of beta-blockers such as atenolol to reduce the velocity of the arterial pulse wave and increase vascular distensibility (Emmanuel & Thorne, 2015; Lim et al., 2017; Yucel & DeFaria Yeh, 2017). Currently, it is recommended that surgical treatment occurs if the diameter of the aorta is greater than or equal to 45 mm in the pregnant woman (Emmanuel & Thorne, 2015). The size of the ascending aorta should be followed regularly throughout pregnancy because surgery may also be recommended if rapid dilation is noted. Vaginal birth is preferred for women with a normal size aorta, and cesarean birth is recommended when the aorta is dilated greater than or equal to 40 mm or is unstable (Lim et al., 2017; Yucel & DeFaria Yeh, 2017).

CHD varies in pathology and symptomatology with various surgical and medical treatments utilized to improve cardiac function. Therefore, it is the responsibility of healthcare providers to carefully assess the risk of pregnancy and be watchful for signs of deterioration of status. Close collaboration between pediatric cardiology and obstetric care providers supports development of a comprehensive, thorough, and individual plan of care (Yucel & DeFaria Yeh, 2017).

ACQUIRED CARDIAC DISEASE IN PREGNANCY

Acquired cardiac disease or disease that develops after birth is a growing contributor to maternal mortality and morbidity. As with CHD, women with acquired cardiac disease need information after diagnosis about the importance of preconception counseling if pregnancy is desired (Thorne et al., 2006). Acquired cardiac lesions that are discussed include valvular disorders, myocardial infarction (MI), and cardiomyopathy.

Valvular Disorders

Infection is a leading cause of acquired valvular disease. Etiology includes diseases such as rheumatic fever and endocarditis. In advanced countries, the incidence of rheumatic cardiac lesions has dropped significantly due to better environmental conditions and medical treatment of infection; however, this has not occurred in developing countries (Emmanuel & Thorne, 2015). In areas with a greater population of women immigrating from developing countries, valvular lesions are commonly seen (Emmanuel & Thorne, 2015). The lesion, typically seen on valves from endocarditis, is described as a mass of cells on the valve or on the surrounding tissue that includes inflammatory cells, microorganisms, fibrin, and platelets. Endocarditis can occur following intravenous (IV) drug abuse, hospital infections, or invasive medical procedures such as central line placement or hemodialysis (Baddour, Freeman, Suri, &

Wilson, 2015). A significant emerging cause of endocarditis is exposure during healthcare, particularly with drug-resistant organisms (Baddour et al., 2015). Due to the variety of presentations of valvular disease and replacement valves, thorough evaluation that includes at minimum an ECG and transthoracic echocardiogram plus risk assessment should be accomplished and discussed with the woman (Nishimura et al., 2014). Women with valvular disease should be referred to a center with cardiologists and maternal-fetal medicine specialists who have experience with valvular disease during pregnancy. Valvular surgery or replacement may be advised before attempting pregnancy depending on the severity of the lesion or during the course of pregnancy if the woman's clinical condition deteriorates (Nishimura et al., 2014; Safi & Tsiaras, 2017). Replacement valves may be mechanical or bioprosthetic. For women with bioprosthetic valves during pregnancy, roughly a third will require another valve replacement within a decade. Currently, the reason for replacement need is not known, but it is possible that bioprosthetic valves deteriorate more rapidly during pregnancy (Emmanuel & Thorne, 2015; Safi & Tsiaras, 2017).

Replacement valves are associated with clot formation and require anticoagulation therapy to decrease this risk. Situations associated with the highest risk of clot formation are presence of older model prosthetic valves such as Starr-Edwards or Björk-Shiley, prior history of clot formation on anticoagulants, or presence of atrial dysrhythmia (Deen et al., 2017). In general, any woman on anticoagulant therapy before pregnancy will need to continue anticoagulation during pregnancy. Unfractionated heparin or low molecular weight heparin are routinely used during pregnancy because they do not cross the placenta and affect the fetus (ACOG, 2018a). However, patients with mechanical heart valves are anticoagulated with warfarin because it is associated with the lowest risk of clot formation (Nishimura et al., 2014). Warfarin does cross the placenta to the fetus. In pregnancy, warfarin is used carefully due to teratogenic effects early in gestation and risk of fetal hemorrhage late in gestation (Nishimura et al., 2014). See Table 9–5 for recommended anticoagulation therapy. In addition, antibiotic prophylaxis should be considered at the time of birth for a previous history of infectious endocarditis, suspicion of infection or for cesarean birth (Emmanuel & Thorne, 2015).

Myocardial Infarction

Acute MI is infrequent during pregnancy with the highest risk of occurrence in the third trimester and postpartum (Emmanuel & Thorne, 2015; Lameijer et al., 2017). Risk factors for MI in pregnancy include typical causes such as hypertension, obesity, diabetes mellitus,

TABLE 9–5. Recommendations for Anticoagulation during Pregnancy

Drug regimens

Aspirin 75 to 100 mg/day with either mechanical or bioprosthetic valve during second and third trimesters

Mechanical valves

Warfarin recommended for all women in second and third trimester with a mechanical valve: therapeutic INR of 3.0
- Planned vaginal birth (more than 1 week before birth)
  - Discontinue warfarin; start **UFH** (aPTT >2 times control).
- Anticoagulation plan for labor
  - UFH is discontinued when labor is active and restarted after bleeding is no longer a risk (usually 6 to 8 hr after birth).
- Postpartum warfarin
  - Warfarin restarted 48 hr after birth depending risk of bleeding

First trimester options

- **Warfarin**: dose of 5 mg/day or less to achieve therapeutic INR
  - Can use during first trimester after counseling woman on risks
- **UFH**: continuous infusion, dose adjusted, aPTT >2 times control
- **LMWH**: administered at least twice daily, dose adjusted, anti-Xa 0.8 to 1.2 U/mL with level drawn 4 to 6 hr after dose

Women who present for birth and are anticoagulated require cesarean birth.

UFH given subcutaneous during pregnancy with mechanical valves is no longer recommended.

aPTT, activated partial thromboplastin time; INR, international normalized ratio; LMWH, low molecular weight heparin; UFH, unfractionated heparin.
From Nishimura, R. A., Otto, C. M., Bonow, R. O., Carabello, B. A., Erwin, J. P., III, Guyton, R. A., . . . Thomas, J. D. (2014). 2014 AHA/ACC guideline for the management of patients with valvular heart disease: Executive summary: A report of the American College of Cardiology/American Heart Association Task Force on Practice Guidelines. *Journal of the American College of Cardiology, 63*(22), 2438–2488. doi:10.1016/j.jacc.2014.02.537; Safi, L. M., & Tsiaras, S. V. (2017). Update on valvular heart disease in pregnancy. *Current Treatment Options in Cardiovascular Medicine, 19*(9), 70. doi:10.1007/s11936-017-0570-2

history of migraines, dyslipidemia, use of tobacco, and age older than 35 years as well as causes specific to pregnancy such as postpartum infection, and blood transfusion (Deen et al., 2017; Kennedy & Baird, 2016). Normal symptoms of pregnancy can mimic those of MI. Any suspicion of MI warrants evaluation with an ECG and laboratory analysis. ECG findings of elevated ST segment are not normal in pregnancy and suggest MI. Cardiac troponin I is unaffected by pregnancy, labor, or birth and therefore is the laboratory measurement of choice in the diagnosis of acute coronary syndrome during pregnancy (Deen et al., 2017; Kennedy & Baird, 2016).

The most important therapy for MI is reperfusion of the cardiac muscle as quickly as possible. This may be accomplished by performing percutaneous coronary intervention with a bare metal stent (Emmanuel & Thorne, 2015). Maternal mortality risk increases if birth occurs within 2 weeks of the MI. Close consultation between obstetric and cardiac providers needs to occur to determine the best course of management including anticoagulation and timing of birth for each individual woman (Deen et al., 2017; Kennedy & Baird, 2016).

Cardiomyopathy

Cardiomyopathy is a disease of the heart muscle resulting in failure. There are different types and causes of cardiomyopathy. Discussion in this chapter is confined to peripartum cardiomyopathy (PPCM). PPCM is defined as cardiac failure with left ventricular ejection fraction <45% occurring in the last month of pregnancy or within 5 months of delivery, in the absence of any identifiable cause of heart failure; thus, PPCM is a diagnosis of exclusion (Johnson-Coyle, Jensen, & Sobey, 2012; Troiano, 2015). The cause of PPCM is unknown but has been attributed to viral disease, autoimmune disorder, inflammatory process mediated by cytokines, abnormal apoptosis, genetic inheritance, and excessive levels of prolactin among others. An occurrence rate of 1:1,300 to 1:15,000, depending on geographic location, makes this condition rare (Troiano, 2015). Risk factors include age older than 30 years, multiparity, twin pregnancy, race (African and African American reported to have higher incidence), and pregnancy-associated hypertension (Johnson-Coyle et al., 2012; Troiano, 2015). Diagnosis requires a careful history and physical, NYHA functional classification, ECG, and echocardiogram. Approximately 30% of women with PPCM will completely recover, with the remaining 70% left with residual effects of varying severity (Johnson-Coyle et al., 2012; Troiano, 2015). Management includes optimization of cardiac function with supportive therapies and pharmacologic treatment using diuretics, beta-blockers, vasodilators, and inotropic agents (Johnson-Coyle et al., 2012; Troiano, 2015). Vaginal birth is generally well tolerated (Troiano, 2015). Due to the delay in disease with occurrence in the third trimester or postpartum, fetal outcomes are usually positive.

CLINICAL MANAGEMENT

The underlying cardiac lesion, functional changes imposed by the lesion, maternal and fetal tolerance, and development of pregnancy-related complications affect perinatal morbidity and mortality. Developing baseline status of cardiac function through careful assessment and diagnostic testing such as echocardiography is crucial. Using this baseline for comparison during ongoing evaluation during pregnancy, labor, and the postpartum period guides the clinical management of women with cardiac disease (ACOG, 2019; Deen et al., 2017; Hameed, Morton, & Moore, 2017; Safi & Tsiaras, 2017; Yucel & DeFaria Yeh, 2017). A summary of common cardiac diseases, risk categories, and clinical management is presented in Table 9–6.

The goals of clinical management for a woman whose pregnancy is complicated by CV disease mirror the goals for optimum uteroplacental perfusion. Stabilization of the mother by maintaining cardiac output required during pregnancy will meet her perfusion needs and those of the fetal compartment. Meeting these goals requires a coordinated multidisciplinary team approach. For women at the highest risk, securing care with providers and hospital facilities experienced in cardiac disease during pregnancy needs to be done preconception or as early in the pregnancy as possible (ACOG, 2019; Canobbio et al., 2017). Management strategies should include estimates of maternal and fetal risk in order for the patient and her family to make an informed decision regarding her pregnancy. The primary practitioner should discuss issues regarding maternal age at the time of pregnancy, estimations of maternal and fetal mortality, potential chronic morbidity, antepartum interventions to minimize risk, and the birth method best suited to her underlying pathology (Canobbio et al., 2017; Deen et al., 2017; Ghandi & Shamshirsaz, 2016).

The primary focus in cardiac management during pregnancy, labor, and birth maximizes cardiac output while limiting metabolic demand. Careful evaluation of the pregnant woman at each prenatal visit with regular evaluation by cardiology and coordination of findings to develop and alter the plan of care is required. Heart failure and arrhythmias are common cardiac events that care providers need to be alert for throughout the pregnancy. Evaluation of the woman for signs of heart failure include assessment for increase in jugular venous distention, adventitious lung sounds, rapid onset of peripheral edema, or reports marked shortness of breath. Assessment for irregular heart rate or report of palpitations may indicate the onset of arrhythmia (ACOG, 2019; Canobbio et al., 2017; Emmanuel & Thorne, 2015; Safi & Tsiaras, 2017).

In the intrapartum period, administration of medications and intravascular volume may be necessary to optimize or minimize preload and afterload in order to maximize cardiac output depending on the underlying cardiac lesion. If any patient experiences heart failure, traditional treatment methods are used during pregnancy with the exception of use of angiotensin-converting enzyme inhibitors or angiotensin receptor blockers. These classes of drugs are associated with fetal and neonatal renal agenesis, failure, and death (Canobbio et al., 2017; Nishimura et al., 2014). See Table 9–7 for CV medications that may be administered to women with cardiac disease.

During the intrapartum period, control of anxiety, pain, and temperature can minimize fluctuation in heart rate. The goal is for labor to be short and pain free (Deen et al., 2017). ECG monitoring is required for women with arrhythmias and pharmacologic

TABLE 9–6. Cardiac Disease in Pregnancy

Cardiac disease/lesion	Risk category	Description	Clinical management
ASD	Small left-to-right shunt = low or minimal risk Large left-to-right shunt = intermediate or moderate risk depending on maternal symptoms	Opening between atria; usually, blood shunts from higher pressure on LA to the right; over time, this can cause enlargement of atria leading to arrhythmias and risk of clot formation	Challenging to diagnose by auscultation; during pregnancy, a pulmonary flow murmur may be heard. Assess for irregular HR/arrhythmias. Common arrhythmias—atrial fibrillation or flutter Assess for change in NYHA functional class. Optimize preload—avoid hypovolemia or hypervolemia. Avoid maternal hypotension—may increase left-to-right shunting. Avoid maternal tachycardia—may increase left-to-right shunting. Oxygen during labor Labor in lateral recumbent position Pain management: Consider narcotic epidural. Anticoagulation if thromboembolism risk
VSD	Small left-to-right shunt = low or minimal risk Large left-to-right shunt = intermediate or moderate risk depending on maternal symptoms	Opening between ventricles: • Small → tolerated well • Larger defects → associated with CHF, arrhythmia, and development of pulmonary hypertension • Left-to-right shunt → burdens pulmonary circulation → can lead to pulmonary hypertension	Physical examination: harsh systolic murmur ECG: normal in most patients Optimize preload—avoid hypovolemia or hypervolemia. Avoid maternal hypotension—may increase left-to-right shunting. Avoid maternal tachycardia—may increase left-to-right shunting. Oxygen during labor Labor in lateral recumbent position Pain management: Consider narcotic epidural.
Eisenmenger syndrome	High or major risk	Left-to-right congenital shunt that reverses to right side volume moving through shunt to the left side of the heart resulting in cyanosis	Physiologic changes of pregnancy contribute to shunt reverse in women with larger shunts. Careful, ongoing assessment of blood pressure, HR, respiratory rate, and SaO_2 Avoid hypotension—decrease in systemic vascular resistance causes massive right-to-left shunting leading to hypoxia. Avoid excessive blood loss. Consider arterial line and central line placement. Continuous oxygen therapy: SaO_2 >90% Avoid conditions that increase PVR. • Metabolic acidosis • Excess catecholamine • Hypoxemia • Hypercapnia • Vasoconstrictors • Lung hyperinflation High risk for thromboembolism—consider anticoagulation. Pain management: Consider narcotic epidural. Vigilant monitoring for up to 10 days postpartum
Aortic coarctation	Corrected associated with lower risk of complications Uncorrected, uncomplicated = intermediate or moderate risk Complicated = high or major risk	Congenital narrowing of aorta; most common site is the origin of the left subclavian artery. Associated anomalies: • VSD, PDA, aortic aneurysm. Intracranial aneurysms of the Circle of Willis are relatively common.	Avoid hypotension. Blood pressure in upper extremities may not correlate with adequate placental perfusion. Assisted second stage of labor (vacuum or forceps) and/or "labor down" technique Avoid Valsalva's maneuver during pushing. Oxygen therapy during labor Pain management: Consider epidural anesthesia. Consider cesarean birth for complicated coarctations with risk of aneurysm rupture.
Tetralogy of Fallot	Corrected = low or minimal risk Uncorrected = intermediate or moderate risk	Congenital complex of VSD, overriding aorta, right ventricular hypertrophy, and pulmonary stenosis; surgical correction by young adulthood common	Maintain preload and blood volume. Pain management: Consider epidural anesthesia.

TABLE 9–6. Cardiac Disease in Pregnancy *(Continued)*

Cardiac disease/lesion	Risk category	Description	Clinical management

Mitral stenosis	Risk based on severity of stenosis and maternal symptoms
	Assess for arrhythmias and pulmonary edema.
		Most commonly from rheumatic heart disease
		Scarring and fusion of valve apparatus
		Area (cm^2)
		  Normal: 4 to 6
		  Mild: 1.5 to 2.5
		  Moderate: 1 to 1.5
		  Severe: ≤1.5
		Left arterial obstruction results in enlargement of LA and RV, and possibly pulmonary hypertension.
		Atrial fibrillation possibility
		Fixed cardiac output
		Ventricular diastolic filling obstruction
			Physical examination: S1 is accentuated and snapping; low-pitch diastolic rumble at the apex: presystolic accentuation
			Invasive hemodynamic monitoring based on severity of lesion and maternal response to management
			Avoid hypotension—consider arterial line for blood pressure for severe disease or maternal instability.
			• Avoid maternal tachycardia—may decrease cardiac output by decreasing left ventricular filling time.
			• Consider beta-blocker for pulse >90 to 100 bpm.
			• Avoid beta-adrenergic tocolytics and/or other medications that increase HR.
			Atrial fibrillation—anticoagulation, digoxin, antiarrhythmics
			Assist second stage with vacuum or forceps; consider "labor down" technique.
			Pain management: Consider narcotic epidural.

Aortic stenosis	Risk based on severity of stenosis and maternal symptoms Assess for signs of heart failure and arrhythmias.	Mean pressure gradient (mm Hg) • Mild: <20 • Moderate: 20 to 39 • Severe: ≥40	Physical examination: harsh systolic ejection murmur in second right intercostal space ECG: left ventricular hypertrophy and left atrial enlargement Invasive hemodynamic monitoring based on severity of lesion and maternal response to management Optimize preload—avoid hypovolemia. Avoid hypotension—decreased venous return will increase the valvular gradient and decrease cardiac output. • Avoid/anticipate hemorrhage. • Avoid supine position—risk of vena cava syndrome. • Avoid maternal tachycardia—may decrease cardiac output by decreasing left ventricular filling time. • Consider beta-blocker for pulse >90 to 100 bpm. • Avoid beta-adrenergic tocolytics and/or other medications that increase HR. Oxygen during labor Pain management: Consider narcotic epidural; avoid spinal block. Vaginal birth preferred with assisted second stage, cesarean birth for obstetric indications
Marfan syndrome	Normal aortic root = low or minimal risk Enlarged aortic root ≥40 mm or valve involvement = severe risk	Autosomal dominant; generalized connective tissue weakness Can result in aneurysm formation, rupture, and dissection Sixty percent may also have mitral or aortic regurgitation.	Echocardiogram needed to determine aortic root involvement Avoid maternal tachycardia—may increase shearing force on the aorta. • Consider beta-blocker if maternal HR >90 to 100 bpm. • Avoid beta-adrenergic tocolytics and/or other medications that increase HR. Avoid hypertension. Avoid positive inotropic medications. Pain management: Consider epidural anesthesia.
Peripartum cardiomyopathy	High or major risk with persistent left ventricular dysfunction	Cardiac failure developing in pregnancy or in the first 5 months postpartum without identifiable cause Higher incidence among older gravidas, multiparas, African American race, multiple gestations, and the patients with preeclampsia Return of ventricular function and normal heart size associated with better prognosis	Optimize cardiac output. Typically requires use of diuretics, antihypertensive agents, and beta-blockers in conjunction with a cardiologist Repeat measurement of ejection fraction should be done if change in patient status detected. Consider serial B-type natriuretic peptide measurements. Consider serial renal and electrolyte measurements. Oxygen therapy during labor; vaginal birth preferred Pain management: Consider narcotic epidural; keep patient comfortable to decrease oxygen utilization.

(continued)

TABLE 9–6. Cardiac Disease in Pregnancy *(Continued)*

Cardiac disease/lesion	Risk category	Description	Clinical management
MI	Previous MI = intermediate or moderate risk MI during pregnancy = high or major risk	Diagnosis during pregnancy is determined by ECG findings, angina, and elevated cardiac enzymes (troponin I). Cardiac troponin I levels are unaffected by pregnancy, labor, and delivery.	MI during pregnancy—attempt to delay delivery for at least 2 weeks. Previous MI—advise patients to wait at least 1 year after infarction; follow-up coronary angiography recommended. Optimize cardiac output. Labor in left or right lateral position Consider assisted second stage of labor (vacuum or forceps) and/or "labor down" technique. Avoid Valsalva's maneuver during pushing. Avoid maternal tachycardia and hypertension. Pain management: Consider narcotic epidural; keep the patient comfortable to decrease oxygen utilization.

ASD, atrial septal defect; CHF, congestive heart failure; ECG, electrocardiogram; HR, heart rate; LA, left atrium; MI, myocardial infarction; NYHA, New York Heart Association; PDA, patent ductus arteriosus; PVR, pulmonary vascular resistance; RV, right ventricle; SaO$_2$, oxygen saturation; VSD, ventricular septal defect.

Adapted from Arafeh, J. M., & Baird, S. M. (2006). Cardiac disease in pregnancy. *Critical Care Nursing Quarterly, 29*(1), 32–52.

Additional references:

Canobbio, M. M., Warnes, C. A., Aboulhosn, J., Connolly, H. M., Khanna, A., Koos, B. J., . . . Stout, K. (2017). Management of pregnancy in patients with complex congenital heart disease: A scientific statement for healthcare professionals from the American Heart Association. *Circulation, 135*(8), e50–e87. doi:10.1161/CIR.0000000000000458

Deen, J., Chandrasekaran, S., Stout, K., & Easterling, T. (2017). Heart disease in pregnancy. In S. G. Gabbe, J. R. Niebyl, J. L. Simpson, M. B. Landon, H. L. Galan, E. R. M. Jauniaux, . . . W. A. Grobman (Eds.), *Obstetrics: Normal and problem pregnancies* (7th ed., pp. 803–827). Philadelphia, PA: Elsevier.

Johnson-Coyle, L., Jensen, L., & Sobey, A. (2012). Peripartum cardiomyopathy: Review and practice guidelines. *American Journal of Critical Care, 21*(2), 89–98. doi:10.4037/ajcc2012163

treatment may be needed if the rhythm affects cardiac output. Cardioversion, direct pacing, and defibrillation may be required to correct serious arrhythmias (Canobbio et al., 2017; Emmanuel & Thorne, 2015).

Intrapartum care and birth options need thoughtful consideration to decrease maternal and fetal risk. An interdisciplinary team approach to planning intrapartum care is essential. In the past, cesarean birth under general anesthesia was often chosen as the birth option with the least risks to the mother with heart disease. However, elective cesarean birth increases the risk of hemorrhage, thrombosis, and infection when compared to vaginal birth. Current practice for most cardiac lesions includes a well-planned labor and vaginal birth unless there is a specific obstetric indication for cesarean birth (ACOG, 2019; Canobbio et al., 2017; Emmanuel & Thorne, 2015; Ghandi & Shamshirsaz, 2016). See Display 9–3 for key aspects of intrapartum management and care. The pain of labor can be managed with epidural anesthesia under the guidance of an anesthesiologist knowledgeable of cardiac disease during pregnancy (ACOG, 2019; Canobbio et al., 2017; Emmanuel & Thorne, 2015; Ghandi & Shamshirsaz, 2016). Initiation of epidural anesthesia early in labor inhibits or minimizes the sympathetic response to pain. Labor pain has potentially significant side effects that should be avoided. Cardiac output can be abruptly increased with the pain and tension associated with labor (Antony et al., 2017). Quality pain management has the benefit of helping avoid tachycardia (important for cardiac lesions that require adequate diastolic filling or systolic ejection time), reducing myocardial workload, and providing pain relief for operative vaginal birth (Canobbio et al., 2017; Ghandi & Shamshirsaz, 2016).

Spontaneous labor is preferred to induction of labor; however, in selected cases, labor induction with a favorable cervix may be the most feasible option to ensure that the required team members are available and present (Canobbio et al., 2017; Deen et al., 2017). Planned labor also may be chosen for women who live remote from the hospital and thus may not be able to arrive on the labor unit in a timely manner after the initiation of spontaneous labor. Controlled labor or birth may also be necessary due to deterioration of the maternal or fetal condition. Labor should progress at a reasonable pace without tachysystole that may lead to fetal intolerance and the risk of an urgent surgical birth. A lateral position during labor will minimize the effects of the hemodynamic fluctuations associated with uterine contractions for most women, but position should be individualized to the specific cardiac lesion (Canobbio et al., 2017; Ghandi & Shamshirsaz, 2016). See Table 9–8 for changes in cardiac output during labor and birth.

The American College of Cardiology and the American Heart Association do not recommend routine antibiotic prophylaxis appropriate for infective endocarditis for all women with heart disease having an otherwise uncomplicated vaginal or cesarean birth unless infection is suspected (Canobbio et al., 2017; Nishimura et al., 2014). Routine prophylaxis given

TABLE 9–7. Cardiovascular Medications (Doses, Nursing Care, and Maternal–Fetal Implications)

	Generic name (Trade name)	Dose	Nursing care specific for pregnancy	Fetal/neonatal effects
Antiarrhythmics	Adenosine	6 mg IV bolus over 1 to 3 sec followed by 20-mL saline bolus; may repeat with 12 mg in 1 to 2 min × 2		No observed fetal or newborn effects reported
	Amiodarone	5 mg/kg IV over 3 min and then 10 mg/kg/day	Observe for prolonged QT.	EFM: Observe for fetal bradycardia. • Potential for congenital hypothyroidism • May cause IUGR • Observe for transient bradycardia and prolonged QT in the newborn.
	Procainamide	100 mg over 30 min and then 2 to 6 mg/min infusion: total dose 17 mg/kg		None reported
	Quinidine	15 mg/kg IV over 60 min and then 0.02 mg/kg/min infusion	Potential oxytocic properties with high doses	Potential for eighth cranial nerve damage and thrombocytopenia
Beta-blockers	Atenolol	5 mg IV over 5 min: Repeat in 5 min: total dose 15 mg.	Observe for maternal hypotension.	EFM: Observe for fetal bradycardia. • May cause IUGR and persistent beta-blockade in the newborn
	Labetalol	10 to 20 mg IV followed by 20 to 80 mg IV every 10 min: total dose of 150 mg	Observe for maternal hypotension.	EFM: Observe for fetal bradycardia. • May cause IUGR
	Metoprolol	5 mg IV over 5 min: Repeat in 10 min.		Rapidly enters fetal circulation; fetal serum levels equal to maternal levels: may cause persistent beta-blockade in the newborn
	Propranolol	1 mg IV every 2 min PRN	Observe for maternal hypotension.	EFM: Observe for fetal bradycardia. • May cause IUGR
Calcium channel blockers	Diltiazem	20 mg IV bolus over 2 min: Repeat in 15 min.		Possible teratogenic effects
	Nifedipine	10 mg PO: Repeat every 6 hr.	Observe for maternal hypotension and tachycardia. May cause severe hypotension and neuromuscular blockade when given with magnesium sulfate	
	Verapamil	2.5 to 5 mg IV bolus over 2 min: Repeat in 5 min and then every 30 min PRN to a maximum dose of 20 mg.	Observe for maternal hypotension (5% to 10% of patients).	Potential for reduced uterine blood flow and fetal hypoxia
Inotropic agents	Dobutamine	Initial dose of 5.0 mcg/kg/min: Titrate up to 20 mcg/kg/min.		
	Digoxin	Loading dose 0.5 mg IV over 5 min and then 0.25 IV every 6 hr × 2 Maintenance dose: 0.125 to 0.375 mg IV/PO every day	Because of increased maternal volume and elimination, increased doses are required to obtain therapeutic levels.	Fetal toxicity and neonatal death have been reported.
	Dopamine	Initial dose 5 mcg/kg/min; titrate by 5–10 mcg/kg/min up to 20 mcg/kg/min		
	Epinephrine	Initial bolus 0.5 mg: Follow with 2 to 10 mcg/kg/min infusion: endotracheal 0.5 to 1.0 mg every 5 min.		

(continued)

TABLE 9–7. Cardiovascular Medications (Doses, Nursing Care, and Maternal–Fetal Implications) *(Continued)*

	Generic name (Trade name)	Dose	Nursing care specific for pregnancy	Fetal/neonatal effects
Vasoconstrictors	Ephedrine sulfate	10 to 25 mg slow IV push: Repeat every 15 min PRN × 3.	First-line medication in pregnancy (causes peripheral vasoconstriction without reducing uterine blood flow)	EFM: Observe for fetal tachycardia and decreased baseline variability following administration.
	Norepinephrine	Initial dose of 0.05 mcg/kg/min: Titrate to maximum dose of 1.0 mcg/kg/min.	Use only with severe maternal hypotension unresponsive to other agents.	May compromise uterine blood flow and cause fetal hypoxia and bradycardia
	Phenylephrine	Initial dose of 0.1 mcg/kg/min: Titrate up to 0.7 mcg/kg/min.	May interact with oxytocics and ergot medications to produce severe maternal hypertension	Potential for reduced uterine blood flow and fetal hypoxia
Vasodilators	Hydralazine	5 to 10 mg IV every 20 min: total dose 30 mg	Frequent, small doses preferred to avoid maternal hypotension	EFM: potential for fetal tachycardia
	Nitroglycerine	IV infusion 10 mcg/min: Titrate up by 10 to 20 mcg/min PRN: 0.4 to 0.8 mg sublingual; 1 to 2 in of dermal paste.		
	Nitroprusside	Initial dose 0.3 mcg/kg/min: Titrate to 10 mcg/kg/min.	Monitor serum pH levels.	Avoid prolonged use: potential for fetal cyanide toxicity.

EFM, electronic fetal monitoring; IUGR, intrauterine growth restriction; IV, intravenous; PO, orally; PRN, as needed.
From Arafeh, J. M., & Baird, S. M. (2006). Cardiac disease in pregnancy. *Critical Care Nursing Quarterly, 29*(1), 32–52.

for any cesarean birth should be continued for women with cardiac disease. As well, if high-risk women are already receiving antibiotic therapy comparable to endocarditis prophylaxis, then an additional antibiotic is not required. Antibiotic prophylaxis should be considered for women with the following: prosthetic heart valves or prosthetic material from cardiac repair, a previous history of endocarditis, complex CHD, or a surgically constructed systemic-pulmonary conduit (ACOG, 2018b; Nishimura et al., 2014). Nonetheless, the decision to administer antibiotic therapy should be based on the individual risks of the woman (Canobbio et al., 2017; Yucel & DeFaria Yeh, 2017). Antibiotic prophylaxis is given in one dose. The dose is given 30 to 60 minutes before birth. The dosage is 2.0 g of ampicillin (IV or orally) or 1.0 g of cefazolin or ceftriaxone IV. Clindamycin 600 mg IV is given for those who are allergic to penicillins. If there is a possibility of an enterococcus infection, vancomycin should be used (ACOG, 2018b). If prophylaxis is not used, the woman should be evaluated carefully for fever, particularly those with no clear etiology (Safi & Tsiaras, 2017)

During the second stage of labor, passive fetal descent, also known as *laboring down*, in a lateral position increases oxygenation, limits maternal metabolic demands, and increases uteroplacental perfusion (Osborne & Hanson, 2014). The management plan for birth should include if the woman will be allowed to attempt open glottis pushing and how operative birth will be accomplished (by forceps or vacuum)

(Canobbio et al., 2017; Deen et al., 2017). Most cardiac conditions are well tolerated with proper anesthesia, minimal or no pushing, and an operative vaginal birth.

It is important to consider the changes that occur immediately at birth due to relief of caval obstruction and transfusion of blood previously held in the maternal placental bed. This return of blood to the central circulation has the potential to overwhelm the patient's ability to cope with the extra volume load. On the other hand, failure of the uterus to contract may result in hemorrhage and blood loss. Risks of cardiac decompensation and obstetric complications continue during the postpartum period, most notably during the first few hours after birth, but depend on the severity of cardiac disease. A period of careful monitoring should follow birth for at least 48 to 72 hours, depending on the type of cardiac disease and maternal condition (ACOG, 2019; Canobbio et al., 2017; Emmanuel & Thorne, 2015).

Maternal death remains a risk during the postpartum period. The most common complications women with cardiac disease experience after birth include development of pulmonary edema and hemorrhage (Deen et al., 2017). Risk of pulmonary edema can persist for up to 3 to 5 days postpartum due to mobilization of interstitial fluid to the vascular space during the normal diuresis that occurs after birth (Canobbio et al., 2017; Deen et al., 2017). Risk of hemorrhage is increased for women who have required anticoagulation during the pregnancy. Because of the large amount

DISPLAY 9–3

Intrapartum Care for Women with Cardiac Disease

An interdisciplinary team should plan and participate in care (nurse and physician representatives from the following specialties: obstetrics, maternal–fetal medicine, anesthesia, cardiology, neonatology, and pediatrics). Social services and chaplain services should be consulted and available as necessary. Topics for discussion include current status of cardiac disease, risk during pregnancy, anticipated plan of care, insurance coverage, and transportation needs.

The unit where labor and birth occurs is based on maternal status. Most women can be managed in the labor unit with personnel from the intensive care unit (ICU) assisting with assessment of maternal hemodynamic status if invasive hemodynamic monitoring is indicated. Selected women may labor and give birth in the ICU. Personnel with expertise in labor management, fetal assessment, and birth are essential.

Labor is the most complex period for many pregnant women with cardiac disease because there are periods of great increases in cardiac output. Therefore, careful monitoring of maternal–fetal status is essential with at least a one-to-one nurse to patient ratio. Patient status and type of cardiac disease provides the basis for selection of monitoring methods.

Invasive hemodynamic monitoring should be considered for women with impaired left ventricular function, New York Heart Association (NYHA) class III and class IV, severe mitral stenosis, and pulmonary hypertension.

Noninvasive monitoring includes oxygen saturation via pulse oximetry, blood pressure, heart rate, respirations, careful monitoring of fluid status, reassessment of NYHA functional status, fetal status, and use of electrocardiogram monitoring for women susceptible to arrhythmias.

Fetal status should be monitored continuously via electronic fetal monitoring. Fetal status can be an indicator of maternal status. A normal fetal heart rate (FHR) can be reflective of adequate maternal perfusion. Use of external or internal monitoring of FHR and uterine activity is based on obstetric considerations.

Lateral positioning should be encouraged in most women to avoid risk of venocaval compression.

Adequate and early pain management (usually via epidural anesthesia) will minimize negative effects of pain, anxiety, and tension on maternal hemodynamic parameters. Patients with severe stenotic heart defects will not tolerate sudden decreases in systemic vascular resistance; therefore, epidural anesthesia must be administered by a provider with experience in cardiac disease during pregnancy.

Supportive nursing care along with support from the patient's partner can minimize anxiety. Appropriate preparation with realistic expectations for how the labor and birth will proceed, including potential complications and resultant interventions, can also minimize stress and anxiety.

Labor and vaginal birth is preferred over cesarean birth for most patients because there is less risk of blood loss, fewer postpartum infections, and earlier ambulation with less risk of thrombosis and pulmonary complications.

The second stage should be managed with passive fetal descent, minimal maternal expulsive efforts, and operative (forceps or vacuum) birth as needed.

Uterine contraction after birth should be maintained to prevent postpartum hemorrhage. Women who have received anticoagulation therapy are at greater risk for hemorrhage. Oxytocic drugs have marked hemodynamic effects and should be used at the lowest effective dose. Postpartum hemorrhage should be managed aggressively to prevent hypovolemia, especially important for patients who are preload dependent such as those with severe aortic stenosis or mitral stenosis. Postpartum hemorrhage should be treated with volume replacement, blood products, and plasma.

Support maternal–infant attachment by encouraging holding, touching, and breastfeeding (if the woman has chosen breastfeeding) as soon as possible.

From Canobbio, M. M., Warnes, C. A., Aboulhosn, J., Connolly, H. M., Khanna, A., Koos, B. J., . . . Stout, K. (2017). Management of pregnancy in patients with complex congenital heart disease: A scientific statement for healthcare professionals from the American Heart Association. *Circulation, 135*(8), e50–e87. doi:10.1161 /CIR.0000000000000458; Gaddipati, S., & Troiano, N. H. (2013). Cardiac disorders in pregnancy. In N. H. Troiano, C. J. Harvey, & B. F. Chez (Eds.), *AWHONN's high-risk & critical care obstetrics* (3rd ed., pp. 125–143). Philadelphia, PA: Lippincott Williams & Wilkins; Safi, L. M., & Tsiaras, S. V. (2017). Update on valvular heart disease in pregnancy. *Current Treatment Options in Cardiovascular Medicine, 19*(9), 70. doi:10.1007/s11936-017-0570-2; and Yucel, E., & DeFaria Yeh, D. (2017). Pregnancy in women with congenital heart disease. *Current Treatment Options in Cardiovascular Medicine, 19*(9), 73. doi:10.1007/s11936-017-0572-0

of blood flow to the uterus at term, significant blood loss can occur in a relative short period if uterine contraction is not maintained during the immediate postpartum period. Postpartum hemorrhage should be treated aggressively by efforts to promote hemostasis and with replacement volume, blood products, and plasma to avoid hypovolemia (Canobbio et al., 2017; Deen et al., 2017). See Chapter 6 for a detailed discussion of postpartum hemorrhage.

All women with known underlying cardiac disease and dysfunction should receive care from clinicians who specialize in cardiac disease during pregnancy in a level III/IV facility due to the risks of preterm labor and birth, small-for-gestational-age fetus, intrauterine growth restriction (IUGR), and potential for fetal or maternal compromise. Although most women with cardiac disease tolerate pregnancy and have a successful outcome, the potential exists to develop significant hemodynamic decompensation requiring comprehensive management to survive the pregnancy, labor, and birth. If this occurs, a plan needs to be in place to address obstetric, cardiac, and intensive care needs of the woman (Safi & Tsiaras, 2017). All women with cardiac disease need to have clear education about symptoms of cardiac decompensation before discharge and follow-up with a cardiologist.

TABLE 9–8. Increases in Cardiac Output during Labor and Birth

Labor phase or stage	Increase above pre-labor values
First stage	10% to 30%
Second stage	Up to 50%
Immediately at birth	60% to 80%

From Canobbio, M. M., Warnes, C. A., Aboulhosn, J., Connolly, H. M., Khanna, A., Koos, B. J., . . . Stout, K. (2017). Management of pregnancy in patients with complex congenital heart disease: A scientific statement for healthcare professionals from the American Heart Association. *Circulation, 135*(8), e50–e87. doi:10.1161/CIR.0000000000000458

NURSING CARE

Arrhythmias may accompany pregnancy and often occur with cardiac disease having an impact on cardiac output if repetitive and prolonged (Canobbio et al., 2017; Deen et al., 2017). Nurses have the most frequent and lengthy patient encounters. Therefore, they must have keen assessment techniques and skills to differentiate normal pregnancy adaptations from cardiac dysfunction and disease. Table 9–3 compares normal adaptations of pregnancy to severe heart disease or heart failure. At any time during the antepartum, intrapartum, or postpartum periods up until 6 months following birth, the nurse should be vigilant for symptoms signaling deterioration. If the pregnant woman reports progressive limitation of physical activity because of worsening dyspnea, chest pain that occurs during exercise or increased activity, or syncope that is preceded by palpitations or physical exertion, underlying cardiac disease should be suspected (Gaddipati & Troiano, 2013). As a part of the multidisciplinary team, the perinatal nurse should maintain knowledge of the unique condition of the woman and the current plan of care prior to each patient encounter.

The woman's history and current physical status are analyzed in relation to CV physiology and function. The nurse should perform an initial review to include examination of the patient's specific medical, surgical, social, and family history. A current understanding of basic pathophysiology regarding the patient's underlying CV disorder, previous therapies (e.g., past hospital admissions for medical stabilization or surgery), current medications, and current NYHA classification are particularly pertinent (Gaddipati & Troiano, 2013). The woman's occupation can also provide useful information about functional status and environmental risk factors.

Knowledge of various methods and tools for cardiac assessment are prerequisites for a complete CV evaluation. Physical assessments will include a head-to-toe inspection with specific focus on cardiorespiratory indicators. A CV assessment minimally includes auscultation of the heart and lungs (count both heart rate and respiratory rate with stethoscope for a full minute);

identification of pathologic edema; evaluation of respiratory rate and rhythm; evaluation of cardiac rate and rhythm; body weight assessed at the same time of day and on the same scale; assessment of skin color, temperature, and turgor; and capillary refill check. Trending of vital sign data is important because tachypnea, tachycardia, and anxiety are often early signs of edema and may be present before a cough or abnormal breath sounds appear (Mason & Dorman, 2013). Abnormal skin and mucous membrane color may indicate problems with oxygenation and perfusion. Assessment of the central nervous system may reveal signs of inadequate blood flow. Restlessness, apprehension, anxiety, or changes in level of consciousness may indicate compromised blood flow and oxygenation of the brain.

Observation for secondary obstetric-specific complications is a primary goal in the treatment of cardiac dysfunction during pregnancy. Hypertension, alone, may be a secondary complication of pregnancy or may signal worsening of the underlying cardiac disease. Proper and consistent blood pressure assessment is crucial. Changing from a supine to a left side-lying position increases blood flow enhancing cardiac output. Maternal positioning, cuff size, device, and timing alter maternal blood pressure results during pregnancy. It is imperative that the entire perinatal team is consistent in blood pressure technique to ensure accuracy and correct interpretation of data.

Any maternal position that causes aortocaval compression may negatively influence maternal cardiac output and blood pressure; avoidance during all phases of pregnancy, labor, and birth is indicated. Vena caval syndrome may significantly limit maternal cardiac output and promote maternal symptomatology (Ghandi & Shamshirsaz, 2016). Therefore, if improved cardiac output is indicated, lateral recumbent position is optimal in most cases.

Additional noninvasive assessment techniques and equipment necessary for the treatment of cardiac disease in pregnancy should include oxygen saturation via a pulse oximetry, urinary output, and electronic fetal monitoring (EFM) (in most cases). Other techniques that should be considered include arrhythmia assessment via 5- or 12-lead ECG. Pulse oximetry should not be used as the only diagnostic tool if hypoxemia is present. Blood gases offer more complete information when severe pulmonary compromise and systemic color changes exist (Mason & Dorman, 2013). Assessment and documentation of baseline vital signs and condition prior to pregnancy is optimal. All pregnant women with preexisting cardiac disease should have a baseline 12-lead ECG and may require 5-lead cardiac monitoring during labor and birth. Kidney function is also assessed for adequacy of peripheral perfusion. An indwelling Foley catheter with an urometer can assist with assessment of fluid balance and indicate signs of inadequate renal and uterine perfusion (Ghandi & Shamshirsaz, 2016). Urinary output should be maintained at least 25 to 30 mL/hr.

Fetal assessment is a sensitive indicator of adequate cardiac function by affording the perinatal team a means for assessing uteroplacental perfusion. Antenatal testing (e.g., fetal movement counting, nonstress test, or biophysical profile) may assist in the diagnosis of uteroplacental insufficiency during the antepartum period with evidence of small for gestational age, IUGR, or oligohydramnios. Prior to 23 weeks' gestation, EFM may be used to screen for an early indicator of deterioration in maternal status. Once viability is established, category II or III fetal heart rate patterns warrant prompt intervention in most cases.

Certain disorders and advanced degrees of CV illness may require invasive hemodynamic monitoring using pulmonary artery catheters, peripheral arterial catheters, or CVP monitors (Gaddipati & Troiano, 2013). Invasive hemodynamic monitoring may be recommended for women designated in the NYHA class III or IV experiencing labor. Many women require continuous cardiac rhythm monitoring during acute events and during prolonged hospitalization (Gaddipati & Troiano, 2013).

Heightened vigilance is warranted in women with cardiac disease throughout pregnancy. Understanding and assessing for variances in normal pregnancy adaptations may signal deterioration. An interdisciplinary approach assists in overall reduction of maternal, fetal, and neonatal morbidity and mortality.

SUMMARY

It is likely that morbidity and mortality from cardiac disease in pregnancy is increasing in either real numbers or awareness, particularly in the postpartum period. Preconception counseling, careful planning of care, and vigilance throughout pregnancy is essential. Use of risk assessment tools are necessary to ensure women at high risk are cared for by a team experienced in cardiac disease during pregnancy at a hospital with access to diagnostic and laboratory testing. While many women with cardiac disease have favorable outcomes, a low threshold should be established for follow-up of signs and symptoms indicating deteriorating status. The plan of care needs to be flexible to reflect alterations dictated by change in the woman's condition as she continually adapts to the physiologic changes of pregnancy (Kuklina & Callaghan, 2011).

REFERENCES

American College of Obstetricians and Gynecologists. (2018a). *Thromboembolism in pregnancy* (Practice Bulletin No. 196). Washington, DC: Author.

American College of Obstetricians and Gynecologists. (2018b). *Use of prophylactic antibiotics in labor and delivery* (Practice Bulletin No. 199). Washington, DC: Author.

American College of Obstetricians and Gynecologists. (2019). *Pregnancy and heart disease* (Practice Bulletin No. 212). Washington, DC: Author.

Antony, K. M., Racusin, D. A., Aagaard, K., & Dildy, G. A. (2017). Maternal physiology. In S. G. Gabbe, J. R. Niebyl, J. L. Simpson, M. B. Landon, H. L. Galan, E. R. M. Jauniaux, . . . W. A. Grobman (Eds.), *Obstetrics: Normal and problem pregnancies* (7th ed., pp. 38–63). Philadelphia, PA: Elsevier.

Arafeh, J. M., & Baird, S. M. (2006). Cardiac disease in pregnancy. *Critical Care Nursing Quarterly*, 29(1), 32–52.

Arif, S., & Thorne, S. A. (2014). Heart disease in pregnancy. *Medicine*, 42(11), 644–649. doi:10.1016/j.mpmed.2014.08.011

Baddour, L. M., Freeman, W. K., Suri, R. M., & Wilson, W. R. (2015). Cardiovascular infections. In D. L. Mann, D. P. Zipes, P. Libby, & R. O. Bonow (Eds.), *Braunwald's heart disease: A textbook of cardiovascular medicine* (10th ed., pp. 1524–1550). Boston, MA: Saunders.

Balci, A., Sollie-Szarynska, K. M., van der Bijl, A. G. L., Ruys, T. P., Mulder, B. J., Roos-Hesselink, J. W., . . . Pieper, P. G. (2014). Prospective validation and assessment of cardiovascular and offspring risk models for pregnant women with congenital heart disease. *Heart (British Cardiac Society)*, 100(17), 1373–1381. doi:10.1136/heartjnl-2014-305597

Balint, O. H., Siu, S. C., Mason, J., Grewal, J., Wald, R., Oechslin, E. N., . . . Silversides, C. K. (2010). Cardiac outcomes after pregnancy in women with congenital heart disease. *Heart*, 96(20), 1656–1661. doi:10.1136/hrt.2010.202838

Bamfo, J. E., Kametas, N. A., Turan, O., Khaw, A., & Nicolaides, K. H. (2006). Maternal cardiac function in fetal growth restriction. *BJOG*, 113(7), 784–791. doi:10.1111/j.1471-0528.2006.00945.x

Canobbio, M. M., Warnes, C. A., Aboulhosn, J., Connolly, H. M., Khanna, A., Koos, B. J., . . . Stout, K. (2017). Management of pregnancy in patients with complex congenital heart disease: A scientific statement for healthcare professionals from the American Heart Association. *Circulation*, 135(8), e50–e87. doi:10.1161/CIR.0000000000000458

Centers for Disease Control and Prevention. (2017). *Pregnancy Mortality Surveillance System*. Retrieved from https://www.cdc.gov/reproductivehealth/maternalinfanthealth/pregnancy-mortality-surveillance-system.htm

Clark, S. L., Cotton, D. B., Lee, W., Bishop, C., Hill, T., Southwick, J., . . . Tolley, D. T. (1989). Central hemodynamic assessment of normal term pregnancy. *American Journal of Obstetrics & Gynecology*, 161(6, Pt. 1), 1439–1442. doi:10.1016/0002-9378(89)90900-9

Criteria Committee of the New York Heart Association. (1979). *Nomenclature and criteria for diagnosis of diseases of the heart and great vessels* (8th ed.). Boston, MA: Little, Brown.

Darovic, G. O. (2002a). Cardiovascular anatomy and physiology. In G. O. Darovic (Ed.), *Hemodynamic monitoring: Invasive and noninvasive clinical application* (3rd ed., pp. 57–90). Philadelphia, PA: Saunders.

Darovic, G. O. (2002b). Pulmonary artery pressure monitoring. In G. O. Darovic (Ed.), *Hemodynamic monitoring: Invasive and noninvasive clinical application* (3rd ed., pp. 191–243). Philadelphia, PA: Saunders.

Darovic, G. O., Graham, P. G., & Pranulis, M. A. (2002). Monitoring cardiac output. In G. O. Darovic (Ed.), *Hemodynamic monitoring: Invasive and noninvasive clinical application* (3rd ed., pp. 245–262). Philadelphia, PA: Saunders.

Darovic, G. O., & Kumar, A. (2002). Monitoring central venous pressure. In G. O. Darovic (Ed.), *Hemodynamic monitoring: Invasive and noninvasive clinical application* (3rd ed., pp. 177–190). Philadelphia, PA: Saunders.

Deen, J., Chandrasekaran, S., Stout, K., & Easterling, T. (2017). Heart disease in pregnancy. In S. G. Gabbe, J. R. Niebyl, J. L. Simpson, M. B. Landon, H. L. Galan, E. R. M. Jauniaux, . . . W. A. Grobman (Eds.), *Obstetrics: Normal and problem pregnancies* (7th ed., pp. 803–827). Philadelphia, PA: Elsevier.

Drenthen, W., Boersma, E., Balci, A., Moons, P., Roos-Hesselink, J. W., Mulder, B. J., . . . Pieper, P. G. (2010). Predictors of pregnancy complications in women with congenital heart disease. *European Heart Journal*, 31(17), 2124–2132. doi:10.1093/eurheartj/ehq200

Emmanuel, Y., & Thorne, S. A. (2015). Heart disease in pregnancy. *Best Practice & Research. Clinical Obstetrics & Gynaecology*, 29(5), 579–597. doi:10.1016/j.bpobgyn.2015.04.002

Gaddipati, S., & Troiano, N. H. (2013). Cardiac disorders in pregnancy. In N. H. Troiano, C. J. Harvey, & B. F. Chez (Eds.), *AWHONN's high-risk & critical care obstetrics* (3rd ed., pp. 125–143). Philadelphia, PA: Lippincott Williams & Wilkins.

Gelson, E., Curry, R., Gatzoulis, M. A., Swan, L., Lupton, M., Steer, P., & Johnson, M. (2011). Effect of maternal heart disease on fetal growth. *Obstetrics & Gynecology*, 117(4), 886–891. doi:10.1097/AOG.0b013e31820cab69

Ghandi, M., & Shamshirsaz, A. A. (2016). Cardiac lesions in the critical care setting. *Obstetrics and Gynecology Clinics of North America*, 43(4), 709–728. doi:10.1016/j.ogc.2016.07.003

Hameed, A. B., Morton, C. H., & Moore, A. (2017). *Improving health care response to cardiovascular disease in pregnancy and postpartum*. Sacramento, CA: California Department of Public Health.

Januzzi, J. L., & Mann, D. L. (2015). Clinical assessment of heart failure. In D. L. Mann, D. P. Zipes, P. Libby, & R. O. Bonow (Eds.), *Braunwald's heart disease: A textbook of cardiovascular medicine* (10th ed., pp. 473–483). Boston, MA: Saunders.

Johnson-Coyle, L., Jensen, L., & Sobey, A. (2012). Peripartum cardiomyopathy: Review and practice guidelines. *American Journal of Critical Care*, 21(2), 89–98. doi:10.4037/ajcc2012163

Kampman, M. A. M., Balci, A., van Veldhuisen, D. J., van Dijk, A. P. J., Roos-Hesselink, J. W., Sollie-Szarynska, K. M., . . . Pieper, P. G. (2014). N-terminal pro-B-type natriuretic peptide predicts cardiovascular complications in pregnant women with congenital heart disease. *European Heart Journal*, 35(11), 708–715. doi:10.1093/eurheartj/eht526

Kennedy, B. B., & Baird, S. M. (2016). Acute myocardial infarction in pregnancy: An update. *The Journal of Perinatal & Neonatal Nursing*, 30(1), 13–24. doi:10.1097/JPN.0000000000000145

Knight, M., Nair, M., Tuffnell, D., Kenyon, S., Shakespeare, J., Brocklehurst, P., & Kurinczuk, J. J. (Eds.). (2016). *Saving lives, improving mothers' care—Surveillance of maternal deaths in the UK 2012–14 and lessons learned to inform maternity care from the UK and Ireland Confidential Enquiries into Maternal Deaths and Morbidity 2009–14*. Oxford, United Kingdom: National Perinatal Epidemiology Unit, University of Oxford.

Kuklina, E. V., & Callaghan, W. M. (2011). Chronic heart disease and severe obstetric morbidity among hospitalisations for pregnancy in the USA: 1995–2006. *BJOG*, 118(3), 345–352. doi:10.1111/j.1471-0528.2010.02743.x

Lameijer, H., Lont, M. C., Buter, H., van Boven, A. J., Boonstra, P. W., & Pieper, P. G. (2017). Pregnancy-related myocardial infarction. *Netherlands Heart Journal*, 25(6), 365–369. doi:10.1007/s12471-017-0989-9

Lim, J. C. E.-S., Cauldwell, M., Patel, R. R., Uebing, A., Curry, R. A., Johnson, M. R., . . . Swan, L. (2017). Management of Marfan syndrome during pregnancy: A real world experience from a Joint Cardiac Obstetric Service. *International Journal of Cardiology*, 243, 180–184. doi:10.1016/j.ijcard.2017.05.077

Lima, F. V., Yang, J., Xu, J., & Stergiopoulos, K. (2017). National trends and in-hospital outcomes in pregnant women with heart disease in the United States. *The American Journal of Cardiology*, 119(10), 1694–1700. doi:10.1016/j.amjcard.2017.02.003

Mason, B. A., & Dorman, K. (2013). Pulmonary disorders in pregnancy. In N. H. Troiano, C. J. Harvey, & B. F. Chez (Eds.), *AWHONN's high-risk & critical care obstetrics* (3rd ed., pp. 144–162). Philadelphia, PA: Lippincott Williams & Wilkins.

Nishimura, R. A., Otto, C. M., Bonow, R. O., Carabello, B. A., Erwin, J. P., III, Guyton, R. A., . . . Thomas, J. D. (2014). 2014 AHA/ACC guideline for the management of patients with valvular heart disease: Executive summary: A report of the American College of Cardiology/American Heart Association Task Force on Practice Guidelines. *Journal of the American College of Cardiology*, 63(22), 2438–2488. doi:10.1016/j.jacc.2014.02.537

Osborne, K., & Hanson, L. (2014). Labor down or bear down: A strategy to translate second-stage labor evidence to perinatal practice. *The Journal of Perinatal & Neonatal Nursing*, 28(2), 117–126. doi:10.1097/JPN.0000000000000023

Pijuan-Domènech, A., Galian, L, Goya, M., Casellas, M., Merced, C., Ferreira-Gonzalez, I., . . . Garcia-Dorado, D. (2015). Cardiac complications during pregnancy are better predicted with the modified WHO risk score. *International Journal of Cardiology*, 195, 149–154. doi:10.1016/j.ijcard.2015.05.076

Pillutla, P., Nguyen, T., Markovic, D., Canobbio, M., Koos, B. J., & Aboulhosn, J. A. (2016). Cardiovascular and neonatal outcomes in pregnant women with high-risk congenital heart disease. *The American Journal of Cardiology*, 117(10), 1672–1677. doi:10.1016/j.amjcard.2016.02.045

Rezk, M., Elkilani, O., Shaheen, A., Gamal, A., & Badr, H. (2017). Maternal hemodynamic changes and predictors of poor obstetric outcome in women with rheumatic heart disease: A five-year observational study. *The Journal of Maternal-Fetal & Neonatal Medicine*, 31(12), 1542–1547. doi:10.1080/14767058.2017.1319932

Safi, L. M., & Tsiaras, S. V. (2017). Update on valvular heart disease in pregnancy. *Current Treatment Options in Cardiovascular Medicine*, 19(9), 70. doi:10.1007/s11936-017-0570-2

Salihu, H. M., Salemi, J. L., Aggarwal, A., Steele, B. F., Pepper, R. C., Mogos, M. F., & Aliyu, M. H. (2017). Opioid drug use and acute cardiac events among pregnant women in the United States. *The American Journal of Medicine*. doi:10.1016/j.amjmed.2017.07.023

Siu, S. C., Colman, J. M., Sorensen, S., Smallhorn, J. F., Farine, D., Amankwah, K. S., . . . Sermer, M. (2002). Adverse neonatal and cardiac outcomes are more common in pregnant women with cardiac disease. *Circulation*, 105(18), 2179–2184. doi:10.1161/01.cir.0000015699.48605.08

Siu, S. C., Sermer, M., Colman, J. M., Alvarez, A. N., Mercier, L. A., Morton, B. C., . . . Sorensen, S. (2001). Prospective multicenter study of pregnancy outcomes in women with heart disease. *Circulation*, 104(5), 515–521. doi:10.1161/hc3001.093437

Tanous, D., Siu, S. C., Mason, J., Greutmann, M., Wald, R. M., Parker, J. D., . . . Silversides, C. K. (2010). B-type natriuretic peptide in pregnant women with heart disease. *Journal of the American College of Cardiology*, 56(15), 1247–1253. doi:10.1016/j.jacc.2010.02.076

Thorne, S., MacGregor, A., & Nelson-Piercy, C. (2006). Risks of contraception and pregnancy in heart disease. *Heart*, 92(10), 1520–1525. doi:10.1136/hrt.2006.095240

Troiano, N. H. (2015). Cardiomyopathy during pregnancy. *The Journal of Perinatal & Neonatal Nursing*, 29(3), 222–228. doi:10.1097/JPN.0000000000000113

van Hagen, I. M., Boersma, E., Johnson, M. R., Thorne, S. A., Parsonage, W. A., Escribano Subías, P., . . . Roos-Hesselink, J. W. (2016). Global cardiac risk assessment in the Registry of Pregnancy and Cardiac disease: Results of a registry from the European Society of Cardiology. *European Journal of Heart Failure*, 18(5), 523–533. doi:10.1002/ejhf.501

van Hagen, I. M., Roos-Hesselink, J. W., Donvito, V., Liptai, C., Morissens, M., Murphy, D. J., . . . Johnson, M. R. (2017). Incidence and predictors of obstetric and fetal complications in women with structural heart disease. *Heart*, 103(20), 1610–1618. doi:10.1136/heartjnl-2016-310644

Yucel, E., & DeFaria Yeh, D. (2017). Pregnancy in women with congenital heart disease. *Current Treatment Options in Cardiovascular Medicine*, 19(9), 73. doi:10.1007/s11936-017-0572-0

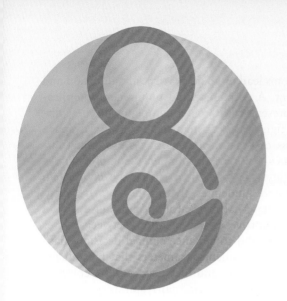

CHAPTER 10

Pulmonary Complications in Pregnancy

Cheryl K. Roth

INTRODUCTION

The frequency and significance of acute and chronic complications in pregnant women are complex and lead to maternal morbidity and mortality (Kuriya et al., 2016). Some of the pulmonary complications are unique to pregnancy (amniotic fluid embolism [AFE], preeclampsia, and tocolytic-induced pulmonary edema), whereas others are preexisting conditions that may worsen or exacerbate (cardiomyopathy, thromboembolic disease, asthma, pneumonia, and HIV-related pulmonary complications). When pulmonary complications occur during pregnancy, an understanding of the normal physiologic changes of pregnancy and their implications for assessing maternal–fetal status is essential for developing appropriate interventions and treatment.

ANATOMIC AND PHYSIOLOGIC CHANGES OF PREGNANCY THAT AFFECT THE RESPIRATORY SYSTEM

Pregnant women are susceptible to respiratory compromise and injury for several reasons, including alterations in the immune system that involve cell-mediated immunity and mechanical and anatomic changes involving the chest and abdominal cavities. The cumulative effect is decreased tolerance to hypoxia and acute changes in pulmonary mechanics.

Upper Airway Changes

Increased hormone levels result in mucosal edema, hyperaemia, mucus hypersecretion, capillary congestion, and greater fragility of the upper respiratory tract (Hemnes et al., 2015; Pacheco, Constantine, & Hankins, 2013). These hormonal changes and mucosal changes

result in rhinitis of pregnancy, characterized by nasal congestion during 6 or more weeks of pregnancy without other symptoms of respiratory tract infection and no known allergic cause. Rhinitis of pregnancy is experienced by 39% of pregnant women and may also include epistaxis, sneezing, voice changes, and mouth breathing (Dzieciolowska-Baran, Teul-Swiniarska, Gawlikowska-Sroka, Poziomkowska-Gesicka, & Zietek, 2013).

Anatomic Changes

Three important changes occur in the configuration of the thorax during pregnancy: (1) an increase of 6 cm in the circumference of the lower chest wall, (2) a 5-cm elevation of the diaphragm, and (3) a 70- to 104-degree widening of the costal angle (Gei & Suarez, 2018). These changes occur to accommodate the increase in uterine size and maternal weight gain, even though they appear in the first trimester prior to significant enlargement of the gravid uterus. The lower rib cage ligaments relax under hormonal influence to allow for a progressive widening of the subcostal angle and increased anterior-posterior and transverse diameters of the chest wall. Increased chest wall circumference accommodates elevation of the diaphragm such that vital lung capacity is not reduced (Gei & Suarez, 2018).

Respiratory Changes

Increased circulating levels of progesterone during pregnancy result in maternal hyperventilation and up to 50% greater tidal volume without corresponding changes in vital capacity or respiratory rate (Gei & Suarez, 2018). Oxygen consumption and minute ventilation increase as functional residual capacity (FRC) and residual volume decreases with expanding abdominal girth (LoMauro & Aliverti, 2015). Total lung capacity is preserved, however, because of rib flaring and unimpaired diaphragmatic excursion. The overall hemoglobin amount increases and allows for an increase in total oxygen-carrying capacity; however, the increase in plasma blood volume is disproportionate to the increase in hemoglobin concentration, thus resulting in a physiologic anemia (Mason & Burke, 2019).

The increase in minute ventilation that is associated with pregnancy is often perceived as a shortness of breath. Dyspnea usually starts in the first or second trimester and is reported by 70% of healthy pregnant women (Gei & Suarez, 2018; Mason & Burke, 2019). An increase of oxygen consumption of 15% to 20% occurs in pregnancy, due to both the needs of the fetoplacental unit and the increased workload of the mother's vital organs (Gei & Suarez, 2018).

Pregnancy is characterized by a state of chronic compensated respiratory alkalosis (LoMauro & Aliverti, 2015). Normal maternal hyperventilation during pregnancy lowers maternal partial pressure of arterial carbon dioxide (P_aCO_2) and minimally increases blood pH. The increase in blood pH increases the oxygen affinity of maternal hemoglobin and facilitates elimination of fetal carbon dioxide but appears to impair release of maternal oxygen to the fetus. The high levels of estrogen and progesterone during pregnancy facilitate a shift in the oxygen dissociation curve back to the right, thereby stimulating oxygen release to a fetus that has an increased affinity for oxygen. These physiologic adaptations ensure fetal advantage from increased oxygen transfer across the placenta and adequate blood gas exchange (Whitty & Dombrowski, 2019).

During labor and birth, hyperventilation is common due to pain, anxiety, and coached breathing techniques. Narcotics administered during labor and birth will act to decrease minute ventilation. In women with marginal placental reserves, hyperventilation and hypocarbia during labor and birth can lead to uterine vessel vasoconstriction and decreased placental perfusion. Decreased placental perfusion can have adverse effects on the fetus. Use of open-glottis pushing during second-stage labor may mediate these effects to some extent. Within 72 hours after birth, the minute ventilation rate decreases significantly with resumption of baseline in a few weeks. Lung volume changes normalize with decompression of the lungs and diaphragm after birth, whereas FRC and residual volume are back to baseline within 48 hours (Hegewald & Crapo, 2011). Chest wall changes of pregnancy return to normal by 24 weeks postpartum, but the subcostal angle remains 20% of pregnancy width (Hegewald & Crapo, 2011).

RECOGNIZING RESPIRATORY COMPROMISE

A significant number of critical events are preceded by early signs of respiratory complications. However, providers and patients may overlook or deny these signs and symptoms leading to delays in communication and management. A woman with a pulmonary complication may present with a chief complaint of chest discomfort or tightness, persistent cough, unusual dyspnea or shortness of breath, or hemoptysis. If clinical history indicates a potential pulmonary complication, a thorough physical assessment should be conducted. Evidence-based guidelines that include early warning signs of maternal respiratory compromise should be used to improve communication between nurses and physicians and to enhance clinical decision making regarding assessment parameters that fall outside defined normal values and that may indicate compromise. Physical signs of maternal respiratory compromise may include anxiety, increasing respiratory rate, wheezing, tachycardia, exertion with minimal activity, decreasing pulse oximetry values (trending below 96%), and/or adventitious breath sounds. Cyanosis, lethargy, agitation, intercostal retractions, and a respiratory rate greater than 30 breaths per minute indicate hypoxia and impending respiratory arrest.

When a patient presents with an elevated respiratory rate, nurses should recognize this trigger as a potential indicator of not only respiratory complications but also undiagnosed or new-onset cardiovascular disease (Hameed, Morton, & Moore, 2017). A respiratory rate of ≥30 breaths per minute and an oxygen saturation of ≤94% should be a "red flag," leading to further evaluation and consultation with specialists such as maternal fetal medicine, primary care, or cardiology.

FETAL SURVEILLANCE WITH MATERNAL PULMONARY COMPLICATIONS

In the presence of maternal respiratory compromise, which may include hypoxia, hypocapnia, or alkalosis, the fetus is at risk for impaired maternal–fetal gas exchange. Impaired gas exchange increases the incidence of fetal compromise and, if prolonged, will lead to intrauterine growth restriction (IUGR), hypoxia, and depletion of fetal oxygen reserves (Garite, 2018). The fetus depends on oxygen from maternal arterial oxygen content, venous return, and cardiac output as well as from uterine artery and placental blood flow. Maternal hypoxia can cause fetal hypoxia directly, or the consequences of poorly controlled pulmonary conditions resulting in hypocapnia and alkalosis can cause fetal hypoxia indirectly by reducing uteroplacental blood flow (Garite, 2018). The fetus is sensitive to changes in maternal respiratory status, and decreases in maternal partial oxygen tension (partial pressure of arterial oxygen [P_aO_2]) may result in decreased fetal PO_2 and cause fetal hypoxia (Vali & Lakshminrusimha, 2017) (Fig. 10–1). Rapid and profound decreases in fetal oxygen saturation and resultant fetal hypoxia occur

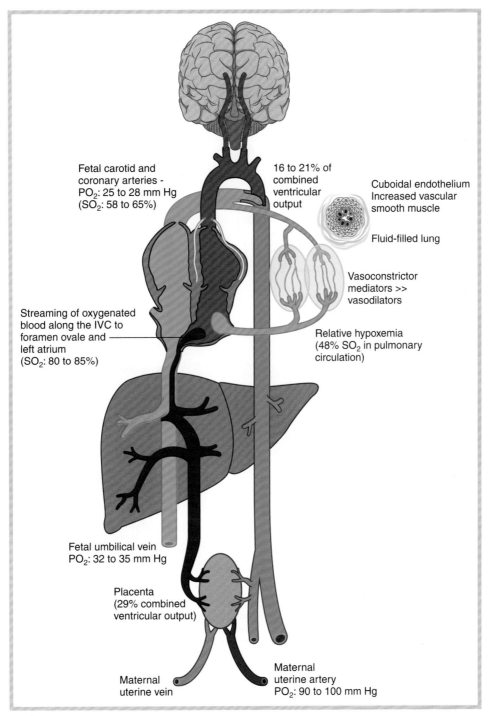

Fetal carotid and
coronary arteries -
PO$_2$: 25 to 28 mm Hg
(SO$_2$: 58 to 65%)

16 to 21% of
combined
ventricular
output

Cuboidal endothelium
Increased vascular
smooth muscle

Fluid-filled lung

Vasoconstrictor
mediators >>
vasodilators

Streaming of oxygenated
blood along the IVC to
foramen ovale and
left atrium
(SO$_2$: 80 to 85%)

Relative hypoxemia
(48% SO$_2$ in pulmonary
circulation)

Fetal umbilical vein
PO$_2$: 32 to 35 mm Hg

Placenta
(29% combined
ventricular output)

Maternal
uterine vein

Maternal
uterine artery
PO$_2$: 90 to 100 mm Hg

FIGURE 10–1. Fetal circulation. The placenta serves as a major buffer in reducing oxygen exposure to the fetus. The partial oxygen tension (PO$_2$) in the maternal uterine artery is 90 to 100 mm Hg compared to 32 to 35 mm Hg in the fetal umbilical vein (UV). The relatively higher oxygenated UV blood does not completely mix with the blood returning from the fetal body in the inferior vena cava (IVC) and is preferentially streamed toward the left atrium (through the foramen ovale). As the lungs do not participate in gas exchange in utero, the fetal pulmonary vascular resistance is very high, and the pulmonary circulation only receives 16% to 21% of the combined ventricular cardiac output (by phase contrast magnetic resonance imaging [MRI] and Doppler studies) in the near-term human fetus. As a result, there is only a small amount of desaturated blood from the pulmonary veins draining into the left atrium, maintaining a relatively high PO$_2$ in the left heart. Therefore, the blood pumped into the aorta supplying the brain and coronaries contains the highest fetal PO$_2$ (25 to 28 mm Hg: saturation 58% in human fetus and 65% in fetal lambs). Desaturated blood returning from the brain and the body into the right heart is pumped through the pulmonary artery and is mostly diverted through the ductus arteriosus to supply the rest of the body. Approximately 29% to 30% of the combined ventricular cardiac output circulates to the placenta. SO$_2$, oxyhemoglobin saturation. (Copyright Satyan Lakshminrusimha.)

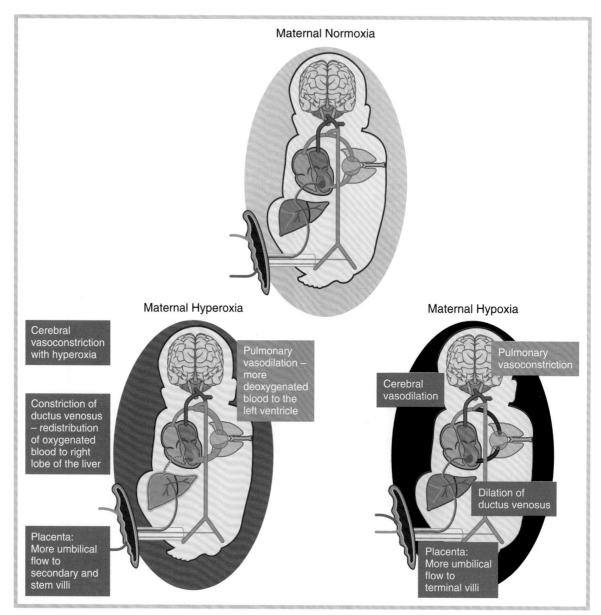

FIGURE 10–2. Fetal adaptation to maternal hypoxia and hyperoxia. The pulmonary circulation plays an important role in maintaining oxygen delivery to the brain. Exposing the mother to supraphysiologic levels of oxygen only slightly raises fetal umbilical venous (UV) partial oxygen tension (PO_2). The higher fetal PO_2 increases blood flow toward the lungs, resulting in more desaturated blood draining into the left atrium from the pulmonary veins, thus lowering the PO_2 in the left heart supplying the brain. With more blood flowing to the lungs, there is decreased blood flow to the brain, effectively counterbalancing the higher UV PO_2 and maintaining constant oxygen delivery to the brain. Other protective mechanisms to avoid oxygen toxicity are highlighted in the red boxes. Conversely, exposing the mother to a hypoxic environment leads to a decrease in UV PO_2, causing increased pulmonary vascular resistance and less blood shunting to the lungs, therefore limiting the amount of desaturated blood returning to the left atrium from the pulmonary veins. Increased umbilical flow, dilation of the ductus venosus, and cerebral vasodilation increase blood flow to the brain to counteract the lower PO_2 to maintain oxygen delivery. (Copyright Satyan Lakshminrusimha.)

with clinically significant decreases in maternal P_aO_2 below 60 mm Hg (Vali & Lakshminrusimha, 2017) (Fig. 10–2). Despite surviving in an environment of low oxygen tension, the fetus has very little oxygen reserve. Administration of oxygen to the mother may produce only small increases in fetal P_aO_2, but this may increase fetal oxygen saturation significantly (Vali & Lakshminrusimha, 2017) (Fig. 10–3). Oxygen should be administered as needed to maintain maternal oxygen saturation at 95% or higher (Garite, 2018).

Fetal status may offer early warning of maternal pulmonary compromise. Because the uterus is physiologically a nonessential organ, when there is decreased

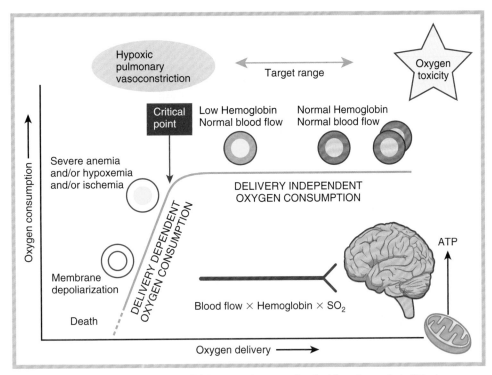

FIGURE 10–3. Relationship between oxygen (O_2) delivery and consumption. O_2 delivery is a product of blood flow and arterial O_2 content. When O_2 delivery decreases below a critical point, O_2 consumption is compromised leading to anaerobic metabolism and lactic acidosis. The driving force for O_2 into mitochondria is PO_2. Increased mitochondrial PO_2 can lead to reactive oxygen species formation, while hypoxia can exacerbate pulmonary vasoconstriction. The optimal target range encompasses oxygenation that guarantees an O_2 delivery higher than the critical point so that oxygen consumption is not dependent on delivery, while also avoiding oxygen toxicity. SaO_2, arterial oxyhemoglobin saturation. (Copyright Satyan Lakshminrusimha.)

blood volume, decreased cardiac output, or significant hypoxia, oxygenated blood flow will be directed to critical organs such as the brain, heart, and adrenal glands at the expense of uterine blood flow and, therefore, fetal well-being (Omo-Aghoja, 2014). Oxygenated blood flow will only be available to the uterus once other critical organs are perfused and oxygenated; therefore, a normal fetal heart rate (FHR) pattern excludes significant maternal hypoxia or hypotension, and an indeterminate or abnormal FHR pattern warrants close evaluation and intervention. Evaluation of the FHR pattern is an important element of assessment of maternal status and clinical decision making in the context of maternal respiratory disease.

The frequency of fetal surveillance should be determined by gestational age, current maternal status, and fetal response to illness. If exacerbations of pulmonary complications occur, vigilant fetal surveillance is important. At each prenatal visit, confirmation that fundal height and fetal size are consistent with expected normal values based on current gestation age is crucial. In conjunction with nonstress testing, serial ultrasounds and biophysical profiles are used to monitor fetal status on an ongoing basis (Garite, 2018; Mason & Burke, 2019). Fetal movement counting may also be initiated based on provider preference.

ASTHMA

Significance and Incidence

Asthma is the most common chronic medical condition affecting up to 4% to 8% of women during pregnancy (American College of Obstetricians and Gynecologists [ACOG], 2008). Up to 6% of women with asthma will be hospitalized with an acute onset of dyspnea (Ali & Ulrik, 2013). Multiple studies have looked at asthma status during pregnancy across the years, resulting in the general thought that about one third of patients improve, one third of patients stay the same, and one third of patients' asthma worsens during pregnancy (Ali & Ulrik, 2013). The underlying severity of the patient's asthma prepregnancy may be an indicator for exacerbation rates during pregnancy. Those with severe asthma are more likely than those with mild asthma to have exacerbations during pregnancy, particularly in the second trimester (de Araujo, Leite, Rizzo, & Sarinho, 2016). History of asthma severity in previous pregnancies may predict the severity of asthma in subsequent pregnancies (Murphy, 2015).

Severe or uncontrolled asthma can be life-threatening for a woman and her fetus during pregnancy. Care for asthma patients should be focused on avoidance of

TABLE 10–1. Classification of Asthma Severity and Control in Person 12 Years of Age or Older

	Mild intermittent	Mild persistent/moderate persistent	Severe persistent
Symptom frequency	≤2 days per week	Mild–2 to 6 days per week Moderate–daily	Throughout day
Use of rescue inhaler	≤2 days per week	Mild–2 to 6 days per week Moderate–daily	Throughout day
Nighttime awakening	≤2 times per month	Mild–≤2 times per month Moderate–>1 time per week	≥4 times per week
Interference with activities of daily living	None	Mild–minor limits Moderate–some limits	Extremely limited
FEV_1	>80% personal best	Mild–>80% personal best Moderate–60%–80% personal best	<60% personal best

FEV_1, forced expiratory volume in 1 second.
Adapted from National Asthma Education and Prevention Program. (2007). *Expert Panel Report No. 3: Guidelines for the diagnosis and management of asthma* (NIH Publication No. 07-4051). Bethesda, MD: National Heart, Lung, and Blood Institute. Retrieved from https://www.nhlbi.nih.gov/sites/default/files/media/docs/asthgdln_1.pdf

viral infections, discontinuation of anti-inflammatory medications, appropriate controller therapy, and adherence to the treatment plan. Women should be clearly informed of their risk for complications of their disease and their pregnancy due to asthma and should be followed closely by both their obstetrician and asthma specialist. Effective control can optimize pregnancy outcomes close to that of the general population (Murphy, 2015). The National Asthma Education and Prevention Program's (NAEPP, 2007) suggested steps for asthma control, as discussed in its publication *Expert Panel Report No. 3: Guidelines for the Diagnosis and Management of Asthma*, are listed in Table 10–1 (Whitty & Dombrowski, 2019).

Pathophysiology

Asthma is a chronic inflammatory disease of the airways characterized by an altered immune response. T helper 2 effector lymphocyte cells produce cytokines (Ali & Ulrik, 2013). Cytokines regulate immunoglobulin synthesis, which in turn activates the production of eosinophils and mast cells. Eosinophil production stimulates a vasomotor response, which might include bronchoconstriction and increased mucus production. The shift away from T helper 1 cells inhibits rejection of the fetus by the maternal immune system (McCracken, Gallery, & Morris, 2004). It is possible that these autoimmune changes could exacerbate maternal asthma (Ali & Ulrik, 2013). Other common triggers of asthma exacerbations are listed in Table 10–2.

The precise cause of airway inflammation and hyperresponsiveness is not well understood. When triggered by external stimuli, inflammatory cells infiltrate bronchial tissue and release chemical mediators such as prostaglandins, histamine, cytokines, bradykinin, and leukotrienes. Narrowing of the airway lumen and airway hyperresponsiveness may be a result of the development of bronchial mucosal edema, excess fluid and mucous, inflammatory cellular infiltrates, and smooth muscle hypertrophy and constriction. During asthma exacerbations, there is decreased expiratory airflow, increased FRC, increased pulmonary vascular resistance, hypoxemia, and hypercapnia. The fetus can be negatively affected during acute episodes of asthma in which there is maternal arterial hypoxemia and the potential for uterine artery vasoconstriction.

Clinical Manifestations

Women may have one or a combination of asthma symptoms, which include shortness of breath, wheezing, nonproductive coughing, flaring nostrils, chest tightness, and use of accessory respiratory muscles. There may be scant or copious sputum, which is usually clear. Reports of nocturnal awakenings with asthma symptoms are common. An increase in cough, the appearance of chest tightness, dyspnea, wheezing, decrease in fetal movement, or a 20% decrease in peak expiratory flow rate may signal worsening of asthma and should warrant immediate clinical attention (Whitty & Dombrowski, 2019).

TABLE 10–2. Common Triggers of Asthma Exacerbations

Allergens	Pollens, molds, animal dander, house-dust mites, cockroach antigen
Irritants	Strong odors, cigarette smoke, wood smoke, occupational dusts and chemicals, air pollution
Medical conditions	Sinusitis, viral upper respiratory infections, esophageal reflux
Drugs, additives	Sulfites, nonsteroidal anti-inflammatory drugs, aspirin, beta-blockers, contrast media
Other	Emotional stress, exercise, cold air, menses

Guidelines for assessing the severity of asthma before initiating therapy have been developed by the NAEPP through the National Institutes of Health (NAEPP, 2007). This classification system, like many others, was developed without specific consideration of pregnancy, but it may be helpful when assessing an adult patient with asthma. Patients are identified as intermittent, mild persistent, moderate persistent, or severe persistent asthmatics (NAEPP, 2007) (Table 10–1). Categories are specific to symptom frequency, use of a beta-agonist, nighttime wakening, interference with normal activities, and forced expiratory volume in 1 second (FEV_1) or peak flow levels.

Identification of the pregnant woman with severe asthma is important, so a plan of care and intensive treatment can be initiated early. See Display 10–1 for a management plan of care for pregnant women with exacerbations of asthma. Characteristics of maternal history that should alert healthcare providers to an increased risk of a potentially fatal asthma exacerbation are listed in Display 10–2. Nursing evaluation of the symptoms of asthma begins with clinical assessment of signs of respiratory distress. Significant findings include dyspnea, cough, wheezing, chest tightness, nasal flaring, presence of sputum, and tachycardia. Intercostal retractions or a respiratory rate greater

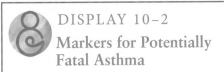

DISPLAY 10–2

Markers for Potentially Fatal Asthma

- Recent history of poorly controlled asthma
  - History of cardiovascular collapse, asthma related
  - History of systemic steroid therapy >4 weeks
- Three recent emergency room visits for asthma
- History of multiple hospitalizations for asthma
- History of hypoxic seizure, hypoxic syncope, or intubation
- History of admission to an intensive care unit for asthma

than 30 breaths per minute indicates moderate to severe asthma. Pulsus paradoxus, an abnormal fall of blood pressure during inspiration, of greater than 15 mm Hg is an indication of severe asthma. If pulsus paradoxus is present, blood pressure is audible only during expiration. To make this assessment, carefully observe the woman's breathing, noting when systole first appears, and the millimeter level of mercury until pulsations are heard during inspiration and expiration. Lung auscultation usually reveals bilateral expiratory wheezing. Occasionally, on inspiration or expiration, only rhonchi are heard. Rales are rarely auscultated in asthmatics. Detailed clinical findings are listed in Display 10–3.

DISPLAY 10–1

Management Plan of Care for Pregnant Women with Exacerbations of Asthma

- Obtain initial blood gas and pulmonary function tests to gather baseline data.
- Continuously monitor maternal pulse oximetry.
- Administer oxygen therapy to maintain SpO_2 >95%
- Monitor fetal status as determined by estimated gestational age.
- Tocolytic of choice for preterm labor management is magnesium sulfate. Use of magnesium sulfate therapy may enhance bronchodilation. Nonsteroidal anti-inflammatory medications, such as indomethacin, may exacerbate asthma and are contraindicated.
- Beta-agonist inhalation therapy is the initial pharmacologic therapy.
- If initial bronchodilator treatments fail to result in adequate response, high-dose intravenous corticosteroids may be considered.
- Antibiotics may be used to cover secondary bacterial infection.
- Measure and record intake and output. Observe for fluid volume imbalances.
- Observe for signs and symptoms of hydrostatic pulmonary edema due to tocolytic therapy and intravenous steroids.
- Provide ongoing care based on response to initial management

DISPLAY 10–3

Clinical Findings in Asthma

Signs and Symptoms
- Shortness of breath, chest tightness, productive or nonproductive cough
- Increased respiratory rate (>20 breaths per minute)
- Tachycardia
- Nasal flaring
- Exertion with minimal activity
- Recurrent episodes of symptoms
- Nocturnal awakenings from symptoms
- Waxing and waning of symptoms

Auscultatory Findings
- Diffuse wheezes
- Diffuse rhonchi
- Longer expiratory phase than inspiratory phase

Signs of Respiratory Distress
- Rapid respiratory rate (>30 breaths per minute)
- Pulsus paradoxus >15 mm Hg
- Retractions intercostally or supraclavicularly
- Lethargy
- Confusion or agitation
- Cyanosis

The most beneficial tools to determine the severity of asthma is a pulmonary function test such as peak expiratory flow. Predicted values of peak expiratory flow rate are unchanged during pregnancy and range from 380 to 550 L/min. An individual baseline value should be established for each woman when her asthma is under control. Evaluation of exacerbations can be made by comparing baseline values with current peak flow values. Peak expiratory flow values that are more than 20% below personal baseline values require immediate attention.

Evaluations of arterial blood gases can help to establish severity of an asthma attack, with attention focused primarily on the pH and PCO_2 to define severity. A mild attack is characterized by an elevated pH and a PCO_2 below normal for pregnancy. The combination of normal pH, low PO_2, and normal PCO_2 for pregnancy indicates a moderate asthma attack. A low PO_2, low pH, and a high PCO_2 are most significant for severe respiratory compromise. When maternal arterial PO_2 falls below 60 mm Hg, the fetus is in severe jeopardy, and risk of fetal demise is increased.

Use of the acronym GARDD will assist the provider in evaluating the need for intubation and mechanical ventilation (Gei & Suarez, 2018):

- Gastropulmonary reflux and aspiration
- Airway obstruction (present or suspected)
- Respiratory arrest (actual or impending)
- Depressed mental status, and
- Difficulty managing secretions (Gei & Suarez, 2018)

Potentially fatal asthma includes a history of any one of the factors listed in Display 10–2. During pregnancy, monthly evaluations of pulmonary function and asthma history are important. These evaluations should include the following assessments: pulmonary function testing, ideally spirometry; detailed symptom history (symptom frequency, nocturnal asthma, interference with activities, exacerbations, and medication use); and physical examination with specific attention paid to the lungs (Mason & Burke, 2019).

Clinical Management

The goals when managing the woman with asthma during pregnancy include educational support, maintaining optimal respiratory status and function, objective assessment of maternal and fetal status, avoiding triggers, and pharmacologic treatment to control symptoms and prevent exacerbations and/or adverse effects of medication (NAEPP, 2007). Fetal surveillance for women with asthma begins early in pregnancy. Women who have moderate or severe asthma during pregnancy should have ultrasound examinations and antenatal fetal testing. If possible, first-trimester ultrasound dating should be performed to assist with subsequent evaluations of fetal growth

restriction and determine risk of preterm birth. Serial ultrasound examinations to monitor fetal activity and growth should be considered (starting at 32 weeks of gestation) for women who have poorly controlled asthma or moderate to severe asthma and for women recovering from a severe asthma exacerbation (Murphy, 2015).

Patient/Family Education

Education should be designed to assist the woman and her family to gain motivation, confidence, and skills to keep asthma symptoms under control and to understand the potential adverse effects of uncontrolled asthma on herself and the fetus. Although some women may be reluctant to take prescribed medications for fear they may harm the developing fetus, the woman needs to be reassured that risks to the fetus from hypoxia-related, untreated asthma are greater than risks of medications (Mason & Burke, 2019). All patients should be taught to be conscientious of fetal activity and to report concerns to their healthcare provider (ACOG, 2008). Also, it is critically important that the pregnant woman be able to recognize symptoms of worsening asthma and have the knowledge of how to treat appropriately. Correct inhaler technique should be taught and return demonstration done. The patient should know how to reduce her exposure to, or control, those factors that exacerbate her asthma (Mason & Burke, 2019). Educational topics (NAEPP, 2007) include the following:

- Signs and symptoms of asthma
- Airway changes
- Avoiding asthma triggers
- Effects of pregnancy on the disease and the disease on pregnancy
- Peak flow meters and metered dose inhalers
- Role of medications
- Correct use of medications
- Adverse effects of medications
- Managing exacerbations
- Emergency care

Individualized education throughout pregnancy should be guided by assessment of the woman's understanding of her asthma assessment management plan and her level of cooperation. It is essential to highlight the changes that pregnancy has on asthma and treatment. When there is active participation by the healthcare provider, the pregnant woman, and her family, asthma control can be maximized.

Nonpharmacologic Control

Identification of triggering factors for asthma in each woman is an important aspect of management that may improve clinical status, prevent acute exacerbations, and decrease the need for pharmacologic intervention. Asthma is associated with allergies, with 75% to 85% of patients reporting positive testing to common allergens (Whitty & Dombrowski, 2019). Historic information and prior skin testing may give important information regarding common triggers such as pollens, molds, house dust mites, animal dander, and cockroach antigens. Other common asthma irritants include air pollutants, strong odors, food additives, and tobacco smoke. It is particularly important for the pregnant asthmatic woman to stop smoking during her pregnancy (ACOG, 2017b; NAEPP, 2007). Education about the risks of smoking, including an increased severity of her asthma, bronchitis, or sinusitis and the need for increased medication, can be helpful in motivating the woman to stop smoking.

Viral respiratory infections, vigorous exercise, and emotional stress may also cause severe asthma exacerbations. Medications such as aspirin, beta-blockers, nonsteroidal anti-inflammatory drugs, radiocontrast media, and sulfites have been implicated as asthma triggers as well. Once the woman has been assisted to identify common asthma triggers, exposure to allergens or irritants can be minimized, thereby lessening exacerbations.

Pharmacologic Therapy

Pharmacologic therapy plays an essential role in optimizing maternal and fetal outcomes by providing protection for the respiratory system from irritant stimuli, prevention of pulmonary and inflammatory response to allergen exposure, relief of bronchospasm, resolution of airway inflammation to reduce airway hyperresponsiveness, and improvement of pulmonary function. Undertreatment is an ongoing problem in the care of pregnant asthmatic women. Medications commonly used in asthma management are generally considered safe and effective during pregnancy and lactation. It is safer for pregnant women with asthma and their fetuses to take prescribed medications than to experience an exacerbation (Mason & Burke, 2019). The effectiveness of medications for the treatment of asthma during pregnancy is assumed to be the same as in nonpregnant women (NAEPP, 2007). Inhalation therapy is usually more effective than systemic treatment because asthma is an airway disease. Aerosolized medications are ideal because they deliver the drug directly to the airways, minimizing systemic side effects and decreasing exposure to the fetus.

Pharmacologic therapy for asthma is divided into two categories: (1) rescue (medications that provide symptomatic relief of acute bronchospasm without treating the cause of the bronchospasm) and (2) maintenance (medications that control airway hyperreactivity and treat underlying inflammation) (Whitty & Dombrowski, 2019). Generally, a stepwise approach to the pharmacologic management of chronic asthma is preferred (see Table 10–1).

Rescue Medications

Short-Acting Beta-Agonists

The use of inhaled beta-2 agonists provides bronchodilation and is recommended for acute and mild intermittent asthma therapy (Bonham, Patterson, & Strek, 2018). The onset of action is rapid with demonstrated safety profiles for mother and fetus, making short-acting beta-2 agonists the preferred rescue medication for acute exacerbations of asthma. Medications in this group include metaproterenol (Alupent) and albuterol (Ventolin, Proventil). This group of drugs has minimal side effects such as maternal tachycardia, tremors, restlessness, anxiety, and palpitations (Lehne, 2010). If symptoms disappear and pulmonary function normalizes, these medications can be used indefinitely. Prolonged use may result in rapid tolerance and limited usefulness. Women are candidates for anti-inflammatory therapy if they require the use of a beta-2 agonist more than three times each week. In the management of moderate to severe persistent asthma, long-acting beta-agonists may be added to a regimen of inhaled corticosteroids for greater asthma control (NAEPP, 2007).

Long-Acting Beta-Agonists

Salmeterol (Serevent Diskus) and formoterol (Foradil) are newer long-acting beta-agonists with limited published data regarding safe use in pregnancy. Therefore, the use of these medications are limited to women with moderate to severe asthma, who report relief of symptoms with use of these agents prior to pregnancy, or as an add-on therapy for women who are currently on inhaled steroids and need additional therapy for symptom relief.

Anticholinergics

Ipratropium (Atrovent) is an anticholinergic medication that may be used in combination with inhaled beta-agonists to promote bronchodilation and limit hypersecretion in patients with bronchitis, pneumonia, and chronic obstructive pulmonary disease (Mason & Burke, 2019). If prescribed during pregnancy, nebulized forms of anticholinergics may be considered in combination with short-acting betamimetics for additional therapy in cases of acute asthma exacerbations in the emergency care setting (Mason & Burke, 2019).

Maintenance Medications

Methylxanthines

Because of the success of inhalation therapy, systemic aminophylline and theophylline are rarely used today.

Sustained-release theophylline may be helpful for the pregnant woman whose symptoms are primarily nocturnal because of its long-acting properties. Although safe at recommended doses during pregnancy, theophylline treatment is associated with a higher incidence of maternal side effects than inhaled beta-agonists (NAEPP, 2007).

Cromolyn Sodium

Cromolyn and nedocromil are nonsteroidal anti-inflammatory agents that work by preventing the release of inflammatory mediators through stabilization of mast cells. Neither produces any side effects. Both are U.S. Food and Drug Administration category B drugs, and cromolyn data have demonstrated long-term safety (NAEPP, 2007). Neither is as effective as inhaled corticosteroids in preventing asthma symptoms and is rarely used due to availability of other treatment options.

Inhaled Corticosteroids

One of the greatest advances in asthma treatment in the past decade has been the availability of inhaled corticosteroids. For women with persistent mild asthma, these medications are currently the treatment of choice because they reduce the risk of asthma exacerbations associated with pregnancy and have not been related to any increase in congenital malformations or other adverse perinatal outcomes (NAEPP, 2007). To minimize systemic effects and improve respiratory tract penetration, inhaled corticosteroids are administered with a spacer. At recommended doses, these medications act without systemic side effects to effectively reduce mucus secretion and airway edema. They may increase bronchodilator responsiveness while inhibiting many of the mediators of inflammation. Studies suggest that budesonide is the inhaled steroid of choice for use during pregnancy due to reassuring safety data (Bonham, Patterson, & Strek, 2018).

Unlike the immediate-acting bronchodilators, the effects of inhaled corticosteroids are gradual. After 2 to 4 weeks of use, full effects of symptom suppression and peak expiratory flow rate improvement are seen. Patient education is vital to ensure that the woman will continue her anti-inflammatory therapy until the medication achieves maximum effectiveness. The most common side effect of inhaled steroids is hoarseness, which disappears when therapy is discontinued. Other uncommon side effects include throat irritation, cough, and oral thrush. Infrequent effects such as easy bruising, skin thinning, and low serum cortisol levels have been reported. Published data have shown no evidence of teratogenicity with use of inhaled corticosteroids. Intranasal corticosteroids have not been studied during human pregnancy, but because their systemic effects are minimal, continued use during pregnancy appears to be safe (NAEPP, 2007).

Systemic Corticosteroids

Due to associated fetal and pregnancy complications, systemic oral corticosteroids may be prescribed when maximum doses of bronchodilators and anti-inflammatory agents fail to control asthma. Conflicting reports show possible association of increased cleft lip and palate formation with exposure (Park-Wyllie et al., 2000; Reinisch, Simon, Karow, & Gandelman, 1978; Robert et al., 1994). Consistently, reports of pregnancy-associated complication have been shown with corticosteroid use. These complications include gestational hypertension, preeclampsia, gestational diabetes or worsening of diabetes mellitus, preterm birth, and low birth weight (NAEPP, 2007). However, if needed for short-term therapy to control exacerbations of acute asthma symptoms or long-term management, the benefits of using oral corticosteroids outweigh the risks and are recommended as needed (Bonham, Patterson, & Strek, 2018; NAEPP, 2007).

Leukotriene Modifiers

Leukotriene modifiers are a class of drugs that limit the inflammatory action of leukotrienes, chemical mediators that cause bronchoconstriction and mucus hypersecretion and stimulate microvascular leakage, edema formation, and eosinophil chemotaxis (Belfort & Herbst, 2010). Examples of these drugs include zileuton (Zyflo), zafirlukast (Accolate), and montelukast (Singulair).

Combination Drugs. Combination drugs, such as Advair Diskus and Combivent, may be prescribed for continued use during pregnancy if symptoms are well controlled. However, because these medications contain a combination of medications, benefits versus risks of the individualized medications contained in these combination formulas must be considered (Bonham, Patterson, & Strek, 2018).

Immunotherapy. Pregnant women with asthma who have allergens responsive to desensitization may benefit from allergen immunotherapy. Pollens, dust mites, and some fungi are aeroallergens that have been effectively suppressed with the use of allergy injections. Maintenance dose injections may continue for a pregnant woman who is not reacting regularly and continues to benefit from the immunotherapy (Blaiss, 2004). Because there is a 6- to 7-month interval before clinical benefits are seen and significant risk of a systemic reaction, pregnancy is not a time for initiation of immunotherapy.

Other Pharmacologic Therapies. Antihistamines may be useful in the woman with a clear allergic stimulus to her asthma. Pseudoephedrine has been routinely used in the treatment of rhinitis, although intranasal corticosteroids are currently the most effective medications for this condition and carry a low risk of systemic effects. Avoidance of oral decongestants in the first trimester is suggested unless absolutely necessary. Pregnant women with asthma should be cautioned about use of over-the-counter medications because many of the medications contain vasoconstrictors that may cause fetal abnormalities and decreased uterine blood flow (NAEPP, 2007). The influenza vaccine is indicated for women with chronic asthma after the first trimester (ACOG, 2018a). Because it is an inactivated virus, the influenza vaccine poses no risk to the fetus.

Labor and Birth

Approximately 10% to 20% of women with asthma experience an exacerbation during the intrapartum period (Gluck & Gluck, 2006; Mason & Burke, 2019). The risk of dyspnea or wheezing can be minimized through ongoing asthma medication during labor and the postpartum period. An exacerbation during labor is treated no differently than at any other time. Control of the asthma is a priority for safety of the mother and her fetus. Intravenous (IV) access should be established on admission (Gardner & Doyle, 2004). A peak flow rate may be taken on admission and then every 12 hours (Gardner & Doyle, 2004). If the woman develops symptoms of asthma, peak flows should be measured after treatments (Gardner & Doyle, 2004). If a systemic steroid has been administered in the past month prior to birth, additional rescue-dosed steroid therapy may be given during labor to prevent maternal adrenal crisis (Belfort & Herbst, 2010). IV hydrocortisone 100 mg every 6 to 8 hours should be administered for 24 hours or until oral medications are tolerated (Belfort & Herbst, 2010).

Air exchange is enhanced through patient positioning in a semi-Fowler or high-Fowler position. Potential for fluid overload can be avoided through strict intake and output measurements. Oxytocin is the drug of choice for the induction of labor because prostaglandin F_2a is a known bronchoconstrictor (Frye, Clark, Piacenza, & Shay-Zapien, 2011; Towers, Briggs, & Rojas, 2004). The use of prostaglandin E2 for cervical ripening intracervically or intravaginally has not been reported to result in a clinical exacerbation of asthma (Mason & Burke, 2019). The pain relief method of choice for women in labor with asthma is epidural analgesia (Gardner & Doyle, 2004). Epidural analgesia can reduce oxygen consumption and may enhance the effects of bronchodilators (NAEPP, 2007). Meperidine and morphine sulfate are contraindicated because of their actions on smooth muscle and the

potential for respiratory depression, and they may result in bronchospasm through histamine release (Belfort & Herbst, 2010). Butorphanol and fentanyl are appropriate substitutes (Belfort & Herbst, 2010).

A vaginal birth is safest for all women but particularly for women with asthma. Open glottis pushing during second stage is optimal. Maternal and fetal hypoxia that is the result of asthma should be managed medically; rarely is cesarean birth indicated. If cesarean birth is necessary for obstetric reasons, regional anesthesia is preferred; however, if general anesthesia is required, propofol is the sedation agent of choice, and ketamine or halogenated anesthetics are preferred due to their bronchodilation effects (Belfort & Herbst, 2010). Use of methylergonovine (i.e., Methergine) and prostaglandin F_2a for postpartum hemorrhage can cause bronchoconstriction and should be avoided (Belfort & Herbst, 2010).

Postpartum

Prepregnancy regimens of inhaled medications should be resumed following birth. Women on oral corticosteroid therapy may require IV dosing until oral medications are tolerated (Belfort & Herbst, 2010). Breastfeeding should be encouraged in women with asthma because breast milk confers some immunity to infection to the baby, especially to respiratory and gastrointestinal infections (Gardner & Doyle, 2004). Although breast milk may contain small amounts of the medications used to treat asthma, in general, they are not known to be harmful to the baby (Gardner & Doyle, 2004). Corticosteroids are approximately 90% protein bound in the blood and not secreted in any significant amounts in breast milk. Inhaled beta-2 agonists (terbutaline, metaproterenol, albuterol) by metered dosage are associated with the lowest exposure to the baby. Theophylline, as with caffeine, can cause irritability and wakefulness in the baby and is no longer considered the primary treatment (Gardner & Doyle, 2004).

PNEUMONIA

Significance and Incidence

Pneumonia is the leading cause of maternal mortality from nonobstetric infection in the peripartum period (Whitty & Dombrowski, 2019). Overall, pneumonia is the primary diagnosis for approximately 4.2% of nonobstetric antepartum hospital admissions (Laibl & Sheffield, 2006). Although pneumonia is not gestational-age dependent, the average gestational age at diagnosis is 32 weeks, and hospital admission for pneumonia is highest between 24 and 31 weeks of gestation (Graves, 2010). Pneumonia during the postpartum period is more than twice as high in women who had a cesarean as compared to vaginal birth (Belfort et al., 2010). The higher incidence may be due to associated pain and decreased activity following the cesarean birth or to a disease process that necessitated cesarean birth and/or predisposed to infection (Brito & Niederman, 2011). The incidence of pneumonia and spectrum of causative pathogens during pregnancy is similar to that of the nonpregnant population. Physiologic changes altering respiratory effort and the immunologic compromise state in pregnancy may contribute to a disease course, which is often more virulent and less tolerated, and the mortality rates from some pathogens are high (Graves, 2010). Unrecognized pneumonia may lead to sepsis and intensive care unit admissions for respiratory compromise.

Pneumonia is seen more frequently in women with poor health and who postpone childbearing. Also, available rates show higher incidence in large urban hospitals than in community settings (Brito & Neiderman, 2011). Pneumonia has been strongly associated with women with a significantly higher risk of preterm birth, low birth weight, small-for-gestational-age infants, low Apgar scores, cesarean section, and preeclampsia/eclampsia (Chen, Keller, Wang, Lin, & Lin, 2012).

Maternal conditions and complications that are associated with pneumonia are listed in Display 10–4. Although the introduction of antimicrobial therapy has significantly decreased maternal mortality from 23% to less than 4%, risk of maternal and fetal morbidity

continues (Whitty & Dombrowski, 2019). Viral pneumonias may be more virulent during pregnancy than in the nonpregnant patient.

Maternal complications of pneumonia include preterm labor, bacteremia, pneumothorax, atrial fibrillation, pericardial tamponade, and respiratory failure requiring intubation (Goodnight & Soper, 2005). Pneumonia has not been related to any congenital syndrome in neonates, but antepartum respiratory infection has been associated with increased incidence of complicated preterm birth. The loss of maternal ventilatory reserve normally seen in pregnancy coupled with maternal fever, tachycardia, respiratory alkalosis, and hypoxemia seen with respiratory infections can be adverse for the fetus. Reports of preterm labor and birth, small-for-gestational-age infants, and fetal death have been attributed to pneumonia during pregnancy (Chen et al., 2012).

Fungal pneumonia from environmental organisms is rare in pregnancy, occurring most often in severely immunocompromised patients (Laibl & Sheffield, 2006). In nonimmunosuppressed patients, this disease is frequently mild, self-limiting, and usually resolves with or without treatment in women without other preexisting illnesses. Disseminated disease from *Pneumocystis carinii* develops occasionally in immunocompromised patients and carries a high risk of preterm birth and perinatal and maternal mortality. Symptoms include fever, anorexia, dry cough, and several weeks of dyspnea. Treatment is prolonged and carries risks to the developing fetus.

Pathophysiology

Pneumonia is an inflammatory infection of the alveoli and distal bronchioles of the lower respiratory tract resulting in consolidation, exudation, and hypoxemia. Pneumonia may be primary or secondary and involve one or both lungs. The microorganisms that give rise to pneumonia are always present in the upper respiratory tract, and unless resistance is lowered, they cause no harm. Most organisms are introduced through inhalation or aspiration of secretions from the nasopharyngeal tract. Bacterial and viral pneumonias and aspiration pneumonitis are the most commonly seen pneumonias during gestation (Display 10–5). Alteration in maternal immune status to prevent rejection of the developing fetus is the major factor predisposing women to severe pneumonic infections during pregnancy. Chronic medical conditions such as obesity and HIV are believed to contribute to the increasing incidence of pneumonia in the general population and consequently in the obstetric population as well (Whitty & Dombrowski, 2019).

Pneumonia develops when host defenses are overwhelmed by an organism invading the lung parenchyma. Although a number of defense mechanisms

---

DISPLAY 10–4
Complications Associated with Pneumonia

- Altered mental status
- Vital sign abnormalities
  - Respirations ≥30 breaths per minute
  - Temperature ≥39°C or ≤35°C
  - Hypotension
  - Heart rate >120 beats per minute
- Laboratory data abnormalities
  - White blood cell count <4,000 mm^3 or 30,000 mm^3 with left shift
  - Room air partial pressure of arterial oxygen (P$_a$O$_2$) <60 mm Hg
  - Room air partial pressure of arterial carbon dioxide (P$_a$CO$_2$) >50 mm Hg
  - Serum creatinine >1.2 mg/dL
- Sepsis leading to multiorgan dysfunction/failure
- Radiologic abnormalities
- Multilobe involvement
- Cavitation
- Pleural effusion

DISPLAY 10–5

Causes of Pneumonia in Pregnancy

- *Streptococcus pneumoniae*
- *Haemophilus influenzae*
- *Legionella* species
- *Mycoplasma pneumoniae*
- *Chlamydia pneumoniae*
- *Pneumocystis carinii*
- Viral pathogens
- Influenza A
- Influenza B
- Varicella-zoster virus
- Coronavirus (severe acute respiratory syndrome)
- Aspiration
- Fungi

protect lower airways from pathogens, infection leads to increased permeability of the capillaries. This causes alveolar and interstitial fluid accumulation, resulting in abnormal chest radiograph findings. Air space pneumonia, interstitial pneumonia, and bronchopneumonia are commonly seen on the chest radiograph of patients with pneumonia. Radiographic patterns differ based on the infective agent and can be helpful in diagnosing the cause of pneumonia.

Clinical Manifestations

Obtaining a detailed history of the illness, including symptoms, and a physical examination are essential. Laboratory and radiologic findings are of primary importance to help diagnose the type of pneumonia present. Chest X-ray on the majority of patients with pneumonia reflects infiltrates, atelectasis, pleural effusions, pneumonitis, or pulmonary edema. Clinical presentation and laboratory data help to determine whether the pneumonia is classic or atypical. Careful questioning about underlying chronic conditions and prior illness can identify risk factors.

Initially, symptoms of pneumonia may mimic common discomforts in pregnancy and may be overlooked and the woman misdiagnosed with rapid progression of the disease course. Clinical manifestations may assist in diagnosis of pneumonia but lack specificity and sensitivity for causative etiology (Graves, 2010). In one study, 9.3% of pregnant women presented with a productive cough, 32% with shortness of breath, and 27.1% with pleuritic chest pain (Ramsey & Ramin, 2001). Physical examination usually reveals tachypnea and use of accessory muscles for respiration. Lung auscultation may identify inspiratory rales, absent breath sounds over the affected lung field, or a pleural friction rub. A sputum sample with secretions from the lower bronchial tree must be collected for Gram stain and culture. These specimens assist in identifying the pathogen responsible for the pneumonia.

Initial arterial blood gases in the pregnant woman with pneumonia usually reflect significant degrees of hypoxia without hypercapnia or acidosis (Laibl & Sheffield, 2006). The nurse should assess each woman closely for symptoms of hypoxia, including irritability and restlessness, tachycardia, hypertension, cool and pale extremities, and decreased urine output. Confusion, disorientation, and loss of consciousness can result if the hypoxia goes untreated.

Differential diagnosis of pneumonia includes pulmonary embolus and pulmonary edema from tocolysis, hypertension, or vascular leak (Graves, 2010).

Bacterial Pneumonia

The leading cause of pneumonia in pregnant women is bacterial (Mason & Burke, 2019). Risks for acquiring bacterial pneumonia include asthma, smoking, positive HIV status, poor nutrition, anemia, immunosuppressive illness, binge drinking, and exposure to viral infections (Laibl & Sheffield, 2006; Whitty & Dombrowski, 2019). The most common causative bacterial pathogen for pneumonia in pregnancy is *Streptococcus pneumoniae*. It is responsible for approximately one half to two thirds of cases of bacterial pneumonia during pregnancy and approximately two thirds of all pneumonias during pregnancy (Laibl & Sheffield, 2006). Women with bacterial pneumonia during pregnancy most often present with a history of malaise and upper respiratory infection. They frequently have abrupt onset of fever above 100°F with rigors and chills. Pleuritic chest pain, productive cough, dyspnea, and rusty sputum are other common symptoms. Blood cultures are positive in approximately 25% of cases (Neu & Sabath, 1993). *Haemophilus influenzae* is the second most common bacterium identified in women with bacterial pneumonia, and symptoms are similar to those caused by to *S. pneumoniae*. Women with chronic obstructive pulmonary diseases and chronic bronchitis are at greatest risk. There are numerous other uncommon pneumonia pathogens that may be seen in childbearing women, including *Mycoplasma pneumoniae*, *Chlamydia pneumoniae*, *Moraxella catarrhalis*, *Klebsiella pneumoniae*, and *Escherichia coli*. These organisms produce an atypical pneumonia syndrome, which is characterized by gradual onset, less toxicity, lower fever, nonproductive cough, malaise, and a patchy or interstitial infiltrate (Maccato, 1991). *Legionella pneumophila* may cause pneumonia with the typical acute course or the atypical symptoms described with the less common pathogens. Underlying chronic illness, advancing age, and cigarette smoking appear to be significant predisposing factors for bacterial pneumonia. When a superimposed pulmonary infection follows a viral pneumonia, *Staphylococcus aureus* is frequently responsible. This organism may also spread by the hematogenous route related to IV catheters, IV drug abuse, or infective endocarditis. The onset of this pneumonia is usually abrupt, and the course is rapid. Pleuritic chest pain and purulent sputum production are evident.

Aspiration can cause a very serious pneumonia that carries a high mortality rate, in spite of respiratory support and aggressive management. Pregnant women are predisposed to gastric aspiration due to the anatomic changes with elevation of the intragastric pressure due to the enlarged gravid uterus, the effect of progesterone influencing relaxation of the gastroesophageal sphincter, and delayed gastric emptying (Brito & Niederman, 2011). Aspiration pneumonia usually occurs during induction or emergence from general anesthesia for a cesarean birth. The aspiration of particulate matter and gastric acid causes an immediate chemical pneumonitis, followed in 24 to 48 hours by a secondary anaerobic or gram-negative bacterial infection. The use of nonparticulate antacids (e.g., sodium citrate), regional anesthesia, and rapid sequence induction of general anesthesia with cricoid pressure dramatically reduces the incidence of aspiration-related maternal mortality. Other causes of aspiration pneumonia include anything that may diminish consciousness, such as seizures and drug or alcohol abuse. Acute symptoms of aspiration include cough, significant bronchospasm, and hypoxia. Signs of chemical pneumonitis begin 6 to 24 hours after aspiration and include tachypnea, tachycardia, hypotension, and frothy pulmonary edema. Mechanical ventilation may be necessary and difficult. Resolution usually occurs over 4 to 5 days unless secondary infection develops (Graves, 2010). Prophylactic antibiotics and corticosteroids are not recommended. However, secondary bacterial infection must be identified and treated promptly with antibiotics to minimize significant perinatal morbidity and mortality (Graves, 2010).

Viral Pneumonias

Varicella pneumonia occurs in up to 20% of adults with varicella (chickenpox) infection. Because 90% of women are immune due to immunization or previous infection, the incidence of varicella pneumonia during pregnancy is rare (0.7 per 1,000) (Pereira & Krieger, 2004). However, the mortality rate for varicella pneumonia is 25% to 55% due to an increased risk for multiple complications such as bacterial superinfection, acute respiratory distress syndrome (ARDS), endotoxin shock, and bronchiolitis obliterans organizing pneumonia (Chandra, Patel, Schiavello, & Briggs, 1998). Intrauterine infections occur in 8.7% to 26%

of cases, exclusively during the first 20 weeks of gestation (Pereira & Krieger, 2004). The neonatal death rate for varicella pneumonia is between 9% and 20% (Grant, 1996). Following the incubation period of 10 to 21 days, symptoms of varicella zoster will begin, which include fever, headache, malaise, and maculopapular-vesicular rash. In a patient with primary varicella symptoms, the diagnosis of varicella pneumonia is confirmed by a chest X-ray that reveals an interstitial, nodular pattern or focal infiltrates. Varicella pneumonia typically presents with fever, dyspnea, tachypnea, dry cough, pleuritic chest pain, oral mucous lesions, and hemoptysis within 2 to 7 days of the vesicular rash (Ramsey & Ramin, 2001). It is not uncommon to see rapid progression to hypoxia and respiratory failure. In addition to maternal complications, intrauterine infection occurs in up to 26% of varicella pneumonia cases (Pereira & Krieger, 2004). Congenital varicella syndrome may occur if infection occurs in the first trimester and is characterized by cutaneous scars, limb hypoplasia, chorioretinitis, cortical atrophy, cataracts, and other anomalies in the neonate (Balducci et al., 1992; Goodnight & Soper, 2005; Laibl & Sheffield, 2005). Second trimester varicella may result in congenital varicella zoster in some infants. Premature labor and perinatal varicella infection are significant adverse effects that may result from varicella infection during pregnancy. Pregnant women with varicella pneumonia should be hospitalized, and infection control precautions should be implemented. Pharmacologic management should be implemented early with IV acyclovir at a dose of 7.5 to 10 mg/kg every 8 hours for 5 days (Graves, 2010; Whitty & Dombrowski, 2019). The addition of corticosteroids may also be given to improve outcomes.

Severe acute respiratory syndrome (SARS) is a viral illness first described in 2002. It is transmitted by respiratory droplets or close personal contact and results in an atypical pneumonia that can progress to hypoxemia and respiratory failure. SARS has been found to be extremely morbid in the pregnant patient, with mortality approaching 30% (Mason & Burke, 2019). Chest X-ray reveals generalized, patchy, interstitial infiltrates in patients with SARS pneumonia (Graves, 2010). Symptoms that are seen 2 to 7 days after exposure include headache, fever, chills, rigors, malaise, myalgia, dyspnea, and a nonproductive cough (Laibl & Sheffield, 2005). Patients are most infectious during the second week of illness (Laibl & Sheffiel, 2005). Based on limited available data, effects on pregnancy from this illness include spontaneous abortion, preterm birth, and small (for gestational age) fetus (Wong et al., 2004). The course of SARS and clinical outcomes are worse for pregnant women when compared to nonpregnant women (Lam et al., 2004; Mason & Burke, 2019). The virus does not appear to cross the placenta and infect the fetus (Wong et al., 2004). Rubeola during pregnancy may lead to spontaneous abortion and preterm birth. Pneumonia can complicate up to 50% of cases, and bacterial superinfection is also common.

The rise of measles in the United States is concerning as pregnant women contracting measles are more likely to be hospitalized, develop pneumonia, and die (Rasmussen & Jamieson, 2015). There does not appear to be a risk of congenital defects related to maternal contraction of the measles (Rasmussen & Jamieson, 2015). Women who are not immune should be offered the MMR vaccine before or after pregnancy.

Influenza and Viral Pneumonia

Physiologic changes cause the pregnant woman to be at increased risk of critical illness from influenza. In 2009, 5% of all U.S. deaths from H1N1, also known as swine flu, occurred in women who were pregnant. Influenza-mediated viral pneumonia is commonly caused by type A influenza, which is the most virulent strain in humans. The February 17, 2017, Morbidity and Mortality Report by the Centers for Disease Control and Prevention (CDC) reported that 59 women of childbearing age (15 to 44 years) in the United States were hospitalized for influenza pneumonia from October 2, 2016, to February 4, 2017, and 20 (33.9%) of these women were pregnant (Blanton et al., 2017). Type A influenza attacks the lung parenchyma and causes edema, hemorrhage, and hyaline membrane formation. Chest X-ray demonstrates unilateral patchy infiltrates. Acute onset of dyspnea, tachypnea, wheezing, malaise, headache, high fever, cough, and myalgias are associated symptoms. Frequently, superimposed bacterial pneumonia develops following resolution of influenza symptoms. During pregnancy, fulminant respiratory failure may develop quickly, requiring extended mechanical ventilation and resulting in significant mortality. In addition, preterm labor and birth risks are increased in women with influenza (ACOG, 2018a). Vaccination in any trimester is safe and recommended during influenza season (October to May) to prevent morbidity and mortality. Pregnant women should receive inactivated vaccine but should not receive the live attenuated nasal mist (ACOG, 2018a; Creanga et al., 2010). Women who are postpartum can receive vaccination. Another benefit of vaccination during pregnancy is protection in the newborn for up to 6 months of age. Infants up to 6 months of age have passive acquired antibodies in mothers who have received the influenza vaccine (ACOG, 2018a). The CDC reports that during the 2016 to 2017 flu season, an estimated 50% of pregnant women protected themselves and their babies by getting the flu vaccine (CDC, 2017a). Obstetric providers should educate and encourage all pregnant and postpartum women to get vaccinated against influenza.

Clinical Management

Prevention of pneumonia in pregnancy has been successful through the administration of seasonal influenza and pneumococcus vaccines. These vaccines are safe for administration in pregnancy and should be given to high-risk women. The varicella vaccine is not safe for administration during pregnancy because it is a live vaccine (Laibl & Sheffield, 2006). In pregnant women diagnosed with pneumonia, regardless of the type of pneumonia, interventions focus on close monitoring; oxygen supplementation; antipyretics; adequate hydration; control of pain, fatigue, and anxiety; and ongoing fetal assessment. Positioning the woman in a semi-Fowler's or high-Fowler's position usually is most comfortable and promotes maximum oxygenation. Oxygen supplementation to maintain oxygen saturation of greater than 95% by pulse oximeter is vital to ensure adequate maternal oxygen delivery to the fetus. The most common method of oxygen administration is 2 to 4 L/min through a nasal cannula. If the woman requires more than 4 L of oxygen to maintain adequate hemoglobin oxygen saturation, the use of a nonrebreather mask is more efficacious in delivering a higher fraction of inspired oxygen (FIO_2) (Simpson & James, 2005). Mechanical ventilation is necessary for women who are unable to maintain a P_aO_2 above 60 mm Hg despite high concentrations of inspired oxygen. For women who are unable to cough effectively, postural drainage and tracheal suctioning can be valuable in mobilizing secretions. The use of incentive spirometry may be helpful as well.

The development of preterm labor as a complication of infection may be the result of the response of the uterus to certain mediators of inflammation and infection. Prompt attention to regular uterine contractions and cervical changes is necessary to minimize the risks of preterm birth as a result of significant maternal illness. Conversely, in patients in whom respiratory and cardiovascular statuses continue to deteriorate despite maximum supportive efforts, birth may be necessary for fetal and maternal survival.

Pharmacologic Therapy

Antibiotic therapy must be specific to the pathogen present, along with consideration for safety during pregnancy (Table 10–3). Until identification of the causative organism, symptoms, sputum Gram stain, and chest radiography can direct initial antibiotic and antiviral use. Erythromycin has proven to be successful in treatment of pneumonia in pregnancy and is often administered initially. Ampicillin may be administered if *S. pneumoniae* or *H. influenzae* is the

TABLE 10–3. Antibiotic Therapy for Pneumonia Pathogens

Pathogen	Amoxicillin	Cephalosporin	Azithromycin/ clarithromycin	Trimethoprim- sulfamethoxazole
Streptococcus pneumoniae	+	+	+	+
Haemophilus influenzae	+	+	+	+
Mycoplasma catarrhalis	−	+	+	+
Chlamydia pneumoniae	−	−	+	−
Legionella pneumophila	−	−	+	−
Mycoplasma pneumoniae	−	−	+	−
Pneumocystis carinii	−	−	−	+

Referral should always be made to culture and sensitivity done on any bacteria identified. +, antibiotic coverage for bacteria; −, antibiotic not effective to treat bacteria.

suspected pathogen. With an increase in ampicillin-resistant pathogens, third-generation cephalosporins and trimethoprim-sulfamethoxazole are other choices for most cases of classic pneumonia. Varicella pneumonia must be treated promptly with acyclovir, with 7.5 to 10 mg/kg given intravenously every 8 hours for 5 days to decrease complications and mortality (Graves, 2010; Whitty & Dombrowski, 2019). Patients who receive acyclovir early in the course of their illness benefit from lower temperatures and respiratory rates and from improved oxygenation without risk to their fetus. Aggressive treatment of hypoxemia and administration of corticosteroids have also shown to improve outcomes in these women (Cheng, Tang, Wu, Chu, & Yuen, 2004; Goodnight & Soper, 2005).

Varicella embryopathy may occur as a result of maternal infection, particularly in the first half of pregnancy, with an incidence of 1% to 2% (Chapman, 1998). Varicella of the newborn is a life-threatening illness that may occur when a newborn is born within 5 days of the onset of maternal illness or after postbirth exposure to varicella. Susceptible newborns should be given VZIG (Chapman, 1998).

Aspiration pneumonia is best treated with broad-spectrum antibiotics to cover gram-negative and gram-positive bacteria that are usually present. Antiviral agents amantadine and ribavirin have been used in the treatment of influenza pneumonia and SARS pneumonia during pregnancy. Although they have shown teratogenicity in some animal studies, both have been effective in decreasing the severity of illness associated with influenza during pregnancy without adverse effects to humans. SARS pneumonia has also been effectively treated with the addition of antibiotics and corticosteroids.

PULMONARY EDEMA

Pulmonary edema is defined as the abnormal accumulation of fluid in the interstitial spaces, alveoli, or cells within the lungs that inhibits adequate diffusion of carbon dioxide and oxygen (Frye et al., 2011). Physiologic changes of the cardiopulmonary system during pregnancy place the pregnant woman at increased risk for developing pulmonary edema (Mason & Burke, 2019). There are two primary types of pulmonary edema: hydrostatic (cardiogenic) and vascular permeability (noncardiogenic, nonhydrostatic).

Hydrostatic

Colloid oncotic pressure (COP) normally pulls excess fluids from the lung tissue into the pulmonary vessels; however, in pulmonary edema, the opposite occurs. Hydrostatic pulmonary edema occurs when the hydrostatic pressure (pushing) within the pulmonary vascular bed exceeds the COP (pulling) of fluid within the vessel, reflected by a high pulmonary capillary wedge pressure (Mason & Burke, 2019). This pressure imbalance causes intravascular fluid to be physically pushed from within the vessel across the semipermeable endothelium; subsequently, interstitial fluid exceeds the pumping capacity of the lymphatic system and alveolar flooding occurs, resulting in interference of gas exchange. Hydrostatic pulmonary edema is related to intravascular hypervolemia. Potential causes in pregnancy include congenital or ischemic heart disease, acquired valvular lesions, tachydysrhythmias, and hypertension, either from chronic disease or preeclampsia. If a woman has systemic hypertension, the outflow of blood from the left ventricle is impaired, resulting in myocardial dysfunction. Systolic dysfunction is one of the most common causes of hydrostatic pulmonary edema during pregnancy. Cardiomyopathy results in systolic dysfunction (defined as an ejection fraction of less than 45%), and diastolic dysfunction results in impaired ventricular contractility and high filling pressures (Mabie, 2010). Hydrostatic pulmonary edema from beta-agonist and/or magnesium sulfate tocolytic therapy for more than 24 hours is well documented but not completely understood. Multifetal pregnancy with increased intravascular volume and reduced COP predisposes this population to hydrostatic changes.

Nonhydrostatic

Vascular permeability (nonhydrostatic) pulmonary edema results from pulmonary capillary or alveolar endothelial injury. The endothelial permeability allows protein-rich (colloid) vascular fluid to leak into the alveoli, pulmonary cells, and interstitial spaces. The resulting hemodynamic values are a decreased COP and decreased intravascular volume (hypovolemia), which results in decreased cardiac output and organ perfusion. The COP in the interstitial spaces increases and will continue to pull intravascular volume (Mason & Burke, 2019). Causes of vascular permeability pulmonary edema in pregnancy include infection leading to sepsis, preeclampsia, blood transfusion reaction, amniotic fluid embolus, aspiration pneumonia, disseminated intravascular coagulopathy, and inhalation injury. Patients with preeclampsia have about a 3% risk of developing pulmonary edema, which occurs in the first 72 hours postpartum 70% of the time, and maternal mortality for this condition is as high as 10% (Mason & Burke, 2019).

Nonhydrostatic pulmonary edema is caused by several mechanisms. Bacterial or viral infection causes release of prostaglandins, cytokines, and complement components, resulting in endothelium injury and myocardial dysfunction (Mabie, 2010). Aspiration and inhaled toxins cause direct chemical injury to the lung tissues and alveoli. Preeclampsia causes endothelial damage, which may lead to leaky capillary syndrome. Combined with the vasospasm caused by preeclampsia, system vascular resistance (afterload) increases, which can lead to significant diastolic dysfunction (Mason & Burke, 2019).

Clinical Manifestations

Clinical manifestations of pulmonary edema are the same, regardless of the type and etiology and may be very subtle at the onset. Symptoms include dyspnea, shortness of breath with a feeling of suffocation. Typically, the woman will want to sit up in bed, demonstrate anxious or agitated behavior, and have tachycardia and tachypnea that progressively increases. Breath sounds may initially be clear but progress to adventitious breath sounds, such as fine crackles, progress to coarse sounds (Mason & Burke, 2019). Wheezing may also be present. Usually, pulmonary edema begins with a nonproductive cough and progresses to a productive state with pink, frothy sputum. As the edema progresses, there will be a downward trend in SaO_2 values along with flaring and retractions. An irregular heart rate may occur if cardiac disease is present.

Clinical Management

Diagnosis of pulmonary edema is confirmed by history, clinical presentation, and diagnostic testing. The woman's history should be reviewed and include assessment of preexisting or pregnancy-related disease (e.g., preeclampsia), medications, fluid balance, chemical exposure, and anesthetic administration. A social history is of importance, to rule out the possibility of cocaine or heroin intoxication, which can lead to pulmonary edema.

Some tests that may be included in the diagnostic process of pulmonary edema are chest X-ray, arterial blood gas measurement, assessment of pulse oximetry trends, and electrocardiogram (ECG) monitoring. Echocardiography may show decreased ejection fraction with intravascular volume changes. Invasive hemodynamic monitoring may be required to determine the type of pulmonary edema and management plan. Acute pulmonary edema treatment may differ if hypertension is involved (Dennis & Solnordal, 2012). For example, a pregnant woman with preeclampsia is at risk of developing both hydrostatic and vascular permeability pulmonary edema, making it difficult to determine the type of pulmonary edema on the basis of noninvasive assessment. Therefore, if traditional, conservative management does not stop the progression of the symptoms and if signs of decreased cardiac output and oxygen availability are present, pulmonary artery catheterization may be considered to make a definitive diagnosis and develop a plan of care to optimize outcomes for the mother and fetus. These critically ill women require a multidisciplinary team approach to determine an individualized plan.

The management plan is not "one-size-fits-all" for pulmonary edema because the pathophysiology may result in intravascular volume extremes. Noninvasive assessment parameters, such as trends in vital signs and pulse oximetry, urine output, pulse pressure, peripheral pulse quality, venous distention, generalized edema, skin color, and temperature, will assist in determining the woman's intravascular volume status and cardiac output (Mason & Burke, 2019).

One of the main goals of managing pulmonary edema includes optimizing oxygen delivery. Humidified oxygen should be administered by a nonrebreather face mask. Because one of the diagnostic tools is the evaluation of the woman's arterial blood gas values, an arterial line may be considered to provide the healthcare team with frequent access and capabilities to determine the woman's response to treatment. Decreasing oxygen consumption is an important component of the management of women who are hypoxic. Limiting the woman's movements and providing pain management are necessary. A P_aO_2 of 70 mm Hg is consistent with early ventilator failure in pregnancy, and a P_aCO_2 greater than 40 mm Hg is strongly suggestive of ventilator insufficiency and possible ventilatory failure (Mason & Burke, 2019). These women should be monitored in an intensive care environment, and hemodynamic monitoring should be considered.

Position of the mother helps to optimize cardiac output, but the ideal position differs depending on the pathophysiology of pulmonary edema. If the mother has hydrostatic pulmonary edema, she should be placed in a high sitting position, preferably with her feet lower than her torso. This position will decrease return from her lower extremities and decrease volume status while still providing for adequate cardiac output. If vascular permeability pulmonary edema is suspected, if tolerated, the woman should lie on her left or right side. This position will optimize return to the right side of the heart and increase cardiac output.

Management of the woman's fluid intake also differs depending on the type of pulmonary edema. If hydrostatic pulmonary edema is suspected, IV and oral fluids should be restricted because the pathophysiology is related to hypervolemia. All IV fluids should be administered via a controlled infusion pump. If vascular permeability pulmonary edema is confirmed, volume resuscitation may be necessary to maintain cardiac output and organ perfusion. A pulmonary artery catheter may be beneficial to guide treatment according to the woman's hemodynamic responses. All intake and output should be monitored closely, documented, and communicated to the obstetrical care provider.

Pharmacologic Therapy

Pharmacologic therapy to treat pulmonary edema and manage the woman's symptoms may be necessary. When hydrostatic, or cardiogenic, pulmonary edema is suspected, furosemide (Lasix) is administered in small doses (10 to 20 mg, IV). A Foley catheter should be placed, and the woman's response to diuretic administration should be observed over the following hour. Serum potassium levels should be monitored closely with repetitive use of diuretics. A woman with left ventricular failure secondary to hypertension may require afterload reduction with antihypertensives to optimize volume status and cardiac output. Hydralazine is the first-line drug of choice to lower systemic vascular resistance. Because of the risk of hydrostatic pulmonary edema, beta-agonist or magnesium sulfate tocolytic therapy should be discontinued. The administration of morphine sulfate in small increments may be beneficial to manage the mother's pain and decrease oxygen consumption. However, morphine sulfate should not be given to women with decreased levels of consciousness or hypotension.

AMNIOTIC FLUID EMBOLISM

AFE, also known as anaphylactoid syndrome of pregnancy, is a rare but devastating condition unique to humans with a mortality rate of 20% to 30% (Benson, 2017; Copper, Otto, & Leighton, 2013;

Leighton, 2013). The incidence of AFE is reported to range from 1:15,200 to 1:53,800 (Thongrong et al., 2013). In women with AFE and cardiac arrest, 10% to 15% survive neurologically intact (Clark, 2014; Leighton, 2013; Shamshirsaz & Clark, 2016). AFE is associated with ruptured membranes 78% of the time (Leighton, 2013).

Understanding of AFE is incomplete; however, AFE classically consists of hypoxia from acute lung injury and transient pulmonary hypertension, hypotension, and cardiac arrest and coagulopathy (Pacheco, Saade, Hankins, & Clark, 2016). Clinically useful risk factors and preventative measures remain elusive, and perinatal morbidity and mortality continues to be significant. Symptoms of sudden dyspnea, hypotension, and cardiac arrest, with evidence of fetal hypoxia during labor, are the classic presentation of AFE, followed by massive fibrinolysis (Clark, 2014). AFE can result in acute lung injury by causing pulmonary vascular endothelial damage, complement activation, and direct platelet aggregation effects of amniotic fluid (Wise, Polito, & Krishnan, 2006).

Historically, AFE was thought to be the result of the infusion of amniotic fluid cells or other debris into the maternal circulation during uterine contractions, and the diagnosis was confirmed by the finding of fetal cells in the maternal pulmonary circulation upon autopsy (Clark, 2014). There has been a shift from this view of the pathophysiology of AFE to understanding the process as a systemic inflammatory response syndrome with inappropriate release of endogenous inflammatory mediators (Pacheco et al., 2016). Diagnosis of AFE is made clinically and should be suspected in any pregnant woman who develops hypotension, coagulopathy, and severe hypoxemic respiratory failure with, during, or immediately after labor. Treatment is mainly supportive with careful monitoring for the development of ARDS and coagulopathy. Basic, advanced, and obstetric cardiac life support protocols are generally followed in initial treatment and resuscitative efforts. Hypoxia is treated with supplemental oxygen and mechanical ventilation, using lung-protective strategies as indicated. Circulatory support is provided with rapid controlled fluid infusion, cardiogenic shock requires use of inotropic and vasoactive agents, and treatment of coagulopathy requires the replacement of coagulation factors (Pacheco et al., 2016). A novel approach to AFE treatment called the A-OK Protocol has been described in the literature in multiple case reports (Copper, Otto, & Leighton, 2013; Leighton, 2013; Rezai, Hughes, Larsen, Fuller, & Henderson, 2017). This approach hypothesizes that three factors contribute to AFE: thromboxane, serotonin, and a vagal response. Amniotic fluid in the maternal circulation stimulates platelet aggregation in the pulmonary vasculature. This triggers thromboxane activation and

serotonin release resulting in severe pulmonary vasoconstriction. The platelet aggregation in the lungs also
stimulates a vagal response, causing bradycardia and
peripheral vasodilation. To treat these effects, a triad
of atropine, ondansetron, and ketorolac (A-OK) were
used. Atropine 1 mg was used to treat the bradycardia
and peripheral vasodilation. Ondansetron 8 mg treated
the serotonin effect, and ketorolac 30 mg treated the
thromboxane effect. These medications are given rapidly upon suspected diagnosis. Case reports show that
the use of these agents are effective in resuscitation of
patients with suspected AFE (Copper et al., 2013).

Fetal or newborn outcomes of AFE are directly
related to the time between maternal cardiac arrest
and birth; however, the relationship is inconsistent
due to the variability in onset and intensity of uterine hypoperfusion and maternal decompensation. In
the presence of viable fetal gestational age, maternal
resuscitative efforts should follow standard cardiac
life support with the addition of consideration of birth
(Pacheco et al., 2016). A perimortem bedside cesarean birth may be indicated in the event of maternal
cardiac arrest. Relieving maternal vena caval compression may theoretically enhance maternal resuscitative
efforts.

VENOUS THROMBOEMBOLISM

The hypercoagulable state and venous stasis increase
the risk for the formation of venous thrombi and pulmonary embolus during pregnancy and the postpartum period (Alhassan et al., 2017; Leung, Sottile, &
Lockwood, 2019). Any type of endothelial injury can
tip the balance to develop a thrombus. Venous thromboembolism (VTE) is both more common and more
complex to diagnose in patients who are pregnant.
The incidence is estimated at 0.76 to 1.72 per 1,000
pregnancies, which is four times greater than in the
nonpregnant population (Alhassan et al., 2017). Deep
venous thrombosis (DVT) and pulmonary embolus are
collectively referred to as thromboembolytic diseases.
Approximately 75% to 80% of cases of pregnancy-
associated venous thrombosis are caused by DVT, and
20% to 25% of cases are caused by pulmonary embolus (James, Jamison, Brancazio, & Myers, 2006).
Regardless of gestational age, VTE may occur at any
time with approximately 40% to 60% of pregnancy-
related pulmonary emboli occurring in the postpartum
period (James et al., 2006). See Display 10–6 for risk
factors for development of VTE during the postpartum
period. It is interesting to note that 88% to 90% of
all DVT during pregnancy will occur in the left lower
extremity, which is thought to be caused by compression from the gravid uterus on the left iliac vein
(Brown & Hiett, 2010).

DISPLAY 10–6
Risk Factors for Development of Venous Thromboembolism during the Postpartum Period

Major risk factors (odds ratio >6)—presence of at least one of the following risk factors suggests a risk of postpartum venous thromboembolism (VTE) >3%:

- Immobility (strict bed rest for >1 week in the antepartum period)
- Postpartum hemorrhage >1,000 mL with surgery
- Previous VTE
- Preeclampsia with fetal growth restriction
- Thrombophilia
  - Antithrombin deficiency
  - Factor V Leiden (homozygous or heterozygous)
  - Prothrombin G20210A (homozygous or heterozygous)
- Medical conditions
  - Systemic lupus erythematosus
  - Heart disease
  - Sickle cell disease
- Blood transfusion
- Postpartum infection

Minor risk factors (odds ratio >6 when combined)—presence of at least two of the following risk factors or one of the following risk factors in the setting of emergency cesarean birth suggests a risk of postpartum VTE of >3%:

- Body mass index >30 kg/m²
- Multiple pregnancy
- Postpartum hemorrhage >1 L
- Smoking >10 cigarettes per day
- Fetal growth restriction (gestational age + sex-adjusted birth weight <25th percentile)
- Thrombophilia
  - Protein C deficiency
  - Protein S deficiency
- Preeclampsia

From Bates, S. M., Greer, I. A., Middeldorp, S., Veenstra, D. L., Prabulos, A. M., & Vandvik, P. O. (2012). VTE, thrombophilia, antithrombotic therapy, and pregnancy: Antithrombotic therapy and prevention of thrombosis, 9th ed: American College of Chest Physicians Evidence-Based Clinical Practice Guidelines. *Chest, 141*(2 Suppl.), e691S–e736S. doi:10.1378/chest.11-2300

Risk Factors for Venous Thromboembolism

There has been inadequate research to validate a specific cause-and-effect relationship between some of the
risk factors and thrombus formation. It is likely that
a combination of several risk factors causes thrombus formation. The most significant risk factor for
VTE in pregnancy is a personal history of thrombosis followed by the presence of an acquired or inherited thrombophilia (ACOG, 2018b). Thrombophilia is
present in 20% to 50% of all women who experience
VTE during pregnancy and postpartum (see Chapter 6

for discussion of thrombophilias). The risk for VTE is higher when multiple risk factors, such as additional abdominal surgery during vaginal delivery or cesarean section, higher parity, prolonged bedrest, infection, dehydration, gross varicosities, sickle cell disease, hypertension, obesity, and heart disease, are present (Witcher & Hamner, 2019). With women delaying childbirth, the risk of VTE may continue to rise. Smoking causes blood vessel constriction that potentially damages the endothelial lining and increases the risk for blood clot formation. The risk of VTE is also present for women with mechanical heart valves or who have certain dysrhythmias (e.g., atrial fibrillation) requiring anticoagulant therapy. In one study, the rate of thromboembolism in black women was 64% higher than that for women of other races (James et al., 2006). Genetics and environmental factors are thought to play a role. A significant decrease in the risk for women of Asian and Hispanic origins was also noted in this study (James et al., 2006). Trauma and infection increase the potential for vessel wall damage, which can lead to clot formation. Prolonged immobilization in any patient increases the likelihood of clot formation because of venous stasis. Antiphospholipid syndrome is an acquired thrombophilic condition associated with an increased risk for both arterial and venous thrombosis, recurrent fetal loss, and other adverse outcomes during pregnancy. Obesity increases risks related to hypertension, heart disease, and venous stasis.

Pathophysiology

A thrombus, which usually arises from a DVT, may dislodge and pass to the lungs. Small thrombi may lodge peripherally in the pulmonary vasculature, preventing blood flow distal to the thrombi and causing the release of inflammatory mediators. These mediators produce a rapid rise in pulmonary vascular resistance, causing symptoms of cough, tachycardia, tachypnea, and rales. If a large thrombus lodges in the pulmonary artery or one of its branches, obstruction of blood flow from the right ventricle occurs. Right ventricular outflow obstruction prevents blood from circulating through the pulmonary vasculature, resulting in deoxygenated blood and hypoxia. The degree of hypoxia and symptoms are related to the size and location of thrombi.

Deep Vein Thrombosis

Appropriate and timely assessments for the symptoms of venous thrombosis are essential for early diagnosis and initiation of treatment. Depending on the size of the thrombus, women may be asymptomatic or have symptoms that mimic common conditions of pregnancy. Symptoms of DVT include pain, swelling, warmth, redness, thickening, and tenderness over vein (Brown & Hiett, 2010). The pregnant woman undergoes several body changes that can mimic some of these symptoms. Lower extremity aches, pain, and swelling are common, especially in the second and third trimesters. Differentiation between normal and abnormal changes may present challenges. The extremity affected by DVT typically demonstrates the cardinal symptoms of inflammation, pain, swelling, warmth, and redness, and should be followed by additional assessment.

Compression ultrasound (CUS) is the primary tool for diagnostics for DVT because there is little radiation exposure. Ultrasound is done from the inguinal region to the deep calf veins, using light compression to determine if the vein is compressible (Khan, Vaillancourt, & Bourjelly, 2017). Although sensitivity and specificity are high, determination of DVT may still require serial ultrasounds. Magnetic resonance imaging (MRI) may also be used, especially in suspected iliac and femoral-popliteal DVT (Witcher & Hamner, 2019). D-dimer assays are not validated in pregnancy and have low negative predictability (Khan et al., 2017; Witcher & Hamner, 2019).

Pulmonary Embolus

Pulmonary embolus is an acute and potentially life-threatening event. Clinical manifestation of pulmonary embolus depends on the number, size, and location of the emboli; therefore, symptoms may be mild to severe (Brown & Hiett, 2010). Often, the woman will be apprehensive or have feelings of "impending doom" before the presentation of other symptoms. Diagnosis of pulmonary embolus may be considered with the presence of clinical signs and symptoms, including the sudden onset of unexplained dyspnea and tachypnea. Pleuritic chest pain, described by patients as "stabbing" in nature, is common following an embolus. The nurse may also find sudden onset of a productive cough and the presence of rales on auscultation. Tachycardia is a common symptom initially and may continue due to the resulting pain or hemodynamic compromise. A "massive" pulmonary embolism (PE) is one in which there is 50% or greater occlusion of the pulmonary artery circulation, severely restricting oxygenation (Witcher & Hamner, 2019). This is often accompanied by hypotension, chest pain, tachycardia, pulmonary crackles, diaphoresis, cyanosis, and syncope, which may mimic a cardiovascular event (Witcher & Hamner, 2019). Following initial assessment, laboratory values and radiologic imaging studies assist the healthcare provider in making the diagnosis.

Because the clinical signs and symptoms are not specific for pulmonary embolus, additional diagnostic testing should be used to rule out other diagnoses, such as pneumonia, myocardial infarction, or pulmonary edema (Leung et al., 2019). Anticoagulation therapy should be initiated upon suspected diagnosis and continued until PE is excluded (Witcher & Hamner, 2019). Continuous ECG is often performed early in the process when the woman reports chest pain. Tachycardia is the most common ECG change. A 12-lead ECG is commonly ordered to rule out other causes of chest pain, such as myocardial infarction. Findings from the 12-lead ECG may include nonspecific T-wave inversion, Q wave changes, and a right-axis shift in women with a large embolus (Leung et al., 2019).

Obtaining an arterial blood gas analysis on room air is one of the first steps in the diagnosis of a pulmonary embolus. Anticipated changes in maternal arterial blood gases associated with a pulmonary embolus are a decrease in P_aO_2, P_aCO_2, and SaO_2. If the woman's P_aO_2 value is greater than 80 mm Hg on room air, a pulmonary embolus is not likely. However, if a woman has persistent signs and symptoms of a pulmonary embolus, even with a P_aO_2 greater than 80 mm Hg, additional testing is needed to make a diagnosis (Leung et al., 2019).

CUS may be used in the lower extremities if there is a need to avoid radiation associated tests. The association between DVT found on CUS and related PE is low, however, and this should not be the primary imaging ordered (Leung et al., 2019). D-dimer assays have a low negative predictability value during pregnancy, and data on use is limited (Leung et al., 2019).

A ventilation-perfusion (V/Q) scan requires IV or bronchial administration of a radioactive substance under fluoroscopy. This substance becomes trapped in perfused lung tissue. The radiologic scan will detect areas of decreased perfusion, which will be suspicious for a pulmonary embolus, and will also detect nonperfused areas that may have appeared normal on a chest X-ray (Witcher & Hamner, 2019). A determination of high probability, moderate probability, low probability, or normal is made following analysis of the testing data. The term *probability* is added to the interpretation of this test because other diagnoses, such as pulmonary tumors, pneumonia, obstructive lung disease, hypoxic vasoconstriction, atelectasis, and emphysema, can also produce perfusion defects (Witcher & Hamner, 2019). Performing this test is considered to be safe during pregnancy, and it usually is the first-line radiologic testing procedure for the diagnosis of pulmonary embolus. The amount of radiation exposure varies but typically remains at levels considered safe during pregnancy (Leung et al., 2019).

Many institutions are using spiral CT as an alternative to the V/Q scan. Spiral CT also requires injection of a contrast media to examine the pulmonary bed. The presence or absence of PE on spiral CT may clarify the need to continue heparin therapy for suspected PE (Witcher & Hamner, 2019).

Pulmonary angiography is the historical definitive procedure to diagnose pulmonary embolus and is advisable when the V/Q scan is indeterminate. For this procedure, contrast dye is injected into lobar or segmental branches of the pulmonary artery, allowing clear visualization of vessels. An emboli would be detected with filling defects or obstructive flow. There is a low risk of an allergic reaction to the contrast dye used for radiographic imaging and vascular damage (pulmonary artery or right ventricular perforation).

Clinical Management

Because pulmonary embolus is such a rare event, but one with potentially devastating outcomes, management requires rapid recognition of symptoms, followed by notification and activation of a multidisciplinary team. The Council on Patient Safety in Women's Health Care has published Alliance for Innovation on Maternal Health (AIM) bundles to promote proven implementation approaches to improve maternal safety and outcomes in the United States, including a bundle on Maternal Venous Thromboembolism Prevention (D'Alton et al., 2016). This bundle promotes readiness, recognition and prevention, responses, and reporting with systems learning. Aspects of care fall into three management categories: respiratory support, cardiovascular support, and anticoagulation therapy.

Nursing assessments and support of respiratory function should focus on optimization of oxygen exchange. If a pulmonary embolus is suspected, warm, humidified oxygen therapy is administered via a nonrebreather face mask at 10 L/min during the acute phase. Arterial blood gases should be assessed frequently to evaluate the maternal response to therapy, degree of hypoxemia, and need for ventilatory support. Follow-up evaluation of blood gases after therapy should also be performed. Therefore, an arterial line may facilitate rapid and easy access for blood gas evaluation. Continuous maternal pulse oximetry should be initiated with the first signs of respiratory compromise. A pulmonary embolus will cause SaO_2 to fall dramatically during the acute event, indicating the need for further assessment. If the pulmonary embolus occurs in the antepartum period, maintenance of SaO_2 at 96% or above is optimal to ensure adequate oxygenation of the fetus (Leung et al., 2019).

Analgesics, such as morphine sulfate, may be used to decrease oxygen consumption in women who have pleuritic chest pain. Analgesics help to reduce the work of breathing in women who are feeling anxious or apprehensive. Other nursing measures to increase comfort include elevating the head of the bed and providing emotional support. The potential need for mechanical ventilation should be anticipated with severe maternal compromise in respiratory function or with cardiopulmonary collapse.

The initial treatment is also focused on restoring maternal cardiopulmonary function. Cardiovascular support should be initiated rapidly and include optimizing maternal preload (volume status), decreasing the workload of the heart, and using a positive inotropic agent to increase maternal cardiac contractility. Continuous ECG monitoring should be initiated with the first signs of maternal cardiovascular changes (Leung et al., 2019).

Noninvasive parameters reflecting maternal preload, such as vital signs, breathe sounds, jugular venous distention, skin color, turgor and color, and urine output, should be assessed frequently according to the woman's condition and facility protocol. Changes in preload values, hypervolemia, or hypovolemia may decrease maternal cardiac output and organ perfusion. Nursing interventions that focus on decreasing the workload of the heart should be initiated, such as decreasing the woman's activity, eliminating unnecessary procedures, administering pain medication for chest pain, and encouraging relaxation techniques. A positive inotrope, such as dopamine or dobutamine, should be considered to support myocardial contractility and cardiac output if symptoms of shock are present (Leung et al., 2019). Cardiopulmonary resuscitation should be initiated as needed.

Venous Thromboprophylaxis and Anticoagulation Therapy

Thromboembolic stockings, use of sequential compression devices (SCDs), and anticoagulation therapy are used for the prevention and treatment of VTE. At present, three types of therapeutic agents are used for anticoagulation in the general population: agents that interfere with platelet aggregation (attraction) and adhesion, agents that interfere with fibrin formation, and agents that facilitate clot lysis (clot breakdown). Anticoagulation during pregnancy requires consideration of both the mother and fetus. The decision for thromboprophylaxis to prevent thrombus formation is based on a previous history of thrombosis; the presence of a diagnosed thrombophilia; and other risk factors, such as race, age, and medical conditions, that may contribute to clot formation. Other risk factors that may indicate treatment to prevent clot formation are age older than 35 years, black race, or medical conditions such as valvular heart disease or antiphospholipid antibodies. Each woman's history should be analyzed to determine the need for thromboprophylaxis.

Heparin

Heparin, also known as unfractionated heparin (UFH), is a large molecule and does not cross the placenta or cause teratogenic effects. Heparin interferes with fibrin formation by binding to AT-III; changing the configuration of AT-III; and neutralizing factors Xa,

thrombin, IXa, XIa, and XIIa. Heparin is not absorbed into the gastrointestinal tract, thereby requiring parenteral administration by IV or subcutaneous injections. Intramuscular injections are contraindicated because of erratic absorption and risk of hematoma formation (Leung et al., 2019). Pregnant women usually require larger doses of heparin to achieve therapeutic anticoagulation because of increases in plasma volume, heparin-binding proteins, renal clearance, and heparin breakdown by the placenta (Leung et al., 2019).

The primary risk of heparin therapy is hemorrhage, which occurs in approximately 2% of patients. The rate of hemorrhage is related to dosing regimens and prolongation of the activated partial thromboplastin time (aPTT). Subcutaneous and intermittent IV bolus doses of heparin are associated with higher risks of bleeding. Thrombocytopenia is an immunologic reaction that occurs in less than 3% of patients undergoing heparin anticoagulation for an extended period of time (Leung et al., 2019). If thrombocytopenia occurs, it is typically 5 to 15 days after initiation of full-dose heparin (Witcher & Hamner, 2019). Patients who undergo prolonged heparin therapy may be at risk for osteoporosis. Changes in bone density have been observed in spine, hip, and femur radiographic tests.

Lack of adequate anticoagulation increases the risk of thromboembolus recurrence by 11- to 15-fold (Leung et al., 2019). Continuous IV administration provides a more consistent therapeutic level and results in fewer hemorrhagic events than intermittent IV bolus. Initial treatments for DVT and pulmonary embolus differ slightly. With a diagnosis of DVT only, an initial IV bolus of 100 U/kg of heparin is usually an appropriate treatment plan. For pulmonary embolus, the initial dose of heparin is 150 U/kg. Following initial IV bolus of heparin, an infusion rate between 15 and 25 U/kg/hr may be initiated, depending on the laboratory values and symptoms (Leung et al., 2019).

Low Molecular Weight Heparin

There are no large trials regarding the use of anticoagulants in pregnancy (ACOG, 2018b). Although for many years, UFH was the standard anticoagulant used during pregnancy and the postpartum period, current guidelines recommend low molecular weight heparin (LMWH) (ACOG, 2018b; Bates, Middeldorp, Rodger, James, & Greer, 2016). LMWH is derived from UFH. Its use in pregnancy is considered safe, and it is now the recommended treatment (ACOG, 2018b; Leung et al., 2019). Compared with UFH, LMWH has increased bioavailability, half-life, and anticoagulant activity (Leung et al., 2019). These characteristics make LMWH an attractive alternative to traditional UFH regimens. Venous thrombosis and pulmonary embolus may be effectively treated with LMWH. The benefits of LMWH are ease of administration; predictable dose-response ratios; less frequent need for monitoring; and fewer complications, such as thrombocytopenia, osteoporosis, and bleeding, compared with UFH. LMWH is four to six times more costly, but the ability to use this medication in the outpatient setting and the decreased need for strict laboratory monitoring decreases the cost of therapy.

Warfarin

Warfarin (Coumadin) is an oral anticoagulant that antagonizes vitamin K and directly inhibits the coagulation cascade. Warfarin crosses the placenta and has been associated with a risk of fetal hemorrhage and of central nervous system and ophthalmologic abnormalities. When administered between 6 and 12 weeks of gestation, warfarin has been associated with nasal and limb hypoplasia as well as stippled chondral calcification. Under most circumstances, warfarin is not the preferred treatment for thromboembolism during pregnancy, and the use of warfarin has been restricted primarily to the postpartum period. However, it may be the drug of choice in high-risk populations, such as women with certain types of mechanical heart valves or with a high risk of thrombosis (ACOG, 2018b).

If there is a desire to convert from heparin to warfarin anticoagulation, this switch should be initiated during the postpartum period while the woman is hospitalized. Following birth and maternal stabilization, full heparin anticoagulation is usually reinstituted. Oral warfarin therapy is usually initiated at 5 mg/day for 2 days and may take 1 to 2 weeks to reach a therapeutic dose. This may require dual therapy of LMWH and warfarin until the therapeutic range is reached (ACOG, 2018b). Maintenance-dose ranges are adjusted per day depending on the woman's international normalized ratio (INR) or prothrombin time. A goal value for the INR is 2.0 to 3.0 (Witcher & Hamner, 2019).

Warfarin anticoagulation is more sensitive to fluctuations and requires close monitoring of clotting-time values. Numerous medications, some foods, and alcohol may augment or interfere with absorption and action of warfarin (Murphy, Meadors, & King, 2011). To avoid common drug interactions, nurses and other healthcare providers should review the woman's medication history, be aware of potential medication interactions, and help educate patients to question or avoid medication (prescription or nonprescription) that is not approved by their primary healthcare provider or physician specialist consultant.

Labor and Birth

Pain management for labor and birth is a concern for patients taking anticoagulants. Potential complications associated with regional anesthesia, including the risk of spinal or epidural hematoma formation, have been linked to use of LMWH. This risk results from the increased half-life of LMWH. The American Society of Regional Anesthesia and Pain Medicine guidelines recommend withholding neuraxial (spinal and epidural anesthesia) blockade for 10 to 12 hours after the last prophylactic dose of LMWH or 24 hours after the last therapeutic dose of LMWH (ACOG, 2018b; Bates et al., 2016). If a woman goes into labor while taking UFH, clearance can be verified with an aPTT. If the aPTT value is prolonged greater than 1 to 1.5 times the control value, protamine sulfate may be required for patients taking UFH near birth to reduce the risk of bleeding (Brown & Hiett, 2010). Cesarean birth increases the risk of VTE; therefore, placement of pneumatic compression devices before birth is recommended for all women not already receiving thromboprophylaxis (ACOG, 2018b). Continued heparin dosing during labor and surgery for high-risk patients, such as those mentioned previously (recent pulmonary embolus, recent ileofemoral thrombosis, and mechanical heart valves), does not significantly increase the risk of hemorrhage during the postpartum period following a normal vaginal birth. Nursing assessments and care should focus on uterine tone and the potential for perineal hematoma following a vaginal birth, according to the healthcare facility's guidelines. If the woman has a cesarean birth, assessments should include signs and symptoms of intra-abdominal bleeding, such as increased abdominal girth, rigid or firm palpation, decreasing blood pressure, and increasing heart rate.

The optimal time to restart anticoagulation therapy in the postpartum period is unclear. A reasonable approach to minimize bleeding complications is to resume UFH or LMWH no sooner than 4 to 6 hours following vaginal birth and 6 to 12 hours following cesarean birth, 12 hours after epidural catheter removal (ACOG, 2018b; Bates et al., 2016). For women who had a thrombotic event during pregnancy, anticoagulation therapy should be continued for 3 to 6 months following birth (James et al., 2006). The woman may continue to use pneumatic compression devices until she is able to ambulate. Clotting factors that had been increased during pregnancy will normalize in approximately 8 weeks following birth (Leung et al., 2019).

Heparin and LMWH have not been found to be secreted in breast milk in clinically significant amounts and can be safely administered to nursing mothers (Rhode, 2011). Research validates the safety of warfarin use in nursing mothers. Warfarin does not induce an anticoagulant effect in the breastfed infant (Orme et al., 1977). Therefore, women who desire to breastfeed their newborn may be safely treated with any of these medications. As a general safety precaution, women receiving anticoagulant therapy should consult their physician or primary healthcare provider to confirm that they may take anticoagulants and other medications while breastfeeding.

CYSTIC FIBROSIS

Cystic fibrosis (CF) is a chronic, hereditary, progressive disease involving the exocrine glands and epithelial cells of the pancreas, sweat glands, and mucous glands in the respiratory, digestive, and reproductive tracts (Whitty & Dombrowski, 2019). CF is a disorder of the CF transmembrane conductance regulator protein that leads to abnormalities of the transport of chloride and sodium ions across membranes (McArdle, 2011). As a result, there can be an increase of viscous secretions in the lungs, pancreas, liver, intestine, and reproductive tract; the most significant morbidity and mortality arising from pulmonary complications (Mason & Burke, 2019).

Significant improvements in the prognosis and health of women with CF, age of survival into the fourth decade, and consistently rising numbers of individuals (men and women) with CF older than 18 years old have led to increasing consideration for management of reproductive issues and pregnancy in this unique group of women. The average age of female survival was predicted to be 54 years based on trends seen in recent years (MacKenzie et al., 2014). As more women with CF achieve pregnancy, taking a multidisciplinary approach to care can optimize maternal and fetal outcomes.

ACOG (2017a) recommends that screening for CF be offered to all pregnant patients. CF is recessive, requiring a mutation from each genetic parent. In couples that are both unaffected but either has a family history of CF, genetic testing for the CFTR gene mutation by DNA sequencing is appropriate. Genetic counseling should follow as needed.

Preconception counseling and planning for pregnancy is optimal for women with CF. Physical and psychosocial issues can be addressed and potential problems identified as well as genetic counseling with investigation of paternal carrier status. The physiologic adaptations of pregnancy may not be tolerated in women with CF. The enlarging uterus causes a change in lung mechanics that may lead to respiratory decompensation in the woman with CF; yet, the majority who were considered safe to undergo pregnancy generally tolerate it well without long-term adverse effects (Whitty & Dombrowski, 2019). However, those women with poor clinical status, malnutrition, hepatic dysfunction, and/or advanced lung disease are at increased risk during pregnancy (Whitty & Dombrowski, 2019).

Lung function is an important predictor of pregnancy outcomes in women with CF. Prepregnancy FEV_1 values are associated with good pregnancy outcomes (Mason & Burke, 2019). In women with moderate to severe lung disease, there is risk for preterm birth and decline in lung function (Patel et al., 2015). CF is associated with pulmonary hypertension (cor pulmonale), which carries high maternal mortality risk in pregnancy. Pulmonary infections are aggressively treated with IV antibiotics. Oral antibiotics are frequently used as chronic therapy, as well as for exacerbations in CF, and are continued in pregnancy with consideration of the type and clearance. Panchaud et al. (2016) published a very comprehensive evaluation of drugs used for CF during pregnancy and breastfeeding that is quite useful. Most routine medications used in CF are safe in pregnancy, but risk of adverse fetal outcomes must be weighed against the benefits. Regular chest physiotherapy and drainage are usual and recommended as components of CF treatment for mucous clearance and are continued in pregnancy. Inhaled dornase alpha is the most frequently used mucolytic, and, although there is no data on safety in pregnancy, it is used in the absence of reported adverse fetal effects (Panchaud et al., 2016).

Malabsorption and pancreatic insufficiency are frequent issues in CF, resulting in difficulty gaining weight and glucose intolerance that may be exacerbated due to the significant increase in energy costs. Poor nutritional status is usually associated with more severe disease and worse outcomes, including premature birth and low birth weight, whereas proper dietary consultation and attention to diet is associated with greater maternal and fetal weight gain (Patel et al., 2015). Ideally, the woman should be at 90% of optimal weight prior to conception if possible but may be difficult to achieve. Enteral and total parenteral feedings have been used to successfully maintain nutritional status and may be considered for support of weight gain (Whitty & Dombrowski, 2019). Rates of nutritional abnormalities, such as pancreatic exocrine insufficiency and diabetes mellitus may be higher in pregnant women with CF (Patel et al., 2015). Risks of gestational diabetes in pregnancy, including polyhydramnios and preeclampsia, are the same in women with CF; thus, careful monitoring of blood glucose values beginning early in pregnancy, along with initiation of diet modification and insulin therapy as needed, is an important component of care. Pancreatic enzyme replacement is required in a large percentage of CF patients and can be continued in pregnancy to optimize nutritional status (Whitty & Dombrowski, 2019).

Antenatal testing is utilized in pregnant women with CF due to the risk for uteroplacental insufficiency and IUGR. Antenatal testing is usually initiated at 32 weeks of gestation and possibly earlier if evidence of fetal compromise is demonstrated (Whitty

& Dombrowski, 2019). Maternal deterioration in lung function may also precipitate early delivery. Vaginal birth is preferable in women with CF, and cesarean birth is reserved for obstetric indications due to higher risk of atelectasis and retained secretions associated with surgery. The physiologic demands of the labor, birth, and postpartum periods stress the respiratory and cardiovascular systems, placing the woman with CF at risk for pulmonary hypertension, cor pulmonale, and right-sided heart failure (Whitty & Dombrowski, 2019). Regional anesthesia to control pain and limiting expulsive efforts is beneficial in reducing the sympathetic response, reducing tachycardia and hyperventilation (Mason & Burke, 2019).

Lung transplantation is a therapeutic option for improved quality of life in CF patients with end-stage lung disease, with 5-year survival rates of 55.5% and 10-year survival rates near 40% (Valapour et al., 2017). Pregnancy should be avoided for 1 to 2 years posttransplant in order to decrease risk of rejection and maximize fetal well-being (Vos et al., 2016). There have been extensive reports of pregnancy after other solid organ transplants with no increased risk of congenital malformation or infections; however, there is a high risk of maternal rejection and mortality (Divithotawela, Chambers, & Hopkins, 2015; Valapour et al., 2017; Vos et al., 2014). Immunosuppression using mycophenolate and rapamycin inhibitors should be avoided due to teratogenic effects (Divithotawela et al., 2015).

SPECIAL CONSIDERATIONS FOR THE RESPIRATORY SYSTEM IN PREGNANCY

Sleep-Disordered Breathing

Sleep disturbances are reported frequently during pregnancy, most notably insomnia and excessive sleepiness associated with the physiologic changes of pregnancy. Sleep-disordered breathing, including obstructive sleep apnea (OSA) and central sleep apnea, periodic breathing, and nocturnal hypoventilation, is uncommon in otherwise healthy women but occurs at rates higher than the general population in pregnant women (Booth & Tonidandel, 2017). Despite protective mechanisms in pregnancy protecting against sleep-disordered breathing, including increased minute ventilation, lateral positioning for sleep, and decreased rapid eye movement sleep, physiologic changes in the upper airway, including mucosal edema and decreased airway patency, may predispose the pregnant woman to sleep-disordered breathing and contribute to adverse outcomes of pregnancy (Booth & Tonidandel, 2017). Weight gain and upper airway resistance due to estrogen effects may cause sleep apnea to develop or worsen during pregnancy.

Although regular snoring is usually underreported, it may occur in 14% to 45% of pregnant women (Bourjeily, Ankner, & Mohsenin, 2011). Snoring during pregnancy is not a benign condition because it has been associated with negative maternal and fetal outcomes such as hypertension, preeclampsia, IUGR, and lower Apgar scores (Bourjeily et al., 2011).

Pregnancy rhinitis may cause OSA in women who are predisposed to sleep apnea but can normally breathe through their nose. Women with rhinitis are at greater risk for snoring and OSA. The increase in nocturnal blood pressure that often accompanies snoring and OSA is associated with gestational hypertensive disorders, particularly preeclampsia (Booth & Tonidandel, 2017), although the underlying mechanism for this increase is not well understood. Pregnant women often have difficulty breathing in the supine position, but they may unintentionally move into this position during sleep. Nasal congestion occurs while the patient is in the supine position because difficult breathing increases the tendency to resort to mouth breathing and snoring.

Pregnancy rhinitis should be identified and treated to minimize risk of potential adverse outcomes. Women should be asked about symptoms of rhinitis routinely during prenatal care. Diagnostic tools for sleep-disordered breathing may be less predictive in pregnancy, but polysomnography is the gold standard for diagnosis (Booth & Tonidandel, 2017). Criteria for diagnosis may be different in pregnancy because total sleep time is increased with decreased efficiency (Bourjeily et al., 2011). With diagnosis and severity firmly established, the pregnant woman must be aware of risks and treatment options. Weight loss, a typical behavioral modification for individuals with OSA, is not appropriate to initiate during pregnancy, but continued usual advice on lateral positioning for sleep and avoidance of alcohol are appropriate components of therapy. Positive airway pressure or oral appliances may be used to reduce the frequency of respiratory events during sleep, surgical procedures not appropriate during pregnancy except in extreme circumstances (Booth & Tonidandel, 2017). It is important to note that most studies of sleep-disordered breathing in pregnancy are based on symptoms rather than confirmed sleep-disordered breathing, and there is currently no evidence on the effects of various treatments and outcomes in pregnancy. Sleep-disordered breathing generally improves in the postpartum period, but repeat sleep-study testing may be indicated in women with preexisting or continuing issues.

Smoking

Although smoking in women of reproductive age in the United States has decreased, it remains a leading preventable cause of adverse maternal and fetal outcomes.

In studies of smoking during pregnancy, prevalence is likely underestimated by as much as 25% because most information is self-reported (CDC, 2017b). The prevalence of smoking is highest in women who are young (adolescents and women aged 18 to 24 years), Caucasian, of lower socioeconomic status, and less educated (CDC, 2017b). Other factors associated with smoking during pregnancy include increased parity and being unmarried, having an unplanned pregnancy, and having a smoking partner (Murin, Rafii, & Bilello, 2011). Pregnancy is usually a strong motivation to quit smoking, but relapse rates both during and after pregnancy are high (ACOG, 2017b; Rockhill et al., 2016). The effects of vaping during pregnancy are unknown and further efforts to determine the outcomes for mothers and babies must be studied. Please refer to Chapter 7 (Preterm Labor and Birth) for further information on the effects and outcomes of smoking in pregnancy.

High Altitude

The compensatory physiologic changes of pregnancy occur in response to the challenges of oxygen transport and maintenance of uteroplacental circulation. In chronic high-altitude conditions with limited oxygen availability and hypoxia, these challenges are magnified. High altitude (greater than 2,500 m, P_aO_2 of 60 to 70 mm Hg) is associated with greater incidence of IUGR and preeclampsia, thus increasing the risk for perinatal morbidity and mortality (Antony, Ehrenthal, Evensen, & Iruretagoyena, 2017).

SUMMARY

The incidence of pulmonary complications during pregnancy has increased over the past few decades and is associated with potentially adverse outcomes for the mother and baby. Perinatal nurses should be able to recognize common pulmonary complications and activate a team response when necessary based on the clinical situation. If the mother continues to show signs of compromise after initial efforts to improve oxygenation, then stabilization and transfer to a higher level of care may be necessary. When the condition of the mother necessitates transfer to an off-service intensive care area, collaboration among healthcare providers is required.

REFERENCES

Alhassan, S., Pelinescu, A., Gandhi, V., Naddour, M., Singh, A. C., & Bihler, E. (2017). Clinical presentation and risk factors of venous thromboembolic disease. *Critical Care Nursing Quarterly, 40*(3), 201–209. doi:10.1097/CNQ.0000000000000159

Ali, Z., & Ulrik, C. S. (2013). Incidence and risk factors for exacerbations of asthma during pregnancy. *Journal of Asthma and Allergy, 6*, 53–60. doi:10.2147/JAA.S43183

American College of Obstetricians and Gynecologists. (2017a). *Carrier screening for genetic conditions* (Committee Opinion No. 691). Washington, DC: Author.

American College of Obstetricians and Gynecologists. (2017b). *Smoking cessation during pregnancy* (Committee Opinion No. 721). Washington, DC: Author.

American College of Obstetricians and Gynecologists. (2018a). *Influenza vaccination during pregnancy* (Committee Opinion No. 732). Washington, DC: Author.

American College of Obstetricians and Gynecologists. (2018b). *Thromboembolism in pregnancy* (Practice Bulletin No. 196). Washington, DC: Author.

American College of Obstetricians and Gynecologists. (2008). *Asthma in pregnancy* (Practice Bulletin No. 90; Reaffirmed 2019). Washington, DC: Author.

Antony, K. M., Ehrenthal, D., Evensen, A., & Iruretagoyena, J. I. (2017). Travel during pregnancy: Considerations for the obstetric provider. *Obstetrical & Gynecological Survey, 72*(2), 97–115. doi:10.1097/OGX.0000000000000398

Balducci, J., Rodis, J. F., Rosengren, S., Vintzileos, A. M., Spivey, G., & Vosseller, C. (1992). Pregnancy outcome following first-trimester varicella infection. *Obstetrics & Gynecology, 79*(1), 5–6.

Bates, S. M., Greer, I. A., Middeldorp, S., Veenstra, D. L., Prabulos, A. M., & Vandvik, P. O. (2012). VTE, thrombophilia, antithrombotic therapy, and pregnancy: Antithrombotic therapy and prevention of thrombosis, 9th ed: American College of Chest Physicians Evidence-Based Clinical Practice Guidelines. *Chest, 141*(2 Suppl.), e691S–e736S. doi:10.1378/chest.11-2300

Bates, S. M., Middeldorp, S., Rodger, M., James, A. H., & Greer, I. (2016). Guidance for the treatment and prevention of obstetric-associated venous thromboembolism. *Journal of Thrombosis and Thrombolysis, 41*(1), 92–128. doi:10.1007/s11239-015-1309-0

Belfort, M. A., Clark, S. L., Saade, G. R., Kleja, K., Dildy, G. A., III, Van Veen, T. R., . . . Kofford, S. (2010). Hospital readmission after delivery: Evidence for an increased incidence of nonurogenital infection in the immediate postpartum period. *American Journal of Obstetrics & Gynecology, 202*(1), 35.e1–35.e7. doi:10.1016/j.ajog.2009.08.029

Belfort, M. A., & Herbst, M. (2010). Severe acute asthma. In M. A. Belfort, G. R. Saade, M. R. Foley, J. P. Phelan, & G. A. Dildy, III (Eds.), *Critical care obstetrics* (5th ed., pp. 327–337). Hoboken, NJ: Wiley-Blackwell.

Benson, M. D. (2017). Amniotic fluid embolism mortality rate. *The Journal of Obstetrics and Gynaecology Research, 43*(11), 1714–1718. doi:10.1111/jog.13445

Blaiss, M. S. (2004). Management of asthma during pregnancy. *Allergy and Asthma Proceedings, 25*(6), 375–379.

Blanton, L., Mustaquim, D., Alabi, N., Kniss, K., Kramer, N., Budd, A., . . . Brammer, L. (2017). Update: influenza activity—United States, October 2, 2016–February 4, 2017. *MMWR Morbidity and Mortality Weekly Report, 66*(6), 159–166. doi:10.15585/mmwr.mm6606a2

Bonham, C. A., Patterson, K. C., & Strek, M. E. (2018). Asthma outcomes and management during pregnancy. *Chest, 153*(2), 515–527. doi:10.1016/j.chest.2017.08.029

Booth, J. M., & Tonidandel, A. M. (2017). Peripartum management of obstructive sleep apnea. *Clinical Obstetrics and Gynecology, 60*(2), 405–417. doi:10.1097/GRF.0000000000000279

Bourjeily, G., Ankner, G., & Mohsenin, V. (2011). Sleep-disordered breathing in pregnancy. *Clinics in Chest Medicine, 32*(1), 175–189. doi:10.1016/j.ccm.2010.11.003

Brito, V., & Neiderman, M. S. (2011). Pneumonia complicating pregnancy. *Clinics in Chest Medicine, 32*(1), 121–132. doi:10.1016/j.ccm.2010.10.004

Brown, H. L., & Hiett, A. K. (2010). Deep vein thrombosis and pulmonary embolism in pregnancy: Diagnosis, complications, and management. *Clinical Obstetrics and Gynecology, 53*(2), 345–359. doi:10.1097/GRF.0b013e3181deb27e

Centers for Disease Control and Prevention. (2017a). *Half of pregnant women protect themselves and their babies against flu. Time to bump it up!* Atlanta, GA: Author.

Centers for Disease Control and Prevention. (2017b). *Tobacco use and pregnancy.* Atlanta, GA: Author.

Chandra, P. C., Patel, H., Schiavello, H. J., & Briggs, S. L. (1998). Successful pregnancy outcome after complicated varicella pneumonia. *Obstetrics & Gynecology, 92*(4, Pt. 2), 680–682. doi:10.1016/S0029-7844(98)00237-3

Chapman, S. J. (1998). Varicella in pregnancy. *Seminars in Perinatology, 22*(4), 339–346. doi:10.1016/S0146-0005(98)80023-2

Chen, Y.-H., Keller, J., Wang, I.-T., Lin, C.-C., & Lin, H.-C. (2012). Pneumonia and pregnancy outcomes: A nationwide population-based study. *American Journal of Obstetrics & Gynecology, 207*, 288.e1–288.e7. doi:10.1016/j.ajog.2012.08.023

Cheng, V. C., Tang, B. S., Wu, A. K., Chu, C. M., & Yuen, K. Y. (2004). Medical treatment of viral pneumonia including SARS in immunocompetent adult. *Journal of Infection, 49*(4), 262–273. doi:10.1016/j.jinf.2004.07.010

Clark, S. L. (2014). Amniotic fluid embolism. *Obstetrics & Gynecology, 123*(2, Pt. 1), 337–348. doi:10.1097/AOG.0000000000000107

Copper, P. L., Otto, M. P., & Leighton, B. L. (2013, April). *Successful management of cardiac arrest from amniotic fluid embolism with ondansetron, metoclopramide, atropine, and ketorolac: A case report.* Paper presented at Society for Obstetric Anesthesia and Perinatology 45th Annual Meeting, San Juan, Puerto Rico.

Creanga, A. A., Johnson, T. F., Graitcer, S. B., Hartman, L. K., Al-Samarrai, T., Schwarz, A. G., . . . Honein, M. A. (2010). Severity of 2009 pandemic influenza A (H1N1) virus infection in pregnant women. *Obstetrics & Gynecology, 115*(4), 717–726. doi:10.1097/AOG.0b013e3181d57947

D'Alton, M. E., Friedman, A. M., Smiley, R. M., Montgomery, D. M., Paidas, M. J., D'Oria, R., . . . Clark, S. L. (2016). National partnership for maternal safety: Consensus bundle on venous thromboembolism. *Obstetrics & Gynecology, 128*(4), 688–698. doi:10.1097/AOG.0000000000001579

de Araujo, G. V., Leite, D. F., Rizzo, J. A., & Sarinho, E. S. (2016). Asthma in pregnancy: Association between the Asthma Control Test and the Global Initiative for Asthma classification and comparisons with spirometry. *European Journal of Obstetrics, Gynecology, and Reproductive Biology, 203*, 25–29. doi:10.1016/j.ejogrb.2016.05.010

Dennis, A. T., & Solnordal, C. B. (2012). Acute pulmonary oedema in pregnant women. *Anaesthesia, 67*, 646–659. doi:10.1111/j.1365-2044.2012.07055.x

Divithotawela, C., Chambers, D., & Hopkins, P. (2015). Pregnancy after lung transplant: Case report. *Breathe, 11*(4), 291–295. doi:10.1183/20734735.008915

Dzieciolowska-Baran, E., Teul-Swiniarska, I., Gawlikowska-Sroka, A., Poziomkowska-Gesicka, I., & Zietek, Z. (2013). Rhinitis as a cause of respiratory disorders during pregnancy. In M. Pokorski (Ed.), *Respiratory regulation—Clinical advances* (pp. 213–220). Dordrecht, Netherlands: Springer. doi:10.1007/978-94-007-4546-9_27

Frye, D., Clark, S. L., Piacenza, D., & Shay-Zapien, G. (2011). Pulmonary complications in pregnancy: Considerations for care. *Journal of Perinatal & Neonatal Nursing, 25*(3), 235–244. doi:10.1097/JPN.0b013e3182230e25

Gardner, M. O., & Doyle, N. M. (2004). Asthma in pregnancy. *Obstetrics and Gynecology Clinics of North America, 31*(2), 385–413. doi:10.1016/j.ogc.2004.03.010

Garite, T. J. (2018). Fetal considerations in the critical care patient. In M. R. Foley, T. H. Strong, & T. J. Garite (Eds.), *Obstetric intensive care manual* (5th ed., pp. 325–336). New York, NY: McGraw-Hill.

Gei, A. F., & Suarez, V. R. (2018). Respiratory emergencies during pregnancy. In M. R. Foley, T. H. Strong, & T. J. Garite (Eds.), *Obstetric intensive care manual* (5th ed., p. 175–200). New York, NY: McGraw-Hill.

Gluck, J. C., & Gluck, P. A. (2006). The effect of pregnancy on the course of asthma. *Immunology and Allergy Clinics of North America, 26*(1), 63–80. doi:10.1016/j.iac.2005.10.008

Goodnight, W. H., & Soper, D. E. (2005). Pneumonia in pregnancy. *Critical Care Medicine, 33*(10 Suppl.), S390–397. doi:10.1097/01.CCM.0000182483.24836.66

Grant, A. (1996). Varicella infection and toxoplasmosis in pregnancy. *Journal of Perinatal & Neonatal Nursing, 10*(2), 17–29.

Graves, C. R. (2010). Pneumonia in pregnancy. *Clinical Obstetrics and Gynecology, 53*(2), 329–336. doi:10.1097/GRF.0b013e3181de8a6f

Hameed, A. B., Morton, C. H., & Moore, A. (2017). *Improving health care response to cardiovascular disease in pregnancy and postpartum* (CMQCC Tool Kit). Stanford, CA: California Maternal Quality Care Collaborative.

Hegewald, M. J., & Crapo, R. O. (2011). Respiratory physiology in pregnancy. *Clinics in Chest Medicine, 32*(1), 1–13. doi:10.1016/j.ccm.2010.11.001

Hemnes, A. R., Kiely, D. G., Cockrill, B. A., Safdar, Z., Wilson, V. J., Al Hazmi, M., . . . Lahm, T. (2015). Statement on pregnancy in pulmonary hypertension from the Pulmonary Vascular Research Institute. *Pulmonary Circulation, 5*(3), 435–465. doi:10.1086/682230

James, A. H., Jamison, M. G., Brancazio, L. R., & Myers, E. R. (2006). Venous thromboembolism during pregnancy and the postpartum period: Incidence, risk factors, and mortality. *American Journal of Obstetrics & Gynecology, 194*(5), 1311–1315. doi:10.1016/j.ajog.2005.11.008

Khan, F., Vaillancourt, C., & Bourjelly, G. (2017). Diagnosis and management of deep vein thrombosis in pregnancy. *BMJ, 357*, j2344. doi:10.1136/bmj.j2344

Kuriya, A., Piedimonte, S., Spence, A. R., Czuzoj-Shulman, N., Kezoug, A., & Abenhaim, H. A. (2016). Incidence and causes of maternal mortality in the USA. *Journal of Obstetric and Gynaecology Research, 42*(6), 661–668. doi:10.1111/jog.12954

Laibl, V. R., & Sheffield, J. S. (2005). Influenza and pneumonia in pregnancy. *Clinics in Perinatology, 32*(3), 727–738. doi:10.1016/j.clp.2005.04.009

Laibl, V. R., & Sheffield, J. S. (2006). The management of respiratory infections during pregnancy. *Immunology and Allergy Clinics of North America, 26*(1), 155–172. doi:10.1016/j.iac.2005.11.003

Lam, C. M., Wong, S. F., Leung, T. N., Chow, K. M., Yu, W. C., Wong, T. Y., . . . Ho, L. C. (2004). A case-controlled study comparing clinical course and outcomes of pregnant and non-pregnant women with severe acute respiratory syndrome. *BJOG, 111*(8), 771–774. doi:10.1111/j.1471-0528.2004.00199.x

Lehne, R. A. (2010). Anticoagulant, antiplatelet, and thrombolytic drugs. In R. A. Lehne (Ed.), *Pharmacology for Nursing Care* (7th ed., pp. 594–618). St. Louis, MO: Saunders Elsevier.

Leighton, B. L. (2013). *Amniotic fluid embolism.* Retrieved from https://www.marchofdimes.org/pdf/missouri/AFE_11-21-13.pdf

Leung, A., Sottile, P., & Lockwood, C. J. (2019). Thromboembolism disease in pregnancy. In R. K. Creasy, C. J. Lockwood, T. R. Moore, M. F. Greene, J. A. Copel, & R. M. Silver (Eds.), *Maternal-fetal medicine principles and practice* (8th ed., pp. 977–990). Philadelphia, PA: Elsevier.

LoMauro, A., & Aliverti, A. (2015). Respiratory physiology of pregnancy: Physiology masterclass. *Breathe, 11*(4), 297–301. doi:10.1183/20734735.008615

Mabie, W. C. (2010). Pulmonary edema. In M. A. Belfort, G. R. Saade, M. R. Foley, J. P. Phelan, & G. A. Dildy (Eds.), *Critical care obstetrics* (5th ed., pp. 348–357). Hoboken, NJ: Wiley-Blackwell.

Maccato, M. (1991). Respiratory insufficiency due to pneumonia in pregnancy. *Obstetrics and Gynecology Clinics of North America, 18*(2), 289–299.

MacKenzie, T., Gifford, A. H., Sabadosa, K. A., Quinton, H. B., Knapp, E. A., Goss, C. H., & Marshall, B. C. (2014).

Longevity of patients with cystic fibrosis in 2000 to 2010 and beyond: Survival analysis of the Cystic Fibrosis Foundation patient registry. *Annals of Internal Medicine, 161*(4), 233–241. doi:10.7326/M13-0636

Mason, B. A., & Burke, C. (2019). Pulmonary disorders in pregnancy. In N. H. Troiano, P. M. Witcher, & S. M. Baird (Eds.), *High-risk and critical care obstetrics* (4th ed., pp. 155–175). Philadelphia, PA: Wolters Kluwer.

McArdle, J. R. (2011). Pregnancy in cystic fibrosis. *Clinics in Chest Medicine, 32*(1), 111–120. doi:10.1016/j.ccm.2010.10.005

McCracken, A., Gallery, E., & Morris, J. M. (2004). Pregnancy-specific down-regulation of NF-kappa B expression in T cells in humans is essential for the maintenance of the cytokine profile required for pregnancy success. *Journal of Immunology, 172*(7), 4583–4591.

Murin, S., Rafii, R., & Bilello, K. (2011). Smoking and smoking cessation in pregnancy. *Clinics in Chest Medicine, 32*(1), 75–91. doi:10.1016/j.ccm.2010.11.004

Murphy, P. J. M., Meadors, B., & King, T. L. (2011). Hematology. In T. L. King & M. C. Brucker (Eds.), *Pharmacology for women's health* (pp. 435–461). Sudbury, MA: Jones and Bartlett.

Murphy, V. E. (2015). Managing asthma in pregnancy. *Breathe, 11*(4), 258–267.

National Asthma Education and Prevention Program. (2007). *Expert Panel Report No. 3: Guidelines for the diagnosis and management of asthma* (NIH Publication No. 07-4051). Bethesda, MD: National Heart, Lung, and Blood Institute.

Neu, H. C., & Sabath, L. D. (1993). Criteria for selecting oral antibiotic therapy for community-acquired pneumonia. *Infections in Medicine, 10*(2 Suppl.), 33S–40S.

Omo-Aghoja, L. (2014). Maternal and fetal acid-base chemistry: A major determinant of perinatal outcome. *Annals of Medical and Health Sciences Research, 4*(1), 8–17. doi:10.4103/2141-9248.126602

Orme, M. L., Lewis, P. J., de Swiet, M., Serlin, M. J., Sibeon, R., Baty, J. D., & Breckenridge, A. M. (1977). May mothers given warfarin breast-feed their infants? *British Medical Journal, 1*(6076), 1564–1565. doi:10.1136/bmj.1.6076.1564

Pacheco, L. D., Constantine, M. M., & Hankins, G. D. V. (2013). Physiologic changes during pregnancy. In D. R. Mattison (Ed.), *Clinical pharmacology during pregnancy* (pp. 5–14). San Diego, CA: Academic Press. doi:10.1016/B978-0-12-386007-1.00002-7

Pacheco, L. D., Saade, G., Hankins, G. D., & Clark, S. L. (2016). Amniotic fluid embolism: Diagnosis and management. *American Journal of Obstetrics & Gynecology, 215*(2), B16–B24. doi:10.1016/j.ajog.2016.03.012

Panchaud, A., DiPaolo, E. R., Koutsokera, A., Winterfeld, U., Weisskopf, E, Baud, D., . . . Csajka, C. (2016). Safety of drugs during pregnancy and breastfeeding in cystic fibrosis patients. *Respiration, 91*, 333–348. doi:10.1159/000444088

Park-Wyllie, L., Mazzotta, P., Pastuszak, A., Moretti, M. E., Beique, L., Hunnisett, L., . . . Koren, G. (2000). Birth defects after maternal exposure to corticosteroids: Prospective cohort study and meta-analysis of epidemiological studies. *Teratology, 62*(6), 385–392. doi:10.1002/1096-9926(200012)62:6<385::AID-TERA5>3.0.CO;2-Z

Patel, E. M., Swamy, G. K., Heine, R. P., Kuller, J. A., James, A. H., & Grotegut, C. A. (2015). Medical and obstetric complications among pregnant women with cystic fibrosis. *American Journal of Obstetrics & Gynecology, 212*(1), 98.e1–98.e9. doi:10.1016/j.ajog.2014.07.018

Pereira, A., & Krieger, B. P. (2004). Pulmonary complications of pregnancy. *Clinics in Chest Medicine, 25*(2), 299–310. doi:10.1016/j.ccm.2004.01.010

Ramsey, P. S., & Ramin, K. D. (2001). Pneumonia in pregnancy. *Obstetrics and Gynecology Clinics of North America, 28*(3), 553–569.

Rasmussen, S. A., & Jamieson, D. J. (2015). What obstetric health care providers need to know about measles and pregnancy. *Obstetrics & Gynecology, 126*(1), 163–170. doi:10.1097/AOG.0000000000000903

Reinisch, J. M., Simon, N. G., Karow, W. G., & Gandelman, R. (1978). Prenatal exposure to prednisone in humans and animals retards intrauterine growth. *Science, 202*(4366), 436–438. doi:10.1126/science.705336

Rezai, S., Hughes, A. C., Larsen, T. B., Fuller, P. N., & Henderson, C. E. (2017). Atypical amniotic fluid embolism managed with a novel therapeutic regimen. *Case Reports in Obstetrics and Gynecology, 2017*, 8458375. doi:10.1155/2017/8458375

Rhode, M. A. (2011). Postpartum. In T. L. King & M. C. Brucker (Eds.), *Pharmacology for women's health* (pp. 1117–1145). Boston, MA: Jones and Bartlett.

Robert, E., Vollset, S. E., Botto, L., Lancaster, P. A., Merlob, P., Mastroiacovo, P., . . . Orioli, I. (1994). Malformation surveillance and maternal drug exposure: The MADRE project. *International Journal of Risk & Safety in Medicine, 6*, 78–118.

Rockhill, K. M., Tong, V. T., Farr, S. L., Robbins, C. L., D'Angelo, D. V., & England, L. J. (2016). Postpartum smoking relapse after quitting during pregnancy: Pregnancy risk assessment monitoring system, 2000-2011. *Journal of Women's Health, 25*(5), 480–488. doi:10.1089/jwh.2015.5244

Shamshirsaz, A. A., & Clark, S. L. (2016). Amniotic fluid embolism. *Obstetrics and Gynecology Clinics of North America, 43*(4), 779–790. doi:10.1016/j.ogc.2016.07.001

Simpson, K. R., & James, D. C. (2005). Efficacy of intrauterine resuscitation techniques in improving fetal oxygen status during labor. *Obstetrics & Gynecology, 105*(6), 1362–1368. doi:10.1097/01.AOG.0000164474.03350.7c

Thongrong, C., Kasemsiri, P., Hofmann, J. P., Bergese, S. D., Papadimos, T. J., Gracias, V. H., . . . & Stawicki, S. P. (2013). Amniotic fluid embolism. *International Journal of Critical Illness and Injury Science, 3*(1), 51–57. doi:10.4103/2229-5151.109422

Towers, C. V., Briggs, G. G., & Rojas, J. A. (2004). The use of prostaglandin E2 in pregnant patients with asthma. *American Journal of Obstetrics & Gynecology, 190*(6), 1777–1780. doi:10.1016/j.ajog.2004.02.056

Valapour, M., Skeans, M. A., Smith, J. M., Edwards, L. B., Cherikh, W. S., Uccellini, K., . . . Kasiske, B. L. (2017). OPTN/SRTR 2015 annual data report: Lung. *American Journal of Transplantation, 17*(Suppl. 1), 357–424. doi:10.1111/ajt.14129

Vali, P., & Lakshminrusimha, S. (2017). The fetus can teach us: Oxygen and the pulmonary vasculature. *Children, 4*(67), 1–12. doi:10.3390/children4080067

Vos, R., Ruttens, D., Verleden, S. E., Vandermeulen, E., Bellon, H., Vanaudenaerde, B. M., & Verleden, G. M. (2014). Pregnancy after heart and lung transplantation. *Best Practice and Research. Clinical Obstetrics & Gynaecology, 28*(8), 1146–1162. doi:10.1016/j.bpobgyn.2014.07.019

Whitty, J. E., & Dombrowski, M. P. (2019). Respiratory diseases in pregnancy. In R. K. Creasy, C. J. Lockwood, T. R. Moore, M. F. Greene, J. A. Copel, & R. M. Silver (Eds.), *Maternal-fetal medicine principles and practice* (8th ed., pp. 1043–1066). Philadelphia, PA: Elsevier.

Wise, R. A., Polito, A. J., & Krishnan, V. (2006). Respiratory physiologic changes in pregnancy. *Immunology and Allergy Clinics of North America, 26*(1), 1–12. doi:10.1016/j.iac.2005.10.004

Witcher, P. M., & Hamner, L. (2019). Venous thromboembolism in pregnancy. In N. H. Troiano, P. M. Witcher, & S. M. Baird (Eds.), *High-risk and critical care obstetrics* (4th ed., pp. 98–112). Philadelphia, PA: Wolters Kluwer.

Wong, S. F., Chow, K. M., Leung, T. N., Ng, W. F., Ng, T. K., Shek, C. C., . . . Tan, P. Y. (2004). Pregnancy and perinatal outcomes of women with severe acute respiratory syndrome. *American Journal of Obstetrics & Gynecology, 191*(1), 292–297. doi:10.1016/j.ajog.2003.11.019

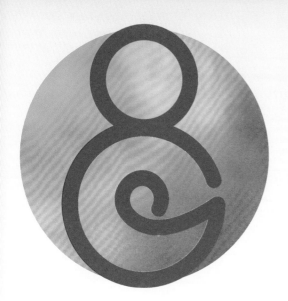

CHAPTER 11

Multiple Gestation

Nancy A. Bowers

INTRODUCTION

Following a stunning 76% rise that began in 1980 and a short period of stabilization after 2009, the rate of twin births in 2014 was the highest ever reported. During that same period, the rate of triplets and other high-order multiples (HOMs) rose more than 500%. That rate has declined 46% since 1998; the 2016, 2017, and 2018 rates are the lowest reported in more than two decades (Martin, Hamilton, Osterman, Driscoll, & Drake, 2018; Martin & Osterman, 2019). In 2017, 1 in every 29 live births was a twin, triplet, or higher multiple (Fig. 11–1).

Trends in delayed childbearing, increased use of infertility therapies, and access to assisted reproductive technologies (ARTs) have contributed greatly to these increased rates (Luke, 2017; Martin et al., 2018). Although multiple births represent only a small percentage of the total live births in the United States, these births contribute disproportionately to the rates of maternal, fetal, and neonatal morbidity and mortality. A key factor is a clear dose–response relationship: Increasing plurality corresponds with higher morbidity and mortality for mothers and their infants. With these high risks, the perinatal team must be alert for potential complications during pregnancy, labor, birth, and the postpartum period.

EPIDEMIOLOGY

Of the nearly 4 million United States live births in 2017, infants born as multiples accounted for 3.4%. Of these multiples, 128,310 (97.0%) were twins, 3,675 (2.7%) were triplets, 193 (0.0015%) were quadruplets, and only 49 infants were born as quintuplets and higher that year (Martin et al., 2018).

Shifts in traditional maternal age patterns have occurred along with the rise in multiple births, mirroring the trend of delayed childbearing. Historically, twin birth rates were low for young women, rose through the age group 35 to 39 years, and then declined for women in their 40s (Martin & Park, 1999). Today, the highest overall multiple birth rates are for women older than age 40 years, particularly in the 45 to 54 years age group (150/1,000; Martin et al., 2018). Regardless of maternal age, use of infertility treatments, a prior multiple pregnancy, and higher parity increase the likelihood for spontaneous dizygotic (DZ) twin conception. Twinning is about 4 times more likely in the fourth or fifth birth than in the first birth (Taffel, 1995).

There are also differences in maternal race patterns. In 2018, twin birth rates for non-Hispanic white women and black women were 34.3 and 40.1 per 1,000 births, respectively, but were much lower for Hispanic women (24.4/1,000; Martin & Osterman, 2019). Race disparities are also present in HOMs. In 2017, the HOM birth rate for non-Hispanic whites was 116.6/100,000 and 119.7/100,000 for blacks but was 68.3/100,000 for Hispanic mothers (Martin et al., 2018) (Fig. 11–2).

PHYSIOLOGY OF TWINNING

Multiple gestations result from either the fertilization of a single ovum that subsequently divides into two or more zygotes (monozygotic [MZ]) or the fertilization of multiple ova (DZ, trizygotic [TZ], etc.).

Among MZ twin pregnancies, about 30% are dichorionic/diamniotic (DCDA; separate placentas and amniotic sacs); about 70% are monochorionic/diamniotic (MCDA; a single placenta with two amniotic sacs); and about 1% are monochorionic/monoamniotic

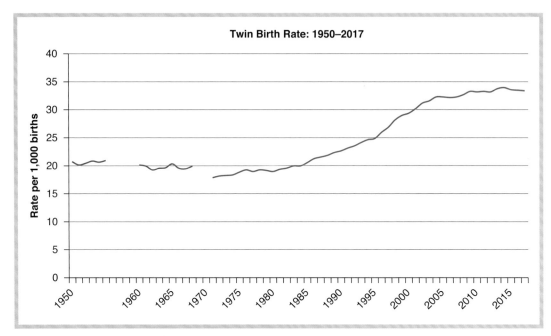

FIGURE 11–1. Twin birth rate: United States, 1950 to 2017. Note: Break in line represents years in which data were not collected. (Based on natality data from the National Center for Health Statistics.)

(MCMA), in which multiple fetuses share a single placenta and one amniotic sac (Smith-Levitin, Skupski, & Chervenak, 1999) (Fig. 11–3). The rate of twinning with ART procedures is increased, and MZ twinning appears to be more likely with assisted hatching procedures where the zona pellucida is breached (Luke, 2017). The degree to which structures are shared is related to the time of zygotic division after conception: Early division (within 72 hours) results in DCDA, division between days 4 and 7 results in MCDA, and later

division results in MCMA. Conjoined twins occur following very late and incomplete zygotic splitting, usually after day 13 (Newman & Unal, 2017). Because they develop from a single fertilized ovum, MZ twins are always of the same sex. DZ twins are always DCDA (even if placentas fuse) and may be the same or different sex. Triplets and other HOMs may have any combination of chorionicity/amnionicity, such as trichorionic/triamniotic, dichorionic/triamniotic, or monochorionic/triamniotic (Figs. 11–4 to 11–6.)

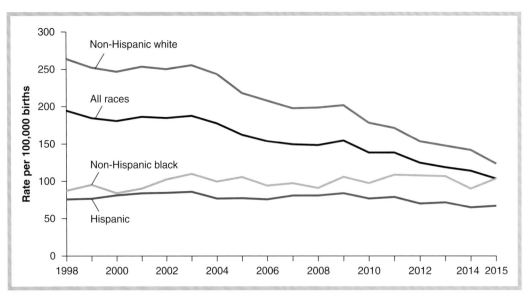

FIGURE 11–2. Triplet and high-order multiple birth rates by race and Hispanic origin of mother: United States, 1998 to 2015. (From Martin, J. A., Hamilton, B. E., Osterman, M. J. K., Driscoll, A. K., & Mathews, T. J. [2017]. Births: Final data for 2015. *National Vital Statistics Reports*, *66*[1], 1–70.

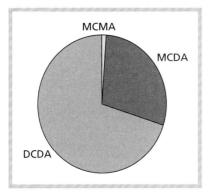

FIGURE 11–3. Monozygotic twinning. DCDA, dichorionic-diamniotic; MCDA, monochorionic-diamniotic; MCMA, monochorionic-monoamniotic.

ROLE OF INFERTILITY AND ASSISTED REPRODUCTIVE TECHNOLOGY

A significant percentage of multiple births today are conceived with some type of infertility therapy, including ART and non-ART treatments (Luke, 2017). ART includes fertility treatments in which both eggs and embryos are handled, such as in vitro fertilization (IVF), but not treatments in which only sperm are handled, such as ovulation induction with intrauterine insemination. Non-ART fertility treatments using ovulation induction and ovarian stimulation with gonadotropins are more likely to result in multiples since there is no control over the number of eggs that

can fertilize. Although the data from the ART National Summary and the ART Fertility Clinic Success Rates Reports provide a fairly accurate estimate of IVF births (Centers for Disease Control and Prevention [CDC], American Society for Reproductive Medicine [ASRM], & Society for Assisted Reproductive Technology [SART], 2017), exact numbers of births from natural conceptions and non-ART procedures are unknown because this information is not reported in a national database. Nineteen percent of twins and 25% of HOMs are attributed to IVF, while 21% of twins and 52% of HOMs are estimated to result from non-IVF procedures (Luke, 2017). Figure 11–7 illustrates the distribution of multiple gestations in ART cycles.

Of concern is not only the higher risk of multiple births with fertility treatments but also the increased rates of poor outcomes for these multiple gestations. Compared with naturally conceived twins, adverse outcomes for mothers and infants are more likely in twin pregnancies from ART and non-IVF fertility treatments (Luke, Gopal, Cabral, Stern, & Diop, 2017). Among IVF births in 2014, 56.8% of twins and 98.7% of HOMs were born preterm and 55.4% of twins and 93.7% of HOMs were low birth weight (LBW) (CDC et al., 2017).

The high risk of multiple births with ART and other infertility therapies has generated policy recommendations and clinical guidelines. Beginning in 1998, the SART and the ASRM affirmed that the goal of ART is to achieve a singleton gestation and issued guidance

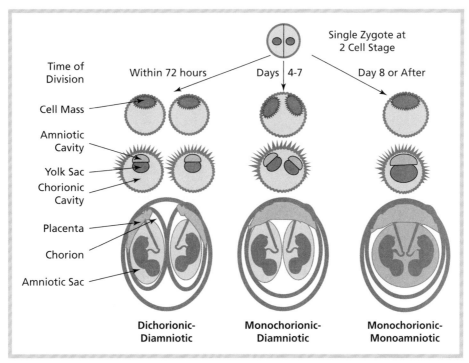

FIGURE 11–4. Monozygotic twins. (Copyright 2006 by Marvelous Multiples, Inc. Used with permission.)

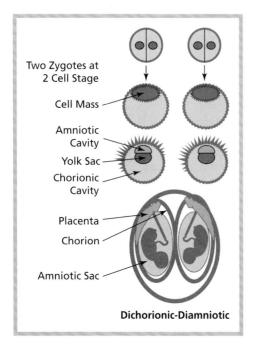

Two Zygotes at
2 Cell Stage

Cell Mass

Amniotic
Cavity

Yolk Sac

Chorionic
Cavity

Placenta

Chorion

Amniotic Sac

Dichorionic-Diamniotic

FIGURE 11–5. Dizygotic twins. (Copyright 2006 by Marvelous Multiples, Inc. Used with permission.)

for women ≥43 years of age. The guidance has been successful: The progressively decreasing number of embryos recommended for transfer have coincided with a fall in HOM birth rates. A recent review of outcomes data from SART found that single embryo transfer decreased the multiple birth rate by 47% while decreasing the live birth rate only 10% to 15% (Mersereau et al., 2017). A continued decrease in the number of iatrogenic multiple births remains challenging due to costs associated with ART, patient desire for multiples, and even competition among infertility practices (Tobias, Sharara, Franasiak, Heiser, & Pinckney-Clark, 2016). Effective tools include personalized patient counseling and education about the risks of multiple births, increased insurance coverage and other financial incentives, IVF success predictor tools such as that developed by SART (https://www.sartcorsonline.com/Predictor/Patient), and using technologies to improve selection of embryos for transfer (Tobias et al., 2016).

Multifetal Pregnancy Reduction

Multifetal pregnancy reduction (MFPR) is a pregnancy termination procedure that reduces the number of fetuses in an HOM pregnancy to a lower and potentially more viable number, with the goal of increasing the chances for a positive pregnancy outcome. Although MFPR is sometimes called selective reduction, the terms are not synonymous. Selective reduction applies to situations in which a specific fetus is targeted for reduction because of a known anomaly, aneuploidy,

to assist ART programs and patients in determining the appropriate number of embryos to transfer (ASRM & SART, 2017). The 2017 recommendations are for transfer of a single euploid embryo in all women, regardless of age, with guidance for other situations depending on embryo ploidy status, stage of development, and use of autologous or donor oocytes. Data are insufficient to recommend a limit

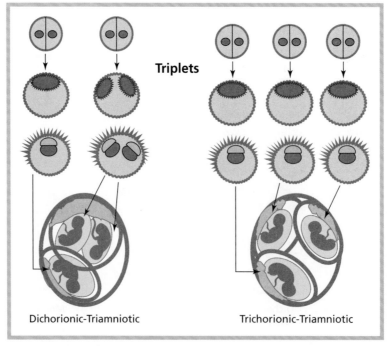

Triplets

Dichorionic-Triamniotic

Trichorionic-Triamniotic

FIGURE 11–6. Triplets. (Copyright 2006 by Marvelous Multiples, Inc. Used with permission.)

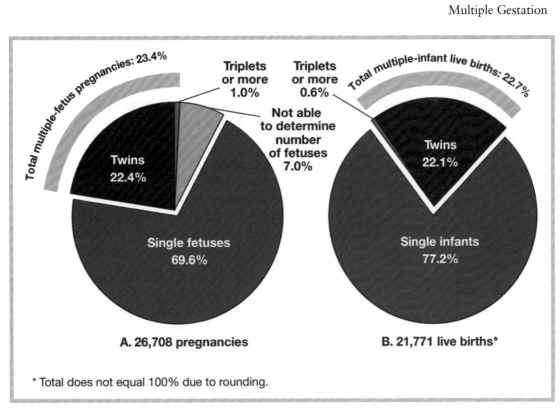

FIGURE 11–7. Distribution of multiple-fetus pregnancies and multiple-infant live births among art cycles using fresh nondonor eggs or embryos, 2015. (From Centers for Disease Control and Prevention, American Society for Reproductive Medicine, & Society for Assisted Reproductive Technology. [2017]. *2015 Assisted reproductive technology national summary report.* Atlanta, GA: U.S. Department of Health and Human Services.

or a risk identified with nuchal translucency (NT) screening. MFPR is typically performed in the late first trimester to terminate one or more fetuses. Transabdominal needle insertion under ultrasound guidance in the late first trimester is used most commonly. Although transvaginal fetal puncture and aspiration between 6 and 8 weeks of gestation is also performed (Lin et al., 2016), this carries a higher loss rate (Evans, Andriole, & Britt, 2014). For the transabdominal procedure, the woman is placed in the lithotomy position, and a 22-gauge needle is inserted transabdominally into the fetal thorax or heart. Asystole is achieved following injection of 2 to 3 mL of potassium chloride and is confirmed by ultrasound. Antibiotics are usually given, and the woman may have abdominal cramping, vaginal spotting, and leaking of amniotic fluid (Little, 2010). Reduction of a single fetus in an MC pair requires occlusion of umbilical cord blood flow to prevent interfetal transfusion. Radiofrequency ablation has been used to destroy cord tissue for selective reduction of an MC twin (Kumar et al., 2014) and of acardiac twins (Lee, Bebbington, & Crombleholme, 2013). Ultrasound-guided laser ablation of the pelvic vessels of one MC twin has also been used in DC triplets but resulted in a 46% loss rate for the remaining co-twin (Chaveeva, Peeva, Pugliese, Shterev, & Nicolaides, 2017).

The most recent Cochrane review on the topic noted that there are no randomized controlled trials (RCTs) comparing maternal and infant outcomes in women treated with expectant management versus MFPR (Dodd, Dowswell, & Crowther, 2015a). The review concluded that while some improved outcomes appear to be associated with MFPR, including decreased rates of pregnancy loss, antenatal complications, birth before 36 weeks, cesarean birth, LBW infants, and neonatal death, and that outcomes appear similar to those of spontaneously conceived or ART multiple gestations, the evidence is based on nonrandomized research with the potential for bias. The literature is also conflicting regarding the outcomes of reduced versus nonreduced twins and the ethics of reducing a normal twin fetus for a nonmedical indication remain in question (Drugan & Weissman, 2017). The American College of Obstetricians and Gynecologists (ACOG) recommends counseling patients that "reduction to a lower-order pregnancy (triplet to twin or twin to singleton) reduces the risk of medical complications associated with maintaining a higher-order multiple pregnancy" but that risks remain higher for reduced pregnancies than those that started at a lower fetal number (ACOG, 2017b, p. e159).

Complications of MFPR include procedural (e.g., infection or incomplete procedure) and a 4% to 5%

risk of total pregnancy loss (Drugan & Weissman, 2017; Evans et al., 2014). Without prenatal diagnostic testing prior to MFPR, there is the possibility of terminating a healthy fetus while leaving an abnormal one. Some centers are using chorionic villus sampling (CVS) and genetic analysis by karyotype and chromosomal microarray prior to MFPR (Evans et al., 2014; Običan, Brock, Berkowitz, & Wapner, 2015). ASRM (2012) recommends that MFPR should be performed only in specialized centers with fetal medicine practitioners experienced in the procedure.

MFPR presents a difficult dilemma for most couples. They often face contradictory values as they consider reduction after years of desiring fertility and must weigh the medical/obstetric/neonatal risks and the psychosocial/moral/economic impact on their family (Elliott, 2005a). The seemingly (and often actual) arbitrary choice as to which fetus should live and which should die is distressing (Bryan, 2005). Furthermore, the decision for reduction must be made in a short time between diagnosis and the optimal timing for the procedure. The decision has been described as highly stressful, psychologically traumatic, frightening, painful, overwhelming, confusing, and a surreal experience (Bergh, Möller, Nilsson, & Wikland, 1999; Bryan, 2005; Collopy, 2004). The following responses from women indicate their inner conflicts about the decision: "I believe reduction saved one of my children. It's the not knowing that kills me." "If I tried to carry all of the babies, I would most definitely lose them all. I also look at my survivor knowing she probably would have been chosen for reduction. This also wracks me with guilt" (from a mother who spontaneously lost some of her fetuses and did not have to reduce) (Pector, 2004, p. 716). There are also indications from interviews with patients that viewing fetuses on ultrasound just prior to or during reduction made the procedure more difficult for them (Maifeld, Hahn, Titler, & Mullen, 2003; Schreiner-Engel, Walther, Mindes, Lynch, & Berkowitz, 1995). Studies have shown that persistent feelings of sadness and guilt may continue after the MFPR procedure; however, most women believe their choice was correct and that reduction was necessary for them to achieve their goal of motherhood (Collopy, 2004). The grief response with MFPR may not fit the classic process and may be more complicated or delayed. H. L. Wang and Yu Chao (2006) interviewed six Taiwanese women undergoing MFPR over 8 to 10 weeks. Although the women could move past the reduction and adjust to a normal pregnancy experience, the researchers found that MFPR created psychosocial distress through exposure to moral and ethical dilemmas. More research is needed to determine long-term psychological outcomes, cultural responses, and effects on parent–child bonding and responses of child survivors.

The reduction debate also can be problematic for clinicians. With the improvements in neonatal care and long-term outcomes for preterm infants, some clinicians may be unwilling to accept that medical risks are sufficient grounds for reducing a triplet pregnancy (Bryan, 2005). Another consideration is the first trimester spontaneous loss rate for multiple gestations, which might make MFPR unnecessary. One study found that spontaneous loss of one or more gestational sacs or embryos occurred before the 12th week of gestation in 65% of quadruplet pregnancies, 53% of triplets, and 36% of twins (Dickey et al., 2002). The controversy is likely to continue. Debates have now moved from reduction of HOMs to the routine offer of reduction for twins to singleton (Evans et al., 2014). ACOG (2017b) recommends offering nondirective patient counseling to all women with high-order multiple gestations with discussion of risks and options of expectant management or reduction. Clinicians are charged with respecting patient autonomy in deciding the best course of action for a woman's individual situation and making appropriate referral to another provider if indicated (ACOG, 2017b).

Nurses have much to contribute in the care of women considering and undergoing MFPR. Establishing a rapport, exploring treatment options, and assisting with decision making with a consistently available primary nurse have been recommended (Collopy, 2004). Patient education includes written instructions, a list of symptoms that would indicate a need for medical care, postprocedure self-care, and grief counseling (Little, 2010).

DIAGNOSIS OF MULTIPLE GESTATIONS

First trimester ultrasound is highly accurate in diagnosing multiple gestations, and women at high risk for multiples, such as those using infertility therapies, should be screened as early as possible. The earliest gestation for determining chorionicity is 5 gestational weeks; for fetal number, 6 weeks; and for amnionicity, as early as 7 weeks. However, careful follow-up is needed as numbers, chorionicity, and amnionicity can change or be misassigned (Newman & Unal, 2017). Counting the gestational sacs establishes the number of chorions and each sac should be evaluated for the presence of a yolk sac, embryo, and cardiac activity (Frates, 2018). A DC pregnancy has two gestational sacs, and an MC pregnancy has a single gestational sac containing two yolk sacs. Later first trimester chorionicity markers include thickness and number of membrane layers seen on ultrasound. The triangular lambda (twin peak) sign predicts DZ chorionicity, a T-shaped junction is present in MC placentas,

TABLE 11–1. First Trimester Ultrasonographic Markers of Chorionicity

Ultrasonographic sign	Chorionicity
T-shaped junction	Monozygotic twins
Lambda (twin peak)	Dizygotic twins
Y-shaped ipsilon	Trizygotic triplets

and a Y-shaped ipsilon zone is characteristic of the three interfetal membranes of TZ triplet gestations, although these markers may not be consistently seen and vary with increasing gestational age (Frates, 2018) (Table 11–1).

First trimester ultrasonography is highly accurate in determining chorionicity, but accuracy decreases as the pregnancy progresses, especially after 14 weeks' gestation when membrane thinning, loss of the lambda sign, and placental fusion may occur (Frates, 2018). Early identification of MC and MA pregnancies is important in planning appropriate management of these high-risk pregnancies. For pregnancies resulting from ART, the embryo transfer date rather than the last menstrual period should be used to establish the gestational age.

Beginning with the initial ultrasound examination, it is critical to identify the location of each fetus to allow consistent and continuous identification until birth. Fetus A is closest to the cervix and should remain Fetus A for the rest of the pregnancy, even if the position changes. Nonpresenting fetuses are labeled Fetus B, C, etc. Specific identification can be added, such as right fundus location, placental location, fetal sex, discordant growth, and anomaly. Labeling systems need to be clear and reproducible for all follow-up examinations (Frates, 2018).

Not all women are psychologically prepared for the diagnosis of twins and even fewer for the discovery of HOMs. Ambivalence is normal, even when a pregnancy has been greatly desired or after years of infertility treatments (Klock, 2001). Revealing the diagnosis of multiple pregnancy should be done with sensitivity to each woman's situation, with a factual nonemotional approach and guarded enthusiasm (Bowers, Gromada, & Wieczorek, 2006). Many are at first overwhelmed with joy by the announcement of multiples and then simply overwhelmed by the physical, emotional, and financial demands ahead.

MATERNAL ADAPTATION

Nearly every maternal structure and body system is affected by the physiologic changes that occur in multiple gestation, with symptoms often more exaggerated than with a singleton pregnancy. General complaints of pregnancy such as urinary frequency, constipation, difficulty sleeping, fatigue, and varicose veins tend to be magnified and occur earlier.

Gastrointestinal

Hyperemesis gravidarum is 2 to 3 times more likely in multiple gestations and may be associated with increased placental mass and rising levels of human chorionic gonadotropin (hCG) (ACOG, 2018; Dypvik, Pereira, Tanbo, & Eskild, 2018; Newman & Unal, 2017). One study found that women carrying a combination of male and female fetuses had the highest risk for hyperemesis, with risks decreasing for all males followed by all females (Fell, Dodds, Joseph, Allen, & Butler, 2006). Women may also complain of gastroesophageal reflux early in multiple pregnancy, which is consistent with decreased lower esophageal sphincter tone of pregnancy, and increasing mechanical pressure due to the rapidly growing uterus and slowed gastrointestinal transit time (Richter, 2003).

Hematologic

Along with increased total body water, plasma volume increases by 50% to 100% with multiple gestations, which results in a dilutional anemia (Goodnight & Newman, 2009). Women carrying twins are 1.7 times more likely to have iron-deficiency anemia (Campbell & Templeton, 2004).

Cardiovascular

Women experience significant cardiovascular changes with a multiple pregnancy. Heart rate and stroke volume are increased over that of singleton gestations, resulting in higher cardiac output and cardiac index (Newman & Unal, 2017). Total vascular resistance has been found to be lower in uncomplicated twin pregnancies from 20 to 34 gestational weeks when compared to singletons (Kuleva et al., 2011). Colloid oncotic pressure is also reduced. Clinically, women have increased dependent edema and together with increased plasma volume, these cardiovascular changes increase the risk of pulmonary edema (Newman & Unal, 2017). Positions that promote aortocaval compression should be avoided as a woman's large uterus may increase her susceptibility to supine hypotension syndrome.

Respiratory

Respiratory changes are similar to that in a singleton pregnancy, but with greater tidal volumes and oxygen consumption, and a more alkalotic arterial pH in women with multiple gestation (Malone & D'Alton, 2014). Increased abdominal distention and loss of abdominal muscle tone may require women to use their accessory muscles during respiration, resulting in greater dyspnea and shortness of breath (Norwitz, Edusa, & Park, 2005).

Musculoskeletal

The rapidly growing uterus of a multiple gestation magnifies typical pregnancy complaints of back and ligament pain, and women often experience symptoms much earlier in their pregnancy. Women may benefit from a pregnancy support garment and many find that increased rest helps relieve back pain. Women also need instructions in good body mechanics, posture, and placement of supportive pillows while sleeping.

Dermatologic

Pruritic urticarial papules and plaques of pregnancy (PUPPP), also known as polymorphic eruption of pregnancy, is a common specific dermatosis of pregnancy that is 10 times more likely in multiple gestations (A. R. Wang & Kroumpouzos, 2017). PUPPP is thought to be related to abdominal distention and presents with redness and itching in the abdominal striae and urticarial papules on the lower abdomen. In severe cases, the papules merge into pruritic plaques, extend to the buttocks and thighs, and may be generalized. PUPPP usually responds to treatment with topical antipruritics, topical steroids, or oral antihistamines or steroids and then typically disappears within 2 weeks after birth. Other causes of abdominal itching should be considered, including normal striae/stretching skin or pruritus secondary to intrahepatic cholestasis, which are both more likely in multiple gestation. Comfort measures to minimize itching include cool baths, oatmeal products in the bath, oatmeal creams or lotions, baking soda baths, and aqueous menthol creams (Gabzdyl & Schlaeger, 2015).

PERINATAL COMPLICATIONS

Despite their overall small numbers and incidence, multiple gestations represent a substantial proportion of poor perinatal outcomes. As will be seen, compared with their counterparts with singleton gestations, women pregnant with multiples are more likely to experience more frequent and severe pregnancy complications and have infants that are smaller, born earlier, less likely to survive the first year of life, and more likely to suffer lifelong disability.

Maternal Morbidity and Mortality

Studies have shown significant increases in adverse maternal outcomes in multiple compared with singleton gestations, often with a dose–response relationship.

The combination of physiologic changes and perinatal pathologies that are unique or more likely in multiple gestations contributes to this increased risk. Increased adverse outcomes include the following (Malone & D'Alton, 2014; Newman & Unal, 2017):

- Abruption
- Acute fatty liver
- Anemia
- Thromboembolism
- Chorioendometritis
- Retained products
- Gestational diabetes
- Gestational hypertension, preeclampsia, and eclampsia
- Hemolysis, elevated liver enzymes, and low platelets (HELLP) syndrome
- Hyperemesis gravidarum
- Manual placental extraction
- Preterm labor (PTL)
- Preterm premature rupture of membranes (PPROM)
- Primary and secondary postpartum hemorrhage
- Postpartum thromboembolism
- Threatened spontaneous abortion

Risks are even higher for many of these adverse outcomes in women carrying HOMs (Wen, Demissie, Yang, & Walker, 2004). A prospective national study in the Netherlands found that women with multiples were 4 times more likely than those with singleton pregnancies to have a severe acute maternal morbidity, which included intensive care unit admission, uterine rupture, eclampsia (including HELLP syndrome), major obstetric hemorrhage, peripartum hysterectomy, or arterial embolization (Witteveen, Van Den Akker, Zwart, Bloemenkamp, & Van Roosmalen, 2016).

There are few studies on maternal deaths in multiple gestations, and national data are likely to be underreported. Recent reports from the CDC (2019b) show increasing rates of maternal deaths since 1987 for all women. Importantly, the most common causes of pregnancy-related deaths are also significant risks with multiple gestations. These include the following, in order of frequency as a cause of death from 2011 to 2015: cardiovascular diseases, 15.1%; medical noncardiovascular diseases, 14.3%; infection or sepsis, 12.4%; hemorrhage, 11.2%; cardiomyopathy, 10.8%; thrombotic pulmonary embolism, 9.2%; and hypertensive disorders of pregnancy, 6.8% (CDC, 2019b). Worldwide, women pregnant with twins were 4 times as likely to die than those with a singleton pregnancy; the risk for a potentially life-threatening condition was more than doubled, and the risk for a maternal near miss (survival of a life-threatening condition) and severe maternal outcomes were each more than 3 times higher. These risks were irrespective of Human Development Index or region (Santana et al., 2016).

TABLE 11-2. Strategies/Interventions for Preterm Birth Prevention or Risk Identification in Multiple Gestation

Strategies/interventions for preterm birth prevention or risk identification	Evidence for effectiveness or recommendations for use in multiple gestations?
Prophylactic bed rest at home or in the hospital	No
Prophylactic 17-alpha-hydroxyprogesterone caproate	No
Cessation of sexual activity	No
Vaginal progesterone administration	Possible in some subgroups of women
Prophylactic beta-mimetic tocolysis	No
Prophylactic cervical cerclage	No
Home uterine activity monitoring	No
Prophylactic pessary use	No
Fetal fibronectin testing	Not in asymptomatic women
Serial transvaginal ultrasound cervical length assessments	Not in asymptomatic women
Course of corticosteroids between 23 and 34 weeks' gestation in women at risk for preterm delivery within 7 days	Yes
Intravenous magnesium sulfate given before anticipated birth <32 weeks' gestation	Yes

Preterm Labor

PTL is a significant and frequent complication for multiple gestations, occurring in 50% of twins, 76% of triplets, and 90% of quadruplets (Elliott, 2005b). Although the exact mechanisms are not understood, it is thought that stimuli, including stretch, placental corticotropin-releasing hormone, and lung maturity factors, may be stronger in multiple gestations due to greater fetal and placental mass (Stock & Norman, 2010). In women with twin pregnancies who have symptoms of PTL, approximately 22% to 29% will deliver within 7 days (Chauhan, Scardo, Hayes, Abuhamad, & Berghella, 2010).

Unfortunately, most strategies effective in preterm birth prevention or identification of risk in singleton pregnancy are not recommended for multiple gestations and are summarized in Table 11-2.

Activity

For many years, prophylactic bed rest was a mainstay in multiple gestation care, but there is no sound evidence to support a policy of routine bed rest at home or in the hospital (da Silva Lopes, Takemoto, Ota, Tanigaki, & Mori, 2017). Recommendations for exercise and physical activity should be individualized and may be limited in women with comorbid obstetric or medical complications. For example, fetal growth restriction is a relative contraindication for exercise during pregnancy (ACOG, 2015). Although some clinicians recommend cessation of sexual activity for women with multiple gestations, particularly those with HOMs, data to support this in the absence of signs of PTL are lacking. One small report of 50 women with twin pregnancy found a decrease in coital frequency from early to late pregnancy. This was especially true in women who had used IVF to achieve pregnancy. There was no association between sexual activity and preterm birth in the report (Stammler-Safar, Ott, Weber, & Krampl, 2010).

Prophylactic Tocolysis

Prophylactic beta-mimetic agents do not reduce the incidence of PTL and birth in multiple gestations. A Cochrane review concluded there was insufficient evidence for or against their use to prevent preterm birth in twin gestations (Yamasmit et al., 2015); however, the ACOG recommendation is clear. ACOG states, "There is no role for the prophylactic use of any tocolytic agent in women with multifetal gestation, including the prolonged use of betamimetics for this indication" (ACOG & Society for Maternal-Fetal Medicine [SMFM], 2016, p. e134). Although home uterine activity monitoring has been used with multiple pregnancies, studies are inconsistent and did not demonstrate an impact on maternal or perinatal outcomes (Urquhart, Currell, Harlow, & Callow, 2017).

Cerclage

ACOG and SMFM (2016) recommend against the use of prophylactic cervical cerclage as an intervention for preterm birth prevention, but existing studies show varying results. Some found cervical cerclage neither prevented preterm birth of multiples (including triplets) nor improved pregnancy or neonatal outcomes (Rafael, Berghella, & Alfirevic, 2014). This includes both prophylactic cerclage and cerclage for transvaginal ultrasound-identified short cervix. In fact, one study found cerclage placement in women with twin gestation and a short cervix doubled the risk of preterm birth (Berghella, Odibo, To, Rust, &

Althuisius, 2005). In contrast, Roman et al. (2015) found that in a planned subgroup, asymptomatic twin pregnancies with transvaginal cervical length (TVCL) ≤15 mm before 24 weeks, ultrasound-indicated cerclage was associated with a significant prolongation of pregnancy by almost 4 weeks, significantly decreased spontaneous preterm birth <34 weeks by 49%, and a decrease in admission to neonatal intensive care units (NICUs) by 58% compared with controls. Houlihan et al. (2016) reported that DCDA gestations with cervical lengths ≤15 mm at 16 to 24 weeks' gestation showed a 60% reduction in the rate of spontaneous birth <32 weeks' gestation. A meta-analysis of three RCTs of women with twins who had TVCL <25 mm before 24 weeks found cerclage did not prevent preterm birth (Saccone, Rust, Althuisius, Roman, & Berghella, 2015). More studies are needed.

Pessary

Use of a pessary has been studied in multiple gestations for both preterm birth prophylaxis and as an intervention for short cervix. A recent small, RCT found that cervical pessary use did not prevent preterm birth in women with twin gestation who also had a short cervix (Berghella, Dugoff, & Ludmir, 2017). Three other RCTs (Goya et al., 2016; Liem et al., 2013; Nicolaides et al., 2016) each addressed the topic of prophylactic pessary placement in twin pregnancies with results showing no benefit of the treatment. Each of these trials also addressed pessary placement in women with short cervical lengths (ranging in cutoffs of ≤25 to <38 mm). The results of this post hoc portion of each study are conflicting. Liem et al. (2013) reported a significant reduction in "poor perinatal outcome" (as defined in the article) and preterm birth in women with multiple pregnancies with a cervical length of <38 mm. In women with short cervix ≤25 mm, the pessary showed no significant benefit (Nicolaides et al., 2016). Goya et al. (2016) found that pessary was associated with a significant reduction in the rate of spontaneous preterm birth in women with a short cervix ≤25 mm.

A recent meta-analysis (Saccone et al., 2017) concluded that Arabin pessary use in twin pregnancies with short transvaginal ultrasound cervical length (TVU-CL) at 16 to 24 weeks may not prevent spontaneous preterm birth or improve perinatal outcome. The analysis suggested potential reasons why the pessary was effective in some trials but not in others and included differences in training of the inserting practitioners and follow-up TVU to confirm correct placement and that study design and patient selection variations may have affected randomization.

In a 10-year retrospective cohort study of twin pregnancies by Fox et al. (2016), the combination of cervical pessary and vaginal progesterone use in twin pregnancies with short cervix <20 mm was reviewed. The researchers found that in twin pregnancies with a short cervix <20 mm, the addition of a cervical pessary with vaginal progesterone was associated with prolonged pregnancy and reduced risk of adverse neonatal outcomes. ACOG and SMFM (2016) currently do not recommend prophylactic pessary use in multiple gestations.

Progesterone

Unlike the positive effects for at-risk singleton pregnancies, 17-alpha-hydroxyprogesterone caproate (17P) has not been shown to be effective for prevention of preterm birth in multiple gestations and is not recommended (ACOG & SMFM, 2016). RCTs with 17P in twin and triplet pregnancies have not shown benefit in prolonging gestation or reducing neonatal morbidity (Awwad et al., 2015; Caritis, Feghali, Grobman, & Rouse, 2016; Lim et al., 2011). In triplet pregnancies, prophylactic treatment with 17P was associated with increased midtrimester fetal loss and did not reduce neonatal morbidity or prolong gestation (Combs, Garite, Maurel, Das, & Porto, 2010). The U.S. Food and Drug Administration (FDA) approval for injectable 17P in the treatment of PTL does not include multiple gestations.

Although use of prophylactic vaginal micronized progesterone did not prevent preterm birth in twin gestations in an RCT (Rode, Klein, Nicolaides, Krampl-Bettelheim, & Tabor, 2011), a meta-analysis of 13 RCTs identified a subgroup of women with twin gestation with a short cervix who may benefit from vaginal progesterone administration (Schuit et al., 2015). A recent updated systematic review and meta-analysis examined individual patient data from six RCTs that compared vaginal progesterone with either a placebo or no treatment in women with twin pregnancies and a sonographic short cervical length of ≤25 mm (Romero et al., 2017). The main finding was that vaginal progesterone administration to asymptomatic women with a twin gestation and a sonographic short cervix in the midtrimester reduces the risk of preterm birth occurring at <30 to <35 gestational weeks, neonatal mortality, and some measures of neonatal morbidity, without any demonstrable harmful effects on childhood neurodevelopment.

Cervical Assessment

Predicting PTL is difficult because most known risk factors for spontaneous preterm birth in singletons are not significantly associated with spontaneous preterm birth of twins (Goldenberg et al., 1996). While it is well known that identification of a short cervix in twin pregnancies, typically using TVU-CL, is a strong predictor of preterm birth, its use in asymptomatic women does not appear to change outcomes

(Berghella, Baxter, & Hendrix, 2013; Gordon et al., 2016). A systematic review and meta-analysis found that using a single TVU-CL measurement between 18 and 24 weeks' gestation appears to be a better predictor of preterm birth in twins than assessing changes with serial measurements (Conde-Agudelo & Romero, 2015). Efficacy of TVU-CL in triplet pregnancies is unclear (Fichera et al., 2018; Rosen, Hiersch, Freeman, Barrett, & Melamed, 2017). TVU-CL use in asymptomatic women pregnant with multiples is not recommended by ACOG and SMFM (2016).

Fetal Fibronectin Testing

Fetal fibronectin (fFN) testing may be an effective tool in predicting preterm birth in symptomatic women, especially in its negative predictive value, but studies are inconsistent (Conde-Agudelo & Romero, 2010), and ACOG and SMFM (2016) do not recommend it as a screening tool in asymptomatic women. However, retrospective cohort studies have shown positive fFN test results combined with short cervical length have higher positive predictive value for preterm birth than either positive test alone (Fox et al., 2009; Matthews et al., 2018).

Management of Preterm Labor

There are several challenges in managing PTL with multiples. These include increased incidence of PTL at earlier gestations, greater tocolytic latency than in singletons, less maternal perceptions of uterine activity, higher risk of tocolytic-related complications, and failure of therapy resulting in multiple infants affected by potential morbidities and mortality of preterm birth (Lam & Gill, 2005b). Twin gestations have been shown to have higher mean uterine contraction frequency than singletons throughout the latter half of pregnancy and between 4:00 pm and 4:00 am, but this did not predict preterm birth prior to 35 weeks' gestation (Newman et al., 2006). Multiple gestations have also been observed to have different uterine activity patterns, including a significant crescendo in uterine activity 24 hours before the development of clinical PTL, and a higher prevalence of low-amplitude, high-frequency (LAHF) contractions (Morrison & Chauhan, 2003). Lam and Gill (2005a) described a characteristic pattern of recurring PTL in twins in Display 11–1.

Treatment of PTL in multiples includes use of tocolytics for short-term intervention to delay delivery and allow time for a corticosteroid regimen. Use of all tocolytic agents is off-label. Calcium channel blockers such as nifedipine, or prostaglandin synthetase inhibitors such as indomethacin, are preferred first-line therapies for a 48-hour course in acute PTL with multiples (ACOG & SMFM, 2016). Side effects of indomethacin include increased fetal pulmonary

DISPLAY 11–1

Pattern of Recurring Preterm Labor in Twins

- Return of excessive levels of LAHF precursor uterine activity patterns
- Return of circadian, nocturnal pattern of organized, high-amplitude uterine contractions
- Rapidly increasing need for increased frequency and dosage of terbutaline
- Acceleration of frequency of uterine contractions 48 to 72 hr before the episode of active recurrent preterm labor

LAHF, low-amplitude, high-frequency.
From Lam, F., & Gill, P. (2005a). Beta-agonist tocolytic therapy. *Obstetrics and Gynecology Clinics of North America, 32*(3), 457–484. doi:10.1016/j.ogc.2005.05.001

vasculature and ductal constriction and should not be used after 32 weeks' gestation or for treatment >72 hours (Lam & Gill, 2005a). Another side effect of indomethacin is decreased fetal renal function, which can lead to oligohydramnios; thus, twin-to-twin transfusion syndrome (TTTS) is a contraindication for this therapy.

There is good evidence that intravenous magnesium sulfate given before anticipated early preterm birth (before 32 weeks) reduces the risk of cerebral palsy (CP) in surviving infants (ACOG & SMFM, 2016; Crowther, Hiller, Doyle, & Haslam, 2003; Marret et al., 2006; Rouse et al., 2008). A 2013 safety alert from the FDA warned not to exceed 5 to 7 days of continuous intravenous (IV) magnesium sulfate in treatment of PTL because it may lead to low fetal calcium levels and bone problems (FDA, 2013). Women receiving magnesium sulfate should be assessed for signs of neurologic depression by evaluating deep tendon reflexes hourly, monitoring of bowel sounds and function, and frequently reviewing the status of each fetal heartbeat. Maternal renal function should also be monitored. Emergency resuscitation equipment should be easily accessible, including calcium gluconate (10 mL in 10% solution) for magnesium toxicity reversal (Lam & Gill, 2005b).

Oral terbutaline should not be used for prevention or any treatment of PTL and injectable terbutaline should not be used in pregnant women for prevention or prolonged treatment (beyond 48 to 72 hours) of PTL in either the hospital or outpatient setting because of the potential for serious maternal heart problems and death (FDA, 2011).

The greatest complication of tocolytic therapy for women with multiple gestation is the high risk for pulmonary edema, particularly when combined with intravenous fluids, corticosteroids, and the increased maternal blood volume (Malone & D'Alton, 2014). Intravenous fluids should be administered cautiously, and a strict intake and output record must be maintained. Nursing assessments should include signs and symptoms of pulmonary edema by observation (shortness of breath, coughing, or wheezing) and auscultation; daily weights; and metabolic evaluations including blood glucose, complete blood count, and electrolyte status (Lam & Gill, 2005b).

A single course of corticosteroids can be given to women pregnant with multiples between 23 and 34 weeks' gestation who are at risk for preterm delivery within 7 days (ACOG & SMFM, 2016). However, the efficacy of steroids is unclear for multiple gestation and dosing requirements have not been evaluated (Roberts, Brown, Medley, & Dalziel, 2017). While there is some evidence that antenatal corticosteroid exposure may not reduce the incidence of respiratory distress syndrome in preterm twins (Viteri et al., 2016), extremely preterm multiples (22 to 28 weeks) whose mothers received a course of antenatal steroids had decreased mortality (Boghossian et al., 2016). An additional single rescue course may be considered if an earlier treatment was given at least 7 to 14 days prior and the gestational age is less than 34 weeks, and delivery is anticipated within 7 days; use of repeated corticosteroid dosing (more than two courses) is not recommended (ACOG & SMFM, 2016). Increases in uterine contractions following corticosteroid administration have been observed in HOM pregnancies (Elliott & Radin, 1995).

Considering the lack of effective preterm birth prevention strategies for multiples, educating women in signs and symptoms of PTL is critical to the early detection of PTL and potential delay of preterm birth. Women should receive formal PTL education by 18 weeks' gestation (Lam & Gill, 2005a) with continual reinforcement at prenatal visits.

Hypertension

Hypertensive disorders of pregnancy, including gestational hypertension and preeclampsia, have a dose–response relationship with plurality, occurring in 11% to 12% of singleton, 18% to 21% of twin, and 23% of triplet gestations (Smith, Merriam, Jung, & Gyamfi-Bannerman, 2018). Maternal age is also a strong contributor, with the greatest impact in women older than age 40 years.

Preeclampsia in a multiple pregnancy tends to develop earlier and become more severe than in singleton gestations. It is thought that fetal number and placental mass are somehow involved in the pathogenesis of preeclampsia (Malone & D'Alton, 2014). Symptoms of severe preeclampsia with laboratory changes may indicate HELLP syndrome. In HOM gestations, the signs and symptoms of hypertensive disorders may be atypical, without the classic elevations of blood pressure or proteinuria. In a review of triplet and quadruplet pregnancies, of 16 women delivered for preeclampsia, only 8 had elevated blood pressure; whereas 10 had epigastric pain, visual disturbances, and/or headache; 9 had elevated liver enzymes; and 7 had low platelet counts (Hardardottir et al., 1996). Careful assessment of maternal signs and symptoms, in addition to laboratory evaluations, is important in the diagnosis and early treatment of hypertensive disease. When magnesium sulfate is used, fluid balance should be carefully monitored because of the increased risk of pulmonary edema.

Preterm Premature Rupture of Membranes

The incidence of PPROM is increased in multiple gestations, with rates of 6% in twins and 9.61% in triplets, compared to 2.68% in singletons (Luke & Brown, 2007). PPROM in twin gestation appears to have a shorter latency to birth than in singletons and chorioamnionitis and placental abruption may be less likely (Kibel et al., 2017). Although membrane rupture usually occurs in the presenting sac, rupture of a nonpresenting sac may occur, especially after invasive procedures such as amniocentesis (Norwitz et al., 2005). It is difficult to assess for PPROM in a nonpresenting sac and intermittent leakage of fluid is the typical clinical presentation. Rupture of the separating membrane in a twin gestation is a unique complication in MCDA twins, creating an MA twin risk scenario. Clinical management of PPROM in multiples is similar to that in singletons; is dependent on gestational age; and may include antibiotics, a single course of corticosteroids, or delivery for nonreassuring fetal status, clinical chorioamnionitis, and significant abruptio placentae (ACOG, 2016).

Gestational Diabetes

The increased placental mass with multiple fetuses and subsequent increase in human placental lactogen that modifies maternal metabolism are thought to influence the incidence of gestational diabetes mellitus (GDM) in multiple gestations (Newman & Unal, 2017). Like other maternal complications, gestational diabetes appears to have a dose–response relationship with increasing plurality. Diagnosis and management of GDM are similar to that in singleton pregnancies (Norwitz et al., 2005). Although twins whose mothers had GDM were more likely to be admitted to the NICU, the incidence of respiratory distress, neonatal hypoglycemia, and low Apgar score was similar to that of GDM singletons (R. T. McGrath et al., 2017).

Intrahepatic Cholestasis

Intrahepatic cholestasis occurs in up to one fourth of women with a twin pregnancy (Mei et al., 2019). The increased risks of preterm birth and fetal death with this condition warrant careful investigation into pruritus, especially on the palms and soles of the feet. Laboratory findings include elevated total serum bile acids in the late second and early third trimesters.

Acute Fatty Liver

In a multicenter review of 16 cases of acute fatty liver of pregnancy (AFLP), 18% were multiple gestations including one triplet pregnancy (Fesenmeier, Coppage, Lambers, Barton, & Sibai, 2005). Nausea and vomiting in the third trimester were the most common symptoms (75%). Although AFLP is very rare, the high associated morbidity and mortality call for careful surveillance. Women with nausea, vomiting, or epigastric pain in the third trimester should be carefully assessed.

Peripartum Cardiomyopathy

The rising rate of peripartum cardiomyopathy (PPCM) (from 1/4,350 live births in 1990 to 1993 to 1/968 in 2003 to 2011) parallels the increases in many of its risk factors: older maternal age, use of ART, multiple gestation, and rate of chronic hypertension associated with multiple gestations (Ersbøll, Damm, Gustafsson, Vejlstrup, & Johansen, 2016). Approximately 13% of cases of PPCM are twins (Elkayam et al., 2005). The condition may occur during late pregnancy or postpartum and may be sudden onset or develop gradually. Women with dyspnea, orthopnea, cough, chest pain, abdominal discomfort, persistent weight retention or weight gain, dizziness, and fatigue should be carefully assessed for this life-threatening condition (Ersbøll et al., 2016). Mortality is as high as 28%.

Antepartum Hemorrhage

Placenta previa does not appear to occur more frequently in multiple gestations, although it has been associated with ART twin pregnancies (Karami, Jenabi, & Fereidooni, 2018). The rate of placental abruption in twins is double that for singletons (Campbell & Templeton, 2004). Risks for abruption, including older maternal age, multiparity, PPROM, anemia, and hypertension, are also common in multiple gestations (Hubinont et al., 2015). Other factors that appear to increase the risks for abruption in twin gestations include low maternal body mass index (BMI) and vaginal bleeding in early pregnancy as well as a potential risk during the delivery interval between the first and second twin (Hubinont et al., 2015).

Pulmonary Embolism

Multiple pregnancy is a risk factor for venous thromboembolism, which may lead to pulmonary embolism (Bates et al., 2012). The mechanical obstruction of the enlarged uterus contributes to venous stasis, particularly for women on bed rest. In addition to the physiologic changes of pregnancy and childbirth, thromboembolism is associated with a personal history of thrombosis, presence of a thrombophilia, obesity, hypertension, smoking, and operative delivery (American Academy of Pediatrics [AAP] & ACOG, 2017). Therapeutic levels of anticoagulation may be more difficult to achieve with multiple gestations because of the larger volume of distribution.

Fetal Morbidity and Mortality

Zygosity, chorionicity, and fetal growth are important predictors of fetal health and survival in multiples. The inherent physiology associated with the twinning process, along with sharing of uterine space and placental resources, increases the risks for fetal morbidity. Perinatal morbidity and mortality rates for MZ twins are estimated to be 3 to 10 times higher than those for DZ twins (Trevett & Johnson, 2005). Perinatal mortality risks increase after 38 completed weeks for all twins (Cheung, Yip, & Karlberg, 2000). Analysis of linked birth and death in U.S. population data found the prospective risk (a proportion of all fetuses still at risk at a given gestational age) of fetal death for singletons, twins, and triplets at 24 weeks' gestation was 0.28/1,000, 0.92/1,000, and 1.30/1,000, respectively (Kahn et al., 2003). In comparison, the corresponding risk was 0.57/1,000 for singletons and 3.09/1,000 for twins at 40 weeks' gestation, and 13.18/1,000 for triplets at ≥38 weeks (Fig. 11–8).

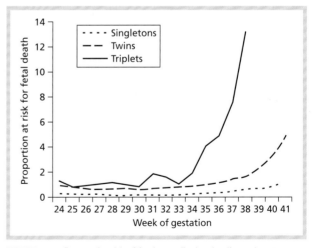

FIGURE 11–8. Prospective risk of fetal mortality by plurality and gestational age. (Data from Kahn, B., Lumey, L. H., Zybert, P. A., Lorenz, J. M., Cleary-Goldman, J., D'Alton, M. E., & Robinson, J. N. [2003]. Prospective risk of fetal death in singleton, twin, and triplet gestations: Implications for practice. *Obstetrics & Gynecology, 102*[4], 685–692. doi:10.1016 /S0029-7844(03)00616-1)

Because of the increased risks for fetal death at late gestational ages in multiple gestations, there are recommendations for delivering earlier (ACOG & SMFM, 2016).

Intrauterine Growth Restriction

Fetal growth and subsequent birth weight are influenced by plurality, zygosity, and chorionicity. Twins and singletons have similar fetal growth rates until about 32 weeks', triplets until 29 to 30 weeks', and quadruplets until approximately 27 weeks' gestation (Garite, Clark, Elliott, & Thorp, 2004). Twin birth weights are highest in DC/DZ, slightly less in DC/MZ, and lowest in MC/MZ (Derom, Derom, & Vlietinck, 1995). There is disagreement on the use of singleton growth curves or twin-specific growth curves for establishing normal fetal growth of twins, but serial evaluations for growth assessment using multiple biometric parameters are recommended (Malone & D'Alton, 2014).

The incidence of intrauterine growth restriction (IUGR) is greater in multiple birth infants than in singletons and is likely due to placental insufficiency and competition for nutrients. IUGR in multiples is associated with increased fetal mortality rates at all gestational ages (Garite et al., 2004) and particularly when it develops in early pregnancy. Studies indicate that slowed or compromised fetal growth in both twins at 20 to 28 weeks' gestation and from 28 weeks to birth is highly associated with very preterm birth (Hediger et al., 2006).

Discordance in estimated fetal weight between co-multiples is also important to monitor, even if there is no IUGR (Newman & Unal, 2017). Discordancy is more common in MC twins and is characteristic of TTTS. In HOMs, two or more fetuses may be concordant but have discordant co-multiple(s). Regardless of chorionicity, increasing degrees of intertwin discordancy in twins born after 34 weeks is associated with increasing perinatal morbidity (D'Antonio, Thilaganathan, Laoreti, & Khalil, 2018). A meta-analysis found that growth discordance in both MC and DC twin pregnancies increased the risk for intrauterine death, and the risk was higher when at least one fetus of the discordant set was also small for gestational age (SGA) (D'Antonio, Odibo, et al., 2018). In the review, the smaller twin was at higher risk for death compared to the larger one for each birth weight discordance group.

Congenital Anomalies

Congenital anomalies are approximately 2 times more likely in twins than singletons, with most anomalies found in MZ twins (Newman & Unal, 2017). Anomalies include structural congenital defects as well as chromosomal and genetic anomalies. The most common are cardiovascular, central nervous systems, ophthalmic, and gastrointestinal. Intrauterine crowding can result in foot deformities, hip dislocation, and skull asymmetry. In DZ twins, it is uncommon for both twins to be affected. Anomalies in MZ twins may result from the twinning process itself or aberrant vascular or placental physiology complications, and the two fetuses may be unequally affected. The rate of anomalies is 3 to 5 times higher in MZ twins (Weber & Sebire, 2010) with midline and neural tube defects being the most common (Newman & Unal, 2017). The risk of congenital heart disease is 9 times higher in MCDA twins and as much as 14 times higher in those with TTTS compared with the general risk of 0.5% (Bahtiyar, Dulay, Weeks, Friedman, & Copel, 2007), and all MC twins should be screened for congenital heart disease (Simpson, 2013).

Conjoined twins occur worldwide at a rate of 1.47/100,000 pregnancies; this rate is 2 times more common in female fetuses than in male fetuses (Mutchinick et al., 2011). The most common type is thoracopagus (42%), where fusion is face-to-face from the upper thorax to upper abdomen and always involves the heart (Mutchinick et al., 2011). Survival of conjoined twins is usually dependent on the extent of shared organs. Congenital anomalies are common in one or both conjoined twins as well as polyhydramnios (Newman & Unal, 2017). Recommendations include extensive counseling regarding survival and potential for separation, use of a tertiary care facility with a team of experienced specialists, and cesarean birth if near term (Newman & Unal, 2017).

Abnormal Vascular/Placental Changes

The presence of multiple placentas and shared placental circulations increase the likelihood of abnormalities such as vascular anastomoses and abnormal cord insertions. Use of ART is also associated with an increased risk of placental and cord insertion abnormalities (Jauniaux, Melcer, & Maymon, 2017).

Vascular anastomoses, or vessel connections, are found in nearly all MC placentas and are categorized as arteriovenous, venovenous, or arterioarterial and may be superficial or deep and balanced or unbalanced (Hubinont et al., 2015). Many MC placentas have anastomoses that allow bidirectional blood flow between the fetuses, resulting in a compensatory and protective balance. Unfortunately, sequelae of shared placental circulations develop in as many as 30% of MC pregnancies (Lewi et al., 2010); TTTS develops in 8% to 10% (Simpson, 2013). Fetal compromise occurs when there is significant single-direction vascular flow without compensatory bidirectional connections. TTTS develops with unequal shunting of blood in an MC placenta from the donor fetus to the co-twin recipient through vascular connections, which are usually arteriovenous and deep. Feto-fetal transfusion can also occur in HOMs with shared placental beds. In TTTS, the recipient twin becomes hypervolemic and polycythemic, progressing to polyhydramnios, congestive heart failure, and death. The donor twin becomes hypovolemic, anemic, and growth restricted. The pathophysiology of TTTS appears to be more complex than just volume shifts between twins. There is evidence that the hypertensive mediators renin and angiotensin also play an important role in TTTS (Harkness & Crombleholme, 2005). A significantly increased risk of TTTS has been associated with the following first trimester ultrasound findings: >10% intertwin discrepancy in crown-rump length, NT >95th percentile in at least one twin, and abnormal ductus venosus flow in at least one twin (Stagnati et al., 2017). Velamentous cord insertion and unequal placental sharing are also more common with discordant fetal growth.

The most severe form of TTTS is the stuck twin, when the donor twin is depleted of amniotic fluid. If left untreated, the mortality rate for TTTS is 80% or more, especially when it presents earlier than 28 weeks' gestation; up to 30% of survivors have associated neurodevelopmental anomalies (Habli, Lim, & Crombleholme, 2009). Because TTTS can develop quickly, SMFM (Simpson, 2013) currently recommends ultrasound evaluations of MCDA twins every 2 weeks from 16 gestational weeks until delivery or more frequently if indicated. Two criteria are required to diagnose TTTS: (1) monochorionicity and (2) discrepancy in amniotic fluid between the amniotic sacs with polyhydramnios in one sac (largest vertical pocket >8 cm) and oligohydramnios in the other sac (largest vertical pocket <2 cm) (Simpson, 2013). Assessment of umbilical artery Doppler flow may also be used, particularly when estimated fetal weights or amniotic fluid amounts are discordant. The Quintero staging system is a standardized tool that is commonly used to describe the severity of TTTS, from stage I (initial diagnostic criteria met) to stage V (fetal death) (Quintero et al., 1999; Simpson, 2013).

The most common treatments for TTTS are amnioreduction and selective fetoscopic laser photocoagulation, sometimes called fetoscopic laser surgery. Other interventions, such as intertwin amniotic membrane septostomy and umbilical cord coagulation, have fallen out of favor due to ineffectiveness or risk. Amnioreduction is an outpatient procedure, performed by a trained obstetrician when the recipient twin's maximum vertical pocket of fluid is >8 cm after 14 gestational weeks (Simpson, 2013). The procedure involves removing large amounts of amniotic fluid,

often more than 1 to 2 L, and may be needed on a recurring basis. In addition to the paradoxical effect of fluid increasing in the oligohydramniotic sac, side benefits of this therapy include prevention of PTL related to polyhydramnios, and improved fetal hemodynamics and uteroplacental blood flow (Harkness & Crombleholme, 2005). Yet, the procedure is not without problems. Survival is approximately 50% to 60%, and there is risk for PTL, PPROM, abruption, and infection (Simpson, 2013).

Laser photocoagulation is now a widely accepted treatment for TTTS. This procedure uses fetoscopy to visualize and laser to coagulate the vascular anastomoses at the intertwin membrane that are contributing to the syndrome. A Cochrane review determined that laser photocoagulation should be considered in the treatment of all stages of TTTS to improve neurodevelopmental outcome (Roberts, Neilson, Kilby, & Gates, 2014). The review found that more infants were alive without neurologic abnormality after laser treatment than with amnioreduction but noted that amnioreduction is the treatment of choice after 26 weeks or without access to skilled experts to perform laser coagulation. Having prior laser treatment also appears to benefit the surviving twin following fetal death of the co-twin. Laser photocoagulation carries risks of PPROM, preterm birth, leaking of amniotic fluid into the maternal peritoneum, abruption, and chorioamnionitis (Simpson, 2013). In one prospective series, PPROM occurred following laser treatment in 39% of the cases at a mean gestational age of 27.2 ± 4.6 weeks with half of those patients delivering in 24 hours (Snowise et al., 2017). Patient education is critical to meet complex learning needs surrounding TTTS, treatment options, and outcome expectations and assist the family in making informed decisions regarding care (Jackson & Mele, 2009).

A variation of TTTS is twin anemia–polycythemia sequence (TAPS), where the donor twin of an MCDA pair is anemic, the recipient twin is polycythemic, but amniotic fluid levels are normal. TAPS is diagnosed by Doppler flow findings of elevated middle cerebral artery peak systolic velocity in the donor and decreased velocity in the recipient. This condition is also a postprocedure complication in up to 13% of TTTS cases treated with laser coagulation (Robyr et al., 2006).

Acardiac malformations are defects in which one twin has no defined cardiac structure and survives using the co-twin's cardiac pump mechanism. This condition is also referred to as twin reversed arterial perfusion (TRAP) sequence because of direct umbilical artery to umbilical artery anastomoses in an MC placenta and reversal of circulation in the acardiac fetus. TRAP sequence occurs in 2.6% of MC twins (van Gemert, van den Wijngaard, & Vandenbussche, 2015), but it has been reported rarely in MC triplets.

The acardiac twin has 100% mortality, but the pump twin is at risk for cardiac failure and preterm birth. Interventions to interrupt the TRAP sequence include fetoscopy with ablation, coagulation, or use of ultrasound scalpel to occlude the acardiac twin's cord (Newman & Unal, 2017).

Abnormal umbilical cords and insertions are common findings in multiple gestations, especially those with MC placentas. Cords with a single umbilical artery are 3 times more common in twins than singletons (Hubinont et al., 2015). Velamentous insertion (directly into the fetal membranes) is 8 times more likely in twins than singletons (Hubinont et al., 2015) and is estimated to occur in 25% of triplet pregnancies (D. M. Feldman et al., 2002). IVF is also associated with an increase in vasa previa (Jauniaux et al., 2017). Velamentous insertions increase the risk for poor uteroplacental perfusion, fetal growth restriction, vascular thrombosis, and TTTS (Hubinont et al., 2015). The coexisting condition of vasa previa increases the risk of rupture of the fetal vessels within the amniotic membranes near the internal cervical os and diagnosis of vasa previa prior to labor onset is essential.

Although MA twins are rare (1% of MZ twins), these fetuses are at risk for cord entanglement and knotting. However, survival is approximately 88% with ultrasound detection of cord entanglement and modern fetal surveillance (Rossi & Prefumo, 2013). Some clinicians recommend daily nonstress testing starting at 24 to 26 weeks' gestation to identify fetal heart rate (FHR) decelerations occurring with cord entanglement (Malone & D'Alton, 2014).

Fetal Loss

Spontaneous loss of gestational sacs or embryos after documentation of FHR in a multiple pregnancy is termed the "vanishing twin" and is estimated to occur in 21% to 30% of twin pregnancies (Landy, Weiner, Corson, Batzer, & Bolognese, 1986; van Oppenraaij et al., 2009). Exact rates are not known, and there may be no visual or pathologic evidence at delivery; the phenomenon is more common in high-order gestations. In known cases, the remaining fetuses are likely to be born preterm, LBW, and SGA, particularly when losses occur after 8 weeks' gestation (van Oppenraaij et al., 2009).

Fetal death at 20 weeks or later occurs in 2.6% of twin and 4.3% of triplet gestations (Johnson & Zhang, 2002). Death of a co-twin does not appear to be an immediate risk to DC survivors, but in MC twins, fetal death results in a sudden drop in vascular resistance across placental anastomoses shunting blood away from the survivor. This is followed by anemia, hypotension, and hypoperfusion of vital organs. Survivors are at risk for fetal death, neonatal death,

and severe long-term morbidity. Risks for MC and DC twins following a co-twin fetal death are, respectively, death, 12% and 4%; neurologic abnormality, 18% and 1%; and preterm birth, 68% and 57% (Ong, Zamora, Khan, & Kilby, 2006). The risk of neurologic abnormality in the survivor appears to be associated with fetal death at any gestational age (Malone & D'Alton, 2014).

Management of single fetal death depends on multiple factors, including chorionicity, gestational age, and condition of the surviving fetus(es), and may include monitoring of the remaining fetuses for evidence of hemodynamic instability and of the mother for coagulopathy, PTL, and preeclampsia (Hillman, Morris, & Kilby, 2010). Ultrasound can reveal sonographic signs of cerebral ischemia in an MC survivor including intracranial hemorrhage, middle cerebral artery infarction, and periventricular white matter injury with subsequent leukomalacia; renal cortical necrosis and limb reduction injuries can also occur (Frates, 2018). Fetal magnetic resonance imaging may provide information about brain abnormalities such as multicystic encephalomalacia in the MC survivor (Newman & Unal, 2017). Immediate delivery in MC twins has not been shown to benefit the survivor, and individualized management based on maternal and fetal wellbeing is recommended (ACOG & SMFM, 2016).

ANTEPARTUM MANAGEMENT

Antepartum management of multiple pregnancy should be a collaborative effort of the members of the perinatal healthcare team, including maternal–fetal specialists, obstetricians, nurse midwives, registered nurses, advanced practice nurses, perinatal educators, ultrasonographers, social workers, genetic counselors, and dietitians.

Prenatal Diagnosis and Genetic Testing

As with all pregnant women, prenatal diagnostic screening should be offered to women with a multiple gestation. However, the assessment and calculations are more complex. The maternal age-related risk for aneuploidy is approximately the same for MZ twins as for singletons (Rustico, Baietti, Coviello, Orlandi, & Nicolini, 2005). However, for DZ twins, the risk of aneuploidy in one of the twins is double that of singletons because the independent risk for each twin is additive. The risk of aneuploidy occurring in both DZ twins is the singleton risk squared (Bush & Malone, 2005). In practical terms, a 33-year-old woman with twins has the same risk of Down syndrome as a 35-year-old woman with a singleton (ACOG & SMFM, 2016). In a 28-year-old woman with triplets, the risk of at least one fetus having Down syndrome is similar to the risk of a 35-year-old with a singleton (Malone & D'Alton, 2014). Referral to a genetic counselor is recommended for women of advanced maternal age who are pregnant with multiples (Cleary-Goldman, Chitkara, & Berkowitz, 2007).

NT screening for aneuploidy at 11 to 14 weeks' gestation is highly sensitive in multiple gestations (Sepulveda, Wong, & Casasbuenas, 2009). For these tests, each fetus is individually assessed and the pregnancy risk is calculated. Increased NT in MC pregnancies may indicate early TTTS rather than increased risk for aneuploidy (Malone & D'Alton, 2014). The use of nasal bone assessment has been shown to lower the false-positive rate of NT screening in triplet pregnancies (Krantz, Hallahan, He, Sherwin, & Evans, 2011).

First trimester maternal serum screening and combined assessments are not as accurate as in singleton pregnancies. For example, free beta-hCG and pregnancy-associated plasma protein A levels are 2 times higher in twins and other factors also affect these levels, including certain ART procedures and chorionicity (Bush & Malone, 2005). Cell-free fetal DNA screening has been shown to accurately detect autosomal trisomies in twin gestations, but further research is needed to validate this test (ACOG & SMFM, 2016; Canick et al., 2012; Huang et al., 2014; Le Conte et al., 2018).

Second trimester maternal serum screening in twin gestations is associated with a high false-positive rate, particularly in ART pregnancies (Maymon, Neeman, Shulman, Rosen, & Herman, 2005), as an unaffected fetus may mask the abnormal maternal serum levels associated with an aneuploid co-twin. Even if screening suggests the presence of an affected fetus, biochemical markers cannot specify which twin is abnormal (Bush & Malone, 2005).

Invasive prenatal diagnostic techniques may be indicated when prenatal screening tests identify increased risks for genetic or chromosomal abnormalities. CVS is often used in follow-up. Accessing multiple chorions can be technically challenging and may require transabdominal and/or transcervical approaches. There are risks for sample cross-contamination, a greater chance of uncertain results compared to singletons, and a procedural loss rate prior to 24 weeks' gestation approximately 1% higher than the background risk (Agarwal & Alfirevic, 2012). Genetic amniocentesis between 15 and 20 weeks has been found to be accurate in twin gestations. Use of a marker dye, such as indigo carmine, helps prevent cross-contamination of fluids when tapping multiple sacs. Amniocentesis appears to have a slightly increased procedure-related loss rate in twins compared to that in singletons (Cahill et al., 2009).

Prenatal diagnosis presents unique challenges for parents, especially if one fetus is abnormal. They may face the dilemma of termination of an abnormal fetus while continuing the pregnancy for the remaining ones. Parents may also worry about the status of the unaffected twin throughout pregnancy, highlighting a potential need for regular pre- and postnatal examination and ongoing reassurance, or invasive prenatal testing in the surviving fetuses after reduction (Bryan, 2005).

Prenatal Care

Women with known infertility-related multiple gestations should be seen as soon as possible and referral of twin gestations to a board-certified obstetrician and consultation with a maternal–fetal specialist if necessary (AAP & ACOG, 2017). It follows that women with HOMs are automatically referred for specialist care. These specialists typically coordinate care with the primary obstetrician or may provide primary obstetric care. Although most clinicians increase the number of antenatal care visits for women with multiple pregnancy, there is no consensus as to the frequency of visits to provide optimal care (Dodd & Crowther, 2005). However, considering the higher risks for perinatal complications in these pregnancies, regular and frequent antenatal visits increase the likelihood for early detection and treatment.

Specialized multiple-birth clinics (twin clinics) have reported improved perinatal morbidity and neonatal outcomes (Henry et al., 2015; Knox & Martin, 2010; Luke et al., 2003; Ruiz, Brown, Peters, & Johnston, 2001). Interventions in such clinics include consistent care providers, intensive education about prevention of preterm birth, individualized modification of maternal activity, increased attention to nutrition, ultrasonography, tracking of clinic nonattendees, and a supportive clinical environment. Cited benefits include improved maternal education; increased maternal weight gain and birth weights; longer gestations; lowered rates of cesarean birth, very LBW (VLBW), late preterm births, and perinatal mortality; decreased NICU admissions; shortened hospital stays; and lower hospital charges. However, the only RCT assessing such interventions found a significant increase in cesarean birth and did not show improved outcomes over standard antenatal care (Dodd, Dowswell, & Crowther, 2015b).

Management of HOM gestations involves more intensive surveillance, attention, and interventions, but there is no consensus as to content or frequency of prenatal care for these high-risk pregnancies.

Prenatal Education

Parents expecting multiples have unique perinatal educational needs. The high-risk nature and extraordinary aspects of their pregnancy, along with the unknowns of parenting multiple infants, present a need for specialized education (Bryan, 2002). The goal of patient education for women with high-risk pregnancies is to assist them in the improvement of their own health (Freda, 2000). Providing education about their condition and healthcare options allows women expecting multiples to make informed decisions concerning treatment. Simkin (2017) noted that shared decision making "requires education and discussion between caregiver and client"; this can be accomplished through appropriate childbirth education where parents can receive "information about birth, care options, and the confidence to offer their opinions or express their concerns" (Simkin, 2017, p. 2).

The increasing number of multiple gestations makes providing specialized multiple birth classes both feasible and practical. Such classes offer detailed information about the differences in multiple pregnancy and birth, educate about potential complications, enhance coping skills, teach parenting skills, and provide an immediate support system for expectant families with other parents of multiples (Bowers et al., 2006). Multiple birth class topics include physical and emotional changes, variations in labor and birth and postpartum care, and detailed education about nutrition. Common pregnancy complications, especially PTL, should also be included with a focus on awareness and actions. Parents will need advice in practical skills for coping with more than one newborn, breastfeeding multiples, and choosing appropriate layette and infant equipment (Bowers et al., 2006). A hospital tour should include the NICU, optimally allowing couples to meet neonatologists and nurses and seeing premature infants in intensive care (Kuhnly, Juliano, & McLarney, 2015). Because so many women with multiples are at risk for complications and potential bed rest, they should attend classes in their early second trimester, by 24 weeks' gestation (Leonard & Denton, 2006). Options include online materials, a mini-class to supplement standard childbirth classes offering tips and practical advice on handling multiple newborns, or a complete multiples-specific prenatal education curriculum (Kuhnly et al., 2015).

Nutrition and Weight Gain

Luke (2015, p. 587) described a multiple pregnancy as "a state of magnified nutritional requirements, resulting in a greater nutrient drain on maternal resources and an accelerated depletion of nutritional reserves." Evidence is growing that optimal maternal nutrition and weight gain are linked with positive perinatal outcomes for multiples, including reduced incidence of LBW and VLBW infants (Luke, 2015). The shortened length of gestation for most multiples limits the time for intrauterine growth, and the more rapid aging of multiple birth placentas shortens the period for effective transfer of nutrients to the developing fetuses.

Thus, higher weight gains during early gestation may influence the structural and functional development of the placenta and subsequently augment fetal growth through more effective placental function as well as the transfer of a higher level of nutrients (Luke, 2015). Four objectives for maternal nutrition in multiple gestations have been described: (1) optimizing fetal growth and development, (2) reducing incidence of obstetric complications, (3) increasing gestational age at delivery, and (4) avoiding excess maternal weight gain that may result in unnecessary weight retention postdelivery (Goodnight & Newman, 2009).

Women pregnant with multiples require additional calories, micronutrient supplementation, and a higher gestational weight gain than women with singletons (Brown & Carlson, 2000; Luke, 2005; Roem, 2003; Roselló-Soberón, Fuentes-Chaparro, & Casanueva, 2005). Maternal energy expenditures are increased as demonstrated by significantly higher resting basal metabolic rates in twin pregnancies compared to singletons ($1,636 \pm 174$ kcal/day and $1,456 \pm 158$ kcal/day, respectively; Shinagawa et al., 2005). The increased body mass in maternal breasts, uterus, body fat, and muscle, along with greater blood volume, can result in a 40% increase in caloric requirements for twin pregnancies (Goodnight & Newman, 2009). Bed rest has a negative effect on maternal weight gain (Maloni, 2010, 2011).

Official dietary standards for nutrient and energy intake for multiple gestations have not been established. The following proposed daily caloric intakes are based on a woman's prepregnant BMI: underweight, 4,000 kcal; normal BMI, 3,000 kcal; overweight, 3,250 kcal; obese, 2,700 to 3,000 kcal (Goodnight & Newman, 2009). One nutritional intervention program for twin and triplet pregnancies recommends a diet with 20% of calories from protein, 40% of calories from carbohydrates, and 40% of calories from fat to provide additional calories with less bulk (Luke, 2004, 2015). This diet emphasizes low glycemic index carbohydrates to prevent wide fluctuations in blood glucose concentrations. Compared to singleton pregnancies, multiple gestations have a faster depletion of glycogen stores and increased metabolism of fat between meals and overnight (Luke, 2005). Women should thus be counseled to eat frequent, small meals, which may also aid digestion as the rapidly growing uterus crowds the stomach. A diet rich in heme iron and animal protein and supplementation with calcium, magnesium, and zinc have also been recommended (Luke, 2015). A recent RCT found that doubling the dose of ferrous sulfate supplements (from 34 to 68 mg) in women with iron deficiency anemia increased serum hemoglobin and ferritin levels at 32 weeks' gestation through 6 weeks' postpartum without increasing gastrointestinal side effects (Shinar, Skornick-Rapaport, & Maslovitz, 2017).

Studies have shown that pregravid maternal weight, weight gain patterns, and total amounts of gain in multiple pregnancy are linked to fetal weight gain, length of gestation, and eventual infant birth weights (Brown & Carlson, 2000; Luke, 2005, 2015; Roselló-Soberón et al., 2005). Early maternal weight gain appears to have a stronger effect on infant birth weights than do mid-pregnancy and late-pregnancy gains for multiple gestations (Luke, 2015). Maternal nutrient stores deposited in early pregnancy are used in late pregnancy for placental growth. This is demonstrated in studies showing that poor early maternal weight gain is associated with inadequate intrauterine growth and increased perinatal morbidity in twins (Newman & Unal, 2017; Roselló-Soberón et al., 2005). A systematic review concluded that lower overall pregnancy weight gains were associated with lower infant birth weights and SGA compared with higher weight gains (Bodnar, Pugh, Abrams, Himes, & Hutcheon, 2014). Pregnancy weight gain was tracked in 1,109 twin pregnancies of normal weight, overweight, and obese women. Total gain was higher compared with singleton pregnancies, and the divergence in weight gain patterns between twin and singleton gestations began after 17 to 19 weeks. The differences were most pronounced in normal weight women and flattened as BMI increased (Hutcheon et al., 2018).

In 2009, the Institute of Medicine (IOM) established provisional guidelines for weight gain in twin pregnancy based on maternal pregravid BMI status. Women with a normal BMI should aim to gain 37 to 54 lb; overweight women, 31 to 50 lb; and obese women, 25 to 42 lb. No recommendations were made for underweight women with twins, but higher gains are prudent for these women (Rasmussen & Yaktine, 2009) (Table 11–3).

One study of nearly 300 women with twin pregnancies and normal starting BMIs found that pregnancy weight gain consistent with the IOM guidelines was significantly associated with improved outcomes, including a decreased risk of prematurity and higher birth weights (Fox et al., 2010). In a subsequent report, the researchers examined a cohort of women with twin pregnancies and normal starting BMIs who delivered at ≥37 weeks' gestation. Those who gained more than 54 lb had significantly larger newborns and a decreased rate of LBW compared to women with normal or poor weight gain. Despite their weight gain exceeding the IOM recommendations, these women did not have a higher incidence of gestational diabetes, gestational hypertension, or preeclampsia (Fox, Saltzman, Kurtz, & Rebarber, 2011). However, studies are conflicting as to whether adverse perinatal outcomes are associated with gaining more than the IOM guidelines and risks appear to differ among groups of women: underweight, normal weight, and overweight/obese (Lal & Kominiarek, 2015; Shamshirsaz et al., 2014). As with all pregnant women, high prepregnancy BMI increases risk for many maternal complications including diabetes and hypertension. A retrospective review of 741 women with twin pregnancy who delivered term infants of normal birth weight found that 43.2% had gestational weight gain within the IOM guidelines (Lutsiv et al., 2017). The researchers reported those who gained above the guidelines had higher odds of labor induction, while those who gained below the guidelines had a greater risk for SGA, LBW, and longer NICU stays.

Few studies have examined weight gain and nutritional recommendations for HOM pregnancies. A 50-lb total weight gain for triplet pregnancy, approximately 1.5 lb/week, has been suggested (Brown & Carlson, 2000). Others have recommended 58 to 75 lb for triplets and 70 to 80 lb for quadruplets (Luke, 2015). Available data indicate that the associations of maternal weight gain with fetal growth and infant birth weights are even more important for these pregnancies, since early pregnancy weight gain and higher total gain in underweight women with HOMs appear to have an even greater effect on outcomes (Luke, 2005). Eddib, Penvose-Yi, Shelton, and Yeh (2007) found that for triplets, higher maternal weight gain is associated with better neonatal outcomes, without an increase in adverse pregnancy outcomes, compared with singleton gestations.

Nutritional care interventions for multiple gestations have focused on targeted diet therapy, monitoring nutritional status and fetal growth, and intensified education and prenatal care (Luke, 2015). Nutrition counseling and weight gain advice is a simple, low-cost, and effective intervention for improving perinatal outcome in multiple gestations (Brown & Carlson, 2000). Surveys showed that more than one fourth of pregnant women, including those with twins, received no advice regarding weight gain, and among women who did receive guidance, more than one third received inappropriate advice (Luke, 2004). A consult with

TABLE 11–3. Institute of Medicine Weight Gain Guidelines for Twin Pregnancies

Prepregnancy BMI	BMI (kg/m²)	Total weight gain twins (lb)
Underweight	<18.5	No recommendation
Normal weight	18.5 to 24.9	37 to 54
Overweight	25.0 to 29.9	31 to 50
Obese	≥30.0	25 to 42

BMI, body mass index.
From Rasmussen, K. M., & Yaktine, A. L. (Eds.). (2009). *Weight gain during pregnancy: Reexamining the guidelines*. Washington, DC: National Academies Press

a registered dietitian specializing in perinatal nutrition is helpful for all expectant mothers of multiples, especially for those who are underweight for height, vegetarian (particularly vegans who consume no animal proteins), and pregnant with HOMs (Bowers et al., 2006; Goodnight & Newman, 2009; Newman & Unal, 2017).

Antepartum Fetal Surveillance

Due to the increased incidence of fetal morbidity and mortality in multiples, assessment of fetal well-being is often incorporated into routine antenatal care. However, there is no defined consensus on the timing or frequency of antenatal testing for multiple gestations. All women with multiple gestation should have first trimester ultrasound to establish chorionicity and a fetal anatomy assessment between 18 and 22 weeks' gestation (ACOG & SMFM, 2016). There are no clear recommendations for frequency of additional ultrasound examinations for DC twins, but surveillance every 4 to 6 weeks is reasonable (ACOG & SMFM, 2016). ACOG and SMFM (2016) also note that umbilical artery Doppler flow should not be routinely offered in uncomplicated twin pregnancies. Antepartum fetal surveillance every 2 weeks beginning at 16 weeks' gestation for MC gestations with signs of TTTS (abnormal growth, abnormal amniotic fluid volumes) should be considered (ACOG & SMFM, 2016). Nonstress testing and biophysical profile assessment can be used as indicated by maternal or obstetric conditions such as hypertension, pregestational diabetes or poorly controlled gestational diabetes, IUGR, or oligohydramnios. Biophysical profile is often preferred for HOMs because it is difficult to accurately record and interpret nonstress tests for more than two fetuses (Newman & Unal, 2017). For all surveillance techniques, fetal positions should be documented consistently beginning in early pregnancy. This allows comparisons with prior assessments and accurate clinical reporting. Fetal movement counting (kick counting) may be a useful adjunct with other antepartum fetal surveillance (AAP & ACOG, 2017). Emphasis should be placed on a woman's perception of a decrease in fetal activity relative to previous levels rather than on a precise number of movements. However, some women may have difficulty differentiating movement among fetuses (Display 11–2).

INTRAPARTUM MANAGEMENT

The high risks of twin and HOM pregnancies require birth in a facility that is capable of emergent cesarean birth and neonatal resuscitation. Antepartum transfer to a specialty or subspecialty level care facility ensures

DISPLAY 11–2
Suggested Plan for Fetal Surveillance of Multiples

- First trimester ultrasound for all women suspected or at risk for multiple gestation, for example, infertility therapies[a]
- First trimester ultrasound for fetal number and chorionicity[a]
- Nuchal translucency assessment between 10 and 13 weeks[a]
- Fetal anatomy assessment between 18 and 22 weeks' gestation[a]
- DC twins: ultrasound examinations every 4 to 6 weeks if no IUGR or complications[a]; weekly NST or BPP beginning at 34 weeks[b]
- MC twins with signs of TTTS: ultrasound every 2 weeks beginning at 16 weeks' gestation[a]; NST or BPP beginning at 32 weeks[b]
- NST or BPP as indicated by other maternal or obstetric conditions[a]
- HOMs: Initiate BPP at 28 weeks.[b]
- Fetal movement (kick counting)[a]
- Umbilical artery Doppler flow should not be routinely offered in uncomplicated twin pregnancies[a]

BPP, biophysical profile; DC, dichorionic; HOMs, high-order multiples; IUGR, intrauterine growth restriction; MC, monochorionic; NST, nonstress test; TTTS, twin-to-twin transfusion syndrome.
[a]From American College of Obstetricians and Gynecologists & Society for Maternal-Fetal Medicine. (2016). *Multifetal gestations: Twin, triplet, and higher-order multifetal pregnancies* (Practice Bulletin No. 169). Washington, DC: Author.
[b]From Newman, R. B., & Unal, E. R. (2017). Multiple gestation. In S. G. Gabbe, J. R. Niebyl, J. L. Simpson, M .B. Landon, H. L. Galan, E. R. M. Jauniaux, . . . W. A. Grobman (Eds.), *Obstetrics: Normal and problem pregnancies* (7th ed., pp. 706–736). Philadelphia, PA: Elsevier.

access to appropriate neonatal care (AAP & ACOG, 2017). This also assures that mother and babies stay together. Obstetric staffing guidelines for multiple gestations are for a 1:1 registered nurse-to-woman ratio (AAP & ACOG, 2017). Ideally, births prior to 34 to 35 weeks' gestation occur in a facility with a level III NICU. All multiple gestations, including twins, are considered absolute contraindications to planned home birth (AAP & ACOG, 2017). Despite some proponents of home birth for multiples, this alternative lacks the obstetric, anesthetic, and surgical care needed for emergency interventions.

On admission, ultrasound should be used to confirm viability, placental location, and fetal presentation. Although there is excellent correlation between fetal presentations at 32 to 36 gestational weeks and those at birth, some twins undergo spontaneous version in the third trimester. Cephalic-presenting twins at 28 weeks tend to be stable, but non–vertex-presenting twins are more likely to spontaneously convert to a vertex presentation before birth (Chasen, Spiro, Kalish, & Chervenak, 2005).

Expectant parents' birth plans and desires should be respected as much as possible, acknowledging the unique aspects of the birth for these families. The mother and support persons should be given anticipatory guidance for all labor and birth procedures. Many are surprised at the large perinatal team that typically attends the birth of multiples. For a preterm cesarean birth of twins, it is not uncommon for as many as 15 people to be present: 2 obstetricians, 2 to 3 labor and delivery nurses, 1 or 2 neonatologists, a NICU team for each infant, 1 or 2 anesthesia staff, and the parents (Bowers et al., 2006). Essential personnel for intrapartum management of multiple births include experienced obstetricians, nurses, anesthesiologists, operating room technicians, and neonatal staff. Women may labor in labor rooms or labor/delivery/recovery rooms, but vaginal births should be performed in a surgical suite with a double setup in case of emergent cesarean birth (Newman & Unal, 2017). The increased risk for cesarean birth of multiples warrants interventions such as withholding oral liquids and solid food (AAP & ACOG, 2017) as well as evaluating the woman's airway and providing an antacid in case of gastric aspiration. Neuraxial analgesia, such as an epidural, should be used to enable conversion of a vaginal birth to cesarean and allow obstetric interventions to be performed rapidly, including operative vaginal birth, external or internal cephalic version, and total breech extraction (ACOG & SMFM, 2016).

Timing of Birth

Since fetal and neonatal morbidity and mortality increase after 37 weeks in twin gestations and after 35 weeks in triplet pregnancies (Kahn et al., 2003), there are recommendations for elective early delivery of multiples. Two randomized trials found that in women with uncomplicated twin pregnancies, elective delivery at 37 weeks' gestation does not appear to increase risk for perinatal or neonatal harm (Dodd, Deussen, Grivell, & Crowther, 2014). A subsequent meta-analysis reported that the risks of cesarean delivery for uncomplicated twin gestation is similar for planned delivery at 37 weeks versus expectant management up to 38 weeks or more (Saccone & Berghella, 2016). The report also concluded that planned delivery at 37 weeks had a significantly lower risk (61%) of serious adverse infant outcomes for these twins. Triplets were not included in these trials. Recommendations for timing of elective delivery of twins are in Display 11–3.

Fetal pulmonary maturity assessment by amniocentesis is not recommended if delivery is medically indicated (ACOG, 2013). If amniocentesis is needed to direct clinical management, both sacs should be

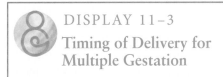

DISPLAY 11–3
Timing of Delivery for Multiple Gestation

Condition at or after 34 Weeks' Gestation

Delivery Timing for Dichorionic (DC) Twins

Uncomplicated DCDA	38 0/7 to 38 6/7 weeks
DCDA with isolated fetal growth restriction	36 0/7 to 37 6/7 weeks
DCDA with fetal growth restriction and coexisting condition (fetal or maternal)	32 0/7 to 34 6/7 weeks

Delivery Timing for Monochorionic (MC) Twins

Uncomplicated MCDA twins	34 0/7 to 37 6/7 weeks
MCDA twins with isolated fetal growth restriction	32 0/7 to 34 6/7 weeks
Uncomplicated MCMA	32 0/7 to 34 0/7 weeks
MC with single fetal death	If death ≥34 weeks, immediate delivery is not of benefit. If death <34 weeks, delivery is based on condition of mother or surviving fetus.

DCDA, dichorionic/diamniotic; MCDA, monochorionic/diamniotic; MCMA, monochorionic/monoamniotic.
Adapted from American College of Obstetricians and Gynecologists & Society for Maternal-Fetal Medicine. (2016). *Multifetal gestations: Twin, triplet, and higher-order multifetal pregnancies* (Practice Bulletin No. 169), Washington, DC: Author; American Academy of Pediatrics & American College of Obstetricians and Gynecologists. (2017). *Guidelines for perinatal care* (8th ed.). Elk Grove Village, IL: American Academy of Pediatrics; and American College of Obstetricians and Gynecologists. (2013). *Medically indicated late-preterm and early-term deliveries* (Committee Opinion No. 560). Washington, DC: Author.

tapped due to inconsistent lecithin/sphingomyelin levels between twins (Cleary-Goldman et al., 2007; Malone & D'Alton, 2014).

Labor with Multiples

Labor in multiple gestations appears to progress differently from that of singletons. Most data are from twin labors, with limited information from triplets. Early studies evaluated cervical dilation on admission and found significant differences between twins and singletons (Friedman & Sachtleben, 1964). However, preterm contractions can lead to advanced cervical dilation long before a woman enters active labor. Later reports evaluated the length of labor from the onset of the active phase at 4 or 5 cm. One study of 1,821 twin births in a single institution found cervical effacements and vertex stations on admission were similar for twins and matched singleton controls (Schiff et al., 1998). Interestingly, women with twins had less cervical dilation on admission. In this study, the time for cervical progression from 4 to 10 cm was less in nulliparous women with twins (3.2 ± 1.3 hours) than those with singletons (4.7 ± 2.6 hours; $p < .001$), but there were no differences for multiparous women. No significant differences in the mean length of the second stage of labor were observed for twins (0.8 hours) and singletons (0.7 hours). Silver et al. (2000) reported similar findings and included triplets in their analysis (32 triplets, 64 twins, and 64 singletons; all at approximately 34 weeks' gestation). The mean rate of cervical dilation in hours from 5 cm to complete was 1.8 ± 1.2 for triplets, 1.7 ± 1.3 for twins, and 2.3 ± 1.5 for singletons ($p < .05$). Factors affecting labor progress may include fetal weights, presentations, and use of epidural anesthesia.

Fetal Monitoring

All women with high-risk conditions such as multiples should have continuous FHR monitoring during labor (Newman & Unal, 2017). Dual-channel electronic fetal monitors allow simultaneous heart rate recordings, eliminating the need to synchronize several monitors for tracing comparisons. Monitors may display each FHR in a different color and/or by printing one in a bold line and the other in a faint line. Each FHR should be clearly labeled to indicate the corresponding ultrasound transducer and fetus that is being monitored. For example, the nurse should monitor one fetus long enough to get a tracing and then identify on the tracing (either electronically or directly on the paper version) and nurses' notes, "Bold line = fetus in LLQ or A" (Bowers et al., 2006). Ultrasound may be helpful in locating fetal hearts for transducer placement. A fetal scalp electrode should be applied to the presenting fetus in early labor if membranes are already ruptured (Cleary-Goldman et al., 2007; Rao, Sairam, & Shehata, 2004).

Eganhouse and Petersen (1998) explained the phenomenon of fetal synchrony in multiples. This is a similarity in frequency and timing of FHR accelerations, baseline oscillations, and periodic changes with contractions that occur in healthy twins more than 50% of the time. Some electronic monitors address synchrony with discrimination technology that uses printing of signal marks on the tracing, separate monitoring scales, or artificial separation of single-scale tracings into two separate tracings (Bowers et al., 2006). However, these system cues do not replace careful nursing assessment of each FHR pattern (Simpson, 2004). Bakker, Colenbrander, Verstraeten, and Van Geijn (2004) reported a higher incidence of signal loss in twins compared to singletons and cited abnormal twin positions, polyhydramnios, and twin–twin interactions as factors contributing to signal loss. Caution is also needed to ensure that maternal heart rate is not mistakenly recorded as the second twin (Hanson, 2010).

Clinicians must be familiar with principles of monitoring preterm fetuses because many multiples present in labor before 37 weeks' gestation. Preterm fetuses typically have baseline FHR in the upper range of normal (150 to 160 beats per minute), and accelerations are shorter in duration and of lower amplitude than in more mature fetuses (Eganhouse & Petersen, 1998). Nonreassuring FHR patterns, including decelerations, bradycardia, tachycardia, and minimal to absent variability may occur in up to 60% of preterm fetuses, and variable decelerations are more common among preterm than term births (ACOG, 2009). Use of betamethasone for fetal lung maturation may temporarily decrease FHR variability in twins as well as decrease the rate of accelerations (ACOG, 2009). However, published data are limited to monitoring preterm twins during antepartum testing, so these conditions and FHR patterns may or may not be applicable to intrapartum monitoring (Simpson, 2004). A full discussion of fetal assessment during labor including specific details regarding monitoring the preterm fetus is presented in Chapter 15.

Labor Induction and Augmentation

There are limited data pertaining to the safety and efficacy of labor induction methods, including prostaglandins, mechanical dilators, and medications to stimulate uterine contractions in twin pregnancies (Healy & Gaddipati, 2005). However, prostaglandin for cervical ripening and labor induction and augmentation with oxytocin appear to be appropriate for twin pregnancies (Malone & D'Alton, 2014). Oxytocin is often used for uterine inertia following the birth of the first twin (Rao et al., 2004).

Mode of Birth

There are three routes for twin birth: vaginal delivery for both, cesarean delivery for both, or a combined vaginal/cesarean birth. The choice varies with fetal presentations, estimated fetal weights, and maternal and fetal health as well as clinician experience and preferences of mother and clinician. Perinatal outcomes for vaginal and cesarean births also vary depending on gestational age and birth weight as well as fetal presentation. Generally, operative vaginal births and cesarean delivery during labor are associated with worse outcomes (Hartley & Hitti, 2017).

ACOG and SMFM (2016) has made recommendations for route of delivery, noting that "a twin gestation in and of itself is not an indication for cesarean delivery" (p. 8). Recommended delivery routes are noted in Display 11–4.

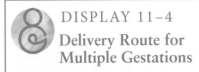

DISPLAY 11–4
Delivery Route for Multiple Gestations

Optimal Route Depends on Type of Twins, Fetal Presentations, Gestational Age, and Clinician Experience

Fetal Characteristics	Delivery Recommendation
MCMA	Cesarean delivery due to cord risk with vaginal route
DCDA and MCDA 32 0/7+ weeks with vertex-presenting fetus	Consider vaginal delivery if obstetrician experienced in internal podalic version and vaginal breech delivery.
Twin A non-vertex-presenting fetus	Cesarean delivery
Uncomplicated triplets with vertex-presenting fetus	Consider planned vaginal delivery if obstetrician is experienced in vaginal delivery of multiples.
Non–vertex-presenting triplet	Cesarean delivery
One previous low transverse cesarean delivery	Candidate for trial of labor

DCDA, dichorionic/diamniotic; MCDA, monochorionic/diamniotic; MCMA, monochorionic/monoamniotic.
Adapted from American College of Obstetricians and Gynecologists & Society for Maternal-Fetal Medicine. (2016). *Multifetal gestations: Twin, triplet, and higher-order multifetal pregnancies* (Practice Bulletin No. 16). Washington, DC: Author; American Academy of Pediatrics & American College of Obstetricians and Gynecologists. (2017). *Guidelines for perinatal care* (8th ed.). Elk Grove Village, IL: American Academy of Pediatrics; Malone, F. D., & D'Alton, M. E. (2014). Multiple gestation: Clinical characteristics and management. In A. H. Jobe & B. D. Kamath-Rayne (Eds.), *Creasy and Resnik's maternal-fetal medicine: Principles and practice.* (7th ed., pp. 578–596). Philadelphia, PA: Elsevier; and Newman, R. B., & Unal, E. R. (2017). Multiple gestation. In S. G. Gabbe, J. R. Niebyl, J. L. Simpson, M .B. Landon, H. L. Galan, E. R. M. Jauniaux, . . . W. A. Grobman (Eds.), *Obstetrics: Normal and problem pregnancies* (7th ed., pp. 706–736). Philadelphia, PA: Elsevier.

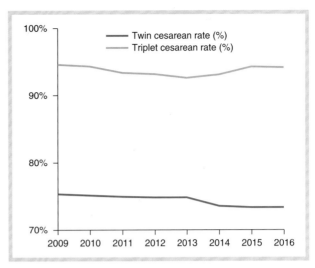

FIGURE 11–9. Cesarean delivery rates per infant for twins and triplets, 2009 to 2016. (Data from U.S. Department of Health and Human Services, National Center for Health Statistics.)

A population-based study found higher rates of cesarean in older mothers and earlier gestational ages and an increasing number of breech-presenting twins (29.1% in 2013) as well as increased rates of cesarean delivery associated with gestational diabetes, gestational hypertension, previous cesarean delivery, and breech presentation. The greatest reduction of risk of cesarean was associated with labor induction (Bateni et al., 2016). The rates of cesarean delivery for twins and triplets in the United States from 2009 to 2016 are shown in Figure 11–9, revealing a slight decline in twin cesarean delivery rates (75.34% to 73.27%), while triplet cesarean rates increased slightly (92.6% to 94.14%) after 2013 (CDC, 2019a).

Twin A Vertex/Twin B Vertex

Approximately 43% to 45% of twins present vertex–vertex, and the ACOG and SMFM (2016) recommendation is for vaginal birth in an otherwise uncomplicated case after 32 0/7 weeks' gestation. An RCT found that a planned cesarean delivery with twin A presenting vertex did not significantly increase or lower the risk of fetal or neonatal death or serious neonatal morbidity compared with planned vaginal delivery (Barrett et al., 2013). Predelivery counseling should include that the presentation of the second twin may change in 5% to 10% of cases (Newman & Unal, 2017).

Twin A Vertex/Twin B Nonvertex

Approximately 34% to 38% of twins present vertex–nonvertex (Cleary-Goldman et al., 2007; Robinson & Chauhan, 2004) and are candidates for vaginal delivery with active management. Attending clinicians must be skilled in performing assisted breech delivery, internal podalic version, and total breech extraction (ACOG & SMFM, 2016). Cesarean delivery may be indicated if twin B is significantly larger than twin A. Following vaginal delivery of twin A, options for twin B include external cephalic version or breech delivery. A change in presentation can occur in up to 20% of vertex-presenting second twins following vaginal birth of twin A (Hofmeyr, Barrett, & Crowther, 2015). Cord prolapse and placental abruption are risks for emergent cesarean of twin B in this scenario. Women who had experienced labor and had a combined delivery (vaginal birth of twin A and cesarean birth of twin B) had an increased risk for maternal endometritis and neonatal sepsis over laboring women who had cesarean delivery for both infants (Alexander et al., 2008).

Twin A Nonvertex

The first twin presents nonvertex in approximately 19% to 21% of cases (Cleary-Goldman, 2007; Robinson & Chauhan, 2004). Although rare, the primary risk is interlocking of the heads of breech–vertex twins during a vaginal birth and cesarean delivery is generally recommended for this presentation (Newman & Unal, 2017).

Triplet Birth

While nearly all triplets (94.14%) and other HOMs (94.01%; quadruplets) are delivered by cesarean (CDC, 2019a), the optimal route is not known and vaginal birth may be an option for select triplet pregnancies in the hands of experienced obstetricians (AAP & ACOG, 2017). Some prospective studies using a standardized protocol have reported improved or similar Apgar scores, cord pH, and length of maternal and neonatal stays compared with cesarean births (Ramsey & Repke, 2003). In addition to standard considerations for a safe birth of multiples, suggested criteria for vaginal birth of triplets include gestational age ≥28 weeks, the presenting triplet is vertex, fetal monitoring for all fetuses, no obstetric contraindications, and informed consent (Ramsey & Repke, 2003). Others have set criteria as viable gestational age, estimated fetal weights >1,800 g, and the first two triplets both presenting cephalic (Newman & Unal, 2017).

However, triplet vaginal delivery is not without consequence. A review of data from the Consortium on Safe Labor reported that of the 80 sets of triplets delivering at ≥28 weeks, 30% (24 sets) had vaginal births (Lappen, Hackney, & Bailit, 2016). The researchers found a statistically higher rate of maternal transfusion (20.8% vs. 3.6%, $p = .01$) and greater risk of neonatal mechanical ventilation in those with attempted vaginal delivery. An earlier study showed increased rates of stillbirth and neonatal and infant death associated with vaginal delivery of triplets (Vintzileos, Ananth, Kontopoulos, & Smulian, 2005). There was no association between birth order and mortality rates, except that the stillbirth rate was increased for the third fetus, regardless of the mode of birth. Cesarean delivery is often recommended as the optimal route for all HOMs (Malone & D'Alton, 2014; Newman & Unal, 2017).

Interdelivery Interval

After birth of the first infant, ultrasound should be used to assess presentation of the second twin and to exclude a funic presentation (cord between the fetal vertex and the internal cervical os; Malone & D'Alton, 2014). Membrane rupture of the second twin should be delayed until contractions are reestablished and the presenting part is engaged in the pelvis to minimize the risk of cord prolapse (Rao et al., 2004). Once the presenting part of the next fetus is accessible and membranes are ruptured, a scalp electrode may be applied. No clear guidelines are established for the interdelivery interval between births of twins, particularly when continuous electronic fetal monitoring is used. However, with increasing time, risks increase in the second twin for complications such as cord prolapse, abruption, and malpresentation (Healy & Gaddipati, 2005). The risk for asphyxia-related mortality increases if the birth interval between twins is greater than 30 minutes (Dodd & Crowther, 2005). Umbilical cord arterial and venous pH of the second twin has been found to decline in a continuous linear fashion with increasing intertwin birth interval time (McGrail & Bryant, 2005). Lengthy interdelivery intervals also increase the chances of a fully dilated cervix to contract down, limiting birth options for the second fetus (Malone & D'Alton, 2014). It has been suggested that with normal fetal status, progressive descent, and stable maternal condition, an interval beyond 30 minutes may be reasonable with judicious oxytocin use (Healy & Gaddipati, 2005). Continuous fetal monitoring of the remaining fetus(es) is essential in the interdelivery interval. In all vaginal delivery scenarios, clinicians should be alert for changes in fetal presentation and maternal and fetal well-being and be ready for emergent cesarean delivery. Combined vaginal–cesarean delivery has been reported in 2.2% to 17% of twin vaginal births (Aviram et al., 2015).

Delayed Interval Birth

Delayed interval birth, or asynchronous birth, occurs when one or more very preterm multiples are vaginally delivered, and births of the remaining fetus(es) are delayed in hopes of improving neonatal survival and decreasing neonatal morbidity. Lengthy interdelivery time intervals (up to 153 days) have been reported in the literature, with a median ranging from 6 to 31 days (Cristinelli, Fresson, André, & Monnier-Barbarino, 2005; Zhang, Hamilton, Martin, & Trumble, 2004). Perinatal outcomes appear to be improved for second twins whose delivery is delayed when the first co-twin is delivered between 20 and 29 weeks' gestation (Arabin & van Eyck, 2009). The optimal clinical management of delayed interval births is unknown. Fetal pathology, monochorionicity, placenta previa, placental abruption, and preeclampsia have been cited as contraindications (Cristinelli et al., 2005). Clinical reports include use of aggressive tocolysis, cervical cerclage, corticosteroids, and prophylactic and therapeutic antibiotics (Arabin & van Eyck, 2009; Oyelese, Ananth, Smulian, & Vintzileos, 2005; Zhang et al., 2004). Although there appear to be benefits for the remaining fetuses, this practice bears substantial risk. Maternal complications frequently associated with delayed interval birth include chorioamnionitis, postpartum hemorrhage, retained placenta, and abruption and neonatal risks of sepsis, anemia, or neurologic development disorders (Benito Vielba et al., 2019). Based on the limited reports on the topic (no RCTs to date), delayed interval delivery may be a reasonable option to preserve the pregnancy and delay delivery for a healthy remaining fetus of a multiple pregnancy (Reinhard et al., 2012; Roman et al., 2011).

Vaginal Birth after Cesarean

A small percentage of twins are delivered by vaginal birth after cesarean (VBAC) (<4%; Bateni et al., 2016). In one study, VBAC was successful in 64.5% of women, but nearly half of those who had a failed trial of labor had a vaginal delivery for twin A and cesarean for twin B. Maternal morbidities were no more likely than with singleton births and fetal and neonatal complications were uncommon in either group at ≤34 weeks' gestation. For women with one prior cesarean birth with a low transverse uterine incision and who meet general criteria for twin vaginal delivery, a trial of labor may be considered (ACOG & SMFM, 2016).

Anesthesia

The choice of anesthesia depends on the potential need for uterine manipulation, operative birth, version of the second twin, emergent cesarean birth, and the increased risks for uterine atony and postpartum hemorrhage (ACOG & SMFM, 2016; Dodd & Crowther, 2005; Ramsey & Repke, 2003). Neuraxial anesthesia is commonly used for vaginal and cesarean births of twins. Both epidural and spinal anesthesia are safely used for triplet cesarean births, but spinal anesthesia has been associated with a larger initial decrease in systolic blood pressure in these pregnancies (Marino, Goudas, Steinbok, Craigo, & Yarnell, 2001). Sublingual or intravenous nitroglycerin may be used for acute uterine relaxation for situations such as head entrapment of the second breech twin or retained placenta (Ramsey & Repke, 2003).

Although nonmedicated vaginal births of twins are uncommon, the woman's preferences must be balanced with potential risks and need for interventions. For example, an option for a woman desiring a nonmedicated birth is to have an epidural catheter placed but not have medication infused through the catheter (Bowers et al., 2006).

Infant Care at Birth

While multiple birth infants might benefit from delayed umbilical cord clamping after birth, there is not enough information to make a clinical recommendation about this procedure for multiples (ACOG, 2017a). Many of the indications for immediate cord clamping or individualized use of the procedure are more common in multiple gestations, including maternal hemorrhage and/or hemodynamic instability, placental abruption or previa, and fetal/neonatal risks including IUGR with abnormal cord Doppler evaluation, cord avulsion, or need for immediate resuscitation; MC gestations are especially at risk (ACOG, 2017a).

Regardless of birth order, each infant should be identified at birth using the system established during antenatal care (fetus A, B, C, etc.) with notation in the medical record of any discrepancies. If this is not possible, fetal identifiers must be correlated with each infant. Likewise, umbilical cords should be identified, such as placing the number of clamps corresponding to the infant's label. Cord blood samples should also be labeled with the correct infant identifier (AAP & ACOG, 2017). Supportive care in the delivery room includes communication with the mother about her infants' health and, when possible, implementing measures such as early skin-to-skin contact.

POSTPARTUM CARE

Hemorrhage

In addition to the larger surface area of an MC twin placenta or two or more placentas, women with multiple gestations often have other risk factors for hemorrhage. These include an overdistended uterus, operative delivery, placental abnormalities, hypertensive disorders, and coagulopathies (ACOG, 2017b; Kramer et al., 2013). Blood loss with twin vaginal births is approximately 1,000 mL; blood loss with triplet cesarean birth is typically much greater than 1,000 mL due to increased risk of uterine atony (Klein, 2002). Blood loss >500 mL in a vaginal delivery warrants investigation (ACOG, 2017b). The relative risk of primary postpartum hemorrhage is 3.4 times higher in twins than in singleton gestations (Campbell & Templeton, 2004). Mothers of multiples were 1.66 times more likely to need blood transfusion than mothers of singletons (Walker, Murphy, Pan, Yang, & Wen, 2004) and the risk of maternal death from hemorrhage is 4 times higher (MacKay, Berg, King, Duran, & Chang, 2006). The risk for placenta accreta and other forms of adherent placenta (increta and percreta) should be considered in any woman who had a previous cesarean delivery due to the risk of uterine rupture and hemorrhage (ACOG, 2012).

Uncontrollable hemorrhage may lead to hysterectomy. A historical review of 100 peripartum hysterectomies performed in one clinical center found a significant increase in risk for twin (0.44%) and HOM (3.48%) gestations compared with singleton pregnancies (0.15%) (Francois, Ortiz, Harris, Foley, & Elliott, 2005). Others have found similar rates (Walker et al., 2004). In the review by Francois et al. (2005), all the hysterectomies in multiple gestations were performed emergently, and all but one were for uterine atony. Hemorrhage prevention includes anticipation of risk, recognition of uterine atony, and use of uterotonic agents in the third stage of labor (AAP & ACOG, 2017; ACOG, 2017c). A comprehensive discussion of risks, prevention, and treatment of postpartum hemorrhage is presented in Chapter 17. Display 11–5 provides recommendations for labor and birth of multiples.

Maternal Recovery

Multiple pregnancy and birth increase stresses on a woman's body, and these are intensified by antepartum, intrapartum, and postpartum complications (Gromada & Bowers, 2005). Having an infant in the NICU or caretaking responsibilities for multiple infants at home can also increase physical and emotional stress. Women who have had extended antepartum bed rest may have difficulty recuperating after birth. A study of 31 women with twins and triplets who had been hospitalized during pregnancy reported a higher mean number and longer duration of postpartum symptoms than women with singleton pregnancies (Maloni, Margevicius, & Damato, 2006). Although many symptoms decreased over the days and weeks after birth, a high percentage persisted at 6 weeks' postpartum, including back muscle soreness, dry skin, fatigue, tenseness, mood changes, and difficulty concentrating. Muscle atrophy also occurs following bed rest, particularly in the weight-bearing muscles of the legs and back (Maloni & Schneider, 2002). These continuing symptoms increase the difficulty for these mothers as they remobilize after birth to care for themselves and their infants. Women need anticipatory guidance that their recovery will be slower than expected. They may also benefit from a physical therapy assessment and rehabilitation plan for their physical limitations due to bed rest–induced muscle atrophy and cardiovascular deconditioning.

MULTIPLE BIRTH INFANTS

Infant Morbidity and Mortality

As in singleton infants, preterm birth and LBW are predictors of infant morbidity and mortality, but the rates are much higher in twins and HOMs (Martin et al., 2018) (Figs. 11–10 and 11–11). Even twins have higher risks of maternal morbidity and mortality and a 10-fold

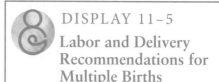

DISPLAY 11–5

Labor and Delivery Recommendations for Multiple Births

- Hospital birth (minimum level I care for term twin gestation) with a level II or III NICU
- Antenatal maternal transport if appropriate maternal or neonatal services are not available
- Two experienced obstetricians or an obstetrician and an obstetrician/gynecologist hospitalist or a certified nurse midwife trained as a surgical first assistant
- Obstetric nurses to circulate and assist and provide support to the woman: 1:1 ratio intrapartum
- Anesthesiologist and assistant to provide neuraxial and general anesthesia
- Neonatal team with nurses and respiratory care personnel sufficient for all infants—pediatricians/neonatologists available if fetal problems occur or birth is preterm or operative
- Delivery in room large enough to accommodate personnel and equipment
- Cesarean birth access immediately available
- Neonatal resuscitation beds available with adequate oxygen, suction, compressed air, and electrical outlets for simultaneous resuscitations of at least twins
- Neonatal transport protocol in place
- Operative delivery equipment immediately available
- Qualified ultrasonographer present with real-time ultrasound
- Continuous electronic fetal monitoring of all fetuses; scalp electrode on each presenting fetus, when possible
- Large-bore (16- to 18-gauge) intravenous access
- Oxytocin infusion, premixed
- Agents for uterine relaxation
- Typed and cross-matched blood/blood products immediately available
- Agents and equipment/supplies for hemorrhage management available (including uterine tamponade balloon)
- Ability to perform emergency uterine artery ligation, embolization, or hysterectomy for uncontrolled hemorrhage
- Cord blood samples for blood gas analysis obtained routinely
- All placentas sent for pathologic examination

NICU, neonatal intensive care unit.
Adapted from American Academy of Pediatrics & American College of Obstetricians and Gynecologists. (2017). *Guidelines for perinatal care* (8th ed.). Elk Grove Village, IL: American Academy of Pediatrics; American College of Obstetricians and Gynecologists & Society for Maternal-Fetal Medicine. (2016). *Multifetal gestations: Twin, triplet, and higher-order multifetal pregnancies* (Practice Bulletin No. 169). Washington, DC: Author; Malone, F. D., & D'Alton, M. E. (2014). Multiple gestation: Clinical characteristics and management. In A. H. Jobe & B. D. Kamath-Rayne (Eds.), *Creasy and Resnik's maternal-fetal medicine: Principles and practice.* (7th ed., pp. 578–596). Philadelphia, PA: Elsevier; Newman, R. B., & Unal, E. R. (2017). Multiple gestation. In S. G. Gabbe, J. R. Niebyl, J. L. Simpson, M .B. Landon, H. L. Galan, E. R. M. Jauniaux, . . . W. A. Grobman (Eds.), *Obstetrics: Normal and problem pregnancies* (7th ed., pp. 706–736). Philadelphia, PA: Elsevier.

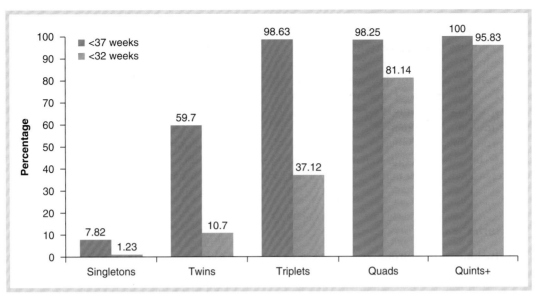

FIGURE 11–10. Preterm and early preterm births by plurality: United States, 2017. (Source: Martin, J. A., Hamilton, B. E., Osterman, M. J. K., Driscoll, A. K., & Drake P. [2018]. Births: Final data for 2017. *National Vital Statistics Reports, 67*[8], 1–50.)

greater risk for preterm birth (<37 weeks' gestation) and (LBW—less than 2,500 g) compared with singletons (Luke, 2017; Santana et al., 2016) (see Figs. 11–10 and 11–11). Compared with only 1% of singletons, 9.4% of twins, 36.7% of triplets, and 67.9% of quadruplets were born VLBW (less than 1,500 g) in 2017 (Martin et al., 2018).

According to national data for 2013, multiples accounted for 3.5% of all live births but 15% of all infant deaths in the United States (Mathews, MacDorman, & Thoma, 2015). The infant mortality rate (IMR) for twins was 24.37/1,000, more than 5 times the rate for singletons (5.25/1,000). The rate increased with plurality; the IMR for triplets was 61.08/1,000 and 137.04/1,000 for quadruplets, more than 12 times and 26 times higher, respectively, than the rate for singleton births. Like singletons, risks for neonatal death and infant morbidity decrease after 28 weeks' gestation. A small percentage (2.5%) of twins are born at periviable gestations (20 to 25 weeks). While there has been improvement in twin neonatal survival rates at 23 and 24 weeks' gestation, neonatal morbidity has increased for these infants, particularly at 23 weeks (Ananth & Chauhan, 2017).

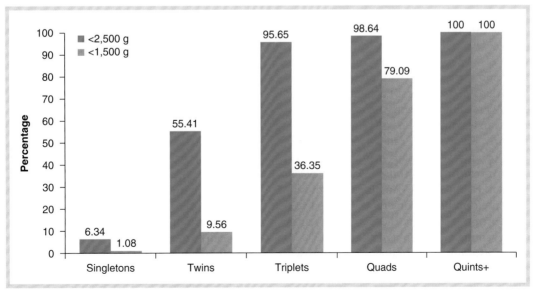

FIGURE 11–11. Low and very low birth weights by plurality: United States, 2017. (Source: Martin, J. A., Hamilton, B. E., Osterman, M. J. K., Driscoll, A. K., & Drake P. [2018]. Births: Final data for 2017. *National Vital Statistics Reports, 67*[8], 1–50.)

IMRs also differ by race. Black infants have the highest IMR for all pluralities compared to whites and Hispanics (Salihu et al., 2005). Hispanic singletons and twins have slightly improved survival over whites, but infant mortality for Hispanic triplets is 20% higher. The association of maternal age with infant mortality in multiple births is a paradox. In singletons, infant mortality is higher at the extremes of maternal age, producing a U-shaped curve, but in multiples, IMRs are highest at young maternal ages but continue to decrease with rising maternal age (Luke & Brown, 2007).

Long-term Morbidities

Not surprisingly, long-term morbidity in twins is inversely related to gestational age; birth at earlier gestational ages was significantly associated with neonatal death and major adverse outcomes (Stern et al., 2018). However, multiple birth infants are more likely than singletons to suffer long-term serious morbidities, including CP, severe learning disabilities, behavioral difficulties, and chronic respiratory disease (Pharoah, 2002; Rand, Eddleman, & Stone, 2005). Although early studies showed lower cognitive abilities of twins compared to singletons, when matched for birth weight and gestation, cognitive abilities of twins are not different (Ingram Cooke, 2010).

The prevalence of CP has been reported as 0.9% in twins, 3.1% in triplets, and 11.1 in quadruplets (Yokoyama, Shimizu, & Hayakawa, 1995). It is thought that multiple birth may be an independent risk factor for CP but is difficult to separate other CP associations that are common in multiple births, including preterm birth, IUGR, and bleeding during pregnancy (O'Callaghan et al., 2011; Wadhawan et al., 2011). The following factors have been associated with increased risk for poor neuromotor outcome among twins: chorionicity (MC > DC), fetal or infant death of one multiple, presence of TTTS, male/female pairs, discordant birth weights, and use of ART (with preterm and multiple births) (Briana & Malamitsi-Puchner, 2019; Rand et al., 2005). A French multicenter prospective cohort study found a single complete course of antenatal steroids significantly reduced the rate of periventricular leukomalacia or intraventricular hemorrhage (IVH) grade III/IV in preterm twins (born 24 to 31 weeks' gestation) (Palas et al., 2018). Antenatal magnesium sulfate before preterm birth (sometimes referred to as magnesium neuroprotection) is the only intervention effective in preventing CP (Shepherd et al., 2017).

Others have examined morbidities associated with poor long-term outcomes in premature infants, including necrotizing enterocolitis (NEC), severe retinopathy of prematurity (ROP), severe IVH, and the need for ventilator use and respiratory support at 28 days of age but found no differences in these morbidities at any gestational age among singletons, twins, and triplets (Blickstein, Shinwell, Lusky, & Reichman, 2005). A complete course of antenatal corticosteroids decreased the risk of short-term respiratory morbidity and neonatal death in twins but did not reduce the risk of bronchopulmonary dysplasia, severe ROP, or NEC (Melamed et al., 2016).

Deformational plagiocephaly (asymmetrically shaped head) has been found to occur more frequently in newborn twins than in singletons (56% vs. 13%; Peitsch, Keefer, LaBrie, & Mulliken, 2002). In utero positioning may be the initial cause of plagiocephaly, with preferential sleep positions worsening the condition. Vertex-presenting first twins, identical twins, and the smaller of a twin pair appear to have more severe involvement (Langkamp & Girardet, 2006). Parent education should include alternating the placement of the infant's head at opposite ends of the crib each night and increasing tummy time when infants are awake and actively observed.

Newborn Hospital Care

Newborn in-hospital care of healthy full-term multiples is similar to the care of singletons. However, meticulous care should be taken to maintain the exact identities of each baby, especially when the babies are MZ, such as double-checking of identification bracelets and crib cards (Gromada & Bowers, 2005).

A sizable proportion of multiple birth infants can be classified as late preterm infants and, like singletons, have increased risks for neonatal mortality and morbidity in the newborn period. Nurses should be alert to the subtle signs of difficulty, including temperature instability, hypoglycemia, need for intravenous infusions, respiratory distress, apnea and bradycardia, symptoms prompting a sepsis evaluation, and clinical jaundice (Medoff-Cooper, Bakewell-Sachs, Buus-Frank, & Santa-Donato, 2005). Additional nursing time, attention, and special skills may be needed to help mothers with breastfeeding, because late preterm infants may have a weak and ineffective suck, resulting in delays in latching on at the breast, establishing successful nutritive breastfeeding, or achieving adequate oral intake from either the breast or bottle (Medoff-Cooper et al., 2005).

Rooming-in with newborn multiples is optimal, if a support person is with the new mother in her hospital room. Because some mothers may not be physically ready or will be overwhelmed with all the infants at once, having only one infant in the room at a time may be helpful at first. However, a mother should be encouraged to assume care for all healthy infants together as soon as she is able before discharge (Gromada & Bowers, 2005).

Developmentally Supportive Care for Multiples

Developmentally supportive care begins at birth, even with a cesarean delivery, with a mother holding two healthy babies skin-to-skin at the same time. With maternal complications, infants can be held skin-to-skin by the other parent or a designated person (Tumblin, 2013). Clinicians are encouraged to recognize the unique needs of multiples and avoid practices to "separate preterm twins and multiples at birth, nest them alone in separate incubators and disconnect them from any familiarity of their own intrauterine experience" (Jarvis & Burnett, 2009, p. 3).

Developmentally supportive care strategies for multiples include simultaneous breastfeeding, shared kangaroo care, and cobedding in the NICU. Simultaneous breastfeeding or breast contact encourages mother–infant attachment and interaction between multiples (Jarvis & Burnett, 2009). It may also enhance effective infant feeding and promote milk production for the mother. Shared kangaroo care, when parents hold their multiple birth infants skin-to-skin, is an appropriate developmentally supportive care strategy (Jarvis & Burnett, 2009). Even with triplets or more, shared kangaroo care can be promoted by holding infants together, sequentially (one after the other), and separately (each parent holding one or more) (Swinth, Nelson, Hadeed, & Anderson, 2000). Maternal breast temperatures have been shown to respond differentially to each infant with shared kangaroo care and were correlated to mean infant skin temperature (Ludington-Hoe et al., 2006).

Cobedding is the practice of placing multiple birth infants together in the same bed based on the concept of continuing the shared intrauterine experience. It is a form of developmentally supportive care and one way to foster the continuity between the intrauterine and extrauterine life of multiple birth infants (Leonard, 2002). Particularly for preterm infants in the NICU, cobedding allows prenatal interaction to continue, thus providing comfort and decreasing stress to the co-multiples. In surveys, nurses and nurse midwives are generally knowledgeable and supportive of the practice, citing benefits to parents and infants (Adams & Gill, 2014).

Cobedding literature and research is growing, but studies are often small and underpowered, typically focusing on preterm multiples in the hospital. A 2016 Cochrane review concluded that while the literature is not sufficient to make practice recommendations, cobedding of stable preterm infants in the neonatal nursery does not appear to affect weight gain, respiratory parameters, or heart rate nor has it been shown to increase risk for poor outcomes such as infection (Lai, Foong, Foong, & Tan, 2016). Since the Cochrane review, there are other reports indicating that cobedding in the NICU can assist with self-regulation and sleep and decrease crying (Hayward et al., 2015). A small RCT found cobedding reduced stress responses of preterm twins undergoing heel lance (Campbell-Yeo et al., 2014), although conclusions were not clear. A single-center French RCT of 32 sets of preterm twins (15 sets cobedded; 17 sets in individual beds) found cobedding in the NICU was associated with reduced delays for birth weight recovery, decreased parenteral weaning delays, and shorter hospital stays, but interestingly, no significant impact on preterm infant weight gain trajectories (Legrand et al., 2017). These researchers reported cobedding as a safe practice, even for infants receiving ventilator support and those with umbilical catheters.

However, there is concern by professional organizations. The National Association of Neonatal Nurses (NANN) states that while the underlying principles of cobedding may be reasonable, cobedding of hospitalized infants cannot be endorsed or rejected until further research is available and that neonatal units choosing to use cobedding should develop a clinical evaluation protocol to assess the safety and benefits of the practice (NANN, 2012). The Task Force on Sudden Infant Death Syndrome of the AAP (2016, p. 5) states, "The safety and benefits of cobedding for twins and higher-order multiples have not been established. It is prudent to provide separate sleep surfaces and avoid cobedding for twins and higher-order multiples in the hospital and at home." The AAP cites the following sudden infant death syndrome (SIDS) risk factors for multiple birth infants: frequency of prematurity and LBW, increased potential for overheating and rebreathing while cobedding, size discordance, frequency of side placement of cobedded twins, and hospital practices of cobedding as an encouragement for parents to continue this practice at home (Moon, 2016).

The concern that in-hospital cobedding translates to cobedding at home has been demonstrated. In addition to mimicking the NICU practice, it appears that parents of multiples may make less-than-optimal choices in infant positioning and other sleep practices for convenience, sleep synchronicity, cost savings, and because of lack of space. In one report, 54% of 109 mothers of twins in New Zealand cobedded their infants at 6 weeks of age with 31% and 10% still cobedding at 4 and 8 months, respectively (Hutchison, Stewart, & Mitchell, 2010). In a British study of 60 twin pairs, 60% of twins were cobedded in eight cobedding configurations (Ball, 2006). No significant differences were found in duration of parent or infant sleep between the cobedded and separate sleeping groups. The study did find that cobedded twins were less likely to be moved from their parents' room than those sleeping separately (9% vs. 33%). A troubling finding was that some parents used potentially hazardous bedding and makeshift barriers between the cobedded infants. Another small study of healthy cobedded twin pairs under 3 months of age used video, behavioral, and physiologic monitoring to assess potential problems with cobedding (Ball, 2007). Cobedded infants in the study did not wake more frequently than separated infants, and there was greater sleep synchrony, no increases in core body temperature, and no evidence of compression or airway obstruction by one twin on the other during cobedding. These researchers advised caution in cobedding babies with fever and with babies of different sizes. In a larger study of 104 sets of twins, 65% were cobedded by their parents at 4 and 9 weeks of age and families did not follow safe sleeping practices to reduce SIDS risk (Damato, Brubaker, & Burant, 2012). A similar report of 14 sets of HOMs found at-home practices included placing a rolled blanket between swaddled, cobedded infants, use of swings for sleep, and not all (<80%) parents placed infants on their backs immediately after discharge (Haas, Dowling, Damato, 2017). A longitudinal study found that the 35 mothers of twins were generally adherent to SIDS reduction strategies, particularly the use of supine sleep position and provision of breast milk (Damato, Haas, Czeck, Dowling, & Barsman, 2016). The researchers reported families used separate cribs for the twins 41% to 75% of the time and room sharing with parents 25% to 57% of the time and noted a trending decline in adherence for most SIDS reduction recommendations during the first 6 months.

AAP notes that all healthcare providers should endorse SIDS risk-reduction recommendations in policy and practice and that these should be modeled from birth or as soon as the infants are medically stable and "significantly" before discharge (Moon, 2016). Parents of multiples should be taught SIDS risk-reduction practices including separate sleeping; supine positioning; firm sleep surface; breastfeeding; parental room sharing; routine immunizations; pacifier use; and avoidance of soft bedding, overheating, and exposure to tobacco smoke, alcohol, and illicit drugs (AAP, 2016).

Discharge Planning

Multiple babies, particularly those born preterm, frequently cannot be discharged at the same time due to illness or differences in growth and feeding abilities. This can place a physical and emotional burden on parents, especially on postpartum mothers recuperating from multiple pregnancy and often a surgical or complicated vaginal birth who must travel back and forth to the hospital (Gromada & Bowers, 2005). Parents will need a place for daytime visits and privacy for breastfeeding, and ideally, rooms are available for overnight stays. Policies should be in place to clarify issues such as bringing the well multiple(s) back to the hospital. Discharging infants separately may be easier for families with HOM. When infants go home one or two at a time, the parents can become acquainted with each infant individually before facing the overwhelming tasks of caring for all the infants together (Gromada & Bowers, 2005). Staggered discharge may also be important in at-risk or fragile family situations to minimize stress (AAP & ACOG, 2017).

Feeding Multiples

Human milk is the ideal food for multiple birth infants, especially those who are born preterm. However, it is common for mothers of multiples to be unaware that breastfeeding is an option, and many question whether they can produce enough milk to meet the needs of two or more infants. Mothers also report that care providers are unaware or discourage breastfeeding multiples. Fortunately, the challenges of managing multiple newborns do not dissuade most mothers of multiples from breastfeeding or expressing their milk. Results from a convenience sample of mothers in a twin support group showed 89.4% initiated breastfeeding or pumping to establish milk production (Damato, Dowling, Madigan, & Thanattherakul, 2005). The investigators reported that mothers who were breastfeeding exclusively or almost exclusively at an average age of about 9 weeks were significantly more likely to still be breastfeeding at about 28 weeks. The same sample also provided information about cessation of breastfeeding in mothers of twins (Damato, Dowling, Standing, & Schuster, 2005). Reasons cited included unique issues related to infants' behaviors, challenges presented by growth and development, and time commitments that interfered with breastfeeding continuation. Inadequate milk production was reported as a leading reason for breastfeeding cessation; however, the survey responses did not clarify whether concerns about milk production were real or perceived. The study authors noted that long-term use of a breast pump, whether to initiate a milk production or to obtain milk to store for future use was beneficial in prolonging the provision of breast milk. However, this practice had the potential to become an extreme burden for a mother who was also breastfeeding or bottle feeding two infants. These reports emphasize the need for ongoing lactation support after birth to manage challenges of new breastfeeding issues with twin growth and development. Unfortunately, there is no good evidence for the effectiveness of breastfeeding education for women with multiples, including how to educate and support mothers, care delivery, timing, or the best person to do so (Whitford, Wallis, Dowswell, West, & Renfrew, 2017). Quality research is needed in this area.

Several breastfeeding principles must be recognized and communicated to mothers of multiples. First, mothers need to be informed early in pregnancy that breastfeeding is not only an option for feeding multiple infants but also the recommended feeding method. Second, establishing adequate milk production for multiple babies begins as soon as possible after birth with babies effectively removing milk at the breast or initiating milk expression/breast pumping when babies are preterm and/or ineffective at adequate milk removal. Third, maintenance of adequate milk production is dependent on frequent feedings or pumping sessions that effectively remove milk from the breasts; infrequent or ineffective milk removal is associated with inadequate milk production. Fourth, meeting a mother's goal of successful breastfeeding requires support from everyone around her, including her care providers. The British Columbia Reproductive Care Program (now Perinatal Services British Columbia, 2007) has developed guidelines for breastfeeding multiples for use by healthcare providers. The guidelines describe best practices based on current research as well as empirical and anecdotal evidence from professionals and multiple birth families and are listed in Display 11–6.

Mothers should also be provided with community breastfeeding support resources, such as International Board Certified Lactation Consultant, mother-to-mother support groups, and parents of multiples clubs.

Breastfeeding management of healthy newborn multiples born at term is much like singleton care but with a focus on meeting the needs of multiple infants. Usually, mothers begin with one infant at a time to monitor for effective breastfeeding behaviors (latch on and active suckling [for ≥10 minutes]) by each infant as both learn to breastfeed. Breasts can be alternated on a per-feeding or daily basis. Once one infant can achieve a deep, comfortable latch and is feeding effectively, the second infant can be positioned for simultaneous feedings. Mothers and/or infants may not be ready for simultaneous feedings in the first few days, or even weeks. However, nurses or lactation consultants should help mothers with positioning options by demonstration before they leave the hospital. These positions include the double football, parallel/cradle–clutch combination, and double cradle/crisscross holds. At home, infants can be fed on cue, feeding each when he or she demonstrates feeding cues, or feeding together, with the mother actively waking the second twin when the first one shows feeding cues. This method of feeding takes less time than feeding the infants separately or based solely on individual infant feeding cues. Many mothers use a combination of individual and simultaneous feedings. For HOMs, a mother may rotate infants and breasts so that each has the optimal time at the breast, or she may have a helper bottle feed one or two infants while she breastfeeds the other two (Gromada & Bowers, 2005).

Breastfeeding premature or sick multiples is more complex, yet there are clear benefits of breast milk for these infants. Some hospitals provide pasteurized donor breast milk to supplement a mother's own supply for multiples who are premature, LBW, or sick. Mothers whose infants are unable to breastfeed should begin expressing milk using a high-quality, multiuser (professional-grade) breast pump and manual (hand) expression ideally within the first hour after birth (Morton et al., 2009; Parker, Sullivan, Krueger, Kelechi, & Mueller, 2012). In 40 mothers of VLBW infants, initiation of milk expression within 6 hours after birth did not improve lactation success unless initiated within the first hour (Parker, Sullivan, Krueger, & Mueller, 2015). Early expression provides sick infants with antibody-rich colostrum, which may have a long-term impact on milk production and volumes obtained, and facilitates the establishment of a pumping routine. Pumped colostrum or milk should be distributed among the infants; however, priority is often given to the sickest of the infants (Gromada & Bowers, 2005). Mothers will need instructions about pumping and storage of breast milk as well as resources for obtaining an appropriate breast pump

DISPLAY 11–6

Guidelines for Breastfeeding Multiples

1. Families need opportunities to become informed about and prepared for breastfeeding term and preterm multiple birth infants.
2. Families require access to multiple-specific and general breastfeeding resources.
3. Families should be supported to initiate lactation and provide breast milk to their infants and the earliest opportunity.
4. Families should be assisted in the ongoing development of a breastfeeding plan that considers the needs of the mother, each infant, and the family as a whole.
5. Families should receive evidence-based and skilled breastfeeding assistance throughout the postpartum and early childhood periods.
6. Families should receive coordinated, comprehensive, consistent, and seamless breastfeeding care throughout pregnancy and early childhood.

Perinatal Services British Columbia. (2007). *Nutrition: Part III. Breastfeeding multiples.* Vancouver, BC, Canada: Author.

TABLE 11–4. Plan for Breastfeeding Multiples (Information for Mothers)

For well newborns	For premature or sick newborns
• After birth (vaginal or cesarean), initiate skin-to-skin contact immediately or as soon as possible to encourage each baby to go to breast within the first 30 to 90 min or as soon as any baby cues to feed. • Avoid using bottles, pacifiers, and other intraoral objects if possible. • Room-in with your babies to allow for frequent breastfeeding of each baby. (You may need a support person to stay with you.) • Ask your nurse or IBCLC to help you the first few times you breastfeed. • Initially feed each baby separately. Make sure each baby can latch on deeply at the breast and actively suckles for 10 or more min. • Nurse each baby when any demonstrates feeding cues, which should be 8 to 12 times over 24 hr by their second 24 hr after birth. • Alternate breasts at each feeding or daily for each baby or offer your fullest breast to the hungriest baby. • If babies are nursing well, you can feed them together. Your nurse or lactation consultant can show you different positions. Practice with all babies before discharge. • If you are concerned about milk production, call an IBCLC or breastfeeding support leader; feed your babies more frequently; and use a double electric breast pump after feedings, between feedings, or as needed to help increase milk production. (If one or more babies is not yet breastfeeding effectively, the rental of a high-quality multiuser breast pump can help you obtain more milk in less time.) • Know the number of your lactation consultant and breastfeeding support leader if you need help at home.	• Begin breast pumping using a combination of hand expression and an electric breast pump with double collection kit setup as soon as possible after delivery (vaginal or cesarean). Ideally, begin within the first hour after your babies' birth. (Rental of a high-quality, multiuser breast pump for home until all babies breastfeed well can help you obtain more milk.) • Apply the pump to both breasts *at least* 8 times each 24 hr. Nighttime pumping can be limited if babies' discharge is unlikely but do not allow more than 5 to 6 hr between pumpings. Pump more often during the day to achieve at least 8 pumping sessions per 24 hr. • Use hands-on pumping techniques during about 5 of the 8 or more pumping sessions each 24 hr. • Learn how to safely collect, store, and transport your breast milk. • Let your babies' nurses and doctors know that you want to start kangaroo care skin to skin as soon as possible. Let each baby have mouth/nose to nipple contact as soon as possible. Allow the babies to progress to breastfeeding as soon as medically possible. • Premature babies must physically mature before they can sustain effective breastfeeding. Gradually, they will improve so you can nurse your babies as with well babies. • Use your breast pump at home after breastfeedings if needed to help with milk production. • Know the number of your IBCLC and breastfeeding support leader if you need help at home.

IBCLC, International Board Certified Lactation Consultant.
From Marvelous Multiples, Inc., used by permission.

after discharge. Mothers should be informed that availability and coverage of specific electric breast pumps depends on the insurance plan. A plan for breastfeeding well and sick or premature multiples is provided in Table 11–4.

Parenting Newborn Multiples

Multiple births have been shown to have a fivefold greater risk of severe parenting stress and double the risk of lower quality of life, social stigma, and maternal depression (Luke & Brown, 2007). In addition to the physical demands of their own recovery, mothers of multiple newborns face challenges in parenting several babies at once. In the first weeks at home, it is essential that tasks of housekeeping, laundry, cooking, grocery shopping, and sibling care are delegated to friends and family so that the mother is permitted time for recovery and interaction with her infants. The first month can be difficult as parents learn skills and routines for infant care, feedings, and sleep. Usually, parents of healthy twins can successfully care for their infants along with occasional help from family and friends. Parents with HOMs or infants with a health problem will need formal help for a much longer time. In simplest terms, one person cannot hold three infants at once. Helpers should assume non–baby care responsibilities, such as household chores and assisting the mother with feedings or diaper changes. Whether helpers are friends, family, or employed, their roles and responsibilities should be clearly outlined.

With the help of their pediatrician, parents can establish routines for feeding, sleep, and activities. This is particularly important for premature infants who may need frequent feedings. Simultaneous feeding can be helpful but requires waking a sleeping infant when another is ready to eat. This may be challenging because the other multiple(s) may not always cooperate, especially when in a deep sleep state. Feeding routines also help develop similar sleep/waking patterns. Nurses should stress flexible routines, allowing for differences in each infant's temperament and needs. Some infants are high need, requiring constant cuddling or touch, whereas others are content with a feeding and a few visual toys. A daily log of feedings and diaper counts for each infant is important until growth and weight gain are well established (Gromada & Bowers, 2005).

Referral of expectant families to both local and national multiple birth support groups provides an

---

---

instant network among other expectant parents of multiples as well as support from experienced parents who have "been there." A list of support groups is provided in Display 11–7.

PSYCHOLOGICAL ISSUES WITH MULTIPLE GESTATIONS

During pregnancy, birth, and the months following the birth of multiples, each family experiences "a constellation of stresses which jeopardize physical and mental health and family functioning" (Malmstrom & Biale, 1990, p. 507). These stresses cut across all socioeconomic and educational levels and include increases in child abuse, marital troubles, and family dysfunction. Having a high-risk pregnancy is associated with significantly higher level of stress and negative emotions and hospitalization increases anxiety (Rodrigues, Zambaldi, Cantilino, & Sougey, 2016). Four interrelated principles have been proposed to guide the care of multiple birth families: interdisciplinary involvement, provision of multiples-focused care, coordinated services, and the building of family competence (Leonard & Denton, 2006). These are illustrated in Figure 11–12.

Prenatal Attachment

The prenatal attachment process for multiples is complex, with maternal–fetal interactions woven together with interfetal interactions. Just as an expectant mother relates to her fetuses through fetal movement, intrauterine tactile stimulation between multiples plays a role in attachment among infants. Each multiple develops an individual temperament and each set of multiples establishes their own patterns of tactile communication.

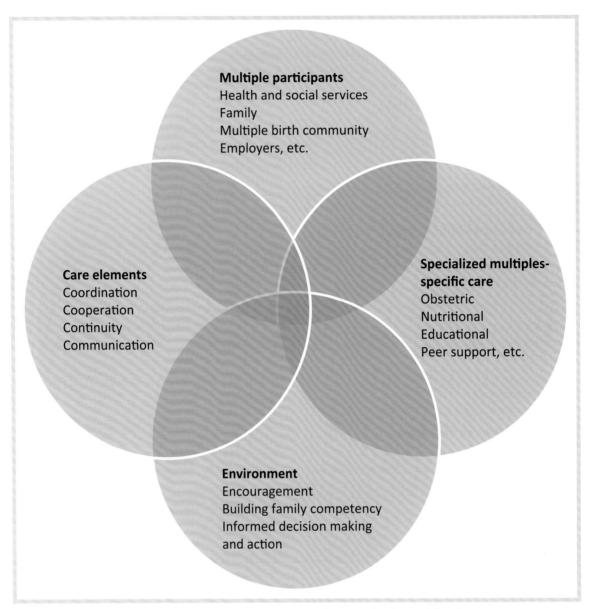

FIGURE 11–12. Framework of care during multiple pregnancy and parenthood. (Leonard, L. G., & Denton, J., [2006]. Preparation for parenting multiple birth children. *Early Human Development, 82*[6], 371–378. doi:10.1016/j.earlhumdev .2006.03.009)

The same behaviors, traits, and intermultiple interactions seen in pregnancy also have been observed in infancy and beyond (Leonard, 2002).

Maternal attachment with multiples is similar to attachment processes in singleton pregnancies. Interestingly, women who were younger, with lower income, a history of infertility, greater self-esteem, who had experienced quickening, and were further along in their pregnancy reported greater prenatal attachment to their twins (Damato, 2004b). However, pregnancy risk factors may affect attachment. Hospitalized women at risk for preterm delivery were shown to have less attachment and higher levels of anxiety and depression compared with controls; however, attachment was independent of emotional state and appeared to be related to the risk of preterm birth (Pisoni et al., 2016). Traumatic diagnoses, such as TTTS, may be associated with a high level of anxiety and signs of post-traumatic stress and may alter prenatal attachment (Beauquier-Maccotta et al., 2016). Postpartum depression, cesarean birth, and the experience of a NICU admission for one or both twins negatively influenced mothers' postnatal attachment compared to their prenatal attachment (Damato, 2004a).

Fetal movements enable a woman expecting multiples to relate to her unborn children, affirm that each one is alive and healthy, and attach to them individually and as a unit (Leonard, 2002). Nurses can promote prenatal attachment by encouraging expectant mothers to observe fetal movements and patterns, differentiate between individual multiples, identify behavioral similarities and differences, recognize inter-multiple contacts (during ultrasound examinations and fetal monitoring), and ask questions during fetal testing (Leonard, 2002). Support and follow-up are especially important for older, higher income women with low self-esteem, and prenatal education and counseling helps build confidence and develop effective parenting strategies (Damato, 2004b).

Prenatal Family Adjustments

Preparation for multiple infants requires significant adjustments for families even before the babies are born. Depending on the presence of complications in the pregnancy, women may need to reduce or stop working, be limited in activities, or be placed on bed rest at home or in the hospital. There is evidence that women on bed rest with multiples may have even greater emotional and physical needs than those with singletons. Women with multiple gestations in one study had many more antepartum symptoms during hospitalization and treatment with bed rest than women with singleton gestations (Maloni et al., 2006). The number of symptoms reported by women with multiples appears to be higher than those reported by women with singleton gestations. Over half of the women in the study had very high depressive symptom scores on admission, and they identified concerns for their family and being separated as major stressors. The average number and persistence of postpartum symptoms reported during the first weeks also appear to be higher than those for women with singleton pregnancies. The authors concluded that women have many physical and psychological discomforts during a multiple gestation and experience continuing symptoms indicative of underlying postpartum morbidity that are not completely recovered by 6 weeks.

Families with a mother on bed rest often have difficulty assuming maternal responsibilities, anxiety about outcomes for mother and infants, and adverse emotional effects on the children (Maloni, Brezinski-Tomasi, & Johnson, 2001). Expectant fathers often receive the brunt of family and household responsibilities during a multiple pregnancy and are often required to "be all things to all family members, including father and mother, financial provider, cook, maid, and the emotional support system" (Bowers et al., 2006, p. 36). In addition to their concerns about the health of the mother and fetuses, fathers must cope with the effects of increased family responsibilities and emotional pressures in their own lives. If a mother's income is eliminated due to pregnancy complications, finances may become a concern, even in economically advantaged families. Fathers may be at increased risk for depression, especially those who have a history of depression, are unemployed, and have an unsupportive partner or one with perinatal depression (Leonard, 1998).

Children in the household may be affected by the strains of a high-risk pregnancy as well. Young children whose mothers are on bed rest may be unable to fully comprehend maternal restrictions, the need to reallocate childcare, or maternal absence during hospitalization (Maloni et al., 2001).

Nurses play an integral role in providing psychosocial support for families expecting multiples. Anticipatory guidance includes the expected physical and emotional changes of a multiple pregnancy; the need for contingency planning at home for children and household management; nutritional assessment and counseling; plans for testing, interventions, and treatment options; referrals to support organizations such as local parents of multiples groups; and information about multiple birth prenatal education classes. It is also important to ensure that hospitalized women and those on bed rest at home have access to education; this may include provision of in-home or online classes, videos, reading materials, and resources. Measures to decrease the stressors of hospitalization may include liberal visitation with family and other children; home-cooked food; provision of technology for in-room videos, music, and Internet access; and opportunities for networking with other expectant mothers of multiples (Bleyl, 2002).

Postnatal Attachment

Postnatal parent–infant attachment with multiple infants is complex and evolves through various processes. Ultimately, parents need to view each infant as an individual with a unique personality and characteristics. Initially, a unit attachment is formed, with parents focusing on the concept of the set of twins or triplets prenatally and after birth (Damato, 2004b). Individual attachments follow, often with brief periods of attachment to one infant before shifting to another (Gromada & Bowers, 2005). Some parents develop preferential feelings for a particular infant. If this is consistently demonstrated, there can be long-term cognitive and behavioral effects for all the infants. Unequal attachments are more likely when one infant is healthier than the other or one is more responsive (Gromada & Bowers, 2005). Postnatal attachment can be supported by implementing measures to increase a mother's opportunities for proximity with her twins such as promotion of breastfeeding, skin-to-skin contact, and encouraging complete access to and participation in her infants' NICU care (Damato, 2004a). Nurses should observe parent–infant interactions noting behaviors indicative of progression toward individualization. Signs of positive attachment/individualization behaviors include acknowledgment and response to each infant's cues; initiating verbalization, touching, soothing, cuddling, and so forth, with each infant; alternating eye contact among infants; and referring to each infant by name (Gromada & Bowers, 2005).

The demands of multiple infants at home can limit parent–infant interactions. Frequent, slow feedings, repeated diaper changes, and constant cries of multiple infants are exhausting. To compensate, parents may focus more on physical care than on their infants' emotional needs. This exposes multiple birth infants to a unique risk—the deprivation of the parents' exclusive focus and involvement (R. Feldman & Eidelman, 2004). A study of preterm twins and singletons found that mothers of twins exhibited fewer initiatives toward their infants and were less responsive to both positive signals and to crying (Ostfeld, Smith, Hiatt, & Hegyi, 2000). The twin mothers lifted or held, touched, patted, and talked to their infants less, and their infants had lower cognitive scores at 18 months than singletons. The child who is less effective in eliciting parental care or who may be less rewarding during interactions appears to be at an especially high risk. A study of social–emotional development of triplets found the infant with birth weight discordance >15% received the lowest levels of parent response and displayed the poorest behavior outcomes among the set. Parenting difficulties appeared to be related to the lack of emotional resources for adapting to each infant's individual patterns (R. Feldman & Eidelman, 2004).

Anxiety and Depression

The very nature of a high-risk pregnancy increases stress and anxiety for expectant mothers and may be intensified by the unknowns of a multiple pregnancy. Once home, the around-the-clock needs of multiple infants, sleep deprivation, inconsistent support, and a sense of isolation may contribute to maternal stress (Gromada & Bowers, 2005). It has been estimated that as many as 25% of multiple birth parents are affected by perinatal depression and anxiety disorders (Leonard, 1998). Compared to parents of singletons, both mothers and fathers of twins experience significantly greater depression, anxiety, sleeping difficulties, and social dysfunction (Vilska et al., 2009). Evidence indicates that stress and depression in pregnant and postpartum women are of considerable concern due to the association with adverse obstetric outcomes, postpartum depression, and emotional and behavioral problems in the children (Mian, 2005). The additive effects of infertility history, multiple birth, and first-time parenting may increase the risk for psychological resource depletion (Klock, 2004). Other

researchers found that regardless of whether multiples were the result of ART or spontaneous conception, families had increased need for material goods, more social stigma, lower marital satisfaction, more depression, and lower quality of life, which included health and social and psychological aspects (Roca-de Bes, Gutierrez-Maldonado, & Gris-Martínez, 2011). Nurses have a key role in identifying parents at risk; early recognition and support of women and families affected by these disorders; and providing prevention-focused health, education, and social support programs at the family and community levels (Leonard, 1998). Uncertainty and stress have been associated with increased risk of preterm birth (Fang, Liu, Day, Chen, & Gau, 2011). This study found positive effects, including higher average birth weights, using nursing care strategies to reduce uncertainty and stress with an educational pamphlet and a telephone health consultation program.

Beck (2002) found that "life on hold" was the basic social psychological problem during the first year for mothers of twins in a multiple birth support group. Mothers in the study experienced four phases: (1) draining power, a demanding, sleep-deprived period, when mothers had no time and were torn between infants' needs; (2) pausing own life, which involved a blurring of days and nights with confinement and self-surrender; (3) striving to reset, when mothers began to develop coping strategies such as routines, schedules, prioritizing tasks, recruiting family help, and problem solving; and (4) resuming own life, which was achieved when mothers felt their lives were more manageable and when milestones such as sleeping through the night or twins beginning to self-feed were reached. It was in this last phase that mothers could relate the blessings of having twins. Beck concluded that the most vulnerable period for these mothers was 3 months' postpartum.

A study of mothers of multiples who conceived with ART identified children's health, unmet family needs, maternal depression, and parental stress as key areas of concern (Ellison & Hall, 2003). The study revealed that the inordinate stresses of raising multiple birth infants strengthened some marriages when there was greater paternal participation in childcare and household tasks. Marriages weakened when couples were unable to equitably divide family and household labor or were unable to work together as a team. The psychosocial risks associated with iatrogenic multiple births appear to increase with plurality. In another study, parents of ART multiples reported significant difficulty in providing basic material needs for their families, decreased quality of life, social stigma, and maternal depression (Ellison et al., 2005). Such distress may decrease their willingness to seek help or admit their distress to their care providers. A review of the research related to parenting after assisted reproduction concluded that supportive nursing interventions should include strategies to reduce parental anxiety, increase parental self-esteem, and foster healthy parent–infant relationships (J. M. McGrath, Samra, Zukowsky, & Baker, 2010). Interventions for improving parenting sense of competence and parenting distress may include attendance at specialized prenatal clinics, postpartum home visits, maternal involvement in neonatal care activities, and assisting women to reframe their expectations for the demands of caring for twins and maintaining a household (Damato, Anthony, & Maloni, 2009).

Child Abuse

The literature has limited information specific to abuse in multiple birth families, but early reports indicated a significant ninefold higher risk of reported abuse/neglect among twins versus singletons (Groothuis et al., 1982). A more recent study of 19 sets of abused multiples (1 set of triplets, 18 twins) found that multiples shared the same mode of abuse; siblings of abused multiples were often abused as well, multiples were significantly more likely to be younger and experience abdominal trauma and fractures, and mothers and fathers were equally likely to be the abuser (Lang, Cox, & Flores, 2013). Case reports show a similar increased risk profile with multiples more likely to have abusive fractures and abdominal trauma and suffer shaken baby syndrome than singletons. Analysis of national cohort linked birth–infant death data of healthy (term, non-LBW) multiples found these infants had a 40% higher risk of death than singletons due to unintentional injuries, assault, and other external causes; this risk increased between 2 and 7 months of age (Ahrens, Thoma, Rossen, Warner, & Simon, 2017). Prevention of injury and maltreatment involves risk assessment and recognition of parenting stress, anticipatory guidance and parenting education, as well as connecting families with supportive resources. Any suspected abuse should prompt an assessment of the co-multiples as well as all children in the household.

Grief and Loss

Parents who experience the death of a complete set of multiples have been found to grieve more intensely than parents who lose a singleton; they are at significant risk for depression, and may experience grief 6 months longer (Pector & Smith-Levitin, 2002). However, the grieving process becomes more complex with the death of part of a set of multiples. The presence of a surviving infant or infants sets multiple birth parents apart in their bereavement process (Cox & Wainwright, 2015). These parents experience the difficult paradox of grieving simultaneously for the infants who died while feeling joy for their living infants. Grieving multiple birth families with a surviving twin have been described as having "special and complex characteristics that affect them in ways greater than, or different from, bereaved single birth families" (Swanson, Kane, Pearsall-Jones, Swanson, & Croft, 2009).

Lee (2012) identified several themes in grieving families after the loss of one or more multiples.

- Conflicting emotions while mourning the loss of their twin while becoming increasingly attached to their living twin; this included ambivalence about the surviving infant(s).
- Difficulty attaching to surviving children and the fear of losing them
- Difficulty returning to the unit to visit their surviving child and concerns of competing attention between the living child and the memory of their lost child
- The need for acknowledgment of the infant who died, regardless of when it occurred—during pregnancy or in the neonatal period

Studies have shown that grief is often delayed for 1 to 3 years while parents focus on survivors, bonding is sometimes impaired, and some parents may even resent the survivors (Pector & Smith-Levitin, 2002). The intensity of grief after a multiple's death equals that with a singleton, yet parents rarely receive as much sympathy (Pector & Smith-Levitin, 2002). In one study, mothers experienced significantly more depression and grief than fathers at the time of loss (Swanson et al., 2009). A fundamental concept with loss in multiple births is that no matter how many infants survive, the parents remain parents of multiples (Gromada & Bowers, 2005). It is important to validate parents' loss with healing actions and responses; parents wished that clinicians had been more sensitive and compassionate to them at the time of the loss (Swanson et al., 2009). Recommendations for clinicians to help grieving parents of multiples are listed in Display 11–8. Peer support can be especially helpful at the time of the loss. Organizations such as Center for Loss in Multiple Birth (CLIMB) have specific information and support to help parents cope with the death of one or more multiples.

Multiple Birth Resources and Support Organizations

Organizations for multiple birth families provide a supportive environment for parents to network and learn from others (see Display 11–7). National organizations often offer free online resources, including e-mail lists and interactive support created especially for expectant parents of multiples.

DISPLAY 11–8

Recommendations to Help Grieving Parents of Multiples

- Provide opportunities for parents to see and/or hold all babies of a set, together, and separately.
- Mementos such as photographs, videos, monitor strips, locks of hair, and footprints should be collected for all babies.
- Do not place beds of surviving multiples beside intact sets in the nursery or NICU.
- After a prenatal loss or multifetal reduction, ask how parents want to refer to the pregnancy: by the number conceived or by the number remaining.
- After neonatal loss, most parents consider living children to be survivors and are comfortable with saying they had triplets or twins.
- Parents should have input into labeling for two or more remaining multiples; generally, triplets B and C should retain their designation of B and C after triplet A's death.

- Allow mothers to wear all their infants' bracelets throughout the hospital stay.
- **Suggested helpful and healing responses include**
  - This must be very hard for you.
  - I'm so sorry your twins died.
  - I have no idea how you must feel.
  - How are you feeling? What would help your family through this?
  - How are you coping with everything?
- **Hurtful responses to be avoided include**
  - You're young, you could have other multiples.
  - You couldn't handle them all.
  - At least it happened before you were too attached.
  - It's for the best. They would have been severely disabled.
  - Set your grief aside. You must be strong for your survivors.
  - At least you have two living babies. Some parents can't have any!
  - Multiples are so expensive. Think of the money you'll save.

NICU, neonatal intensive care unit.

From Pector, E. A., & Smith-Levitin, M. (2002). Mourning and psychological issues in multiple birth loss. *Seminars in Neonatology, 7*(3), 247–256; Gromada, K. K., & Bowers, N. A. (2005). *Care of the multiple-birth family: Postpartum through infancy.* New York, NY: March of Dimes.

SUMMARY

With the high incidence of multiples in the United States, perinatal nurses frequently have the opportunity to care for women pregnant with more than one fetus. Appreciation of the increased obstetric, perinatal, and neonatal risks in multiple gestations enables nurses to identify potential complications and make appropriate care interventions. A thorough knowledge of the special needs of women with multiple gestation is requisite for safe care for these high-risk mothers and their babies. Parent education includes acknowledging the challenges of caring for multiple infants and the importance of adhering to safe practices.

REFERENCES

Adams, C., & Gill, F. J. (2014). Co-bedding of multiples in the neonatal unit: Assessing nurses and midwives attitude and level of understanding. *Journal of Neonatal Nursing, 20*(2), 82–88. doi:10.1016/j.jnn.2013.07.002

Agarwal, K., & Alfirevic, Z. (2012). Pregnancy loss after chorionic villus sampling and genetic amniocentesis in twin pregnancies: A systematic review. *Ultrasound in Obstetrics & Gynecology, 40*(2), 128–134. doi:10.1002/uog.10152

Ahrens, K. A., Thoma, M. E., Rossen, L. M., Warner, M., & Simon, A. E. (2017). Plurality of birth and infant mortality due to external causes in the United States, 2000–2010. *American Journal of Epidemiology, 185*(5), 335–344. doi:10.1093/aje/kww119

Alexander, J. M., Leveno, K. J., Rouse, D., Landon, M. B., Gilbert, S. A., Spong, C. Y., . . . Gabbe, S. G. (2008). Cesarean delivery for the second twin. *Obstetrics & Gynecology, 112*(4), 748–752. doi:10.1097/AOG.0b013e318187ccb2

American Academy of Pediatrics. (2016). SIDS and other sleep-related infant deaths: Updated 2016 recommendations for a safe infant sleeping environment. *Pediatrics, 138*(5), e20162938. doi:10.1542/peds.2016-2938

American Academy of Pediatrics & American College of Obstetricians and Gynecologists. (2017). *Guidelines for perinatal care* (8th ed.). Elk Grove Village, IL: American Academy of Pediatrics.

American College of Obstetricians and Gynecologists. (2009). *Intrapartum fetal heart rate monitoring: Nomenclature, interpretation, and general management principles* (Practice Bulletin No. 106), Washington, DC: Author.

American College of Obstetricians and Gynecologists. (2012). *Placenta accreta* (Committee Opinion No. 529), Washington, DC: Author.

American College of Obstetricians and Gynecologists. (2013). *Medically indicated late-preterm and early-term deliveries* (Committee Opinion No. 560), Washington, DC; Author.

American College of Obstetricians and Gynecologists. (2015). *Physical activity and exercise during pregnancy and the postpartum period* (Committee Opinion No. 650), Washington, DC: Author.

American College of Obstetricians and Gynecologists. (2016). *Premature rupture of membranes* (Practice Bulletin No. 172), Washington, DC: Author.

American College of Obstetricians and Gynecologists. (2017a). *Delayed umbilical cord clamping after birth* (Committee Opinion No. 684), Washington, DC: Author.

American College of Obstetricians and Gynecologists. (2017b). *Multifetal pregnancy reduction* (Committee Opinion No. 719), Washington, DC: Author.

American College of Obstetricians and Gynecologists. (2017c). *Postpartum hemorrhage* (Practice Bulletin No. 183), Washington, DC: Author.

American College of Obstetricians and Gynecologists. (2018). *Nausea and vomiting of pregnancy* (Practice Bulletin No. 189), Washington, DC: Author.

American College of Obstetricians and Gynecologists & Society for Maternal-Fetal Medicine. (2016). *Multifetal gestations: Twin, triplet, and higher-order multifetal pregnancies* (Practice Bulletin No. 169), Washington, DC: Author.

American Society for Reproductive Medicine. (2012). Multiple gestation associated with infertility therapy: An American Society for Reproductive Medicine practice committee opinion. *Fertility and Sterility*, 97(4), 825–834. doi:10.1016/j.fertnstert.2011.11.048

American Society for Reproductive Medicine & Society for Assisted Reproductive Technology. (2017). Guidance on the limits to the number of embryos to transfer: A committee opinion. *Fertility and Sterility*, 107(4), 901–903. doi:10.1016/j.fertnstert.2017.02.107

Ananth, C. V., & Chauhan, S. P. (2017). Epidemiology of periviable births: The impact and neonatal outcomes of twin pregnancy. *Clinics in Perinatology*, 44(2), 333–345. doi:10.1016/j.clp.2017.01.002

Arabin, B., & van Eyck, J. (2009). Delayed-interval delivery in twin and triplet pregnancies: 17 years of experience in 1 perinatal center. *American Journal of Obstetrics & Gynecology*, 200(2), 154.e1–154.e8. doi:10.1016/j.ajog.2008.08.046

Aviram, A., Weiser, I., Ashwal, E., Bar, J., Wiznitzer, A., & Yogev, Y. (2015). Combined vaginal-cesarean delivery of twins: Risk factors and neonatal outcome—A single center experience. *The Journal of Maternal-Fetal & Neonatal Medicine*, 28(5), 509–514. doi:10.3109/14767058.2014.927430

Awwad, J., Usta, I., Ghazeeri, G., Yacoub, N., Succar, J., Hayek, S., . . . Nassar, A. (2015). A randomised controlled double-blind clinical trial of 17-hydroxyprogesterone caproate for the prevention of preterm birth in twin gestation (PROGESTWIN): Evidence for reduced neonatal morbidity. *BJOG*, 122(1), 71–79. doi:10.1111/1471-0528.13031

Bahtiyar, M. O., Dulay, A. T., Weeks, B. P., Friedman, A. H., & Copel, J. A. (2007). Prevalence of congenital heart defects in monochorionic/diamniotic twin gestations. *Journal of Ultrasound in Medicine*, 26(11), 1491–1498. doi:10.7863/jum.2007.26.11.1491

Bakker, P. C., Colenbrander, G. J., Verstraeten, A. A., & Van Geijn, H. P. (2004). Quality of intrapartum cardiotocography in twin deliveries. *American Journal of Obstetrics & Gynecology*, 191(6), 2114–2119. doi:10.1016/j.ajog.2004.04.037

Ball, H. L. (2006). Caring for twin infants: Sleeping arrangements and their implications. *Evidence Based Midwifery*, 4(1), 10–16.

Ball, H. L. (2007). Together or apart? A behavioural and physiological investigation of sleeping arrangements for twin babies. *Midwifery*, 23(4), 404–412. doi:10.1016/j.midw.2006.07.004

Barrett, J. F. R., Hannah, M. E., Hutton, E. K., Willan, A. R., Allen, A. C., Armson, B. A., . . . Asztalos, E. V. (2013). A randomized trial of planned cesarean or vaginal delivery for twin pregnancy. *The New England Journal of Medicine*, 369(14), 1295–1305. doi:10.1056/NEJMoa1214939

Bateni, Z. H., Clark, S. L., Sangi-Haghpeykar, H., Aagaard, K. M., Blumenfeld, Y. J., Ramin, S. M., . . . Shamshirsaz, A. A. (2016). Trends in the delivery route of twin pregnancies in the United States, 2006–2013. *European Journal of Obstetrics, Gynecology, and Reproductive Biology*, 205, 120–126. doi:10.1016/j.ejogrb.2016.08.031

Bates, S. M., Greer, I. A., Middeldorp, S., Veenstra, D. L., Prabulos, A.-M., & Vandvik, P. O. (2012). VTE, thrombophilia, antithrombotic therapy, and pregnancy: Antithrombotic Therapy and Prevention of Thrombosis, 9th ed: American College of Chest Physicians Evidence-Based Clinical Practice Guidelines. *Chest*, 141(2 Suppl.), e691S–e736S. doi:10.1378/chest.11-2300

Beaquier-Maccotta, B., Chalouhi, G. E., Picquet, A.-L., Carrier, A., Bussières, L., Golse, B., & Ville, Y. (2016). Impact of monochorionicity and twin to twin transfusion syndrome on prenatal attachment, post traumatic stress disorder, anxiety and depressive symptoms. *PLoS One*, 11(1), e0145649. doi:10.1371/journal.pone.0145649

Beck, C. T. (2002). Releasing the pause button: Mothering twins during the first year of life. *Qualitative Health Research*, 12(5), 593–608. doi:10.1177/104973202129120124

Benito Vielba, M., De Bonrostro Torralba, C., Pallares Arnal, V., Herrero Serrano, R., Tejero Cabrejas, E. L., & Campillos Maza, J. M. (2019). Delayed-interval delivery in twin pregnancies: Report of three cases and literature review. *The Journal of Maternal-Fetal & Neonatal Medicine*, 32(2), 351–355. doi:10.1080/14767058.2017.1378336

Bergh, C., Möller, A., Nilsson, L., & Wikland, M. (1999). Obstetrical outcome and psychological follow-up of pregnancies after embryo reduction. *Human Reproduction (Oxford, England)*, 14(8), 2170–2175. doi:10.1093/humrep/14.8.2170

Berghella, V., Baxter, J. K., & Hendrix, N. W. (2013). Cervical assessment by ultrasound for preventing preterm delivery. *Cochrane Database of Systematic Reviews*, (1), CD007235. doi:10.1002/14651858.cd007235.pub3

Berghella, V., Dugoff, L., & Ludmir, J. (2017). Prevention of preterm birth with pessary in twins (PoPPT): A randomized controlled trial. *Ultrasound in Obstetrics & Gynecology*, 49(5), 567–572. doi:10.1002/uog.17430

Berghella, V., Odibo, A. O., To, M. S., Rust, O. A., & Althuisius, S. M. (2005). Cerclage for short cervix on ultrasonography: Meta-analysis of trials using individual patient-level data. *Obstetrics & Gynecology*, 106(1):181–189. doi:10.1097/01.AOG.0000168435.17200.53

Bleyl, J. (2002). Familial and psychological reaction in triplet families. In L. G. Keith & I. Blickstein (Eds.), *Triplet pregnancies and their consequences* (pp. 361–369). New York, NY: The Parthenon.

Blickstein, I., Shinwell, E. S., Lusky, A., & Reichman, B. (2005). Plurality-dependent risk of respiratory distress syndrome among very-low-birth-weight infants and antepartum corticosteroid treatment. *American Journal of Obstetrics & Gynecology*, 192, 360–364. doi:10.1016/j.ajog.2004.10.604

Bodnar, L. M., Pugh, S. J., Abrams, B., Himes, K. P., & Hutcheon, J. A. (2014). Gestational weight gain in twin pregnancies and maternal and child health: A systematic review. *Journal of Perinatology*, 34(4), 252–263. doi:10.1038/jp.2013.177

Boghossian, N. S., McDonald, S. A., Bell, E. F., Carlo, W. A., Brumbaugh, J. E., Stoll, B. J., . . . Higgins, R. D. (2016). Association of antenatal corticosteroids with mortality, morbidity, and neurodevelopmental outcomes in extremely preterm multiple gestation infants. *JAMA Pediatrics*, 170(6), 593–601. doi:10.1001/jamapediatrics.2016.0104

Bowers, N. A., Gromada, K. K., & Wieczorek, R. R. (2006). *Care of the multiple-birth family: Pregnancy and birth*. White Plains, NY: March of Dimes.

Briana, D. D., & Malamitsi-Puchner, A. (2019). Twins and neurodevelopmental outcomes: The effect of IVF, fetal growth restriction, and preterm birth. *The Journal of Maternal-Fetal & Neonatal Medicine*, 32(13), 2256–2261. doi:10.1080/14767058.2018.1425834

Brown, J. E., & Carlson, M. (2000). Nutrition and multifetal pregnancy. *Journal of the American Dietetic Association*, 100(3), 343–348. doi:10.1016/S0002-8223(00)00105-X

Bryan, E. (2002). Educating families, before, during and after a multiple birth. *Seminars in Neonatology*, 7(3), 241–246. doi:10.1053/siny.2002.0111

Bryan, E. (2005). Psychological aspects of prenatal diagnosis and its implications in multiple pregnancies. *Prenatal Diagnosis*, 25(9), 827–834. doi:10.1002/pd.1270

Bush, M. C., & Malone, F. D. (2005). Down syndrome screening in twins. *Clinics in Perinatology*, 32(2), 373–386. doi:10.1016/j.clp.2005.03.001

Cahill, A. G., Macones, G. A., Stamilio, D. M., Dicke, J. M., Crane, J. P., & Odibo, A. O. (2009). Pregnancy loss rate after mid-trimester amniocentesis in twin pregnancies. *American Journal of Obstetrics & Gynecology*, 200(3), 257.e1–257.e6. doi:10.1016/j.ajog.2008.09.872

Campbell, D., & Templeton, A. (2004). Maternal complications of twin pregnancy. *International Journal of Gynecology & Obstetrics, 84*(1), 71–73. doi:10.1016/s0020-7292(03)00314-x

Campbell-Yeo, M. L., Johnston, C. C., Joseph, K. S., Feeley, N., Chambers, C. T., Barrington, K. J., & Walker, C.-D. (2014). Co-bedding between preterm twins attenuates stress response following heel lance. *The Clinical Journal of Pain, 30*(7), 598–604. doi:10.1097/AJP.0000000000000015

Canick, J. A., Kloza, E. M., Lambert-Messerlian, G. M., Haddow, J. E., Ehrich, M., Boom, D., . . . Palomaki, G. E. (2012). DNA sequencing of maternal plasma to identify Down syndrome and other trisomies in multiple gestations. *Prenatal Diagnosis, 32*(8), 730–734. doi:10.1002/pd.3892

Caritis, S. N., Feghali, M. N., Grobman, W. A., & Rouse, D. J. (2016). What we have learned about the role of 17-alpha-hydroxyprogesterone caproate in the prevention of preterm birth. *Seminars in Perinatology, 40*(5), 273–280. doi:10.1053/j.semperi.2016.03.002

Centers for Disease Control and Prevention. (2019a). *About natality 2007-2017.* Atlanta, GA; Author.

Centers for Disease Control and Prevention. (2019b). *Pregnancy mortality surveillance system.* Atlanta, GA: Author.

Centers for Disease Control and Prevention, American Society for Reproductive Medicine, & Society for Assisted Reproductive Technology. (2017). *2015 Assisted reproductive technology national summary report.* Atlanta, GA: U.S. Department of Health and Human Services.

Chasen, S. T., Spiro, S. J., Kalish, R. B., & Chervenak, F. A. (2005). Changes in fetal presentation in twin pregnancies. *The Journal of Maternal-Fetal & Neonatal Medicine, 17*(1), 45–48. doi:10.1080/14767050400028592

Chauhan, S. P., Scardo, J. A., Hayes, E., Abuhamad, A. Z., & Berghella, V. (2010). Twins: Prevalence, problems, and preterm births. *American Journal of Obstetrics & Gynecology, 203*(4), 305–315. doi:10.1016/j.ajog.2010.04.031

Chaveeva, P., Peeva, G., Pugliese, S. G., Shterev, A., & Nicolaides, K. H. (2017). Intrafetal laser ablation for embryo reduction from dichorionic triplets to dichorionic twins. *Ultrasound in Obstetrics & Gynecology, 50*(5), 632–634. doi:10.1002/uog.18834

Cheung, Y. B., Yip, P., & Karlberg, J. (2000). Mortality of twins and singletons by gestational age: A varying-coefficient approach. *American Journal of Epidemiology, 152*(12), 1107–1116. doi:10.1093/aje/152.12.1107

Cleary-Goldman, J., Chitkara, U., & Berkowitz, R. L. (2007). Multiple gestations. In S. G. Gabbe, J. R. Niebyl, & J. L. Simpson (Eds.), *Obstetrics: Normal and problem pregnancies* (5th ed., pp. 733–763). Philadelphia, PA: Churchill Livingstone.

Collopy, K. S. (2004). "I couldn't think that far": Infertile women's decision making about multifetal reduction. *Research in Nursing & Health, 27*(2), 75–86. doi:10.1002/nur.20012

Combs, C. A., Garite, T., Maurel, K., Das, A., & Porto, M. (2010). Failure of 17-hydroxyprogesterone to reduce neonatal morbidity or prolong triplet pregnancy: A double-blind, randomized clinical trial. *American Journal of Obstetrics & Gynecology, 203*(3), 248.e1–248.e9. doi:10.1016/j.ajog.2010.06.016

Conde-Agudelo, A., & Romero, R. (2010). Cervicovaginal fetal fibronectin for the prediction of spontaneous preterm birth in multiple pregnancies: A systematic review and meta-analysis. *The Journal of Maternal-Fetal & Neonatal Medicine, 23*(12), 1365–1376. doi:10.3109/14767058.2010.499484

Conde-Agudelo, A., & Romero, R. (2015). Predictive accuracy of changes in transvaginal sonographic cervical length over time for preterm birth: A systematic review and metaanalysis. *American Journal of Obstetrics & Gynecology, 213*(6), 789–801. doi:10.1016/j.ajog.2015.06.015

Cox, A., & Wainwright, L. (2015). The experience of parents who lose a baby of a multiple birth during the neonatal period—A literature review. *Journal of Neonatal Nursing, 21*(3), 104–113. doi:10.1016/j.jnn.2014.11.003

Cristinelli, S., Fresson, J., André, M., & Monnier-Barbarino, P. (2005). Management of delayed-interval delivery in multiple gestations. *Fetal Diagnosis and Therapy, 20*(4), 285–290. doi:10.1159/000085087

Crowther, C. A., Hiller, J. E., Doyle, L. W., & Haslam, R. R. (2003). Effect of magnesium sulfate given for neuroprotection before preterm birth: A randomized controlled trial. *JAMA, 290*(20), 2669–2676. doi:10.1001/jama.290.20.2669

Damato, E. G. (2004a). Predictors of prenatal attachment in mothers of twins. *Journal of Obstetric, Gynecologic, and Neonatal Nursing, 33*(4), 436–445. doi:10.1177/0884217504266894

Damato, E. G. (2004b). Prenatal attachment and other correlates of postnatal maternal attachment to twins. *Advances in Neonatal Care, 4*(5), 274–291. doi:10.1016/j.adnc.2004.07.005

Damato, E. G., Anthony, M. K., & Maloni, J. A. (2009). Correlates of negative and positive mood state in mothers of twins. *Journal of Pediatric Nursing, 24*(5), 369–377. doi:10.1016/j.pedn.2008.05.003

Damato, E. G., Brubaker, J. A., & Burant, C. (2012). Sleeping arrangements in families with twins. *Newborn and Infant Nursing Reviews, 12*(3), 171–178. doi:10.1053/j.nainr.2012.06.001

Damato, E. G., Dowling, D. A., Madigan, E. A., & Thanattherakul, C. (2005). Duration of breastfeeding for mothers of twins. *Journal of Obstetric, Gynecologic, and Neonatal Nursing, 34*(2), 201–209.

Damato, E. G., Dowling, D. A., Standing, T. S., & Schuster, S. D. (2005). Explanation for cessation of breastfeeding in mothers of twins. *Journal of Human Lactation, 21*(3), 296–304. doi:10.1177/0890334405277501

Damato, E. G., Haas, M. C., Czeck, P., Dowling, D. A., & Barsman, S. G. (2016). Safe sleep infant care practices reported by mothers of twins. *Advances in Neonatal Care, 16*(6), E3–E14. doi:10.1097/anc.0000000000000332

D'Antonio, F., Odibo, A. O., Prefumo, F., Khalil, A., Buca, D., Flacco, M. E., . . . Acharya, G. (2018). Weight discordance and perinatal mortality in twin pregnancy: Systematic review and meta-analysis. *Ultrasound in Obstetrics & Gynecology. 2018, 52*, 11–23. doi:10.1002/uog.18966

D'Antonio, F., Thilaganathan, B., Laoreti, A., & Khalil, A. (2018). Birth-weight discordance and neonatal morbidity in twin pregnancies: Analysis of the STORK multiple pregnancy cohort. *Ultrasound in Obstetrics & Gynecology, 52*(5), 586–592. doi:10.1002/uog.18916

da Silva Lopes, K., Takemoto, Y., Ota, E., Tanigaki, S., & Mori, R. (2017). Bed rest with and without hospitalisation in multiple pregnancy for improving perinatal outcomes. *Cochrane Database of Systematic Reviews, (3),* CD012031. doi:10.1002/14651858.cd012031.pub2

Derom, R., Derom, C., & Vlietinck, R. (1995). Placentation. In L. G. Keith, E. Papiernik, D. M. Keith, & B. Luke (Eds.), *Multiple pregnancy: Epidemiology, gestation and perinatal outcome* (pp. 113–128). New York, NY: The Parthenon.

Dickey, R. P., Taylor, S. N., Lu, P. Y., Sartor, B. M., Storment, J. M., Rye, P. H., . . . Matulich, E. M. (2002). Spontaneous reduction of multiple pregnancy: Incidence and effect on outcome. *American Journal of Obstetrics & Gynecology, 186*(1), 77–83. doi:10.1067/mob.2002.118915

Dodd, J. M., & Crowther, C. A. (2005). Evidence-based care of women with a multiple pregnancy. *Best Practice & Research. Clinical Obstetrics & Gynaecology, 19*(1), 131–153. doi:10.1016/j.bpobgyn.2004.11.004

Dodd, J. M., Deussen, A. R., Grivell, R. M., & Crowther, C. A. (2014). Elective birth at 37 weeks' gestation for women with an uncomplicated twin pregnancy. *Cochrane Database of Systematic Reviews, (2),* CD003582. doi:10.1002/14651858.cd003582.pub2

Dodd, J. M., Dowswell, T., & Crowther, C. A. (2015a). Reduction of the number of fetuses for women with a multiple pregnancy. *Cochrane Database of Systematic Reviews, (11),* CD003932. doi:10.1002/14651858.cd003932.pub3

Dodd, J. M., Dowswell, T., & Crowther, C. A. (2015b). Specialised antenatal clinics for women with a multiple pregnancy for improving maternal and infant outcomes. *Cochrane Database of Systematic Reviews*, (11), CD005300. doi:10.1002/14651858 .cd005300.pub4

Drugan, A., & Weissman, A. (2017). Multi-fetal pregnancy reduction (MFPR) to twins or singleton—Medical justification and ethical slippery slope. *Journal of Perinatal Medicine*, 45(2), 181–184. doi:10.1515/jpm-2016-0058

Dypvik, J., Pereira, A. L., Tanbo, T. G., & Eskild, A. (2018). Maternal human chorionic gonadotrophin concentrations in very early pregnancy and risk of hyperemesis gravidarum: A retrospective cohort study of 4372 pregnancies after in vitro fertilization. *European Journal of Obstetrics, Gynecology, and Reproductive Biology*, 221, 12–16. doi:10.1016/j .ejogrb.2017.12.015

Eddib, A., Penvose-Yi, J., Shelton, J. A., & Yeh, J. (2007). Triplet gestation outcomes in relation to maternal prepregnancy body mass index and weight gain. *The Journal of Maternal-Fetal & Neonatal Medicine*, 20(7), 515–519. doi:10.1080/14767050701436247

Eganhouse, D. J., & Petersen, L. A. (1998). Fetal surveillance in multifetal pregnancy. *Journal of Obstetric, Gynecologic, and Neonatal Nursing*, 27(3), 312–321. doi:10.1111/j.1552-6909.1998 .tb02654.x

Elkayam, U., Akhter, M. W., Singh, H., Khan, S., Bitar, F., Hameed, A., & Shotan, A. (2005). Pregnancy-associated cardiomyopathy: Clinical characteristics and a comparison between early and late presentation. *Circulation*, 111(16), 2050–2055. doi:10.1161/01.CIR.0000162478.36652.7E

Elliott, J. P. (2005a). Management of high-order multiple gestations. *Clinics in Perinatology*, 32(2), 387–402. doi:10.1016/j.clp .2005.04.001

Elliott, J. P. (2005b). Preterm labor in twins and high-order multiples. *Obstetrics and Gynecology Clinics of North America*, 32(3), 429–439. doi:10.1016/j.ogc.2005.04.003

Elliott, J. P., & Radin, T. G. (1995). The effect of corticosteroid administration on uterine activity and preterm labor in high-order multiple gestations. *Obstetrics & Gynecology*, 85(2), 250–254. doi:10.1016/0029-7844(94)00355-H

Ellison, M. A., & Hall, J. E. (2003). Social stigma and compounded losses: Quality-of-life issues for multiple-birth families. *Fertility and Sterility*, 80(2), 405–414. doi:10.1016/S0015-0282 (03)00659-9

Ellison, M. A., Hotamisligil, S., Lee, H., Rich-Edwards, J. W., Pang, S. C., & Hall, J. E. (2005). Psychosocial risks associated with multiple births resulting from assisted reproduction. *Fertility and Sterility*, 83(5), 1422–1428. doi:10.1016/j.fertnstert .2004.11.053

Ersbøll, A. S., Damm, P., Gustafsson, F., Vejlstrup, N. G., & Johansen, M. (2016). Peripartum cardiomyopathy: A systematic literature review. *Acta Obstetricia et Gynecologica Scandinavica*, 95(11), 1205–1219. doi:10.1111/aogs.13005

Evans, M. I., Andriole, S., & Britt, D. W. (2014). Fetal reduction: 25 Years' experience. *Fetal Diagnosis and Therapy*, 35(2), 69–82. doi:10.1159/000357974

Fang, H. C., Liu, C. Y., Day, H. L., Chen, C. P., & Gau, M. L. (2011). Uncertainty, stress, and birth outcomes in non-hospitalized, high-risk pregnancy women: The effectiveness of health consultation. *Journal of Nursing and Healthcare Research*, 7, 3–13. doi:10.1177/105477389600500306

Feldman, D. M., Borgida, A. F., Trymbulak, W. P., Barsoom, M. J., Sanders, M. M., & Rodis, J. F. (2002). Clinical implications of velamentous cord insertion in triplet gestations. *American Journal of Obstetrics and Gynecology*, 186(4), 809–811. doi:10.1067/mob.2002.121653

Feldman, R., & Eidelman, A. I. (2004). Parent-infant synchrony and the social-emotional development of triplets. *Developmental Psychology*, 40(6), 1133–1147. doi:10.1037/0012-1649.40.6.1133

Fell, D. B., Dodds, L., Joseph, K. S., Allen, V. M., & Butler, B. (2006). Risk factors for hyperemesis gravidarum requiring hospital admission during pregnancy. *Obstetrics & Gynecology*, 107(2, Pt. 1), 277–284. doi:10.1097/01.AOG.0000195059.82029.74

Fesenmeier, M. F., Coppage, K. H., Lambers, D. S., Barton, J. R., & Sibai, B. M. (2005). Acute fatty liver of pregnancy in 3 tertiary care centers. *American Journal of Obstetrics & Gynecology*, 192(5), 1416–1419. doi:10.1016/j.ajog.2004.12.035

Fichera, A., Pagani, G., Stagnati, V., Cascella, S., Faiola, S., Gaini, C., . . . Prefumo, F. (2018). Cervical-length measurement at mid-gestation to predict spontaneous preterm birth in asymptomatic triplet pregnancies. *Ultrasound in Obstetrics & Gynecology*, 51(5), 614–620. doi:10.1002/uog.17464

Fox, N. S., Gupta, S., Lam-Rachlin, J., Rebarber, A., Klauser, C. K., & Saltzman, D. H. (2016). Cervical pessary and vaginal progesterone in twin pregnancies with a short cervix. *Obstetrics & Gynecology*, 127(4), 625–630. doi:10.1097 /AOG.0000000000001300

Fox, N. S., Rebarber, A., Roman, A. S., Klauser, C. K., Peress, D., & Saltzman, D. H. (2010). Weight gain in twin pregnancies and adverse outcomes: Examining the 2009 Institute of Medicine guidelines. *Obstetrics & Gynecology*, 116(1), 100–106. doi:10.1097/AOG.0b013e3181e24afc

Fox, N. S., Saltzman, D. H., Klauser, C. K., Peress, D., Gutierrez, C. V., & Rebarber, A. (2009). Prediction of spontaneous preterm birth in asymptomatic twin pregnancies with the use of combined fetal fibronectin and cervical length. *American Journal of Obstetrics & Gynecology*, 201(3), 313.e1–313.e5. doi:10.1016 /j.ajog.2009.06.018

Fox, N. S., Saltzman, D. H., Kurtz, H., & Rebarber, A. (2011). Excessive weight gain in term twin pregnancies: Examining the 2009 Institute of Medicine definitions. *Obstetrics & Gynecology*, 118(5), 1000–1004. doi:10.1097/AOG.0b013e318232125d

Francois, K., Ortiz, J., Harris, C., Foley, M. R., & Elliott, J. P. (2005). Is peripartum hysterectomy more common in multiple gestations? *Obstetrics & Gynecology*, 105(6), 1369–1372. doi:10.1097/01.AOG.0000161311.31894.31

Frates, M. (2018). Multifetal pregnancy. In C. M. Rumack & D. Levine (Eds.), *Diagnostic ultrasound* (5th ed., pp. 1115–1132). Philadelphia, PA: Elsevier.

Freda, M. C. (2000). Educational interventions in high-risk pregnancy. In W. R. Cohen (Ed.), *Cherry and Merkatz's complications of pregnancy* (pp. 177–184). Philadelphia, PA: Lippincott Williams & Wilkins.

Friedman, E. A., & Sachtleben, M. R. (1964). The effect of uterine overdistention on labor. I. Multiple pregnancy. *Obstetrics & Gynecology*, 23, 164–172.

Gabzdyl, E. M., & Schlaeger, J. M. (2015). Intrahepatic cholestasis of pregnancy: A critical clinical review. *The Journal of Perinatal & Neonatal Nursing*, 29(1), 41–50. doi:10.1097/jpn .0000000000000077

Garite, T. J., Clark, R. H., Elliott, J. P., & Thorp, J. A. (2004). Twins and triplets: The effect of plurality and growth on neonatal outcome compared with singleton infants. *American Journal of Obstetrics & Gynecology*, 191(3), 700–707. doi:10.1016 /j.ajog.2004.03.040

Goldenberg, R. L., Iams, J. D., Miodovnik, M., Van Dorsten, J. P., Thurnau, G., Bottoms, S., . . . McNellis, D. (1996). The preterm prediction study: Risk factors in twin gestations. National Institute of Child Health and Human Development Maternal-Fetal Medicine Units Network. *American Journal of Obstetrics & Gynecology*, 175(4, Pt. 1), 1047–1053. doi:10.1016/s0002 -9378(96)80051-2

Goodnight, W., & Newman, R. (2009). Optimal nutrition for improved twin pregnancy outcome. *Obstetrics & Gynecology*, 114(5), 1121–1134. doi:10.1097/AOG.0b013e3181bb14c8

Gordon, M. C., McKenna, D. S., Stewart, T. L., Howard, B. C., Foster, K. F., Higby, K., . . . Barth, W. H. (2016). Transvaginal cervical length scans to prevent prematurity in twins: A randomized controlled trial. *American Journal of Obstetrics & Gynecology*, 214(2), 277.e1–277.e7. doi:10.1016/j.ajog.2015.08.065

Goya, M., de la Calle, M., Pratcorona, L., Merced, C., Rodó, C., Muñoz, B., . . . Cabero, L. (2016). Cervical pessary to prevent preterm birth in women with twin gestation and sonographic short cervix: A multicenter randomized controlled trial (PECEP-Twins). *American Journal of Obstetrics & Gynecology*, 214(2), 145–152. doi:10.1016/j.ajog.2015.11.012

Gromada, K. K., & Bowers, N. A. (2005). *Care of the multiple-birth family: Postpartum through infancy*. New York, NY: March of Dimes.

Groothuis, J. R., Altemeier, W. A., Robarge, J. P., O'Connor, S., Sandler, H., Vietze, P., & Luztig, J. V. (1982). Increased child abuse in families with twins. *Pediatrics*, 70(5), 769–773.

Haas, M. C., Dowling, D., & Damato, E. G. (2017). Adherence to safe sleep recommendations by families with higher-order multiples. *Advances in Neonatal Care*, 17(5), 407–416. doi:10.1097/ANC.0000000000000416

Habli, M., Lim, F. Y., & Crombleholme, T. (2009). Twin-to-twin transfusion syndrome: A comprehensive update. *Clinics in Perinatology*, 36(2), 391–416. doi:10.1016/j.clp.2009.03.003

Hanson, L. (2010). Risk management in intrapartum fetal monitoring: Accidental recording of the maternal heart rate. *Journal of Perinatal & Neonatal Nursing*, 24(1), 7–9. doi:10.1097/JPN.0b013e3181cc3a95

Hardardottir, H., Kelly, K., Bork, M. D., Cusick, W., Campbell, W. A., & Rodis, J. F. (1996). Atypical presentation of preeclampsia in high-order multifetal gestations. *Obstetrics & Gynecology*, 87(3), 370–374. doi:10.1016/0002-9378(95)91130-8

Harkness, U. F., & Crombleholme, T. M. (2005). Twin-twin transfusion syndrome: Where do we go from here? *Seminars in Perinatology*, 29(5), 296–304. doi:10.1053/j.semperi.2005.10.001

Hartley, R. S., & Hitti, J. (2017). Please exit safely: Maternal and twin pair neonatal outcomes according to delivery mode when twin A is vertex. *The Journal of Maternal-Fetal & Neonatal Medicine*, 30(1), 54–59. doi:10.3109/14767058.2016.1161748

Hayward, K. M., Johnston, C. C., Campbell-Yeo, M. L., Price, S. L., Houk, S. L., Whyte, R. K., . . . Caddell, K. E. (2015). Effect of cobedding twins on coregulation, infant state, and twin safety. *Journal of Obstetric, Gynecologic, and Neonatal Nursing*, 44(2), 193–202. doi:10.1111/1552-6909.12557

Healy, A. J., & Gaddipati, S. (2005). Intrapartum management of twins: Truths and controversies. *Clinics in Perinatology*, 32(2), 455–473. doi:10.1016/j.clp.2005.02.001

Hediger, M. L., Luke, B., Gonzalez-Quintero, V. H., Martin, D., Nugent, C., Witter, F. R., . . . Newman, R. B. (2006). Fetal growth rates and the very preterm delivery of twins. *American Journal of Obstetrics & Gynecology*, 193(4), 1498–1507. doi:10.1016/j.ajog.2005.03.040

Henry, A., Lees, N., Bein, K. J., Hall, B., Lim, V., Chen, K. Q., . . . Shand, A. W. (2015). Pregnancy outcomes before and after institution of a specialised twins clinic: A retrospective cohort study. *BMC Pregnancy and Childbirth*, 15, 217. doi:10.1186/s12884-015-0654-5

Hillman, S. C., Morris, R. K., & Kilby, M. D. (2010). Single twin demise: Consequence for survivors. *Seminars in Fetal & Neonatal Medicine*, 15(6), 319–326. doi:10.1016/j.siny.2010.05.004

Hofmeyr, G. J., Barrett, J. F., & Crowther, C. A. (2015). Planned caesarean section for women with a twin pregnancy. *Cochrane Database of Systematic Reviews*, (12), CD006553. doi:10.1002/14651858.CD006553.pub3

Houlihan, C., Poon, L. C., Ciarlo, M., Kim, E., Guzman, E. R., & Nicolaides, K. H. (2016). Cervical cerclage for preterm birth prevention in twin gestation with short cervix: A retrospective cohort study. *Ultrasound in Obstetrics & Gynecology*, 48(6), 752–756. doi:10.1002/uog.15918

Huang, X., Zheng, J., Chen, M., Zhao, Y., Zhang, C., Liu, L., . . . Wang, W . (2014). Noninvasive prenatal testing of trisomies 21 and 18 by massively parallel sequencing of maternal plasma DNA in twin pregnancies. *Prenatal Diagnosis*, 34(4), 335–340. doi:10.1002/pd.4303

Hubinont, C., Lewi, L., Bernard, P., Marbaix, E., Debiève, F., & Jauniaux, E. (2015). Anomalies of the placenta and umbilical cord in twin gestations. *American Journal of Obstetrics & Gynecology*, 213(4 Suppl.), S91–S102. doi:10.1016/j.ajog.2015.06.054

Hutcheon, J. A., Platt, R. W., Abrams, B., Braxter, B. J., Eckhardt, C. L., Himes, K. P., & Bodnar, L. M. (2018). Pregnancy weight gain by gestational age in women with uncomplicated dichorionic twin pregnancies. *Paediatric and Perinatal Epidemiology*, 32(2), 172–180. doi:10.1111/ppe.12446

Hutchison, B. L., Stewart, A. W., & Mitchell, E. A. (2010). The prevalence of cobedding and SIDS-related child care practices in twins. *European Journal of Pediatrics*, 169(12), 1477–1485. doi:10.1007/s00431-010-1246-z

Ingram Cooke, R. W. (2010). Does neonatal and infant neurodevelopmental morbidity of multiples and singletons differ? *Seminars in Fetal & Neonatal Medicine*, 15(6), 362–366. doi:10.1016/j.siny.2010.06.003

Jackson, K. M., & Mele, N. L. (2009). Twin-to-twin transfusion syndrome: What nurses need to know. *Nursing for Women's Health*, 13(3), 224–233. doi:10.1111/j.1751-486X.2009.01423.x

Jarvis, M. R., & Burnett, M. (2009). Developmentally supportive care for twins and higher-order multiples in the NICU: A review of existing evidence. *Neonatal, Paediatric and Child Health Nursing*, 12, 2–5.

Jauniaux, E., Melcer, Y., & Maymon, R. (2017). Prenatal diagnosis and management of vasa previa in twin pregnancies: A case series and systematic review. *American Journal of Obstetrics & Gynecology*, 216(6), 568–575. doi:10.1016/j.ajog.2017.01.029

Johnson, C. D., & Zhang, J. (2002). Survival of other fetuses after a fetal death in twin or triplet pregnancies. *Obstetrics & Gynecology*, 99(5, Pt. 1), 698–703. doi:10.1016/S0029-7844(02)01960-9

Kahn, B., Lumey, L. H., Zybert, P. A., Lorenz, J. M., Cleary-Goldman, J., D'Alton, M. E., & Robinson, J. N. (2003). Prospective risk of fetal death in singleton, twin, and triplet gestations: Implications for practice. *Obstetrics & Gynecology*, 102(4), 685–692. doi:10.1016/S0029-7844(03)00616-1

Karami, M., Jenabi, E., & Fereidooni, B. (2018). The association of placenta previa and assisted reproductive techniques: A meta-analysis. *The Journal of Maternal-Fetal & Neonatal Medicine*, 31(14), 1940–1947. doi:10.1080/14767058.2017.1332035

Kibel, M., Barrett, J., Tward, C., Pittini, A., Kahn, M., & Melamed, N. (2017). The natural history of preterm premature rupture of membranes in twin pregnancies. *The Journal of Maternal-Fetal & Neonatal Medicine*, 30(15), 1829–1835. doi:10.1080/14767058.2016.1228052

Klein, V. R. (2002). Maternal complications. In L. G. Keith & I. Blickstein (Eds.), *Triplet pregnancies and their consequences* (pp. 215–224). New York, NY: The Parthenon.

Klock, S. C. (2001). The transition to parenthood. In I. Blickstein & L. G. Keith (Eds.), *Iatrogenic multiple pregnancy: Clinical implications* (pp. 225–234). New York, NY: The Parthenon.

Klock, S. C. (2004). Psychological adjustment to twins after infertility. *Best Practice & Research. Clinical Obstetrics & Gynaecology*, 18(4), 645–656. doi:10.1016/j.bpobgyn.2004.04.015

Knox, E., & Martin, W. (2010). Multiples clinic: A model for antenatal care. *Seminars in Fetal & Neonatal Medicine*, 15(6), 357–361. doi:10.1016/j.siny.2010.07.001

Kramer, M. S., Berg, C., Abenhaim, H., Dahhou, M., Rouleau, J., Mehrabadi, A., & Joseph, K. S. (2013). Incidence, risk factors, and temporal trends in severe postpartum hemorrhage. *American Journal of Obstetrics & Gynecology*, 209(5), 449.e1–449.e7. doi:10.1016/j.ajog.2013.07.007

Krantz, D. A., Hallahan, T., He, K., Sherwin, J., & Evans, M. I. (2011). First-trimester screening in triplets. *American Journal of Obstetrics & Gynecology*, 205(4), 364.e1–364.e5. doi:10.1016/j.ajog.2011.06.107

Kuhnly, J. E., Juliano, M., & McLarney, P. S. (2015). The development and implementation of a prenatal education program for expectant parents of multiples. *The Journal of Perinatal Education*, 24(2), 110–118. doi:10.1891/1946-6560.24.2.110

Kuleva, M., Youssef, A., Maroni, E., Contro, E., Pilu, G., Rizzo, N., . . . Ghi, T. (2011). Maternal cardiac function in normal twin pregnancy: A longitudinal study. *Ultrasound in Obstetrics & Gynecology*, 38(5), 575–580. doi:10.1002/uog.8936

Kumar, S., Paramasivam, G., Zhang, E., Jones, B., Noori, M., Prior, T., . . . Wimalasundera, R. C. (2014). Perinatal- and procedure-related outcomes following radiofrequency ablation in monochorionic pregnancy. *American Journal of Obstetrics & Gynecology*, 210(5), 454.e1–454.e6. doi:10.1016/j.ajog.2013.12.009

Lai, N. M., Foong, S. C., Foong, W. C., & Tan, K. (2016). Co-bedding in neonatal nursery for promoting growth and neurodevelopment in stable preterm twins. *Cochrane Database of Systematic Reviews*, (4), CD008313. doi:10.1002/14651858.CD008313.pub3

Lal, A. K., & Kominiarek, M. A. (2015). Weight gain in twin gestations: Are the Institute of Medicine guidelines optimal for neonatal outcomes? *Journal of Perinatology*, 35(6), 405–410. doi:10.1038/jp.2014.237

Lam, F., & Gill, P. (2005a). Beta-agonist tocolytic therapy. *Obstetrics and Gynecology Clinics of North America*, 32(3), 457–484. doi:10.1016/j.ogc.2005.05.001

Lam, F., & Gill, P. (2005b). Inhibition of preterm labor and subcutaneous terbutaline therapy. In I. Blickstein & L. G. Keith (Eds.), *Multiple pregnancy: Epidemiology, gestation, and perinatal outcome* (2nd ed., pp. 601–620). New York, NY: CRC Press.

Landy, H. J., Weiner, S., Corson, S. L., Batzer, F. R., & Bolognese, R. J. (1986). The "vanishing twin": Ultrasonographic assessment of fetal disappearance in the first trimester. *American Journal of Obstetrics & Gynecology*, 155(1), 14–19. doi:10.1016/0002-9378(86)90068-2

Lang, C. A., Cox, M. J., & Flores, G. (2013). Maltreatment in multiple-birth children. *Child Abuse & Neglect*, 37(12), 1109–1113. doi:10.1016/j.chiabu.2013.03.002

Langkamp, D. L., & Girardet, R. G. (2006). Primary care for twins and higher order multiples. *Current Problems in Pediatric and Adolescent Health Care*, 36(2), 47–67. doi:10.1016/j.cppeds.2005.10.005

Lappen, J. R., Hackney, D. N., & Bailit, J. L. (2016). Maternal and neonatal outcomes of attempted vaginal compared with planned cesarean delivery in triplet gestations. *American Journal of Obstetrics & Gynecology*, 215(4), 493.e1–493.e6. doi:10.1016/j.ajog.2016.04.054

Le Conte, G., Letourneau, A., Jani, J., Kleinfinger, P., Lohmann, L., Costa, J.-M., & Benachi, A. (2018). Cell-free fetal DNA analysis in maternal plasma as screening test for trisomies 21, 18 and 13 in twin pregnancy. *Ultrasound in Obstetrics & Gynecology*, 52(3), 318–324. doi:10.1002/uog.18838

Lee, H., Bebbington, M., & Crombleholme, T. M. (2013). The North American Fetal Therapy Network registry data on outcomes of radiofrequency ablation for twin-reversed arterial perfusion sequence. *Fetal Diagnosis and Therapy*, 33(4), 224–229. doi:10.1159/000343223

Lee, K. E. (2012). Critical review of the literature: Parental grief after the loss of a multiple. *Journal of Neonatal Nursing*, 18(6), 226–231. doi:10.1016/j.jnn.2011.12.002

Legrand, A., Frondas, A., Aubret, F., Corre, A., Flamant, C., Simon, L., . . . Rozé, J.-C. (2017). Randomised controlled trial shows that co-bedding twins may reduce birthweight recovery delay, parenteral nutrition weaning time and hospitalisation. *Acta Paediatrica (Oslo, Norway: 1992)*, 106(12), 2055–2059. doi:10.1111/apa.13885

Leonard, L. G. (1998). Depression and anxiety disorders during multiple pregnancy and parenthood. *Journal of Obstetric, Gynecologic, and Neonatal Nursing*, 27(3), 329–337. doi:10.1111/j.1552-6909.1998.tb02656.x

Leonard, L. G. (2002). Prenatal behavior of multiples: Implications for families and nurses. *Journal of Obstetric, Gynecologic, and Neonatal Nursing*, 31(3), 248–255. doi:10.1111/j.1552-6909.2002.tb00046.x

Leonard, L. G., & Denton, J. (2006). Preparation for parenting multiple birth children. *Early Human Development*, 82(6), 371–378. doi:10.1016/j.earlhumdev.2006.03.009

Lewi, L., Gucciardo, L., Van Mieghem, T., de Koninck, P., Beck, V., Medek, H., . . . Deprest, J. (2010). Monochorionic diamniotic twin pregnancies: Natural history and risk stratification. *Fetal Diagnosis and Therapy*, 27(3), 121–133. doi:10.1159/000313300

Liem, S., Schuit, E., Hegeman, M., Bais, J., de Boer, K., Bloemenkamp, K., . . . Bekedam, D. (2013). Cervical pessaries for prevention of preterm birth in women with a multiple pregnancy (ProTWIN): A multicentre, open-label randomised controlled trial. *Lancet (London, England)*, 382(9901), 1341–1349. doi:10.1016/S0140-6736(13)61408-7

Lim, A. C., Schuit, E., Bloemenkamp, K., Bernardus, R. E., Duvekot, J. J., Erwich, J. J., . . . Bruinse, H. W. (2011). 17α-hydroxyprogesterone caproate for the prevention of adverse neonatal outcome in multiple pregnancies. *Obstetrics & Gynecology*, 118(3), 513–520. doi:10.1097/AOG.0b013e31822ad6aa

Lin, H., Wen, Y., Li, Y., Chen, X., Yang, D., & Zhang, Q. (2016). Early fetal reduction of dichorionic triplets to dichorionic twin or singleton pregnancies: A retrospective study. *Reproductive Biomedicine Online*, 32(5), 490–495. doi:10.1016/j.rbmo.2016.02.011

Little, C. M. (2010). Nursing considerations in the case of multifetal pregnancy reduction. *MCN: The American Journal of Maternal Child Nursing*, 35(3), 166–171. doi:10.1097/NMC.0b013e3181d765bc

Ludington-Hoe, S. M., Lewis, T., Morgan, K., Cong, X., Anderson, L., & Reese, S. (2006). Breast and infant temperatures with twins during shared kangaroo care. *Journal of Obstetric, Gynecologic, and Neonatal Nursing*, 35(2), 223–231. doi:10.1111/j.1552-6909.2006.00024.x

Luke, B. (2004). Improving multiple pregnancy outcomes with nutritional interventions. *Clinical Obstetrics and Gynecology*, 47, 146–162. doi:10.1097/00003081-200403000-00018

Luke, B. (2005). Nutrition and multiple gestation. *Seminars in Perinatology*, 29(5), 349–354. doi:10.1053/j.semperi.2005.08.004

Luke, B. (2015). Nutrition for multiples. *Clinical Obstetrics and Gynecology*, 58(3), 585–610. doi:10.1097/GRF.0000000000000117

Luke, B. (2017). Pregnancy and birth outcomes in couples with infertility with and without assisted reproductive technology: With an emphasis on US population-based studies. *American Journal of Obstetrics & Gynecology*, 217(3), 270–281. doi:10.1016/j.ajog.2017.03.012

Luke, B., & Brown, M. B. (2007). Contemporary risks of maternal morbidity and adverse outcomes with increasing maternal age and plurality. *Fertility and Sterility*, 88(2), 283–293. doi:10.1016/j.fertnstert.2006.11.008

Luke, B., Brown, M. B., Misiunas, R., Anderson, E., Nugent, C., van de Ven, C., . . . Gogliotti, S. (2003). Specialized prenatal care and maternal and infant outcomes in twin pregnancy. *American Journal of Obstetrics & Gynecology*, 189(4), 934–938. doi:10.1067/s0002-9378(03)01054-8

Luke, B., Gopal, D., Cabral, H., Stern, J. E., & Diop, H. (2017). Adverse pregnancy, birth, and infant outcomes in twins: effects of maternal fertility status and infant gender combinations; the Massachusetts outcomes study of assisted reproductive technology. *American Journal of Obstetrics & Gynecology*, 217(3), 330.e1–330.e15. doi:10.1016/j.ajog.2017.04.025

Lutsiv, O., Hulman, A., Woolcott, C., Beyene, J., Giglia, L., Armson, B. A., . . . McDonald, S. D. (2017). Examining the provisional guidelines for weight gain in twin pregnancies: A retrospective cohort study. *BMC Pregnancy and Childbirth, 17*(1), 330. doi:10.1186/s12884-017-1530-2

MacKay, A. P., Berg, C. J., King, J. C., Duran, C., & Chang, J. (2006). Pregnancy-related mortality among women with multifetal pregnancies. *Obstetrics & Gynecology, 107*(3), 563–568. doi:10.1097/01.AOG.0000200045.91015.c6

Maifeld, M., Hahn, S., Titler, M. G., & Mullen, M. (2003). Decision making regarding multifetal reduction. *Journal of Obstetric, Gynecologic, and Neonatal Nursing, 32*(3), 357–369. doi:10.1177/0884217503253493

Malmstrom, P. M., & Biale, R. (1990). An agenda for meeting the special needs of multiple birth families. *Acta Geneticae Medicae et Gemellologiae, 39*(4), 507–514. doi:10.1017/S0001566000003755

Malone, F. D., & D'Alton, M. E. (2014). Multiple gestation: Clinical characteristics and management. In A. H. Jobe & B. D. Kamath-Rayne (Eds.), *Creasy and Resnik's maternal-fetal medicine: Principles and practice* (7th ed., pp. 578–596). Philadelphia, PA: Elsevier.

Maloni, J. A. (2010). Antepartum bed rest for pregnancy complications: Efficacy and safety for preventing preterm birth. *Biological Research for Nursing, 12*(2), 106–124. doi:10.1177/1099800410375978

Maloni, J. A. (2011). Lack of evidence for prescription of antepartum bed rest. *Expert Review of Obstetrics & Gynecology, 6*(4), 385–393. doi:10.1586/eog.11.28

Maloni, J. A., Brezinski-Tomasi, J. E., & Johnson, L. A. (2001). Antepartum bedrest: Effect upon the family. *Journal of Obstetric, Gynecologic, and Neonatal Nursing, 30*(2), 165–173. doi:10.1111/j.1552-6909.2001.tb01532.x

Maloni, J. A., Margevicius, S. P., & Damato, E. G. (2006). Multiple gestations: Side effects of antepartum bed rest. *Biological Research for Nursing, 8*(2), 115–128. doi:10.1177/1099800406291455

Maloni, J. A., & Schneider, B. S. (2002). Inactivity: Symptoms associated with gastrocnemius muscle disuse during pregnancy. *AACN Clinical Issues, 13*(2), 248–262. doi:10.1097/00044067-200205000-00010

Marino, T., Goudas, L. C., Steinbok, V., Craigo, S. D., & Yarnell, R. W. (2001). The anesthetic management of triplet cesarean delivery: A retrospective case series of maternal outcomes. *Anesthesia and Analgesia, 93*(4), 991–995. doi:10.1097/00000539-200110000-00039

Marret, S., Marpeau, L., Zupan-Simunek, V., Eurin, D., Lévêque, C., Hellot, M.-F., & Bénichou, J. (2006). Magnesium sulphate given before very-preterm birth to protect infant brain: The randomised controlled PREMAG trial. *BJOG, 114*(3), 310–318. doi:10.1111/j.1471-0528.2006.01162.x

Martin, J. A., Hamilton, B. E., Osterman, M. J. K., Driscoll, A. K., & Drake, P. (2018). Births: Final data for 2017. *National Vital Statistics Reports, 67*(8), 1–50.

Martin, J. A., Hamilton, B. E., Osterman, M. J. K., Driscoll, A. K., & Mathews, T. J. (2017). Births: Final data for 2015. *National Vital Statistics Reports, 66*(1), 1–70.

Martin, J. A., & Park, M. M. (1999). Trends in twin and triplet births: 1980–97. *National Vital Statistics Reports, 47*(24), 1–16.

Martin, J. A., & Osterman, M. J. K. (2019). *Is twin childbearing on the decline? Twin births in the United States, 2014–2018* (NCHS Data Brief No. 351). Hyattsville, MD: National Center for Health Statistics.

Mathews, T. J., MacDorman, M. F., & Thoma, M. (2015). Infant mortality statistics from the 2013 period linked birth/infant death data set. *National Vital Statistics Reports, 64*(9), 1–30.

Matthews, K. C., Gupta, S., Lam-Rachlin, J., Saltzman, D. H., Rebarber, A., & Fox, N. S. (2018). The association between fetal fibronectin and spontaneous preterm birth in twin pregnancies with a shortened cervical length. *The Journal of Maternal-Fetal & Neonatal Medicine, 31*(19), 2564–2568. doi:10.1080/14767058.2017.1347627

Maymon, R., Neeman, O., Shulman, A., Rosen, H., & Herman, A. (2005). Current concepts of Down syndrome screening tests in assisted reproduction twin pregnancies: Another double trouble. *Prenatal Diagnosis, 25*(9), 746–750. doi:10.1002/pd.1259

McGrail, C., & Bryant, D. (2005). Intertwin time interval: How it affects the immediate neonatal outcome of the second twin. *American Journal of Obstetrics & Gynecology, 192*(5), 1420–1422. doi:10.1016/j.ajog.2005.02.079

McGrath, J. M., Samra, H. A., Zukowsky, K., & Baker, B. (2010). Parenting after infertility: Issues for families and infants. *MCN: The American Journal of Maternal Child Nursing, 35*(3), 156–164. doi:10.1097/NMC.0b013e3181d7657d

McGrath, R. T., Hocking, S. L., Scott, E. S., Seeho, S. K., Fulcher, G. R., & Glastras, S. J. (2017). Outcomes of twin pregnancies complicated by gestational diabetes: A meta-analysis of observational studies. *Journal of Perinatology, 37*(4), 360–368. doi:10.1038/jp.2016.254

Medoff-Cooper, B., Bakewell-Sachs, S., Buus-Frank, M. E., & Santa-Donato, A. (2005). The AWHONN Near-Term Infant Initiative: A conceptual framework for optimizing health for near-term infants. *Journal of Obstetric, Gynecologic, and Neonatal Nursing, 34*(6), 666–671. doi:10.1177/0884217505281873

Mei, Y., Gao, L., Lin, Y., Luo, D., Zhou, X., & He, L. (2019). Predictors of adverse perinatal outcomes in intrahepatic cholestasis of pregnancy with dichorionic diamniotic twin pregnancies. *The Journal of Maternal-Fetal & Neonatal Medicine, 32*(3), 472–476. doi:10.1080/14767058.2017.1384461

Melamed, N., Shah, J., Yoon, E. W., Pelausa, E., Lee, S. K., Shah, P. S., & Murphy, K. E. (2016). The role of antenatal corticosteroids in twin pregnancies complicated by preterm birth. *American Journal of Obstetrics & Gynecology, 215*(4), 482.e1–482.e9. doi:10.1016/j.ajog.2016.05.037

Mersereau, J., Stanhiser, J., Coddington, C., Jones, T., Luke, B., & Brown, M. B. (2017). Patient and cycle characteristics predicting high pregnancy rates with single-embryo transfer: An analysis of the Society for Assisted Reproductive Technology outcomes between 2004 and 2013. *Fertility and Sterility, 108*(5), 750–756. doi:10.1016/j.fertnstert.2017.07.1167

Mian, A. I. (2005). Depression in pregnancy and the postpartum period: Balancing adverse effects of untreated illness with treatment risks. *Journal of Psychiatric Practice, 11*(6), 389–396.

Moon, R. Y. (2016). SIDS and other sleep-related infant deaths: Evidence base for 2016 updated recommendations for a safe infant sleeping environment. *Pediatrics, 138*(5), e20162940. doi:10.1542/peds.2016-2940

Morrison, J. C., & Chauhan, S. P. (2003). Current status of home uterine activity monitoring. *Clinics in Perinatology, 30*(4), 757–801. doi:10.1016/S0095-5108(03)00112-X

Morton, J., Hall, J. Y., Wong, R. J., Thairu, L., Benitz, W. E., & Rhine, W. D. (2009). Combining hand techniques with electric pumping increases milk production in mothers of preterm infants. *Journal of Perinatology, 29*(11), 757–764. doi:10.1038/jp.2009.87

Mutchinick, O. M., Luna-Muñoz, L., Amar, E., Bakker, M. K., Clementi, M., Cocchi, G., . . . Arteaga-Vázquez, J. (2011). Conjoined twins: A worldwide collaborative epidemiological study of the International Clearinghouse for Birth Defects Surveillance and Research. *American Journal of Medical Genetics. Part C, Seminars in Medical Genetics, 157*(4), 274–287. doi:10.1002/ajmg.c.30321

National Association of Neonatal Nurses. (2012). Cobedding of twins or higher-order multiples (Position Statement No. 3053). *Advances in Neonatal Care, 2012, 12*(1), 61–67.

Newman, R. B., Iams, J. D., Das, A., Goldenberg, R. L., Meis, P., Moawad, A., . . . Fischer, M. (2006). A prospective masked observational study of uterine contraction frequency in twins. *American Journal of Obstetrics & Gynecology, 195*(6), 1564–1570. doi:10.1016/j.ajog.2006.03.063

Newman, R. B., & Unal, E. R. (2017). Multiple gestation. In S. G. Gabbe, J. R. Niebyl, J. L. Simpson, M .B. Landon, H. L. Galan, E. R. M. Jauniaux, . . . W. A. Grobman (Eds.), *Obstetrics: Normal and problem pregnancies* (7th ed., pp. 706–736). Philadelphia, PA: Elsevier.

Nicolaides, K. H., Syngelaki, A., Poon, L. C., de Paco Matallana, C., Plasencia, W., Molina, F. S., . . . Conturso, R. (2016). Cervical pessary placement for prevention of preterm birth in unselected twin pregnancies: A randomized controlled trial. *American Journal of Obstetrics & Gynecology, 214*(1), 3.e1–3.e9. doi:10.1016/j.ajog.2015.08.051

Norwitz, E. R., Edusa, V., & Park, J. S. (2005). Maternal physiology and complications of multiple pregnancy. *Seminars in Perinatology, 29*(5), 338–348. doi:10.1053/j.semperi.2005.08.002

Običan, S., Brock, C., Berkowitz, R., & Wapner, R. J. (2015). Multifetal pregnancy reduction. *Clinical Obstetrics and Gynecology, 58*(3), 574–584. doi:10.1097/GRF.0000000000000119

O'Callaghan, M. E., MacLennan, A. H., Gibson, C. S., McMichael, G. L., Haan, E. A., Broadbent, J. L., . . . Dekker, G. A. (2011). Epidemiologic associations with cerebral palsy. *Obstetrics & Gynecology, 118*(3), 576–582. doi:10.1097/AOG.0b013e31822ad2dc

Ong, S. S., Zamora, J., Khan, K. S., & Kilby, M. D. (2006). Prognosis for the co-twin following single-twin death: A systematic review. *BJOG, 113*(9), 992–998. doi:10.1111/j.1471-0528.2006.01027.x

Ostfeld, B. M., Smith, R. H., Hiatt, M., & Hegyi, T. (2000). Maternal behavior toward premature twins: Implications for development. *Twin Research, 3*(4), 234–241. doi:10.1375/136905200320565201

Oyelese, Y., Ananth, C. V., Smulian, J. C., & Vintzileos, A. M. (2005). Delayed interval delivery in twin pregnancies in the United States: Impact on perinatal mortality and morbidity. *American Journal of Obstetrics & Gynecology, 192*(2), 439–444. doi:10.1016/j.ajog.2004.07.055

Palas, D., Ehlinger, V., Alberge, C., Truffert, P., Kayem, G., Goffinet, F., . . . Vayssière, C. (2018). Efficacy of antenatal corticosteroids in preterm twins: The EPIPAGE-2 cohort study. *BJOG, 125*(9), 1164–1170. doi:10.1111/1471-0528.15014

Parker, L. A., Sullivan, S., Krueger, C., Kelechi, T., & Mueller, M. (2012). Effect of early breast milk expression on milk volume and timing of lactogenesis stage II among mothers of very low birth weight infants: A pilot study. *Journal of Perinatology, 32*(3), 205–209. doi:10.1038/jp.2011.78

Parker, L. A., Sullivan, S., Krueger, C., & Mueller, M. (2015). Association of timing of initiation of breastmilk expression on milk volume and timing of lactogenesis stage II among mothers of very low-birth-weight infants. *Breastfeeding Medicine, 10*(2), 84–91. doi:10.1089/bfm.2014.0089

Pector, E. A. (2004). How bereaved multiple-birth parents cope with hospitalization, homecoming, disposition for deceased, and attachment to survivors. *Journal of Perinatology, 24*(11), 714–722. doi:10.1038/sj.jp.7211170

Pector, E. A., & Smith-Levitin, M. (2002). Mourning and psychological issues in multiple birth loss. *Seminars in Neonatology, 7*(3), 247–256. doi:10.1053/siny.2002.0112

Peitsch, W. K., Keefer, C. H., LaBrie, R. A., & Mulliken, J. B. (2002). Incidence of cranial asymmetry in healthy newborns. *Pediatrics, 110*(6), e72. doi:10.1542/peds.110.6.e72

Perinatal Services British Columbia. (2007). *Nutrition: Part III. Breastfeeding multiples.* Vancouver, BC, Canada: Author.

Pharoah, P. O. (2002). Neurological outcome on twins. *Seminars in Neonatology, 7*(3), 223–230. doi:10.1053/siny.2002.0109

Pisoni, C., Garofoli, F., Tzialla, C., Orcesi, S., Spinillo, A., Politi, P., . . . Stronati, M. (2016). Complexity of parental prenatal attachment during pregnancy at risk for preterm delivery. *The Journal of Maternal-Fetal & Neonatal Medicine, 29*(5), 771–776. doi:10.3109/14767058.2015.1017813

Quintero, R., Morales, W., Allen, M., Bornick, P. W., Johnson, P. K., & Kruger, M. (1999). Staging of twin-twin transfusion syndrome. *Journal of Perinatology, 19*(8, Pt. 1), 550–555. doi:10.1038/sj.jp.7200292

Rafael, T. J., Berghella, V., & Alfirevic, Z. (2014). Cervical stitch (cerclage) for preventing preterm birth in multiple pregnancy. *Cochrane Database of Systematic Reviews,* (9), CD00916. doi:10.1002/14651858.CD009166.pub2

Ramsey, P. S., & Repke, J. T. (2003). Intrapartum management of multifetal pregnancies. *Seminars in Perinatology, 27*(1), 54–72. doi:10.1053/sper.2003.50009

Rand, L., Eddleman, K. A., & Stone, J. (2005). Long-term outcomes in multiple gestations. *Clinics in Perinatology, 32*(2), 495–513. doi:10.1016/j.clp.2005.03.002

Rao, A., Sairam, S., & Shehata, H. (2004). Obstetric complications of twin pregnancies. *Best Practice & Research. Clinical Obstetrics & Gynaecology, 18*(4), 557–576. doi:10.1016/j.bpobgyn.2004.04.007

Rasmussen, K. M., & Yaktine, A. L. (Eds.). (2009). *Weight gain during pregnancy: Reexamining the guidelines.* Washington, DC: National Academies Press.

Reinhard, J., Reichenbach, L., Ernst, T., Reitter, A., Antwerpen, I., Herrmann, E., . . . Louwen, F. (2012). Delayed interval delivery in twin and triplet pregnancies: 6 Years of experience in one perinatal center. *Journal of Perinatal Medicine, 40*(5), 551–555. doi:10.1515/jpm-2011-0267

Richter, J. E. (2003). Gastroesophageal reflux disease during pregnancy. *Gastroenterology Clinics of North America, 32*(1), 235–261. doi:10.1016/S0889-8553(02)00065-1

Roberts, D., Brown, J., Medley, N., & Dalziel, S. R. (2017). Antenatal corticosteroids for accelerating fetal lung maturation for women at risk of preterm birth. *Cochrane Database of Systematic Reviews,* (3), CD004454. doi:10.1002/14651858.CD004454.pub3

Roberts, D., Neilson, J. P., Kilby, M. D., & Gates, S. (2014). Interventions for the treatment of twin-twin transfusion syndrome. *Cochrane Database of Systematic Reviews,* (1), CD002073. doi:10.1002/14651858.CD002073.pub3

Robinson, C., & Chauhan, S. P. (2004). Intrapartum management of twins. *Clinical Obstetrics and Gynecology, 47*(1), 248–462.

Robyr, R., Lewi, L., Salomon, L. J., Yamamoto, M., Bernard, J.-P., Deprest, J., & Ville, Y. (2006). Prevalence and management of late fetal complications following successful selective laser coagulation of chorionic plate anastomoses in twin-to-twin transfusion syndrome. *American Journal of Obstetrics and Gynecology, 194*(3), 796–803. doi:10.1016/j.ajog.2005.08.069

Roca-de Bes, M., Gutierrez-Maldonado, J., & Gris-Martínez, J. M. (2011). Comparative study of the psychosocial risks associated with families with multiple births resulting from assisted reproductive technology (ART) and without ART. *Fertility and Sterility, 96*(1), 170–174. doi:10.1016/j.fertnstert.2011.05.007

Rode, L., Klein, K., Nicolaides, K., Krampl-Bettelheim, E., & Tabor, A. (2011). Prevention of preterm delivery in twin gestations (PREDICT): A multicenter, randomized placebo-controlled trial on the effect of vaginal micronized progesterone. *Ultrasound in Obstetrics & Gynecology, 38*(3), 272–280. doi:10.1002/uog.9093

Rodrigues, P. B., Zambaldi, C. F., Cantilino, A., & Sougey, E. B. (2016). Special features of high-risk pregnancies as factors in development of mental distress: A review. *Trends in Psychiatry and Psychotherapy, 38*(3), 136–140. doi:10.1590/2237-6089-2015-0067

Roem, K. (2003). Nutritional management of multiple pregnancies. *Twin Research, 6*(6), 514–519. doi:10.1375/136905203322686518

Roman, A., Fishman, S., Fox, N., Klauser, C., Saltzman, D., & Rebarber, A. (2011). Maternal and neonatal outcomes after delayed-interval delivery of multifetal pregnancies. *American Journal of Perinatology, 28*(2), 91–96. doi:10.1055/s-0030-1262513

Roman, A., Rochelson, B., Fox, N. S., Hoffman, M., Berghella, V., Patel, V., . . . Fleischer, A. (2015). Efficacy of ultrasound-indicated cerclage in twin pregnancies. *American Journal of Obstetrics & Gynecology, 212*(6), 788.e1–788.e6. doi:10.1016/j.ajog.2015.01.031

Romero, R., Conde-Agudelo, A., El-Refaie, W., Rode, L., Brizot, M. L., Cetingoz, E., . . . Nicolaides, K. H. (2017). Vaginal progesterone decreases preterm birth and neonatal morbidity and mortality in women with a twin gestation and a short cervix: An updated meta-analysis of individual patient data. *Ultrasound in Obstetrics & Gynecology, 49*(3), 303–314. doi:10.1002/uog.17397

Roselló-Soberón, M. E., Fuentes-Chaparro, L., & Casanueva, E. (2005). Twin pregnancies: Eating for three? Maternal nutrition update. *Nutrition Reviews, 63*(9), 295–302. doi:10.1111/j.1753-4887.2005.tb00144.x

Rosen, H., Hiersch, L., Freeman, H., Barrett, J., & Melamed, N. (2017). The role of serial measurements of cervical length in asymptomatic women with triplet pregnancy. *The Journal of Maternal-Fetal & Neonatal Medicine, 31*(6), 713–719. doi:10.1080/14767058.2017.1297402

Rossi, A. C., & Prefumo, F. (2013). Impact of cord entanglement on perinatal outcome of monoamniotic twins: A systematic review of the literature. *Ultrasound in Obstetrics & Gynecology, 41*(2), 131–135. doi:10.1002/uog.12345

Rouse, D. J., Hirtz, D. G., Thom, E., Varner, M. W., Spong, C. Y., Mercer, B. M., . . . Roberts, J. M. (2008). A randomized, controlled trial of magnesium sulfate for the prevention of cerebral palsy. *The New England Journal of Medicine, 359*(9), 895–905. doi:10.1056/nejmoa0801187

Ruiz, R. J., Brown, C. E., Peters, M. T., & Johnston, A. B. (2001). Specialized care for twin gestations: Improving newborn outcomes and reducing costs. *Journal of Obstetric, Gynecologic, and Neonatal Nursing, 30*(1), 52–60. doi:10.1111/j.1552-6909.2001.tb01521.x

Rustico, M. A., Baietti, M. G., Coviello, D., Orlandi, E., & Nicolini, U. (2005). Managing twins discordant for fetal anomaly. *Prenatal Diagnosis, 25*(9), 766–771. doi:10.1002/pd.1260

Saccone, G., & Berghella, V. (2016). Planned delivery at 37 weeks in twins: A systematic review and meta-analysis of randomized controlled trials. *The Journal of Maternal-Fetal & Neonatal Medicine, 29*(5), 685–689. doi:10.3109/14767058.2015.1016423

Saccone, G., Ciardulli, A., Xodo, S., Dugoff, L., Ludmir, J., D'Antonio, F., . . . Berghella, V. (2017). Cervical pessary for preventing preterm birth in twin pregnancies with short cervical length: A systematic review and meta-analysis. *The Journal of Maternal-Fetal & Neonatal Medicine, 30*(24), 2918–2925. doi:10.1080/14767058.2016.1268595

Saccone, G., Rust, O., Althuisius, S., Roman, A., & Berghella, V. (2015). Cerclage for short cervix in twin pregnancies: Systematic review and meta-analysis of randomized trials using individual patient-level data. *Acta Obstetricia et Gynecologica Scandinavica, 94*(4), 352–358. doi:10.1111/aogs.12600

Salihu, H. M., Garces, I. C., Sharma, P. P., Kristensen, S., Ananth, C. V., & Kirby, R. S. (2005). Stillbirth and infant mortality among Hispanic singletons, twins, and triplets in the United States. *Obstetrics & Gynecology, 106*(4), 789–796. doi:10.1097/01.AOG.0000177975.61197.ae

Santana, D. S., Cecatti, J. G., Surita, F. G., Silveira, C., Costa, M. L., Souza, J. P., . . . Vogel, J. P. (2016). Twin pregnancy and severe maternal outcomes: The World Health Organization multicountry survey on maternal and newborn health. *Obstetrics & Gynecology, 127*(4), 631–641. doi:10.1097/AOG.0000000000001338

Schiff, E., Cohen, S. B., Dulitzky, M., Novikov, I., Friedman, S. A., Mashiach, S., & Lipitz, S. (1998). Progression of labor in twin versus singleton gestations. *American Journal of Obstetrics & Gynecology, 179*(5), 1181–1185. doi:10.1016/s0002-9378(98)70128-0

Schreiner-Engel, P., Walther, V. N., Mindes, J., Lynch, L., & Berkowitz, R. L. (1995). First-trimester multifetal pregnancy reduction: Acute and persistent psychologic reactions. *American Journal of Obstetrics & Gynecology, 172*(2, Pt. 1), 541–547. doi:10.1016/0002-9378(95)90570-7

Schuit, E., Stock, S., Rode, L., Rouse, D., Lim, A., Norman, J. E., . . . Mol, B. W. (2015). Effectiveness of progestogens to improve perinatal outcome in twin pregnancies: An individual participant data meta-analysis. *BJOG, 122*(1), 27–37. doi:10.1111/1471-0528.13032

Sepulveda, W., Wong, A. E., & Casasbuenas, A. (2009). Nuchal translucency and nasal bone in first-trimester ultrasound screening for aneuploidy in multiple pregnancies. *Ultrasound in Obstetrics & Gynecology, 33*(2), 152–156. doi:10.1002/uog.6222

Shamshirsaz, A. A., Haeri, S., Ravangard, S. F., Sangi-Haghpeykar, H., Gandhi, M., Ozhand, A., . . . Shamshirsaz, A. A. (2014). Perinatal outcomes based on the Institute of Medicine guidelines for weight gain in twin pregnancies. *The Journal of Maternal-Fetal & Neonatal Medicine, 27*(6), 552–556. doi:10.3109/14767058.2013.836177

Shepherd, E., Salam, R. A., Middleton, P., Makrides, M., McIntyre, S., Badawi, N., & Crowther, C. A. (2017). Antenatal and intrapartum interventions for preventing cerebral palsy: An overview of Cochrane systematic reviews. *Cochrane Database of Systematic Reviews,* (8), CD012077. doi:10.1002/14651858.CD012077.pub2

Shinagawa, S., Suzuki, S., Chihara, H., Otsubo, Y., Takeshita, T., & Araki, T. (2005). Maternal basal metabolic rate in twin pregnancy. *Gynecologic and Obstetric Investigation, 60*(3), 145–148. doi:10.1159/000086132

Shinar, S., Skornick-Rapaport, A., & Maslovitz, S. (2017). Iron supplementation in twin pregnancy—The benefit of doubling the iron dose in iron deficient pregnant women: A randomized controlled trial. *Twin Research and Human Genetics, 20*(5), 419–424. doi:10.1017/thg.2017.43

Silver, R. K., Haney, E. I., Grobman, W. A., MacGregor, S. N., Casele, H. L., & Neerhof, M. G. (2000). Comparison of active phase labor between triplet, twin, and singleton gestations. *Journal of the Society for Gynecologic Investigation, 7*(5), 297–300. doi:10.1016/S1071-5576(00)00067-8

Simkin, P. (2017). Should ACOG support childbirth education as another means to improve obstetric outcomes? Response to ACOG Committee Opinion # 687: Approaches to limit intervention during labor and birth. *Birth, 44*(4), 293–297. doi:10.1111/birt.12306

Simpson, K. R. (2004). Monitoring the preterm fetus during labor. *MCN: The American Journal of Maternal/Child Nursing, 29*(6), 380–388. doi:10.1097/00005721-200411000-00008

Simpson, L. L. (2013). Twin-twin transfusion syndrome. *American Journal of Obstetrics & Gynecology, 208*(1), 3–18. doi:10.1016/j.ajog.2012.10.880

Smith, D., Merriam, A., Jung, J., & Gyamfi-Bannerman, C. (2018). Effect of maternal age and fetal number on the risk of hypertensive disorders of pregnancy. *American Journal of Perinatology, 35*(3), 311–316. doi:10.1055/s-0037-1607297

Smith-Levitin, M., Skupski, D. W., & Chervenak, F. A. (1999). Multifetal pregnancies: Epidemiology, clinical characteristics and management. In E. A. Reece & J. C. Hobbins (Eds.), *Medicine of the fetus and mother* (2nd ed., pp. 243–264). Philadelphia, PA: Lippincott-Raven.

Snowise, S., Mann, L. K., Moise, K. J., Jr., Johnson, A., Bebbington, M. W., & Papanna, R. (2017). Preterm prelabor rupture of membranes after fetoscopic laser surgery for twin-twin transfusion syndrome. *Ultrasound in Obstetrics & Gynecology, 49*(5), 607–611. doi:10.1002/uog.15958

Stagnati, V., Zanardini, C., Fichera, A., Pagani, G., Quintero, R. A., Bellocco, R., & Prefumo, F. (2017). Early prediction of twin-to-twin transfusion syndrome: Systematic review and meta-analysis. *Ultrasound in Obstetrics & Gynecology, 49*(5), 573–582. doi:10.1002/uog.15989

Stammler-Safar, M., Ott, J., Weber, S., & Krampl, E. (2010). Sexual behaviour of women with twin pregnancies. *Twin Research and Human Genetics, 13*(4), 383–388. doi:10.1375/twin.13.4.383

Stern, E., Cohen, N., Odom, E., Stroustrup, A., Gupta, S., Saltzman, D. H., . . . Fox, N. S. (2018). Long-term outcomes of twins based on gestational age at delivery. *The Journal of Maternal-Fetal & Neonatal Medicine*, *31*(23), 3102–3107. doi:10.1080/14767058.2017.1364725

Stock, S., & Norman, J. (2010). Preterm and term labour in multiple pregnancies. *Seminars in Fetal & Neonatal Medicine*, *15*(6), 336–341. doi:10.1016/j.siny.2010.06.006

Swanson, P. B., Kane, R. T., Pearsall-Jones, J. G., Swanson, C. F., & Croft, M. L. (2009). How couples cope with the death of a twin or higher order multiple. *Twin Research and Human Genetics*, *12*(4), 392–402. doi:10.1375/twin.12.4.392

Swinth, J. Y., Nelson, L. E., Hadeed, A., & Anderson, G. C. (2000). Shared kangaroo care for triplets. *MCN: The American Journal of Maternal Child Nursing*, *25*(4), 214–216. doi:10.1097/00005721-200007000-00010

Taffel, S. M. (1995). Demographic trends: USA. In L. G. Keith, E. Papiernik, D. M. Keith, & B. Luke (Eds.), *Multiple pregnancy: Epidemiology, gestation and perinatal outcome* (pp. 133–144). New York, NY: The Parthenon.

Tobias, T., Sharara, F. I., Franasiak, J. M., Heiser, P. W., & Pinckney-Clark, E. (2016). Promoting the use of elective single embryo transfer in clinical practice. *Fertility Research and Practice*, *2*, 1. doi:10.1186/s40738-016-0024-7

Trevett, T., & Johnson, A. (2005). Monochorionic twin pregnancies. *Clinics in Perinatology*, *32*(2), 475–494. doi:10.1016/j.clp.2005.02.007

Tumblin, A. (2013). A family-centered cesarean birth story. *The Journal of Perinatal Education*, *22*(3), 130–132. doi:10.1891/1058-1243.22.3.130

Urquhart, C., Currell, R., Harlow, F., & Callow, L. (2017). Home uterine monitoring for detecting preterm labour. *Cochrane Database of Systematic Reviews*, (2), CD006172. doi:10.1002/14651858.CD006172.pub4

U.S. Food and Drug Administration. (2011). *FDA drug safety communication: New warnings against use of terbutaline to treat preterm labor*. Retrieved from http://www.fda.gov/Drugs/DrugSafety/ucm243539.htm

U.S. Food and Drug Administration. (2013). *FDA drug safety communication: FDA recommends against prolonged use of magnesium sulfate to stop pre-term labor due to bone changes in exposed babies*. Retrieved from https://www.fda.gov/Drugs/DrugSafety/ucm353333.htm

van Gemert, M. J. C., van den Wijngaard, J. P. H. M., & Vandenbussche, F. P. H. A. (2015). Twin reversed arterial perfusion sequence is more common than generally accepted. *Birth Defects Research. Part A, Clinical and Molecular Teratology*, *103*(7), 641–643. doi:10.1002/bdra.23405

van Oppenraaij, R. H., Jauniaux, E., Christiansen, O. B., Horcajadas, J. A., Farquharson, R. G., & Exalto, N. (2009). Predicting adverse obstetric outcome after early pregnancy events and complications: A review. *Human Reproduction Update*, *15*(4), 409–421. doi:10.1093/humupd/dmp009

Vilska, S., Unkila-Kallio, L., Punamäki, R. L., Poikkeus, P., Repokari, L. M., Sinkkonen, A., . . . Tulppala, M. (2009). Mental health of mothers and fathers of twins conceived via assisted reproduction treatment: A 1-year prospective study. *Human Reproduction (Oxford, England)*, *24*(2), 367–377. doi:10.1093/humrep/den427

Vintzileos, A. M., Ananth, C. V., Kontopoulos, E., & Smulian, J. C. (2005). Mode of delivery and risk of stillbirth and infant mortality in triplet gestations: United States, 1995 through 1998. *American Journal of Obstetrics & Gynecology*, *192*(2), 464–469. doi:10.1016/j.ajog.2004.08.012

Viteri, O. A., Blackwell, S. C., Chauhan, S. P., Refuerzo, J. S., Pedroza, C., Salazar, X. C., & Sibai, B. M. (2016). Antenatal corticosteroids for the prevention of respiratory distress syndrome in premature twins. *Obstetrics & Gynecology*, *128*(3), 583–591. doi:10.1097/AOG.0000000000001577

Wadhawan, R., Oh, W., Vohr, B. R., Wragem, L., Dasm, A., Bellm, E. F., . . . Higgins, R. D. (2011). Neurodevelopmental outcomes of triplets or higher-order extremely low birth weight infants. *Pediatrics*, *127*(3), e654–e660. doi:10.1542/peds.2010-2646

Walker, M. C., Murphy, K. E., Pan, S., Yang, Q., & Wen, S. W. (2004). Adverse maternal outcomes in multifetal pregnancies. *BJOG*, *111*(11), 1294–1296. doi:10.1111/j.1471-0528.2004.00345.x

Wang, A. R., & Kroumpouzos, G. (2017). Skin disease and pregnancy. In S. G. Gabbe, J. R. Niebyl, J. L. Simpson, M. B. Landon, H. L. Galan, E. R. M. Jauniaux, . . . W. A. Grobman (Eds.), *Obstetrics: Normal and problem pregnancies* (7th ed., pp. 1075–1088). Philadelphia, PA: Elsevier.

Wang, H. L., & Yu Chao, Y. M. (2006). Lived experiences of Taiwanese women with multifetal pregnancies who receive fetal reduction. *The Journal of Nursing Research*, *14*(2), 143–154. doi:10.1097/01.JNR.0000387572.20856.9e

Weber, M. A., & Sebire, N. J. (2010). Genetics and developmental pathology of twinning. *Seminars in Fetal & Neonatal Medicine*, *15*(6), 313–318. doi:10.1016/j.siny.2010.06.002

Wen, S. W., Demissie, K., Yang, Q., & Walker, M. C. (2004). Maternal morbidity and obstetric complications in triplet pregnancies and quadruplet and higher-order multiple pregnancies. *American Journal of Obstetrics & Gynecology*, *191*(1), 254–258. doi:10.1016/j.ajog.2003.12.003

Whitford, H. M., Wallis, S. K., Dowswell, T., West, H. M., & Renfrew, M. J. (2017). Breastfeeding education and support for women with twins or higher order multiples. *Cochrane Database of Systematic Reviews*, (2), CD012003. doi:10.1002/14651858.CD012003.pub2

Witteveen, T., Van Den Akker, T., Zwart, J. J., Bloemenkamp, K. W., & Van Roosmalen, J. (2016). Severe acute maternal morbidity in multiple pregnancies: A nationwide cohort study. *American Journal of Obstetrics & Gynecology*, *214*(5), 641.e1–641.e10. doi:10.1016/j.ajog.2015.11.003

Yamasmit, W., Chaithongwongwatthana, S., Tolosa, J. E., Limpongsanurak, S., Pereira, L., & Lumbiganon, P. (2015). Prophylactic oral betamimetics for reducing preterm birth in women with a twin pregnancy. *Cochrane Database of Systematic Reviews*, (12), CD004733. doi:10.1002/14651858.CD004733.pub4

Yokoyama, Y., Shimizu, T., & Hayakawa, K. (1995). Prevalence of cerebral palsy in twins, triplets and quadruplets. *International Journal of Epidemiology*, *24*(5), 943–948. doi:10.1093/ije/24.5.943

Zhang, J., Hamilton, B., Martin, J., & Trumble, A. (2004). Delayed interval delivery and infant survival: A population-based study. *American Journal of Obstetrics & Gynecology*, *191*(2), 470–476. doi:10.1016/j.ajog.2004.03.002

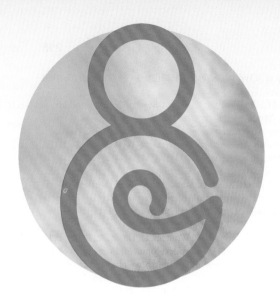

CHAPTER 12

Obesity in Pregnancy

Mary Ann Maher

SIGNIFICANCE AND INCIDENCE

Obesity is a medical condition characterized by excessive body fat that may impair a person's health. A crude population screening tool used to measure body fat is the body mass index (BMI), which is defined as a person's weight in kilograms divided by height in meters squared (kg/m²). The National Heart, Lung, and Blood Institute (NHLBI, 2013) of the National Institutes of Health and the World Health Organization (WHO, 2000) organize BMI in six classifications: underweight, <18.5; normal range, 18.5 to 24.9; overweight (preobese), 25.0 to 29.9; obese class I, 30.0 to 34.9; obese class II, 35.0 to 39.9; and obese class III, ≥40. The term *superobesity* is used in bariatric literature to describe individuals who weigh more than 225% of their ideal body weight or a BMI of greater than 50 kg/m². One study noted this subgroup of individuals has grown 5 times faster than other groups observed (Marshall, Guild, Cheng, Caughey, & Halloran, 2012). The American College of Obstetricians and Gynecologists (ACOG, 2015) recommends that at the first prenatal visit, prepregnancy weight and height be recorded for all women to allow calculation of BMI. See Table 12–1 for a summary of BMI criteria for classifying weight status.

Worldwide obesity has nearly tripled between 1975 and 2016 (WHO, 2018). In 2016, more than 1.9 billion adults aged 18 years and older were overweight, and of these, over 650 million were obese, representing 39% and 13%, respectively (WHO, 2018). In 2016, WHO estimated 41 million children aged younger than 5 years were overweight or obese and over 340 million children and adolescents aged 5 to 19 years were overweight or obese (WHO, 2018). Globally, overweight and obesity are responsible for more deaths than underweight (WHO, 2018).

In the United States, estimated prevalence of obesity during the year 2015 to 2016 was 38.9% in adults and 18.5% in youth (Hales, Carroll, Fryar, & Ogden, 2017). Results from the 2011 to 2012 National Health and Nutrition Examination Survey estimated 33.9% of U.S. adults aged 20 years and older are overweight, 35.1% are obese, and 6.4% are extremely obese (Fryar, Carroll, & Ogden, 2014). Among children and youth, the prevalence of obesity was least among children aged 2 to 5 years (13.9%) compared with youth aged 6 to 11 years (18.4%) and adolescents aged 12 to 19 years (20.6%) (Hales et al., 2017). Both non-Hispanic black and Hispanic adults and youth had the highest prevalence of obesity compared with other race and Hispanic-origin groups, whereas the lowest was among non-Hispanic Asian men and women (Hales et al., 2017). Women had a higher prevalence of obesity than men among non-Hispanic black, non-Hispanic Asian, and Hispanic adults, however, not among non-Hispanic white adults (Hales et al., 2017). There was no significant difference in obesity between girls and boys of the same race and Hispanic origin. Overall, the obesity prevalence increased in both adults and youth during the 18 years between 1999 to 2000 and 2015 to 2016 (Hales et al., 2017). Colorado, Massachusetts, Hawaii, and the District of Columbia have the lowest prevalence of adult obesity (20% to <25%); Alabama, Arkansas, Louisiana, Mississippi, and West Virginia have the highest (≥35%) (Hales et al., 2017).

For childbearing women, prepregnancy BMI is used to recommend weight gain during pregnancy and determine a woman's risk for obesity complications during pregnancy, labor, birth, and postpartum. Among U.S. women giving birth in 2014, 45.9% were normal weight, 25.6% were overweight, 24.8% were obese, and 3.8% were underweight based on prepregnancy

TABLE 12–1. Body Mass Index (BMI) Criteria for Classifying Weight Status in Adults

BMI formulas

weight (kg) / height (m²) or weight (lb) × 703 / height (in²)

Weight classification	BMI (kg/m²)
Underweight	<18.5
Normal range	18.5 to 24.9
Overweight (preobese)	25.0 to 29.9
Obese	≥30
Obese class I	30.0 to 34.9
Obese class II	35.0 to 39.9
Obese class III	≥40

Adapted from National Heart, Lung, and Blood Institute. (2013). *Managing overweight and obesity in adults: Systematic evidence review from the obesity expert panel, 2013.* Washington, DC: National Institutes of Health; World Health Organization. (2000). *Obesity: Preventing and managing the global epidemic* (WHO Technical Report Series, 894). Geneva, Switzerland: Author. Retrieved from http://www .who.int/nutrition/publications/obesity/WHO_TRS_894/en/

BMI calculations (Branum, Kirmeyer, & Gregory, 2016). The prevalence of prepregnancy obesity and overweight was lowest among women younger than 20 years, non-Hispanic Asian women, women with at least a college degree, primiparous women, and women using self-payment, whereas women with prepregnancy obesity were more likely to be older (aged 40 to 54 years), non-Hispanic black or non-Hispanic Native American or Alaska Native, to have had at least three prior births, or use Medicaid for payment (Branum et al., 2016).

Although the etiology of obesity may be very basic, for example, an energy imbalance due to taking in more calories than energy expended, there are multiple complex factors contributing to the increase in obesity in the United States. These factors occur at all social, economic, and environmental levels (Centers for Disease Control and Prevention [CDC], 2011). Body weight is the result of genes, metabolism, behavior, environment, culture, and socioeconomic status (Chescheir, 2011). A significant factor related to the current prevalence of obesity is the evolution of the human species, which occurred in an environment where few calories were available and a significant expenditure of energy was needed to acquire those calories (Phelan, 2010). To ensure survival of the species, humans needed to store fat for times when resources were limited. Women specifically needed to have adequate stores of fat to sustain a pregnancy and breast-feed their newborns (Phelan, 2010). As a result, the human body is quite efficient in using calories and has no limit in storing excessive caloric intake in the form of fat. Humans may be predisposed to preferring sweet foods that are calorie dense

and require a relatively low expenditure of energy to obtain (Phelan, 2010). Some scientists hypothesize that certain DNA are responsible for consumption of sugary foods and are linked to obesity-related illnesses such as diabetes (Daniels, 2006). Storing unlimited amounts of fat may have been a useful trait in the early days of evolution when humans were hunters and gatherers but has not been shown to be advantageous in today's environment where many occupations are sedentary, physical activity is limited, and minimal energy is required to acquire high-calorie food (Phelan, 2010). American society has become characterized by environments that promote physical inactivity and increased consumption of less healthy food (CDC, 2011; Chescheir, 2011). The increased intake of energy-dense foods that are high in fat, salt, and sugars but low in vitamins, minerals, and other micronutrients combined with the decrease in physical activity due to the increasingly sedentary nature of many forms of work, changing modes of transportation, and increasing urbanization have not been beneficial in promoting human health (WHO, 2018).

Among women, obesity prevalence increases as income decreases, but the majority of women with obesity in the United States are not low income (below the 130% poverty level) (Ogden, Lamb, Carroll, & Flegal, 2010). However, 42% of low-income women (incomes below 130% of the poverty level) are obese (ACOG, 2014; Ogden, Lamb, et al., 2010). Women in low-income areas often face multiple challenges including limited safe areas for walking or exercise and limited healthy food selections. Small grocery stores located in the most economically depressed areas often lack access to affordable fruits, vegetables, whole grains, low-fat milk, and other foods that make a healthy diet (ACOG, 2014; CDC, 2011). Transportation to larger supermarkets with a variety of food choices may be too expensive or require long bus or car rides. However, fast-food restaurants are often easily accessible and offer quick, low-cost meals. These high-caloric, high-fat, and high-glucose meals can easily exceed 1,000 calories for $5 or less, further contributing to obesity among women and their families.

As a chronic disease, obesity represents a significant economic burden to society. The total economic cost of overweight and obesity in the United States and Canada caused by medical costs, loss of productivity due to excess mortality and disability is approximately $300 billion per year (Society of Actuaries [SOA], 2010). Approximately $80 billion is due to overweight, whereas $220 billion is due to obesity (SOA, 2010). The United States accounts for 90 percent of overweight and obesity whereas Canada accounts for only 10 percent (SOA, 2010). People who have obesity, compared to normal weight individuals, are at

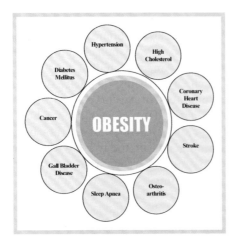

FIGURE 12–1. Obesity: a vicious cycle. (From Reece, E. A. [2008]. Perspectives on obesity, pregnancy and birth outcomes in the United States: The scope of the problem. *American Journal of Obstetrics & Gynecology*, *198*[1], 23–27.)

increased risk for all causes of death, hypertension, dyslipidemia, coronary heart disease, type 2 diabetes, stroke, gallbladder disease, osteoarthritis, sleep apnea, certain cancers (endometrial, breast, colon, kidney, gallbladder, and liver), and psychological disorders such as depression (Flegal, Carroll, Ogden, & Curtin, 2010; NHLBI, 2013; Reece, 2008; Vallejo, 2007) (Fig. 12–1). Pregnant women who are obese use more healthcare dollars, resources, equipment, and hospital days than their nonobese counterparts (Ghaffari, Srinivas, & Durnwald, 2015).

During the reproductive years, women are usually at peak health, which can accommodate the dramatic physiologic changes of pregnancy and the physical challenges of birth. However, more women are becoming pregnant who have preexisting medical conditions such as obesity. Pregnancy can exacerbate obesity-related comorbidities such as hypertension and/or diabetes as well as result in the development of additional maternal complications during pregnancy, labor, and birth (ACOG, 2015). Maternal morbidity and mortality increase with increasing BMI (Hemond, Robbins, & Young, 2016; Lisonkova et al., 2017; Mantakas & Farrell, 2010; Marshall et al., 2012; Vallejo, 2007). Women may develop lifelong obesity as a result of excessive pregnancy weight gain and postpartum weight retention (ACOG, 2015; Kirkegaard et al., 2014).

OBESITY-RELATED RISKS TO THE MOTHER AND FETUS

Obesity during pregnancy increases the risk or morbidity and mortality for both the mother and baby (Display 12–1). Compared with normal weight women, women who are obese are at increased risk for

cardiac dysfunction, proteinuria, nonalcoholic fatty liver disease, gestational diabetes mellitus (GDM), preeclampsia, spontaneous abortion, recurrent miscarriage, stillbirth, protracted labor, medically indicated preterm birth, multiple gestation, postterm pregnancy, operative vaginal or cesarean birth, anesthesia complications, wound infections, wound rupture or dehiscence, deep vein thrombosis, respiratory complications such as asthma and obstructive sleep apnea, urinary tract infections, maternal death, birth trauma related to macrosomic infants, early termination of breastfeeding, postpartum anemia, depression, and postpartum weight retention (ACOG, 2015; Blomberg, 2011; Catalano, 2007; Chescheir, 2011; Ehrenberg, 2011; Hendler et al., 2005; Jungheim & Moley, 2010; Kominiarek et al., 2010; Marchi, Berg, Dencker, Olander, & Begley, 2015; Ovesen, Rasmussen, & Kesmodel, 2011; Stream & Sutherland, 2012; Tan & Sia, 2011; Thornburg, 2011; Weiss et al., 2004). Pregnant adolescents who are obese, when compared to normal weight adolescents, are at increased risk for many of the same comorbidities as adult obese pregnant women (ACOG, 2017).

A pregnant woman who is obese is much more likely to develop GDM than a woman of normal weight (Chu et al., 2007; Saldana, Siega-Riz, Adair, & Suchindran, 2006; Weiss et al., 2004). Hypertensive disorders of pregnancy are more common in women with obesity. With each 5 to 7 kg/m^2 increase in prepregnancy BMI, the risk of preeclampsia doubles (Gunatilake & Perlow, 2011). Comorbidities associated with obesity, such as preeclampsia, predispose women who are overweight and obese to medically indicated preterm birth and their babies to the sequelae of prematurity. The Maternal-Fetal Medicine Units Network Preterm Prediction study found a strong inverse association between prepregnancy BMI and spontaneous preterm birth at less than 37 weeks' gestation. Obesity before pregnancy is associated with a lower rate of spontaneous preterm birth (Hendler et al., 2005). Women who are obese and have cesarean birth are at increased risk of significant operative and postoperative complications, including increased blood loss, anesthesia complications, surgical technical difficulties, prolonged time from incision to birth of the baby, and wound infection and healing complications (ACOG, 2015; Gunatilake & Perlow, 2011). In a large retrospective population-based cohort study, pregnant women with low and high prepregnancy BMI, compared to normal BMI, were associated with a significant but small absolute increase in severe maternal morbidity or mortality (Lisonkova et al., 2017).

Women with obesity compared to normal weight women are at increased risk of pregnancies affected by neural tube defects, spina bifida, cardiovascular

DISPLAY 12–1

Risks Associated with Maternal Obesity during Pregnancy, Labor, and Birth

Maternal	Fetal and infant
Spontaneous abortion	Congenital anomalies (neural tube defects, cardiovascular anomalies, diaphragmatic hernia, cleft lip and palate, anorectal atresia, hydrocephaly, limb reduction)
Antepartum hospitalization	
Hypertensive diseases, both preexisting and gestational, preeclampsia	
Diabetes, both preexisting and gestational	Intrauterine growth restriction
Ischemic heart disease	Prematurity related to medically indicated preterm birth due to maternal complications and comorbidities
Sleep apnea	
Multiple pregnancy	Conditions associated with prematurity (intracranial hemorrhage, respiratory distress, vision, gastrointestinal, and cardiac problems)
Medically indicated preterm birth	
Postterm pregnancy	
Labor and birth abnormalities (labor dystocia, prolonged labor, labor induction and augmentation, unsuccessful vaginal birth after cesarean, fetal compromise, shoulder dystocia, operative vaginal birth, fourth-degree lacerations, postpartum hemorrhage, cesarean birth)	Neonatal macrosomia
	Fetal death
	Stillbirth
	Low Apgar scores
	Birth trauma
Labor anesthesia complications (difficult epidural catheter placement, inadvertent dural puncture, failure to establish regional anesthesia, insufficient duration of regional anesthesia, hypotension, postdural headaches)	Neonatal acidemia
	Neonatal intensive care unit admission
	Neonatal respiratory complications
	Childhood, adolescent, and adult obesity
Complications of cesarean birth (increased time from decision to incision, increased time from incision to birth, increased intraoperative time, general anesthesia, failed intubation, aspiration, intraoperative hypotension, increased blood loss, venous thromboembolism, surgical site infection, wound dehiscence)	
Infection (urinary tract infection, episiotomy infection, endometritis, wound infection)	
Increased length of stay	
Breastfeeding difficulties	
Short duration of breastfeeding	
Postpartum maternal rehospitalization	
Maternal death	

From American College of Obstetricians and Gynecologists. (2015). *Obesity in pregnancy* (Practice Bulletin No. 156). Washington, DC: Author; Blomberg, M. I. (2011). Maternal obesity and risk of postpartum hemorrhage. *Obstetrics & Gynecology, 118*(3), 561–568. doi:10.1097/AOG.0b013e31822a6c59; Chescheir, N. (2011). Global obesity and the effect on women's health. *Obstetrics & Gynecology, 117*(5), 1213–1222. doi:10.1097/AOG.0b013e3182161732; Ehrenberg, H. M. (2011). Intrapartum considerations in perinatal care. *Seminars in Perinatology, 35*(6), 324–329. doi:10.1053/j.semperi.2011.05.016; Gunatilake, R. P., & Perlow, J. H. (2011). Obesity and pregnancy: Clinical management of the obese gravida. *American Journal of Obstetrics & Gynecology, 204*(2), 106–119. doi:10.1016/j.ajog.2010.10.002; Jungheim, E. S., & Moley, K. H. (2010). Current knowledge of obesity's effects in the pre- and periconceptional periods and avenues for future research. *American Journal of Obstetrics & Gynecology, 203*(6), 525–530. doi:10.1016/j.ajog.2010.06.043; Marchi, J., Berg, M., Dencker, A., Olander, E. K., & Begley, C. (2015). Risks associated with obesity in pregnancy, for the mother and baby: A systematic review. *Obesity Reviews, 16*(8), 621–638. doi:10.1111/obr.12288; Ovesen, P., Rasmussen, S., & Kesmodel, U. (2011). Effect of prepregnancy maternal overweight and obesity on pregnancy outcome. *Obstetrics & Gynecology, 118*(2, Pt. 1), 305–312. doi:10.1097/AOG.0b013e3182245d49; Tan, T., & Sia, A. T. (2011). Anesthesia considerations in the obese gravida. *Seminars in Perinatology, 35*(6), 350–355. doi:10.1053/j.semperi.2011.05.021; and Thornburg, L. L. (2011). Antepartum obstetrical complications associated with obesity. *Seminars in Perinatology, 35*(6), 317–323. doi:10.1053/j.semperi.2011.05.015

anomalies, septal anomalies, cleft palate, cleft lip and palate, anorectal atresia, hydrocephaly, and limb reduction anomalies (ACOG, 2015; Blomberg & Källén, 2010; Gunatilake & Perlow, 2011; Stothard, Tennant, Bell, & Rankin, 2009). However, the risk of gastroschisis is significantly reduced (Stothard et al., 2009). Whereas maternal obesity is associated with an increased risk of structural anomalies, the absolute risk of a pregnancy affected by neural tube defect or serious heart anomaly is small (Stothard et al., 2009). All women who are planning or able to become pregnant are encouraged to take a daily supplement containing 400 to 800 mcg of folic acid (American Academy of Pediatrics [AAP] & ACOG, 2017). Compared with pregnant women of normal BMI at their first prenatal visit, obese pregnant women have lower median serum folate measurements (O'Malley et al., 2018). Although the protective effect of 400 mcg of folic acid daily for women planning a pregnancy to protect against neural tube defects is well recognized, higher doses of folic acid periconceptually should be recommended for women with obesity (da Silva et al., 2013; O'Malley et al., 2018).

Maternal obesity predisposes the fetus to macrosomia, which can increase the risk for shoulder dystocia and associated birth trauma, including perinatal lacerations, fetal injury, and postpartum hemorrhage (ACOG, 2015). While overweight and obesity, excessive gestational weight gain above the Institute of Medicine (IOM) (Rasmussen & Yaktine, 2009) recommendations, and GDM all are associated with large-for-gestational-age (LGA) infants, preventing excessive gestational weight gain has the greatest potential to reduce LGA risk (Kim, Sharma, Sappenfield, Wilson, & Salihu, 2014).

Excessive weight gain during pregnancy appears to create an intrauterine environment that promotes larger babies with more fat cells, which in turn puts the baby at higher risk for obesity during childhood and as an adult with all the long-term consequences (Phelan, 2010). There is evolving evidence about the developmental origins of disease that has implications for fetuses of women who gain excessive weight during pregnancy. When the fetus is subjected to an environment during pregnancy characterized by nutritional factors contributing to excessive maternal weight gain, fetal programing, for example, the process in which a stimulus in utero establishes a permanent response in the fetus can lead to increased susceptibility to disease in childhood and throughout life (Catalano, 2007). Children born to obese mothers are twice as likely to develop obesity at 2 to 4 years of age (Whitaker, 2004). Primarily due to the obesity epidemic, U.S. children born now are projected to have a shorter life span than their parents (Phelan, 2010). Excessive weight gain during pregnancy results in a negative cycle of adverse health as women who are obese give birth to macrosomic daughters who are more likely to become obese themselves and have large babies (Artal, Lockwood, & Brown, 2010).

The risk for offspring of women with obesity extends past the pregnancy. Children born of obese mothers are at increased risk for diabetes, heart disease, and long-term obesity (Ghaffari et al., 2015; Gunatilake & Perlow, 2011; Hemond et al., 2016). Several studies have noted an association between birth weight and childhood obesity (Baird et al., 2005; Hui et al., 2008; Phelan et al., 2011). Research has shown a close association between LGA babies and childhood obesity in African American, inner-city single mothers of low income and education, putting this population at high risk (Mehta, Kruger, & Sokol, 2011). The United States has launched programs to address childhood obesity. These efforts are aimed at school foods and activity level of school children, food marketing, taxation, and reducing sedentary time at a computer or television (Ogden, Carroll, Curtin, Lamb, & Flegal, 2010). Because the antenatal period is further implicated in contributing to the obesity of children, more emphasis is needed on counseling mothers on the association between the effects of pregnancy and obesity to address some of the modifiable risk factors before pregnancy occurs (Mehta et al., 2011).

PRECONCEPTION CARE

Weight loss and modification of nutritional intake before pregnancy reduce risk of obesity and the related potential complications for the mother and baby (AAP & ACOG, 2017; Johnson et al., 2006). Preconception care that includes risk screening, health promotion counseling, and interventions based on individual patient status enables women to enter pregnancy in optimal health (Johnson et al., 2006). Therefore, *all* pregnant women including those who are overweight or obese should have a preconception visit to their obstetrical care provider to assess health status, evaluate physical, emotional and nutritional readiness for pregnancy, and allow for modification of potential risk factors and behaviors (Johnson et al., 2006). Women with obesity should be counseled that achieving a successful pregnancy may be more difficult because obesity can increase the risk of early miscarriage by two- to threefold and decrease success of fertility treatments (Jungheim & Moley, 2010; Thornburg, 2011). Women who have had bariatric surgery are encouraged to wait 12 to 24 months before conceiving to achieve their full weight loss goals and to lessen the exposure of their fetuses to an environment of rapid maternal weight loss (ACOG, 2009). While no prospective or randomized studies have tested these time periods, a small retrospective study of women who conceived during the first year after bariatric surgery compared to women who conceived more than a year following bariatric surgery found no significant increase in bariatric complications and no differences in maternal comorbidities, pregnancy-related complications, delivery mode, or neonatal outcomes (Sheiner, Edri, Balaban, & Aricha-Tamir, 2011). However, the recommendation still stands to wait 12 to 18 months postbariatric surgery for the woman's habits and nutrition to stabilize (Monson & Jackson, 2016).

Counseling a woman with obesity who is planning pregnancy should include information regarding maternal and fetal risks associated with obesity, screening for diabetes and hypertension, nutrition counseling, encouragement of exercise, and consultation with a weight loss specialist before attempting pregnancy. This counseling should take into consideration the woman's food preferences, eating patterns, cultural beliefs, and accessibility to healthy food (AAP & ACOG, 2017). Referral to a dietitian may be indicated for women who are overweight or obese. Women with obesity considering pregnancy should be encouraged to follow an exercise program (AAP & ACOG, 2017). Follow-up visits with healthcare providers to monitor lifestyle changes in nutrition and physical activity prior to pregnancy may be warranted.

Preconception weight loss with possible resolution of hypertension, hyperlipidemia, and diabetes most likely will improve both maternal and fetal outcomes during pregnancy, labor, birth, and the postpartum period (AAP & ACOG, 2017). Establishing a healthy diet and physical activity program prior to pregnancy may translate into maintaining these beneficial lifestyle changes during the pregnancy and beyond. The fetus and newborn may have less risk of maternal obesity–related problems when the mother adopts a healthier lifestyle. Weight loss will also decrease the lifelong disease burden for the woman (Gunatilake & Perlow, 2011).

ANTENATAL CARE

Healthcare providers caring for pregnant women should determine a woman's BMI at the initial prenatal visit to provide diet and exercise counseling (AAP & ACOG, 2017; ACOG, 2015). The IOM (now known as the Health and Medicine Division of the National Academies of Science, Engineering, and Medicine) (Rasmussen & Yaktine, 2009) guidelines for maternal weight gain are based on a woman's prepregnancy BMI. See Table 12–2 for IOM recommendations for weight gain during pregnancy. These recommendations are inclusive for all women regardless of race, ethnicity, height, or age. Women with a prepregnancy BMI of 30 or greater are classified as obese and recommended to gain weight within a narrow window of 11 to 20 lb. Data were insufficient to offer specific guidelines for women with class I versus class II versus class III obesity; therefore, the recommendation for gaining 11 to 20 lb includes all classes of obesity (Rasmussen & Yaktine, 2009). Among women with extreme obesity, weight loss, or restricted weight gain during pregnancy has been associated with

small-for-gestational-age (SGA) infants and, therefore, should not be encouraged (ACOG, 2015). More research is needed regarding optimal weight gain targets for women with obesity.

Generally, women can be expected to gain 3 to 6 lb during the first trimester and 0.5 to 1 lb each week thereafter until birth; however, for women with obesity, it is important to try to avoid gaining more than the recommended weight. Proper maternal nutrition can have a positive influence on improving the woman's overall health and birth of healthy baby of an appropriate weight (AAP & ACOG, 2017). Weight gain during pregnancy should be assessed and recorded at each prenatal visit to allow for immediate feedback to the woman regarding potential modifications in diet and exercise. As during the preconception period, prenatal nutrition counseling should take into consideration the woman's food preferences, eating patterns, cultural beliefs, and accessibility to healthy food (AAP & ACOG, 2017). If financial resources are a barrier to proper nutritional needs, the woman should be referred to federal food and nutrition programs such as the Special Supplemental Nutrition Program for Women, Infants, and Children (AAP & ACOG, 2017).

Nutrition counseling is an essential component of prenatal care for all women (AAP & ACOG, 2017). Dietitians and nutritionists may be enlisted to help the woman who is overweight or obese achieve appropriate gestational weight goals. It may be advisable for some women with obesity to participate in a session with a dietitian during each prenatal visit to offer suggestions for success, answer questions, and monitor progress. Obese pregnant women can benefit from a healthy well-balanced nutrition monitoring program (Thornton, Smarkola, Kopacz, & Ishoof, 2009). If there are no medical or obstetric contraindications, 30 minutes or more of exercise per day is recommended for pregnant women (AAP & ACOG, 2017). Moderate exercise is safe during pregnancy: however, each activity should be reviewed with the woman by the healthcare provider for potential risk of injury, and those with high risk of falling or abdominal trauma

TABLE 12–2. Recommendations for Total and Rate of Weight Gain during Pregnancy, by Prepregnancy Body Mass Index (BMI)

Prepregnancy weight classification	BMI (kg/m²)	Total weight gain range (lb)	Rates of weight gain second and third trimester (Mean range in lb/week)
Underweight	<18.5	28 to 40	1 (1 to 1.3)
Normal range	18.5 to 24.9	25 to 35	1 (0.8 to 1)
Overweight	25.0 to 29.9	15 to 25	0.6 (0.5 to 0.7)
Obese (including all classes)	≥30	11 to 20	0.5 (0.4 to 0.6)

Adapted from American College of Obstetricians and Gynecologists. (2015). *Obesity in pregnancy* (Practice Bulletin No. 156). Washington, DC: Author and Rasmussen, K. M., & Yaktine, A. L. (Eds.). (2009). *Weight gain during pregnancy: Reexamining the guidelines.* Washington, DC: National Academies Press.

should be avoided (AAP & ACOG, 2017; Szymanski & Satin, 2012).

While all pregnant women should be screened for GDM with laboratory-based screening test(s) using blood glucose levels, women with BMI 25 or greater, known impaired glucose metabolism, or previous GDM should have early screening for glucose intolerance (ACOG, 2018). Overweight and obesity exacerbate insulin resistance often leading to high blood glucose levels when metabolism does not respond properly to insulin. Obese and overweight pregnant women are 6 times more likely to have GDM than normal weight women (Davis & Olson, 2009; Saldana et al., 2006). If the initial early diabetes screening is negative, a repeat diabetes screening is generally performed at 24 to 28 weeks' gestation (ACOG, 2015; ACOG, 2018). First-trimester aneuploidy screening should not be postponed because of obesity. In addition to routine prenatal laboratory tests, serum chemistries, including uric acid, liver enzymes, creatinine, and a 24-hour urine for proteinuria, are recommended for class III obesity to serve as a baseline (Gunatilake & Perlow, 2011).

Ultrasound should be performed at the first prenatal visit to confirm viability and estimated gestational age because ovulatory dysfunction and oligomenorrhea are more common with obesity (Gunatilake & Perlow, 2011). Assessment for multiple gestations should be made given the increased chance of twins in women with obesity. Detailed fetal anatomy ultrasound may be more difficult in early gestation due to the abdominal contour resulting in suboptimal visualization of detailed fetal anatomy (Khoury, Ehrenberg, & Mercer, 2009). For this reason, some experts have reported better results when this examination was done at 20 to 22 weeks of gestation (Gunatilake & Perlow, 2011; Society of Obstetricians and Gynaecologists of Canada [SOGC], 2010).

Obese pregnant women are at risk for developing sleep-disordered breathing, including the most severe form, obstructive sleep apnea, which is characterized by repeated episodes of partial or complete upper airway obstruction accompanied by oxygen desaturation during sleep (ACOG, 2015). Obstructive sleep apnea can result in disruption of normal ventilation, intermittent hypoxemia, and arousals from sleep (Izci-Balserak & Pien, 2010). Physiologic and hormonal changes occur during pregnancy that increase the likelihood of developing sleep-disordered breathing and exacerbate its effects, including pregnancy weight gain, pregnancy-associated nasopharyngeal edema, decreased functional reserve capacity, and increased arousals from sleep (Izci-Balserak & Pien, 2010). The mother may experience pauses in breathing for several seconds followed by gasps of air while she is sleeping during the night. The nighttime breathing disturbances can result in daytime sleepiness, chronic fatigue, and difficulty concentrating. Risk of sleep apnea is higher for those who are overweight because of excess fat stored in the neck area, which may make the airway smaller and make breathing difficult, loud such as snoring, or stop intermittently (Facco, 2011). If the woman is symptomatic, a sleep apnea study should be conducted. Treatment often leads to improved sleep quality and daytime functioning. The most common treatment for obstructive sleep apnea is continuous positive airway pressure via a device worn while sleeping, which appears to be a safe treatment with minimal adverse effects (Chen et al., 2012; Facco, 2011). Obstructive sleep apnea during pregnancy has been linked to an increased risk of developing gestational hypertension, preeclampsia, and GDM (Bourjeily, Ankner, & Mohsenin, 2011; Chen et al., 2012; Izci-Balserak & Pien, 2010; Olivarez et al., 2011).

Healthcare providers should be aware of the tendency to have implicit bias toward women with obesity and that this bias may result in disrespectful or inadequate care (ACOG, 2019). Care should be provided in a nonjudgmental manner, being cognizant of the medical and social implications of obesity (ACOG, 2019).

INTRAPARTUM CARE

Potential peripartum complications for obese pregnant women are numerous (Table 12–3); however, advance planning and anticipation of problems may be able to mitigate risk of an adverse outcome. If an anesthesia consultation was not obtained during the prenatal period, it should be conducted early in labor to allow adequate time for the development of an anesthesia care plan (AAP & ACOG, 2017). Women with obesity may have inadequate anesthesia due to technical difficulties (Gaiser, 2016). Early catheter placement should be considered after discussing risks and benefits with the woman (ACOG, 2015). Women with class III obesity have a higher risk of hypotension and prolonged fetal heart rate (FHR) decelerations compared with normal weight pregnant women from regional analgesia due to the often inability to relieve aortocaval compression (ACOG, 2015; Gaiser, 2016; Vricella, Louis, Mercer, & Bolden, 2011). However, for obese pregnant women regional analgesia is preferred compared to general anesthesia, which can have difficulties with endotracheal intubation due to excessive tissue and edema (AAP & ACOG, 2017; ACOG, 2015). Anesthesia consultation should also be considered for obese women with obstructive sleep apnea as these women are at increased risk for hypoxemia, hypercapnia, and sudden death (ACOG, 2015).

TABLE 12–3. Obesity-Related Peripartum Complications and Possible Interventions

Obesity-related peripartum complications	
Problem/risk potential intervention	Problem/risk potential intervention
Increased respiratory work and myocardial oxygen requirement	Epidural anesthesia, supplemental oxygen, lateral laboring position
Difficult peripheral intravenous access	Central intravenous catheter
Inaccurate blood pressure monitoring	Appropriate-sized cuff, arterial line
Increased risk of general anesthesia	Anesthesia consultation, early epidural
Anticipated difficulty with intubation	Capability for awake/fiber-optic intubation
Difficulty with patient transfers	Bariatric lifts and inflatable mattresses, additional personnel
Prolonged cesarean operative time	Combined spinal-epidural anesthesia
Poor operative exposure	Evaluation of maternal anthropometry, panniculus retraction, periumbilical skin incision, atraumatic self-retaining retractor
Enhanced risk of hemorrhage	Blood typed and crossed for transfusion, ligate large subcutaneous vessels, meticulous surgical technique
Enhanced aspiration risk	Prophylactic epidural, H_2 antagonist, sodium citrate with citric acid, metoclopramide, nothing by mouth in labor
Enhanced thromboembolic risk	Early postoperative ambulation, sequential pneumatic compression, heparin until fully ambulatory
Enhanced risk of infectious morbidity	Thorough skin preparation, adequate antimicrobial prophylaxis, avoidance of subpannicular incision, meticulous surgical technique, consideration of subcutaneous drain
Enhanced risk of cesarean delivery	Informed consent, monitoring of labor curve, and intervention for labor dystocia
Enhanced risk of shoulder dystocia	Near-term sonographic fetal weight, caution with operative delivery

From Gunatilake, R., & Perlow, J. H. (2011). Obesity and pregnancy: Clinical management of the obese gravida. *American Journal of Obstetrics & Gynecology*, *204*(2), 106–119. doi:10.1016/j.ajog.2010.10.002.

Due to the increased rate of complications associated with obesity such as diabetes, hypertension, and postdates, women with obesity are more likely to have an induction or augmentation of labor. However, excessive maternal weigh and obesity have a negative effect on uterine contractility and can therefore, increase the length of the labor induction (Josefsson, Blomberg, Bladh, Frederidsen, & Sydsjo, 2011; Zhang, Bricker, Wray, & Quenby, 2007). Wolfe, Rossi, and Warshak (2011) found that women with obesity experience 2 times the rate of failure of induction of labor as mothers of normal weight. The rate of induction failure is associated with the degree of obesity. Women in obesity class III who are nulliparous with a macrosomic fetus and obese women without a prior successful vaginal birth had the highest rate of failed induction at 80% (Wolfe et al., 2011). Labor proceeds more slowly as BMI increases, as well as labor lengthens, suggesting that labor management be altered to allow longer time for these differences (Kominiarek et al., 2011; Polonia Valente, Santos, Ferraz, Montenegro, & Rodrigues, 2019; Vahratian, Zhang, Troendle, Savitz, & Siega-Riz, 2004). Uterine contractility may be diminished in women who are overweight and obese (Zhang et al., 2007), which can cause prolonged or dysfunctional labor, and may be attributed to an increased level of serum cholesterol, which is more common in women with obesity than in their normal weight counterparts (Wolfe et al., 2011; Zhang et al., 2007). Other factors might be related to a decreased responsiveness of uterine muscle to oxytocin (Kominiarek et al., 2011).

Obese pregnant women are at increased risk of operative vaginal birth (ACOG, 2015; Gunatilake & Perlow, 2011). Maternal obesity also increases a woman's risk of having a fetus with macrosomia (ACOG, 2015; Dai, He, & Hu, 2018; Mazouni et al., 2006). Intrapartum risks of shoulder dystocia and inherent birth trauma, including perinatal lacerations, fetal injury, and postpartum atonic hemorrhage, are increased in a woman with obesity carrying an appropriately grown or macrosomic fetus (Gunatilake & Perlow, 2011; Johnson, Longmate, & Frentzen, 1992; Mazouni et al., 2006; Robinson, Tkatch, Mayes, Bott, & Okun, 2003; Vidarsdottir, Geirsson, Hardardottir, Valdimarsdottir, & Dagbjartsson, 2011; Weiss et al., 2004). A large population-based study examined the association of maternal overweight and obesity, excessive gestational weight gain (above the IOM recommendations), and GDM, stratified by race, with fetal overgrowth and LGA infants (Kim et al., 2014). Although maternal overweight and obesity, excessive gestational weight gain, and gestational diabetes are all associated with women birthing LGA infants, preventing excessive gestational weight gain has the greatest potential to reducing LGA risk (Kim et al., 2014).

Advance planning for birth for women who are extremely obese is prudent. Ideally, the obstetric care provider will notify the nursing clinical leadership team well in advance of the woman's due date. Earlier notification is warranted if complications are developing that may result in preterm labor and birth. Advance notice will give the perinatal team in the inpatient setting time to evaluate the unit's capability to provide safe care by planning for additional personnel as needed and ordering special equipment to accommodate the woman's excess weight. Advance evaluation of the unit's capabilities may reveal that the patient's needs for labor and birth may be best served elsewhere, which should prompt instructions to the patient regarding where to go when labor begins and plans for transfer if she presents to the unit in early labor but is stable enough for transport. When the facility or care providers cannot safely and effectively care for the patient because of lack of specialized training, experience, or institutional resources, transfer to a tertiary facility should be considered to provide the safest care possible for both the mother and the baby (ACOG, 2019) (see Chapter 13). However, there may be times when the best plans do not become reality as may be the situation when an extremely obese pregnant patient presents for care but is unstable for transport due to labor status or her clinical condition. In this case, necessary resources and equipment need to be assembled as quickly as possible based on availability.

After notification from the obstetrical care provider and determination that the perinatal service can safely handle care of the extremely obese pregnant patient for her labor and birth, clinical care conferences can be scheduled so all members of the team can be involved and develop a plan to provide the best care possible. Participation by the obstetric and anesthesia care providers is very useful in anticipating special clinical needs and securing adequate resources. See Display 12–2 for suggestions for clinical, operational,

---

DISPLAY 12–2

Advance Preparations for a Woman with Extreme Obesity Who Will Be Admitted to the Hospital for Childbirth

The following factors should be evaluated and considered for advance unit preparations for pregnant women with extreme obesity:

Evaluation of Unit Capabilities

What is the best location for patient's care?

Can the facility manage these special needs?

Is referral to a tertiary or other center necessary?

Preadmission Planning

Develop plan of care for labor, vaginal and cesarean birth, and postpartum period.

Conduct pre-anesthesia evaluation and airway evaluation.

Develop plans for pain relief during labor, birth, and postoperative period.

Practice drills for using and moving special equipment.

Conduct tabletop rehearsals before and during the mother's stay.

Plan for additional time for epidural placement, repositioning for intrauterine resuscitation, and emergent movement to OR and/or birthing suite.

Equipment and Supplies Needs and Evaluation
Bariatric scale

Extra-wide wheelchair

Evaluate weight limits of labor bed, OR table in the perinatal unit, and OR table in the main surgical department in flat and in semi-Fowler position and with use of stirrups.

Evaluate need to order a bariatric bed and/or hover mat.

Evaluate weight limits of LDR and MB room furniture including visitor chairs if partner or family members are persons of size.

Evaluate weight limits of commode in LDR and MB rooms.

Obtain extra large gowns, appropriate-size blood pressure cuffs, extra large pneumatic compression devices.

Practice use of hover mat for transfer of patient to OR table.

Practice application of stirrups to bariatric bed.

Practice application and removal of bed extenders.

Practice movement of a large bed throughout department, for example, from labor room to the OR (conduct drills for emergent cesarean birth).

Practice positioning for possible shoulder dystocia.

Plan for supplies and equipment for potential cesarean birth including extra deep abdominal instruments and Montgomery straps for visualization.

Obtain bariatric OR table extensions that provide an additional 6 to 8 inches on each side of the table, if needed based on patient size.

Contact information for equipment suppliers for each item needed should be included in the patient's file and readily available to the clinical leadership team.

Roles of Additional Personnel

At a minimum, anticipate one to one nursing care; however, more than one nurse may be needed at various stages of labor, birth, and the immediate postpartum period.

Assisting with holding external ultrasound transducer and TOCO for continuous EFM during labor

Assisting with positioning during epidural placement

Assisting with repositioning during labor

Assisting with holding legs during vaginal birth

Retraction during vaginal birth

Assisting with transfer

Assisting with holding extra tissue and the panniculus adiposus away from the field during cesarean birth

---

EFM, electronic fetal monitoring; LDR, labor, delivery, and recovery; MB, mother-baby; OR, operating room.

Adapted from James, D. C., & Maher, M. (2009). Caring for the extremely obese woman during pregnancy and birth. *MCN: The American Journal of Maternal Child Nursing, 34*(1), 24–30. doi:10.1097/01.NMC.0000343862.72237.62

and equipment issues that should be considered in planning for inpatient care of the extremely obese pregnant woman (James & Maher, 2009). Extra time and attention is necessary to make sure appropriate specialty equipment is ordered and available, including a bariatric bed with 1,000-lb weight capacity and an expandable frame, lift equipment, a lateral transfer device to assist with transfer after regional anesthesia, a commode and/or toilet that will support 500+ lb, extra large gowns, appropriate-size blood pressure cuffs, extra large pneumatic compression devices, extra wide wheelchairs, and a method to weigh a person who is extremely obese. Surgical equipment to care for the extremely obese person should be available, including an operating room (OR) table with a 1,000-lb capacity, extension devices to increase the width of the table and extra long surgical instruments and retractors.

There can be many challenges for nurses caring for women with extreme obesity during labor. Intravenous (IV) access may be more difficult. External fetal monitoring may be more complex due to abdominal girth, so frequent adjustments may be necessary to continually assess both the mother and fetus. One-to-one nursing care may be necessary to maintain a continuous FHR and uterine activity tracing if electronic fetal monitoring (EFM) is used (Association of Women's Health, Obstetric and Neonatal Nurses, 2010). Some of the newer types of fetal monitors are designed to detect FHR and uterine activity of women with obesity with better accuracy. It is important to avoid confusing the maternal heart rate with the FHR. Clinical conditions that increase risk of confusion include low FHR baseline, maternal pushing efforts during second-stage labor, maternal repositioning, maternal obesity, and maternal tachycardia, which may be associated with an elevated temperature, anxiety, or medications (Neilson, Freeman, & Mangan, 2008; Simpson, 2011). An abrupt change in the characteristics of the FHR tracing or FHR accelerations consistently coincident with uterine contractions or coincident with maternal pushing efforts warrant evaluation of the mother's pulse to confirm that the tracing is of fetal origin. In the case of fetal demise, the recording may be of the maternal heart rate either via the external ultrasound transducer detecting maternal aortic pulsations or via the fetal spiral electrode (FSE) detecting the maternal electrocardiogram. When there are two sources of data, for example, maternal heart rate via pulse oximetry or via external tocodynamometer and fetal or maternal heart rate via external ultrasound or via FSE, the fetal monitor may display coincident alerts to suggest that both data sources are detecting the same heart rate. When these alerts are displayed, confirmation of two distinct heart rates, one from the fetus and one from the mother, should be undertaken. Coincident alerts may not be displayed if the data from the automatic blood pressure device indicates a maternal pulse in the same range as the FHR. It may be helpful to confirm maternal heart rate by palpation of maternal pulse during initiation of EFM and compare it periodically to the FHR during both first and second stages of labor when caring for an obese laboring woman (Simpson, 2011).

More nurses may be needed for prolonged periods of time because the mother who is overweight or obese may have a longer labor. The unit will likely need to provide additional personnel to transfer the patient, to position and turn her and to assist with her legs for procedures such as catheterization, internal lead placement, and during the active pushing phase of the second stage of labor. Adequate personnel are required for both for the woman's safety and the safety of the staff. Caregivers should be mindful of proper body mechanics to protect themselves from injury; however, good body mechanics may not be sufficient to prevent injury. Equipment for transfer and moving the woman with extreme obesity is required. Transporting the extremely obese mother will take more time than usual, so it may be necessary to rehearse with unfamiliar equipment and practice movement through the department in order to provide safe care, especially in the case of an unplanned cesarean birth.

A sensitive and empathetic environment should be provided for the mother and her partner. When there are challenges in care due to the patient's weight status, for example, IV access, epidural catheter placement, and external fetal monitoring and extra steps or equipment are required for patient transfer and anesthesia management, it important to avoid reminding the woman that these additional clinical issues are related to her obesity. The woman and her support person will appreciate the time and effort devoted to her special needs in the context of a care environment that does not cause embarrassment, guilt, or self-esteem problems. The focus of care should be centered on her safety and clinical needs as it is with women with other chronic diseases.

INTRAOPERATIVE CARE

Multiple studies have shown that women with obesity have an increased risk for either elective or emergent cesarean birth (ACOG, 2015; Dietz, Callaghan, Morrow, & Cogswell, 2005; Ehrenberg, 2011; Fyfe et al., 2011; Kominiarek et al., 2010; Ovesen et al., 2011; Sarkar et al., 2007; SOGC, 2010; Weiss et al., 2004). A cesarean birth rate of nearly 50% has been reported for women with extreme obesity (Ehrenberg, 2011; Gunatilake & Perlow, 2011). Excessive weight gain in pregnancy above the IOM recommendations is also an independent risk factor for cesarean birth even in women with normal weight (Johnson et al., 2013;

Stotland, Hopkins, & Caughey, 2004). It is estimated that over 20% of cesarean births of nulliparous women could be prevented if all pregnant women limited their gestational weight gain to within the IOM recommendations (Stotland et al., 2004).

Women with obesity should be counseled prior to birth that cesarean birth for emergent conditions may be more difficult (ACOG, 2015). The time interval from decision to incision may be longer for the obese mother due to difficulty with anesthesia and challenges with transfer and transport. The time from incision to birth may also be prolonged due to operative difficulty as a result of excessive abdominal adipose tissue. Prolonged time from incision to birth may result in a depressed baby at birth if the medications given to the mother for induction anesthesia or sedation are transferred to the baby before birth and/or if the fetus becomes hypoxemic due to difficulties in getting the baby out of the uterus in a timely manner because of excess maternal fat and tissue. Inability to achieve an appropriate tilt of the pelvis due to maternal size could also be a factor in the status of the baby at birth (Gaiser, 2016). The challenge may be increased with extremely obese mothers, as pressure on the fundus to assist in delivering the baby may dissipate due to the adipose tissue. If operative table width extenders are used, it may be more difficult for the surgeon to reach the operative site. Therefore, presence of a neonatal resuscitation team at the birth involving a woman with extreme obesity is advised.

All women undergoing cesarean birth are recommended to receive broad-spectrum antimicrobial prophylaxis unless the woman is already receiving antibiotics for conditions such as chorioamnionitis (AAP & ACOG, 2017; ACOG, 2015). For women with a BMI of 30 or greater, consideration may be given to providing a higher preoperative dose (AAP & ACOG, 2017; ACOG, 2015). However, in a recent randomized trial comparing 2 g cefazolin to 3 g cefazolin, adipose tissue concentrations did not significantly differ; therefore, the trial did not support the use of 3 g cefazolin in women with obesity (Maggio, Nicolau, DaCosta, Rouse, & Hughes, 2015). Wound breakdown and dehiscence is also more common in the obese mother who has had a cesarean birth. A major determinant of cesarean wound morbidity is likely due to depth of the incision (Ehrenberg, 2011). Suture closure of the subcutaneous layer has been found to decrease postoperative wound dehiscence and is recommended (AAP & ACOG, 2017; ACOG, 2015; Gunatilake & Perlow, 2011). Depending on the abdominal contour and deposition of fat in the extremely obese mother, there may be variations in the type of cesarean incision (ACOG, 2015). Choice of incision direction is based on individual clinical situations and surgeon preference. Vertical skin incision is often used for the more profoundly obese patient, although there is no conclusive evidence supporting use of either the Pfannenstiel or vertical skin incision for obese patients requiring cesarean birth. In one study, risk of postoperative complications requiring the reopening of the wound were found to be 12-fold greater in vertical skin incisions than in the Pfannenstiel incision; however, in this study, patients who had a vertical incision had higher BMIs than those with the Pfannenstiel incision (Ehrenberg, 2011). Vertical abdominal incisions and closed suction subcutaneous drains are commonly used to reduce postoperative wound complications for obese patients having cesarean birth, although evidence suggests that these two practices have a negligible or even negative impact on the incidence of wound complications (Alanis, Villers, Law, Steadman, & Robinson, 2010). Each type of incision holds separate theoretic benefits and risks to the patient, but these risks have not yet been adequately studied (Ehrenberg, 2011). Typically, low transverse incisions afford less pain postoperatively, which can improve postoperative mobility and prevent atelectasis and respiratory complications, which are more common in this population. There are generally fewer cases of wound breakdown with this type of incisions. Exposure may be difficult with low transverse approach and a dependent panniculus. Montgomery straps may be used to retract the panniculus superiorly, but this maneuver can cause difficulties in ventilation, hypotension, cardiovascular, and respiratory compromise from the weight of the tissue on the chest. The fetus may be negatively affected as well due to maternal compromise related to cephalad retraction of the panniculus for surgical access (Tan & Sia, 2011). Depending on the abdominal contour, the panniculus can be retracted downward as well. A low transverse incision could lead to wound infection as the surgical wound is covered by tissue and maintains moisture. A vertical skin incision, placed in a periumbilical fashion, can accommodate rapid entry into the abdomen and allow for extension of the incision if necessary, but it is also associated with more hernias, increased operative time, increased blood loss, increased postoperative discomfort, and more wound separation (Alanis et al., 2010; Gunatilake & Perlow, 2011). There are no studies comparing the safety of the cesarean incision in morbidly obese women nor has the risk and benefit of pannus retraction been studied (Smid et al., 2016). In a 2015 survey of obstetricians, most practitioner preferred the Pfannenstiel incision and most considered exposure, infection and wound breakdown as the most important factors to consider (Smid et al., 2016). Maintaining normothermia intraoperatively may help reduce incidence of postoperative wound complications for women with obesity after cesarean birth (Tipton, Cohen, & Chelmow, 2011).

There are multiple anesthesia risks for the obese pregnant woman both for general and regional anesthesia.

These include difficulties in epidural catheter placement, failure to establish regional anesthesia, insufficient duration of regional anesthesia, postdural headaches, a higher rate of general anesthesia, and intraoperative hypotension (Gaiser, 2016; Vricella, Louis, Mercer, & Bolden, 2010). Regional anesthesia may be difficult due to decreased ability to identify landmarks because of adipose tissue and difficulty with positioning, so adequate time should be allowed as multiple attempts at catheter placement may be necessary. Morbidly obese women not only have a higher initial epidural failure rate but also have a higher rate of catheter migration probably from increased subcutaneous tissue causing the skin to slide and dislodge the catheter (Vallejo, 2007). For these reasons and because of the increased risk of cesarean, early epidural placement in labor is suggested (ACOG, 2015; SOGC, 2010).

Aspiration is the number one cause of anesthesia-related death in the obstetric population (Tan & Sia, 2011). Obese pregnant women are at increased risk for aspiration and should ideally be given nothing by mouth in active labor and 8 hours prior to cesarean birth (Gunatilake & Perlow, 2011). Physiologic changes in pregnancy that increase the risk of aspiration such as relaxed esophageal sphincter, increased abdominal pressure, increased acidity and decreased gastrointestinal motility considerations with normal gravida as well as the morbidly obese patient (Gaiser 2016; Vallejo, 2007). There is a higher rate of difficult intubation with obese mothers (Gaiser, 2016). During the pre-anesthesia assessment, particular attention must be devoted to neck circumference rather BMI alone when evaluating a patient with respect to intubation (Bell & Rosenbaum, 2005; Vallejo, 2007). The patient's Mallampati score should be evaluated along with ability to open the mouth, neck range of motion and any difficulties with airway should be assessed (Ghaffari et al., 2015). Plans for intubation while awake may be necessary along with other tools to secure a difficult airway (Gunatilake & Perlow, 2011; SOGC, 2010) if general anesthesia is planned. Unintentional awareness can be a problem with the obese patient during cesarean birth if the patient was underdosed with general anesthesia due to concern for slow emergence because of drug affinity for lipid in these women (Gaiser, 2016). As women with obesity require additional resources for safe care, a cesarean birth might best be performed in the main OR. If adequate resources for safe and timely care are not available, referral to a more appropriate center may be necessary (Ghaffari et al., 2015).

POSTPARTUM CARE

Obese mothers are at increased risk postoperatively for atelectasis, pneumonia, hypoxemia, postpartum cardiomyopathy, surgical site infections, venous thromboembolism (VTE), uterine atony, and postpartum hemorrhage (ACOG, 2015; Blomberg, 2011; Wloch et al., 2012). Compared with women of normal weight, obese women have an increased risk of surgical site infections after cesarean birth (Wloch et al., 2012) even after adjusting for diabetes and emergent or elective cesarean birth (Leth, Uldbjerg, Nørgaard, Møller, & Thomsen, 2011). Depending on the depth of the surgical site infection, management may include the use of antibiotics or wound exploration and debridement (Fitzwater & Tita, 2014). Postoperative morbidity is high in obese women after cesarean birth; thus, postoperative care issues, such as supplementary monitoring, thromboprophylaxis, and additional respiratory support devices, must be planned for in advance (Tan & Sia, 2011). Mothers with a history of obstructive sleep apnea should have oxygen administered continuously and be monitored closely until they can maintain oxygen saturation on room air. A lateral or upright position is advised rather than supine, which can exacerbate obstructive sleep apnea. Opioids given for pain relief may blunt the arousal response and result in hypoxemia while sleeping; therefore, alternative analgesics such as nonsteroidal anti-inflammatory medications should be considered. For extremely obese mothers who have had a cesarean birth, it may be more appropriate to observe them in the post-anesthesia care unit (American Society of Anesthesiologists, 2014). If the woman is cared for on the postpartum unit after being discharged from post-anesthesia care, careful monitoring is required. Placing patient in a monitored bed with specific vital signs observed at a central station with 24-7 surveillance rather than relying on in-room alarms may allow any negative changes in patient status to be identified in a timely manner. End-tidal carbon dioxide monitoring during postoperative pain relief with narcotics is possible with use of smart pumps with this option.

Careful assessment of the wound for signs of infection, use of incentive spirometry to prevent respiratory complications and accurate assessment of vital signs and intake and output are warranted. Precise assessment of bleeding and uterine tone may be difficult due to maternal size. Due to the increased risk for atonic postpartum hemorrhage, administration of prophylactic postpartum uterotonic drugs should be considered for women with obesity in the immediate postpartum period (Blomberg, 2011). Since the risk of venous VTE is increased with obesity above the risks related to pregnancy (ACOG, 2011; SOGC, 2010; Vallejo, 2007), use of intermittent pneumatic pressure stockings prior to cesarean birth and continued until the mother is fully ambulatory is recommended (ACOG, 2011; Gunatilake & Perlow, 2011). Adequate fluid intake and early ambulation after cesarean birth can decrease risk of VTE (Bates et al., 2012).

Women with obesity should be encouraged to breast-feed for the health benefits to themselves as well as their babies, yet obese women tend to have more difficulties. Women with obesity are less likely to initiate breastfeeding, experience delayed lactogenesis more frequently, and breast-feed for shorter durations than women of normal weight (Baker, Michaelsen, Rasmussen, & Sørensen, 2004; Denison et al., 2018; Donath & Amir, 2008). Because women who breast-feed tend to lose their pregnancy weight gain more quickly than nonbreastfeeding mothers and breast-fed infants are less likely to become obese as adults every effort should be given to support breastfeeding (Chescheir, 2011).

Generally, carbohydrate intolerance and insulin resistance related to GDM resolves in the postpartum period; however, up to one third of women with GDM will have evidence of abnormal glucose metabolism during postpartum screening and up to 70% of those women may develop diabetes (predominantly type 2) in the decades after the pregnancy (ACOG, 2018). Therefore, all women with GDM should be screened at 4 to 12 weeks postpartum (ACOG, 2018).

One of the most important interventions in the later postpartum period is discussion of prevention strategies. Excessive pregnancy weight gain, retention of gestational weight, and high prepregnancy weight are predictors of obesity during the postpartum period and into the midlife years with associated comorbidities of diabetes, hypertension, and heart disease (Gore, Brown, & Smith, 2003; Rooney, Schauberger, & Mathiason, 2005; Viswanathan et al., 2008). Excessive postpartum weight retention is especially prevalent among minority women (Gore et al., 2003). Women who gain more than the IOM (Rasmussen & Yaktine, 2009) recommended weight are more likely to retain that excessive weight both short term and long term (Viswanathan et al., 2008). Furthermore, it is estimated that up to 40% of women who were not obese prior to pregnancy retain at least 14 lb past the postpartum period (Ohlendorf, Weiss, & Ryan, 2012). More than 60% of women become overweight in subsequent pregnancies (Artal et al., 2010). Women should be supported to lose the weight gained in pregnancy and offered referral to weight management services where these are available (Denison et al., 2018). Excessive gestational weight gain and the effect on the next pregnancies cause a permanent increase in weight for every BMI category and is a significant contributor to the obesity epidemic and associated comorbidities in the United States (Artal et al., 2010).

For women with obesity, the ideal time for interventions to optimize their health and the health of their future children is preconception (ACOG, 2015; Davis & Olson, 2009; Gunatilake & Perlow, 2011; Johnson et al., 2006); however, the interconception period prior to the next pregnancy is an additional opportunity to develop healthy behaviors and eating patterns that will promote well-being (Ohlendorf et al., 2012). During the postpartum hospitalization and postpartum outpatient visit, it is important to discuss plans for postpartum weight loss offering specific examples and resources as to how this might be accomplished (Ohlendorf et al., 2012). Many postpartum women are seeking quality information on this topic during their hospital stay. In one study, over 50% of normal weight women, 75% of overweight women, and 82% of obese postpartum women indicated they were planning to search for information about losing their pregnancy weight (Ohlendorf et al., 2012). Referral to weight management healthcare professionals including hospital or community-based services is appreciated by postpartum women (Ohlendorf et al., 2012). Hospitals may consider offering postpartum exercise classes as part of their women's services program.

BARIATRIC SURGERY AND PREGNANCY

A number of women with class III obesity choose to have bariatric surgery to lose weight and control their obesity. Patients are considered eligible for weight-loss surgery if they have a BMI >40 kg/m^2 or a BMI >35 kg/m^2 with other comorbid conditions (Kominiarek, 2011). Indications for bariatric surgery have also included persons with a BMI of greater than or equal to 30 kg/m^2 plus a metabolic comorbid condition such as type 2 diabetes. There was an 800% increase in bariatric procedures in the United States from 1998 to 2005 (Maggard et al., 2008; Shekelle et al., 2008). According to the United States Census Bureau projection for 2015, the total population for the United States was 321 million, of whom 247 million individuals were adults aged 18 years or older (Ponce et al., 2016). Using obesity prevalence data (BMI >40), an estimated 15.8 million individuals qualified for bariatric surgery (Ponce et al., 2016). As of 2014, approximately 200,000 bariatric surgeries are performed in the United States per year. Approximately 80% of these surgeries are performed on women (Ponce, Nguyen, Hutter, Sudan, & Morton, 2015). More than one half of bariatric surgeries are performed on reproductive age women (ACOG, 2009; Josefsson et al., 2011). Although bariatric surgery is considered an aggressive intervention, it carries a very low morbidity and mortality rate in the United States (Dolin, Ude Welcome, & Caughey, 2016). It is estimated that bariatric surgery costs in the United States are at least $1.5 billion annually (Livingston, 2010); however, over time, healthcare costs are lowered due to reduction in morbidity (Borisenko, Lukyanov, & Ahmed, 2018; Krishna et al., 2018). There are variations in insurance coverage for bariatric surgery; all costs may not be covered under some plans.

There are various methods for bariatric surgery. In general, bariatric surgery is either purely restrictive in nature, for example, reducing the size of the stomach or a combination of restrictive and malabsorptive methods in which in addition to a smaller stomach, a bypass of part of the intestine adds the aspect of less area for food to be absorbed. These procedures can be performed either via laparoscopy or laparotomy based on the method selected and the individual clinical situation (Kominiarek, 2011). The sleeve gastrectomy (SG) is the most common type of procedure in 2014 in the United States. The greater curvature of the stomach is surgically removed, which results in 20% to 25% of the stomach remaining. This restricts food intake but does not affect the absorptive capabilities of the small intestine. New observations suggest there may be secretory changes that affect hormones related to hunger (Dolin et al., 2016). The second most common type of bariatric surgery done in the United States is the Roux-en-Y gastric bypass (RYGB) comprising 25% of all bariatric procedures (Dolin et al., 2016). With this approach, a small section of the stomach is sectioned off to contain <30 mL and is reconnected to the jejunum (Conrad, Russell, & Keister, 2011; Kominiarek, 2011). Food bypasses a large portion of the stomach and the duodenum, thereby allowing a smaller area of the intestine for absorption of calories and also stimulating a full feeling so patients eat less (Conrad et al., 2011). The laparoscopic adjustable gastric band (LAGB) is the third most common bariatric surgery in the United States, accounting for 10%. With the LAGB procedure, an adjustable ring is placed around the stomach and restricts food intake. Although this is the least invasive procedure, this does not result in the same weight loss as the SG or the RYGB (Dolin et al., 2016). Nutritional deficiencies are less common with LAGB surgery when compared to procedures that involve restrictive and malabsorption techniques. Bariatric surgeries in isolation are not guaranteed to produce long-term results. To maintain weight loss, it is important that patients are aware that significant lifestyle changes including modifications of eating habits and exercise are required. Close supervision before, during, and after pregnancy that follows bariatric surgery and nutrition supplementation adapted to the individual needs of the woman is necessary to prevent nutrition-related complications (Magdaleno, Pereira, Chaim, & Turato, 2012).

The woman contemplating pregnancy after bariatric surgery has special nutritional needs. Preconception counseling is especially important for these patients because deficiencies in vitamins B_{12}, A, and K; iron; folate; and calcium may occur and can result in maternal and fetal complications (Magdaleno et al., 2012). Vitamin supplementation is recommended (ACOG, 2009). Laboratory tests to evaluate potential deficiencies should be considered each trimester and, if identified, treated with oral or parental therapy (ACOG, 2009). Recommendations for the nutritional management including supplementation and laboratory testing of the postbariatric surgery patient from a task force of the American Association of Clinical Endocrinologists, the Obesity Society, and the American Society for Metabolic and Bariatric Surgery (Mechanick et al., 2009) are listed in Table 12–4. Most obstetric care providers recommend waiting at least 1 to 2 years after bariatric

TABLE 12–4. Guidelines for Supplementation and Laboratory Testing of the Postbariatric Surgery Patient

Deficiency	Laboratory testing	Treatment if deficient or not responsive to oral supplements	Routine supplementation in pregnancy
Protein	Serum albumin	Protein supplements	60-g protein/day in balanced diet
Calcium	Total and ionized calcium, parathyroid hormone		1,200 mg/d calcium citrate in addition to prenatal vitamin 400 μg/d contained in prenatal vitamin
Folic acid	Complete blood count, folic acid level	Oral folate 1,000 μg/d	400 μg/d contained in prenatal vitamin
Iron	Complete blood count, serum, iron, ferritin, total iron binding capacity	Parental iron; consult with nutritionist or hematologist	Ferrous sulfate, 300 mg two to three times per day with vitamin C in addition to prenatal vitamin 4,000 IU/d contained in prenatal vitamin
Vitamin A	Vitamin A levels	Vitamin A supplements should not exceed 10,000 IU/d in pregnancy	4,000 IU/d contained in prenatal vitamin
Vitamin B_{12}	Complete blood count, vitamin B_{12} levels	Oral crystalline B_{12} 350 μg/d or 1,000–2,000 μg intramuscularly every 2–3 mo; consult with nutritionist or hematologist	4 μg/d contained in prenatal vitamin
Vitamin D	25-hydroxy vitamin D	Calcitriol oral vitamin D 1,000 IU/d	400-800 IU/d contained in prenatal vitamin

Adapted from Mechanick, J. I., Kushner, R. F., Sugerman, H. J., Gonzalez-Campoy, J. M., Collazo-Clavell, M. L., Spitz, A. F., . . . Guven, S. (2009). American Association of Clinical Endocrinologists, the Obesity Society, and American Society for Metabolic & Bariatric Surgery medical guidelines for clinical practice for the perioperative nutritional, metabolic, and nonsurgical support of the bariatric surgery patient. *Obesity, 17*(Suppl. 1), S1–S70. doi:10.1038/oby.2009.28

surgery to conceive because the resultant initial rapid weight loss can be harmful to the growing fetus (ACOG, 2009). This waiting period may allow for the woman to fully meet her weight loss goal. Women who have had bariatric surgery but are not planning immediate pregnancy should be aware that there is an increased risk of failure of oral contraceptives due to gastric malabsorption (ACOG, 2009). Other types of contraceptives rather than oral hormones should be considered for this patient population (ACOG, 2009).

Small, frequent meals consisting of calorie-dense foods high in protein and low in fat and carbohydrates are advised (James & Maher, 2009). Generally, 60 g of protein per day is recommended (Kominiarek, 2011). After RYGB bariatric surgery, it is important to minimize or eliminate intake of simple carbohydrate-dense foods and beverages because their ingestion can result in dumping syndrome (a group of symptoms, including abdominal pain, cramping, nausea, diarrhea, light-headedness, flushing, tachycardia, and syncope) thought to be caused as gut peptides are released when food bypasses the stomach and enters the small intestine directly (Kominiarek, 2011). This potential problem has implications for screening for GDM during pregnancy. A substitute for the 50 g of Glucola for GDM screening is home glucose monitoring with fasting and post-prandial values during 1 week in the 24- to 28-week period (ACOG, 2009; Kominiarek, 2011; Monson & Jackson, 2016). When a woman has had LAGB surgery, one concern is how to manage the band during pregnancy. Some experts advocate deflating the band either before or early in the pregnancy to lessen complications, such as band migration and nausea and vomiting in pregnancy, while others prefer to wait and see if complications such as vomiting or lack of weight gain occur before releasing the band (Kominiarek, 2011). If complications arise, care should be individualized and provided in consultation with a bariatric surgeon.

Bariatric surgery is associated with several health benefits to the mother and fetus, mainly, reduced risk for maternal GDM and LGA infants, respectively (Johansson et al., 2015). In addition, bariatric surgery appears to decrease the risk of maternal hypertensive disorders, postpartum hemorrhage, and postpartum infection, however, increase the risk for maternal anemia (Monson & Jackson, 2016). Of special concern are the studies demonstrating an increased risk SGA infants in women who have had bariatric surgery (Johansson et al., 2015; Kjær, Lauenborg, Breum, & Nilas, 2013; Roos et al., 2013; Rottenstreich et al., 2018).

Bariatric surgery can increase the risk for gallstones, abdominal hernias, herniation of the bowel, changes in metabolism, and organ displacement caused by increased uterine size (National Institute of Diabetes and Digestive and Kidney Diseases, 2004). Both bariatric surgery and previous abdominal surgery are risk factors for intestinal obstruction (Stuart & Källen, 2017). During pregnancy, diagnosis of bariatric-related operative complications may be delayed (ACOG, 2009). These include anastomotic leaks, bowel obstruction, internal hernias, ventral hernias, band erosion, and band migration. Care providers should be alert for complaints of abdominal pain, nausea, vomiting, and fever, which could signify intestinal obstruction or other complication in pregnant women with a history of bariatric surgery. When these types of patients present with abdominal pain, a high index of suspicion of a surgical complication should exist and consultation with the bariatric surgeon is indicated because the underlying pathology may be related to the bariatric surgery (ACOG, 2009).

SUMMARY

Obesity is an epidemic that affects women of child-bearing age. This population has a significantly greater chance for complications during pregnancy labor, birth, and the postpartum period. Obesity is a preventable disease with lifelong implications for both the mother and her baby. Preconception counseling may encourage changes in nutrition and lifestyle modifications that can mitigate risks by promoting weight loss prior to pregnancy. Care of the woman with obesity during childbirth can be challenging. Advance planning by the interdisciplinary perinatal team, knowledge of how to manage complications, and adequate resources can promote safe care for the woman with obesity and her baby.

REFERENCES

Alanis, M. C., Villers, M. S., Law, T. L., Steadman, E. M., & Robinson, C. J. (2010). Complications of cesarean delivery in the massively obese parturient. *American Journal of Obstetrics & Gynecology*, 203(3), 271.e1–271.e7. doi:10.1016/j.ajog.2010.06.049

American Academy of Pediatrics & American College of Obstetricians and Gynecologists. (2017). *Guidelines for perinatal care* (8th ed.). Elk Grove Village, IL: American Academy of Pediatrics.

American College of Obstetricians and Gynecologists. (2009). *Bariatric surgery and pregnancy* (Practice Bulletin No. 105). Washington, DC: Author.

American College of Obstetricians and Gynecologists. (2011). *Thromboembolism in pregnancy* (Practice Bulletin No. 123). Washington, DC: Author.

American College of Obstetricians and Gynecologists. (2014). *Challenges for overweight and obese women* (Committee Opinion No. 591). Washington, DC: Author.

American College of Obstetricians and Gynecologists. (2015). *Obesity in pregnancy* (Practice Bulletin No. 156). Washington, DC: Author.

American College of Obstetricians and Gynecologists. (2017). *Obesity in adolescents* (Committee Opinion No. 714). Washington, DC: Author.

American College of Obstetricians and Gynecologists. (2018). *Gestational diabetes mellitus* (Practice Bulletin No. 190). Washington, DC: Author.

American College of Obstetricians and Gynecologists. (2019). *Ethical considerations for the care of patients with obesity* (Committee Opinion No. 763). Washington, DC: Author.

American Society of Anesthesiologists. (2014). Practice guidelines for the perioperative management of patients with obstructive sleep apnea: An updated report by the American Society of Anesthesiologists Task Force on Perioperative Management of patients with obstructive sleep apnea. *Anesthesiology, 120,* 268–286. doi:10.1097/ALN.0000000000000053

Artal, R., Lockwood, C. J., & Brown, H. L. (2010). Weight gain recommendations in pregnancy and the obesity epidemic. *Obstetrics & Gynecology, 115*(1), 152–155. doi:10.1097/AOG .0b013e3181c51908

Association of Women's Health, Obstetric and Neonatal Nurses. (2010). *Guidelines for professional registered nurse staffing for perinatal units.* Washington, DC: Author.

Baird, J., Fisher, D., Lucas, P., Kleijnen, J., Roberts, H., & Law, C. (2005). Being big or growing fast: Systematic review of size and growth in infancy and later obesity. *BMJ, 331*(7522), 929–915. doi:10.1136/bmj.38586.411273.E0

Baker, J. L., Michaelsen, K. F., Rasmussen, K. M., & Sørensen, T. I. (2004). Maternal prepregnant body mass index, duration of breastfeeding, and timing of complementary food introduction are associated with infant weight gain. *American Journal of Clinical Nutrition, 80*(6), 1579–1588. doi:10.1093 /ajcn/80.6.1579

Bates, S. M., Greer, I. A., Middeldorp, S., Veenstra, D. L., Prabulos, A. M., & Vandvik, P. O. (2012). VTE, thrombophilia, antithrombotic therapy, and pregnancy: Antithrombotic Therapy and Prevention of Thrombosis, 9th ed: American College of Physicians Evidence-Based Clinical Practice Guidelines. *Chest, 141*(2 Suppl.), e691S–e736S. doi:10.1378/chest.11-2300

Bell, R. L., & Rosenbaum, S. H. (2005). Postoperative considerations for patients with obesity and sleep apnea. *Anesthesiology Clinics of North America, 23*(3), 493–500. doi:10.1016/j.atc .2005.03.007

Blomberg, M. I. (2011). Maternal obesity and risk of postpartum hemorrhage. *Obstetrics & Gynecology, 118*(3), 561–568. doi:10.1097/AOG.0b013e31822a6c59

Blomberg, M. I., & Källén, B. (2010). Maternal obesity and morbid obesity: The risk for birth defects in the offspring. *Birth Defects Research: Part A. Clinical and Molecular Teratology, 88*(1), 35–40. doi:10.1002/bdra.20620

Borisenko, O., Lukyanov, V., & Ahmed, A. R. (2018). Cost-utility analysis of bariatric surgery. *British Journal of Surgery, 105*(10), 1328–1337. doi:10.1002/bjs.10857

Bourjeily, G., Ankner, G., & Mohsenin, V. (2011). Sleep-disordered breathing in pregnancy. *Clinics in Chest Medicine, 32*(1), 175–189. doi:10.1016/j.ccm.2010.11.003

Branum, A. M., Kirmeyer, S. E., & Gregory, E. C. W. (2016). Prepregnancy body mass index by maternal characteristics and state: Data from the birth certificate, 2014. *National Vital Statistics Reports, 65*(6), 1–11.

Catalano, P. M. (2007). Management of obesity in pregnancy. *Obstetrics & Gynecology, 109*(2, Pt. 1), 419–433. doi:10.1097/01 .AOG.0000253311.44696.85

Centers for Disease Control and Prevention. (2011). *Obesity: Halting the epidemic by making health easier. At a glance.* Atlanta, GA: Author.

Chen, Y. H., Kang, J. H., Lin, C. C., Wang, I. T., Keller, J. J., & Lin, H. C. (2012). Obstructive sleep apnea and the risk of adverse pregnancy outcomes. *American Journal of Obstetrics & Gynecology, 206*(2), 136.e1–136.e5. doi:10.1016/j.ajog .2011.09.006

Chescheir, N. (2011). Global obesity and the effect on women's health. *Obstetrics & Gynecology, 117*(5), 1213–1222. doi:10.1097 /AOG.0b013e3182161732

Chu, S. Y., Callaghan, W. H., Kim, S. Y., Schmid, C. H., Lau, J., England, L. J., & Dietz, P. M. (2007). Maternal obesity and risk of gestational diabetes mellitus. *Diabetes Care, 30*(8), 2070–2076. doi:10.2337/dc06-2559a

Conrad, K., Russell, A. C., & Keister, K. J. (2011). Bariatric surgery and its impact on childbearing. *Nursing for Women's Health, 15*(3), 226–234. doi:10.111/j.1751-486X.2011.01637.x

Dai, R. X., He, X. J., & Hu, C. L. (2018). Maternal pre-pregnancy obesity and the risk of macrosomia: A meta-analysis. *Archives of Gynecology and Obstetrics, 297*(1), 139–145. doi:10.1007 /s00404-017-4573-8

Daniels, J. (2006). Obesity: America's epidemic. *American Journal of Nursing, 106*(1), 40–50.

da Silva, V. R., Hausman, D. B., Kauwell, G. P. A., Sokolow, A., Tackett, R. L., Rathbun, S. L., & Bailey, L. B. (2013). Obesity affects short-term folate pharmacokinetics in women of childbearing age. *International Journal of Obesity, 37,* 1608–1610. doi:10.1038/ijo.2013.41

Davis, E., & Olson, C. (2009). Obesity in pregnancy. *Primary Care, 36*(2), 341–356. doi:10.1016/j.pop.2009.01.005

Denison, F. C., Aedla, N. R., Keag, O., Hor, K., Reynolds, R. M., Milne, A., & Diamond, A. (2018). Care of women with obesity in pregnancy: Green-top Guideline No. 72. *BJOG, 126*(3), e62–e106. doi:10.1111/1471-0528.15386

Dietz, P. M., Callaghan, W. M., Morrow, B., & Cogswell, M. E. (2005). Population-based assessment of the risk of primary cesarean delivery due to excess pre-pregnancy weight among nulliparous women delivering term infants. *Maternal and Child Health Journal, 9*(3), 237–244. doi:10.1007/s10995-005 -0003-9

Dolin, C., Ude Welcome, A. O., & Caughey, A. (2016). Management of pregnancy in women who have undergone bariatric surgery. *Obstetrical & Gynecological Survey, 71*(12), 734–740. doi:10.1097/OGX.0000000000000378

Donath, S. M., & Amir, L. H. (2008). Maternal obesity and initiation and duration of breastfeeding: Data from the longitudinal study of Australian children. *Maternal & Child Nutrition, 4*(3), 163–170. doi:10.1111/j.1740-8709.2008.00134.x

Ehrenberg, H. M. (2011). Intrapartum considerations in perinatal care. *Seminars in Perinatology, 35*(6), 324–329. doi:10.1053 /j.semperi.2011.05.016

Facco, F. L. (2011). Sleep-disordered breathing and pregnancy. *Seminars in Perinatology, 35*(6), 335–339. doi:10.1053/j.semperi .2011.05.018

Fitzwater, J. L., & Tita, A. T. (2014). Prevention and management of cesarean wound infection. *Obstetrics and Gynecology Clinics of North America, 41,* 671–689. doi:10.1016/j.ogc.2014.08.008

Flegal, K. M., Carroll, M. D., Ogden, C. L., & Curtin, L. R. (2010). Prevalence and trends in obesity among US adults, 1999-2008. *JAMA, 303*(3), 235–241. doi:10.1001/jama.2009.2014

Fryar, C. D., Carroll, M. D., & Ogden, C. L. (2014). *Prevalence of overweight, obesity, and extreme obesity among adults: United States, 1960-1962 through 2011-2012.* Atlanta, GA: National Centers for Disease Control and Prevention.

Fyfe, E. M., Anderson, N. H., North, R. A., Chan, E. H. Y., Taylor, R. S., Dekker, G. A., & McCowan, L. M. E. (2011). Risk of first-stage and second-stage cesarean delivery by maternal body mass index among nulliparous women in labor at term. *Obstetrics & Gynecology, 117*(6), 1315–1322. doi:10.1097/AOG .0b013e318217922a

Gaiser, R. (2016). Anesthetic considerations in the obese parturient. *Clinical Obstetrics and Gynecology, 59*(1), 193–203. doi:10.1097/GRF.0000000000000180

Ghaffari, N., Srinivas, S. K., & Durnwald, C. P. (2015). The multidisciplinary approach to the care of the obese parturient. *American Journal of Obstetrics & Gynecology, 213*(3), 318–325. doi:10.1016/j.ajog.2015.03.001

Gore, S. A., Brown, D. M., & West, D. S. (2003). The role of post-partum weight retention in obesity among women: A review of the evidence. *Annals of Behavioral Medicine, 26*(2), 149–159. doi:10.1207/S15324796ABM2602_07

Gunatilake, R. P., & Perlow, J. H. (2011). Obesity and pregnancy: Clinical management of the obese gravida. *American Journal of Obstetrics & Gynecology, 204*(2), 106–119. doi:10.1016/j.ajog.2010.10.002

Hales, C. M., Carroll, M. D., Fryar, C. D., & Ogden, C. L. (2017). *Prevalence of obesity among adults and youth: United States, 2015-2016* (CDC/NCHS Data Brief No. 288). Hyattsville, MD: National Center for Health Statistics.

Hemond, J., Robbins, R. B., & Young, P. C. (2016). The effects of maternal obesity on neonates, infants, children, adolescents, and adults. *Clinical Obstetrics & Gynecology, 59*(1), 216–227. doi:10.1097/GRF.0000000000000179

Hendler, I., Goldenberg, R. L., Mercer, B. M., Iams, J. D., Meis, P. J., Moawad, A. H., . . . Sorokin, Y. (2005). The preterm prediction study: Association between maternal body mass index and spontaneous and indicated preterm birth. *American Journal of Obstetrics & Gynecology, 192*(3), 882–886. doi:10.1016/j.ajog.2004.09.021

Hui, L. L., Schooling, C. M., Leung, S. S., Mak, K. H., Ho, L. M., Lam, T. H., & Leung, G. M. (2008). Birth weight, infant growth, and childhood body mass index: Hong Kong's children of 1997 birth cohort. *Archives of Pediatric & Adolescent Medicine, 162*(3), 212–218. doi:10.1001/archpediatrics.2007.62

Izci-Balserak, B., & Pien, G. W. (2010). Sleep-disordered breathing and pregnancy: Potential mechanisms and evidence for maternal and fetal morbidity. *Current Opinion in Pulmonary Medicine, 16*(6), 574–582. doi:10.1097/MCP.Ob013e32833f0d55

James, D. C., & Maher, M. (2009). Caring for the extremely obese woman during pregnancy and birth. *MCN: The American Journal of Maternal Child Nursing, 34*(1), 24–30. doi:10.1097/01.NMC.0000343862.72237.62

Johansson, K., Cnattingius, S., Näslund, I., Roos, N., Lagerros, Y. T., Granath, F., . . . Neovius, M. (2015). Outcomes of pregnancy after bariatric surgery. *The New England Journal of Medicine, 372*(9), 814–824. doi:10.1056/NEJMoa1405789

Johnson, J. W., Clifton, R. G., Roberts, J. M., Myatt, L., Hauth, J. C., Spong, C. Y., . . . Sorokin, Y. (2013). Pregnancy outcomes with weight gain above or below the 2009 Institute of Medicine Guidelines. *Obstetrics & Gynecology, 121*(5), 969–975. doi:10.1097/AOG.0b013e31828aea03

Johnson, J. W., Longmate, J. A., & Frentzen, B. (1992). Excess maternal weight and pregnancy outcome. *American Journal of Obstetrics & Gynecology, 167*(2), 353–372. doi:10.1016/S0002-9378(11)91414-8

Johnson, K., Posner, S. F., Biermann, J., Cordero, J. F., Atrash, H. K., Parker, C. S., . . . Curtis, M. G. (2006). Recommendations to improve preconception health and health care—United States. A report of the CDC/ATSDR preconception care work group and the select panel on preconception care. *MMWR Morbidity and Mortality Weekly Report, 55*(RR-6), 1–23.

Josefsson, A., Blomberg, M., Bladh, M., Frederidsen, S. G., & Sydsjo, G. (2011). Bariatric surgery in a national cohort of women: Sociodemographics and obstetric outcomes. *American Journal of Obstetrics & Gynecology, 205*(3), 206.e1–206.e8. doi:10.1016/j.ajog.2011.03.025

Jungheim, E. S., & Moley, K. H. (2010). Current knowledge of obesity's effects in the pre- and periconceptional periods and avenues for future research. *American Journal of Obstetrics & Gynecology, 203*(6), 525–530. doi:10.1016/j.ajog.2010.06.043

Khoury, F. R., Ehrenberg, H. M., & Mercer, B. M. (2009). The impact of maternal obesity on satisfactory detailed anatomic ultrasound image acquisition. *The Journal of Maternal-Fetal & Neonatal Medicine, 22*(4), 337–341. doi:10.1080/14767050802524586

Kim, S. Y., Sharma, A. J., Sappenfield, W., Wilson, H. G., & Salihu, H. M. (2014). Association of maternal body mass index, excessive weight gain, and gestational diabetes mellitus with large-for-gestational age births. *Obstetrics & Gynecology, 123*(4), 737–744. doi:10.1097/AOG.0000000000000177

Kirkegaard, H., Stovring, H., Rasmussen, K. M., Abrams, B., Sorensen, T. I. A., & Nohr, E. A. (2014). Maternal weight change from prepregnancy to 7 years postpartum—The influence of behavioral factors. *Obesity, 23*(4), 870–878. doi:10.1002/oby.21022

Kjær, M. M., Lauenborg, J., Breum, B. M., & Nilas, L. (2013). The risk of adverse pregnancy outcome after bariatric surgery: A nationwide register-based matched cohort study. *American Journal of Obstetrics & Gynecology, 208*(6), 464.e1–464.e5. doi:10.1016/j.ajog.2013.02.046

Kominiarek, M. A. (2011). Preparing for and managing a pregnancy after bariatric surgery. *Seminars in Perinatology, 35*(6), 356–361. doi:10.1053/j.semperi.2011.05.022

Kominiarek, M. A., VanVeldhuisen, P., Hibbard, J., Landy, H., Haberman, S., Learman, L., . . . Zhang, J. (2010). The maternal body mass index: A strong association with delivery route. *American Journal of Obstetrics & Gynecology, 203*(3), 264.e1–264.e7. doi:10.1016/j.ajog.2010.06.024

Kominiarek, M. A., Zhang, J., Vanveldhuisen, P., Troendle, J., Beaver, J., & Hibbard, J. (2011). Contemporary labor patterns: The impact of maternal body mass index. *American Journal of Obstetrics & Gynecology, 205*(3), 244.e1–244.e8. doi:10.1016/j.ajog.2011.06.014

Krishna, S. G., Rawal, V., Durkin, C., Modi, R. M., Hinton, A., Cruz-Monserrate, Z., . . . Hussan, H. (2018). Weight loss surgery reduces healthcare resource utilization and all-cause inpatient mortality in morbid obesity: A propensity-matched analysis. *Obesity Surgery, 28*(10), 3213–3220. doi:10.1007/s11695-018-3345-2

Leth, R. A., Uldbjerg, N., Nørgaard, M., Møller, J. K., & Thomsen, R. W. (2011). Obesity, diabetes, and the risk of infections diagnosed in hospital and post-discharge infections after cesarean section: A prospective cohort study. *Acta Obstetricia et Gynecologica Scandinavica, 90*, 501–509. doi:10.1111/j.1600-0412.2011.01090.x

Lisonkova, S., Muraca, G. M., Potts, J., Liauw, J., Chan, W., Skoll, A., & Lim, K. (2017). Association between prepregnancy body mass index and severe maternal morbidity. *JAMA, 318*(18), 1777–1786. doi:10.1001/jama.2017.16191

Livingston, E. H. (2010). The incidence of bariatric surgery has plateaued in the U.S. *American Journal of Surgery, 200*(3), 378–385.

Magdaleno, R., Jr., Pereira, B. G., Chaim, E. A., & Turato, E. R. (2012). Pregnancy after bariatric surgery: A current view of maternal, obstetrical and perinatal challenges. *Archives of Gynecology and Obstetrics, 285*(3), 559–566. doi:10.1007/s00404-011-2187-0

Maggard, M. A., Yermilov, I., Li, Z., Maglinone, M., Newberry, S., Suttorp, M., . . . Shekelle, P. G. (2008). Pregnancy and fertility following bariatric surgery: A systematic review. *JAMA, 300*(19), 2286–2296. doi:10.1001/jama.2008.641

Maggio, L., Nicolau, D. P., DaCosta, M., Rouse, D. J., & Hughes, B. L. (2015). Cefazolin prophylaxis in obese women undergoing cesarean delivery: A randomized controlled trial. *Obstetrics & Gynecology, 125*(5), 1205–1210. doi:10.1097/AOG.0000000000000789

Mantakas, A., & Farrell, T. (2010). The influence of increasing BMI in nulliparous women on pregnancy outcome. *European Journal of Obstetrics & Gynecology and Reproductive Biology, 153*(1), 43–46. doi:10.1016/j.ejogrb.2010.06.021

Marchi, J., Berg, M., Dencker, A., Olander, E. K., & Begley, C. (2015). Risks associated with obesity in pregnancy, for the mother and baby: A systematic review. *Obesity Reviews, 16*(8), 621–638. doi:10.1111/obr.12288

Marshall, N. E., Guild, C., Cheng, Y. W., Caughey, A. B., & Halloran, D. R. (2012). Maternal superobesity and perinatal outcomes. *American Journal of Obstetrics & Gynecology, 2012*(206), 417. e1–417.e6. doi:10.1016/j.ajog.2012.02.037

Mazouni, C., Porcu, G., Cohen-Solal, E., Heckenroth, H., Guidicelli, B., Bonnier, P., & Gamerre, M. (2006). Maternal and anthropomorphic risk factors for shoulder dystocia. *Acta Obstetricia et Gynecologica Scandinavica, 85*(5), 576–570. doi:10.1080/00016340600605044

Mechanick, J. I., Kushner, R. F., Sugerman, H. J., Gonzalez-Campoy, J. M., Collazo-Clavell, M. L., Spitz, A. F., . . . Guven, S. (2009). American Association of Clinical Endocrinologists, the Obesity Society, and American Society for Metabolic & Bariatric Surgery medical guidelines for clinical practice for the perioperative nutritional, metabolic, and nonsurgical support of the bariatric surgery patient. *Obesity, 17*(Suppl. 1), S1–S70. doi:10.1038/oby.2009.28

Mehta, S. H., Kruger, M. S., & Sokol, R. J. (2011). Being too large for gestational age precedes childhood obesity in African Americans. *American Journal of Obstetrics & Gynecology, 204*(3), 265.e1–265.e5. doi:10.1016/j.ajog.2010.12.009

Monson, M., & Jackson, M. (2016). Pregnancy after bariatric surgery. *Clinical Obstetrics & Gynecology, 59*(1), 158–171. doi:10.1097/GRF.0000000000000178

National Heart, Lung, and Blood Institute. (2013). *Managing overweight and obesity in adults: Systematic evidence review from the obesity expert panel, 2013.* Washington, DC: National Institutes of Health.

National Institute of Diabetes and Digestive and Kidney Diseases. (2004). *Gastrointestinal surgery for severe obesity.* Bethesda, MD: Author.

Neilson, D. R., Jr., Freeman, R. K., & Mangan, S. (2008). Signal ambiguity resulting in unexpected outcome with external fetal heart rate monitoring. *American Journal of Obstetrics & Gynecology, 198*(6), 717–724. doi:10.1016/j.ajog.2008.02.030

Ogden, C. L., Carroll, M. D., Curtin, L. R., Lamb, M. M., & Flegal, K. M. (2010). Prevalence of high body mass index in US children and adolescents, 2007-2008. *JAMA, 303*(3), 242–249. doi:10.1001/jama.2009.2012

Ogden, C. L., Lamb, M. M, Carroll, M. D., & Flegal, K. M. (2010). *Obesity and socioeconomic status in adults: United States, 2005-2008* (National Center for Health Statistics Data Brief No. 50). Atlanta, GA: National Centers for Disease Control and Prevention.

Ohlendorf, J. M., Weiss, M. E., & Ryan, P. (2012). Weight-management information needs of postpartum women. *MCN: The American Journal of Maternal Child Nursing, 37*(1), 56–63. doi:10.1097/NMC.0b013e31823851ee

Olivarez, S. A., Ferres, M., Antony, K., Mattewal, A., Maheshwari, B., Sangi-Haghpeykar, H., & Aagaard-Tillery, K. (2011). Obstructive sleep apnea screening in pregnancy, perinatal outcomes, and impact of maternal obesity. *American Journal of Perinatology, 28*(8), 651–658. doi:10.1055/s-0031-1276740

O'Malley, E. G., Reynolds, C. M. E., Cawley, S., Woodside, J. V., Molloy, A. M., & Turner, M. (2018). Folate and vitamin B12 levels in early pregnancy and maternal obesity. *European Journal of Obstetrics, Gynecology, and Reproductive Biology, 231*, 80–84.

Ovesen, P., Rasmussen, S., & Kesmodel, U. (2011). Effect of prepregnancy maternal overweight and obesity on pregnancy outcome. *Obstetrics & Gynecology, 118*(2, Pt. 1), 305–312. doi:10.1097/AOG.0b013e3182245d49

Phelan, S. (2010). Obesity in the American populations: Calories, cost, and culture. *American Journal of Obstetrics & Gynecology, 203*(6), 522–524. doi:10.1016/j.ajog.2010.07.026

Phelan, S., Hart, C., Phipps, M., Abrams, B., Schaffner, A., Adams, A., & Wing, R. (2011). Maternal behaviors during pregnancy impact offspring obesity risk. *Experimental Diabetes Research, 2011*, 985139. doi:10.115/2011/985139

Polonia Valente, R., Santos, P., Ferraz, T., Montenegro, N., & Rodrigues, T. (2019). Effect of obesity on labor duration among nulliparous women with epidural analgesia. *The Journal of Maternal-Fetal & Neonatal Medicine.* doi:10.1080/14767058.2018.1543655

Ponce, J., DeMaria, E. J., Nguyen, N. T., Hutter, M., Sudan, R., & Morton, J. M. (2016). American Society for Metabolic and Bariatric Surgery estimation of bariatric surgery procedures in 2015 and surgeon workforce in the United States. *Surgery for Obesity and Related Diseases, 12*, 1637–1639. doi:10.1016/j.soard.2016.08.488

Ponce, J., Nguyen, N. T., Hutter, M., Sudan, R., & Morton, J. M. (2015). American Society for Metabolic and Bariatric Surgery estimation of bariatric surgery procedures in the United States, 2011-2014. *Surgery for Obesity and Related Diseases, 11*(6), 1199–1200. doi:10.1016/j.soard.2015.08.496

Rasmussen, K. M., & Yaktine, A. L. (Eds.). (2009). *Weight gain during pregnancy: Reexamining the guidelines.* Washington, DC: National Academies Press.

Reece, E. A. (2008). Perspectives on obesity, pregnancy and birth outcomes in the United States: The scope of the problem. *American Journal of Obstetrics & Gynecology, 198*(1), 23–27. doi:10.1016/j.ajog.

Robinson, H., Tkatch, S., Mayes, D.C., Bott, N., & Okun, N. (2003). Is maternal obesity a predictor of shoulder dystocia? *Obstetrics & Gynecology, 101*(1), 24–27.

Rooney, B. L., Schauberger, C. W., & Mathiason, M. A. (2005). Impact of perinatal weight change on long-term obesity and obesity-related illnesses. *Obstetrics & Gynecology, 106*(6), 1349–1356.

Roos, N., Neovius, M., Cnattingius, S., Lagerros, Y. T., Saaf, M., Granath, F., & Stephansson, O. (2013). Perinatal outcomes after bariatric surgery: Nationwide population based matched cohort study. *BMJ, 347*, f6460. doi:10.1136/bmj.f6460

Rottenstreich, A., Elchalal, U., Kleinstern, G., Beglaibter, N., Khalaileh, A., & Ram, E. (2018). Maternal and perinatal outcomes after laparoscopic sleeve gastrectomy. *Obstetrics & Gynecology, 131*(3), 451–456. doi:10.1097/AOG.0000000000002481

Saldana, T. M., Siega-Riz, A. M., Adair, L. S., & Suchindran, C. (2006). The relationship between pregnancy weight gain and glucose tolerance status among black and white women in central North Carolina. *American Journal of Obstetrics & Gynecology, 195*(6), 1629–1635. doi:10.1016/j.ajog.2006.05.017

Sarkar, R., Cooley, S., Donnelly, J., Walsh, T., Collins, C., & Geary, P. (2007). The incidence and impact of increased body mass index on maternal and fetal morbidity in the low-risk primigravid population. *The Journal of Maternal-Fetal & Neonatal Medicine, 20*(120), 879–883. doi:10.1080/14767050701713090

Sheiner, E., Edri, A., Balaban, E., & Aricha-Tamir, B. (2011). Pregnancy outcome of patients who conceive during or after the first year following bariatric surgery. *American Journal of Obstetrics & Gynecology, 204*(1), 50.e1–50.e6. doi:10.1016/j.ajog.2010.08.027

Shekelle, P. G., Newberry, S., Maglione, M., Li, Z., Yermilov, I., Hilton, L., . . . Chen, S. (2008). Bariatric surgery in women of reproductive age: Special concerns for surgery. *Evidence Report/Technology Assessment, 11*(169), 1–51.

Simpson, K. R. (2011). Avoiding confusion of maternal heart rate with fetal heart rate during labor. *MCN: The American Journal of Maternal Child Nursing, 36*(4), 272. doi:10.1097/NMC.0b013e318217a61a

Smid, M. C., Smiley, S. G., Schulkin, J., Stamilio, D. M., Edwards, R. K., & Stuebe, A. M. (2016). The problem of the pannus: Physician preference survey and a review of the literature on cesarean skin incision in morbidly obese women. *American Journal of Perinatology, 33*(5), 463–472. doi:10.1055/s-0035 -1566000

Society of Actuaries. (2010). *Obesity and its relation to mortality and morbidity costs.* Schaumburg, IL: Author.

Society of Obstetricians and Gynaecologists of Canada. (2010). *Obesity in pregnancy* (Clinical Practice Guideline No. 239). Vancouver, Canada: Author.

Stothard, K. J., Tennant, P. W., Bell, R., & Rankin, J. (2009). Maternal overweight and obesity and the risk of congenital anomalies: A systematic review and meta-analysis. *JAMA, 301,* 636–650. doi:10.1001/jama.2009.113

Stotland, N. E., Hopkins, L. M., & Caughey, A. B. (2004). Gestational weight gain, macrosomia, and risk of cesarean birth in nondiabetic nulliparas. *Obstetrics & Gynecology, 104*(4), 671–677. doi:10.1097/01.AOG.0000139515.97799.f6

Stream, A. R., & Sutherland, E. R. (2012). Obesity and asthma disease phenotypes. *Current Opinion in Allergy and Clinical Immunology, 12*(1), 76–81. doi:10.1097/ACI.0b013e32834eca41

Stuart, A., & Kälen, K. (2017). Risk of abdominal surgery in pregnancy among women who have undergone bariatric surgery. *Obstetrics & Gynecology, 129*(5), 887–895. doi:10.1097/AOG .0000000000001975

Szymanski, L. M., & Satin, A. J. (2012). Exercise in pregnancy: Fetal responses to current public health guidelines. *Obstetrics & Gynecology, 119*(3), 603–610. doi:10.1097/AOG .0b013e31824760b5

Tan, T., & Sia, A. T. (2011). Anesthesia considerations in the obese gravida. *Seminars in Perinatology, 35*(6), 350–355. doi:10.1053/j.semperi.2011.05.021

Thornburg, L. L. (2011). Antepartum obstetrical complications associated with obesity. *Seminars in Perinatology, 35*(6), 317–323. doi:10.1053/j.semperi.2011.05.015

Thornton, Y. S., Smarkola, C., Kopacz, S. M., & Ishoof, S. B. (2009). Perinatal outcomes in nutritionally monitored obese pregnant women: A randomized trial. *Journal of the National Medical Association, 101*(6), 569–577. doi:10.1016/s0027-9684(15) 30942-1

Tipton, A. M., Cohen, S. A., & Chelmow, D. (2011). Wound infection in the obese pregnant woman. *Seminars in Perinatology, 35*(6), 345–349. doi:10.1053/j.semperi.2011.05.020

Vahratian, A., Zhang, J., Troendle, J. F., Savitz, D. A., & Siega-Riz, A. M. (2004). Maternal prepregnancy overweight and obesity and the pattern of labor progression in term nulliparous women. *Obstetrics & Gynecology, 104*(5, Pt. 1), 943–951. doi:10.1097/01.AOG.0000142712.53197.91

Vallejo, M. C. (2007). Anesthetic management of the morbidly obese parturient. *Current Opinion in Anaesthesiology, 20*(3), 175–180. doi:10.1097/ACO.0b013e328014646b

Vidarsdottir, H., Geirsson, R. T., Hardardottir, H., Valdimarsdottir, U., & Dagbjartsson, A. (2011). Obstetric and neonatal risks among extremely macrosomic babies and their mothers. *American Journal of Obstetrics & Gynecology, 204*(5), 423.e1–423.e6. doi:10.1016/j.ajog.

Viswanathan, M., Siega-Riz, A. M., Moos, M. K., Deierlein, A., Mumford, S., Knaack, J., . . . Lohr, K. N. (2008). *Outcomes of maternal weight gain* (Evidence Report/Technology Assessment No. 168). Rockville, MD: Agency for Healthcare Research and Quality.

Vricella, L. K., Louis, J. M., Mercer, B. M., & Bolden, N. (2010). Anesthesia complications during scheduled cesarean delivery for morbidly obese women. *American Journal of Obstetrics & Gynecology, 203*(3), 276.e1–276.e5. doi:10.1016/j.ajog.2010.06.022

Vricella, L. K., Louis, J. M., Mercer, B. M., & Bolden, N. (2011). Impact of morbid obesity on epidural anesthesia complications in labor. *American Journal of Obstetrics & Gynecology, 205*(4), 370.e1–370.e6. doi:10.1016/j.ajog.2011.06.085

Weiss, J. L., Malone, F. D., Emig, D., Ball, R. H., Nyberg, D. A., Comstock, C. H., . . . D'Alton, M. (2004). Obesity, obstetric complications and cesarean delivery rate: A population-based screening study. *American Journal of Obstetrics & Gynecology, 190,* 1091–1097. doi:10.1016/j.ajog.2003.09.058

Whitaker, R. C. (2004). Predicting preschooler obesity at birth: The role of maternal obesity in early pregnancy. *Pediatrics, 114*(1), 29–36. doi:10.1542/peds.114.1.e29

Wloch, C., Wilson, J., Lamagni, T., Harrington, P., Charlett, A., & Sheridan, E. (2012). Risk factors for surgical site infection following caesarean section in England: Results from a multicenter cohort study. *BJOG, 119,* 1324–1333. doi:10.1111/j.1471 -0528.2012.03452.x

Wolfe, K. B., Rossi, R. A., & Warshak, C. (2011). The effect of maternal obesity on the rate of failed induction of labor. *American Journal of Obstetrics & Gynecology, 205*(2), 128.e1–128.e7. doi:10.1016/j.ajog.2011.03.051

World Health Organization. (2000). *Obesity: Preventing and managing the global epidemic* (WHO Technical Report Series, 894). Geneva, Switzerland: Author. Retrieved from http://www.who .int/nutrition/publications/obesity/WHO_TRS_894/en/

World Health Organization. (2018). *Obesity and overweight.* Geneva, Switzerland: Author.

Zhang, J., Bricker, L., Wray, S., & Quenby, S. (2007). Poor uterine contractility in obese women. *BJOG, 114*(3), 343–348. doi:10.1111/j.1471-0528.2006.01233.x

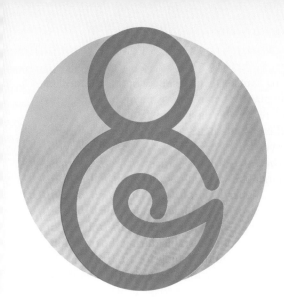

CHAPTER 13

Maternal–Fetal Transport

Judy Wilson-Griffin

INTRODUCTION

Maternal transport is a fundamental component of regionalized care. Perinatal regionalization through a structured designated method guarantees that hospitals and healthcare systems provide a full range of services for pregnant women and their babies within a specified geographic region (American Academy of Pediatrics [AAP] & American College of Obstetricians and Gynecologists [ACOG], 2017). ACOG and the Society for Maternal-Fetal Medicine have published levels for maternal care that systematically support the idea of appropriate care at the right site (ACOG, 2019b). In a seminal document published in 1976, and repeated in the third version, *Toward Improving the Outcome of Pregnancy*, the March of Dimes (MOD, 1976, 2010) proposed a model system for regionalization of perinatal care including definitions for levels of care (e.g., levels I to III) in hospitals that provided perinatal services. The goal was to promote transfer of high-risk mothers to hospitals with the appropriate level of care based on gestational age of the fetus. This model was adopted across the United States and resulted in perinatal regionalization and improved perinatal outcomes as more preterm babies and babies with high-risk conditions were born at centers that had skilled personnel and additional resources for their stabilization and ongoing care (MOD, 2010). High-risk pregnant women also benefited by being cared for in level II and level III perinatal centers. Since the 1970s, regionalized care has proven to be a useful service that can improve both maternal and/or fetal outcomes (AAP & ACOG, 2017; ACOG, 2019b). Due to evidence of significant improvements in outcomes for these patients when stabilized and transferred appropriately, the National Quality Forum (2009), in their *National Voluntary Consensus Standards for Perinatal Care*, recommended using "babies under 1,500 g be born at a hospital with the appropriate level of care" as a quality care indicator. Today, every facility and region should include maternal transport as part of their emergency plan. This can be essential in caring for the perinatal population during natural or man-made emergencies (AAP & ACOG, 2017; ACOG, 2019b).

Neonatal transport has been active in the United States since the 1960s, after the establishment of neonatal intensive care units (AAP & ACOG, 2017). However, even with the development of well-trained neonatal transport teams, evidence has shown that in most cases, the mother proves to be the best transport vehicle for the fetus (AAP & ACOG, 2017; MOD, 2010). Thus, maternal, instead of neonatal transport, is preferred when feasible. As with any procedure, transport has advantages and disadvantages. While there may be advantages to the health of both the mother and her unborn fetus, it can be less than ideal to have women give birth potentially far from their home, family, and friends, and without their primary obstetrician who they have become accustomed to for continued care. Indications for maternal–fetal transport are listed in Display 13–1.

EMERGENCY MEDICAL TREATMENT AND ACTIVE LABOR ACT

When discussing maternal–fetal transport, it is important to review the Emergency Medical Treatment and Active Labor Act (EMTALA) regulations as they relate to appropriate transfers. EMTALA originated in 1985 as part of the Consolidated Omnibus Budget Reconciliation Act to protect patients during an emergency regardless of their ability to pay for care or insurance status.

DISPLAY 13–1

Indications for Maternal–Fetal Transport

Medical
- Anemia
- Autoimmune
- Cardiac disease
- Diabetes
- Hematologic disorder
- Infection/sepsis
- Liver disease
- Malignancy
- Neurologic disorder
- Obesity
- Psychiatric disorder
- Pulmonary disease
- Renal disease
- Substance disorder
- Surgical emergencies
- Thromboembolic disease

Obstetric
- Amniotic fluid abnormalities
- Fetal demise
- Hemorrhagic disorders of pregnancy
- Hypertensive disorders in pregnancy
- Multiple gestation
- Premature labor
- Premature rupture of membranes
- Vaginal bleeding

Fetal/Newborn
- Fetal anomalies
- Fetal growth restriction
- Placental abnormalities
- Congenital abnormalities
- Isoimmunization

Contraindication or May Not Be Advisable for Reason Listed
- Lack of an appropriate method for safe transfer
- Weather and road conditions to hazardous for safety
- Maternal or fetal condition unstable
- Patient who declines transfer

The law requires that all patients, including those in labor, be assessed, stabilized, and treated at the hospital where they present regardless of their ability to pay for care or insurance status. EMTALA requires that hospitals perform a medical screening exam for anyone who presents with an emergency medical condition (EMC) (AAP & ACOG, 2017; Angelini & LaFontaine, 2017). The goal for the patient who presents is to either be stabilized, treated, or transferred to a facility that can better meet the medical needs of the patient based on her individual clinical situation (AAP & ACOG, 2017; Angelini & LaFontaine, 2017). Pregnant women who present contracting and/or who may be in labor are considered unstable. The question then becomes when it is

appropriate to transfer a pregnant woman to another facility. A pregnant woman who is having contractions is not considered to be having an EMC if it is determined that there is adequate time to safely transfer her before she gives birth, or if the transfer will not pose a threat to the safety of the patient. Caregivers must evaluate whether the woman and her fetus will be better served at a higher level of care. This is not always a straightforward or clear clinical judgment (Wade & Greenwood, 2018). A woman who appears stable prior to transport may become unstable during the transport. Unanticipated birth could occur prior to arrival at the receiving facility. Transfer might also be feasible based on the patient's request. Using a triage tool to determine the urgency of a women's complaint can assist in appropriate management and disposition. The Association of Women's Health, Obstetric and Neonatal Nurses (AWHONN) developed the Maternal Fetal Triage Index tool that can be an adjunct tool when time is essential in obtaining information and planning for next steps (AAP & ACOG, 2017; Angelini & LaFontaine, 2017, AWHONN, 2016; Wade & Greenwood, 2018).

Whenever maternal transport is an option, the risks and benefits must be thoroughly considered. Several procedures must be completed to be compliant with EMTALA regulations. A conversation between the referring physician and accepting physician at the receiving location should occur prior to transfer. The receiving location should have adequate space and staff to accommodate the woman being transferred and the baby anticipated to be born. A copy of the medical record should accompany the mother on transfer. Prior to the transport, consent is required from the mother regarding the transfer, the destination, and method of transport. It is important to avoid violating the spirit, intent, and rules of the EMTALA law when transferring a pregnant woman. EMTALA violations can result in significant fines and can have negative implications for the reputation of the transferring facility. Common EMTALA violations include the following (AAP & ACOG, 2017; Angelini & LaFontaine, 2017):

- Lack of or inadequate assessment
- Lack of patient stabilization prior to transfer to another facility
- Failure to obtain patient consent for the transfer
- No documented accepting physician
- Transferring with inappropriate equipment and personnel
- Failure to stabilize the patient prior to transfer

TYPES OF INTER–MATERNAL–FETAL TRANSPORT

One-Way Transport

One-way transport is the most common type of transport. The referring institution makes arrangements for the patient transfer, usually by local ambulance or helicopter service, which provides transportation to the accepting facility. The advantages of one-way transport are that the patient may be transported by staff they are familiar with from the referring hospital, potentially facilitating a more rapid transport process. The referring facility assumes responsibility and direction of care until a formal handoff is given at the accepting institution. A disadvantage is limited availability of transport vehicles and appropriately skilled personnel in transport and emergency procedures at the originating facility. Often, personnel at level I facilities are not trained in maternal transport, or they may not receive ongoing training in prehospital care and safety in transport vehicles, which could potentially pose additional safety concerns (AAP & ACOG, 2017; Drummond, 2017; Wade & Greenwood, 2018).

Two-Way Transport

In a two-way transport, the receiving facility accepts the patient and then sends a team to transport the patient to their facility. That facility accepts medical and legal responsibility for the patient once report has been received by the team upon arrival. The advantage of two-way transport is that it allows the receiving institution to bring its highly skilled service directly to the bedside and begin that level of care immediately. The transport team should explain what the patient can expect once they arrive at the receiving institution. The two-way transport team has been trained in the prehospital management and care of the pregnant patient. A disadvantage may include delay in transfer because travel of the team from the receiving facility to the referring facility adds time to the process (AAP & ACOG, 2017; ACOG, 2019a; MOD, 2010).

MODE OF TRANSPORT

Fixed Wing (Airplane)

Airplanes can be a viable option for long-distance and possible weather-affected maternal transports. It also provides a more spacious mode of air transport. Compared to the cost of a rotor wing (helicopter), it may be a less expensive option for air transport. Fixed wing flights require access to a runway, along with an additional method of transport to the receiving facility. This transport method many times can become a major challenge when time is a factor in moving a patient from one location to another. Finding airplanes that come equipped with personnel ready to deal with obstetric emergencies can also be a disadvantage for some programs. Potential side effects during flight may include nausea and vomiting, increase in contractions, worsening hypertension or hypotension, decrease in respiratory effort, and unplanned changes in the intravenous (IV) flow rate (AAP & ACOG, 2017; Scott, 2016; Vyas & Menghani, 2016).

Rotor Wing (Helicopter)

Helicopters are usually used for shorter distances or when the patient has a more urgent need. When speed is important, use of a helicopter offers advantages in accessing timely care for the perinatal patient (AAP & ACOG, 2017). The helicopter is staffed with critical care personnel experienced in airway management and acute conditions. Long distance by ground can affect outcomes for the pregnant patient, thus making air a more attractive option.

Challenges for use of helicopters include aircraft availability. Concerns are for appropriate landing zones at either the referring or receiving location. Weather may be problematic for air transport. The cost of helicopter transport may also be a disadvantage for using this as a means for moving the patient from one location to another. Ability to adequately assess labor status and monitor the fetus continuously may be of concern due to the noise and vibration. Despite the advantage of air transport, flight teams are often concerned about in-flight birth.

Ground (Ambulance)

Ambulances are used for urgent or interfaculty patient transport based on patient condition, distance, and provider request. The major advantage to using ground transport is that it is usually easy to access and there may be different types of units readily available. Ambulances are less affected by weather when compared to air transport. Ground transport is also more economical than other forms of patient transport. Equipment in an ambulance varies depending on whether the ambulance is a basic or critical care unit. Ambulances are equipped with medical supplies, telemetry monitors, and portable oxygen. Maternal–fetal transport team composition may include nurses, respiratory therapists, paramedics, and emergency medical technicians (EMTs). Team composition may be driven by location resources, provider contacts, and governmental oversight. Some states have specialized maternal–fetal transport units equipped and used exclusively for transports of the mother or baby.

TRANSPORT EQUIPMENT

The transport team requires equipment to adequately monitor the patient during transport and for emergency treatment if necessary. When planning a maternal–fetal transport, it is important to check to make sure everything that is needed is available in the transport vehicle. The following equipment is suggested regardless of the method of transport. Other equipment may be necessary based on the individual clinical situation.

- Vital sign monitoring equipment
- Doppler/fetal monitor for fetal heart rate assessment

- IV administration setup and infusion device (smart pumps)
- Respiratory equipment
- Medications
- Emergency birth equipment
- Latex-free supplies
- Infant resuscitation equipment
- Documentation method (electronic or manual) (AAP & ACOG, 2017; Huwe et al., 2019; Scott, 2016)

TRANSPORT PERSONNEL

Well-trained personnel who can manage obstetric patients in the prehospital environment are essential for a successful program. Composition of the team may vary depending on resources, regulatory requirements, patient condition, and vehicle used during transport. When transporting a patient by ground, the team may consist of an EMT or paramedic, respiratory therapist, labor and delivery nurse, and/or neonatal nurse. For patients requiring air transport, the team may be composed of critical care flight nurses and flight paramedics, a labor and delivery nurse, and/or neonatal nurse. Clinical experience needed to care for perinatal patients during transport includes annual prehospital safety training, leadership skills, advanced cardiac life support skills, knowledge of how to care for high-risk labor conditions and emergent birth, and neonatal resuscitation skills. Requirements for joining a maternal-fetal transport team are determined by each program. It is important to establish clear guidelines and medical control once the team has received report and assumes care of the patient until arriving at the receiving location. During transport, a well-prepared team will be able to respond to possible complications or risks in the prehospital environment.

COMMUNICATION PLAN

Care team communication requires complete, current, and reasonable dialogue to decrease the risk of errors. Communication tools found in TeamSTEPPS can assist in effectively communicating key information at a critical time. The use of checklists and mnemonics are other useful aides (ACOG, 2017; Wade & Greenwood, 2018).

Patient communication and involvement can be essential in addressing concerns related to the reason for the transport and her personal well-being. Patients should understand not only the reason for the transport but also what to expect during and after they arrive at the receiving location.

Family should be provided information regarding where the patient is being transferred, directions, estimated time of arrival, and contact numbers.

TRANSPORT PLAN AND PATIENT PREPARATION

Once the need for maternal transport has been identified, a discussion with the patient and her family regarding the reason for transfer must occur. The pregnant woman must agree to transfer to another facility by providing written consent. A copy of the transfer consent should accompany the patient to the receiving location. The referring physician will contact the accepting location and review the reason for referral. Both physicians will decide on the mode of transport based on the distance, weather, patient condition, safety, and cost, in most cases. Information should be provided to the family regarding where the patient is being transferred, directions, and contact numbers. All pertinent medical records should accompany the patient to the receiving location (AAP & ACOG, 2017; ACOG, 2019b; MOD, 2010).

Basic preparations prior to departing the facility include establishing IV access, supplemental oxygen as needed, monitoring pulse oximetry levels, and assessing the patient's bladder. Pretransport assessment including vital signs, fetal well-being, labor status, and current state of initial reason for transport should be documented prior to departure (AAP & ACOG, 2017; Drummond, 2017; Huwe et al., 2019; Wade & Greenwood, 2018). When securing the patient to the stretcher, it is important to encourage uterine displacement to promote blood flow during transport. Care should be taken to maintain physical safety while maintaining respiratory and hemodynamic stability during maternal–fetal transport. Once the woman arrives at the new location, a direct patient handoff from the transport team with the receiving staff is ideal to promote patient safety. Patient handoff information includes any significant events during transport, along with the reason for the referral, vital signs, and response to any medications and treatments (see Fig. 13–1 for a sample documentation form to be used for maternal transport to record these types of data). This report should include information about emergency contacts and the family that is en route to the hospital. Figures 13–2 and 13–3 provide examples of physician orders that can be used for maternal transport, with Figure 13–3 specific to a woman in early preterm labor. It is important that the receiving physician keep the sending provider updated on the status of his or her patient and the plan following discharge.

MATERNAL TRANSPORT FORM

Please check (✓) the appropriate box (□) and fill in the blank(s) as needed.

Date: _____ Initiational call time: _____ □ Airplane □ Helicopter □ Ground Miles	RN:		Trip accepted
	Accepting MD	Phone number	
Trip No.	Departed	Arrive Location	Depart	Arrive
Location		Phone	
Referring MD	Phone number	
Patient name	Age	DOB	Weight
Transport Diagnosis		Height

CURRENT LABOR HISTORY

Gravida	Para	Abortion	Living children	Gestational age	
Estimated date of confinement	Last menstrual period	Time □ Sterile speculum	Time □ Vaginal exam	
Dilation ___ cm	Effacement	Station	Membranes □ intact	Time PROM	Location of scars x Location of fetal heart tones

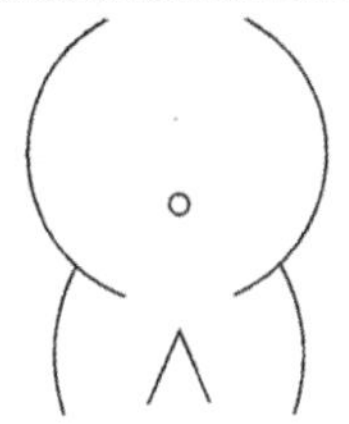

Antenatal testing: □ Ultrasound □ Amniocentesis □ Non stress test

Fetal status / Strip review
Date: _____   Time: _____

PATIENT ASSESSMENT

Allergies/Sensitivities □ NKDA □ Latex □ Other:	Blood Glucose Time _____ Results _____	Circulatory: □ WNL □ Heart disease □ MVP □ Chest pain □ Blood transfusions
Respiratory □ 02 _____ □ Asthma □ Smoker	Sensory □ Visual changes □ Glasses □ Contacts □ Headaches	LOC □ Seizure □ WNL □ Alert	Pain score (1-10)
Reflexes □ 4+ □ 3+ □ 2+ □ 1+ □ Absent	Urinalysis □ Protein □ Ketones	Abdomen □ Soft □ Tender □ Rigid	Edema □ Face □ Hands □ Feet

Complications of pregnancy:

Support person	Contact number
Status update to referring hospital	
Status update to referring hospital	
Date	Time	Call report to RN: _____

RN Signature: _____

PATIENT LABEL

FIGURE 13–1. Maternal transport form. (From SSM St. Mary's Health Center, Richmond Heights, MO.)

MATERNAL TRANSPORT FORM

PRE-TRANSPORT NOTES

Date: _____ Time: _____

INTRA-TRANSPORT NOTES

Date: _____ Time: _____

Transfer of care to: Name _____   Date: _____   Time: _____

| MEDICATIONS/IV FLUIDS | | | | | VITAL SIGNS | | | | | | | |
TIME	MEDICATION/FLUID TYPE	DOSE RATE	ROUTE SITE	GIVEN BY REFER HOSP.	TIME	T	HR	RR	BP	SpO2	FHT	CTX

PATIENT LABEL

FIGURE 13–1. *(Continued)*

MATERNAL TRANSPORT PHYSICIAN ORDERS

DRUG MAY BE DISPENSED IN ACCORDANCE WITH THE
HOSPITAL FORMULARY SYSTEM UNLESS CHECKED HERE ⇨ ☐

ALLERGIES: ☐ NO KNOWN ALLERGIES

			IMPORTANT REMINDERS	
			1. "Daily" instead of "qd"	5. "Morphine" instead of "MSO4"
			2. "Units" instead of "u"	6. "Magnesium sulfate" instead of "MgSO4"
			3. No trailing zeros (1mg, not 1.0mg)	7. "Every other day" instead of "Q.O.D."
			4. Always use leading zeros	8. "MCG" instead of "µg"
			(0.1mg, not .1mg)	9. "International Units" instead of "IU"

PATIENT WEIGHT ⇨ _____   ☐ Kgs ☐ Lbs   PATIENT HEIGHT ⇨ _____

✓	DATE ORDERED	TIME	√	INITIAL HERE TO INDICATE TELEPHONE ORDER READ BACK FOR ACCURACY	ORDERS

Accepting physician: Dr. _____   Contact #

IUP:

Monitoring

- Vital signs on arrival at referral hospital and review fetal monitor strip before transfer
- Obtain maternal vital signs and FHR just prior to transport 5-15 minutes prior to departure. Vitals Q 15 minutes during transport. Temperature Q 4 hours, if membranes ruptured then Q 2 hours.
- EKG monitoring as needed
- Assess level of consciousness
- Assess abdominal tenderness and for bladder distention.
- Position patient to provide for uterine displacement.
- If indicated to assess cervical dilation, sterile vaginal exam if membranes intact, sterile speculum exam if membranes ruptured
- Call physician for:
  - Temperature greater than 99.9°F
  - RR greater than 22 or less than 12
  - Pulse greater than 120
  - Systolic BP greater than 160 or less than 80
  - Diastolic BP greater than 100 or less than 40
  - Tetanic contractions and or non reassuring FHT's

Labs

☐ GBS culture, bring specimen back to St. Mary's laboratory

☐ Fern test to rule out ROM

☐ Fetal fibronectin if no vaginal exam in the past 24 hours

Intake & Output

- Foley for bladder distention prn
- Intake and output prior to departure

Fluids

- IV with 18 gauge needle: (not necessary to restart IV if adequate 18 gauge line in place)
- 1000 ml Lactated Ringers at 125 ml per hour

Respiratory

- O2 at 10L/min per non-rebreather mask for fetal intolerance or maternal oxygen saturation level less than 95%

NPO

PATIENT LABEL

FIGURE 13–2. Maternal transport physician orders. (From SSM St. Mary's Health Center, Richmond Heights, MO.)

MATERNAL TRANSPORT PHYSICIAN ORDERS

DRUG MAY BE DISPENSED IN ACCORDANCE WITH THE
HOSPITAL FORMULARY SYSTEM UNLESS CHECKED HERE ⇨ ☐

ALLERGIES:

	IMPORTANT REMINDERS
1. "Daily" instead of "qd" 2. "Units" instead of "u" 3. No trailing zeros (1mg, not 1.0mg) 4. Always use leading zeros (0.1mg, not .1mg)	5. "Morphine" instead of "MSO4" 6. "Magnesium sulfate" instead of "MgSO4" 7. "Every other day" instead of "Q.O.D." 8. "MCG" instead of "μg" 9. "International Units" instead of "IU"

PATIENT WEIGHT ⇨ _____   ☐ Kgs ☐ Lbs   PATIENT HEIGHT ⇨ _____

✓	DATE ORDERED	TIME	↓	INITIAL HERE TO INDICATE TELEPHONE ORDER READ BACK FOR ACCURACY	ORDERS
				Medications:	
				Antiemetic	
				☐ Zofran 8 mg IVP one time for nausea	
				Fetal Lung Maturity	
				☐ Betamethasone 12 mg IM x 1 if 24 to 34 weeks gestation, for fetal lung maturity	
				☐ Finger stick per portable blood glucose monitor prior to administration of medication. If blood glucose greater than 200 contact medical control before administration.	
				GBS Prophylaxis for positive on unknown status	
				☐ Penicillin 5 million units IVPB x 1	
				If allergic to Penicillin:	
				☐ Clindamycin 900 mg IVPB x 1	
				Additional Orders:	
				Nurse Signature: Date: Time:	
				Physician Signature: Date: Time:	

PATIENT LABEL

FIGURE 13–2. *(Continued)*

MATERNAL TRANSPORT PREMATURE LABOR/PROM PHYSICIAN ORDERS

DRUG MAY BE DISPENSED IN ACCORDANCE WITH THE
HOSPITAL FORMULARY SYSTEM UNLESS CHECKED HERE ⇒ ☐

ALLERGIES: ☐ NO KNOWN ALLERGIES

	IMPORTANT REMINDERS
1. "Daily" instead of "qd"	5. "Morphine" instead of "MSO4"
2. "Units" instead of "u"	6. "Magnesium sulfate" instead of "MgSO4"
3. No trailing zeros (1mg, not 1.0mg)	7. "Every other day" instead of "Q.O.D."
4. Always use leading zeros	8. "MCG" instead of "μg"
(0.1mg, not .1mg)	9. "International Units" instead of "IU"

PATIENT WEIGHT ⇒ _____ ☐ Kgs ☐ Lbs   PATIENT HEIGHT ⇒ _____

✓	DATE ORDERED	TIME	✓ INITIAL HERE TO INDICATE TELEPHONE ORDER READ BACK FOR ACCURACY	ORDERS
				Accepting physician: Dr. _____ Contact #
				IUP:
				Monitoring
				• Vital signs on arrival at referral hospital and review fetal monitor strip before transfer
				• Obtain maternal vital signs and FHR 5-15 minutes prior to departure. Vitals Q 15 minutes during transport.
				Temperature Q 4 hours, if membranes ruptured then Q 2 hours.
				• EKG monitoring as needed
				• Assess abdominal tenderness and for bladder distention.
				• Position patient to provide for uterine displacement.
				• Assess level of consciousness
				• Check deep tendon reflexes (DTR) prior to departure and following loading dose of Magnesium Sulfate
				• If indicated to assess cervical dilation, sterile vaginal exam if membranes intact, sterile speculum exam if membranes ruptured
				• Call physician for:
				• Temperature greater than 99.9°F
				• RR greater than 22 or less than 12
				• Pulse greater than 120
				• Systolic BP greater than 160 or less than 80
				• Diastolic BP greater than 100 or less than 40
				• Tetanic contractions and or non reassuring FHT's
				• Active vaginal bleeding
				NPO
				Intake & Output
				• Foley for bladder distention prn
				• Intake and output prior to departure
				Labs
				☐ GBS culture, bring specimen back to St. Mary's laboratory
				☐ Fern test to rule out ROM
				☐ Fetal fibronectin if no vaginal exam in the past 24 hours
				☐ Finger stick blood glucose prior to administration of medication. If blood glucose greater than 200 contact medical control before administration of Terbutaline and/or Betamethasone
				Fluids
				• IV with 18 gauge needle: (not necessary to restart IV if adequate 18 gauge line in place)
				☐ 125mL/hr 1000 ml Lactated Ringers
				☐ 75 mL/hr 1000 ml Lactated Ringers if receiving Magnesium Sulfate IV
				Respiratory
				• O2 at 10L/min per non-rebreather mask for fetal intolerance or maternal oxygen saturation level less than 95%

PATIENT LABEL

FIGURE 13–3. Maternal transport physician orders for premature labor/premature rupture of membranes. (From SSM St. Mary's Health Center, Richmond Heights, MO.)

MATERNAL TRANSPORT PREMATURE LABOR/PROM PHYSICIAN ORDERS

DRUG MAY BE DISPENSED IN ACCORDANCE WITH THE HOSPITAL FORMULARY SYSTEM UNLESS CHECKED HERE ⇒ ☐

ALLERGIES:

PATIENT WEIGHT ⇒ _____ ☐ Kgs ☐ Lbs   PATIENT HEIGHT ⇒ _____

IMPORTANT REMINDERS

1. "Daily" instead of "qd"
2. "Units" instead of "u"
3. No trailing zeros (1mg, not 1.0mg)
4. Always use leading zeros (0.1mg, not .1mg)
5. "Morphine" instead of "MSO4"
6. "Magnesium sulfate" instead of "MgSO4"
7. "Every other day" instead of "Q.O.D."
8. "MCG" instead of "μg"
9. "International Units" instead of "IU"

✓	DATE ORDERED	TIME	▼	INITIAL HERE TO INDICATE TELEPHONE ORDER READ BACK FOR ACCURACY	ORDERS

Medications

IV tocolytic medications for preterm labor:

Choose one: ☐ 2 gm Magnesium Sulfate in 50 mL Sterile Water over 20 minutes

☐ 4 gm Magnesium Sulfate in 100 mL Sterile Water over 30 minutes

☐ 6 gm bolus of Magnesium Sulfate (2 gm plus 4 gm dosage noted above)

☐ Magnesium Sulfate 20 grams in 500 mL Sterile Water run at 2gm/hour (2gm in 50mL) maintenance infusion.

Increase every 30 minutes by 0.5 grams per hour until contractions less than Q 15 minutes to a maximum dose of 4 grams per hour.

- *For absent DTR or change in level of consciousness discontinue Magnesium Sulfate and contact medical control.*
- *If patient unresponsive and RR less than 8 administer calcium gluconate and contact medical control.*

Sub-Q or IVP Terbutaline medications in nondiabetic patients

Choose one: ☐ 0.25 mg Terbutaline IVP every 10 minutes times 2 for non-reassuring fetal heart tones. Hold if maternal heart rate over 120 beats per minutes.

☐ 0.25 mg Terbutaline Sub-Q every 20 minutes times 2 for preterm labor if contractions more frequent than Q 15 minutes. Hold if maternal heart rate over 120 beats per minutes

PO tocolytic medications for preterm labor

Choose one: ☐ 50 mg Indocin PO times one

☐ 20 mg Procardia PO times one

Magnesium Sulfate toxicity

☐ 10% Calcium gluconate 10 mL IVP over 5 minutes

Antiemetic

☐ Zofran 8 mg IVP times 1 for nausea

Fetal Lung Maturity

☐ Betamethasone 12 mg IM times 1 if 24 to 34 weeks gestation, for fetal lung maturity

GBS Prophylaxis for positive on unknown status

☐ Penicillin 5 million units IVPB x 1

If allergic to Penicillin:

☐ Clindamycin 900 mg IVPB x 1

Additional Orders:

Nurse Signature: Date: Time:

Physician Signature: Date: Time:

PATIENT LABEL

FIGURE 13–3. *(Continued)*

SUMMARY

Maternal transport is an adjunct therapy that can enhance a region's ability to meet the demands for perinatal care and yet be fiscally responsible and improve maternal and fetal outcomes. A critical systematic interdisciplinary review of referrals can be an effective tool to further identify ways to improve the care provided to perinatal patients. Feedback to the referring hospital from the receiving hospital regarding the patient preparation process can be valuable in promoting quality care, as is feedback from the referring hospital to the receiving hospital when it is focused on how patient needs were met and the timeliness and courtesy of response. Together, the teams can assist each other in providing the best care possible during maternal referral and transport.

REFERENCES

American Academy of Pediatrics & American College of Obstetricians and Gynecologists. (2017). *Guidelines for perinatal care* (8th ed.). Elk Grove Village, IL: American Academy of Pediatrics.

American College of Obstetricians and Gynecologists. (2017). *Hospital disaster preparedness for obstetricians and facilities providing maternity care* (Committee Opinion No. 726). Washington, DC: Author.

American College of Obstetricians and Gynecologists. (2019a). *Critical care in pregnancy* (Practice Bulletin No. 211). Washington, DC: Author.

American College of Obstetricians and Gynecologists. (2019b). Levels of maternal care (Obstetric Care Consensus No. 9). *Obstetrics & Gynecology, 134*(2), e41–e55. doi:10.1097/AOG.0000000000003383

Angelini, D. J., & LaFontaine, D. (Eds.). (2017). *Obstetric triage and emergency care protocols* (2nd ed.). New York, NY: Springer.

Association of Women's Health, Obstetric and Neonatal Nurses. (2016). *Maternal Fetal Triage Index*. Washington, DC: Author.

Drummond, S. (2017). Maternal transport. In M. Kennedy (Ed.), *Intrapartum management modules: A perinatal education program* (5th ed., pp. 501–514). Philadelphia, PA: Wolters Kluwer.

Huwe, V. Y., Puck, A. L., Vasher, J., Baird, S. M., Witcher, P. M., & Troiano, N. H. (2019). Maternal transport clinical care guidelines. In N. H. Troiano, P. M. Witcher, & S. M. Baird (Eds.), *High-risk & critical care obstetrics* (4th ed., pp. 405–409). Philadelphia, PA: Wolters Kluwer.

March of Dimes. (1976). *Toward improving the outcomes of pregnancy I*. White Plains, NY: Author.

March of Dimes. (2010). *Toward improving the outcome of pregnancy III*. White Plaines, NY: Author.

National Quality Forum. (2009). *National voluntary consensus standards for perinatal care 2008: A consensus report*. Washington, DC: Author.

Scott, J. (2016). Obstetric transport. *Obstetrics and Gynecology Clinics of North America, 43*(4), 821–840. doi:10.1016/j.ogc.2016.07.013

Vyas, L., & Menghani, R. (2016). Transport of the critically ill obstetric patient. In A. Gandhi, N. Malhotra, J. Malhotra, N. Gupta, & N. M. Bora (Eds.), *Principles of critical care in obstetrics* (pp. 337–344). doi:10.1007/978-81-322-2686-4_36

Wade, K., & Greenwood, T. (2018). Gynecologic and obstetric emergencies. Critical care transport. In R. S. Holleran, A. C. Wolfe, & M. A. Frakes (Eds.), *Patient transport: Principles & practice* (5th ed., pp. 429–466). St. Louis, MO: Elsevier.

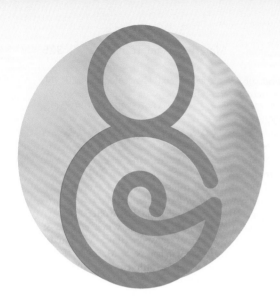

CHAPTER 14

Labor and Birth

Kathleen Rice Simpson • Nancy O'Brien-Abel

INTRODUCTION

Labor and birth are natural processes. Most women do well with support and minimal selected intervention. The minimal intervention philosophy acknowledges that most pregnancies, labors, and births are normal and that intervention creates the potential for iatrogenic maternal–fetal injuries. Interventions should move forward on a continuum from noninvasive to least invasive and from nonpharmacologic to pharmacologic according to the wishes of the woman and the discretion of healthcare providers based on individual clinical situations. A philosophy of minimal intervention works best in the context of a well-designed safety net, allowing for intervention when necessary, in a clinically timely manner. During the intrapartum period, nurses use knowledge of physiologic and psychosocial aspects of birth and selected pharmacologic therapies to provide comprehensive care for women and families. The focus of this chapter is on nursing interventions that enable the labor and birth process.

OVERVIEW OF LABOR AND BIRTH

Onset of Labor

Multiple theories have been proposed to explain the biophysiologic factors that initiate labor; however, this process is not yet fully understood. A combination of maternal–fetal factors influence labor onset (Display 14–1). It is likely that a parturition cascade occurs in humans that results in the removal of the mechanisms that maintain uterine quiescence and the initiation of factors that promote uterine activity (Buckley, 2015; Liao, Buhimschi, & Norwitz, 2005). Labor and birth are multifactorial processes that involve interconnected positive feedforward and negative feedback loops that are linked in a carefully time-regulated fashion (Nathanielsz, 1998; Smith, 2007). These pathways in the fetus, placenta, and mother require sequential initiation and include redundancy that can prevent a single factor from prematurely initiating labor or preventing the initiation of labor (Liao et al., 2005). Ongoing research related to preterm birth prevention has suggested that there is a genetic component to the timing of labor (Plunkett et al., 2011; Zhang et al., 2017), which may help to explain why some women experience preterm birth and others remain pregnant until 41 weeks or more.

A complex series of events must occur during labor and birth that represent a reversal of role for the uterus and cervix during pregnancy. The myometrium, which has remained relatively quiet for many months, has to become active, and the cervix, which has functioned to prevent birth, must lose its resistance. This involves an integrated set of changes within the maternal tissues (myometrium, decidua, and cervix) that occur gradually over a period of days to weeks (Buckley, 2015; Liao et al., 2005; Smith, 2007). Despite extensive research, knowledge of the exact mechanism for spontaneous labor remains incomplete. Most of what is known is from animal studies and in vitro investigations of biopsies obtained from the myometrium and cervix at cesarean birth (Bernal, 2003; Hurd, Gibbs, Ventolini, Horowitz, & Guy, 2005; Liao et al., 2005).

The forces of labor are uterine contractions acting on the resistance of the cervix. The uterine walls are flexible, expanding over time until the onset of labor, when the myometrium converts from a quiet state to a highly active contractile organ. The cervix, composed of connective tissue, remains firmly closed until it is time for labor to begin; then it undergoes

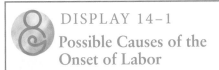

rapid, dramatic changes, including ripening, effacement, and dilation (Liao et al., 2005). The conditions and processes that result in term labor are regulated by several compounds and biochemical systems, including progesterone withdrawal and prostaglandin synthesis (Bernal, 2003; Buckley, 2015). Activation of the myometrium requires receptor sites, an increased production of prostaglandin, and the formation of gap junctions. Gap junctions are specialized protein units located within the cell membrane that connect neighboring cells and provide communication channels (Ulmsten, 1997). The number of gap junctions, as well as their permeability and performance, has a direct influence on myometrial function during labor (Bernal, 2003).

It is theorized that after the preparation and activation period, the myometrium is ready to be stimulated for contractions (Buckley, 2015; Liao et al., 2005). Prostaglandin and oxytocin are the most important biochemical factors in stimulating term myometrial activity (Oláh & Gee, 1996; Slater, Zervou, & Thornton, 2002). Prostaglandin synthesis during the cervical ripening period also prepares the myometrium to respond to oxytocin (Sheehan, 2006). It is known that oxytocin alone cannot induce the formation of gap junctions. The oxytocin hormone is synthesized by the hypothalamus and then transported to the posterior lobe of the pituitary gland, where it is released into maternal circulation (Blackburn, 2018).

The release of oxytocin is caused by stimuli such as breast stimulation, sensory stimulation of the lower genital tract, and cervical stretching (Blackburn, 2018). The milk-ejection reflex results from oxytocin released due to breast stimulation. Oxytocin released in response to vaginal and cervical stretching results in uterine contractions through Ferguson reflex. Differences in reported plasma concentrations of oxytocin during pregnancy and spontaneous labor can be attributed in part to individual variations among pregnant women and methodologies used to measure levels of oxytocin; however, it is generally accepted that in addition to a tonic baseline release of oxytocin, there is a pulsatile release action that may increase in amplitude and frequency during labor (Fuchs et al., 1991).

Two types of oxytocin receptors have been identified and quantified in the human uterus: myometrial and decidual (Liao et al., 2005). Both play an important part in the initiation of spontaneous labor and birth. Oxytocin receptors are present in low concentrations until the later part of the third trimester, during which their numbers increase dramatically (Buckley, 2015). This lack of receptors until late pregnancy probably contributes to the lack of uterine response to oxytocin earlier than during the third trimester (Sultatos, 1997). Oxytocin receptors in the myometrium and decidua reach their peak levels at slightly different times during pregnancy and labor. During pregnancy, as weeks of gestation increase, there is a steady increase in the number of oxytocin receptors in the myometrium (Buckley, 2015; Caldeyro-Barcia & Poseiro, 1960). As pregnancy progresses, the number of oxytocin receptor sites in the myometrium increases by 100-fold at 32 weeks and by 300-fold at the onset of labor (Arias, 2000). This rise in receptor concentration is paralleled by an increase in uterine sensitivity to circulating oxytocin. Myometrial receptors are thought to peak in early spontaneous labor and significantly contribute to the initiation of uterine activity (Fuchs, Fuchs, Husslein, & Soloff, 1984). It is likely that the concentration of myometrial receptors plays a dominant role in uterine response to endogenous and exogenous oxytocin. Over an approximate 2-week period before the onset of labor, contraction frequency and intensity increase in a pre-labor synchronization of uterine activity. However, these contractions are usually not perceived by the pregnant woman because they are less than 20 mm Hg in intensity (Newman, 2005). As intensity increases beyond 20 to 30 mm Hg, the woman gradually becomes aware of uterine activity, especially via palpation, although these contractions are not noted as painful by most women (Newman, 2005). When contraction intensity is above 30 mm Hg, some women may perceive discomfort. This type of contraction pattern is usually characterized by infrequent contractions and periodic episodes until active labor begins (Newman, 2005). Early labor contractions are concentrated in the lower and middle uterine segments, whereas active labor contractions originate in the fundal area of the uterus (Newman, 2005).

Oxytocin receptors in the decidua are thought to increase as labor progresses and reach peak levels during birth (Fuchs, Husslein, & Fuchs, 1981). During labor, oxytocin stimulates the production and release of arachidonic acid and prostaglandin F_2 by the decidua that has been sensitized to oxytocin, thus potentiating oxytocin-induced uterine activity (Husslein, Fuchs, & Fuchs, 1981). All oxytocin receptor site interactions do not result in uterine muscle contraction. Although oxytocin does occupy myometrial and decidual receptor sites during labor, the uterus is not in a constant state of contraction. Labor contractions are rhythmic and coordinated, providing evidence that some smooth muscle cells have their oxytocin receptor site occupied without stimulating contraction (Bernal, 2003; Sultatos, 1997).

The exact mechanism of muscle cell coordination during labor remains unknown (Blackburn, 2018; Buckley, 2015). One theory is that a signal from pacemaker cells, possibly located in the uterine fundus, is transmitted to other myometrial cells by cell-to-cell communication through gap junctions (Sultatos, 1997). Another theory is that although there is a tonic baseline release of oxytocin from the posterior lobe of the pituitary gland, it is the pulsatile release action that may increase in amplitude and frequency during labor, which could be responsible for the rhythmic nature of uterine contractions (Fuchs et al., 1991). More data are needed to confirm or dispute these theories.

Premonitory signs, such as lightening, urinary frequency, pelvic pressure, changes in vaginal discharge, bloody show, loss of mucous plug, and irregular contractions, are frequently reported several weeks before actual labor begins. Some women also describe changes in sleep patterns and increased energy levels in the final weeks of pregnancy. True labor is characterized by regular uterine contractions resulting in progressive cervical effacement and dilation accompanied by fetal descent into the maternal pelvis (Display 14–2).

Duration of Labor

There are significant variations in normal labor progress and duration among childbearing women. Classic research by Friedman (1955) described characteristics of normal labor progression in nulliparous women in the 1950s. This research was later expanded to include

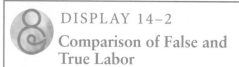

DISPLAY 14–2
Comparison of False and True Labor

False Labor
- Regular contractions
- Decrease in frequency and intensity; longer intervals
- Discomfort in lower abdomen and groin
- Activity has no effect or decreases contractions; disappears with sleep
- No appreciable change in cervix
- Sedation decreases or stops contractions.
- Show usually not present

True Labor
- Regular contractions
- Progressive frequency and intensity; closer intervals
- Discomfort begins in back, radiating to the abdomen.
- Activity such as walking increases contractions; continues even when sleeping
- Progressive effacement and dilation of cervix
- Sedation does not stop contractions.
- Show usually present

a series of definitions of labor protraction and arrest (Friedman, 1978). Friedman's work made major contributions to what was known about normal labor progress. His findings that changes in cervical dilatation and fetal station over time were the most useful parameters for the assessment of the progress of labor were novel at the time (Cohen & Friedman, 2018). Evidence that normal labors had similar patterns of dilatation and descent, differing only in the durations and slopes of their component parts, led to development of criteria that changed the way labor was assessed in the United States and across the world (Caughey, 2017; Cohen & Friedman, 2018).

The Friedman (1955, 1978) curve likely represented the ideal labor progression of women during the time these data were collected and analyzed rather than the average labor progression (Zhang, Troendle, & Yancey, 2002). Historically, the Friedman labor curve was widely used in the clinical setting to assess normal labor progression (Cohen & Friedman, 2018). However, both maternal characteristics and obstetric practices have changed considerably over the past 50 years (American College of Obstetricians and Gynecologists [ACOG] & Society for Maternal-Fetal Medicine [SMFM], 2014; Caughey, 2017; Laughon, Branch, Beaver, & Zhang, 2012). Women are older and have higher body mass indices, both of which are associated with longer labor duration (Hilliard, Chauhan, Zhao, & Rankins, 2012; Hirshberg, Levine, & Srinivas, 2014; Kominiarek et al., 2011; Laughon et al., 2012; Treacy, Robson, & O'Herlihy, 2006; Vahratian, Zhang, Troendle, Savitz, & Siega-Riz, 2004; Zaki, Hibbard,

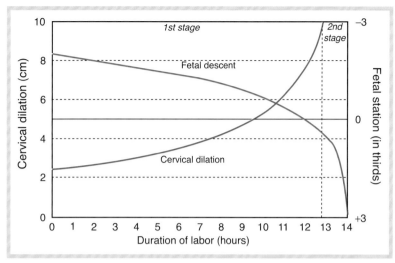

FIGURE 14–1. Patterns of cervical dilation (*left*) and fetal descent (*right*) in nulliparous women based on contemporary clinical conditions. (From Zhang, J., Troendle, J. F., & Yancey, M. K. [2002]. Reassessing the labor curve in multiparous women. *American Journal of Obstetrics & Gynecology, 187*[4], 824–828.)

& Kominiarek, 2013). Oxytocin induction and epidural use are also more common, and each has been shown to contribute to longer labors (Harper, Caughey et al., 2012; Laughon et al., 2012; Osmundson, Ou-Yang, & Grobman, 2010). Figure 14–1 represents data on patterns of cervical dilation and fetal descent for nulliparous women in spontaneous labor based on clinical conditions occurring in the present obstetric environment (Zhang et al., 2002). These data are averages; each woman progresses in labor based on individual factors and clinical conditions.

Data from pregnancies at term, in spontaneous active labor, with cephalic, singleton fetuses were compared between the *Collaborative Perinatal Project* (labors during 1959 to 1966) and the *Consortium on Safe Labor* (labors during 2002 to 2008) (Laughon et al., 2012). Based on review of these data, active labor (4 to 10 cm) is longer by a median of 2.6 hours for nulliparous women and active labor (5 to 10 cm) is longer by median of 2 hours for multiparous women in the modern obstetric cohort when compared to women who labored in the 1950s and 1960s (Laughon et al., 2012). Figures 14–2 A and B represent data comparing active labors of nulliparous and multiparous women from the *Collaborative Perinatal Project* to the *Consortium for Safe Labor*. Due to limited data about cervical dilation before 4 cm in nulliparous women and before 5 cm in multiparous women, the labor curves begin at 4 cm and 5 cm for nulliparous and multiparous women, respectively (Laughon et al., 2012). It is unclear why these differences have developed; however, they likely have been influenced by changes in obstetric practice over the last 50 years because after adjusting for changes in maternal and pregnancy characteristics, researchers found the increase in length

of labor remained significantly longer in the modern cohort compared to the older cohort (Laughon et al., 2012). The modern cohort also experienced dramatic changes in obstetric practices including more oxytocin for labor induction and augmentation, more epidurals, and a fourfold increase in cesarean births, along with less episiotomies and operative vaginal births (Laughon et al., 2012).

Therefore, based on available data (Abalos et al., 2018; Harper, Caughey, et al., 2012; Laughon et al., 2012; Neal, Lowe, Ahijevych, et al., 2010; Neal, Lowe, Patrick, Cabbage, & Corwin, 2010; Oladapo et al., 2018; Tilden et al., 2019; Zhang, Landy, et al., 2010; Zhang, Troendle, Reddy, et al., 2010; Zhang et al., 2002), previously held arbitrary time frames for duration of labor (Friedman, 1955, 1978; Friedman, Niswander, Bayonet-Rivera, & Sachtleben, 1966; Hellman & Prystowsky, 1952) are no longer valid for all women. Multiple factors, including parity, timing, and dosage of epidural analgesia/anesthesia; use of oxytocin or misoprostol; amniotomy; fetal size, position, and gender; and maternal psyche, age, body mass, labor positions, and pelvic structure, influence progress of labor (ACOG, 2009a; ACOG & SMFM, 2014; Cahill, Roehl, Odibo, Zhao, & Macones, 2012; Harper, Caughey, et al., 2012; Hoffman, Vahratian, Sciscione, Troendle, & Zhang, 2006; Laughon et al., 2012; Rhoades & Cahill, 2017; Zhang et al., 2002). Reconsidering the expected duration of labor based on these data from a contemporary obstetric population has significant clinical indications for potentially avoiding unnecessary interventions.

Labor dystocia (i.e., slow abnormal progression of labor) is the leading indication for primary cesarean birth in the United States (American Academy of

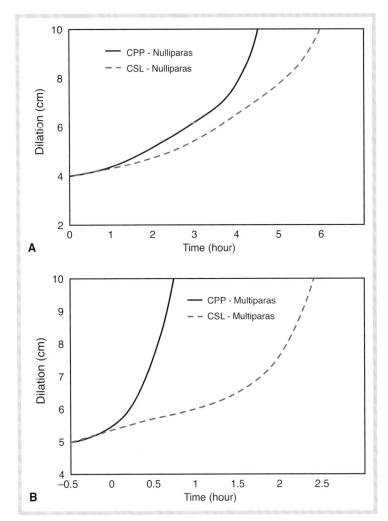

FIGURE 14–2. Comparison of active labor of nulliparous **(A)** and multiparous **(B)** women using data from the Collaborative Perinatal Project (CPP) and the Consortium for Safe Labor (CSL). Due to limited data about cervical dilation before 4 cm in nulliparous women and before 5 cm in multiparous women, the labor curves begin at 4 and 5 cm for nulliparous and multiparous women, respectively. (From Laughon, S. K., Branch, D. W., Beaver, J., & Zhang, J. [2012]. Changes in labor patterns over 50 years. *American Journal of Obstetrics & Gynecology, 206*[5], 419.e1–419.e9. doi:10.1016/j.ajog.2012.03.003)

Pediatrics [AAP] & ACOG, 2017; ACOG & SMFM, 2014; Zhang, Troendle, Reddy, et al., 2010). According to AAP and ACOG (2017), a prolonged latent phase (e.g., greater than 20 hours in nulliparous women or greater than 14 hours in multiparous women) should not be an indication for cesarean birth. Contemporary labor patterns suggest the active phase of first stage spontaneous labor likely does not start until 6 cm for nulliparous women and until 5 cm for multiparous women (Zhang, Landy, et al., 2010). A 2-hour threshold without cervical change for diagnosing labor arrest is too short before 6-cm dilation (Zhang, Troendle, Mikolajczk, et al., 2010). Progress of labor from 4 to 6 cm is far slower than previously thought based on contemporary labor patterns (Zhang, Landy, et al., 2010). Labor takes more than 6 hours to progress from 4 to 5 cm and more than 3 hours to progress

from 5 to 6 cm for both nulliparous and multiparous women (Zhang, Landy, et al., 2010). See Table 14–1 for duration of labor in hours by parity for women in spontaneous labor based on the work of Zhang, Landy, et al. (2010).

Nulliparous women likely have cervical dilation less than 0.5 cm/hr in earlier active labor and faster in later active labor (Neal, Lowe, Patrick, et al., 2010). Unrealistic expectations of faster labor based on outdated evidence is a problem contributing to excessive unnecessary interventions such as labor augmentation techniques as well as primary and repeat cesarean birth in the United States (ACOG, 2019a; ACOG & SMFM, 2014; Neal & Lowe, 2012; Oladapo et al., 2018). Based on data about cesarean birth from the *Consortium for Safe Labor*, Zhang, Troendle, Reddy, et al. (2010) found that one half of women who had a

TABLE 14–1. Duration of Spontaneous Labor by Parity

Cervical dilation (cm)	Parity 0 (cm/hr; n = 25,624)	Parity 1 (cm/hr; n = 16,755)	Parity 2+ (cm/hr; n = 16,219)
3 to 4	1.8 (8.1)	—	—
4 to 5	1.3 (6.4)	1.4 (7.3)	1.4 (7.0)
5 to 6	0.8 (3.2)	0.8 (3.4)	0.8 (3.4)
6 to 7	0.6 (2.2)	0.5 (1.9)	0.5 (1.8)
7 to 8	0.5 (1.6)	0.4 (1.3)	0.4 (1.2)
8 to 9	0.5 (1.4)	0.3 (1.0)	0.3 (0.9)
9 to 10	0.5 (1.8)	0.3 (0.9)	0.3 (0.8)
Second stage with epidural analgesia	1.1 (3.6)	0.4 (2.0)	0.3 (1.6)
Second stage without epidural analgesia	0.6 (2.8)	0.2 (1.3)	0.1 (1.1)

Data are median (95th percentile).

From Zhang, J., Landy, H. J., Branch, D. W., Burkman, R., Haberman, S., Gregory, K. D., . . . Reddy, U. M. (2010). Contemporary patterns of spontaneous labor with normal neonatal outcomes. *Obstetrics & Gynecology, 116*(6), 1281–1287. doi:10.1097/AOG.0b013e3181fdef6e

cesarean birth for labor dystocia had not yet reached 6-cm cervical dilation. There are significant differences in length of spontaneous labor and induced labor (Grobman, Bailit, et al., 2018; Grobman, Rice, et al., 2018; Harper, Caughey, et al., 2012; Hoffman et al., 2006; Incerti et al., 2011; Rouse, Owen, Savage, & Hauth, 2001; Simon & Grobman, 2005; Vahratian, Zhang, Troendle, Sciscione, & Hoffman, 2005; Zhang, Landy, et al., 2010). Spontaneous labor is generally shorter.

A latent phase as long as 18 hours during labor induction for nulliparous women is not unusual, and most of these women will give birth vaginally if time is allowed to achieve active labor (ACOG, 2009a; ACOG & SMFM, 2014; Harper, Caughey, et al., 2012; Simon & Grobman, 2005; Zhang, Landy, et al., 2010). Regional analgesia/anesthesia lengthens the active phase of labor by approximately 60 to 90 minutes (Alexander, Sharma, McIntire, & Leveno, 2002; ACOG, 2019b). Labor progression for nulliparous and multiparous women appears to be at a similar pace before 6 cm; however, after 6 cm, labor accelerates much faster in multiparous compared to nulliparous women (Zhang, Landy, et al., 2010).

Although multiparous women usually experience faster active labor than nulliparous women, additional childbearing generally has no further effect on labor progression (Vahratian, Hoffman, Troendle, & Zhang, 2006). There also is a relationship between parity and type of labor progression variances. It is known that women in labor with their first child are more likely to experience hypertonic uterine dysfunction, primary inertia, or a prolonged latent phase in early labor (Friedman, 1978). During second and subsequent labors, deviations from the Friedman criteria during active labor, such as hypotonic uterine dysfunction, secondary inertia, and protraction or arrest of the active phase, are more common (Ness, Goldberg, & Berghella, 2005).

Based on the evidence, an arbitrary 2-hour time frame is not clinically valid for evaluating second stage labor progress. As long as the fetal heart rate (FHR) is normal and there is evidence of fetal descent, there is no risk to the fetus in waiting a reasonable time for spontaneous birth (ACOG & SMFM, 2014; Cheng & Caughey, 2017; Cheng, Hopkins, & Caughey, 2004; Le Ray, Audibert, Goffinet, & Fraser, 2009). A prolonged second stage beyond 4 hours may increase maternal risk of operative vaginal birth and perineal trauma (Cheng et al., 2004; Myles & Santolaya, 2003). The length of first-stage labor can be a predictor of length of second-stage labor in nulliparous women (Nelson, McIntire, Leveno, 2013). There is an association between long first-stage labor and long second-stage labor (Nelson et al., 2013).

Recommendations from AAP and ACOG (2017) include consideration of operative vaginal birth for nulliparous women when there is lack of continuing progress for 3 hours with regional anesthesia or for 2 hours without regional anesthesia. For multiparous women, operative vaginal birth should be considered after lack of continuous progress for 2 hours with regional anesthesia or for 1 hour without regional anesthesia (AAP & ACOG, 2017). These recommendations are for consideration and not an absolute necessity for operative vaginal birth. In other words, after these time periods, a complete evaluation of the woman's progress, maternal–fetal status, and the likelihood that more pushing will safely accomplish vaginal birth should be undertaken.

The recommendations from AAP and ACOG (2017) are based on timing of determination of complete cervical dilation and fetal head engagement. Supportive evidence is based on when women were noted to be completely dilated via vaginal examination, rather than when they were actually 10 cm, so these data are inexact. Frequency of vaginal examinations during labor has a significant effect on accuracy of determination of the beginning of second-stage labor. Other maternal factors, such as length of active pushing and efficacy of maternal pushing efforts, should be considered as well when determining the safest method of birth. Some women may need to individualize pushing efforts based on the fetal response (e.g., pushing with every other or every third contraction or discontinuing pushing temporarily to maintain a normal FHR pattern). Other women may become fatigued after sustained pushing efforts and request a period of rest. Therefore, maternal–fetal status and individual clinical situations provide the best data for labor assessment and management.

Stages of Labor and Birth

Labor and birth are divided into stages. The first stage has been subdivided into the latent and active phases of labor. Cervical changes are used in assessing progression through each phase: latent phase, 0 to 5 cm; active phase, 6 to 10 cm. Women laboring for the first time usually experience complete cervical effacement prior to dilation. Increasing effacement usually occurs simultaneously with dilation in multiparous women. The second stage of labor begins at complete cervical dilation and ends with the birth of the baby. This stage of labor is subdivided into the initial latent phase (passive fetal descent) and the active pushing phase (Association of Women's Health, Obstetric and Neonatal Nurses [AWHONN], 2019b; Roberts, 2002, 2003). The third stage of labor begins with the birth of the baby and ends with the delivery of the placenta. The fourth stage of labor begins with the delivery of the placenta and lasts until the woman is stable in the immediate postpartum period, usually within the first hour after birth. The immediate postpartum recovery period extends beyond the fourth stage of labor and includes at least the first 2 hours after birth based on maternal status (AAP & ACOG, 2017).

Nursing Assessments

Admission Assessment of Maternal–Fetal Status

Major roles of the perinatal nurse caring for laboring women include a thorough admission assessment and ongoing maternal–fetal assessments. The focus of this assessment is on prior obstetric history, current pregnancy, and labor symptoms. Usually, a complete history and physical examination has been conducted by the primary care provider during the prenatal period and is included in the prenatal records that become part of the hospital's medical record. By 36 weeks of gestation, a copy of the prenatal record should be on file in the perinatal unit or available in the electronic medical record, so pertinent data can easily be accessed when the woman presents in labor. If the woman has

received prenatal care and if data on a recent history and physical examination confirming normal progress of pregnancy are available for review, the admission evaluation may be limited to an interval history and a physical examination directed at the presenting condition. If the woman has not had prenatal care, or if no prenatal care records are available, a more comprehensive assessment including appropriate laboratory data is advised. *Guidelines for Perinatal Care* (AAP & ACOG, 2017) provide recommendations for the components of a comprehensive admission assessment for pregnant women.

Whereas most pregnant women come to the hospital's labor and birth unit for perinatal care, some women may be seen for an evaluation and treatment of nonobstetric illnesses. Department policies will help determine conditions best treated in the labor and birth unit and those that should be treated in other hospital-care units. Any pregnant woman presenting to a hospital for care should, at a minimum, be assessed for the following: FHR (as appropriate for gestational age), maternal vital signs, and uterine contractions. The responsible perinatal healthcare provider should be informed promptly if any of the following findings are present or suspected: vaginal bleeding, acute abdominal pain, temperature of 100.4°F or higher, abnormal maternal heart rate or respiratory rate, preterm labor, preterm premature rupture of membranes, hypertension, category II or III FHR pattern, signs of imminent birth, or inability to detect FHR (AAP & ACOG, 2017). When a pregnant woman is evaluated for labor, the following factors should be assessed and recorded: estimated due date, blood pressure (BP), pulse, temperature, frequency and duration of uterine contractions, fetal well-being, cervical dilation and effacement (unless contraindicated [e.g., placenta previa]), preterm rupture of membranes, fetal presentation and station of the presenting part, status of the membranes, date and time of the woman's arrival, and notification of the provider (AAP & ACOG, 2017). The provider should assess and document the maternal pelvic examination, cervical length, as ascertained by transvaginal ultrasonography, if performed, and estimated fetal weight (AAP & ACOG, 2017). Previously identified risk factors should be recorded in the prenatal record. If no new risk factors are found, attention may be focused on the following historical factors: time of onset and frequency of contractions; status of the membranes; presence or absence of bleeding; fetal movement; history of allergies; the time, content, and amount of the most recent food or fluid ingestion; and use of any medication (AAP & ACOG, 2017).

At times, pregnant women may come to the hospital before labor is established. They may be experiencing uterine contractions that have not yet resulted in cervical changes or they may be in very early labor.

Onset of labor is established by observing progressive cervical change; thus, differentiation between true and false labor status may require two or more cervical examinations that are separated by an adequate period to observe change (AAP & ACOG, 2017). Admission to the labor and birth unit may be deferred during the latent phase of labor for women who have been evaluated and deemed stable and the FHR tracing indicates fetal well-being (ACOG, 2019a). They should be offered frequent contact, support, and nonpharmacologic pain management measures (ACOG, 2019a). A policy that allows for the adequate evaluation of labor and prevents unnecessary admissions to the perinatal unit is advisable (AAP & ACOG, 2017; ACOG, 2016b, 2019a; AWHONN, 2015). When false or early labor is diagnosed, the woman should be given instructions for when to return to the hospital. Fetal status should be determined prior to discharge, ideally using a reactive nonstress test. If a thorough maternal–fetal assessment results in the decision to discharge the woman, it is important to ensure that assessment and discharge processes are consistent with federal regulations as per the Emergency Medical Treatment and Active Labor Act. The leadership teams in some perinatal units have found it helpful to require that two clinicians review fetal data and verify their agreement on fetal status prior to the discharge of a pregnant woman from the hospital.

A Maternal Fetal Triage Index (MFTI) has been developed by AWHONN (2015) as a tool that can be helpful in assessing pregnant women who present to the hospital for care and making sure they are seen and treated in a timely manner based on maternal and fetal condition. The tool has been tested for validity and reliability in a number of hospitals in the United States (Ruhl, Scheich, Onokpise, & Bingham, 2015a, 2015b) and is suggested by AAP and ACOG (2017) and ACOG (2016b) as a good option for assessing pregnant women who present to the hospital for care (Fig. 14–3).

When women are observed or admitted for pain or fatigue in latent labor, techniques such as education and support, oral hydration, positions of comfort, and nonpharmacologic pain management techniques such as massage or hydrotherapy may be helpful (ACOG, 2019a). The initial interaction during the admission process is used to develop rapport with the woman and her family and to get a sense of their expectations for their birth experience. Ideally, the amount of childbirth preparation and type of pain management anticipated during labor is covered during the admission assessment. A review of preferences for childbirth, including a discussion of options that are available at the institution, works best to facilitate a positive experience. Although some labor nurses, physicians, and other members of the perinatal team may have negative feelings toward written birth plans, a birth plan can be valuable in helping the nurse meet the couple's expectations and indicates that the woman has given considerable thought to how she would like the labor and birth to proceed. Birth plans that have been discussed previously with the woman's primary healthcare provider can promote her participation in and satisfaction with her care (AAP & ACOG, 2017). See Display 17–1 in Chapter 17 for a family preference plan for childbirth.

Ongoing Assessment of Maternal–Fetal Status

Limited data are available to support prescribed frequencies of maternal–fetal assessments during labor and birth. No prospective studies have been published concerning how often to assess the mother and fetus during labor. Therefore, a reasonable approach to determining the frequency of assessment is based on individual clinical situations, guidelines, and standards from professional organizations and unit policies. According to AAP and ACOG (2017), maternal temperature, pulse, respirations, and BP should be assessed and recorded at least every 4 hours. This frequency may be increased, particularly as active labor progresses and in the presence of complications such as infection or preeclampsia.

Frequency of FHR and uterine activity assessment and documentation are guided by professional nursing and medical organizations, unit guidelines, and the clinical situation (AAP & ACOG, 2017; American College of Nurse-Midwives [ACNM], 2015a; ACOG, 2009b, 2010; AWHONN, 2011, 2018b, 2019b; Liston, Sawchuck, Young, 2018; National Institute for Health and Care Excellence, 2014; Wisner & Holschuh, 2018). Generally, the assessment and documentation of fetal status during labor includes FHR baseline, variability, the presence or absence of accelerations and decelerations, and pattern evolution over time. Generally, the assessment and documentation of uterine activity during labor includes contraction frequency, duration, and intensity along with uterine resting tone between contractions. If oxytocin is infusing, the rate in milliunits per minute (mU/min) should be included.

When using electronic fetal monitoring (EFM), if no risk factors are present at the time of admission or none develop during labor, the FHR should be determined and evaluated at 30-minute intervals during the latent phase of labor from 4 up to 6 cm and the active phase of the first stage of labor (6 to 10 cm) and at 15-minute intervals during the active pushing phase of the second stage of labor, unless fetal risk status or response to labor indicates the need for more frequent assessment (AAP & ACOG, 2017; ACOG, 2009b; AWHONN, 2018b, 2019b). Low risk in this context

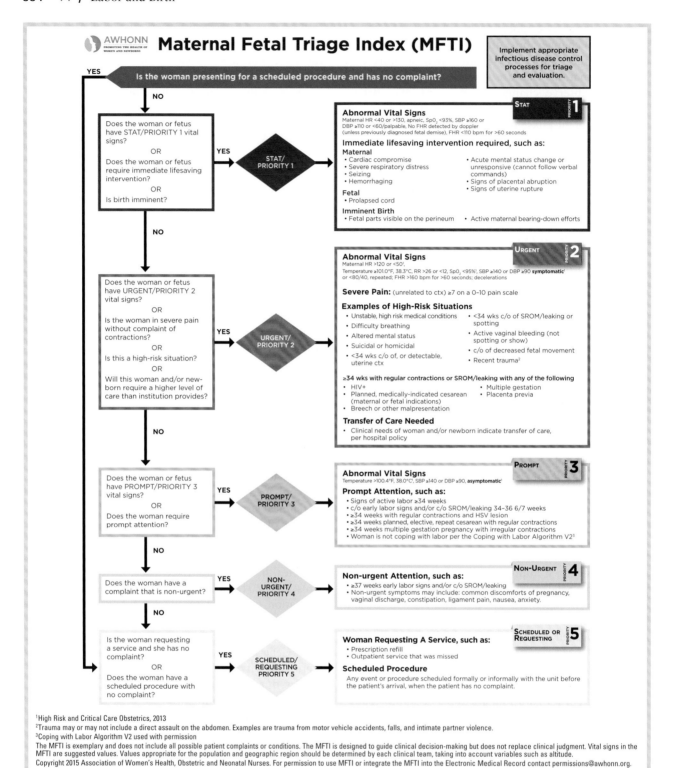

FIGURE 14–3. The Maternal Fetal Triage Index (MFTI) is exemplary and does not include all possible patient complaints or conditions. The MFTI is designed to guide clinical decision making but does not replace clinical judgment. Vital signs in the MFTI are suggested values. Values appropriate for the population and geographic region should be determined by each clinical team, taking into account variables such as altitude.

has been variously defined. Per AAP and ACOG (2017), low risk generally includes women who have

- No meconium staining, intrapartum bleeding, or abnormal or undetermined fetal test results before birth or at initial admission
- No increased risk of developing fetal acidemia during labor (e.g., congenital anomalies, intrauterine growth restriction)
- No maternal condition that may affect fetal well-being (e.g., prior cesarean scar, diabetes, hypertensive disease)
- No requirement for oxytocin induction or augmentation of labor

If risk factors or complications are present on admission or develop during the course of labor, the FHR should be determined and evaluated every 15 minutes during the latent phase of labor from 4 up to 6 cm and the active phase of the first stage of labor (6 to 10 cm) and every 5 minutes during the active pushing phase of the second stage of labor (AAP & ACOG, 2017; ACOG, 2009b; AWHONN, 2018b, 2019b). There are insufficient data from clinical trials to make a firm recommendation for how often to assess fetal status via EFM during latent phase labor from 0 up to 4 cm (AWHONN, 2018b). Data are available to guide suggestions from latent phase labor from 4 up to 6 cm and for active phase of labor (AWHONN, 2018b). Continuous EFM is recommended for women with complications (e.g., suspected fetal growth restriction, preeclampsia) and those that require oxytocin for induction or augmentation of labor (AAP & ACOG, 2017; ACOG, 2009b). During oxytocin administration, the FHR should be determined and evaluated every 15 minutes during the first stage of labor and the latent or passive fetal descent phase of the second stage of labor, then every 5 minutes during the active pushing phase of the second stage of labor (AAP & ACOG, 2017; AWHONN, 2018b, 2019b).

When EFM is used to record FHR data permanently, periodic documentation can be used to summarize fetal status during second-stage labor maternal pushing efforts, as outlined by unit protocol (AWHONN, 2018b, 2019a). For example, it may be appropriate for a nurse who is at the bedside continually assessing FHR and supporting the woman during the active pushing phase of the second stage of labor to document FHR interpretation in a summary note approximately every 30 minutes (AWHONN, 2018b, 2019b).

To facilitate the option of intermittent auscultation of the FHR, healthcare providers and hospitals should consider adopting protocols and educating nurses to use a handheld Doppler device for low-risk women desiring such monitoring during labor (ACOG, 2019a). When using intermittent auscultation, if no risk factors or complications are present at the time of admission or none develop during labor, AAP and ACOG (2017) recommend that the FHR should be determined, evaluated, and recorded at least every 30 minutes (preferably before, during, and after a contraction) during the active phase of the first stage of labor and at least every 15 minutes during the active pushing phase of the second stage of labor. If risk factors or complications are present on admission or develop during the course of labor, the FHR should be determined, evaluated, and recorded at least every 15 minutes during the active phase of the first stage of labor and every 5 minutes during the active pushing phase of the second stage of labor (AAP & ACOG, 2017). Frequency ranges of every 15 to 30 minutes during the active phase of the first stage of labor and every 5 to 15 minutes during the active pushing phase of the second stage of labor are recommended by AWHONN based on an evaluation of factors including patient preferences, the phase and stage of labor, maternal response to labor, an assessment of maternal–fetal condition and risk factors, and facility rules and procedures (AWHONN, 2018b; Wisner & Holschuh, 2018). Either protocol (AAP & ACOG, 2017, or AWHONN, 2018b) is acceptable for intermittent auscultation of the FHR during labor. The AWHONN practice monograph *Fetal Heart Rate Auscultation* (Wisner & Holschuh, 2018) provides a comprehensive discussion about technique, rationale, interpretation, and clinical decision making when using intermittent auscultation during labor.

When auscultation or EFM is used, FHR and uterine activity are documented according to unit protocol. A reasonable approach is to document findings each time they are determined, except when assessing the FHR at 5-minute intervals, due to the difficulty of documenting and concurrently providing labor support to the woman. In these cases, summary documentation is acceptable, and the individual hospital policy should be followed (AWHONN, 2018b). Summary documentation of fetal status every 30 minutes during the active pushing phase of second stage labor, while indicating continuous nursing bedside attendance and evaluation, seems reasonable. For AWHONN's (2018b) recommendation for frequency of assessment of fetal status using EFM and intermittent auscultation, see Tables 15–4 and 15–8. When a woman is receiving oxytocin for labor induction or augmentation, recommendations are for the assessment of maternal and fetal status every 5 to 15 minutes (first stage labor) and every 5 minutes (active pushing phase of second stage labor) (AAP & ACOG, 2017). Nurse staffing of one nurse to one woman receiving oxytocin is recommended (AWHONN, 2010) and should allow for the ability to document these data in the medical record in a timely manner. When nurse staffing is not as recommended (e.g., the labor nurse is caring for more than one woman receiving oxytocin), the documentation of maternal and fetal status every 5 to 15 minutes in real time is a challenge.

Guidelines for ongoing labor assessments are described in AWHONN's Practice Monographs *Cervical Ripening, Labor Induction and Labor Augmentation* (Simpson, 2020) and *Fetal Heart Rate Auscultation* (Wisner & Holschuh, 2018) and Evidence-Based Clinical Practice Guidelines *Nursing Care and Management of the 2nd Stage of Labor* (AWHONN, 2019b) and *Nursing Care of the Woman Receiving Regional Analgesia/Anesthesia in Labor* (AWHONN, 2011). *Guidelines for Perinatal Care* (AAP & ACOG, 2017); the ACOG Practice Bulletins *Intrapartum Fetal Heart Rate Monitoring: Nomenclature, Interpretation, and General Management Principles* (ACOG, 2009b) and *Management of Intrapartum Fetal Heart Rate Tracings* (ACOG, 2010); and the American Society of Anesthesiologists (ASA) publication "Practice Guidelines for Obstetric Anesthesia" (ASA, 2016). Perinatal nursing textbooks and some state board of health publications are other resources that provide guidelines for initial and ongoing nursing assessments of women in labor. Based on these standards and guidelines, each perinatal center should have expectations for maternal–fetal assessment during labor in the form of clinical policies, protocols, or algorithms. See Display 14–3 and Table 14–2 for suggested guidelines for maternal and fetal assessment during labor, birth, and immediately postpartum (see Chapters 17 and 18 for more detailed information about postpartum and newborn assessment).

Maternal–fetal assessment should occur at the bedside by laying hands on the pregnant woman rather than using data obtained from viewing screens at the central monitoring station. Characteristics of FHR patterns may be different when obtained by direct observation of the EFM tracing at the bedside. Direct observation allows for the assessment of maternal anxiety or pain, contractions, and positioning, all of which have the potential to affect vital signs. For example, maternal anxiety or pain can result in increases in BP, pulse, and respirations, while maternal supine positioning can result in hypotension. Repositioning from a semi-Fowler position to a lateral position may result in a decrease in diastolic BP of up to 10 mm Hg. During second-stage pushing, maternal heart rate accelerations have the potential to overlap with FHR decelerations, resulting in signal ambiguity and confusion (Neilson, Freeman, & Mangan, 2008). Maternal pushing efforts that involve the Valsalva maneuver result in an initial increase and then a decrease in BP (Caldeyro-Barcia et al., 1981).

When assessing FHR via EFM, make sure the heart rate that is tracing is indeed of fetal origin rather than maternal (Simpson, 2011b). If coincident alerts are being displayed, an assessment of the source of the heart rate tracing is indicated. Confirm maternal heart rate by palpation of maternal pulse during initiation of EFM and compare with FHR; repeat this confirmation periodically during labor. Be aware of abrupt changes in FHR that may indicate maternal heart rate is tracing.

Be knowledgeable about fetal physiology (it is unlikely that an FHR baseline with tachycardia, minimal variability, intermittent late decelerations, and no accelerations will spontaneously improve to a normal baseline rate, moderate variability, and accelerations during second-stage pushing; what appear to be FHR accelerations during pushing are often maternal heart rate). Be aware that maternal tachycardia could be tracing as FHR; if the mother is tachycardic, pay close attention to distinguishing between maternal heart rate and FHR. Recognize other clinical situations that could result in maternal heart rate being recorded as FHR including contractions, maternal movement such as walking with the cordless transducer or telemetry, inaccurate transducer placement, maternal weight/size, fetal position, number of fetuses, and placental location (Simpson, 2011b).

There is insufficient evidence to support a definitive recommendation for the frequency of BP monitoring prior to, during, and after the initiation of epidural analgesia/anesthesia. However, there is evidence that maternal BP can decrease significantly 5 to 15 minutes after initiation or rebolus of anesthetic/analgesic agents and up to one third of women may develop hypotension within 1 hour of regional anesthetic injection (AWHONN, 2011). Therefore, a reasonable approach is to assess maternal BP after the initiation or rebolus of a regional block, including patient-controlled epidural analgesia (AWHONN, 2011). BP may be assessed every 5 minutes for the first 15 minutes and then repeated at 30 minutes and at 1 hour after the procedure (AWHONN, 2011). More or less frequent monitoring may be indicated based on a consideration of factors such as the type of analgesia/anesthesia, route and dose of medication used, the maternal–fetal response to medication, the maternal–fetal condition, the stage of labor, and unit protocol (AWHONN, 2011). Frequency of subsequent BP assessment while epidural analgesia/anesthesia is in place should be based on a consideration of these variables. Absent evidence from clinical trials to support a specific time frame for the reassessment of BP for this patient population, a reasonable approach is BP assessment approximately every hour.

In many institutions, routine care for healthy women during epidural analgesia/anesthesia includes pulse oximetry and frequent BP assessment using an automatic BP device. The continuous use of these monitoring devices is not required (AAP & ACOG, 2017; ACOG, 2019b; AWHONN, 2011) and may lead to increased cost and unnecessary technologic interventions for women without identified risk factors. Automatic BP devices often cause considerable discomfort. There is no need to leave the cuff in place during labor. Periodic assessment of maternal BP should be based on the individual maternal-fetal situation and involve the caregiver at the bedside placing the BP cuff for the assessment and removing the cuff once the procedure is completed. Continuous maternal oxygen saturation (SpO_2) monitoring should be discouraged

DISPLAY 14–3

Maternal–Fetal–Newborn Assessments during Labor, Birth, and the Immediate Postpartum Period

Risk Status as a Determinate of Timing and Type of Assessment

Low risk in this context generally includes women who have no meconium staining, intrapartum bleeding, or abnormal or undetermined fetal test results before birth or at initial admission; no increased risk of developing fetal acidemia during labor (e.g., congenital anomalies, intrauterine growth restriction); no maternal condition that may affect fetal well-being (e.g., prior cesarean scar, diabetes, hypertensive disease); and no requirement for oxytocin induction or augmentation of labor (American Academy of Pediatrics [AAP] & American College of Obstetricians and Gynecologists [ACOG], 2017).

Maternal Vital Signs

Maternal vital signs should be assessed and recorded at regular intervals, at least every 4 hours. This frequency may be increased, particularly as active labor progresses according to clinical signs and symptoms (AAP & ACOG, 2017).

Intermittent Auscultation of Fetal Heart Rate/Palpation of Uterine Activity

In the absence of risk factors:

- A standard approach is to determine, evaluate, and record the fetal heart rate (FHR) every 30 minutes during the active phase of the first stage of labor and at least every 15 minutes during the active pushing phase of the second stage of labor, unless fetal risk status or response to labor indicates the need for more frequent assessment (AAP & ACOG, 2017). Uterine activity is generally assessed at the same frequency as FHR.

When risk factors or complications are present:

- AAP and ACOG (2017) recommend determining, evaluating, and recording the FHR at least every 15 minutes during the active phase of the first stage of labor and at least every 5 minutes during the active pushing phase of the second stage of labor, preferably before, during, and after a uterine contraction. Uterine activity is generally assessed at the same frequency as FHR.

- AWHONN (2018b) suggests auscultation of FHR within the range of every 15 to 30 minutes during the latent phase (4 to 5 cm) and the active phase (≥6 cm) of the first stage of labor, every 15 minutes during the passive fetal descent phase of the second stage of labor, and every 5 to 15 minutes during the active pushing phase of the second stage of labor. Uterine activity is generally assessed at the same frequency as FHR.

- Either protocol is acceptable and should be based on the individual clinical situation.

Electronic Fetal Heart Rate and Uterine Activity Monitoring

Periodic review and documentation of the electronic fetal monitoring (EFM) tracing during active labor should be accomplished based on clinical status and underlying risk factors (ACOG, 2010).

- A standard approach is to evaluate/review the FHR every 30 minutes during the latent phase (4 to 5 cm) and the active phase (≥6 cm) of the first stage of labor, every 30 minutes during the passive fetal descent phase of the second stage of labor, and every 15 minutes during the active pushing phase of the second stage of labor FHR, unless fetal risk status or response to labor indicates the need for more frequent assessment (AAP & ACOG, 2017; ACOG, 2009b; Association of Women's Health, Obstetric and Neonatal Nurses [AWHONN], 2018b, 2019b). Uterine activity is generally assessed at the same frequency as FHR.

When risk factors or complications are present:

- Generally, it is recommended to evaluate/review the FHR every 15 minutes during the latent phase (4 to 5 cm) and the active phase (≥6 cm) of the first stage of labor, every 15 minutes during the passive fetal descent phase of the second stage of labor, and every 5 minutes during the active pushing phase of the second stage of labor (AAP & ACOG, 2017; ACOG, 2009b; AWHONN, 2018b, 2019b). The exact nature of the risk factor and/or complication will guide the frequency of assessment. Uterine activity is generally assessed at the same frequency as FHR.

Cervical Ripening, Labor Induction, and Labor Augmentation

- Prostaglandin preparations for cervical ripening (e.g., misoprostol, or vaginal insert) should be administered where FHR and uterine activity can be monitored continuously for an initial observation period (4 hours after misoprostol intravaginally and 2 hours after misoprostol orally). With the dinoprostone vaginal insert (Cervidil [prostaglandin E_2]), FHR, and uterine activity should be monitored continuously while in place and for at least 15 minutes after removal. Further monitoring of fetal status and uterine activity during cervical ripening can be governed by individual indications for induction and fetal status (ACOG, 2009a).

- When pharmacologic agents are used for cervical ripening, an assessment of FHR and uterine activity every 30 minutes seems reasonable (AWHONN, 2010).

- During oxytocin induction or augmentation, FHR monitoring should be as per high-risk patients (AAP & ACOG, 2017). When using EFM, the FHR should be evaluated/reviewed every 15 minutes during the first stage of labor and during the passive fetal descent phase of the second stage of labor, and every 5 minutes during the active pushing phase of the second stage of labor (AAP & ACOG, 2017; ACOG, 2009b; AWHONN, 2018b, 2019b). Uterine activity is generally assessed at the same frequency as FHR.

Special Considerations for Second-Stage Labor

When EFM is used to record FHR data permanently, periodic documentation can be used to summarize an evaluation of fetal status as outlined by unit protocols. Thus, while an evaluation of the FHR may be occurring every 5 minutes or every 15 minutes based on risk status, a summary including findings of fetal status may be documented in the medical record less frequently. It is challenging to simultaneously record FHR and uterine activity data during second-stage labor while providing support and encouragement related to maternal pushing efforts. Continuous bedside attendance by the nurse is required during second-stage labor maternal pushing efforts (AAP & ACOG, 2017; AWHONN, 2010, 2019b). During the active pushing phase of the second stage of labor, summary documentation of fetal status approximately every 30 minutes while indicating continuous nursing bedside attendance and evaluation seems reasonable (AWHONN, 2018b, 2019b).

(continued)

DISPLAY 14–3

Maternal–Fetal–Newborn Assessments during Labor, Birth, and the Immediate Postpartum Period (Continued)

Monitoring and Assessment during Regional Analgesia/Anesthesia

Women who receive epidural analgesia should be monitored in a manner similar to that used for any woman in labor. When regional anesthesia is administered during labor, maternal vital signs should be monitored at regular intervals by a qualified member of the healthcare team (AAP & ACOG, 2017). Neuraxial (regional) anesthesia for labor and/or vaginal birth requires maternal vital signs and FHR be monitored and documented by a qualified individual (American Society of Anesthesiologists [ASA], 2016).

- Assess maternal blood pressure (BP) after the initiation or rebolus of regional block, including patient-controlled epidural anesthesia (PCEA). BP may be assessed every 5 minutes for the first 15 minutes and then repeated at 30 minutes and at 1 hour after the procedure. More or less frequent monitoring may be indicated based on a consideration of factors (e.g., type of analgesia/anesthesia, route and dose of medication used, maternal–fetal response to medication, maternal–fetal condition, stage of labor, facility protocol) (AWHONN, 2011).
- Assess pulse and respiratory rates consistent with frequency of BP assessment (AWHONN, 2011).
- Consider periodic assessment of maternal oxygen saturation for selected women at high risk or those who receive neuraxial opioids as indicated and per institution protocol (AWHONN, 2011).
- The FHR should be monitored by a qualified individual before and after the administration of neuraxial analgesia for labor. Continuous electronic recording of FHR may not be necessary in every clinical setting and may not be possible during initiation of the block (ASA, 2016).
- Assess the FHR and uterine activity after the initiation or rebolus of regional block, including PCEA. FHR and uterine activity may be assessed every 5 minutes for the first 15 minutes. More or less frequent monitoring may be indicated based on a consideration of factors (e.g., type of analgesia/anesthesia, route and dose of medication used, maternal–fetal response to medication, maternal–fetal condition, stage of labor, facility protocol) (AWHONN, 2011).

Labor Progress

For women who are at no increased risk for complications, an evaluation of the quality of uterine contractions and vaginal examinations should be sufficient to detect abnormalities in the progress of labor (AAP & ACOG, 2017).

- Vaginal examinations include an assessment of dilation and effacement of the cervix and station of the fetal presenting part.
- Generally, uterine activity should be assessed each time the FHR is assessed because uterine activity has implications for fetal status.

Additional Parameters during Labor

Assess character and amount of amniotic fluid (e.g., clear, bloody, meconium stained, odorous).

Assess character and amount of bloody show/vaginal bleeding.

Assess maternal and fetal response to labor.

Assess level of maternal discomfort, coping, and effectiveness of pain management/pain relief measures.

Assess labor support person(s) interactions with the woman and contributions to labor support as indicated.

Assessments during the Immediate Postpartum Period
Maternal Assessments

- During the period of observation immediately after birth, maternal vital signs and additional signs or events should be monitored and recorded as they occur. Maternal BP and pulse should be assessed and recorded immediately after birth and at least every 15 minutes for 2 hours or more frequently and of longer duration if complications are encountered (AAP & ACOG, 2017). Assess fundal height, tone and position, amount of lochia, condition of the perineum, incision and drainage from incision, and pain. The woman's temperature should be taken at least every 4 hours for 8 hours after birth and then at least every 8 hours (AAP & ACOG, 2017).

Newborn Assessments

- Apgar scores should be obtained at 1 and 5 minutes after birth. If the 5-minute Apgar score is less than 7, additional scores should be assigned every 5 minutes up to 20 minutes. Temperature, heart and respiratory rates, skin color, adequacy of peripheral circulation, type of respiration, level of consciousness, tone, and activity should be monitored and recorded at least once every 30 minutes until the newborn's condition has remained stable for at least 2 hours (AAP & ACOG, 2017). Some babies may lack ability to move their head to maintain normal breathing during skin-to-skin care and attempts at breastfeeding processes, so all babies being held by their mothers during the 2-hour transition and recovery process require frequent assessment by the nurse to assure safety.

Summary

When determining frequency of maternal–fetal assessments during labor, factors such as stage of labor; maternal–fetal risk status; and institutional policies, procedures, and protocols should be taken into consideration. As new standards and guidelines are published from professional organizations, these assessment parameters will need to be reviewed and updated.

Adapted from Killion, M. M. (2019). Enhanced recovery after cesarean birth. *MCN: The American Journal of Maternal Child Nursing, 44*(6), 296. doi:10.1097/NMC.0000000000000572

because it often produces inaccurate data due to maternal movement and dislocation of the device. Often, long periods of erroneous recordings of low SpO$_2$ are automatically entered into the electronic medical record and printed on the paper version of the FHR tracing without nursing confirmation that these data accurately reflect maternal condition. Pulse oximeters are designed to measure SpO$_2$ rather than heart rate. Continuous tracing of maternal heart rate on the FHR tracing often obscures the FHR, particularly during second-stage pushing. Spot

TABLE 14–2. Maternal–Fetal Assessment and Documentation Suggested Guidelines

	Labor	Oxytocin	Cervidil/Cytotec	Second-stage labor (active pushing phase)	First hour of magnesium sulfate and any change in dose	Magnesium sulfate maintenance dose	All other patients
Assessment and documentation	Every 30 min	Assessment each time rate is increased or at least every 15 min if rate is unchanged	Every 30 min	Assessment every 5 to 15 min based on risk status; summary notes every 30 min	Every 15 min	At least every hour	At least every hour
Maternal vital signs	P, R, BP every hour; T every 2 hr unless ROM, then every hour	P, R, BP every hour; T every 2 hr unless ROM, then every hour	P, R, BP every 4 hr; T every 4 hr unless ROM, then every hour	P, R, BP every hour; T every 2 hr unless ROM, then every hour	P, R, BP every 15 min; T every hour	P, R, BP every hour; T every 2 hr unless ROM, then every hour	T, P, R, BP every 4 hr
FHR and uterine activity	Every 30 min	Assessment each time rate is increased or at least every 15 min if rate is unchanged	Every 30 min	Assessment every 5 to 15 min based on risk status; summary notes every 30 min	Every 15 min	At least every hour	At least every hour
Pain status	Every 30 min	Assessment each time rate is increased or at least every 15 min if rate is unchanged	Every 30 min	Assessment every 5 to 15 min based on risk status; summary notes every 30 min	Every 15 min	At least every hour	At least every hour
Response to labor	Every 30 min	Every 30 min	Every 30 min if applicable	Assessment every 5 to 15 min based on risk status; summary notes every 30 min	Every 15 min if applicable	At least every hour if applicable	At least every hour if applicable
Comfort measures	Every 30 min if applicable	Every 30 min	Every 30 min if applicable	Assessment every 5 to 15 min based on risk status; summary notes every 30 min	Every 15 min if applicable	At least every hour if applicable	At least every hour if applicable
Position	Every 30 min	Every 30 min	Every 30 min	Assessment every 5 to 15 min based on risk status; summary notes every 30 min	Every 15 min	At least every hour	At least every hour
Oxytocin rate (mU/min)		Assessment each time rate is increased or at least every 15 min if rate is unchanged					
Vaginal exam/fetal station/progress in descent	As needed	As needed	As needed	As needed, at least every 30 min			
Magnesium sulfate rate (g/hr)					Every 15 min	At least every hour	
Any signs and symptoms of side effects of magnesium sulfate					Every 15 min	At least every hour	
Intake and output	Every 8 hr	Every 8 hr	Every 8 hr		Every hour	Every hour	Every 8 hr

Fetal heart rate (FHR) characteristics include baseline rate, variability, and presence or absence of accelerations and decelerations. Uterine activity includes contraction frequency, duration, intensity, and uterine resting tone.
BP, blood pressure; P, pulse; R, respirations; ROM, rupture of membrane; T, temperature.

checks of maternal SpO_2 are more appropriate if there is a concern regarding maternal oxygen status. Manual assessment of maternal pulse is more appropriate for differentiating between maternal heart rate and FHR if there is a concern regarding the origin of heart rate tracing as maternal versus fetal. Unless risk factors have been identified, care for a woman with epidural analgesia/anesthesia may be similar to that of any other woman in labor.

Vaginal Examinations

Nurses should develop proficiency in performing vaginal examinations to assess labor progress and to determine the need for nursing interventions such as position change and timing of medication. They must first be able to identify situations in which a vaginal examination is required and also recognize when a vaginal examination is contraindicated, such as with unexplained vaginal bleeding or with premature rupture of the membranes. Developing clinical proficiency in performing vaginal examinations requires practice and assistance from a knowledgeable preceptor. Because a full assessment may require more time than usual during the period when vaginal examination skills are being acquired, an ideal patient for nurses to learn the technique has adequate regional analgesia/anesthesia and intact membranes, so she can tolerate the potentially longer vaginal examination and there is less risk of infection with the confirmation examination by the preceptor. Usually, patients who are fully informed that the examiner is learning will consent to this type of examination.

Women undergoing a vaginal examination should be minimally exposed, advised of the necessity of the examination before it is performed, have given permission, and be informed of the findings. The woman should be positioned on her back with her head slightly elevated. The vaginal examination should be as quick as possible, but systematic, beginning with an assessment of dilation and effacement and then fetal presentation, station, and position. The normal length of the pregravid cervix is 3.5 to 4 cm. The length of the cervix may vary in women who have had any cervical surgery, such as conization or laser excision procedures. As labor progresses and as the fetal presenting part descends, the cervix shortens and dilates, changing from long, thick, and closed to thin and 10 cm (Fig. 14–4).

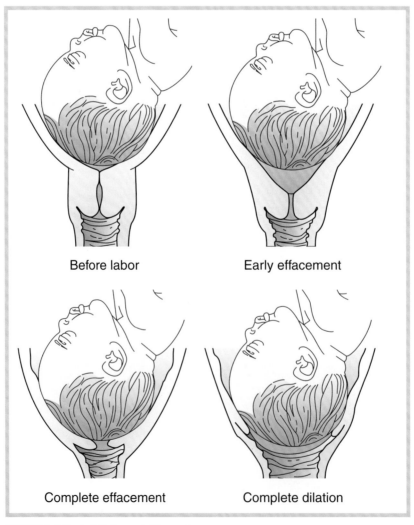

Before labor

Early effacement

Complete effacement

Complete dilation

FIGURE 14–4. Cervical dilation and effacement.

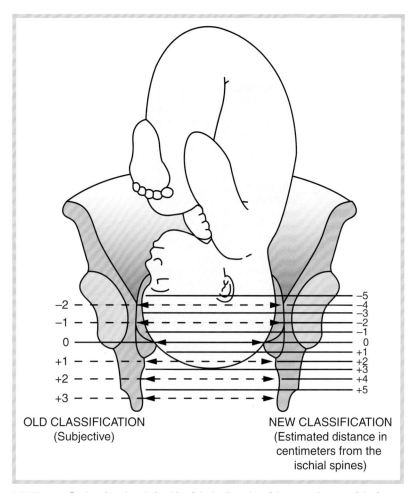

OLD CLASSIFICATION
(Subjective)

NEW CLASSIFICATION
(Estimated distance in
centimeters from the
ischial spines)

FIGURE 14–5. Fetal station: the relationship of the leading edge of the presenting part of the fetus to the plane of the maternal ischial spines determines the station. Station +1/+3 or +2/+5 is illustrated. (From Kilpatrick, S., & Garrison, E. [2017]. Normal labor and delivery. In S. G. Gabbe, J. R. Niebyl, J. L. Simpson, M. B. Landon, H. L. Galan, E. R. M. Jauniaux, D. A. Driscoll, B. Vincenzo, & W. A. Groban [Eds.]. *Obstetrics: Normal and problem pregnancies* [7th ed., pp. 246–270]. Philadelphia, PA: Elsevier.)

An assessment of station and position of the fetal head requires more skill. The ischial spines must be identified to assess station in relation to the biparietal diameter of the fetal head. The ischial spines may be identified by pressing in the sidewall of the vagina approximately 1 inch, with the examining fingers at approximately 3 and 9 o'clock, respectively. It is not necessary to identify both spines to assess station. The occiput of the fetal head should be at the level of the ischial spines, to be engaged or zero station (Fig. 14–5). The examiner should not be confused by caput formation but should instead identify the fetal skull for this assessment.

Often, the most difficult determination to make is that of fetal head position: occiput anterior (OA) or occiput posterior (OP). The examining nurse must be familiar with the location of the suture lines in the fetal skull more so than the shape of the anterior or posterior fontanelle because distortion or overlapping bones will alter fontanelle shape. Figure 14–6 is a drawing of the fetal fontanelles, which can be used as a reference when assessing fetal head position during vaginal examination. The nurse should first identify the sagittal suture and then slide fingers to a fontanelle and count the number of suture lines extending from it exclusive of the sagittal suture (Fig. 14–7). This can be accomplished by sweeping the examining finger 180 degrees at a right angle to the sagittal suture. The anterior fontanelle has three suture lines extending from it, and the posterior fontanelle has two suture lines. It is not necessary to palpate the posterior fontanelle to determine the position of the fetal head. Determination of the position of the fetal head becomes necessary primarily during the second stage when descent is slow. Repositioning the woman to a squatting, side-lying, or hands-and-knees position to push or using the towel-pull technique during pushing may facilitate rotation of the fetal head.

Perineal hygiene is important during periodic vaginal examinations. Attention to clean technique is critical, particularly if membranes are ruptured. Sterile, water-soluble lubricants may be used to decrease discomfort during vaginal examinations; however, antiseptics such as povidone-iodine and hexachlorophene should be avoided. These antiseptics have not been shown to decrease infections acquired during the intrapartum period, but they may

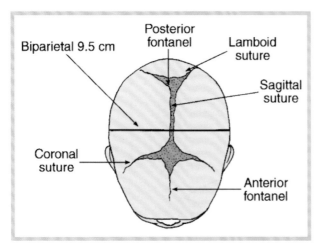

FIGURE 14–6. Fetal fontanelles: fetal presentation, vertex, fetal skull showing the bony segments of the fetal skull important for determining the baby's position and station for birth.

cause local irritation and are absorbed through maternal mucous membranes (AAP & ACOG, 2017).

Leopold Maneuvers

Leopold maneuvers provide a systematic assessment of fetal position and presentation and should be performed prior to application of EFM as part of the admission assessment. Information obtained while performing these maneuvers supports assessments made during vaginal examinations and assists in determining the best position to locate the FHR (Fig. 14–8). Leopold maneuvers may be difficult with women who are obese, have tense or guarded abdominal muscles, or have polyhydramnios. In these situations, an ultrasound may be necessary to determine fetal position and presentation.

Fetal Heart Rate Assessment

Systematic assessment of the FHR via EFM includes a determination of the baseline rate, variability, and presence or absence of accelerations and decelerations. Intermittent auscultation of the FHR via stethoscope or handheld ultrasound device includes a determination of the rate and whether the rhythm is regular or irregular, and presence or absence of increases or decreases in the FHR. If decreases are noted, further assessment to clarify FHR findings is required. Clinical interventions are based on a comprehensive assessment of all the characteristics of the FHR pattern depicted via EFM or noted during auscultation and the individual clinical situation of the mother and fetus including, but not limited to, gestational age and medications administered to the mother. The FHR can be determined by use of the external ultrasound device of the EFM in most situations. If the clinical situation is such that a continuous external tracing of the FHR is ordered but

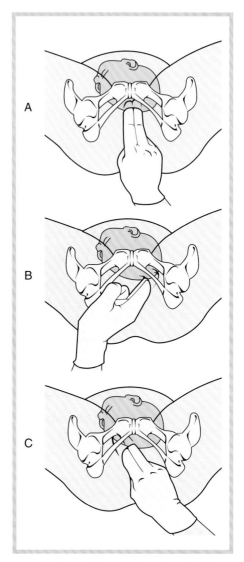

FIGURE 14–7. Vaginal examination. **A,** Determining the station and palpating the sagittal suture. **B,** Identifying the posterior fontanelle. **C,** Identifying the anterior fontanelle. (From Nettina, S. M. [2010]. *Lippincott manual of nursing practice* [9th ed.]. Philadelphia, PA: Lippincott, Williams & Wilkins.)

presents challenges (e.g., a woman with obesity at term undergoing a medically indicated labor induction with oxytocin), an internal fetal scalp electrode (FSE) may be applied. See Chapter 15 for a comprehensive discussion about FHR assessment.

Uterine Activity Assessment

During labor, interpretation of FHR patterns cannot occur in isolation of evaluation of uterine activity, which includes a complete assessment of four components of uterine contractions: frequency, duration, intensity of contractions, and the uterine resting tone between contractions. These assessments can be made by either palpation alone or by palpation in conjunction with an external tocodynamometer (TOCO) or with an intrauterine pressure catheter (IUPC). Contraction frequency

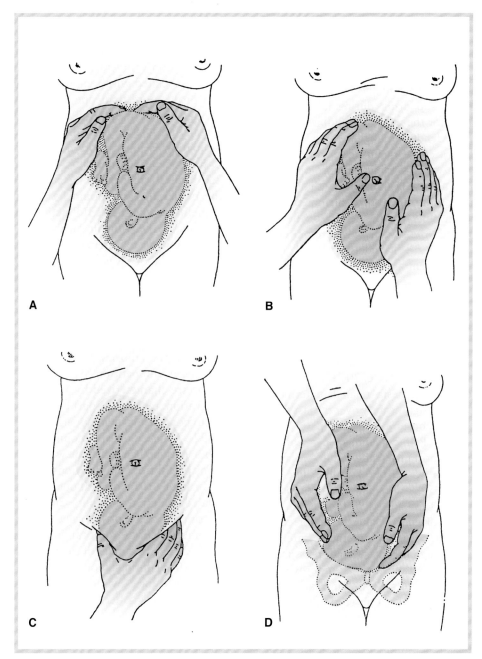

FIGURE 14–8. Leopold maneuvers. **A**, First maneuver. **B**, Second maneuver. **C**, Third maneuver. **D**, Fourth maneuver.

is measured from the beginning of one contraction to the beginning of the next and is described in minutes. Duration is assessed by the length of the contraction and is described in seconds. Intensity refers to the strength of the contraction and is described as mild, moderate, or strong by palpation, or millimeters of mercury (mm Hg) of intraamniotic pressure if an IUPC is used. Uterine resting tone is assessed in the absence of contractions or between contractions. By direct palpation, resting tone is described as soft or hard, and by IUPC is measured in mm Hg of intraamniotic pressure.

The external TOCO detects changes in abdominal wall shape during contractions and uterine relaxation.

This method provides information about frequency and duration; however, resting tone and intensity must be determined by palpation. Contraction frequency, duration, intensity, and uterine resting tone can be evaluated by both palpation and an IUPC. The IUPC is more accurate because a direct measurement of intraamniotic pressure is recorded but requires ruptured membranes for insertion. The cervix should be at least 2 to 3 cm dilated before insertion of an IUPC or FSE. As with any procedure, the least invasive approach is preferred unless maternal–fetal status indicates a clear indication for internal monitoring. See Chapter 15 for a comprehensive discussion about uterine activity.

Oral Intake and Intravenous Fluids during Labor and Birth

Oral Intake

Before the 1940s, women in the United States were encouraged to eat and drink during labor to maintain their stamina for the work of childbirth (ACNM, 2016). In 1946, Mendelson suggested that maternal aspiration of gastric contents during general anesthesia for cesarean birth was a significant cause of maternal morbidity. This was based on his theory that the delay in gastric emptying during labor contributed to aspiration pneumonitis and that the acidity of the gastric contents determined the severity of maternal complications and risk of death (Mendelson, 1946). For the next 50 years, to prevent aspiration should a cesarean birth be necessary, fasting became the norm for laboring women in most hospitals in the United States. It is now known that regardless of the time of the woman's last meal, the stomach is never completely empty and that fasting stimulates acid secretion, thereby augmenting rather than solving the risk of aspiration (ACNM, 2016; Singata, Tranmer, & Gyte, 2013).

Risks of general anesthesia–related maternal morbidity have decreased significantly over the last 50 years but have remained constant over the past 20 years (Hawkins, Chang, Palmer, Gibbs, & Callaghan, 2011). Maternal mortality ratios due to anesthesia are estimated to be 1.0 per 1 million live births, which represents a 59% decrease when compared to the period between 1979 and 1990 (Lim et al., 2018). The decreased use of general anesthesia for cesarean birth, published standards for anesthesia care, better anesthesia monitoring, use of cricoid pressure, and routine tracheal intubation with an improved technique have contributed to a decline in maternal mortality (Hawkins et al., 2011; Lim et al., 2018). In the cases of anesthesia-related maternal deaths that have been reported in the literature, complications such as advanced maternal age, poor physical status, obesity, emergent procedures, delay in response, high neuraxial block, hypertension, embolism, and hemorrhage appear to be coexisting factors (ACNM, 2016; Davies, Posner, Lee, Cheney, & Domino, 2009; Hawkins et al., 2011). Most women in the United States who have a cesarean birth are given regional anesthesia. The case fatality rate for regional anesthesia between 1997 and 2002 was reported to be 3.8 per million regional anesthetics during cesarean birth (Hawkins et al., 2011). The case fatality rate for general anesthesia during the same period was 6.5 per million general anesthetics for cesarean birth (Hawkins et al., 2011). The leading causes of anesthesia-related pregnancy deaths for 1991 to 2002 were intubation failure or anesthesia induction problems (23%), respiratory failure (20%), and high spinal or epidural block (16%) (Hawkins et al., 2011).

Causes of death varied by type of obstetric anesthesia; approximately two thirds of deaths associated with general anesthesia were caused by intubation failure or induction problems, but for women whose deaths were associated with regional anesthesia during cesarean birth, more than one fourth (26%) were caused by high spinal or epidural block, followed by respiratory failure (19%), and drug reaction (19%). Failed intubation is much more common in obstetrics than in the general population (1 in 280 obstetrics vs. 1 in 2,230 in all other patients); therefore, all members of the perinatal team should be familiar with the ASA (Apfelbaum et al., 2013) Practice Guidelines for Management of the Difficult Airway.

Physiologic requirements for glucose increase during active labor (Wasserstrum, 1992). Fasting depletes the carbohydrates available; thus, women in labor who are not allowed oral intake may have to metabolize fat for energy (Keppler, 1988). Although there has been limited research about specific nutritional needs during labor, it has been suggested that the energy requirements of the laboring woman are similar to those of athletes in competition (ACNM, 2016). Pregnancy and labor are characterized by an exaggerated response to starvation, reflected in part by more rapid development of hypoglycemia and hyperketonemia (Wasserstrum, 1992). Thus, modest amounts of oral intake during labor may be beneficial for women without complications or risks of complications.

In light of the data about the rarity of anesthesia-related maternal mortality and other evidence about nutritional needs of laboring women, ASA revised its recommendations for oral intake during labor (Lim et al., 2018). Examples of clear liquids recommended by ASA (2016) during labor include, but are not limited to, water, fruit juices without pulp, carbonated beverages, clear tea, black coffee, and sports drinks. Flavored gelatin, fruit ice, popsicles, and broth are also often offered. The volume of liquid is less important than the presence of particulate matter in the ingested liquid. The ASA recommends restricting oral fluids on a case-by-case basis for women who are at risk for aspiration (e.g., women with obesity, diabetes, or difficult airway) and for women at increased risk for operative birth (e.g., indeterminate or abnormal FHR patterns). Although the literature does not quantify modest amounts of fluid, some experts have suggested that the volume of fluid intake may be determined by maternal thirst.

While there seems to be a consensus that selected oral fluids during labor are generally not harmful in low-risk women, controversy exists regarding solid foods. In a randomized controlled trial of 2,426 nulliparous, nondiabetic women in labor at term, with a cervical dilatation of less than 6 cm, consumption of a light diet was compared to consumption of water (O'Sullivan, Liu, Hart, Seed, & Shennan, 2009).

Consumption of a light diet during labor did not influence obstetric or neonatal outcomes nor did it increase the incidence of vomiting. Women who were allowed to eat in labor had similar lengths of labor and operative birth rates as those allowed water only (O'Sullivan et al., 2009). A review of the literature from 1986 to 2009 on oral intake during labor found that foods high in fat slow gastric emptying during labor and that solid food intake is associated with vomiting and increased labor duration, without adverse maternal or neonatal effects (Sharts-Hopko, 2010). The most recent Cochrane Review reports a lack of evidence to support restricting fluids and food during labor in women at low risk for complications (Singata et al., 2013). Neither benefit nor harm associated with eating during labor was found. Women who ate lightly, compared with those who only consumed water, were no more likely to vomit and had similar lengths of labor and cesarean birth rates (Singata et al., 2013). One randomized controlled trial found no cases of aspiration among women in labor who consumed only liquids and those who consumed low-fat, low-residue foods during labor (O'Sullivan et al., 2009). The pooled data of the five studies in the Cochrane Review ($N = 3,130$) were of insufficient power to assess the incidence of aspiration of gastric contents during general anesthesia. Aspiration of gastric contents among women who have cesarean birth is so rare that a randomized clinical trial to determine if oral intake is related to maternal mortality is not feasible (Sharts-Hopko, 2010).

Most pertinent professional organizations such as ACOG (AAP & ACOG, 2017; ACOG, 2019a), ASA (2016), and Canadian Anesthesiologists' Society (Merchant et al., 2012) recommend avoiding solid food intake during labor. Risk for aspiration of gastric contents during emergency cesarean birth is the basis for their recommendations. A fasting time for solid food that is predictive of maternal anesthesia complications has not been determined; thus, there is insufficient evidence to support safe recommendations for solid intake during labor (ASA, 2016). A fasting time for solid food of at least 6 to 8 hours prior to elective cesarean birth is recommended (ACOG, 2009c; ASA, 2016). A risk assessment of women in labor is the basis of determining whether oral fluid and/or solid intake is appropriate (ACNM, 2016).

Each institution should have a policy for oral nutrition during labor that has been developed in collaboration with anesthesia providers. This policy should not arbitrarily restrict oral and solid intake during labor but rather should be based on what is known about complications that increase the risk of general anesthesia. Women should be informed of the small, but potentially serious, risks of aspiration related to oral intake during labor (ACNM, 2016). It should be made clear that it is the anesthesia that is the risk, not the oral intake, and if labor deviates from the normal, she may be asked to refrain from oral intake (ACNM, 2016).

Intravenous Fluids

Normal healthy women at term have at least 2 L of water stored in their extravascular spaces and have accumulated fat and fluids over the course of the pregnancy. A long labor with the woman fasting may deplete those energy resources. Maternal fluid loss occurs with perspiration, use of various breathing techniques, and vomiting. When fasting during labor became the norm after the 1940s, administration of intravenous (IV) fluids became routine practice. Prophylactic IV access was advocated in anticipation of the administration of rapid volume expanders and blood products in the case of emergencies that can result in maternal hypovolemia and hemorrhage, such as uterine rupture, abruptio placentae, regional anesthesia complications, and immediate postpartum hemorrhage.

IV fluids are thought to increase maternal blood volume, leading to increased blood flow (oxygen) to the placenta and resulting in more oxygen available at the placenta site for maternal–fetal exchange. Therefore, non–glucose-containing IV fluid boluses are often given during an indeterminate or abnormal FHR pattern (Garite & Simpson, 2011). In one study, fetuses of mothers who were given an IV fluid bolus of either 500 mL or 1,000 mL of lactated Ringer's (L/R) solution over 20 minutes had significant increases in fetal SpO_2 that persisted at least 30 minutes after the IV fluid bolus was completed (Simpson & James, 2005b). The greatest increase occurred in the fetuses of mothers who received 1,000 mL. The women in this study were normotensive and adequately hydrated, and their fetuses had normal FHR patterns. Therefore, an IV fluid bolus can result in a transfer of maternal oxygen to the fetus even if the woman is not experiencing hypotension or dehydration (Simpson & James, 2005b). It is likely that the benefits of an IV fluid bolus would be greater if the FHR pattern were indeterminate or abnormal because of the transfer of oxygen through the placenta by passive diffusion from high concentration to low concentration, but more data are needed regarding this common intervention.

The administration of IV solutions containing glucose during labor is controversial. In theory, the administration of glucose averts maternal hypoglycemia and starvation ketosis; however, there is evidence to suggest that maternal IV administration of glucose can have potentially detrimental effects on the fetal status, including increased fetal lactate and decreased fetal pH (ACNM, 2016; Philipson, Kalhan, Riha, & Pimentel, 1987). If the fetus is hypoxic, relatively small elevations in glucose can lead to lactate acidosis (Philipson et al., 1987; Wasserstrum, 1992). IV solutions with glucose can cause fetal hyperglycemia and subsequent reactive hypoglycemia, hyperinsulinism, hyponatremia, acidosis, jaundice, and transient tachypnea in the newborn after birth (ACNM, 2016; Carmen, 1986; Grylack, Chu, & Scanlon, 1984; Mendiola, Grylack, & Scanlon, 1982; Singhi, 1988; Sommer, Norr, & Roberts, 2000). A bolus of IV solution containing glucose can cause marked maternal hyperglycemia (Mendiola et al., 1982; Wasserstrum, 1992). Thus, when the clinical situation is such that a bolus of IV fluids may be necessary to expand plasma volume (e.g., initial treatment for preterm labor, before administration of epidural analgesia/anesthesia, or during hypovolemic maternal emergencies), IV fluids should not contain glucose (ACNM, 2016; Garite & Simpson, 2011).

Despite the controversy about IV glucose administration during labor, occasionally L/R solution with 5% dextrose (D5L/R) may be administered during labor. One liter of D5L/R IV solution provides 180 calories. It is possible that a maintenance rate (125 mL/hr) of glucose-containing IV fluids during labor may be beneficial in shortening labor, although more data are needed before recommendations can be made for the adoption of this type of protocol for routine care. In a double-blind, randomized controlled trial comparing IV normal saline (NS) with and without dextrose on the course of labor in nulliparous women, patients in active labor were randomized into one of three groups receiving either NS, NS with 5% dextrose, or NS with 10% dextrose at 125 mL/hr (Shrivastava et al., 2009). The administration of a dextrose solution, regardless of concentration, was associated with a shortened labor duration in term vaginally delivered nulliparous women in active labor, while there were no significant differences observed in the cesarean section rates between groups or in neonatal outcomes (Shrivastava et al., 2009). Glucose requirements vary depending on weight, use of analgesia/anesthesia, phase of labor, fetal status, and other factors, so it is difficult to determine the optimal rate of glucose infusion during labor.

The most common IV solution used during labor is L/R. An isotonic IV solution should be used to dilute oxytocin during induction and augmentation of labor (ACOG, 2009a). Two randomized controlled trials suggest that the usual amount of IV fluids during labor (125 mL/hr) may be insufficient to meet the needs of women and that inadequate hydration during labor may cause complications of labor (Eslamian, Marsoosi, & Pakneeyat, 2006; Garite, Weeks, Peters-Phair, Pattillo, & Brewster, 2000). These researchers found that women who received 125 mL/hr of L/R solution had longer labors, more oxytocin, and higher rates of cesarean birth when compared with women who received 250 mL/hr of L/R IV fluids. A study of pregnant women comparing different amounts of oral intake considering the same outcome variables would add to what is known about how much and what method of hydration during labor is appropriate.

Individual clinical situations should guide the selection of IV fluids during labor. It is important to avoid boluses of glucose-containing IV solutions during labor, especially in the context of intrauterine resuscitation when the FHR pattern suggests fetal compromise. Thus, if glucose-containing solutions are administered as the main line IV fluids, L/R solution should be available as a piggyback IV solution in case an IV fluid bolus is needed for intrauterine resuscitation or pre-epidural hydration.

More data are needed about the appropriate amount and type of IV fluids during labor. This area of intrapartum care has not been well researched, so practice is based on tradition rather than solid evidence. Current resources for guidelines about IV fluids and oral intake during labor include the Committee Opinion *Oral Intake during Labor* (ACOG, 2009c), *Practice Guidelines for Obstetric Anesthesia* (ASA, 2016), the Clinical Bulletin *Providing Oral Nutrition to Women in Labor* (ACNM, 2016), and the Evidence-Based Clinical Practice Guideline *Nursing Care of the Woman Receiving Regional Analgesia/Anesthesia in Labor* (AWHONN, 2011).

Maternal Positioning during Labor and Birth

Unit culture, clinician preferences, and patient cultural background often determine the position women assume during labor and childbirth, such as lying down, squatting, sitting, standing, kneeling, or on all fours. Recumbency, a Western cultural tradition for the convenience of obstetricians, began when more women were hospitalized for childbirth. Early medical research challenging the recumbent position was ignored (Mengert & Murphy, 1933; Vaughn, 1937). Many women today are confined to the bed during the majority of labor as a result of the widespread use of EFM, IVs, oxytocin, and regional analgesia/anesthesia. However, even while in bed, women may be assisted to various positions for labor and birth that may improve maternal and fetal outcomes. Policies that encourage women to walk or change position in labor may result in shorter labors, more efficient contractions, greater comfort, and less need for pain medicine in labor (Bick et al., 2017; Shilling, Romano, & DiFranco, 2007). Choices in positioning offer women control and empowerment and enhance satisfaction with the birth experience (Holvey, 2014; Nieuwenhuijze, de Jonge, Korstjens, Budé, & Lagro-Janssen, 2013; Nieuwenhuijze, Low, Korstjens, & Lagro-Janssen, 2014).

Ambulation during labor has been shown to decrease the rate of operative birth by 50% (Albers et al., 1997). Women who are encouraged to be mobile during labor report greater comfort and ability to tolerate labor as well as decreased use of analgesia and anesthesia

(Bloom et al., 1998). Although the tradition in the United States is to confine women in active labor to the bed, there is no greater risk of adverse maternal–fetal outcomes when women are encouraged to ambulate during labor (Bloom et al., 1998). If continuous EFM has been selected as the method of fetal assessment during labor, use of EFM via telemetry can allow the woman to ambulate while being monitored, even while Cervidil is in place or oxytocin is being administered.

An upright position shortens labor (Chang et al., 2011; Deliktas & Kukulu, 2017; DiFranco, Romano, & Keen, 2007; Gupta, Sood, Hofmeyr, & Vogel, 2017; Lawrence, Lewis, Hofmeyr, & Styles, 2013). Duration of both first- and second-stage labor are shorter in women who labor 30 degrees upright as compared to those in a flat recumbent position (Chang et al., 2011; Liu, 1989; Terry, Westcott, O'Shea, & Kelly, 2006). An upright position can also decrease the use of pain medication and the need for oxytocin (Bodner-Adler et al., 2003). In one study, the second stage of labor was decreased when women were in a squatting position, and there was less use of oxytocin, fewer mechanically assisted births, and fewer and less severe lacerations and episiotomies compared to semirecumbent births (Golay, Vedam, & Sorger, 1993). Both AWHONN (2019b) and ACOG (2019a) recommend upright positioning and frequent repositioning during labor as per the woman's desires and her individual clinical situation.

Evidence suggests that any upright or lateral position during second-stage labor results in less pain, less fatigue, less perineal trauma, fewer episiotomies, fewer operative-assisted births, and fewer FHR abnormalities (Bodner-Adler et al., 2003; Chang et al., 2011; da Silva et al., 2012; de Jong et al., 1997; De Jonge, Van Diem, Scheepers, Buitendijk, & Lagro-Janssen, 2010; Downe, Gerrett, & Renfrew, 2004; Gupta et al., 2017; Kettle & Tohill, 2011; Ragnar, Altman, Tydén, & Olsson, 2006; Roberts, Algert, Cameron, & Torvaldsen, 2005; Schiessl et al., 2005). Sitting on the toilet may be an acceptable and comfortable alternative to squatting for women who are fatigued (Shermer & Raines, 1997). Perineal edema and pelvic congestion can be prevented when using the toilet for first- or second-stage labor by position changes every 10 to 15 minutes (Shermer & Raines, 1997).

It is important to avoid the supine position during labor because of the relationship between lying flat and maternal hypotension and impedance of uteroplacental blood flow. When the woman in labor is supine, the pressure of the uterus against the spine causes compression of the inferior vena cava, aorta, and iliac arteries (AWHONN, 2019b). If the woman prefers to lie down, a left or right lateral position promotes maternal–fetal exchange at the placental level and enhances fetal well-being (Simpson & James, 2005b). During the second stage of labor, there are fewer indeterminate FHR patterns and a decreased risk of fetal acidemia when women

are positioned upright or lateral compared to supine positioning (De Jonge, Teunissen, & Lagro-Janssen, 2004; Gupta et al., 2017; Scholz, Benedicic, Arikan, Haas, & Petru, 2001). Research has been done to enhance fetal rotation from OP to OA because there is an association between adverse neonatal outcomes and a persistent OP position (Cheng, Shaffer, & Caughey, 2006). A hands-and-knees position for at least 30 minutes during labor may be beneficial in promoting rotation from OP to OA (Stremler et al., 2005). Other methods that may be beneficial are lateral positioning during labor and using the towel-pull technique during second-stage pushing efforts (AWHONN, 2006). The hands-and-knees position can help to reduce back pain for women in labor and may be useful during both first- and second-stage labor (Stremler et al., 2005). Women are often assisted to hands-and-knees position for certain indeterminate or abnormal FHR patterns but returned to a more standard position for birth. A last-minute change of maternal position for birth may be unwarranted because birth may be just as easily accomplished in hands-and-knees position (Bruner, Drummond, Meenan, & Gaskin, 1998; Gannon, 1992). Some women may benefit from the use of a birthing ball for relieving pressure and facilitating a more comfortable position during labor. Figures 14–9 A–V depict positions for labor and birth.

(text continues on page 352)

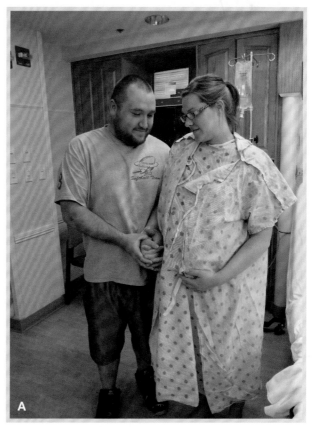

FIGURE 14–9A. Physiologic positions during labor: walking.

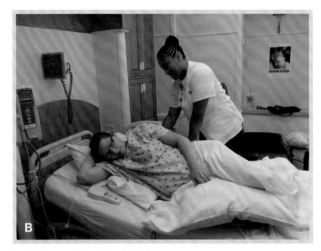

FIGURE 14–9B. Side lying with pillow support.

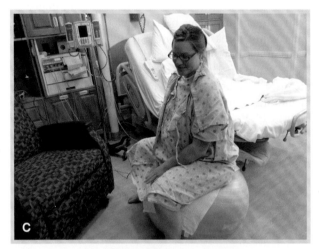

FIGURE 14–9C. Sitting on a birthing ball.

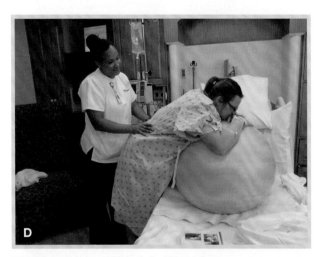

FIGURE 14–9D. Using a birthing ball while standing.

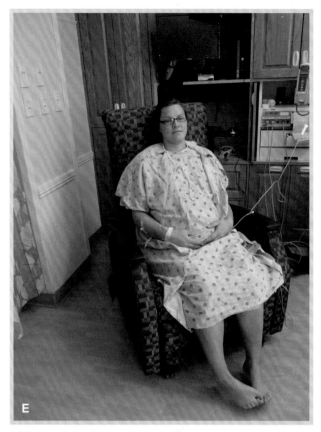

FIGURE 14–9E. Rocking.

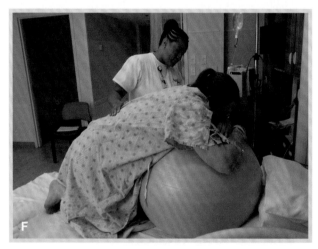

FIGURE 14–9F. Kneeling in bed using a birthing ball.

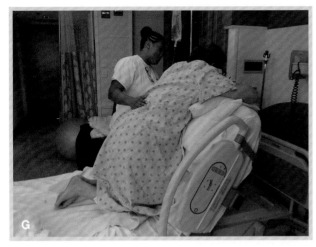

FIGURE 14–9G. Kneeling in bed with head of bed elevated and chest supported.

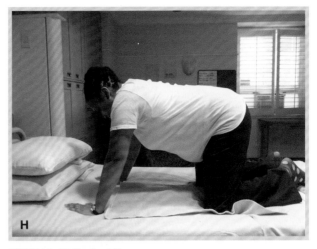

FIGURE 14–9H. Hands and knees.

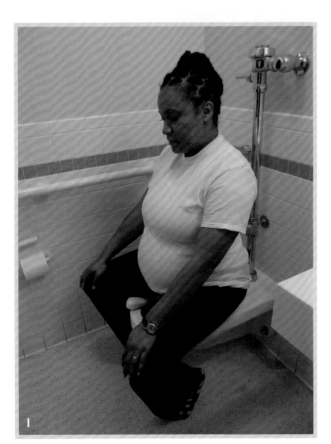

FIGURE 14–9I. Sitting on toilet; also can be used for pushing.

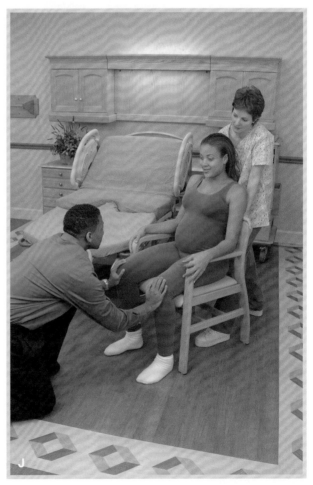

FIGURE 14–9J. Sitting with partner massaging legs. (Courtesy of Hill-Rom.)

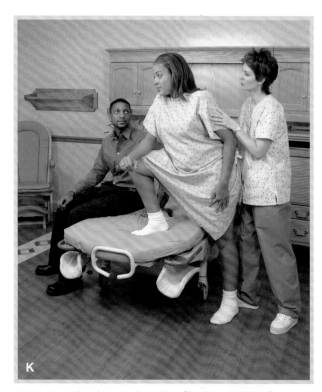

FIGURE 14–9K. Lunging using foot of bed. (Courtesy of Hill-Rom.)

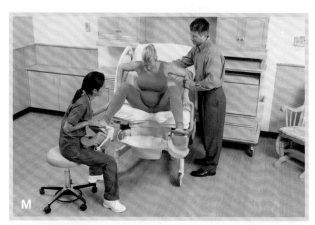

FIGURE 14–9M. Pushing using foot rests as support. (Courtesy of Hill-Rom.)

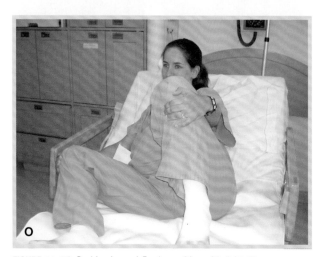

FIGURE 14–9O. Pushing in semi-Fowler position with right tilt.

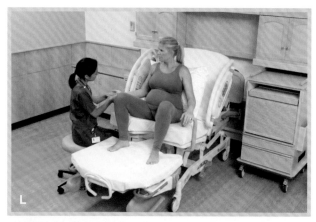

FIGURE 14–9L. Sitting with foot of bed lowered; also can be used for pushing. (Courtesy of Hill-Rom.)

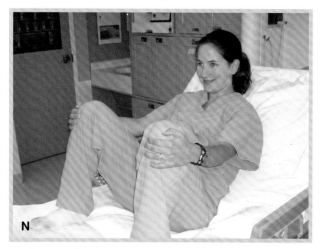

FIGURE 14–9N. Pushing in semi-Fowler position with feet flat on bed.

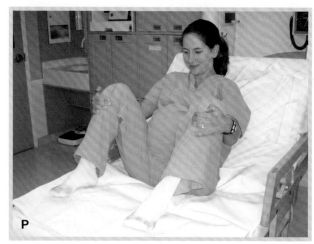

FIGURE 14–9P. Pushing in semi-Fowler position with mother holding knees back slightly.

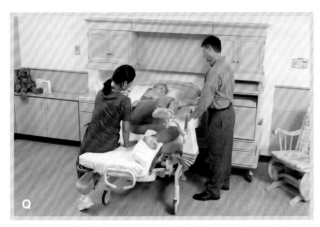

FIGURE 14–9Q. Pushing in side-lying position. (Courtesy of Hill-Rom.)

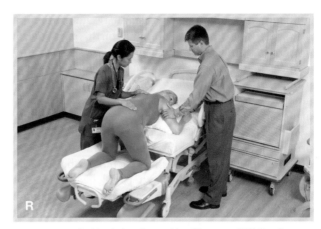

FIGURE 14–9R. Pushing in kneeling position. (Courtesy of Hill-Rom.)

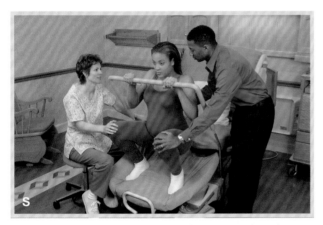

FIGURE 14–9S. Pushing using squatting bar. (Courtesy of Hill-Rom.)

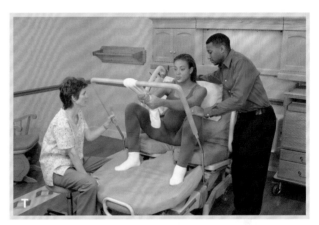

FIGURE 14–9T. Pushing using towel-pull technique with squatting bar and feet flat on bed. (Courtesy of Hill-Rom.)

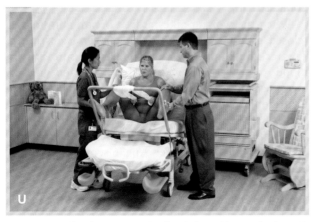

FIGURE 14–9U. Pushing using towel-pull technique with squatting bar and feet supported against bar. (Courtesy of Hill-Rom.)

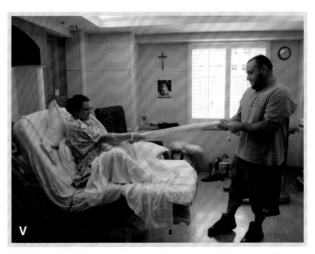

FIGURE 14–9V. Pushing using towel-pull technique with counterpull of partner.

Regional analgesia/anesthesia may limit the use of some positions for labor and birth, particularly if there is significant enough motor blockade to prevent easy repositioning or ambulation. Epidurals that produce less motor block intrathecal narcotics are more efficient because they can provide excellent pain management without as much of a limit to mobility (AWHONN, 2011). Using medication dosages that provide an analgesic rather than an anesthetic level of epidural allow the woman to move about more freely and feel pressure as the fetal head descends (AWHONN, 2011). Feeling pressure will facilitate spontaneous maternal bearing down efforts during the second stage of labor (Roberts, 2002). Nurses should be innovative with the use as well of positioning techniques for women with epidurals to as well facilitate birth while maintaining maternal safety. If the mother is confined to the bed, sitting may still be accomplished by adjusting the birthing bed to a more upright position, dropping the lower section, or by helping the mother sit on the side of the bed with a stool for support. When assisting women with epidural analgesia/anesthesia to various positions during labor and/or lowering bed side rails, ensure that the woman is well supported and there are precautions to minimize the risk of patient falls.

Upright positioning during labor is a safe and effective measure that can be encouraged by the perinatal nurse (ACOG, 2019a; AWHONN, 2019b; da Silva et al., 2012; Gupta et al., 2017; Lawrence et al., 2013). Women should be supported in assuming positions of comfort per their choice during labor. Supportive care techniques during labor and interventions to manage the pain most women experience related to labor and birth are covered in detail in Chapter 16.

Care during Second–Stage Labor

Evidence-based guidelines for nursing care during second-stage labor are available from AWHONN (2019b). The second stage of labor begins when the cervix is completely dilated. However, women often begin to have an involuntary urge to push prior to complete cervical dilation (Roberts, 2002). This urge to push is triggered by the Ferguson reflex as the presenting fetal part stretches pelvic floor muscles (Ferguson, 1941). Stretch receptors are then activated, releasing endogenous oxytocin, supporting the hypotheses that the urge to push is dependent more on station than dilation (Cosner & deJong, 1993). Women report well-defined urges to push that occur before, during, and after complete dilation (McKay, Barrows, & Roberts, 1990). These findings suggest that "when to push" should be individualized to the maternal response rather than labor routines that dictate pushing at complete dilation (AWHONN, 2006, 2019b; Lemos et al., 2015; Roberts, 2002). The goals during the second stage of labor

should be to support, rather than direct, the woman's involuntary pushing efforts leading to movement of the fetus down and out of the pelvis and to minimize the use of the Valsalva maneuver with its associated negative maternal hemodynamic effects and resultant adverse implications for the fetus (AWHONN, 2006, 2019b; Simpson & James, 2005a). Preparing women who attend childbirth classes to anticipate and actively participate in a physiologic-based second stage of labor may be beneficial in promoting optimal care. Physiologic-based second-stage labor includes delaying pushing until the woman feels the urge to push. Delayed pushing is waiting for fetal descent and or the initiation of the Ferguson reflex before pushing begins in the second stage of labor. Delayed pushing is also referred to as "laboring down," "passive fetal descent," and "rest and descend" (AWHONN, 2019b).

There are generally two approaches to coaching women to push during the second stage of labor: open- and closed-glottis pushing. The closed-glottis pushing approach often includes encouraging the woman to begin pushing and offering bearing down instructions at complete dilation whether or not she feels the urge to push. This technique can have a negative affect on the fetus (Aldrich et al., 1995; AWHONN, 2019b; Caldeyro-Barcia, 1979; Langer et al., 1997; Simpson & James, 2005a; Thomson, 1993). Typically, women are coached to take a deep breath and hold it for at least 10 seconds while bearing down three to four times during each contraction. Women are instructed not to make a sound and to bring their knees up toward their abdomen with their elbows outstretched while pushing. Many clinicians will assist by holding the woman's legs back against her abdomen and counting to 10 with each pushing effort. These approaches are outdated and physiologically inappropriate (AWHONN, 2006, 2019b).

When the woman takes a deep breath and holds it (closed glottis), the Valsalva maneuver is instituted. This technique increases intrathoracic pressure, impairs blood return from lower extremities, and initially increases and then decreases BP, resulting in a decrease in uteroplacental blood flow (Barnett & Humenick, 1982; Bassell, Humayun, & Marx, 1980; Caldeyro-Barcia et al., 1981). In the newborn, iatrogenic hypoxemia, acidemia, and lower Apgar scores may result. Sustained pushing of 9 to 15 seconds can result in significant decelerations in the FHR (Caldeyro-Barcia et al., 1981) and decreases in fetal SpO_2 (Aldrich et al., 1995; Langer et al., 1997; Simpson & James, 2005a) (Fig. 14–10). Based on the results of a randomized clinical trial, when compared to spontaneous pushing, Valsalva pushing can have significant adverse effects including an increase in the length of the second stage of labor, a decrease in Apgar scores at 1 minute and 5 minutes, and a decrease in umbilical cord pH and PO_2 (Yildirim & Beji, 2008).

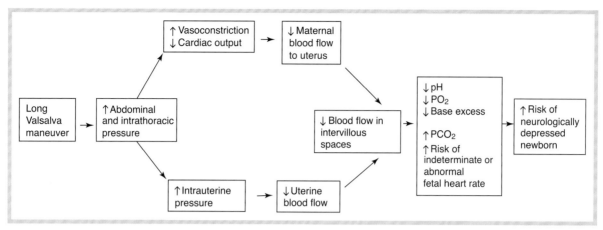

FIGURE 14–10. Coached closed-glottis (Valsalva) pushing during second stage: effect on maternal hemodynamics and fetal status. (From Barnett, M. M., & Humenick, S. S. [1982]. Infant outcome in relation to second stage labor pushing method. *Birth, 9*[4], 221–229.)

Transient and permanent peroneal nerve damage have been reported following prolonged periods of coached pushing with the woman in the supine lithotomy position. When the woman and/or care provider applies pressure to the peroneal nerve during pushing over a prolonged period, nerve damage resulting in numbness and tingling of the legs, inability to bear weight, and transient loss of feeling may result (Colachis, Pease, & Johnson, 1994; Tubridy & Redmond, 1996; Wong et al., 2003). This type of iatrogenic injury can be prevented by encouraging the woman to keep her feet flat on the bed during second-stage pushing. Healthcare providers should avoid forcibly pushing the woman's legs against her abdomen and placing the woman's legs in stirrups while pushing, because these techniques increase the risk of peroneal nerve damage (Colachis et al., 1994; Tubridy & Redmond, 1996; Wong et al., 2003).

The length and type of pushing, as well as maternal position during pushing, has a direct impact on the fetal response to the second stage of labor and newborn transition to extrauterine life. Avoid sustained closed-glottis pushing if at all possible. The practice of the caregiver counting to 10 with each pushing effort to encourage prolonged breath holding should be abandoned. There are strategies that can be used to decrease the impact of pushing on fetal well-being. If the fetus is not responding well to maternal pushing efforts, as evidenced by recurrent late and/or variable FHR decelerations, the most appropriate intervention is to modify pushing efforts, which can include pushing with every other or every third contraction and repositioning (Freeman, Garite, Nageotte, & Miller, 2012; Simpson, 2015). If modification of pushing efforts does resolve the FHR pattern, consider stopping pushing temporarily and assisting the woman to a lateral position to allow the fetus to recover (AWHONN, 2006, 2019b). It may be necessary to encourage the woman to push with every other contraction or every third contraction to maintain a normal FHR pattern. A baseline FHR

should be identified between contractions. If the fetus does not tolerate pushing and the woman has an epidural, the passive fetal descent approach works best. In the context of recurrent late, variable, or prolonged decelerations, oxytocin should be discontinued. Avoid tachysystole during the active pushing phase. Tachysystole in second-stage labor is associated with adverse neonatal outcomes such as need for hypothermic treatment (e.g., head cooling), need for ventilatory support, meconium aspiration, seizures, suspected sepsis, and death (Zahedi-Spung et al., 2019). Discuss concerns with the physician/certified nurse midwife (CNM) if there is pressure or a sense of urgency (unrelated to maternal or fetal status) to get the baby delivered.

At present, there is no reliable method to know which fetuses can tolerate continued physiologic stress of sustained coached closed-glottis pushing. Therefore, the FHR pattern must be used as the indicator as to how well the fetus is responding. It is known that recurrent late and/or variable decelerations during the second stage are associated with respiratory acidemia at birth (Kazandi, Sendag, Akercan, Terek, & Gundem, 2003). Some fetuses may develop metabolic acidemia if this type of pattern continues over a long period (Parer, King, Flanders, Fox, & Kilpatrick, 2006; Schifrin & Ater, 2006). These babies are difficult to resuscitate and may not transition well to extrauterine life. Sustained pushing efforts in the presence of an indeterminate or abnormal FHR pattern during second-stage labor characterized by recurrent late and/or variable decelerations, a rising baseline rate, and decreasing variability increase the risk of fetal harm, such as fetal hypoxic and ischemic injuries (Hamilton, Warrick, Knox, O'Keeffe, & Garite, 2012; Schifrin & Ater, 2006).

In contrast, physiologic second-stage management is based on the principles that the second stage of labor is a normal physiologic event and that women should push spontaneously and give birth with minimal intervention (Adams, Stark, & Low, 2016; AWHONN, 2006, 2019b).

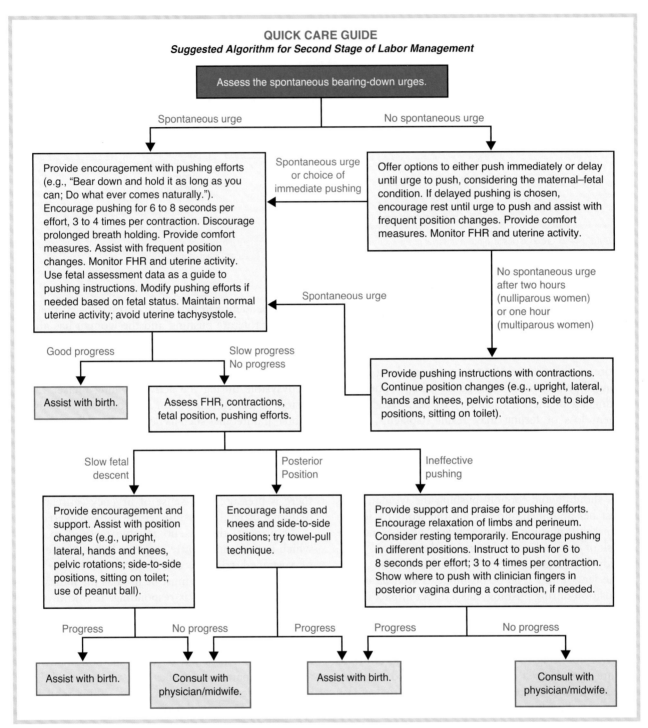

FIGURE 14–11. Suggested algorithm for second stage of labor. FHR, fetal heart rate. (Adapted from Association of Women's Health, Obstetric and Neonatal Nurses. [2019b]. *Nursing care and management of the 2nd stage of labor* [Evidence-Based Clinical Practice Guideline, 3rd ed.]. Washington, DC: Author; Cosner, K. R., & deJong, E. [1993]. *Physiologic second-stage labor. MCN: The American Journal of Maternal Child Nursing, 18*[1], 38–43.)

Second-stage labor has been divided into two phases (latent phase and active pushing phase) with the first described as the period from complete dilatation to spontaneous bearing down during which the fetus passively descends until the woman feels the urge to push (Roberts, 2002). The second phase is characterized by vigorous expulsive efforts based on the woman feeling pressure and the urge to push (Roberts & Woolley, 1996). More effective expulsive efforts are associated with delaying pushing until the mother feels the urge to do so (Roberts, 2002). Figure 14–11 provides an algorithm from AWHONN (2019b) for physiologic second-stage management. Display 14–4 lists suggestions from AWHONN for optimal second-stage labor care.

DISPLAY 14-4
Nursing Management of the Second Stage of Labor

Preparation of the Woman for the Second Stage of Labor

A woman's sense of self-efficacy, empowerment, and satisfaction with her labor and birth experience may increase when she receives patient-centered, realistic information prenatally and throughout the course of labor. In preparation for the second stage of labor, the woman should receive information about:

- The phases and estimated duration of the second stage of labor
- The sensations she might experience
- Options for initiation of pushing (immediate or delayed), including advantages and disadvantages of each option
- Options for physiologically based positions she might assume, such as sitting, kneeling, squatting, or standing
- Benefits of having a support person present during labor and birth whenever available

Supportive Care: Physical, Emotional, Instructional, and Advocacy

Assessment of the woman and her partner throughout pregnancy and labor to evaluate the need for physical, emotional, instructional, or psychosocial supportive care may contribute to positive birth outcomes:

- Encourage ambulation and frequent position changes whenever possible.
- Promote physical comfort by applying cool or warm compresses, changing linens, performing vaginal exams only as needed, offering fluids as tolerated, and providing massage and touch as the mother desires.
- Provide emotional support through caring, reassurance, empathy, acceptance, and encouragement.
- Provide information and instruction throughout labor to help reduce stress caused by fear of the unknown.
- Act as an advocate for the laboring woman and her partner to support preferences whenever possible and promote maternal–fetal safety.

Positioning

Changing maternal positions frequently may align the fetus in a better position in the pelvis and promote comfort. If a woman is unable to maintain an upright position, facilitate lateral positioning. Benefits of upright and lateral positioning for the second stage of labor include the following:

- The pelvic diameter may be increased by up to 30%, and fetal descent may be facilitated.
- The duration of the second stage of labor may be decreased.
- Fetal oxygenation may be enhanced, and there may be fewer abnormal fetal heart rate patterns.
- The intensity of pain and discomfort experienced during the second stage of labor may be minimized.

- Perineal trauma may be decreased, provided the pelvis and perineum are given adequate support.
- Upright and lateral positioning may result in fewer episiotomies and operative-assisted births.

Options for Initiation of Pushing and Nondirected Pushing Techniques

Provide information to the woman about options for immediate or delayed pushing. Include discussion of potential advantages and disadvantages based on maternal and fetal status.

- If delayed pushing until urge to push is chosen as an option, these time frames are considered: up to 2 hours for nulliparous women and up to 1 hour for multiparous women with regional anesthesia.
- Assess the woman's knowledge of pushing techniques, expectations for pushing, presence of Ferguson reflex, and readiness to push as well as the fetal presentation, position, and station.
- Encourage open-glottis pushing for 6 to 8 seconds, repeating this pattern for three to four pushes per contraction, or as tolerated by the woman.
- Discourage prolonged breath holding. Avoid counting to 10 with each contraction.
- Provide aids such as peanut balls, birthing balls, squat bars, birthing stools, and pillows to support the woman and the pelvis.

Evaluation of Physiologic Processes of the Second Stage of Labor

Continuous assessment of the woman's progress and evaluation of individualized nursing interventions during the second stage of labor are important. Clinical practice recommendations for evaluating and facilitating progress through the second stage of labor include, but are not limited to, the following:

- Evaluate the effectiveness of pushing efforts and descent of the presenting part.
- Support and facilitate the woman's spontaneous pushing efforts.
- Evaluate effectiveness of upright or other positions on fetal descent, rotation, and maternal–fetal condition.
- Assess and document fetal status every 30 minutes during the passive fetal descent phase and every 5 to 15 minutes during the active pushing phase. More frequent assessment may be needed depending on maternal–fetal condition. Evaluate effectiveness of upright or other positions on fetal descent, rotation, and maternal–fetal condition. Summary documentation indicating continuous bedside attendance and assessment by the nurse may be appropriate at less frequent intervals during the active phase of the second stage of labor.
- If fetal descent is too rapid, assist the woman to maintain a lateral position and avoid sitting or squatting.
- If fetal descent is delayed, provide the woman with continuous feedback and encouragement regarding her progress, change maternal position to facilitate rotation and descent, discourage lithotomy or semirecumbent position to facilitate rotation and descent, discourage lithotomy or semirecumbent positions whenever possible, and help the woman maintain an empty bladder.

Adapted from Association of Women's Health, Obstetric and Neonatal Nurses. (2019b). *Nursing care and management of the 2nd stage of labor* (Evidence-Based Clinical Practice Guideline, 3rd ed.). Washington, DC: Author. Used with permission.

With involuntary pushing, women are observed to hold their breath for 6 seconds while bearing down and take several breaths in between bearing-down efforts (Roberts, Goldstein, Gruener, Maggio, & Mendez-Bauer, 1987). When pushing spontaneously without instructions, women do not instinctively take a deep breath; they do not start expulsive efforts at the beginning of the contraction, and they use both open- and closed-glottis pushing (Thomson, 1995). This is in contrast to second-stage coaching instructions that encourage breath-holding for 10 seconds while bearing down and allowing only one quick breath between pushes. Open-glottis or gentle pushing avoids fetal stress, has less impact on uteroplacental blood flow, allows for perineal relaxation, and is more physiologically appropriate (AWHONN, 2006, 2019b; Caldeyro-Barcia et al., 1981; Hanson, 2009; Simpson & James, 2005a). The woman is more in control and responding to her body's own pushing cues, enhancing maternal confidence and satisfaction with the birth experience. Open-glottis pushing as compared to closed-glottis pushing can shorten the length of the second stage of labor (Chang et al., 2011; Parnell, Langhoff-Roos, Iversen, & Damgaard, 1993). Encourage the woman to bear down as long as she can or to do whatever comes naturally (Bloom, Casey, Schaffer, McIntire, & Leveno, 2006). Supporting the woman's voluntary pushing efforts is the best approach (Prins, Boxem, Lucas, & Hutton, 2011). Randomized clinical trials have found that women prefer spontaneous voluntary pushing efforts over directed Valsalva pushing (Chang et al., 2011; Prins et al., 2011; Yildirim & Beji, 2008). Women push with an open glottis when not coached to breathe in a specific way (ACOG, 2019a). Each woman should be encouraged to use her preferred and most effective technique (ACOG, 2019a).

Delayed Pushing (Laboring Down/Passive Fetal Descent) for Women with Regional Analgesia/Anesthesia

When women have regional analgesia/anesthesia, they may not feel the urge to push when they are completely dilated. In this situation, one approach to the second stage is to delay pushing while the fetus descends passively. Various researchers have described success with a protocol allowing nulliparous women to wait 2 hours or until the urge to push and allowing multiparous women 1 hour or until the urge to push (Brancato, Church, & Stone, 2008; Chang et al., 2011; Hansen, Clark, & Foster, 2002; Simpson & James, 2005a). A lateral position will facilitate passive fetal descent until the presenting part is low enough to stimulate the Ferguson reflex. There are significantly fewer FHR decelerations when the fetus is allowed to descend spontaneously when compared to coached

closed-glottis pushing (Hansen et al., 2002; Simpson & James, 2005a). Maternal fatigue is less when women are allowed a period of passive descent when compared to immediate pushing when there is no urge to push (Chang et al., 2011; Hansen et al., 2002; Lai, Lin, Li, Shey, & Gau, 2009).

Results of a recent multicenter randomized controlled trial have contributed more evidence to what is known about how to best advise nulliparous women with epidural analgesia when they reach 10-cm cervical dilation (Cahill et al., 2018). Nulliparous women with epidural analgesia were randomized to immediate pushing at 10 cm or delayed pushing for up to 1 hour. There were no differences between groups on cesarean versus vaginal birth or on the composite of neonatal morbidity (Cahill et al., 2018). As earlier studies have found, there are advantages and disadvantages to either approach. Advantages of immediate pushing include a shorter overall second stage (Cahill et al., 2018; Fraser et al., 2000; Hansen et al., 2002; Simpson & James, 2005a; Tuuli, Frey, Odibo, Macones, & Cahill, 2012), lower risk of postpartum hemorrhage as per visually estimated blood loss defined as >500 mL for vaginal birth and >1,000 mL for cesarean (immediate: 2.3% vs. delayed: 4%), and a lower risk of chorioamnionitis (immediate: 6.7% vs. delayed: 9.1%) defined as diagnosed clinically by the physician during second stage and treated with antibiotics (Cahill et al., 2018). Advantages of delayed pushing include shorter pushing time (Cahill et al., 2018; Fraser et al., 2000; Hansen et al., 2002; Simpson & James, 2005a; Tuuli et al., 2012), fewer variable decelerations (Hansen et al., 2002; Simpson & James, 2005a), lower risk of a negative effect on fetal oxygen status (Simpson & James, 2005a), and less third- and fourth-degree lacerations (Cahill et al., 2018). It is important to note in the Cahill study, there were no significant differences between the groups in estimated blood loss (immediate: 419.0 mL vs. delayed: 424.4 mL), rate of blood transfusions (immediate: 1.2% vs. delayed: 1.3%), or severe postpartum hemorrhage (immediate: 1.8% vs. delayed: 2.7%) defined as estimated blood loss >1,000 mL for vaginal birth and >2,000 mL for cesarean. There were no differences between groups on endometritis (immediate: 0.6% vs. delayed: 0.3%).

Risk of operative vaginal birth is less with delayed pushing until urge to push when compared to pushing immediately at 10 cm (Brancato et al., 2008; Fraser et al., 2000; Roberts, Torvaldsen, Cameron, & Olive, 2004). Injuries to the structure and function of the pelvic floor are less likely when a passive second stage results in a decreased period of maternal expulsive efforts. Delaying pushing and avoiding closed-glottis pushing has been shown to decrease the risk of perineal injuries (Albers, Sedler, Bedrick, Teaf, & Peralta, 2006; Sampselle & Hines, 1999; Simpson & James, 2005a).

When compared to spontaneous bearing down efforts, coached pushing results in a greater risk of urodynamic stress incontinence, decreased bladder capacity, decreased first urge to void, and detrusor overactivity (Schaffer et al., 2005).

Allowing a variable period of rest with spontaneous fetal descent may be beneficial for mother and fetus (AWHONN, 2019b; Bloom et al., 2006; Brancato et al., 2008; Grobman et al., 2016; Handa, Harris, & Ostergard, 1996; Hansen et al., 2002; Maresh, Choong, & Beard, 1983; Mayberry, Hammer, Kelly, True-Driver, & De, 1999; Roberts & Hanson, 2007; Simpson & James, 2005a; Tuuli et al., 2012; Vause, Congdon, & Thornton, 1998). The active pushing phase is the most physiologically stressful part of labor for the fetus, so shortening pushing time can promote fetal well-being (Roberts, 2002; Simpson & James, 2005a). Longer duration of active pushing is associated with an increased relative risk for neonatal complications, such as mechanical ventilation, sepsis, brachial plexus palsy, encephalopathy, and death (Grobman et al., 2016). Laboring down avoids maternal fatigue and the indeterminate or abnormal FHR patterns associated with sustained coached closed-glottis pushing. Allowing maternal rest and passive fetal descent will not result in a clinically significant increase in the duration of the second stage of labor (Fraser et al., 2000; Hansen et al., 2002). Active pushing time is significantly decreased with delayed pushing (Brancato et al., 2008; Gillesby et al., 2010; Kelly et al., 2010; Simpson & James, 2005b; Tuuli et al., 2012). Throughout passive and active second stage, a periodic assessment of descent of the fetal presenting part via vaginal examination will provide important information about progress and will assist in guiding subsequent care.

Include the woman as a full partner in her care by offering her information based on the most recent evidence. The conversation should include the context of her individual clinical situation (maternal–fetal condition such as maternal vital signs, FHR tracing; risk of postpartum hemorrhage, maternal fatigue; urge to push, fetal station/position, etc.), answering any questions and encouraging her to discuss options for timing of pushing with the other members of the healthcare team. The woman's preferences can be informed by a thoughtful, thorough discussion and should be the basis for her care (Simpson, 2019a, 2019b).

Applying the clinical practices described in the AWHONN (2019b) evidence-based guidelines can be beneficial for overall outcomes. In one health system, the AWHONN guidelines were adopted in 34 birthing hospitals with significant improvements in using spontaneous mother-initiated pushing, a lower rate of cesarean births for nulliparous women at term with a singleton fetus, and a decrease in unexpected complications in the newborn (Garpiel, 2018). There were no negative effects on maternal or newborn outcomes and patient satisfaction significantly increased (Garpiel, 2018).

Maintaining Adequate Pain Relief while Pushing for Women with Labor Epidurals

In the past, some care providers have discontinued the labor epidural infusion when women are unable to push effectively and/or do not feel an adequate urge to push. The efficacy and ethics of this practice should be questioned (Roberts, 2002). There has been an erroneous assumption by some care providers that the discontinuation of epidural analgesia/anesthesia could speed the second-stage process and avoid an operative vaginal birth or cesarean birth. However, often, the opposite occurs. Women who have been receiving adequate regional pain relief and then have discontinuation of the epidural infusion experience significant pain and are at risk for fetal malrotations, dysfunctional uterine activity, a longer second stage, and forceps- or vacuum-assisted birth (Phillips & Thomas, 1983; Roberts, 2002). The increased catecholamine levels related to severe pain can adversely affect uterine activity and fetal status as well as prolong the second stage (Roberts, 2002). There is no evidence to support the hypothesis that discontinuing epidural analgesia/anesthesia late in labor benefits the mother or baby (Torvaldsen, Roberts, Bell, & Raynes-Greenow, 2004). The effect of epidural analgesia/anesthesia on length of second-stage labor is clinically negligible (ASA, 2016); therefore, withholding pain relief via epidural is not appropriate. If women have difficulty feeling the urge to push and effectively working with the pressure as the baby descends, review the level of motor block and type and amount of medications routinely used for regional labor analgesia/anesthesia in the perinatal unit. Consult with anesthesia providers to develop a more appropriate combination of medications that will result in adequate pain relief without an overly dense motor block. As per ASA (2016), the goal of modern labor epidural analgesia favors minimizing motor blockade by initiating and maintaining analgesia using low-concentration local anesthetic solutions.

Shoulder Dystocia

Shoulder dystocia is an uncommon and unpredictable obstetric emergency typically diagnosed when attempts at gentle, downward traction on the fetal head fails to result in delivery of the impacted anterior shoulder. The classic "turtle sign," in which the head appears to retract into the perineum, may or may not occur simultaneously. The reported incidence of shoulder dystocia among vaginal births of vertex presenting infants ranges from 0.2% to 3% (ACOG, 2017; Bingham, Chauhan, Hayes, Gherman, & Lewis, 2010;

Hoffman et al., 2011; Leung et al., 2011; Ouzounian, Gherman, Chauhan, Battista, & Lee, 2012). These data are based on retrospective studies. Data based on prospective studies suggest a higher incidence of 3.3% to 7% of vaginal births (Gurewitsch & Allen, 2011). Recurrent shoulder dystocia occurs in approximately 3.7% to 12% of women who experienced shoulder dystocia during a prior birth (Bingham et al., 2010; Ouzounian et al., 2012). Challenges in determining the actual incidence of shoulder dystocia include variations in the definition of shoulder dystocia among providers and in the literature, not all shoulder dystocia cases are documented as such in medical records, and shoulder dystocia as a birth complication is unable to be collected from certificates of live births in the United States. In addition, the head-to-body time interval during a shoulder dystocia is often not documented in the medial record (Gherman, Chauhan, & Lewis, 2012). A universally used definition of shoulder dystocia would enhance the ability of researchers to advance science and knowledge about risk factors and appropriate interventions.

During shoulder dystocia, the umbilical cord may be partially or completely occluded between the fetal body and maternal pelvis. Compression of the fetal neck, resulting in cerebral venous obstruction, excessive vagal stimulation, and bradycardia, may be combined with reduced arterial oxygen supply to cause clinical deterioration out of proportion to the duration of hypoxia (Kwek & Yeo, 2006). The normally oxygenated fetus can tolerate several minutes of cord compression without significant adverse effects. However, most experts note that a >5-minute head-to-body interval may result in acid–base deterioration in a fetus whose condition was normal prior to the onset of shoulder dystocia (Benedetti, 1995; Leung et al., 2011). Leung et al. (2011) found that pH dropped at a rate of 0.011 per minute of head-to-body interval during birth complicated by shoulder dystocia. When the head-to-body interval exceeds 4 minutes, there is greater risk of neonatal depression (Lerner, Durlacher, Smith, & Hamilton, 2011). If fetal status was not normal prior to the shoulder dystocia, the fetus may have less physiologic reserve (Kwek & Yeo, 2006; Schifrin & Ater, 2006). Constant provider-coached pushing efforts for a prolonged period with recurrent late and variable decelerations can result in fetal oxygen desaturation, fetal metabolic acidemia, and risk of fetal hypoxic and ischemic injuries (Hamilton et al., 2012; Parer et al., 2006; Schifrin & Ater, 2006; Simpson & James, 2005a). In this context, the fetus may have less ability to tolerate an additional insult such as shoulder dystocia. In one study using neonatal brain injury as the outcome, brain injury cases were associated with a significantly prolonged head-to-body interval >10 minutes, and ≥7 minutes had a sensitivity of 67% and specificity of 74% in predicting brain injury (Ouzounian, Korst, Ahn, & Phelan, 1998).

The most commonly reported immediate neonatal injuries associated with shoulder dystocia include brachial plexus injuries and fractures of the clavicle and humerus (ACOG, 2017). While the rate of transient brachial plexus injuries varies, most studies report a 10% to 20% injury rate immediately after birth (ACOG, 2017). However, since most shoulder dystocia studies lack long-term neonatal follow-up and a uniform definition for recovery from injury, it is difficult to determine the true rate of persistent or permanent neonatal brachial plexus injuries (ACOG, 2017). Not all brachial plexus injuries are related to shoulder dystocia and the injury is multifactorial (ACOG, 2017). Severe brachial plexus injuries have been documented in the absence of shoulder dystocia and identifiable risk factors (ACOG, 2017; Torki, Barton, Miller, & Ouzounian, 2012). Slightly more than one half of brachial plexus injuries are associated with uncomplicated vaginal births (ACOG, 2017). Brachial plexus injuries have been found to occur in vertex-presenting fetuses birthed by a traumatic cesarean (ACOG, 2017).

Numerous antepartum and pregnancy risk factors associated with shoulder dystocia have been discussed in the literature, including fetal macrosomia (past and/ or present pregnancy), preexisting or gestational diabetes mellitus, a previous pregnancy complicated by gestational diabetes, a history of a prior shoulder dystocia, maternal obesity, excessive maternal weight gain, multiparity, postterm pregnancy, and disproportionate fetal growth with increased abdominal and chest circumference relative to occipitofrontal diameter (ACOG, 2016a, 2017; Belfort, White, & Vermeulen, 2012; Gurewitsch & Allen, 2011; Larson & Mandelbaum, 2012; Overland, Vatten, & Eskild, 2012; Tsur, Sergienko, Wiznitzer, Zlotnik, & Sheiner, 2012). Intrapartum risk factors that have been reported include labor induction; abnormal labor progress, including prolonged second-stage labor; and operative vaginal birth (ACOG, 2017; Gurewitsch & Allen, 2011; Okby & Sheiner, 2012; Tsur et al., 2012). While increasing fetal birth weight and maternal diabetes have been associated with an increased risk of shoulder dystocia, most cases occur in nondiabetic women with normal-sized newborns (ACOG, 2017). Elective cesarean birth should be considered for women without diabetes who are carrying fetuses with suspected macrosomia with an estimated fetal weight of at least 5,000 g and for women with diabetes whose fetuses are estimated to weigh at least 4,500 g (ACOG, 2017). Clinicians should be aware of these risk factors for shoulder dystocia in order to anticipate those births at risk and should be prepared to manage shoulder dystocia in all births (ACOG, 2017). However, many women have one or more of these risk factors and do not experience shoulder dystocia.

Prompt intervention is necessary to decrease the risk of maternal and neonatal complications and long-term sequelae. While most cases of shoulder dystocia are unpredictable, reasonable steps can be undertaken once shoulder dystocia is identified. A thorough knowledge of what to do should this crisis occur is essential to ensure the best possible outcomes for the mother and baby. Key nursing interventions include calling for additional help; calm, supportive actions; and working in sync with the physician or CNM who is directing the maneuvers to deliver the impacted shoulder.

Simulation exercises and shoulder dystocia protocols to improve team communication and maneuver use to reduce the incidence of brachial plexus palsy associated with shoulder dystocia are recommended by ACOG (2017). The Joint Commission's Sentinel Event Alert *Preventing Infant Death and Injury during Delivery* recommends conducting periodic drills for obstetric emergencies such as shoulder dystocia (The Joint Commission, 2004). Reported reductions in obstetric brachial plexus injuries related to shoulder dystocia after training include from 30% pretraining to 11% after training (Inglis et al., 2011), from 10% pretraining to 4% during training to 2.6% after training (Grobman, Miller, Burke, Hornbogen, Tam, & Costello, 2011), and from 9.3% pretraining to 2.3% after training (Draycott et al., 2008). An evaluation of force applied during simulated shoulder dystocia can be helpful in illustrating the need for changes in practice related to the safe amount of force when an actual shoulder dystocia is encountered (Deering, Weeks, & Benedetti, 2011). The simulation process, including practicing how to respond effectively to shoulder dystocia, can be useful in introducing and improving concepts of teamwork and interdisciplinary interactions that are necessary for success during an obstetric emergency (Grobman, Hornbogen, Burke, & Costello, 2010; Grobman et al., 2011).

When shoulder dystocia is suspected, nursing, obstetric, anesthesia, and pediatric staff should be called to attend the birth if not already present. The time the shoulder dystocia is diagnosed should be documented as well as the time the birth is complete (ACOG, 2017). The mother is instructed about when and how to push and is positioned with her buttocks at the edge of the bed while preparations and maneuvers to disimpact the shoulder are made under the direction of the physician or CNM. Calmly assisting the woman to the appropriate positions during the maneuvers will help her feel confident that necessary interventions are being done as quickly as possible by competent healthcare providers. If possible, an assessment of fetal status via EFM or handheld ultrasound devices will provide information about how the fetus is tolerating the interventions. However, time should not be lost attempting to locate the FHR if it is not readily identified. It is better to direct attention to dislodging the fetal shoulder by assisting the woman to the appropriate positions and following the direction of the physician or CNM.

Interventions described in the literature to relieve the impacted shoulder include the McRoberts maneuver (Fig. 14–12), suprapubic pressure (Fig. 14–13), delivery of the posterior arm, Rubin technique, Woods screw maneuver, Gaskin all-fours maneuver, clavicular fracture, Zavanelli maneuver, and symphysiotomy. While there is no clear evidence-based order of these maneuvers, most clinicians use McRoberts as the initial intervention, followed by suprapubic pressure (ACOG, 2017; Hoffman et al., 2011). The *Consortium on Safe Labor* (Hoffman et al., 2011) found delivery of the posterior arm following the McRoberts maneuver and suprapubic pressure to be associated with highest rate of vaginal birth when compared to other maneuvers. Although suprapubic pressure and McRoberts are often used prophylactically for women considered to be at high risk for shoulder dystocia, there is no evidence that these interventions reduce the incidence of shoulder dystocia or neonatal adverse outcomes (Beall, Spong, & Ross, 2003). The essential issue during shoulder dystocia is to continue to intervene using an organized expeditious series of steps until the baby has been delivered. If an injury occurs as a result of shoulder dystocia despite the best efforts of the obstetric providers, it is likely that litigation will follow (Gherman, 2002). Birth injuries associated with a shoulder dystocia are the most common reason for obstetric malpractice claims (Colombara, Soh, Menacho, Schiff, & Reed, 2011).

The McRoberts maneuver is usually the first maneuver initiated (Hoffman et al., 2011), and it involves hyperflexion of the woman's thighs against her abdomen (see Fig. 14–12). This position can ease delivery of the shoulder by changing the relationship of the maternal pelvis to the lumbar spine. This maneuver may not actually increase birth canal dimensions, but it does result in flattening of the sacrum relative to the maternal lumbar spine (Gherman, Tramont, Muffley, & Goodwin, 2000). In many cases, the McRoberts maneuver alone or along with suprapubic pressure will result in birth. If the McRoberts maneuver is not immediately successful, the next approach is usually suprapubic pressure (Hoffman et al., 2011).

Firm suprapubic pressure (see Fig. 14–13) using the palm of the hand or fist may be used to dislodge the impacted anterior shoulder. The physician or CNM may request the nurse to apply suprapubic pressure posteriorly or laterally to either the right or left side depending on which direction the fetus is facing. Posterior pressure is used to dislodge the anterior shoulder and push it under the symphysis. Lateral pressure to the posterior surface of the anterior shoulder may be used to push the fetal anterior shoulder toward the fetal chest, thereby decreasing shoulder-to-shoulder distance.

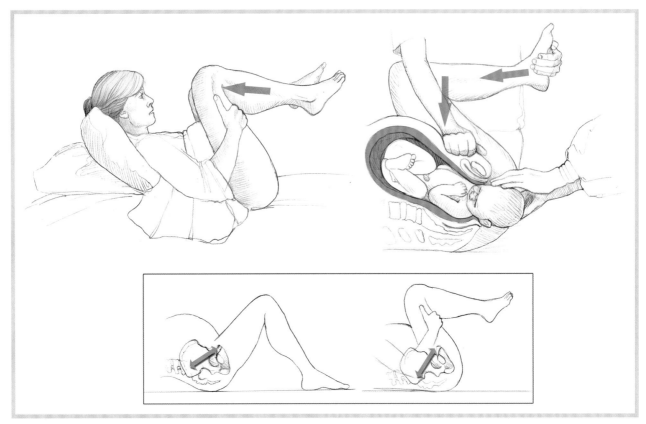

FIGURE 14–12. McRoberts maneuver.

Fundal pressure (Fig. 14–14) should be avoided during shoulder dystocia because it can further impact the fetal shoulder, resulting in an inability to deliver the fetal body as well as contributing to fetal brachial plexus injuries and fractures of the humerus and clavicle (ACOG, 2017; Gherman et al., 2006). Gross, Shime, and Farine (1987) reported a 77% fetal injury rate when fundal pressure was the only maneuver used to relieve shoulder dystocia. Fundal pressure during shoulder dystocia has been associated with a high rate of permanent brachial plexus injuries (Phelan, Ouzounian, Gherman, Korst, & Goodwin, 1997).

If birth does not occur immediately with McRoberts and suprapubic pressure, an appropriate next maneuver is delivery of the posterior arm (Hoffman et al., 2011). Physicians or CNMs gently insert their hand along the

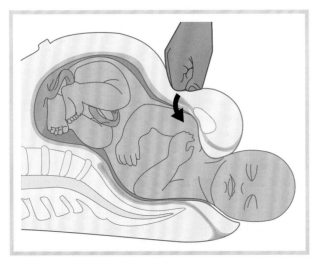

FIGURE 14–13. Suprapubic pressure. (From Penney, D. S., & Perlis, D. W. [1992]. When to use suprapubic or fundal pressure. *MCN: The American Journal of Maternal Child Nursing, 17*, 34–36.)

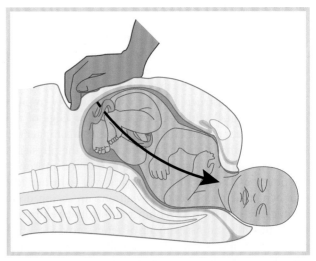

FIGURE 14–14. Fundal pressure. (From Penney, D. S., & Perlis, D. W. [1992]. When to use suprapubic or fundal pressure. *MCN: The American Journal of Maternal Child Nursing, 17*, 34–36.)

curvature of the maternal sacrum, and their fingers follow along the humerus to the antecubital fossa. The fetal forearm is flexed and swept across the chest and face and out the vagina. Ideally, the anterior shoulder will slide under the symphysis after the posterior arm is delivered. This technique may result in fracture of the humerus or clavicle.

In the Rubin technique, the fetal shoulders are adducted and displaced into the oblique position, thereby allowing the posterior arm to enter the pelvis. Initially, the Rubin technique described both external and internal maneuvers (Rubin, 1964). During the external maneuver, fetal shoulders are rocked side to side by applying force to the maternal abdomen. If the shoulder dystocia persists, the physician or CNM inserts fingers of one hand vaginally behind the most accessible fetal shoulder and pushes the fetal shoulder toward the anterior surface of the fetal chest in the direction of the fetal face. This most often results in abduction of the shoulders, a smaller shoulder-to-shoulder diameter, and displacement of the anterior shoulder from behind the symphysis pubis.

The Woods screw maneuver involves placing pressure on the anterior surface of the fetal posterior shoulder and gently rotating the shoulder anteriorly. The concern about this maneuver is that it can result in abduction of the shoulders, resulting in increased shoulder-to-shoulder diameter. As a result, the Rubin technique, which adducts the fetal shoulders and rounds them into a decreased shoulder-to-shoulder diameter, is often preferred.

The Gaskin all-fours maneuver (Fig. 14–15) involves assisting the laboring woman to her hands and knees (not a knee–chest position). In a study of 82 consecutive cases of shoulder dystocia, 83% of the women birthed using the Gaskin all-fours maneuver without the need for any additional maneuvers (Bruner et al., 1998). Position change and the effects of gravity appear to provide a rapid, safe, and effective method for reducing shoulder dystocia. The women in the Bruner et al. (1998) study received no anesthesia for labor or birth. For women with epidural analgesia or anesthesia, it may be difficult, but not impossible, to assist the woman to this position.

Episiotomy, as an intervention for shoulder dystocia, is controversial. Because shoulder dystocia is considered a "bony dystocia" and therefore not caused by obstructing soft tissue, its use may not be helpful (ACOG, 2017). Episiotomy or proctoepisiotomy has been associated with nearly a sevenfold increase in the rate of severe perineal trauma without the benefit of reducing the occurrence of neonatal depression or brachial plexus injury (Gherman et al., 2006). In one large U.S. perinatal service, an analysis of 94,842 births from 1999 to 2009 found the rate of episiotomy during shoulder dystocia decreased from 40% to 4%;

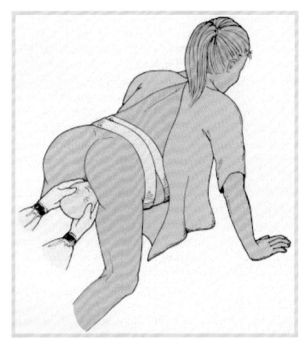

FIGURE 14–15. Gaskin all-fours maneuver. (From Bruner, J. P., Drummond, S. B., Meenan, A. L., & Gaskin, I. M. [1998]. All-fours maneuver for reducing shoulder dystocia during labor. *Journal of Reproductive Medicine, 43*[5], 439–443.)

however, there was no change in the rate of obstetric brachial plexus injuries (Paris, Greenberg, Ecker, & McElrath, 2011).

While the performance of a symphysiotomy is described in the literature, most practitioners have not had experience with this procedure (Gherman et al., 2006). Risks to the mother include major bladder and urethra damage, long-term pain, and difficulty walking. This procedure is rarely used in the United States (ACOG, 2017). The deliberate fracture of the clavicles is also described as a method to reduce shoulder width; however, many practitioners find this procedure technically difficult (Gherman et al., 2006).

If these or other maneuvers do not result in birth, the physician or CNM may attempt to replace the fetal head into the vagina and proceed with cesarean birth. This is known as the Zavanelli maneuver or cephalic replacement. It is important that the head be returned to the occipitoanterior or occipitoposterior position, then flexed, and slowly pushed back into the birth canal. A review of 103 published cases of the Zavanelli maneuver from 1985 to 1997 revealed a 92% success rate, with no reports of fetal injuries in those eventually born via cesarean section (Sandberg, 1999). Others have reported fetal injuries such as Erb palsy, paresis of the lower extremities, seizures, brain damage, delayed motor development, quadriplegia, cerebral palsy, and death as a result of the Zavanelli maneuver (Gherman et al., 2006). If the Zavanelli maneuver is successful, when possible, an assessment of fetal status via EFM or a handheld ultrasound device is desired while preparing for an emergent cesarean birth. Personnel skilled in neonatal resuscitation should be in attendance at the cesarean birth. The Zavanelli maneuver is not used often. A 2009 survey of obstetricians in the United States revealed that 85% had never used this procedure (Gherman et al., 2012).

Once the shoulder has been disimpacted and birth has occurred, the nurse can direct attention to newborn care and assessment. After the newborn and mother are stabilized, documentation about the events surrounding the birth involving shoulder dystocia is possible. Use of a standardized checklist in the birth note after a shoulder dystocia can improve documentation of key elements (ACOG, 2012b; Clark, Belfort, Byrum, Meyers, & Perlin, 2008; Deering, Tobler, & Cypher, 2010). Team training and unit protocol implementation can provide similar positive effects on medical record documentation (Grobman et al., 2011; Moragianni, Hacker, & Craparo, 2011; Nguyen, Fox, Friedman, Sandler, & Rebarber, 2011). Ideally, each care provider documents his or her specific actions and interventions. For example, the nurse may record the application of suprapubic pressure and repositioning the woman using the McRoberts maneuver, while the physician or CNM may record the techniques and maneuvers used to disimpact the shoulder and birth the baby. There is no need for duplicate notes by both the nurse and the healthcare provider who delivered the baby of the same components of the procedure.

Support and communication with the family is important after birth. The woman and her family will likely be concerned about the condition of the baby and will have questions about what occurred. Debriefing with the family soon after the shoulder dystocia can maximize communication and provide support. As part of the discussion, the woman should be informed that she is at risk of a recurrent shoulder dystocia in subsequent birth.

The Perineum

Episiotomy

Episiotomy is a surgical enlargement of the posterior wall of the vagina by an incision into the perineum just prior to birth. In the United States, the midline or median episiotomy is more common, while in Europe, the mediolateral episiotomy is more frequently performed. However, based on existing evidence, there are no clinical situations in which episiotomy is essential; rather, the decision to perform an episiotomy should be based on clinical factors (ACOG, 2018). Restrictive episiotomy use is recommended over routine episiotomy (ACOG, 2018). Routine use of episiotomy is not necessary and may lead to an increase in the risk of third- and fourth-degree perineal lacerations and a delay in the woman's resumption of sexual activity. Episiotomy is only done for a specific medical indication (AAP & ACOG, 2017).

Those who consider routine episiotomy to be beneficial cite the following advantages: prevention of perineal tearing; ease of repair when compared to lacerations; reduction in the time and stress of the second stage of labor; decreased compression of fetal head, especially for preterm infants; and allowance of easier manipulation during breech or operative vaginal birth. However, the benefits of routine episiotomy have not been demonstrated by rigorous research (ACOG, 2018; Eason & Feldman, 2000; Eason, Labrecque, Wells, & Feldman, 2000; Hartmann et al., 2005; Jiang, Qian, Carroli, & Garner, 2017). It appears that personal beliefs, education, and experience of the practitioner, rather than evidence, influence clinical judgment about whether to perform an episiotomy (ACOG, 2018; Low, Seng, Murtland, & Oakley, 2000).

Based on available data, giving birth over an intact perineum results in less blood loss, less risk of infection, and less perineal pain postpartum (ACOG, 2018; Eason & Feldman, 2000). Methods to prevent perineal trauma during birth include upright positioning, avoidance of episiotomy, avoidance of forceps or vacuum extractors, passive fetal descent, avoidance of Valsalva pushing, slowing the birth of the fetal head to allow the perineum time to stretch, and birth between contractions (Albers et al., 2006; Andrews, Sultan, Thakar, & Jones, 2006; da Silva et al., 2012; De Jonge et al., 2010; Eason & Feldman, 2000; FitzGerald, Weber, Howden, Cundiff, & Brown, 2007; Gupta et al., 2017; Hastings-Tolsma, Vincent, Emeis, & Francisco, 2007; Kudish et al., 2006; Mayerhofer et al., 2002; Sampselle & Hines, 1999; Schaffer et al., 2005; Simpson & James, 2005a).

Episiotomy is often performed when the physician or CNM feels that there is a risk of lacerations of the perineum or vagina during birth. The goal is to protect the perineum and to maintain future perineal function and integrity; however, supportive evidence is lacking that these goals can be achieved with routine episiotomy (ACOG, 2018; Scott, 2005). Episiotomy is associated with significant risks such as increased risk of third- and fourth-degree lacerations, anal sphincter injuries, severe lacerations and injuries in subsequent births, infection, delayed healing, breakdown in repair, increased blood loss, scarring, increased pain, and sexual dysfunction.

Episiotomy does not protect against problems with perineal muscle function postpartum (Fleming, Newton, & Roberts, 2003). Data from *Mothers' Outcome after Delivery*, a longitudinal cohort study of pelvic floor disorders after childbirth, found that forceps and perineal lacerations, but not episiotomies, were associated with pelvic floor disorders 5 to 10 years after first delivery (Handa, Blomquist, McDermott, Friedman, & Muñoz, 2012). Lacerations of the vagina and perineum are classified according to degree as listed

DISPLAY 14–5

Classification of Perineal Lacerations

Type of laceration	Classification
First degree	Injury to perineal skin only
Second degree	Injury to perineum involving perineal muscles but not involving anal sphincter
Third degree	Injury to perineum involving anal sphincter complex:
	3a: less than 50% of external anal sphincter thickness torn
	3b: more than 50% external anal sphincter thickness torn
	3c: both external anal sphincter and internal anal sphincter torn
Fourth degree	Injury to perineum involving anal sphincter complex (external anal sphincter and internal anal sphincter) and anal epithelium

Adapted from American College of Obstetricians and Gynecologists. (2018). *Prevention and management of obstetric lacerations at vaginal delivery* (Practice Bulletin No. 198). Washington, DC: Author.

in Display 14–5. Risk factors for third- and fourth-degree lacerations are nulliparity (a 7.2-fold risk), episiotomy (a 2.4-fold risk for nulliparous women and a 4.4-fold risk for multiparous women), increasing gestational age, increasing birth weight, oxytocin, epidural analgesia/anesthesia, operative vaginal birth, and increasing length of the second stage of labor (Landy et al., 2011). In the *Consortium on Safe Labor* database of 228,668 births from 2002 to 2008, third- or fourth-degree lacerations occurred in 2,516 women (2,223 nulliparous [5.8%], 293 [0.6%] multiparous) (Landy et al., 2011).

Nursing interventions during labor can have a direct impact on the use and perceived need for episiotomy. Upright position and open-glottis, gentle pushing that coincide with the woman's natural urges and sensations, aids gradual perineal stretching with less pain, thus avoiding the need for episiotomy and resultant perineal trauma (Eason et al., 2000; Sampselle & Hines, 1999; Simpson & James, 2005a). Women who give birth in the lithotomy position are more likely to have an episiotomy than women who give birth in squatting, on hands-and-knees, standing, or in sitting positions (Bodner-Adler et al., 2003; da Silva et al., 2012; de Jong et al., 1997; Gupta et al., 2017; Terry et al., 2006). Passive fetal descent and spontaneous bearing down efforts versus directed Valsalva pushing result in fewer episiotomies and perineal lacerations (Albers et al., 2006; Sampselle & Hines, 1999; Simpson & James, 2005a).

EMOTIONAL AND PHYSICAL SUPPORT DURING LABOR AND BIRTH

Impact of the Psyche on Childbirth

The psyche plays a major role in the process of labor and birth. A high level of anxiety has been associated with increased catecholamine secretion that can result in ineffective uterine activity and longer and dysfunctional labor (Buckley, 2015; Lederman, Lederman, Work, & McCann, 1985). Anxiety, uncertainty, loss of control, loss of self-confidence, patterns of coping, support systems, fatigue, optimism, fatalism, and aloneness are some of the psychosocial factors to consider when caring for women in labor. Previous birth experiences, present support systems, concerns or questions, anxiety or fear, and cultural considerations further contribute to attitudes and expectations for the current pregnancy experience.

Facilitating Labor and Birth

Nursing care during childbirth includes providing information so the woman knows what to expect, interpreting physical sensations, encouraging maternal position changes, reinforcing breathing and other relaxation efforts, support during the second stage, and continued pain management. Women expect that their nurse will provide physical comfort and informational and emotional support as well as technical nursing care and ongoing monitoring of maternal–fetal status during labor (Lyndon, Simpson, & Spetz, 2017; Tumblin & Simkin, 2001). Women appreciate the nurse being there for them (Hodnett et al., 2002; MacKinnon, McIntyre, & Quance, 2005). Women rank attentive, caring maternity nurses as an important aspect of high-quality maternity care (Declercq, Sakala, Corry, Applebaum, & Herrlick, 2014; Sakala, Declercq, Turon, & Corry, 2018). Some women experience increased anxiety and fear when the labor and birth unit is so busy that they do not have as much nursing contact and support as they had expected (Larkin, Begley, & Devane, 2012). Women value personal control during childbirth, and this is an important factor related to the woman's satisfaction with the childbirth experience (Christiaens & Bracke, 2007; Goodman, Mackey, & Tavakoli, 2004). When women experienced the birth they planned (e.g., vaginal or cesarean), they expressed satisfaction with childbirth, whereas an unplanned cesarean birth is associated with a less favorable view of the experience (Blomquist, Quiroz, Macmillan, McCullough, & Handa, 2011). Helping women to increase their personal control during labor and birth may increase the woman's childbirth satisfaction. Some hospitals offer birth plans for women so they can select options they would like to include as part of their labor and birth. See Display 17–1 in Chapter 17 for a family preference plan for childbirth.

Nurse Staffing

In a systematic review of women's satisfaction with their childbirth experience, women whose experiences were better than expected and women with high expectations were more likely to be satisfied, whereas women with low expectations that were subsequently met had lower levels of satisfaction (Hodnett, 2002). One-to-one nursing care during labor is a significant patient satisfier (Hodnett et al., 2002). When there is inadequate nurse staffing, nurses report they are unable to provide all intended care for women in labor. Some nurses reported that labor support and bedside attendance were the first to be missed in times of short staffing (Simpson & Lyndon, 2017a). Labor support by nurses should include thorough assessment of labor progress, facilitation of physiologic processes such as position changes and ambulation, provision of comfort measures, advocacy, information, evaluation of maternal–fetal status and coping, role modeling, and collaboration with other members of the healthcare team (Adams et al., 2016; AWHONN, 2018a, 2019b). In a recent study, the majority of labor nurses reported nurse staffing in their units was frequently or always consistent with the AWHONN (2010) nurse staffing guidelines (Simpson, Lyndon, Spetz, Gay, & Landstrom, 2019). The results reflect an improvement since 2011 and 2012 soon after the staffing guidelines were published in the fall of 2010 when Scheich and Bingham (2015) surveyed birthing hospitals as part of the AWHONN perinatal staffing data collaborative.

Nurse staffing guidelines from AWHONN (2010) delineate types of patients and clinical situations that require one nurse to one woman staffing, thus they are based on various patient acuities commonly encountered during labor, birth, and postpartum. Patient acuity is dynamic over the course of labor, birth, and postpartum. Nurse staffing should be adjusted accordingly. Women initially assessed as low risk on admission can develop complications or significant changes in maternal or fetal status that require 1 to 1 nursing care, at times including continuous bedside attendance. Nursing behaviors that demonstrate valuing and respecting childbearing women are essential in enhancing the quality of the birth experience (Matthews & Callister, 2004). Women appreciate nurses being supportive during labor and advocating for them, including keeping them informed, cheerleading, avoiding a cesarean, and following their wishes (Lyndon et al., 2017).

Recommendations for nurse staffing for women during labor and birth include the following:

- Women receiving pharmacologic agents for cervical ripening such as Cervidil (prostaglandin E_2 [PGE_2] vaginal insert) or Cytotec (misoprostol) require a minimum of one nurse to two women with assessment of maternal–fetal status at least every 30 minutes.

- One nurse to one woman for women choosing to labor with minimal to no pharmacologic pain relief or medical interventions (Timing of the 1 to 1 assignment is based on the woman's level of comfort and overall maternal–fetal status).
- One nurse to one woman when using intermittent auscultation for fetal assessment starting at 4 cm during the first stage of labor and the entire second-stage labor.
- Women using birthing balls or undergoing hydrotherapy in the shower or tub should not be left unattended. If no support person or ancillary personnel is available, the nurse should stay with the woman.
- Patient assignment for women receiving oxytocin for labor induction or augmentation should be one nurse to one woman to be able to assess maternal and fetal status every 15 minutes in the first stage of labor and the passive descent phase of the second stage of labor, and every 5 minutes in the active pushing phase of the second stage of labor.
- If a nurse cannot clinically evaluate the effects of medication at least every 15 minutes in the first stage of labor and maintain continuous bedside attendance during the active pushing phase of the second stage of labor, the oxytocin infusion should be discontinued until that level of maternal and fetal nursing care can be provided.
- Elective procedures should be deferred until there are adequate nurses to safely meet the needs of the service.
- One nurse to one woman with labor complications.
- Women in labor who are receiving magnesium sulfate should have one nurse in continuous bedside attendance for the first hour of administration and one nurse to one woman thereafter.
- Two nurses should attend every birth, one for the mother and one for the baby. In the case of multiples, there should be one nurse for each baby.
- One person capable of initiating newborn resuscitation (including positive pressure ventilation and chest compressions) should attend every birth. That person or someone else who is immediately available should have the skills required to perform complete resuscitation, including endotracheal intubation and the use of medications. It is not sufficient to have someone at home or "on call" (either at home or in a remote area of the hospital) for newborn resuscitation in the delivery room.
- If the birth is anticipated to be high risk, a neonatal resuscitation team should be assembled according to the Neonatal Resuscitation Program (AAP & American Heart Association [AHA], 2016) guidelines.

Supportive Care by Partners, Family, and Friends

Attention also should be given to the woman's partner/support person, family members, and friends in attendance. Every effort should be made to support and encourage those in attendance to assist the woman during labor and to allow as many support persons as the woman desires. Arbitrary rules prohibiting more than one support person during labor are contrary to the philosophy that the birth experience belongs to the woman and her family, rather to those providing clinical care. Although healthcare providers are sometimes inclined to attempt to control this aspect of the birth process using various arguments for safety and convenience, when examined critically, these arguments have little scientific merit. Women should be able to choose who will be with them during this special and unique life experience. Family-centered care supports the concept that the "family" is defined by the childbearing woman.

Women who have continuous labor support when compared to women who have the usual labor care are more likely to have a spontaneous vaginal birth and are less likely to have a cesarean birth, intrapartum analgesia/anesthesia, operative vaginal birth, a baby with a low 5-minute Apgar score, or to report dissatisfaction with their childbirth experiences (Bohren, Hofmeyr, Sakala, Fukuzawa, & Cuthbert, 2017; McGrath & Kennell, 2008). Labor is shorter for women with continuous labor support (Bohren et al., 2017). Continuous labor support is associated with greater benefits when the provider of that support is not a member of the hospital staff (Bohren et al., 2017; Campbell, Lake, Falk, & Backstrand, 2006; Hodnett et al., 2002; Kozhimannil, Hardeman, Attanasio, Blauer-Peterson, & O'Brien, 2013). Doulas and other support persons may enhance the childbirth process (ACOG, 2019a; AWHONN, 2018a). See Chapter 16 for a more detailed discussion of labor support.

Families should be free to take pictures and make video and/or audio recordings during labor and birth. Policies restricting cameras are in conflict with the philosophy that the birth experience should be what the woman and her family desire within reason. There is no evidence that videos of labor and birth later produced as part of a legal claim increase liability. Videos or pictures showing that the perinatal team provided excellent care in a challenging situation could prove to be beneficial to a situation known to suffer from hindsight bias. Concerns about safety, liability, privacy, and space limitations can be adequately addressed without restrictive policies about visitors and pictures/videos during labor and birth if care providers are committed to meeting the needs of childbearing women and their support persons.

Supporting Maternal and Family Attachment

At birth, skin-to-skin contact between mother and baby has many positive benefits. Although babies were traditionally separated from their mothers immediately after birth for assessment and temperature stabilization and regulation by placing babies in warmers in the delivery room, this practice is not necessary for newborn well-being. Immediate skin-to-skin contact with the baby on the mother's chest after birth and continued contact during the first few days of life can promote normal temperature stabilization and regulation in the newborn and can decrease the risk of neonatal hypothermia and hypoglycemia.

While some may perceive challenges in providing skin-to-skin contact between the mother and baby immediately after cesarean birth, it can be accomplished by collaboration of the perinatal team including nurses, obstetrics, pediatricians, and anesthesia providers (Fig. 14–16) (Hung & Berg, 2011). The baby nurse in the surgical suite should remain immediately next to the mother while she is holding the newborn, and maintain direct observation of mother and baby to promote their safety. Healthy babies should be placed on their mother and remain in direct skin-to-skin contact with their mothers immediately after birth until the first feeding is accomplished (AAP & ACOG, 2017; AWHONN, 2016). The alert, healthy newborn infant is capable of latching on to a breast without specific assistance within the first hour after birth. The baby should be dried, Apgar scores assigned, and initial physical assessment performed while the baby is with the mother (AAP & ACOG, 2017; AWHONN, 2016). The mother is an optimal heat source for the infant (Fig. 14–17). Weighing, measuring, bathing, needle-sticks, and eye prophylaxis can be delayed until after the first feeding is completed (AAP & ACOG, 2017). Babies affected by maternal medications may require assistance for effective latch on. Except under unusual circumstances, the newborn should remain with the mother throughout the recovery period (AAP & ACOG, 2017). Immediate skin-to-skin contact after birth has considerable benefits because it requires minimal financial resources, is not associated with adverse effects among healthy babies, shows an overall positive effect on breastfeeding, and appears to improve newborn stabilization during transition (Hung & Berg, 2011). See Chapter 17 for more details on skin-to-skin contact during the immediate postpartum period.

Women's expectations and desires regarding who will be present at the birth vary widely. Some women prefer that their partner be the sole participant, while others choose to have more family members and friends share this important event. The desires of the woman should guide this process rather than arbitrarily determined visitor policies. As long as space permits and the safety of the mother and baby are not a consideration, the woman should be able to have as many family members and support persons as she requests. Every effort should be made to have the woman's partner next to her as she is giving birth and to be able to see and touch the baby immediately after birth. If newborn resuscitation is required, encourage the partner to be close to the baby as soon as possible. As the baby's condition is stabilized, encourage the woman and her partner to hold and examine their baby.

Sibling presence during labor and birth also presents a unique opportunity for nurses to promote

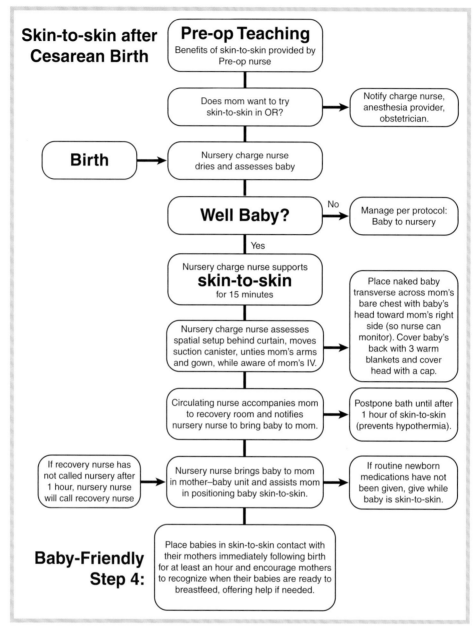

FIGURE 14–16. Protocol for providing skin-to-skin contact in the surgical suite during cesarean birth. (Adapted from Hung, K. J., & Berg, O. [2011]. Early skin-to-skin after cesarean to improve breastfeeding. *MCN: The American Journal of Maternal Child Nursing, 36*[5], 318–324. doi:10.1097/NMC.0b013e3182266314)

family attachment. Sibling classes to prepare children for the birth experience are sometimes offered by hospitals to facilitate a positive experience. Children need to be aware of potential maternal behavior and sounds in labor, and reassurance that pain experienced by the mother is temporary. Each child needs a support person to accompany the child and to be familiar with the child's developmental level so that both the child's curiosity and concerns for his or her mother and new brother or sister are answered.

As the family is introduced to their newborn immediately at birth, an explanation of umbilical cord clamping/cutting and inspection of the placenta help

the family understand the final physiologic separation of the newborn from the mother's life-support system. During skin-to-skin contact, allow the family, support persons, and siblings to be close to the mother to see and touch the baby. After stabilization, if the baby has been wrapped, the nurse can unwrap the newborn and describe normal physical characteristics. Siblings can count fingers and toes. Encouraging interaction with the newborn sets the stage for successful attachment and integration into the family unit. All family members can hold the newborn after birth as desired, and opportunities for photographs and videos should be provided.

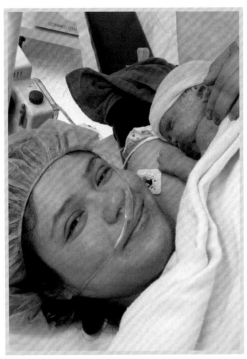

FIGURE 14–17. Skin-to-skin contact of mother and baby in the surgical suite during cesarean birth. (From Hung, K. J., & Berg, O. [2011]. Early skin-to-skin after cesarean to improve breastfeeding. *MCN: The American Journal of Maternal Child Nursing, 36*[5], 318–324. doi:10.1097 /NMC.0b013e3182266314)

CLINICAL INTERVENTIONS FOR WOMEN IN LABOR

The majority of pregnancies, labors, and births are normal, requiring little or no intervention. However, some women require clinical interventions to optimize outcomes in pregnancies with identified maternal or fetal risk factors. Risk status for the woman and fetus may increase at any time during the pregnancy, labor and birth, or the postpartum period (AAP & ACOG, 2017). Nurses in perinatal settings must be able to quickly assess and identify changes in maternal–fetal status and adjust nursing care accordingly. For example, nursing management during labor may require intrauterine resuscitation techniques when an indeterminate or abnormal FHR is noted, or plans for vaginal birth may be quickly changed when an emergent cesarean birth becomes the safest option for the mother and baby. Knowledge of appropriate nursing interventions for common maternal–fetal complications during labor is essential. The nurse must also be aware of changes in maternal–fetal status requiring physician or CNM notification and those requiring bedside evaluation by the physician or CNM. The next section focuses on the clinical interventions of cervical ripening, labor induction and augmentation, operative vaginal birth, and amnioinfusion. Implications for nursing care are presented with key points for assessment and intervention.

Cervical Ripening and Induction and Augmentation of Labor

Definition of Terms

Cervical ripening is the process of effecting physical softening and distensibility of the cervix in preparation for labor and birth. Cervical ripening can occur naturally or by use of mechanical or pharmacologic methods. *Induction of labor* is the stimulation of uterine contractions to initiate labor. Examples of methods include, but are not limited to, artificial rupture of membranes, balloons, oxytocin, prostaglandin, laminaria, or other cervical ripening agents (ACOG, 2014b). *Augmentation of labor* is the stimulation of uterine contractions using pharmacologic methods or artificial rupture of membranes to increase their frequency and/or strength following the onset of spontaneous labor or contractions following spontaneous rupture of membranes (ACOG, 2014b). *Tachysystole* is excessive uterine activity, which can be either spontaneous or induced. Tachysystole is defined as more than five contractions in 10 minutes (averaged over 30 minutes) by the National Institute of Child Health and Human Development (NICHD) expert group on EFM that met in 2008 (Macones, Hankins, Spong, Hauth, & Moore, 2008).

Incidence

According to the National Center for Health Statistics (Martin, Hamilton, Osterman, Driscoll, & Drake, 2018), in 2017 (the most recent year for which natality data on induction are available), the rate of induction of labor in the United States was approximately 25.7% of all births. Data on augmentation are usually similar to the induction rate (Menacker & Martin, 2008); thus, based on reported data, approximately one half of women laboring in the United States receive labor stimulation. The 2017 induction rate is 170% higher than the rate in 1990 (9.5%). The latest natality data can be accessed at http://www.cdc.gov/nchs/births.htm. Most clinicians would note that these data seem low when compared to actual clinical practice. The induction rate is calculated based on all women who give birth. If women who had a planned or repeat cesarean birth are excluded from the denominator and the figures are calculated based on all others who potentially could have had labor induction, the reported rate of induction would be significantly higher. It is likely that data on induction and augmentation are significantly underreported on birth certificates.

Indications

According to AAP and ACOG (2017) and ACOG (2009a), induction of labor has merit as a therapeutic option when the benefits of expeditious birth outweigh the risks of continuing the pregnancy. Therefore, benefits of labor induction must be weighed against the associated potential maternal and fetal risks (ACOG, 2009a). The various opinions among providers and patients about the exact nature and intensity of some risks and benefits are reflected in clinical practice. Multiple factors influence the decision to induce labor. Not all of the indications are clinical; some are primarily based on convenience (Simpson, 2010). Display 14–6 lists commonly cited convenience issues related to elective induction of labor. Figures 14–18 and 14–19 illustrate differences in birth time when labor and births are scheduled rather than occur spontaneously (Matthews & Curtin, 2015). The data in Figure 14–18 demonstrate timing of birth based on the hour and day of birth. Peak periods artificially occur Monday to Friday before office hours and during lunch breaks. Fewer births occur between 8 pm and 7 am when compared to the rest of the day. The data in Figure 14–19 show the distribution of births by hour of the day based on whether the birth was a cesarean, induced vaginal birth, or vaginal birth via spontaneous labor. Peaks in birth time are noted for cesarean birth and induced vaginal birth, while birth via spontaneous labor occurs generally evenly over the course of the day.

DISPLAY 14–6

Commonly Cited Convenience Issues for Patients, Physicians, and Institutions Related to Elective Induction of Labor

Patients

Timing of birth to coincide with personal schedules; availability of partners, support persons, and family; babysitting issues

Desire for preferred midwife or physician to attend the birth rather than a partner in the group practice

Wish to "get the pregnancy over with"

Relief from pregnancy discomforts; feeling "miserable"

Avoidance of certain dates such as holidays, preference for certain dates with personal meaning

Physicians

Quality-of-life issues (labor and birth occurs during a weekday, during the day shift, while on call; avoidance of interruptions of office hours, weekends, and evenings; ability to schedule more than one patient on the same day)

Patient satisfaction

Liability concerns

Desire to attend birth of primary patient for reimbursement issues or per patient request

Institutions

Ability to plan for scheduling and staffing

Patient satisfaction

Provider satisfaction

Market share issues

Display 14–7 lists criteria, indications, and contraindications for cervical ripening and induction of labor based on recommendations from ACOG (2009a). For recommendations from the NICHD expert group (Spong et al., 2011) on timing of birth when conditions complicate pregnancy at or after 34 weeks of gestation, see Table 7–1 in Chapter 7 Preterm Labor and Birth. These publications can be used to guide unit policy on elective births.

According to ACOG (2009a), labor may be induced for logistic reasons, such as a history of rapid labor, distance from the hospital, or "psychosocial indications." The interpretation of psychosocial indications varies widely among providers and is most commonly noted for an elective (i.e., nonmedical indication) induction of labor. When labor is induced for logistic reasons or psychosocial indications, the pregnant woman should be at least 39 completed weeks of gestation to avoid the risk of iatrogenic prematurity (ACOG, 2009a; AWHONN, 2019a). Use of checklists for labor induction and planned cesarean birth (ACOG, 2011a, 2011b) can be helpful in ensuring that the appropriate gestational age has been confirmed.

Risk–Benefit Analysis and Informed Consent

Labor induction is not an isolated intervention. The decision for labor induction often results in a cascade of other interventions and activities that have the potential to negatively affect the childbirth process. Labor induction in the United States leads to an IV line, bed rest, and continuous EFM, and often amniotomy, significant discomfort, epidural analgesia/anesthesia, and a prolonged stay on the labor unit, and cesarean birth. Nulliparous women should be informed that electively induced labor may last significantly longer than spontaneous labor (ACOG, 2009a).

Avoiding associated complications can be accomplished by allowing labor to begin on its own when the mother and baby are healthy (AWHONN, 2012). Women can be encouraged by nurses to await spontaneous labor by providing education regarding potential risks of elective induction during prepared childbirth classes and prenatal encounters during the third trimester (AWHONN, 2012, 2019a; Simpson, Newman, & Chirino, 2010a, 2010b). Although there is some concern that requests by pregnant women to have their labor induced electively are a major reason for the steady increase in elective induction in the United States, in a study of over 3,300 nulliparous women, 70% were offered the option of elective induction by their obstetrician; this discussion occurred in most cases before the estimated date of birth (Simpson et al., 2010a). It is possible that women perceive the offer of elective induction by their obstetrician as a recommendation. In this study, women who were offered the option of elective induction by their obstetrician

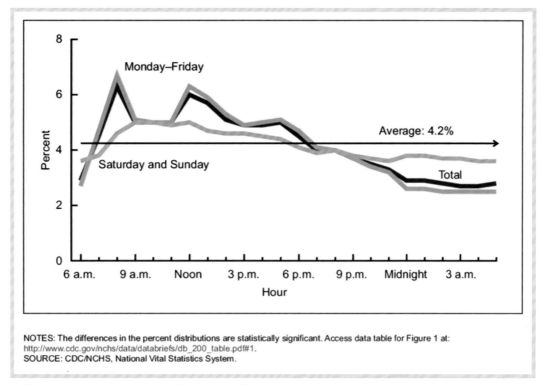

NOTES: The differences in the percent distributions are statistically significant. Access data table for Figure 1 at: http://www.cdc.gov/nchs/data/databriefs/db_200_table.pdf#1.
SOURCE: CDC/NCHS, National Vital Statistics System.

FIGURE 14–18. Percent distribution of births, by hour and day of the week of delivery: 41 states and the District of Columbia, 2013. (From Mathews, T. J., & Curtin, S. C. [2015]. *When are babies born: Morning, noon, or night? Birth certificate data for 2013* [NCHS Data Brief No. 200]. Hyattsville, MD: National Center for Health Statistics.)

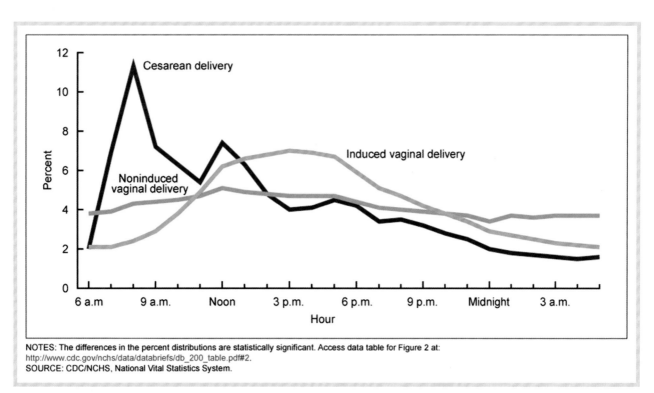

NOTES: The differences in the percent distributions are statistically significant. Access data table for Figure 2 at: http://www.cdc.gov/nchs/data/databriefs/db_200_table.pdf#2.
SOURCE: CDC/NCHS, National Vital Statistics System.

FIGURE 14–19. Percent distribution of births, by hour and method of delivery and induction status: 41 states and the District of Columbia, 2013. (From Mathews, T. J., & Curtin, S. C. [2015]. *When are babies born: Morning, noon, or night? Birth certificate data for 2013* [NCHS Data Brief No. 200]. Hyattsville, MD: National Center for Health Statistics.)

DISPLAY 14-7

Criteria, Indications, and Contraindications for Cervical Ripening, Labor Induction, and Labor Augmentation

Criteria for Cervical Ripening and Induction of Labor

Generally, induction of labor has merit as a therapeutic option when the benefits of expeditious delivery outweigh the risks of continuing the pregnancy. The benefits of labor induction need to be weighed against the potential maternal and fetal risks associated with this procedure. Before 41 0/7 weeks of gestation, induction of labor generally should be performed based on maternal and fetal medical indications. Inductions at 41 0/7 weeks of gestation and beyond should be performed to reduce the risk of cesarean birth and the risk of perinatal morbidity and mortality.

- Gestational age, cervical status, pelvic adequacy, fetal size, and fetal presentation should be assessed.
- Any potential risks to the mother and fetus should be considered.
- The medical record should document that a discussion was held between the pregnant woman and her healthcare provider about the indications; the agents and methods of labor induction, including the risks, benefits, and alternative approaches; and the possible need for repeat induction or cesarean birth.
- Cervical ripening and induction agents should be administered by trained personnel familiar with the effects on mother and fetus.
- Prostaglandin preparations should be administered where uterine activity and fetal heart rate (FHR) can be monitored continuously for an initial observation period. FHR monitoring should be continued if regular uterine contractions persist.
- FHR and uterine contractions should be monitored closely during induction and augmentation as for any high-risk patient in active labor.
- A physician capable of performing a cesarean birth should be readily available.
- For women undergoing trial of labor after a cesarean, induction of labor for maternal or fetal indications remains an option.
- Misoprostol should not be used for third trimester cervical ripening or labor induction in women who have had a cesarean birth or major uterine surgery.

Indications for Cervical Ripening and Induction of Labor

Indications for the induction of labor are not absolute but should consider maternal and fetal conditions, gestational age, cervical status, and other factors. Following are examples of maternal or fetal conditions that may be indications for the induction of labor:

- Abruptio placentae
- Chorioamnionitis (intraamniotic infection)
- Fetal demise
- Gestational hypertension
- Preeclampsia, eclampsia
- Premature rupture of membranes
- Postterm pregnancy
- Maternal medical conditions (e.g., diabetes mellitus, renal disease, chronic pulmonary disease, chronic hypertension, or antiphospholipid syndrome)
- Fetal compromise (e.g., severe fetal growth restriction, isoimmunization, oligohydramnios)

Labor may also be induced for logistic reasons (e.g., risk of rapid labor, distance from the hospital, or psychosocial indications). In such circumstances, at least one of the following criteria should be met or fetal lung maturity should be established:

- Ultrasound measurement at less than 20 weeks of gestation supports gestational age of 39 weeks or greater.
- Fetal heart tones have been documented as present for 30 weeks by Doppler ultrasonography.
- It has been 36 weeks since a positive serum or urine human chorionic gonadotropin pregnancy test result.
- Testing for fetal lung maturity should not be performed, and is contraindicated, when delivery is mandated for fetal or maternal indications. Conversely, a mature fetal lung maturity test result before 39 weeks of gestation, in the absence of appropriate clinical circumstances, is not an indication for elective labor induction.

Contraindication to Induction of Labor

Generally, the contraindications for labor induction are the same as those for spontaneous labor and vaginal birth. They include, but are not limited to, the following:

- Vasa previa or complete placenta previa
- Transverse fetal lie
- Umbilical cord prolapse
- Previous classical cesarean birth
- Active genital herpes infection
- Previous myomectomy entering the endometrial cavity

American Academy of Pediatrics & American College of Obstetricians and Gynecologists. (2017). *Guidelines for perinatal care* (8th ed.). Elk Grove Village, IL: American Academy of Pediatrics; American College of Obstetric and Gynecology. (2009a). *Induction of labor* (Practice Bulletin No. 107; Reaffirmed, 2019). Washington, DC: Author; American College of Obstetricians and Gynecologists & Society for Maternal-Fetal Medicine. (2014). Safe prevention of the primary cesarean delivery (Obstetric Care Consensus No. 1). Obstetrics & Gynecology, *123*(3), 693–711. doi:10.1097/01.AOG.0000444441.04111.1d

were significantly more likely to have an elective induction. However, the education did have a positive effect as 63% of women who chose not to have an elective induction indicated that information about the risks of the procedures presented in prepared childbirth classes was a factor in their choice (Simpson et al., 2010a).

Because of known risks, a risk–benefit analysis is recommended before the procedure as well as a discussion by the provider with the patient of the agents, methods, advantages, disadvantages, and alternative approaches, including the risk of cesarean birth and a repeat induction (ACOG, 2009a; National Quality Forum, 2018). Following this discussion, when the woman has enough information to participate in the decision-making process, the provider should obtain informed consent. The medical record should contain documentation that this discussion occurred and that the woman consented to proceed (AAP & ACOG, 2017; ACOG, 2009a; AWHONN, 2019a). It is not the nurse's responsibility to provide the required information to the woman undergoing induction or to obtain informed consent; however, advocating for the woman and fetus includes ensuring that the woman has been fully informed by her primary healthcare provider before beginning the procedure.

The Nurse's Role

The primary role of the labor nurse during cervical ripening, labor induction, or labor augmentation is ongoing maternal and fetal assessment to support safe care. The goal is labor progression without excessive uterine activity or fetal compromise. The nurse providing care for the woman during cervical ripening and induction of labor must be aware of appropriate indications for the use of each mechanical method and pharmacologic agent as well as their actions, expected results, and potential risks. Before any cervical ripening or labor induction agent is used, maternal status and fetal well-being should be established, and cervical status should be assessed and documented in the medical record. Nurses can evaluate cervical status by vaginal examination prior to the induction process. Cervical ripening, labor induction, and labor augmentation are processes that require care by several members of the perinatal team working together to promote patient well-being and successful vaginal birth. Indications for preinduction cervical ripening and induction of labor also should be documented by the provider. Ongoing maternal–fetal assessments during cervical ripening, labor induction, and labor augmentation are presented in Display 14–3. During oxytocin induction or augmentation, FHR monitoring should be as per high-risk patients (AAP & ACOG, 2017) and therefore via continuous EFM. The FHR should be evaluated every 15 minutes during the first stage of labor and every 5 minutes during the active pushing phase of the second stage of labor (AAP & ACOG, 2017; ACOG, 2009b; AWHONN, 2018b, 2019b). Uterine activity is generally assessed at the same frequency as FHR. The absence of fetal well-being necessitates direct bedside evaluation by a physician or CNM, interdisciplinary discussion, and written documentation of further clinical management plans.

Clinical Protocol and Unit Policy Development

Healthcare providers at each institution should develop a policy or protocol for cervical ripening, labor induction, and labor augmentation (AAP & ACOG, 2017; ACOG, 2009a; Simpson, 2020). Suggestions for key concepts to be included are presented in Display 14–8.

Ideally, physicians, CNMs, and nurses together develop these policies or protocols on the basis of current evidence and published guidelines from professional organizations such as ACOG, AAP, AWHONN, and ACNM. The best approach is to develop a single unit policy or protocol rather than allowing each provider to have his or her own protocol with individual variations. For example, the group should come to consensus on the IV concentrations, rate of dosage increases, and interval between increases in dosage rate on the basis of available evidence and published guidelines. There should be established processes in place for addressing and preventing elective induction before 39 weeks' gestation. Once the interdisciplinary team agrees on a policy or protocol, it should be expected that all providers will practice within the established unit parameters. Standardization of an oxytocin policy for induction and augmentation of labor among hospitals within a healthcare system can be beneficial in promoting patient safety by selecting appropriate candidates and avoiding tachysystole (Jackson, Wickstrom, & Anderson, 2019; Krening, Rehling-Anthony, & Garko, 2012; O'Rourke et al., 2011; Simpson, Knox, Martin, George, & Watson, 2011; Sundin, Mazac, Ellis, & Garbo, 2018). A systematic review of the potential benefits of establishing an elective induction policy found that their implementation resulted in lower rates of labor induction, cesarean birth, operative/instrumental vaginal births, and maternal/neonatal morbidity in part because women spontaneously gave birth before the scheduled elective induction date after policies were implemented, thereby resulting in lower rates of elective labor induction (Akinsipe, Villalobos, & Ridley, 2012). Each unit should develop processes to periodically evaluate the incidence of oxytocin-induced tachysystole and how the team responds to this clinical situation.

Resource Allocation Considerations for Cervical Ripening and Induction of Labor

The number of women who are scheduled for cervical ripening and induction of labor influences nursing staff requirements for labor and birth units. Because inductions of labor are likely to occur during the day, more nurses may be needed during this time than during the late evening or early morning. A record maintained on the unit of women who are scheduled for labor induction is essential to plan nurse staffing and ancillary personnel needs based on expected volume. Many units place a limit on the number of scheduled labor inductions that can be performed on any given day to ensure that adequate nurses and rooms are available to provide the appropriate level of care. Patient safety is at risk when scheduled procedures such as elective

DISPLAY 14-8

Suggestions for Key Concepts to Include in Clinical Protocols and Unit Policies for Cervical Ripening, Labor Induction, and Labor Augmentation

Prioritization and Documentation

- Criteria for designating patient priority for cervical ripening and induction based on the nature and intensity of the indication that can be used as a framework for decision making during periods of limited staffing, rooms, or other resources
- Documentation of indication by primary care provider
- Documentation of risk–benefit analysis discussion with the pregnant woman by the primary healthcare provider and informed decision-making process
- Specific recommendations for the care of women with a prior history of cesarean birth or uterine scar

Staffing Considerations

- Experience of registered nurse
- Availability of registered nurses to meet recommended nurse-to-patient ratios (one nurse to two women undergoing cervical ripening with pharmacologic agents; one nurse to one woman undergoing labor induction or augmentation with oxytocin)
- Acuity of patient (e.g., medical or obstetric complications)
- Ongoing evaluation of labor status
- Availability and skill level of support personnel
- Contingency plans such as on-call list

Patient Assessment

- Establishment of maternal and fetal well-being
- Establishment of at least 39 completed weeks of gestation if procedure is being performed without a medical indication

- Documentation of cervical status, including Bishop score
- Documentation of pelvic examination
- Method of fetal assessment
- Frequency of maternal–fetal assessments
- Assessment of specific patient needs and requests

Methods and Dosages

- Cervical ripening agents to be used
- Initial oxytocin or misoprostol dosage
- Intervals and amounts for oxytocin dosage increases
- Intervals and amounts for misoprostol dosages
- Orders for oxytocin and documentation in milliunits per minute
- Titration of oxytocin dosage based on progress of labor and maternal–fetal response
- Dosage of misoprostol based on progress of labor and maternal–fetal status
- Maintenance or decrease in oxytocin dosage if labor is progressing

Complications

- Definition of tachysystole
- Interventions for tachysystole
- Interventions for indeterminate or abnormal fetal status
- Criteria for CNM or physician notification
- Criteria for bedside evaluation by the CNM or physician

Unit Policy

- Algorithm/chain of consultation for addressing clinical disagreements
- Methods for documenting all of the key concepts and interventions outlined in the policy/protocol
- An expectation that the policy will be followed by all members of the healthcare team

---

labor induction and cesarean birth are clustered on one or two weekdays for provider convenience without concurrent changes in nurse staffing. This is especially a potential problem in small-volume units where there may not be enough nurses to safely handle these artificial peaks in census on busy days and not enough volume on other days to earn productive nursing hours required by the budget while maintaining at least two nurses with obstetric skills in-house at all times.

The development of criteria for designating patient priority for inductions of labor based on the nature and intensity of the indication can provide a useful decision-making framework when conflicts arise. Ideally, these criteria are developed jointly by physician, CNM, and nurse members of a unit practice committee. Requiring documentation of indications and having these data available on the unit may be helpful in designating patient priority when resources are limited. Elective inductions of labor may need to be postponed or rescheduled at times, especially if there are not enough resources available.

The establishment of a perinatal nurse on-call system may facilitate securing staffing resources as needed in a timely manner.

The appropriate number of qualified professional registered nurses should be in attendance during cervical ripening and induction or augmentation of labor (AWHONN, 2010). Current recommendations for the nurse-to-woman ratio for women undergoing cervical ripening with pharmacologic agents is 1 to 2 (AWHONN, 2010). Current recommendations for the nurse-to-woman ratio during induction or augmentation of labor with oxytocin is 1 to 1 (AAP & ACOG, 2017; AWHONN, 2010, 2019a; Society of Obstetricians and Gynaecologists of Canada [SOGC], 2001). If a nurse cannot clinically evaluate the effects of the medication at least every 15 minutes or a physician who has privileges to perform a cesarean birth is not readily available, oxytocin should not be initiated or if infusing, the oxytocin infusion should be discontinued, until this level of maternal–fetal nursing care can be provided (AAP & ACOG, 2017; Simpson, 2020).

TABLE 14–3. Bishop Score for Assessing Readiness for Induction

Factor	Assigned value			
	0	1	2	3
Cervical dilation	0	1 to 2 cm	3 to 4 cm	5 cm or more
Cervical effacement	0% to 30%	40% to 50%	60% to 70%	80% or more
Fetal station	−3	−2	−1, 0	+1, +2
Cervical consistency	Firm	Moderate	Soft	
Cervical position	Posterior	Midposition	Anterior	

From Bishop, E. H. (1964). Pelvic scoring for elective induction. *Obstetrics & Gynecology, 24,* 266.

Cervical Status

Cervical assessment includes documentation of the Bishop score (Bishop, 1964) and the presence or absence of uterine activity. Cervical status is the most important factor predicting the success of an induction of labor. It is assessed most commonly by using the Bishop pelvic scoring system (Bishop, 1964) (Table 14–3). Perinatal nurses are qualified to assess and document cervical status based on the Bishop score. A score of 6 or less is associated with a higher probability of failed induction (ACOG, 2009a). If the total score is more than 8, the probability of vaginal birth following an induction of labor is similar to that of spontaneous labor (ACOG, 2009a). Despite efforts by many researchers to modify the Bishop score, it remains the most reliable and cost-effective method of predicting the likelihood of successful induction. The risk of cesarean birth after labor induction is inversely related to the Bishop score; a higher rate of cesarean birth is consistently observed in women with a lower Bishop score when compared to women with a more favorable cervix (Caughey et al., 2009). The factor with the strongest association with successful induction seems to be cervical dilation; however, all components collectively can be quite useful in selecting appropriate candidates for labor induction. Other factors that have been shown to influence successful labor inductions are maternal age, parity, weight, and height. Younger women, women who are normal weight, women who are tall, and women who are multiparous are more likely to have success with labor induction (Caughey et al., 2009; Crane, 2006). Display 14–9 provides information about mechanical methods of cervical ripening and labor induction. Table 14–4 provides information about pharmacologic methods of cervical ripening and induction of labor and augmentation of labor.

Cervical Ripening

Cervical ripening is a complex process that results in physical softening and distensibility of the cervix, eventually leading to beginning cervical effacement and dilation. Cervical ripening agents facilitate the process of cervical softening, thinning, and dilating and can result in reduction in the rate of failed induction and induction-to-birth time (AAP & ACOG, 2017). A number of mechanical and pharmacologic methods have been used to induce cervical ripening (Penfield & Wing, 2017). Effective methods include mechanical cervical dilators and administration of synthetic prostaglandin E_1 (PGE_1) and PGE_2 (AAP & ACOG, 2017). Mechanical methods are less likely to result in tachysystole and have similar rates of success when compared to pharmacologic agents for cervical ripening (Cromi et al., 2012; Fox et al., 2011; Jozwiak et al., 2012). Based on the most recent Cochrane Review, when compared with oxytocin, mechanical methods for labor induction have less risk of cesarean birth (Jozwiak et al., 2012).

Pharmacologic Methods of Cervical Ripening

Various hormonal preparations are available to induce cervical ripening. These agents include PGE_1 such as misoprostol (Cytotec) and PGE_2 preparations such as the dinoprostone (Cervidil insert). Cervidil and misoprostol are approved by the U.S. Food and Drug Administration (FDA) for cervical ripening. Nurses caring for women receiving any of these agents should be aware that they may lead to the onset of labor, particularly if the cervix is favorable. When the cervix is unfavorable, cervical softening and thinning are more likely to occur.

Prostaglandin E_2. Dinoprostone (PGE_2) is one of the most frequently prescribed medications for cervical ripening. The mechanism of action is similar to the natural ripening process, and women often go into spontaneous labor following administration. The prostaglandin preparations used successfully for cervical ripening today produce the desired cervical changes, but all tend to increase myometrial contractility. For this reason, prostaglandins for cervical ripening must be viewed as the first step in labor induction. Dinoprostone induces cervical ripening by directly softening the cervix, relaxing the cervical smooth muscle, and producing uterine contractions. Dinoprostone preparations appear to be as efficacious as other methods of cervical ripening.

DISPLAY 14-9
Mechanical Methods of Cervical Ripening and Labor Induction

Membrane Stripping

- Digital separation of the chorioamniotic membrane from the wall of the cervix and lower uterine segment by inserting the examiner's gloved finger beyond the internal cervical os and then rotating the finger 360 degrees along the lower uterine segment
- Typically performed during an office visit for a pregnant woman ≥39 weeks of gestation with a partially dilated cervix who wants to hasten the onset of spontaneous labor
- Routine membrane stripping is not recommended given no evidence of improved maternal and neonatal outcome.
- The woman should call her certified nurse midwife (CNM)/physician or come to the hospital if the membranes rupture, bleeding occurs, fetal activity decreases, fever develops, regular contractions begin, or discomfort persists between uterine contractions.

Amniotomy

- For women with normally progressing labor and no evidence of fetal compromise, routine amniotomy is not necessary unless required to facilitate monitoring
- Artificial rupture of membranes involves the perforation of the chorioamniotic membranes with a plastic hook performed by a qualified physician or CNM.
- Typically requires cervical dilation of at least 2–3 cm
- Effective method of labor induction for multiparous women with favorable cervices
- Essential to confirm that the fetal vertex, not the umbilical cord or other fetal part, is presenting and well applied to the cervix
- Artificial rupture of membranes should only be performed when the fetal vertex is well applied to the cervix.
- Risks include the possibility of umbilical cord prolapse, cesarean birth, variable decelerations, intraamniotic infection, fetal injury, bleeding from an undiagnosed vasa previa, and commitment to labor with an uncertain outcome.
- Early amniotomy is contraindicated when maternal infection, such as HIV, an active perineal herpes simplex viral infection, and possibly viral hepatitis, is present.
- Medical record documentation should include the indication for amniotomy; amount, color, and odor of amniotic fluid; fetal heart rate characteristics before amniotomy; fetal response following the procedure; cervical status; and fetal station.

Transcervical Balloon Catheters

- A deflated Foley catheter, #16 to 18 French with a 30-mL balloon, is inserted into the extra-amniotic space and then inflated above internal os with 30 to 60 mL of sterile water.
- The inflated balloon is then retracted to rest against the internal os.
- Appears to be effective for preinduction cervical ripening by causing direct pressure and overstretching of the lower uterine segment and cervix as well as local prostaglandin release
- Balloon catheter usually falls out when cervical dilation occurs.
- A double-balloon device specifically designed for cervical ripening can be used.
- Extra-amniotic saline infusion (e.g., continuous infusion of isotonic fluid into the extra-amniotic space at rates of 30 to 40 mL/hr) can be used, although this technique has not been found to improve induction outcomes when compared to balloon catheter alone.
- Remove the catheter after 24 hours if it has not fallen out on its own.
- Minimal risk of infection with use

Hygroscopic/Osmotic Dilators

- Natural: laminaria tents (made from cold water seaweed)
- Synthetic product: *Dilapan-S*
- Absorb fluid from cervical tissue
- Allow for controlled dilation by mechanical pressure and prostaglandin release
- Used primarily during pregnancy termination rather than for cervical ripening in term pregnancies
- Synthetic dilators are more expensive than laminaria; however, they work more quickly.
- Insertion of a large number of small diameter laminaria (2 or 3 mm) preferable to using a few larger ones (6 mm)
- Progressively placed until the cervix is "full"
- The "tails" are allowed to fall into the vagina for ease of identification and removal.
- Laminaria are kept in place with a couple 4 × 4 gauze sponges tucked into the fornix.
- The number of laminaria inserted is documented in medical record.

Advantages of mechanical methods of cervical ripening include low risk of tachysystole, few maternal systemic side effects, low cost, and convenient storage.

Disadvantages of mechanical methods include some maternal discomfort, small increase risk of maternal and neonatal infection, and potential disruption of a low-lying placenta.

Cervidil. The Cervidil vaginal insert is a thin, flat, rectangular-shaped, cross-linked polymer hydrogel that releases dinoprostone from a 10-mg reservoir at a controlled rate of approximately 0.3 mg/hr in vivo (Ferring Pharmaceuticals, 2017). The reservoir chip is encased within a pouch of knitted polyester with a removal cord. The entire system comes preassembled and prepackaged in sterile foil packets.

Cervidil may be inserted by the perinatal nurse when the nurse has demonstrated competence in insertion and the activity is within the scope of practice as defined by state and provincial regulations. Institutional guidelines should be established for the nurse's role related to the use of Cervidil. The insert is placed into the posterior fornix of the vagina, with its long axis transverse to the long axis of the vagina. The ribbon end of the retrieval system may be allowed to extrude distally from the vagina or tucked into the vagina. Once placed, Cervidil absorbs moisture, swells, and releases dinoprostone at a controlled rate. The system makes Cervidil relatively simple to insert and requires only a single digital examination.

TABLE 14–4. Pharmacologic Agents Used for Cervical Ripening/Labor Induction and Augmentation

Factor	Pitocin (oxytocin)	Cervidil (dinoprostone)	Cytotec (misoprostol)
Storage and preparation	Room temperature storage Available in 20-unit ampules Several variations in the dilution rate exist. Some protocols suggest adding 10 units of oxytocin to 1,000 mL of an isotonic electrolyte IV solution, resulting in an infusion dosage rate of 1 mU/min = 6 mL/hr. Other commonly reported dilutions are 20 units of oxytocin to 1,000 mL IV fluid (1 mU/min = 3 mL/hr) and 30 units of oxytocin to 500 mL of IV fluid or 60 units of oxytocin to 1,000 mL IV fluid (1 mU/min = 1 mL/hr). One advantage to using 30 units in 500 mL IV fluid or 60 units in 1,000 mL IV fluid is that they result in a 1:1 solution (1 mU/min = 1 mL/hr); therefore, no calculations are needed. The key issue is consistency in practice within each institution.	Keep frozen (−20°C) until immediately before use. No warming required.	Available in 100 and 200 mcg tablets 100-mcg tablet is not scored; dose should be prepared (cut in four equal pieces) by hospital pharmacy.
Initial administration	Administered IV in an isotonic electrolyte solution, piggybacked into the main IV line at port most proximal to venous site Start at 1 to 2 mU/min.	10-mg dinoprostone in a controlled-release vaginal insert with removable cord	25 mcg (one-fourth tablet) placed in the posterior vaginal fornix should be considered for the initial dose. Adverse effects can be minimized by using the lowest dose (25 mcg) no more than every 3 to 6 hr. Oral administration at equivalent doses to vaginal route is not as efficacious; generally, the dose should not exceed 50 mcg.
Patient considerations	Bedrest is not required during infusion. EFM telemetry can be used during ambulation or sitting on a chair or birthing ball. Careful close monitoring for women with history of prior cesarean birth or uterine scar; use lowest dose possible to achieve labor progress.	Contraindicated in women with history of prior cesarean birth or uterine scar Supine positioning with a lateral tilt for 2 hr following insertion Continuous monitoring of FHR and uterine activity is indicated while insert is in place. Ambulation is an option if continuous EFM telemetry is available.	Contraindicated in women with history of prior cesarean birth or uterine scar Baseline uterine activity is a relative contraindication to the use of prostaglandins because the addition of an exogenous uterotonic agent could lead to excessive uterine activity. Continuous monitoring of FHR and uterine activity is indicated for 4 hr after intravaginal dose and 2 hr after oral dose.
Effects	Wide variations in time from initial dose to uterine activity. The biologic half-life is approximately 10 to 12 min. Three to four half-lives are need to reach physiologic steady state (30 to 60 min) at which time full effect of dosage on the uterine response can be assessed.	Uterine contractions usually occur within 5 to 7 hr.	Wide variations exist in time of onset of uterine contractions. Peak action is approximately 1 to 2 hr when administered intravaginally but can be up to 4 to 6 hr for some women. Peak action is approximately 30 min when administered orally; half-life is 90 min.

(continued)

TABLE 14–4. Pharmacologic Agents Used for Cervical Ripening/Labor Induction and Augmentation (Continued)

Factor	Pitocin (oxytocin)	Cervidil (dinoprostone)	Cytotec (misoprostol)
Adjusting dosage	Advance by 1 to 2 mU/min at intervals no less than every 30 to 60 min until adequate labor progress is achieved. Titrate dose to maternal–fetal response to labor. Use lowest dose possible to achieve adequate progress of labor (progressive cervical effacement and cervical dilation of approximately 0.5 to 1.0 cm/hr once active labor has been achieved expectation for labor progress is based on maternal parity). Reevaluate clinical situation if oxytocin dosage rate reaches 20 mU/min. Contractions should not be more frequent than every 2 min. Avoid tachysystole. When uterine tachysystole occurs with a normal (category I) FHR tracing, reposition mother and consider an IV fluid bolus. If these interventions do not resolve tachysystole, decrease dose of oxytocin. When tachysystole occurs with either an indeterminate or abnormal (category II or III) FHR tracing, decrease or stop oxytocin and initiate intrauterine resuscitative measures. If intrauterine resuscitative measures are not successful, discontinue oxytocin.	Remove after 12 hr or at onset of active labor. Remove if uterine tachysystole and/or abnormal (category III) FHR occurs. Removal may be indicated for some types of indeterminate (category II) FHR.	Redosing is permissible if (1) cervical condition remains unfavorable, (2) uterine activity is minimal, (3) FHR is normal (category I), and (4) it has been at least 3 hr since last dose. Consider observation for up to 2 hr after spontaneous rupture of membranes before redosing. Consider delaying or avoiding administration in a woman with frequent, low-amplitude, painless contractions or 2 or more painful contractions per 10 minutes, particularly if a uterotonic has already been administered. Redosing is *withheld* if the FHR is indeterminate or abnormal (category II or III) because increased uterine activity can further compromise fetal status.
Monitoring	Administer in labor and birth suite, where uterine activity and FHR can be recorded continuously via EFM and evaluated at a minimum every 15 min during the first stage of labor and every 5 min during the second stage of labor.	Administer at or near the labor and birth suite, where uterine activity and FHR can be monitored continuously while in place and for at least 15 min after removal. Ambulation is an option after initial 2 hr if continuous EFM telemetry is available.	Administer at or near labor and birth suite, where uterine activity and FHR can be monitored as appropriate based on route of administration. Continuous monitoring of FHR and uterine activity is indicated for 4 hr after intravaginal dose and 2 hr after oral dose.
Use with oxytocin, if needed	N/A	Oxytocin should be delayed for at least 30 to 60 min after removal of insert. Previous exposure to PGE$_2$ potentiates contractile response to oxytocin, so careful maternal–fetal monitoring of FHR and uterine activity is warranted.	Oxytocin should be delayed until at least 4 hr after last dose. Previous exposure to misoprostol potentiates contractile response to oxytocin, so careful maternal–fetal monitoring of FHR and uterine activity is warranted.
Complications	Risk of uterine tachysystole is dose related. Approximately 50% of cases of tachysystole will result in an indeterminate or abnormal (category II or III) FHR. Terbutaline, 0.25 mg subcutaneously, can be used in an attempt to correct indeterminate or abnormal FHR pattern or uterine tachysystole if intrauterine resuscitative measures and discontinuation of oxytocin are not successful in resolving the FHR pattern and/or uterine tachysystole.	Rate of uterine tachysystole is about 5%; usually occurs within 1 hr of administration but may occur up to 9.5 hr after administration. Terbutaline, 0.25 mg subcutaneously, can be used in an attempt to correct indeterminate or abnormal FHR pattern or uterine tachysystole if removal of insert has not been successful in resolving the FHR pattern and/or uterine tachysystole. Side effects of prostaglandins include tachysystole, fever, chills, vomiting, and diarrhea.	Uterine tachysystole is more common with misoprostol as compared to Cervidil and oxytocin. Rates of uterine tachysystole are lower with lower dosages (25 mcg) and when dosed less frequently (i.e., less problems when dosed every 6 hr instead of every 3 hr). Terbutaline, 0.25 mg subcutaneously, can be used in an attempt to correct indeterminate or abnormal FHR pattern or uterine tachysystole. Side effects of prostaglandins include tachysystole, fever, chills, vomiting, and diarrhea.

EFM, electronic fetal monitoring; FHR, fetal heart rate; IV, intravenous; N/A, not available; PGE$_2$, prostaglandin E$_2$.

Adapted from Simpson, K. R. (2020). *Cervical ripening and labor induction and augmentation* (AWHONN Practice Monograph) (5th ed.). Washington, DC: Association of Women's Health, Obstetric and Neonatal Nurses. Used with permission.

Cervidil is removed after 12 hours, or when active labor begins (Ferring Pharmaceuticals, 2017). Regular contractions (three in 10 minutes lasting 60 seconds or more with moderate patient discomfort) will occur in approximately 25% of women after Cervidil placement (Rayburn, Tassone, & Pearman, 2000). One major advantage of Cervidil is that the system can be easily and quickly removed in the event of uterine tachysystole or other complications. Tachysystole usually occurs within 1 hour after insertion but can occur up to 9.5 hours after the insert has been placed (ACOG, 2009a). If uterine tachysystole occurs, complete reversal of the prostaglandin-induced uterine pattern usually occurs within 15 minutes of removal. If necessary, the woman may be given tocolytic therapy (0.25 mg of terbutaline subcutaneously). Previous exposure to PGE_2 potentiates the contractile response to oxytocin (Ferring Pharmaceuticals, 2017; Maul, Macray, & Garfield, 2006), so careful maternal–fetal monitoring is warranted when oxytocin is administered after Cervidil has been used for cervical ripening. Oxytocin administration should be delayed until at least 30 to 60 minutes after removal of the Cervidil insert (ACOG, 2009a). Continuous monitoring of the FHR and uterine activity is indicated while Cervidil is in place (Ferring Pharmaceuticals, 2017). Ambulation while Cervidil is in place is an option if continuous EFM via telemetry is available. There have been no studies using methods other than continuous EFM for maternal–fetal assessment. There is risk of initiation of regular contractions progressing to active labor and an approximate 5% rate of tachysystole with Cervidil (ACOG, 2009a; Ferring Pharmaceuticals, 2017). Cervidil is not appropriate for outpatient cervical ripening as its use in the outpatient setting has not been studied (ACOG, 2009a). There is a risk of uterine rupture when prostaglandins are used for women attempting vaginal birth after cesarean birth (VBAC); thus, Cervidil is not recommended for these patients (Ferring Pharmaceuticals, 2017).

Prostaglandin E₁. Misoprostol (PGE_1) is a synthetic PGE_1 analogue that has been used for cervical ripening and induction of labor. Misoprostol was originally approved by the FDA for the prevention of peptic ulcers, not for cervical ripening or induction of labor. In April 2002, the FDA removed the contraindication for the use of misoprostol for women during pregnancy because it was widely used for cervical ripening and labor induction and was part of an FDA-approved regime for use with mifepristone to induce abortion in pregnancies of 49 days or less. The FDA (2002) included warnings about potential adverse effects of misoprostol when used for cervical ripening, labor induction, and treatment of serious postpartum hemorrhage in the presence of uterine atony. According to the FDA, a major adverse effect of the obstetric use of misoprostol is uterine tachysystole, which may progress to uterine tetany with marked impairment of uteroplacental blood flow, uterine rupture, or amniotic fluid embolism. The FDA further noted that pelvic pain, retained placenta, severe genital bleeding, shock, fetal bradycardia, and fetal and maternal death have been reported. As more data are published from ongoing clinical research studies, a clearer understanding of safety and appropriate dosages will emerge.

When used for cervical ripening or induction of labor, 25 mcg placed in the posterior vaginal fornix should be considered for the initial dose (ACOG, 2009a). Higher dosages have been associated with an increased rate of tachysystole (ACOG, 2009a; McMaster, Sanchez-Ramos, Kaunitz, 2015; Penfield & Wing, 2017). However, it is important to consider that tachysystole and indeterminate or abnormal FHR changes are associated with both the 25- and 50-mcg doses (Crane, Young, Butt, Bennett, & Hutchens, 2001; Keirse, 2006). Tachysystole with and without indeterminate or abnormal FHR changes is significantly higher with the use of misoprostol when compared with Cervidil and oxytocin (Hofmeyr, Gülmezoglu, & Pileggi, 2010; Penfield & Wing, 2017). A recent meta-analysis and systematic review on the efficacy and safety of intravaginal misoprostol found 25 mcg, as compared to 50 mcg, had a better safety profile with lower rates of tachysystole, fewer cesarean births for "nonreassuring" fetal status, less admissions to the neonatal intensive care unit, and less meconium passage (McMaster et al., 2015). A 3- to 6-hour interval between doses has been associated with less uterine tachysystole than the 3-hour interval (ACOG, 2009a; Penfield & Wing, 2017).

Misoprostol is contraindicated in women with a history of or prior uterine surgery or cesarean birth because of the risk of uterine rupture (ACOG, 2009a, 2019c; Lydon-Rochelle, Holt, Easterling, & Martin, 2001; Penfield & Wing, 2017; Weeks, Navaratnam, & Alfirevic, 2017). However, it is important to consider that uterine rupture after misoprostol (or oxytocin) can occur in the unscarred uterus, although the risk is lower than for women with a previous uterine scar (Akhan, Iyibozkurt, & Turfanda, 2001; Bennett, 1997; Catanzarite, Cousins, Dowling, & Daneshmand, 2006).

Because the 100-mcg tablet is unscored, there is no assurance that the PGE_1 is uniformly dispersed throughout the tablet. It is possible that one quarter of a tablet may contain more or less than 25 mcg of PGE_1. The hospital pharmacist should prepare the tablet in four equal parts before administration of a quarter of a tablet intravaginally (Simpson, 2020). Individual providers attempting to break or cut the small tablet into four equal parts increases the risk of inaccurate dose administration.

If uterine tachysystole and an indeterminate or abnormal FHR pattern occur with misoprostol and there is no response to routine corrective measures (e.g., maternal repositioning, supplemental oxygen, IV fluid bolus), consider cesarean birth (ACOG, 2009a). Terbutaline, 0.25 mg subcutaneously, also can be used in an attempt to correct the indeterminate or abnormal FHR pattern or the uterine tachysystole (ACOG, 2009a).

If induction or augmentation of labor is required after cervical ripening with misoprostol, some providers opt to use oxytocin. The plasma concentration of misoprostol after vaginal administration of misoprostol rises gradually, reaching peak levels between 1 and 2 hours and declining slowly to an average of 61% of peak level at 4 hours (Arias, 2000; Goldberg, Greenberg, & Darney, 2001; Zeiman, Fong, Benowitz, Bankster, & Darney, 1997). Some women will have increased plasma concentrations 4 to 6 hours after vaginal administration (Zeiman et al., 1997). Based on these pharmacologic data, the administration of oxytocin should be delayed for at least 4 hours after the last dose of misoprostol (ACOG, 2009a). Baseline uterine activity is a relative contraindication to the use of prostaglandins because the addition of an exogenous uterotonic agent can lead to excessive uterine activity (Penfield & Wing, 2017). Delaying or avoiding administration in a woman with frequent, low-amplitude, painless contractions or two or more painful contractions per minute, particularly if a uterotonic has already been administered, is recommended (Penfield & Wing, 2017).

Some providers opt to use oral misoprostol, which, at equivalent doses to the vaginal route of administration, is not as efficacious but is associated with fewer indeterminate or abnormal FHR patterns and episodes of tachysystole when compared to vaginal administration (ACOG, 2009a). Pharmacokinetic studies show that oral misoprostol reaches its peak serum level within 30 minutes, but that its half-life is only 90 minutes, as misoprostol acid is rapidly metabolized by the liver and excreted by the kidneys (Weeks et al., 2017). With oral misoprostol, sustained uterine activity is achieved in 90 minutes and the duration of action is approximately 2 hours. Oral administration may offer more patient comfort, satisfaction, and convenience of administration. There is a clear, positive dose–response relationship seen between the dosage of oral misoprostol and the rate of tachysystole; 25- and 50-mcg dosages are associated with a lower tachysystole rate (Alfirevic, Aflaifel, & Weeks, 2014; Weeks et al., 2017). Based on the most recent Cochrane Review, generally, misoprostol 25 mcg orally is recommended over 50 mcg if oral misoprostol is used (Alfirevic, Aflaifel, & Weeks, 2014).

Misoprostol can be administered intravaginally by perinatal nurses; however, in many institutions, this practice is deferred to CNMs or physicians. If vaginal misoprostol administration is delegated to perinatal nurses, they must have demonstrated competence in insertion and the activity must be within the scope of practice as defined by state and provincial regulations. Misoprostol orally can be administered by perinatal nurses as ordered by the CNM or physician.

Pharmacologic Methods of Induction of Labor

Oxytocin

Oxytocin is the most commonly used induction agent in the United States (ACOG, 2009a). Although oxytocin is an effective means of labor induction in women with a favorable cervix, it is not efficacious as a cervical ripening agent based on multiple randomized trials comparing oxytocin with other methods of cervical ripening (Penfield & Wing, 2017). Oxytocin following preinduction cervical ripening prostaglandin agents appears to be more efficacious than oxytocin alone as a method of induction (ACOG & SMFM, 2014; Penfield & Wing, 2017). An unfavorable cervix generally has been defined as a Bishop score of 6 or less in most randomized trials. If the total score is more than 8, the probability of vaginal delivery after labor induction is similar to that after spontaneous labor (ACOG, 2009a). Cervical ripening should be used when labor is induced in women with an unfavorable cervix (ACOG & SMFM, 2014).

Oxytocin is a peptide consisting of nine amino acids. Endogenous oxytocin is synthesized by the hypothalamus and then transported to the posterior lobe of the pituitary gland, where it is released into maternal circulation. It is released in response to breast stimulation, sensory stimulation of the lower genital tract, and cervical stretching. Oxytocin released in response to vaginal and cervical stretching results in uterine contractions. Minimal change occurs in myometrial sensitivity to oxytocin from 34 weeks' gestation until term; however, when spontaneous labor is initiated, uterine sensitivity to oxytocin increases rapidly (ACOG, 2009b). Therefore, based on this physiologic mechanism, oxytocin is more effective in augmenting labor than in inducing labor. Synthetic oxytocin is chemically and physiologically identical to endogenous oxytocin (Page, McCool, & Guidera, 2017).

Oxytocin circulates in the blood as a free peptide and has a molecular weight of 1,007 d (Zeeman, Khan-Dawood, & Dawood, 1997). Volume of distribution is estimated to be 305 ± 46 mL/kg; thus, oxytocin is distributed into both the intravascular and extravascular compartments (Zeeman et al., 1997). Plasma clearance of oxytocin is through the maternal kidneys and liver by the enzyme oxytocinase, with only a small amount excreted unchanged in the urine. Maternal metabolic clearance rate of oxytocin at term is 19 to 21 mL/kg/min and is unaffected by pregnancy (Zeeman et al., 1997).

During the first stage of spontaneous labor, maternal circulating concentrations of endogenous oxytocin are approximately that which would be achieved with a continuous infusion of exogenous oxytocin at 2 to 4 mU/min (Dawood, Ylikorkala, Trivedi, & Fuchs, 1979). The fetus is thought to secrete oxytocin during labor at a level similar to an infusion of oxytocin at approximately 3 mU/min (Dawood, Wang, Gupta, & Fuchs, 1978). Thus, the combined effects of maternal–fetal contributions to maternal plasma oxytocin concentration are equivalent to a range of about 5 to 7 mU/min (Shyken & Petrie, 1995).

Although there are considerable variations in reports of the biologic half-life of oxytocin, it is now generally agreed that the half-life is between 10 and 12 minutes (Arias, 2000; Dawood, 1995a; Page et al., 2017). Early data based on in vitro studies estimated a plasma half-life of 3 to 4 minutes, but Seitchik, Amico, Robinson, and Castillo (1984) used in vivo methods to study oxytocin pharmacokinetics and found half-life was probably closer to 10 to 15 minutes.

Oxytocin concentration and saturation follow first-order kinetics with a progressive, linear, stepwise increase with each increase in the infusion rate (Arias, 2000). Three to four half-lives of oxytocin are generally needed to reach a steady-state plasma concentration (Stringer, 1996). Therefore, with a half-life of 10 to 15 minutes, steady state is reached in approximately 30 to 60 minutes. Uterine response to oxytocin usually occurs within 3 to 5 minutes of IV administration. There is an incremental phase of uterine activity when oxytocin is initiated during which contractions progressively increase in frequency and strength, followed by a stable phase, during which time any further increase in oxytocin will not lead to further normal changes in uterine contractions (Dawood, 1995b; Phaneuf, Rodríguez Liñares, TambyRaja, MacKenzie, & López Bernal, 2000). Instead, abnormal uterine activity such as frequent low-intensity contractions, coupling or tripling of contractions, or uterine tachysystole may be produced with further increases in oxytocin rates. There has long been a myth that these types of abnormal uterine activity patterns are best treated with oxytocin rate increases (i.e., "pit through the pattern"); however, an understanding of their genesis (excessive oxytocin and oxytocin receptor site desensitization) should guide clinicians to reduce the rate or discontinue oxytocin until uterine activity returns to normal. Often, a 30- to 60-minute rest period along with an IV fluid bolus of L/R solution will allow oxytocin receptors to be sensitive to artificial oxytocin and produce uterine contractions that will result in normal uterine activity and labor progress (Dawood, 1995b; Phaneuf et al., 2000; Zeeman et al., 1997).

There appears to be no advantage to continuing oxytocin once active labor is established. Reducing or discontinuing oxytocin may result in an equal or shorter length of labor compared to labor for women for whom oxytocin is continued or incrementally increased after active labor is achieved (Daniel-Spiegel, Weiner, Ben-Shlomo, & Shalev, 2004). Continued increases in oxytocin rates over a prolonged period can result in oxytocin receptor desensitization or down-regulation, making oxytocin less effective in producing normal uterine contractions and having the opposite than intended result (Page et al., 2017). There is a direct inverse relationship between the duration and dosage of oxytocin and the number of oxytocin receptor sites available for oxytocin uptake during labor (Phaneuf et al., 1998; Phaneuf et al., 2000; Robinson, Schumann, Zhang, & Young, 2003). Prolonged oxytocin infusion at higher-than-appropriate doses can result in oxytocin side effects such as dysfunctional uterine activity patterns and uterine tachysystole (Dawood, 1995b; Phaneuf et al., 2000). Once active labor is established, oxytocin rates should be discontinued to avoid receptor down-regulation, especially in cases of long labor induction. A recent meta-analysis and systematic review found discontinuation of oxytocin once 5-cm cervical dilation is reached reduces the risk of uterine tachysystole and cesarean birth when compared to continuing oxytocin (Saccone et al., 2017). Risk of excessive uterine activity and FHR abnormalities are decreased with oxytocin regimens that include discontinuation of oxytocin at 5 cm (Boie et al., 2018; Bor, Lederfoug, Boie, Knoblauch, & Stornes, 2016). Prolonged high-dose oxytocin infusions are counterproductive to the augmentation of established labor (Robinson et al., 2003).

Tachysystole is the most concerning side effect of oxytocin. Use of oxytocin for induction or augmentation of labor doubles the risk of tachysystole (Heuser et al., 2013). There is a dose–response relationship between oxytocin and tachysystole, with approximately one fourth of those tracings reflecting "unfavorable" FHR changes (Heuser et al., 2013). In a study of over 50,000 births, tachysystole increases risk of operative vaginal birth, admission to the neonatal intensive care unit, a composite neonatal adverse outcome (sepsis, intraventricular hemorrhage, necrotizing enterocolitis, pneumothorax, and low Apgar scores) by approximately 30% (Heuser et al., 2013). In a study of 7,319 women, tachysystole in second-stage labor was found to be associated with adverse neonatal outcomes per a composite neonatal morbidity outcome variable that included need for hypothermic treatment, need for ventilatory support, meconium aspiration, seizures, suspected sepsis, and death (Zahedi-Spung et al., 2019). The researchers concluded that neonatal resuscitation teams should be notified and neonatal resuscitation be anticipated following second-stage labor tachysystole.

Normal uterine contractions produce intermittent diminution of blood flow to the intervillous space where oxygen exchange occurs. The decreased intervillous blood flow associated with tachysystole ultimately leads to decreased oxygen transfer to the fetus (Simpson & James, 2008). When fetal oxygenation is sufficiently impaired to produce fetal metabolic acidosis from anaerobic glycolysis, direct myocardial depression occurs (King, 2018). If the intermittent interruption in blood flow caused by excessive uterine activity exceeds a critical level, the fetus responds with evolving hypoxia, acidosis, and ultimately asphyxia (King, 2018). Therefore, every effort should be made to avoid tachysystole and treat it appropriately when identified (Simpson & Knox, 2009). Waiting until the FHR is indeterminate or abnormal to treat tachysystole is not consistent with fetal safety (Simpson, 2020). When tachysystole occurs during induced or augmented labor and the FHR pattern is normal, ACOG (2010) recommends decreasing oxytocin. If there are changes in the FHR pattern, further interventions such as discontinuation of oxytocin, maternal repositioning, and an IV fluid bolus should be considered (ACOG, 2010; Simpson, 2020). A simultaneous initiation of maternal repositioning, an IV fluid bolus and discontinuation of oxytocin will usually resolve oxytocin-induced tachysystole within 6 to 10 minutes (Simpson & James, 2008). See Display 14–10 for a suggested protocol for the treatment of tachysystole.

While oxytocin is the most frequently used medication for labor induction and augmentation, it is also the drug most commonly associated with preventable adverse events during childbirth (Clark, Belfort, Dildy, & Meyers, 2008). The risks of oxytocin are generally dose related and, in addition to tachysystole, include fetal compromise, neonatal acidemia, abruptio placentae, and uterine rupture (ACOG, 2009a; Bakker, Kurver, Kuik, & Van Geijin, 2007). Other types of oxytocin errors involve mistaken administration of IV fluids with oxytocin for IV fluid resuscitation during indeterminate or abnormal FHR patterns and/or maternal hypotension and inappropriate elective administration of oxytocin to women who are less than 39 completed weeks of gestation (Simpson & Knox, 2009). Oxytocin is also often implicated in professional liability claims and thus poses a dual concern for individual clinicians and the organizations in which they practice (Clark, Simpson, Knox, & Garite, 2009). Approximately half of all paid obstetric litigation claims involve allegations of oxytocin misuse (Clark, Belfort, Dildy, et al., 2008). Oxytocin administration is a significant source of clinical conflict between nurses and physicians during labor (Simpson, James, & Knox, 2006; Simpson & Lyndon, 2009). Standardized policies for oxytocin are helpful in avoiding conflict as agreed upon dosing for oxytocin and definitions and interventions for oxytocin-induced tachysystole are available for guiding the perinatal team (Jackson et al., 2019; Krening et al., 2012; O'Rourke et al., 2011; Simpson et al., 2011; Sundin et al., 2018).

In 2007, oxytocin was added to the Institute for Safe Medication Practices (2007) list of high-alert

DISPLAY 14–10

Suggested Clinical Protocol for Oxytocin-Induced Uterine Tachysystole

Oxytocin-Induced Tachysystole (Normal [Category I] Fetal Heart Rate)

- Assist the mother to a lateral position.
- Give IV fluid bolus of at least 500 mL lactated Ringer's (L/R) solution as indicated.
- If uterine activity has not returned to normal after 10 to 15 minutes, decrease oxytocin rate by at least half; if uterine activity has not returned to normal after 10 to 15 more minutes, discontinue oxytocin until uterine activity is normal.
- Resume oxytocin after the resolution of tachysystole: If oxytocin has been discontinued for less than 20 to 30 minutes, the fetal heart rate (FHR) is normal, and contraction frequency, intensity, and duration are normal, resume oxytocin at no more than half the rate that caused the tachysystole and gradually increase the rate as appropriate based on unit protocol and maternal–fetal status. If the oxytocin is discontinued for more than 30 to 40 minutes, resume oxytocin at the initial dose ordered.

Oxytocin-Induced Tachysystole (Indeterminate [Category II] or Abnormal [Category III] Fetal Heart Rate)

- Discontinue oxytocin.
- Assist the mother to a lateral position.
- Give IV fluid bolus of at least 500 mL of L/R solution as indicated.
- Consider oxygen at 10 L/min via a nonrebreather face mask (discontinue as soon as possible based on the FHR pattern).
- If no response, consider 0.25-mg terbutaline subcutaneous.
- Resume oxytocin after the resolution of tachysystole: If oxytocin has been discontinued for less than 20 to 30 minutes, the FHR is normal, and contraction frequency, intensity, and duration are normal, resume oxytocin at no more than half the rate that caused the tachysystole and gradually increase the rate as appropriate based on unit protocol and maternal–fetal status. If the oxytocin is discontinued for more than 30 to 40 minutes, resume oxytocin at the initial dose ordered.

medications. High-alert medications are defined as those bearing a heightened risk of harm when they are used in error and that may require special safeguards to reduce the risk of error. While oxytocin administered using pharmacologic principles can be therapeutic during labor, inappropriate timing or excessive doses can have a potentially negative effect on the mother and baby (Clark et al., 2009).

DOSAGE AND RATE INCREASE INTERVALS

Based on physiologic and pharmacokinetic principles, Seitchik et al. (1984) recommended at least a 40-minute interval between oxytocin dosage increases because the full effect of oxytocin on the uterine response to increases in dosage cannot be evaluated until steady-state concentration has been achieved. Seitchik et al. used a sensitive oxytocin radioimmunoassay to show that approximately 40 minutes was required to reach steady-state plasma concentration. Their data suggested that increasing the infusion rate before steady-state concentrations were achieved resulted in laboring women receiving higher doses of oxytocin than necessary. The works of Seitchik and Castillo (1982, 1983) and Seitchik et al. were the basis of oxytocin protocols with intervals in oxytocin dosage increases between 30 and 60 minutes.

There is no consensus in the literature on the ideal oxytocin dosage regimen, although available data support a lower dosage rate of infusion (Crane & Young, 1998; SOGC, 2001). The most commonly used regime in the United States includes starting at 1 to 2 mU/min with incremental doses of 1 to 2 mU/min every 30 to 60 minutes, which is based on the work of Seitchik et al. (1984) who advocated for a *physiologic* approach to oxytocin dosage and rate increase intervals.

Most researchers noted that higher doses and shorter dose increase intervals led to more uterine tachysystole and indeterminate or abnormal FHR patterns and did not result in a clinically significant decrease in length of labor (Crane & Young, 1998). The most recent Cochrane review found high-dose oxytocin, when compared to low-dose oxytocin, did not increase the rate of vaginal birth within 24 hours, but did increase the rate of "hyperstimulation" (Budden, Chen, & Henry, 2014). There have been a number of randomized trials of low-dose versus high-dose oxytocin; however, most were conducted over two decades ago. In a 2018 multicenter randomized trial, high-dose oxytocin was found to increase risk of tachysystole and "fetal distress" with no benefit to reducing cesarean births (Selin et al., 2019), similar to the cumulative results of the earlier studies (Crane & Young, 1998).

In spontaneous active labor, the unripe cervix is not a significant factor, and oxytocin receptor sites are thought to be increased in number and sensitivity (Buckley, 2015; Carbillon, Seince, & Uzan, 2001; Dawood, 1995a; Page et al., 2017). Other factors that may influence the dose response to oxytocin include maternal body surface area, parity, week of pregnancy duration, and cervical status (Dawood, 1995a). Although these factors may be significant, to date, there are no practical predictive models for determining the required oxytocin dosage for successful labor induction. Until more is known about the pharmacokinetics of oxytocin, each pregnant woman receiving oxytocin will continue to represent an individual bioassay.

Generally, starting doses of 1 to 2 mU/min with increases in 1 to 2 mU/min increments every 30 to 60 minutes are most appropriate and commonly used. Shorter intervals between dosage increases are associated with a greater risk of tachysystole, somewhat

shorter duration of labor, and no reduction in the cesarean birth rate (Crane & Young, 1998). Multiple clinical studies and current data based on physiologic and pharmacologic principles have shown that 90% of pregnant women at term will have labor successfully induced with 6 mU/min or less of oxytocin (Dawood, 1995a, 1995b; Seitchik et al., 1984).

Although higher doses of oxytocin and short intervals between dosage increments have generally not been found to be beneficial (Crane & Young, 1998), some providers intuitively believe that this approach is better. According to ACOG (2009a), protocols that involve high-dose oxytocin are acceptable; however, ACOG cautions that high-dose oxytocin is associated with more uterine tachysystole. Conversely, SOGC (2001) recommends using the minimum dose to achieve active labor, increasing the dosage no more frequently than every 30 minutes, and reevaluating the clinical situation if the oxytocin dosage rate reaches 20 mU/min.

ADMINISTRATION

Oxytocin is administered intravenously and piggy-backed into the mainline solution at the port most proximal to the venous site (see Table 14–4 for a summary of oxytocin administration). There are many variations in the dilution rate. Some protocols suggest adding 10 units of oxytocin to 1,000 mL of an isotonic electrolyte IV solution, resulting in an infusion dosage rate of 1 mU/min = 6 mL/hr. However, other commonly reported dilutions are 20 units of oxytocin to 1,000 mL IV fluid (1 mU/min = 3 mL/hr) and 30 units of oxytocin to 500 mL IV fluid or 60 units of oxytocin to 1,000 mL IV fluid (1 mU/min = 1 mL/hr). One advantage to the dilution rates of 30 units of oxytocin to 500 mL IV fluid or 60 units of oxytocin to 1,000 mL IV fluid is that they result in a 1:1 solution (1 mU/min = 1 mL/hr); therefore, no calculations are needed for the dosage increases, an important consideration for medication safety. The key issues are knowledge of how many mU/min are administered and consistency in clinical practice within each institution. To enhance communication among members of the perinatal healthcare team and to avoid confusion, oxytocin administration rates should always be ordered by the physician or CNM as milliunits per minute and documented in the medical record as milliunits per minute.

Nursing responsibility during oxytocin infusion involves careful titration of the drug to the maternal–fetal response. The titration process includes decreasing the dosage rate or discontinuing the medication when contractions are too frequent, discontinuing the medication when fetal status is indeterminate or abnormal, and increasing the dosage rate when uterine activity and labor progress are inadequate. Often, during oxytocin infusion, physicians and nurses are focused on the rate increase section of the protocol while ignoring the clinical criteria for dosage increases. For example, if cervical effacement is occurring or if the woman is progressing in labor as expected based on parity and other individual clinical factors, there is no need to increase the oxytocin rate, even if contractions appear to be mild and infrequent. Labor progress and maternal–fetal response to the medication should be the primary considerations.

When uterine tachysystole occurs or fetal status is such that oxytocin is discontinued, data are limited to guide the decision about the timing and dosage of subsequent IV oxytocin administration. Physiologic and pharmacologic principles may be used to determine the most appropriate dosage. If oxytocin has been discontinued for less than 20 to 30 minutes, the FHR is normal and contraction frequency, intensity, and duration are normal, a suggested protocol may include restarting oxytocin at half the rate that caused the tachysystole and gradually increase the rate as appropriate based on unit protocol and maternal–fetal status. However, if the oxytocin is discontinued for more than 30 to 40 minutes, most of the exogenous oxytocin is metabolized and plasma levels are similar to that of a woman who has not received IV oxytocin. In this clinical situation, a suggested protocol may include restarting the oxytocin at the initial dose ordered. There are individual differences in myometrial sensitivity and the response to oxytocin during labor (Arias, 2000; Ulmsten, 1997). It may be necessary to use a lower dose and increase the interval between dosages when there is evidence of the patient's previous sensitivity to the drug. See Display 14–10 for a suggested protocol for managing oxytocin infusion during tachysystole with and without an indeterminate or abnormal FHR pattern.

Misoprostol

Misoprostol is also used for induction of labor. See the section "Cervical Ripening" for a full discussion of misoprostol.

Augmentation of Labor

For some women, labor progresses more slowly than expected. The terms *dystocia* and *failure to progress* are sometimes used to characterize an abnormally long labor. However, this diagnosis is often mistakenly made before the woman has entered the active phase of labor and, therefore, before an adequate trial of labor has been achieved. Some women have a cesarean birth because of "failure to progress in labor" for the diagnosis of lack of labor progress; yet, active labor has not begun or labor has not been abnormally

long (ACOG & SMFM, 2014). *Cephalopelvic disproportion* is another common term used when labor has not progressed. This condition can rarely be diagnosed with certainty and is usually related to malposition of the fetal head.

Wide variations in labor progress and duration exist among childbearing women (see previous section "Duration of Labor") (ACOG & SMFM, 2014; Spong, Berghella, Wenstrom, Mercer, & Saade, 2012). From a physiologic and pharmacologic standpoint, less oxytocin is needed for labor augmentation than for labor induction, but most studies and clinical protocols report higher doses of oxytocin administration during the augmentation of labor. For women in spontaneous active labor, cervical resistance is less than in women who have not yet experienced cervical effacement and dilation. The response to oxytocin seems to depend on preexisting uterine activity and sensitivity rather than the amount given (Arias, 2000).

Clinical Implications of Labor Induction

Multiple methods of cervical ripening, labor induction, and labor augmentation are currently in use in the United States and Canada. Each method has pros and cons as well as risks and benefits to the mother and fetus. Clearly, the state of the cervix is an important clinical indicator for likelihood of induction success. There is enough evidence to suggest that cervical ripening can increase the chances of success if the indication for induction allows time for cervical ripening. Oxytocin has been used for many years and has proven safe and effective for induction and augmentation. A physiologic dosage regimen for labor induction appears to be the best approach for most women because the risks of higher doses and increasing the doses at more frequent intervals (such as uterine tachysystole and cesarean birth for indeterminate or abnormal fetal status) do not outweigh the benefits (if any) of a slightly shorter labor. Misoprostol is sometimes used for cervical ripening and labor induction. Uterine tachysystole and indeterminate or abnormal FHR patterns related to tachysystole are more common with misoprostol than with oxytocin. Lower doses of misoprostol and increased intervals between doses will decrease the risk to the mother and fetus. Women who are attempting VBAC are at increased risk for uterine rupture with subsequent catastrophic results for both the mother and fetus if pharmacologic agents are used for cervical ripening or labor induction (ACOG, 2019c).

The increase in the elective induction rate over the past two decades has profoundly changed the practice of perinatal nursing. Instead of predominately caring for patients who present in spontaneous active labor, many labor nurses spend a significant portion of their time titrating an oxytocin infusion and managing the side effects of oxytocin. Nurses often are pressured by physician colleagues to increase the oxytocin rate to "keep labor on track" and speed the labor process when labor is otherwise proceeding normally or there is evidence of excessive uterine activity (Simpson et al., 2006; Simpson & Lyndon, 2009). Although nurses report that they usually resist these types of requests for patient safety reasons, these ongoing clinical conflicts are a source of dissatisfaction for both nurses and physicians (Simpson et al., 2006; Simpson & Lyndon, 2009). Oxytocin mismanagement has become a significant factor in perinatal liability (Clark, Belfort, Dildy, et al., 2008; Knox & Simpson, 2011).

In 2018, results of a multicenter randomized trial on elective induction of labor at 39 weeks' gestation (ARRIVE Trial) were published (Grobman, Rice, et al., 2018). The primary purpose of the study was to see if expectant management (e.g., waiting for labor to begin on its own) was safe for the mother and baby. In this study, 6,101 low-risk nulliparous women were randomized to elective induction of labor between 39 weeks and 39 weeks and 4 days or to expectant management, which included an agreement not to have an elective induction before 40 weeks and 5 days and to give birth no later than 42 weeks and 2 days. There were no differences between groups for the primary study outcome, which was a composite of perinatal adverse events. There was a difference in one of the key secondary outcomes: method of birth. The rate of cesarean birth was lower (18.6%) in the induction of labor group than the expectant management group (22.2%) (Grobman, Rice, et al., 2018). This finding has led some to conclude that elective induction of labor at 39 weeks is an ideal way to decrease risk of cesarean birth for healthy women. However, the answer to the main question posed by the trial that it is safe for the mother and baby to await spontaneous labor has been largely ignored (Breedlove, 2019).

On close examination, there are several limitations of the ARRIVE trial (Grobman, Rice, et al., 2018) including low interest to enroll as recruitment occurred at 41 hospitals over 3 years. Of the 22,533 eligible low-risk nulliparous women, only 27% agreed to participate, suggesting selection bias (Breedlove, 2019). Unavailable data include epidural or narcotic use, childbirth education classes, presence of a doula, and 1 to 1 care by a registered nurse for women receiving oxytocin. Variances to care include admitting provider approach and management style (94% physician and 6% midwife), type of induction method (left to discretion), and oxytocin protocol. An inability to generalize findings is due to participants' characteristics such as average age ~24 years old, 44% white, 59% single, 48% nonemployed, and 45% without private insurance. Inductions were conducted in academic teaching centers compared to community-based or rural hospitals. Women were queried via the Labor Agentry Scale (LAS) and a Likert assessment of labor pain. The LAS, developed in 1980s, elicits one dimension, perceived personal control during pregnancy and childbirth. It is not surprising that the labor induction group scored high positive on perceived control as they desired induction compared to 16,427 eligible women that chose not to participate in the study. Labor pain scores were not correlated to epidural or narcotic use.

A response by SMFM (2019), endorsed by ACOG, was soon released. They conclude it is reasonable to offer elective induction of labor to low-risk, nulliparous women at or beyond 39 weeks for women meeting eligibility criteria used in the trial and recommend against offering elective induction of labor to women inconsistent with the study protocol unless part of research or quality improvement activity. It is important to remember that the study protocol did not consider an induction of labor to have "failed" unless at least 12 hours had elapsed since both rupture of membranes and use of a uterine stimulant, and the woman remained in the latent phase of the first stage of labor (Grobman, Rice, et al., 2018). Thus, cesarean birth was not done until after ample time for labor progress based on the study protocol. Adherence to study protocols in the context of a clinical trial is not likely to be the same in community hospitals offering elective induction.

Of significant concern about potential routine elective induction for nulliparous women are institutional implications, unit operations, and financial resources. What costs are associated with increase need for labor beds and surgical rooms to accommodate potential physician and consumer demand for 39-week elective induction of labor (Breedlove, 2019)? If requested and the labor unit is at capacity, is there increased professional liability since findings suggest decreased incidence of cesarean birth, less maternal hypertension, and fewer newborn respiratory consequences? What is the cost for an increase in nurse staffing to provide 1 to 1 nursing care for women in labor being induced with oxytocin as recommended by AWHONN (2010) and AAP and ACOG (2017)? Will there be increased legal risk related to imprudent use of oxytocin, the most common obstetric medication associated with harm (Clark, Belfort, Byrum, et al., 2008)? Grobman, Rice, et al. (2018) note that 28 nulliparous women would need to have elective induction of labor at 39 weeks to avoid one cesarean birth. If elective induction of labor were applied to the 1.6 million women in the United States who are considered low risk, Hersh, Skeith, Sargent, and Caughey (2019) estimated it would lead to an additional $2.26 billion of healthcare costs.

It is important to consider women's experience with induction (Breedlove, 2019). In the Listening to Mothers III survey, 15% of mothers reported experiencing pressure from a care provider to have labor induced without a medical indication, 53% experienced attempted labor induction, and 30% had a medically induced labor (Declercq et al., 2014). It is likely this situation will become more common because pregnant women are vulnerable to making uninformed decisions about induction when there is not a medical reason. In a study of 3,337 nulliparous women, physicians offered the option of elective induction to 69.5% of survey participants (Simpson et al., 2010a). This was a factor in women's decisions; 43.2% of those offered the option had elective induction, whereas 90.8% of those not offered the option did not have elective induction. Women were given explicit information in prepared childbirth classes about the potential risks and associated interventions involved with elective induction of labor; however, many women felt their physician would not be offering the option of elective induction unless it was in their best interests; the offer was generally interpreted to be a recommendation (Simpson et al., 2010a). Women often describe induction as an exhausting and disempowering experience (Declercq et al., 2014). Much more data are needed before, if ever, elective induction of labor can be recommended as routine for low-risk women (Breedlove, 2019).

There are clinical practices based on the best available evidence that promote the safest care possible for mothers and babies during labor induction. These include, but are not limited to, the following:

- Awaiting spontaneous labor until 41 weeks' gestation
- Informed consent with the woman and her family as true partners in care (Information should be at the appropriate literacy level, in understandable language, evidence based, unbiased, and individualized and include potential benefits and risks.)
- If elective, not performing labor induction before 39 completed weeks of gestation
- Cervical readiness before labor induction achieved without pharmacologic agents (if induction is elective)
- Standard physiologic oxytocin protocol including a standard concentration and standard dosing regime
- Agreed upon definition of tachysystole
- Appropriate and timely interventions for tachysystole
- One nurse for each woman undergoing induction of labor
- Assessment of fetal well-being based on national guidelines for interpretation and frequency of assessment
- Common understanding among members of the perinatal team regarding how labor induction will be conducted and an agreement that all team members will participate

Much work lies ahead to provide education to pregnant women, so they have enough information to make an informed decision about labor induction (Simpson, 2019b). Multiple factors contribute to the steady increase in the rate of induction of labor in the United States. This is a complex issue that involves all participating parties: the pregnant woman, her family, her healthcare provider, the institution, and the intrapartum nurse. More data are needed to fully evaluate the risks and benefits of artificial induction and stimulation of labor. On the basis of what is known, a cautious process that allows for individualization to each clinical situation should be outlined by each institution to ensure the best outcomes for mothers and babies.

Operative Vaginal Birth

Operative vaginal birth is performed to expedite a safe vaginal birth for either maternal or fetal indications. Operative vaginal births are accomplished by applying direct traction on the fetal scull with of forceps or by applying traction to the fetal scalp with a vacuum extractor with or without the assistance of maternal pushing (AAP & ACOG, 2017; ACOG, 2015). The rate of operative vaginal birth has slowly decreased over recent years from 9% of all births in 1990 (the first year, these data were collected from certificates of live births) to 3.1% in 2017 (Martin et al., 2018). However, operative vaginal rates vary widely across the United States, suggesting almost random decision making and the need for outcomes-based data to assist in clinical decision making (Clark, Belfort, Hankins, Meyers, & Houser, 2007). Some predictors of operative vaginal birth are maternal age, parity, previous cesarean birth, diabetes, gestational age, gender, estimated birth weight, induction of labor, oxytocin augmentation, intrapartum fever, prolonged rupture of membranes, meconium-stained amniotic fluid, and epidural anesthesia (Schuit et al., 2012). Nonoperative interventions such as 1 to 1 labor support by nurses, doulas, monitoring labor progress, using oxytocin when labor is not progressing adequately, and delayed pushing in women using epidurals can decrease the need for operative vaginal birth (AWHONN, 2018a; Hodnett, Gates, Hofmeyr, & Sakala, 2013; SOGC, 2004). Flexibility in the management of second stage including upright positioning, adequate analgesia/anesthesia, and delaying pushing until the woman has the urge to push may be beneficial in reducing the risk of operative vaginal birth (SOGC, 2004). The rate of operative vaginal birth is reduced when the arbitrary time limit of 2 hours for second stage is abandoned if progress is being made (Fraser et al., 2000; SOGC, 2004).

While no indications are absolute, according to ACOG (2015) and AAP and ACOG (2017), indications for operative vaginal birth, when the fetal head is engaged and the cervix is fully dilated, include prolonged second stage of labor, suspicion of immediate or potential fetal compromise, or shortening of the second stage for maternal benefit (e.g., maternal cardiac disease).

Prolonged second-stage labor for nulliparous women, as defined by ACOG and AAP is lack of continuing progress for 3 hours with regional anesthesia or 2 hours without regional analgesia/anesthesia and for multiparous women as a lack of continuing progress for 2 hours with regional anesthesia or 1 hour without regional anesthesia. Multiparous women experiencing a second stage of 3 hours or longer are at increased risk for operative birth, peripartum morbidity, and adverse neonatal outcomes (Cheng, Hopkins, Laros, & Caughey, 2007; Laughon et al., 2014). Fetal station indicates the level of the leading bony point of the fetal presenting part in centimeters at or below the maternal ischial spines (0 to 5 cm) and is important in the evaluation of fetal progress or descent (AAP & ACOG, 2017; ACOG, 2015) (see Fig. 14–6).

According to the *Guidelines for Perinatal Care* (AAP & ACOG, 2017), the clinician should ensure that the following prerequisites are met before resorting to an operative vaginal birth: The cervix is fully dilated and retracted; the membranes are ruptured; the fetal head is engaged in the pelvis; the position of the fetal head has been determined; the fetal weight has been estimated; the maternal pelvis has been assessed and is thought to be adequate for vaginal birth; there is an adequate level of anesthesia; the maternal bladder has been emptied; the woman has agreed to operative vaginal delivery after being informed of the risks and benefits of the procedure; the operator is willing to abandon the trial of operative vaginal delivery; and a backup plan is in place in case of failure to deliver.

The choice of instrument is determined by the clinical circumstance and the training and clinical experience of the obstetric provider. The vacuum extractor is believed to be easier to learn and may be used when asynclitism prevents the proper application of forceps (AAP & ACOG, 2017). The vacuum extractor is associated with an increased risk of neonatal cephalohematoma, retinal hemorrhage, and jaundice when compared to forceps (AAP & ACOG, 2017). In contrast, forceps may provide a more secure application and are appropriate for rotation of the fetal head to OA or OP (AAP & ACOG, 2017). The use of forceps is associated with higher rates of third- and fourth-degree perineal tears (AAP & ACOG, 2017; ACOG, 2015). Routine use of episiotomy is not recommended with operative vaginal birth due to poor healing and increased maternal injuries (AAP & ACOG, 2017; ACOG, 2015). When there is a failed trial, the obstetric care provider must be willing to abandon the attempt if appropriate descent does not occur (ACOG, 2015). Sequential use of vacuum extractor and forceps should not be performed due to increased rates of neonatal complications (ACOG, 2015).

Although sometimes necessary, operative vaginal birth is not without complications for the woman and baby. Perineal trauma is the main injury risk for women including vaginal and perineal lacerations, extension of the episiotomy, hematoma, and anal sphincter disruption (Aukee, Sundström, & Kairaluoma, 2006; Caughey et al., 2005; Dandolu et al., 2005; FitzGerald et al., 2007; Kudish et al., 2006; Laughon et al., 2014). Operative vaginal birth significantly increases the risk for all pelvic floor disorders, especially prolapse, 5 to 10 years after a first birth (Handa et al., 2012). Among women with operative vaginal birth, there are significant risks for rehospitalization for postpartum hemorrhage, perineal wound infection complications, and pelvic injuries when compared to women who had spontaneous vaginal birth (Liu et al., 2005; Lydon-Rochelle, Holt, Martin, & Easterling, 2000). The most common reason for rehospitalization for women after operative vaginal birth is perineal wound infection (Lydon-Rochelle et al., 2000). Maternal injuries appear to be more common with forceps as compared to vacuums, whereas fetal injuries are more common with vacuums as compared to forceps (AAP & ACOG, 2017; Johnson, Figueroa, Garry, Elimian, & Maulik, 2004; Mollberg, Hagberg, Bager, Lilja, & Ladfors, 2005). Comparing neonatal outcome between forceps- and vacuum-assisted birth, babies delivered with forceps have more facial nerve palsy, while babies born with vacuums have more cephalohematomas, scalp lacerations, seizures, and 5-minute Apgar scores less than 7 (Werner et al., 2011). Sequential use of vacuum extractor and forceps should not be performed as it increases the risk of neonatal complications (ACOG, 2015; Castro, Hoey, & Towner, 2003; Towner, Castro, Eby-Wilkens, & Gilbert, 1999; Vacca, 2002). There are several manufacturers of vacuum devices, each with detailed instructions for users. Following the instructions from the manufacturer contributes to safe practice, minimizing risk of adverse outcomes, and decreases liability exposure.

Forceps

Forceps are used to assist delivery of the fetal head when birth must be facilitated for the health of the mother or fetus. Piper forceps are sometimes used during vaginal breech births to assist in delivery of the fetal head after the body has been delivered. Maternal conditions that may necessitate use of forceps are medical complications such as cardiac or pulmonary disease, maternal exhaustion, or high level of regional analgesia/anesthesia that diminishes the woman's expulsive efforts. Additional factors associated with use of forceps are birth weight greater than 4,000 g, an OP position, epidural analgesia/anesthesia, maternal age over 35 years, and a prolonged first- or second-stage labor (Mazouni et al., 2006). The fetus may demonstrate signs of compromise via EFM or FHR auscultation during second-stage labor, such as minimal or absent variability associated with bradycardia, tachycardia, or recurrent late or variable decelerations, or prolonged decelerations, suggesting that attempts at assisted birth may be warranted.

The classification of forceps procedures is listed in Table 14–5. All perinatal nurses should be familiar with this classification so that documentation of the procedure is accurate if they are entering these data in the medical record. Consultation with the provider who applied the forceps before medical record documentation is appropriate to ensure accuracy. The number of forceps applications and attempts with traction are usually documented. Ultimately, the responsibility for complete documentation of the operative birth procedure rests with the provider who performed the procedure. There is no need for duplicative documentation about the procedure in the medical record by the nurse.

Use of forceps are associated with pain, vaginal and cervical lacerations, extension of the episiotomy, anal sphincter injuries, perineal wound infection, uterine rupture, bladder trauma, fracture of the coccyx, hemorrhage, increased vaginal bleeding, uterine atony, anemia, and pelvic floor disorders (ACOG, 2015; Benavides, Wu, Hundley, Ivester, & Visco, 2005; Caughey et al., 2005; Christianson, Bovbjerg, McDavitt, & Hullfish, 2003; FitzGerald et al., 2007; Handa et al., 2012; Hudelist

---

TABLE 14–5. Criteria for Forceps-Assisted Birth According to Station and Rotation

Types of procedure	Criteria
Outlet forceps	• Leading point of the fetal skull has reached the pelvic floor, and at or on the perineum, the scalp is visible at the introitus without separating the labia. • Sagittal suture is in the anteroposterior diameter or a right or left occiput anterior or posterior position. • Rotation does not exceed 45 degrees.

Low forceps	• Leading point of the fetal skull is ≥2 cm beyond the ischial spines but not on the pelvic floor (i.e., station is at least +2/5 cm).
	• Low forceps have two subdivisions:
	  • Without rotation: Rotation is <45 degrees (i.e., right or left occiput anterior to occiput anterior or right or left occiput posterior to occiput posterior).
	  • With rotation: Rotation is greater than 45 degrees.

Midforceps	• The fetal head is engaged (i.e., at least 0 station), but the leading point of the fetal skull is not ≥2 cm beyond the ischial spines (i.e., station is 0 to +1/5 cm).
High forceps	• Not included in the classification

Fetal station is measured using the −5 to +5-centimeter classification system.
Adapted from American College of Obstetricians and Gynecologists. (2015). *Operative vaginal delivery* (Practice Bulletin No. 154; Reaffirmed, 2018). Washington, DC: Author.

---

et al., 2005; Johnson et al., 2004). Babies delivered by forceps are at risk for skin markings, lacerations, bruising, nerve injuries, skull fractures, cephalohematoma, ocular trauma, and intracranial hemorrhage (Doumouchtsis & Arulkumaran, 2006; Dupuis et al., 2005; Towner et al., 1999; Uhing, 2005) and should be observed closely in the immediate newborn period. The incidence of subarachnoid hemorrhage is estimated to be 3.3 per 10,000 forceps-assisted births and subdural hemorrhage 9.8 per 10,000 forceps-assisted births (Doumouchtsis & Arulkumaran, 2006). However, when compared with vacuum-assisted vaginal births or cesarean birth, a forceps-assisted birth is associated with a reduced risk of neonatal seizures and 5-minute Apgar scores less than 7 (Werner et al., 2011). The condition of the mother and newborn at birth should be documented in the medical record. The complete details of the procedure should be documented by the healthcare provider who delivered the baby. Neonatal care providers should be made aware of the forceps-assisted vaginal birth (AAP & ACOG, 2017).

Vacuum Extraction

Some physicians and CNMs use vacuum extraction in lieu of forceps, usually dependent on their education, experience, and privileges. A vacuum extractor consists of a soft or rigid cup available in various sizes that has a suction device attached. The cup is placed on the fetal head, and suction is increased gradually until a seal is formed. Gentle traction is then applied to deliver the fetal head. Recommendations from the manufacturer of the vacuum extractor device being used should be followed. Indications and prerequisites for vacuum extraction or for the use of forceps are generally the same; however, most experts agree that rotation is not appropriate via vacuum extraction (ACOG, 2015). Proponents of vacuum extraction feel that its advantages include easier application, less force applied to the fetal head, less analgesia/anesthesia needed, less maternal soft tissue injury, fewer fetal injuries, and fewer parental concerns (ACOG, 2015; Caughey et al., 2005).

Complications from both vacuum- and forceps-assisted births are dependent primarily on skill of the practitioner. Neonatal injuries reported from the use of vacuum extractor include scalp lacerations, cephalohematoma formation, subgaleal (subaponeurotic) hemorrhage, intracranial hemorrhage, retinal hemorrhage, and increased rates of hyperbilirubinemia (ACOG, 2015). With increased duration of vacuum application, exceeding 5 minutes, the incidence of cephalohematoma in neonates increases to 28% (ACOG, 2015; Bofill et al., 1997). The incidence of subarachnoid hemorrhage after vacuum is estimated to be 2.2 per 10,000 vacuum-assisted births; subdural hemorrhage, 8.0 per 10,000 vacuum-assisted births; and subgaleal hemorrhage, 59 per 10,000 vacuum-assisted births

(Doumouchtsis & Arulkumaran, 2006; Towner et al., 1999). Avoiding difficult vacuum-assisted births and avoiding the use of forceps to complete a failed vacuum will likely minimize the risk of subgaleal hemorrhages (ACOG, 2015). Vacuum devices should not be used to assist births prior to 34 weeks' gestation because of the increased risk of fetal intraventricular hemorrhage (ACOG, 2015).

There have been reports of neonatal subgaleal hematoma and intracranial hemorrhage after the vacuum extractor has been used. The FDA issued a warning letter to providers in 1998 alerting them to these risks (FDA, 1998). A subgaleal hematoma occurs when emissary veins are damaged and blood accumulates in the potential space between the galea aponeurotica (epicranial aponeurosis) and the periosteum of the skull (pericranium). Because the subaponeurotic space has neither containing membranes nor boundaries, the subgaleal hematoma may extend from the orbital ridges to the nape of the neck. This condition is dangerous because of the large potential space for blood accumulation and the possibility of life-threatening hemorrhage (FDA, 1998). Signs and symptoms of subgaleal hematoma include diffuse swelling of the fetal head and evidence of hypovolemic shock (e.g., pallor, hypotension, tachycardia, and increased respiration rate). These signs and symptoms may be present immediately after birth or may not become clinically apparent until several hours or up to a few days after birth (FDA, 1998). The swelling is usually diffuse, shifts when the newborn's head is repositioned, and indents easily on palpation. In some cases, the swelling is difficult to distinguish from edema of the scalp. On occasion, the hypotension and pallor are the dominant signs, while the cranial signs are unremarkable (FDA, 1998). Intracranial hemorrhage includes subdural, subarachnoid, intraventricular, and/or intraparenchymal hemorrhage. Signs and symptoms of intracranial hemorrhage include indications of cerebral irritation such as seizures, lethargy, obtundation, apnea, bulging fontanelle, poor feeding, increased irritability, bradycardia, and/or shock. These signs and symptoms are sometimes delayed until several hours after birth (FDA, 1998). Mortality with subgaleal hemorrhage approaches 25% (Doumouchtsis & Arulkumaran, 2006). A decrease in hematocrit that is greater than 25% of the baseline value at birth in association with significant birth asphyxia is the most important risk factor for newborn mortality (Doumouchtsis & Arulkumaran, 2006).

As with forceps, there should be a willingness to abandon attempts at a vacuum-assisted birth if satisfactory progress is not made (ACOG, 2015; SOGC, 2004). A unit policy about the use of vacuum devices and forceps, including a list of those credentialed in these procedures, facilitates safe maternal–fetal care

and avoids clinical controversies at the bedside if there is disagreement between healthcare professionals regarding the amount of pressure, length of application, number of pop-offs and pull attempts, and the need to abandon the procedure. Documentation of fetal station, the duration of application, pressure, number of pulls, and number of pop-offs should be included in the medical record by the provider performing the procedure. Neonatal care providers should be made aware of a vacuum-assisted vaginal birth in order to observe the neonate for potential complications (AAP & ACOG, 2017; ACOG, 2015).

The Nurse's Role

The healthcare provider who delivers the baby is responsible for explaining the procedure to the patient and discussing potential risks and benefits. Nurses have a role in educating and reassuring the woman when an assisted vaginal birth is anticipated. Maternal comfort level should be assessed prior to the application of forceps or a vacuum extractor. The urinary bladder may be emptied by the provider or the nurse to decrease the risk of trauma if necessary. If the FHR pattern is the indication for the immediate birth, then the nurse must be prepared for newborn resuscitation ensuring that appropriate equipment, supplies, and personnel are available. Nurses should also be aware of potential complications related to the use of forceps and vacuums and observe both the mother and baby for associated signs and symptoms. Some complications may be life-threatening for the mother and baby, so the prompt identification and initiation of appropriate treatment is necessary. Parents should be prepared for and shown any forceps or vacuum extraction marks on their baby and be reassured that they should disappear in a few days.

Complete and accurate medical record documentation of any adverse effects of operative vaginal birth is required. Responsibility for the documentation of station, the position prior to application of the vacuum or forceps, and the complete procedure rests with the provider who performs the operative birth. There is no need for nurses to enter duplicate data in the medical record. The nurse may indicate in the medical record that forceps- or vacuum-assisted birth was performed and any related nursing interventions.

Amnioinfusion

Amnioinfusion is the transcervical instillation of fluid into the amniotic cavity to alleviate umbilical cord compression resulting from decreased amniotic fluid or oligohydramnios (ACOG, 2006, 2010). Amnioinfusion is a reasonable and effective measure used to treat recurrent variable FHR decelerations during the first stage of labor that have not been resolved with maternal repositioning. Amnioinfusion has been found to significantly resolve patterns of "moderate" or "severe" variable decelerations but does not affect late decelerations or patterns with absent variability (Hofmeyr & Lawrie, 2012; Miño, Puertas, Miranda, & Herruzo, 1999; Miyazaki & Nevarez, 1985). For women with oligohydramnios and a normal FHR tracing, prophylactic amnioinfusion offers no benefit (Novikova, Hofmeyr, & Essilfie-Appiah, 2010). However, when amnioinfusion is used in women with recurrent variable decelerations, the number of cesarean births performed for FHR abnormalities is reduced

(Hofmeyr & Lawrie, 2012). Amnioinfusion is not recommended for treatment of meconium-stained amniotic fluid (AAP & ACOG, 2017). Because recurrent variable decelerations may be a sign of impending uterine rupture during a trial of labor after a cesarean (TOLAC), careful consideration should be made prior to amnioinfusion. Additional contraindications may include vaginal bleeding, placenta previa, uterine anomalies, and active infection such as human immunodeficiency virus or herpes virus (Simpson, 2015). An amnioinfusion procedure is presented in Display 14–11.

DISPLAY 14–11
Amnioinfusion

Amnioinfusion is a reasonable therapeutic option when there are recurrent variable decelerations during the first stage of labor that are unresolved with maternal position changes. Ruptured membranes are required.

An institutional protocol may include the following:
- Contraindications (e.g., vaginal bleeding, uterine anomalies, active infections such as HIV or herpes, impending birth, trial of labor after a cesarean)
- Who can perform amnioinfusion?
- Who can insert the intrauterine pressure catheter?
- What type of fluid may be used (normal saline or lactated Ringer's solution)?
- What instillation method may be used (gravity flow or infusion pump)?
- What infusion techniques may be used (bolus, continuous, or a combination of both)?
- When and why the procedure should be altered (e.g., loss of large amount of fluid resulting from position change or coughing, increased uterine resting tone, reappearance of recurrent variable decelerations, or no fluid return)?

General guidelines for the procedure are as follows:
- The amnioinfusion procedure and the indication should be explained to the woman and her support persons prior to initiation.
- During amnioinfusion, room temperature normal saline or lactated Ringer's solution is infused into the uterus transcervically via an intrauterine pressure catheter.
- The initial bolus is usually 250 to 500 mL given over a 20- to 30-min period using either an infusion pump or gravity flow. Both methods are appropriate and seem to be equally efficacious.
- Some protocols allow for a continuous infusion of 2 to 3 mL/min (120 to 180 mL/hr) after the bolus until resolution of the variable decelerations. Usually, the maximum amount of fluid infused is 1,000 mL.
- If recurrent variable decelerations have not resolved after the infusion of 800 to 1,000 mL, the infusion may be discontinued and alternative approaches used.
- During bolus of the infusion and maintenance rate, the approximate amount of fluid returning should be noted and recorded to avoid iatrogenic polyhydramnios.

- An assessment of fluid return can be accomplished by weighing the underpads (1 mL of fluid equals = 1 g of weight).
- As a general consideration, if 250 mL has infused with no return, the amnioinfusion is discontinued until the fluid has returned.
- Overdistention is more likely when the presenting part obstructs flow, thus releasing the fluid by gently elevating the presenting part may be a successful intervention.
- A dual-lumen intrauterine catheter is preferred so that an estimate of uterine resting tone can be assessed during the infusion.
- The uterine resting tone may appear higher than normal during the procedure (from 25 to 40 mm Hg). If there is a concern about an elevated uterine resting tone (>40 mm Hg), temporarily discontinue the infusion to attempt a more accurate assessment. If the uterine resting tone exceeds 25 mm Hg while the infusion is temporarily discontinued for an assessment of uterine resting tone, consider discontinuing the infusion.
- Warming of the solution may not be necessary for full-term fetuses but may be appropriate for preterm or growth-restricted fetuses. Fetal bradycardia may occur if the solution is colder than room temperature and/or is infused too rapidly. Some providers prefer to warm the solution to body temperature. If the solution is warmed, acceptable temperatures are 93° to 96°F (34° to 37°C). The safest method to warm the solution is by use of an electronic blood/fluid warmer. Microwaves and other types of warming techniques should not be used to heat the solution.
- Assessment and documentation
  - Contraction intensity and frequency should be continually assessed during the procedure.
  - In addition to assessments appropriate for the first stage of labor, additional assessments may include the following:
    - Fundal height and leakage of fluids
    - Amount, color, and odor of fluid leaking from vagina
    - Fetal response such as resolution of the variable decelerations
  - Documentation may include the maternal and fetal response; uterine resting tone; fluid output; duration of the procedure; and the type, rate, and amount of solution infused.

Adapted from Simpson, K. R. (2015). Physiologic interventions for fetal heart rate patterns. In A. Lyndon & L. U. Ali (Eds.). *AWHONN's fetal heart monitoring principles and practices* (5th ed.) Dubuque, IA: Kendall Hunt.

VAGINAL BIRTH

Although cesarean birth is at an all-time high in the United States, most (68.1%) women have a vaginal birth (Hamilton, Martin, Osterman, & Rossen, 2019). The cesarean birth rate was 31.9% in 2018; the low-risk cesarean rate decreased to 25.9% (the last year for which these data are available). Routine episiotomy is no longer recommended as a result of the evidence of risks of perineal trauma and its associated sequelae, and its use has greatly decreased over the past decade (ACOG, 2018). Healthy women should be allowed and encouraged to give birth in an upright (rather than supine lithotomy) position with minimal intervention. The woman should be allowed and encouraged to have family and support persons at her birth as per her desire in the context of space limitations and clinical conditions (AAP & ACOG, 2017). The birth process should be conducted as a celebration of a natural life event rather than a medical intervention as much as possible based on the clinical situation. At least one registered nurse should attend every birth to assist the healthcare provider delivering the baby and assess maternal–fetal status. At least one additional person attending the birth should be solely responsible for the newborn and capable of initiating resuscitation including the administration of positive-pressure ventilation and assisting with chest compressions (AAP & AHA, 2016). Either this person or an additional person immediately available to the birthing area should have the additional skills required to perform a complete resuscitation, including endotracheal intubation and the administration of medications (AAP & AHA, 2016). Having someone on-call (either at home or in a remote area of the hospital) for newborn resuscitation is not sufficient (AAP & AHA, 2016). When resuscitation is needed, it must be initiated without delay (AAP & AHA, 2016). If the birth is anticipated to be high risk (e.g., meconium staining of the amniotic fluid), at least two persons should be present solely to manage the neonate: one with completed resuscitation skills and one or more to assist (AAP & AHA, 2016). A comprehensive discussion of the newborn's transition to extrauterine life and neonatal resuscitation is presented in Chapter 18.

CESAREAN BIRTH

Incidence

According to the latest data available in 2018, the cesarean birth rate in the United States was 31.9% (Hamilton et al., 2019). Labor dystocia (i.e., slow abnormal progression of labor) is the leading indication for primary cesarean birth in the United States (AAP & ACOG, 2017; ACOG & SMFM, 2014). In response to cumulative data on average length of labor and concern about the rising cesarean birth rate, an expert workshop sponsored by the NICHD, SMFM, and ACOG was held to review evidence and develop strategies for preventing cesarean birth in low-risk women (Spong et al., 2012). In 2014, ACOG and SMFM published guidelines for labor management with the intent of encouraging clinicians to allow more time for labor progress within the context of careful assessment of fetal well-being (ACOG & SMFM, 2014). The goal was to potentially decrease risk of primary cesarean births. The Alliance for Innovation on Maternal Health (2017) Program of the Council on Patient Safety in Women's Health Care, which has partnered with most of the leading professional organizations for maternal health in the United States including AWHONN, ACNM, ACOG, SMFM, the American Academy of Family Physicians, and the Health Resources and Services Administration Maternal and Child Health Bureau of the United States Department of Health and Human Services, is a coalition working to collectively promote safe maternity care for all women through maternal patient safety research, programs and tools, education, dissemination, and promotion of a culture of respect transparency and accountability. They have published a patient safety bundle on reducing primary cesarean birth that includes evidence on what to expect for normal labor process (Lagrew et al., 2018). Free access to the bundle is available at https://safehealthcareforeverywoman.org/patient-safety-bundles/safe-reduction-of-primary-cesarean-birth/. BirthTOOLS is an initiative sponsored by ACNM (2015b) to help clinicians and birthing hospitals work together to reduce the cesarean birth rate. The California Maternal Quality Care Collaborative has a toolkit on supporting vaginal birth preventing primary cesareans (Smith, Peterson, Lagrew, & Main, 2016). Free access to this toolkit is available at https://www.cmqcc.org/VBirthToolkit. These efforts can be successful in reducing cesarean birth rates for low-risk nulliparous women (Main et al., 2019).

Nurses have an important influence on whether a woman has a cesarean or vaginal birth. In one study, nurses reported the following aspects of care that they routinely offered to avoid a cesarean birth: emotional support, labor support (including ambulation, frequent repositioning, hydrotherapy, peanut ball, birthing ball, passive fetal descent in second-stage labor, appropriate titration of oxytocin for induction and augmentation of labor), sharing adequate and accurate information about what to expect, advocating on behalf of women, preparing and encouraging women to advocate for themselves, and communicating with physician colleagues on positive aspects of labor progress (Simpson & Lyndon, 2017b). More data are needed to quantify the effect of nursing care on birth outcomes.

The risk of cesarean birth is not increased with the initiation of early neuraxial analgesia when compared to IV opioid analgesia (ACOG, 2019b). Cesarean births are associated with significant morbidity such as blood transfusion, ruptured uterus, unplanned hysterectomy, and admission to the intensive care unit as well as increased risk for future pregnancies such placenta previa, placenta accreta, hysterectomy, and mortality when compared to vaginal births (ACOG & SMFM, 2014; Curtin, Gregory, Korst, & Uddin, 2015; Korb, Goffinet, Seco, Chevret, & Deneux-Tharaux, 2019; National Institutes of Health [NIH], 2010; Sargent & Caughey, 2017).

Perioperative Standards and Guidelines for Cesarean Birth

Perioperative perinatal nursing incorporates the skills of the specialties of obstetrics, surgery, and post-anesthesia care to provide comprehensive care to women who have a cesarean birth. Patients with the same health status and condition should receive a comparable level of quality care regardless of where that care is provided within the hospital. This standard ensures that women having cesarean births with regional or general anesthesia should have perioperative care consistent with those patients who have had general surgical procedures. It is important to distinguish between the concepts of comparable care and equivalent care. Comparable care to that which is provided in the main hospital surgical department is recommended (ASA, 2016); however, equivalent care is not required. The special needs of obstetric patients, their babies, and their families must be considered when planning care and designing protocols and clinical practices. For example, care during cesarean birth should include the woman's support person and family. In the main hospital surgical suite, family members are rarely allowed to be with patients during surgery. However, women having cesarean birth should be allowed to have a support person with them prior to and during the procedure and the recovery period. Some facilities allow more than one support person. Skin-to-skin contact between the healthy mother and baby is recommended after birth while the patient is in the surgical suite (AWHONN, 2016). Patient desires and patient safety should guide practice. During the recovery period, the newborn should be allowed to stay with the mother as long as the condition of the mother and baby are stable. Support should be provided so that breast-feeding can be initiated as soon as possible if the woman has chosen to breast-feed (AAP & ACOG, 2017).

When unplanned cesarean birth occurs, and the decision is made to proceed, the surgical team should be notified so they can begin preparations. In some facilities, this will involve calling in a surgical team whose members are not in-house, while other facilities maintain a full surgical team around the clock. A full surgical team includes a surgeon, anesthesia provider, surgical first assistant, scrub tech, circulating nurse, and person whose sole responsibility is for potential neonatal resuscitation. All hospitals offering labor and birth services should be equipped to perform an emergency cesarean birth (AAP & ACOG, 2017). In general, the consensus has been that hospitals should have the capacity of beginning a cesarean birth within 30 minutes of the decision to operate (AAP & ACOG, 2017). However, the scientific evidence to support this threshold is lacking (AAP & ACOG, 2017; ACOG, 2010). The decision-to-incision interval should be based on the timing that best incorporates maternal and fetal risks and benefits (AAP & ACOG, 2017; ACOG, 2010). Some high-risk conditions (e.g., morbid obesity, eclampsia, cardiopulmonary compromise, hemorrhage) may require maternal stabilization time before performing emergent cesarean birth (AAP & ACOG, 2017; ACOG, 2010). On the other hand, some clinical situations require more expeditious birth because they can directly or indirectly cause fetal death or other adverse maternal–fetal outcomes. These include hemorrhage from placenta previa, placental abruption, umbilical cord prolapse, uterine rupture, and an abnormal EFM tracing (AAP & ACOG, 2017; ACOG, 2010; Silver, 2007).

When the indication for cesarean is an abnormal (category III) EFM tracing, preparation often requires an assessment of several logistic issues depending on the setting and clinical circumstances (ACOG, 2010) (Display 14–12). Sterile materials and supplies needed for emergent cesarean birth are kept sealed but properly arranged and available so that the instrument table can be made ready at once for an obstetric emergency (AAP & ACOG, 2017). Whenever possible, a surgical suite should be kept available for emergent cases. If keeping at least one surgical suite continuously available to handle emergencies is not possible, at a minimum, elective or nonemergent cases should be staggered to allow rapid readiness if an emergency occurs that requires expeditious cesarean birth.

Plans should be in place to call in backup team members, such as surgeons and anesthesia providers, when those providers primarily responsible for covering the service for obstetric emergencies are not readily available. A list of emergency backup team members and the quickest method to reach each of them should be available at all times to the labor and delivery charge nurse. Access to direct telephone numbers of those on-call is more likely to result in the fastest communication rather than beepers, which require additional time to send the signal and await response. If the attending physician is notified of an obstetric emergency likely to require emergent cesarean birth while not in-house, including, but not limited to, fetal bradycardia, umbilical cord prolapse, significant bleeding, suspected placental abruption, or uterine rupture, and he or she

DISPLAY 14-12

Potential Logistical Considerations in Preparation for Operative Birth in the Context of an Abnormal (Category III) Fetal Heart Rate Tracing

- Obtain informed consent from the woman (verbal or written as feasible).
- Provide information to the woman and her support person/family about what is being recommended and the urgency based on maternal and/or fetal status.
- Assemble the surgical team (surgeon, anesthesia personnel, scrub technician, circulating nurse, and baby nurse).
- Assess transit time to the surgical suite and location for operative birth.
- Ensure IV access.
- Review the status of laboratory tests (e.g., complete blood type and screen) and assess the need for availability of blood products.
- Assess the need for preoperative placement of an indwelling Foley catheter and insert if feasible.
- Assemble personnel for neonatal resuscitation, notify members of the neonatal team in-house or on-call, and request their immediate attendance at the birth.

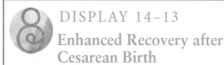

DISPLAY 14-13

Enhanced Recovery after Cesarean Birth

Preoperative Care (Wilson et al., 2018)
The preoperative pathway begins up to 60 minutes before incision, where allowed. If the cesarean is an emergency, some aspects of the pathway may be done postoperatively. Ideally, teaching the woman and her family or support persons about the entire care process, including her role as a team member, should occur preoperatively. When possible, the pregnant woman should have nothing to eat for at least 6 hours before surgery. Clear fluids are encouraged up until 2 hours before surgery, including oral carbohydrate fluid drinks in women without diabetes. All women should be premedicated with an antacid and histamine H2 receptor antagonist.

Intraoperative Care (Caughey et al., 2018)
The intraoperative care pathway focuses on the period in the operating room (OR). The first recommendation is for intravenous (IV) cephalosporin antibiotics to be given 60 minutes before incision for all women to decrease risk of surgical site infection, with the addition of azithromycin advised for women who were in labor or with ruptured membranes. For skin preparation, chlorhexidine-alcohol is preferred over povidone-iodine; however, vaginal cleansing with povidone-iodine may be protective against surgical site infection. Avoidance of hypothermia via temperature monitoring and treatment with forced air warming, IV fluid warming, and increasing OR temperature are strong recommendations. Ensuring euvolemia both peri- and intraoperative have shown improvement in maternal and fetal outcomes after cesarean birth. Neonatal care is covered with recommendations to delay cord clamping (1 minute at term and at least 30 seconds for preterm), ensure temperature management to maintain the newborn between 36.5°C and 37.5°C, resuscitation with room air over oxygen supplementation, and ability to initiate immediate neonatal resuscitation in all settings performing cesareans.

Postoperative Care (Macones et al., 2019)
The postoperative pathway covers avoidance of postoperative nausea and vomiting through fluid and blood pressure management, with addition of lower limb compression, which may provide benefit in length of stay and patient satisfaction. Gum chewing may provide benefit but is likely redundant if early feeding (a regular diet within 2 hours after surgery) is implemented. Management and tight control of blood glucose are important to aid in wound healing. Regular and scheduled use of nonsteroidal anti-inflammatory medications paired with acetaminophen can help control pain while limiting need for opiates. Early ambulation, removal of any urinary catheter placed during surgery immediately after, and use of pneumatic compression stockings can help decrease complications.

Adapted from Killion, M. M. (2019). Enhanced recovery after cesarean birth. *MCN: The American Journal of Maternal Child Nursing, 44*(6), 296. doi:10.1097/NMC.0000000000000572

orders preparations for the surgery, hospital policy should allow preparations to begin prior to the arrival of the attending physician. Hospital policies requiring that the physician be in-house to order preparations for emergent cesarean birth or to move the patient to the surgical suite can delay the process and potentially contribute to an adverse maternal or fetal outcome. In July 2004, The Joint Commission, in their Sentinel Event Alert *Preventing Infant Death and Injury during Delivery*, recommended conducting periodic drills for emergent cesarean birth (The Joint Commission, 2004). Similar recommendations for drills in emergent situations were offered by ACOG (2011a, 2014a).

Comprehensive information about perioperative care of the woman having a cesarean birth can be found in the evidence-based clinical practice guideline *Perioperative Care of the Pregnant Woman* (AWHONN, 2019c). See Table 14–6 for a summary of perioperative, intraoperative, and postoperative care of the pregnant woman (AWHONN, 2019c).

Enhanced recovery after surgery (ERAS) pathways using standardized perioperative care have been associated with positive postoperative outcomes including decreased length of stay, surgical complications, readmissions, and costs (Caughey et al., 2018; Macones et al., 2019; Wilson et al., 2018). These principles are being applied to care for women having cesarean birth in some institutions (Killion, 2019). See Display 14–13 for a summary of ERAS procedures for cesarean birth.

Detailed clinical practice recommendations, referenced rationales, and ratings supporting information on perioperative care summarized here are presented in the Guideline.

Preoperative care	Intraoperative care	Postoperative care
Family Support	**Maternal Positioning during Surgery**	**Immediate Post-anesthesia Care and Postpartum Assessment**
1. Individualize care to meet the needs of the woman and her family. Include the family members and support persons in decisions, as applicable.	1. Maintain maternal uterine displacement using one or more of the following approaches:	1. Assess maternal status according to facility and professional organization guidelines. Assessments include but may not be limited to the following:
• Allow at least one support person to be present during the entire surgical time frame.	a. Use a 12-cm (4.7-inch) wedge under the right lumbar region, above the iliac crest, and below the lower costal region to achieve a 12- to 15-degree lateral tilt.	• Level of consciousness
Assessment for Pain Management	b. Position the woman in a left lateral position with a wedge under the right pelvis. Use a wedge, pillow, or rolled blanket to achieve a 12- to 15-degree tilt.	• Blood pressure and pulse (every 15 min for 2 hr)
1. Screen for anesthesia and analgesia alternatives for women diagnosed with chronic pain, opioid use disorder, or opioid dependence.	c. Tilt the OR bed 15 to 45 degrees to the left.	• Color
2. Consider the use of intravenous (IV) paracetamol (acetaminophen) prior to anesthesia whenever possible.	**Fetal Heart Monitoring**	• Oxygen saturation
Prevention of Infection	1. For scheduled cesarean births, document fetal status (baseline heart rate, presence of regular vs. irregular rhythm, presence of increases or decreases in rate) prior to the scheduled procedure and according to facility guidelines.	• Cardiac monitoring for rate and rhythm
A. Group B Streptococcus Prophylaxis	2. If electronic fetal monitoring is being used as the method of fetal surveillance for the laboring woman transitioning to a surgical birth, continue monitoring until the abdominal preparation begins.	• Pain
1. Collaborate with the primary health care provider to determine the need for intrapartum prophylaxis in the case of unplanned cesarean or planned cesarean with rupture of membranes.	3. If a fetal spiral electrode is being used to monitor the fetal heart rate for the laboring woman transitioning to a surgical birth, the electrode should remain in place until the abdominal preparation is completed and should be removed just prior to the start of the surgical procedure.	• Dressing condition
B. Vaginal cleansing		• Intake and output
1. Consider vaginal cleansing immediately prior to the cesarean birth, especially for women with ruptured membranes and those who have labored prior to surgery.	**Skin Antisepsis**	• Sensory and motor function
C. Vaginal seeding	1. Assess women having **scheduled** cesarean birth for preoperative skin cleansing by bathing or showering.	• Temperature at least hourly; if hypothermic, every 15 min
1. Facilitate a discussion with the healthcare provider for women requesting vaginal seeding.	2. Cleanse the lower abdomen to clear the surgical site of soil, debris, and exudate if needed.	• Fundal height and lochia
D. Antibiotic prophylaxis	a. Consider using preoperative skin cleansing wipes prior to OR transfer.	2. Assess for side effects of anesthesia and provide interventions, if indicated.
1. Identify women at higher risk for postoperative infection. Administer prophylactic antibiotics prior to surgery according to provider orders.	3. Use a safe, effective, antiseptic agent for preoperative abdominal preparation according to healthcare provider orders and facility guidelines. Ideally, alcohol-based products should be used.	3. Initiate interventions according to facility protocols and provider orders to prevent potential gastrointestinal complications in the postoperative period.
a. Ideally, the administration of prophylactic antibiotics should occur 60 min prior to skin incision whenever possible.	4. Do not remove hair unless it will interfere with the surgical incision. If hair must be removed:	a. Early oral nutrition within 2 hr of birth
• Otherwise, antibiotics may be administered during the procedure, after cord clamp, or immediately after the procedure.	a. Use hair clippers before moving into the operative suite.	b. Gum chewing during the first 12 hr of the postoperative period
b. The antibiotic of choice is generally a first-generation cephalosporin, such as cefazolin. For women with penicillin and cephalosporin allergy, alternative antibiotics may include clindamycin with an aminoglycoside.	b. In an emergency situation, wet clipping with the use of a suction device is recommended.	4. Use a facility-approved scoring system to determine the appropriate timing for transition from phase I to phase II post-anesthesia care. Examples of scoring systems include the Aldrete Scoring System, the Modified Aldrete Scoring System, and the Post Anesthetic Discharge Scoring System.
• Some providers may use azithromycin in addition to cefazolin to extend the coverage.	5. Implement safety measures to protect the skin and prevent injury from skin preparation agents.	**Skin-to-Skin (STS) Contact and Breastfeeding Support**
c. Additional doses of antibiotics or higher doses of antibiotics may be indicated in certain conditions, such as procedures lasting longer than 3 to 4 hr, women with obesity, and excessive blood loss.	a. Protect sheets, padding, and positioning equipment from dripping or pooling of antiseptic agents.	1. Place all full-term and late-preterm, stable newborns in immediate STS contact.
	b. Remove excess linens if pooling is noted.	• If the mother is unable to participate in STS contact, place the newborn STS with the father or partner if feasible.
	c. Allow skin antiseptics to dry completely and fumes to dissipate before application of surgical drapes.	2. Ensure proper maternal and newborn positioning as well as appropriate staff availability, during STS contact.
	d. Remove antiseptic soaked materials from the room. Alcohol-based products are flammable and present a fire hazard.	3. Ensure appropriately skilled healthcare personnel are available to monitor the mother and newborn during STS contact throughout the recovery period.
		4. Encourage uninterrupted STS contact for at least the first hour of life or until completion of the first breastfeeding.
		• When possible, delay routine care practices until the completion of the first STS session.
		5. Recognize that STS contact facilitates newborn feeding behaviors including rooting and sucking.
		• Ideally, breastfeeding should occur within the first hour of life.
		6. Be aware that cesarean birth is a risk factor for failed breastfeeding.

Hypothermia Prevention

1. Recognize that intraoperative hypothermia may lead to an increase in maternal morbidity.
2. Individualize active (conductive or convective) and passive (insulative) hypothermia prevention measures for the pregnant woman prior to the administration of anesthesia and throughout surgery whenever possible.
   a. Establish normothermia prior to transferring the woman to the operative suite.
   b. Consider the use of forced air warming devices or under-body carbon polymer mattresses.
   c. Apply additional blankets or warmed blankets for maternal comfort.
   d. Administer warmed IV fluids and boluses, whenever possible. (Inline IV fluid warming may also be considered.)
   e. Maintain operating room (OR) temperature at 20 to 23°C (68 to 73°F).

Aspiration Prophylaxis

1. Assess the woman for conditions that may increase the risk of aspiration.
2. Document the time of the woman's last solid and liquid intake.
   a. Last solid intake should be 6 to 8 hours prior to the procedure.
   b. Last liquids should be clear liquids only up to 2 hours prior to the procedure.
3. Administer medications to reduce the risk of aspiration according to anesthesia orders and facility guidelines.

Anesthesia

A. Practice considerations

1. Ensure that basic and advanced life support equipment and appropriately trained personnel are available to assist the anesthesia care provider as indicated.
2. Obtain baseline vital signs prior to the initiation of anesthesia, including temperature, pulse, respiratory rate, blood pressure, and baseline pulse oximeter reading.
3. Monitor and document the fetal heart rate before and after the administration of regional anesthesia.
   • Monitor fetal heart tones during the initiation of anesthesia as indicated and whenever possible.
4. The anesthesia care provider should conduct a history and physical examination prior to the administration of anesthesia.
5. Facilitate preoperative blood work, if indicated and according to anesthesia provider orders and facility guidelines.

B. Regional anesthesia

1. Identify women at risk for hypotension following the initiation of regional anesthesia.
2. Administer preload or coload or both according to anesthesia provider orders and facility guidelines.
   a. Administer preload approximately 20 to 30 min prior to initiation of anesthesia to ensure optimal prophylactic efficacy.
   b. Administer coload immediately after the initiation of regional anesthesia.
3. Assist the mother into the appropriate position for administration of regional anesthesia, which may include sitting, pendant position, or side lying with head elevation.
4. Conduct a time-out prior to the administration of anesthesia and document completion of the time-out.
5. Assess for complications after regional anesthesia has been administered and throughout the surgical procedure.
6. If indicated, administer medications to improve spinal-induced hypotension according to anesthesia provider orders and facility guidelines. Medications may include ephedrine, phenylephrine, or 5-HT3 receptor antagonist.

Newborn Safety

1. An appropriately trained healthcare provider should be present during all initial STS contacts for the first 2 hr of life, with frequent observation of mother and newborn.
2. Implement measures to recognize and prevent newborn falls.
3. Be aware of risk factors leading to newborn falls or drops, such as the following:
   • Cesarean birth
   • Maternal use of pain medication within 4 hr
   • Second or third postpartum night, specifically around mid-night to early morning hours
   • Breastfeeding
4. Consider the use of a falls risk assessment tool relevant to the newborn population.

Urinary Catheters and Bladder Care

1. If an indwelling urinary catheter was used, remove it in a timely manner during the postoperative period according to assessment of the woman's condition, healthcare provider orders, and facility guidelines.
   • Ideally, the urinary catheter should be removed in the immediate postoperative period.
2. Assess for urinary output and bladder distension at least every 4 to 6 hr after removal of the urinary catheter.
   • Encourage the woman to void spontaneously.
   • Consider the use of a bladder scanner to detect bladder distension.
3. Assess for potential damage to the bladder or ureters demonstrated by inability to void.

(continued)

TABLE 14–6. Quick Care Guide: Perioperative Care of the Pregnant Woman (Continued)

Preoperative care	Intraoperative care	Postoperative care

Urinary Catheters and Bladder Care
1. Recognize the benefits and risks to the use of indwelling urinary catheters during cesarean.
2. Empty urinary bladder prior to cesarean while considering maternal preference and provider order. Methods may include the following:
  • Indwelling urinary catheter
  • Ambulation to bathroom
  • Intermittent catheterization prior to surgery
 	
Safe Staffing for Cesarean Birth
1. Implement safe registered nurse (RN)-to-patient staffing ratios when providing care to women having cesarean birth including:
a. One RN per patient in the role of the circulator in the OR with no other responsibilities.
b. Two RNs in attendance at every cesarean birth in the following roles:
  • One RN for the mother (circulating nurse)
  • One RN for the newborn (newborn nurse)
  • In the case of multiples, one RN for each newborn
c. Two RNs should be present during the initial admission to the post-anesthesia care unit. One RN should be assigned solely to the care of the mother and one RN should be assigned solely to the care of each newborn until the critical elements for the mother and the newborn have been met.
 	
Note: The mother and newborn should be under continuous observation for at least the first 2 hours and longer if complications to either are encountered.
	C. General Anesthesia
	1. Recognize potential complications associated with general anesthesia for pregnant women.
	2. Assist with proper positioning for intubation. The ramped position may be indicated for the woman with obesity.
	3. Assist with cricoid pressure as requested by the anesthesia care provider.
	4. In the case of failed intubation, assist the anesthesia care provider with laryngeal mask ventilation, if indicated.
	
	Urinary Catheters and Bladder Care
	1. Recognize that damage to the bladder or ureters may occur during surgery.
	2. Assist with diagnostic equipment used in detection of injury, if indicated, which may include cystoscopy or the instillation of methylene blue/indigo carmine.
		Pain Management
		1. Individualize pain management based on preoperative pain management plan, maternal assessment, healthcare provider orders, and facility guidelines.
		2. Provide pharmacologic pain relief measures according to obstetric healthcare provider orders, maternal request, and maternal history.
		3. Use an individualized multimodal approach to pain management in the postoperative period according to provider orders.
		a. Encourage the use of scheduled nonsteroidal anti-inflammatory drugs (NSAIDs) and acetaminophen postoperatively.
		b. Administer opioids sparingly for breakthrough pain and as indicated based on pain scores.
		4. Recognize that standard pain protocols may not be sufficient for some women with comorbidities, including anxiety, history of chronic pain, and opioid use disorders.
		5. Use nonpharmacologic interventions in conjunction with pharmacologic agents whenever possible.
		6. Be aware of maternal and fetal risks associated with pain management medications.
		a. Monitor for side effects related to administration of IV and intrathecal opioids.
		b. Ensure analgesics are safe for women who choose to breastfeed.
		c. Increase staffing as needed to provide safe monitoring for women using opioid analgesics in the postpartum period.

Adapted from Association of Women's Health, Obstetric and Neonatal Nurses. (2019c). *Perioperative care of the pregnant woman* (Evidence-Based Clinical Practice Guideline, 2nd ed.). Washington, DC: Author.

Advanced cardiac life support (ACLS) competence validation for perinatal nurses who provide post-anesthesia care for obstetric patients is not required (AWHONN, 2017). However, each hospital must ensure that teams capable of providing ACLS care (e.g., a code team) and the means to provide invasive monitoring or extensive ventilatory support to obstetric patients are available at all times (AWHONN, 2017). Because the need to implement ACLS skills during the care of obstetric patients is rare, perinatal nurses lack opportunity to use ACLS knowledge and skills and, therefore, to maintain proficiency (AWHONN, 2019c). Mobilizing the code team when maternal resuscitation requiring ACLS care is needed during the perioperative period may be more appropriate (AWHONN, 2017, 2019c).

Phase I post-anesthesia recovery focuses on providing post-anesthesia nursing in the immediate post-anesthesia period, transitioning to phase II in the inpatient setting, or to an intensive care setting for continued care (AWHONN, 2019c). Basic life-sustaining needs are of the highest priority; therefore, constant vigilance is required during phase I (AWHONN, 2019c). It is important to consider that phase I post-anesthesia recovery is a level of care rather than a location or time frame. During postoperative recovery, the nurse-to-patient ratio on the perinatal unit should be comparable to that of the main hospital post-anesthesia care unit (PACU). Phase I recovery for general surgical patients usually occurs in the PACU; however, obstetric patients may be cared for during phase I in a labor and delivery room or a labor/delivery/recovery/postpartum room if there is the availability of continuous one nurse–to–one woman care and one nurse for the baby until the critical elements are met when the baby remains with the mother (AWHONN, 2010).

Critical elements for the mother's post-anesthesia care after cesarean birth before the mother's nurse accepts the baby as part of the patient care assignment are defined as (1) the report has been received from the anesthesia provider, questions answered, and the transfer of care has taken place; (2) the woman is conscious, with adequate respiratory status; (3) the initial assessment is completed and documented; and (4) the woman is hemodynamically stable (AWHONN, 2010). Critical elements for the baby's care before the mother's nurse accepts the baby as part of the patient care assignment are defined as (1) the report has been received from the baby nurse, questions answered, and the transfer of care has taken place; (2) the initial assessment and care are completed and documented; (3) identification bracelets have been applied; and (4) the baby's condition is stable (AWHONN, 2010). Post-anesthesia recovery care for the mother is as follows: BP levels and maternal pulse should be monitored every 15 minutes for 2 hours and more frequently and of longer duration if complications are encountered; maternal postpartum observation should be designed for the timely identification of excessive blood loss, including hypotension and tachycardia; the amount of vaginal bleeding should be evaluated continuously and the uterine fundus identified, massaged, and assessed for size and degree of contraction; and there should be timely response to changes in maternal vital signs and clinical condition as this is critical to patient safety (AAP & ACOG, 2017; AWHONN, 2010). Care for the baby at birth is as follows: the baby's airway should be cleared, tactile stimulation provided, and respirations and heart rate evaluated. An Apgar score should be determined at 1 minute and 5 minutes after birth. If the 5-minute Apgar score is less than 7, additional scores should be assigned every 5 minutes for up to 20 minutes. Temperature, heart and respiratory rates, skin color, adequacy of peripheral circulation, type of respiration, level of consciousness, tone, and activity should be monitored and recorded at least once every 30 minutes until the newborn's condition has remained stable for 2 hours (AAP & ACOG, 2017). If the mother has chosen to breast-feed, the baby should be placed at the breast within the first hour after birth (AAP & ACOG, 2017). The mother and baby should be monitored continuously by the nurse during the immediate recovery period (AWHONN, 2010; Feldman-Winter & Goldsmith, 2016).

A PACU discharge scoring tool is helpful in conducting a systematic assessment and determining readiness for discharge from post-anesthesia care (AWHONN, 2019c). Whenever a patient is transferred from one level of care to another level of care requiring a change in caregivers, communicate all pertinent information to the next caregiver. The handoff should be interactive, encouraging questions, with limited interruptions and include a process for verification and an opportunity to review all relevant patient data (ACOG, 2012a). Transfers or patient handoffs present a risk of missing key information with the potential to adversely affect patient status; thus, development of a checklist for important clinical content to be included in the hand-off report can be beneficial (Simpson, 2005). Suggested components of a comprehensive transfer report are included in Display 14–14. These components may vary based on the type of care model. In some perinatal units, discharge from post-anesthesia care will not result in the physical transfer of the patient; rather, care will continue in the same room. Transfer of care from one caregiver to another may or may not occur at this time. In other units, discharge from post-anesthesia care will result in a physical transfer of the patient from the obstetric PACU to the mother–baby unit, and care will be transferred to another nurse.

DISPLAY 14–14

Suggested Components of Communication Handoff during Transfer from Post-Anesthesia Recovery Care to Postpartum Care for Women after Cesarean Birth

- Vital signs
- Level of consciousness
- Muscular strength and ability to move lower extremities
- Allergies
- Condition of the operative site and dressing
- Fundal height
- Lochia characteristics and amount
- Condition of the perineum if vaginal birth was attempted
- Location and patency of any tubes and/or drains including indwelling urinary catheter
- Intake and output (e.g., IV fluids, oral fluids, estimated blood loss, urinary output)
- Type of analgesia/anesthesia and response
- Medications given and response to those medications (e.g., antibiotics, narcotics)
- Venous thromboembolism prophylaxis
- Pain level, interventions for pain, and response to those interventions
- Nausea and vomiting
- Tests ordered with pertinent results, if available
- Initiation of breastfeeding and quality of first breastfeeding experience (e.g., successful latch-on; mother's confidence), if applicable
- Status of the baby (e.g., admitted to special care nursery or neonatal intensive care unit and preliminary diagnosis)
- Condition of the baby during skin-to-skin contact if applicable
- Psychosocial status
- Involvement of the significant other and family
- Plans for immediate care of the baby (e.g., rooming-in if support person will be continuously available to assist the mother during the first few hours)
- If the baby is being relinquished for adoption, the mother's wishes for handling newborn care
- If the mother does not want any publicity or it to be known that she is a patient at the hospital or has given birth
- Discharge orders
- Attending midwife or physician

Supporting Mother–Baby Attachment after Cesarean Birth

Whether anticipated or unexpected, the need for surgical birth increases the family's anxiety, places additional strain on the maternal–newborn relationship, makes postpartum recovery more difficult for the woman and family, and creates a need for accepting the altered birth experience. Women who give birth via cesarean have special needs for information, the presence of the partner throughout cesarean birth, and sustained contact

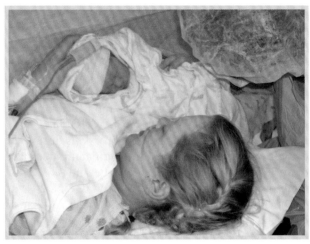

FIGURE 14–20. Promoting mother–baby attachment during cesarean birth.

with their newborn (Fig. 14–20). An unplanned emergent cesarean birth can result in significant stress for the new mother. Continuity in caregivers, choice where possible, and control over specific aspects of care can reduce stress. To facilitate a positive birth experience and attachment to the newborn, consideration should be given to the ongoing attention of the family's understanding of cesarean birth, ways to maintain the father or support person's presence throughout the birth experience, and early and sustained contact with the newborn (Fig. 14–21). Support and encouragement in the surgical suite and immediately postpartum are key indicators of breastfeeding success after a cesarean birth. Encouraging sibling interaction promotes the attachment and integration of the baby into the family (Fig. 14–22). See Chapter 17 for details of immediate postoperative care.

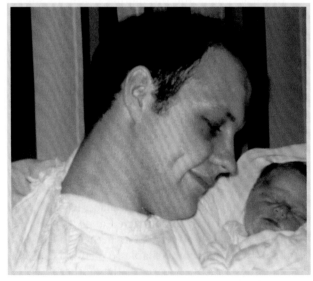

FIGURE 14–21. Promoting father involvement.

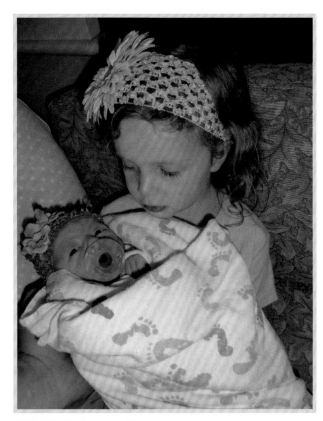

FIGURE 14–22. Promoting sibling attachment.

Vaginal Birth after Previous Cesarean

A TOLAC offers these women the opportunity of having a VBAC. The VBAC rate (VBACs per 100 women with a prior cesarean birth) increased from approximately 5% in 1985 to a high of 28.3% by 1996, at which time the total cesarean birth rate dipped to 20.7%. Over the next 10 years, the VBAC rate fell dramatically to 8.5% in 2006, while the overall cesarean birth rate increased to 32.8% (Hamilton et al., 2011; Martin et al., 2012). The rate of cesarean birth for 2018 was 31.9% (Hamilton et al., 2019). The steep decline in the VBAC rate corresponds with an increasing repeat cesarean birth rate. Once a woman has a cesarean, she has approximately a 90% chance of having a cesarean for her next birth (Hamilton et al. 2012; Rhoades & Cahill, 2017). The continuing decrease in the VBAC rate, and subsequent increase in the repeat cesarean rate, may be related to reports of associate risks, physician or maternal preference, more conservative practice guidelines such as the requirement for immediate availability of a surgical team during a TOLAC, legal pressures, as well as the continuing debate regarding the potential risks and benefits of vaginal birth compared to cesarean birth (Sargent & Caughey, 2017).

In March 2010, the NICHD and Office of Medical Application of NIH convened a Consensus Development Conference on VBAC to evaluate evidence regarding the safety and outcome of TOLAC and VBAC. The NIH panel recognized TOLAC as a reasonable option for many pregnant women with one prior low transverse uterine incision (NIH, 2010). Overall benefits of TOLAC are directly related to having a VBAC, which provides women the lowest morbidity (ACOG, 2019c; NIH, 2010). Women who successfully achieve VBAC avoid major abdominal surgery, resulting in lower rates of hemorrhage, thromboembolism, and infection, and have a shorter recovery compared with elective repeat cesareans (ACOG, 2019c). For women considering future pregnancies, VBAC may avoid consequences of multiple cesarean births including hysterectomy, bowel or bladder injury, transfusion, infection, placenta previa, and placenta accreta (ACOG, 2019c). Therefore, a successful VBAC is associated with less complications compared with elective repeat cesarean; however, a failed TOLAC is associated with more complications. Uterine rupture or dehiscence associated with TOLAC results in the most significant increase in maternal and neonatal morbidity (ACOG, 2019c).

Multiple studies of women attempting TOLAC have shown that 60% to 80% will result in successful vaginal births (ACOG, 2019c; Guise et al., 2010). However, an individual woman's chance for VBAC success varies depending on her demographic and obstetric characteristics (ACOG, 2019c). Favorable influences for a successful VBAC are a previous vaginal birth and spontaneous labor (ACOG, 2019c; Scott, 2011). Most women with one prior cesarean birth with a low transverse incision are candidates for and should be counseled about and offered TOLAC (ACOG, 2019c). Women with two prior low transverse cesarean births may be candidates for TOLAC and should be counseled based on the combination of other factors that affect their probability of achieving a successful VBAC (ACOG, 2019c).

Waiting for spontaneous labor, thus avoiding cervical ripening agents and oxytocin, appears to significantly decrease the risk of uterine rupture for women attempting VBAC (ACOG, 2019c; Shanks & Cahill, 2011). There are enough data to suggest that prostaglandins and high rates of oxytocin infusion increase the risk for rupture (ACOG, 2019c; Cahill et al., 2007). Uterine ruptures at the scar site and sites remote from the previous scar site have been reported with high doses of oxytocin. It has been theorized that prostaglandins induce local biochemical modifications that weaken the prior uterine scar, thus predisposing it to rupture. Misoprostol should not be used for third trimester cervical ripening or labor induction in women who have had a cesarean birth or major uterine surgery (ACOG, 2019c).

Women attempting TOLAC require close surveillance and continuous electronic monitoring of the

FHR and uterine activity. Because FHR abnormality is the most common sign of uterine rupture, associated with up to 70% of cases of uterine rupture, continuous FHR monitoring is recommended (ACOG, 2019c). Careful assessment during recurrent variable decelerations may signal the beginning of a uterine rupture rather than the need for amnioinfusion. There are no data to suggest FSEs or IUPCs are superior to external monitoring (ACOG, 2019c). The IUPC does not assist in the diagnosis of uterine rupture (ACOG, 2019c). IV access is a reasonable precaution because of the risk of uterine rupture, which would require the administration of rapid volume expanders and blood products. Rate of cervical dilation and fetal descent should be assessed frequently, and abnormal labor progress reported to the primary care provider. Epidural analgesia for labor may be provided during TOLAC (ACOG, 2019c). Clinical suspicion for uterine rupture should be high for women during TOLAC who require frequent epidural dosing (Cahill, Odibo, Allsworth, & Macones, 2010). Women undergoing a trial of labor require comprehensive care by an interdisciplinary perinatal team. The patient and family need reassurance and support.

Most maternal morbidity that occurs during TOLAC happens when a repeat cesarean birth becomes necessary (ACOG, 2019c; NIH, 2010). While VBAC is associated with fewer complications than elective repeat cesareans, a failed TOLAC is associated with more complications than an elective repeat cesarean (ACOG, 2019c). Uterine rupture or dehiscence significantly increases the risk of maternal and or neonatal morbidity (ACOG, 2019c). Therefore, ACOG recommends that TOLAC be attempted only in facilities capable of performing immediate cesarean births (ACOG, 2019c). In some cases, benefits for the mother may come as a price for the fetus, or vice versa, posing an ethical dilemma for the woman and her caregiver (NIH, 2010). When TOLAC and an elective repeat cesarean are medically equivalent options, the woman's preferences should be honored in a shared decision-making process (NIH, 2010).

Uterine rupture or dehiscence associated with TOLAC can be life-threatening to both the mother and the neonate. The terms *uterine rupture* and *uterine dehiscence* are not clinically distinguished from each other and often used interchangeably in the literature (ACOG, 2019c). The risk of clinically determined uterine rupture during TOLAC in women with low transverse uterine incision is approximately 0.5% to 0.9% (ACOG, 2019c), although absolute risk varies based on the type of previous uterine scar, the number of prior cesarean births, whether the mother had a prior vaginal birth, whether labor was spontaneous or induced, the cervical ripening/induction agent, a history of postpartum fever after a previous cesarean

birth, a previous preterm cesarean birth, a single-layer uterine closure, an interval between pregnancies of less than 24 months, body mass index, race, and maternal age over 30 years (ACOG, 2019c; Cahill et al., 2007; Cahill et al., 2008; Cahill, Tuuli, Odibo, Stamilio, & Macones, 2010; Hibbard et al., 2006; Scifres, Rohn, Odibo, Stamilio, & Macones, 2011; Shanks & Cahill, 2011). Labor dystocia after 7 cm for women having TOLAC may be associated with uterine rupture (Harper, Cahill, et al., 2012).

The most common presenting sign associated with uterine rupture is FHR abnormality, which has been found in 70% of the cases of uterine ruptures (ACOG, 2019c; Leung, Farmer, Leung, Medearis, & Paul, 1993). Acute signs of uterine rupture are variable and may include fetal bradycardia, increased uterine contractions, vaginal bleeding, loss of station, or new onset of intense uterine pain (ACOG, 2019c; Leung, Farmer, et al., 1993; Ridgeway, Weyrich, & Benedetti, 2004; Scott, 2011; Yap, Kim, & Laros, 2001). Uterine or abdominal pain in the area of the previous incision may be described as mild to "tearing" in nature (Scott, 2011). Bleeding, either vaginal or intraabdominal, may produce anxiety, restlessness, weakness, dizziness, gross hematuria, shoulder pain, and shock (Scott, 2011). Because uterine rupture is often sudden and may be catastrophic, any of these findings warrant rapid laparotomy (Scott, 2011). If complete cord occlusion occurs or the fetus is extruded from the uterus, the outcome may be poor. In a classic study, Leung, Leung, and Paul (1993) evaluated 78 cases of uterine rupture in a large tertiary medical center and reported significant neonatal morbidity when 18 minutes or more elapsed between the onset of prolonged deceleration and birth. When the prolonged deceleration was preceded by "severe" late or variable decelerations, fetal asphyxia occurred as early as 10 minutes from the onset of prolonged deceleration. An evaluation of 36 cases of uterine rupture by Holmgren, Scott, Porter, Esplin, and Bardsley (2012) found that babies born within 18 minutes after uterine rupture had normal umbilical pH levels or 5-minute Apgar scores greater than 7, whereas a longer time frame was associated with adverse outcomes. Prompt intervention does not always prevent severe, fetal metabolic acidosis or neonatal death. Even in facilities with immediate access to cesarean birth, uterine rupture can result in catastrophic outcome.

Although the actual numbers of adverse fetal or neonatal outcomes are low with VBAC, risks to the baby associated with uterine rupture are significant and can be catastrophic. They include hypoxemia, neurologic depression, pathologic fetal acidosis, seizures, asphyxia, hypoxic ischemic encephalopathy, cerebral palsy, and death (Chauhan, Martin, Hendrichs, Morrison, & Magann, 2003; Guise et al., 2004;

Holmgren et al., 2012; Smith, Pell, Cameron, & Dobbie, 2002; Yap et al., 2001).

Common sequelae associated with uterine rupture include excessive hemorrhage requiring surgical exploration; the need for hysterectomy; the need for blood product transfusion; hypovolemia; hypovolemic shock; injury to the bladder or ureters; bowel laceration; extrusion of any part of the fetus, cord, or placenta through the disruption; emergent cesarean birth for suspected rupture; emergent cesarean birth for indeterminate or abnormal fetal status; and general anesthesia (Guise et al., 2004; Hibbard et al., 2001; Kirkendall, Jauregui, Kim, & Phelan, 2000; Paré, Quiñones, & Macones, 2006). Many women with uterine rupture experience more than one of these complications.

Because of the risks associated with TOLAC and the unpredictable nature of uterine rupture and other complications, ACOG (2019c) has made recommendations for healthcare providers and facilities offering TOLAC:

- A TOLAC should be attempted at facilities capable of emergency surgery.
- A TOLAC should be undertaken in facilities with staff immediately available to provide emergency care.
- When resources for immediate cesarean birth are not available, healthcare providers and patients considering TOLAC should discuss the hospital's resources and availability of obstetric, pediatric, anesthetic, and operating room staffs.
- The decision to offer and pursue TOLAC in a setting in which the option of emergency cesarean birth is more limited should be carefully considered by patients and their healthcare providers. In such situations, the best alternative may be to refer patients to a facility with available resources.
- Healthcare providers and insurance carriers should do all they can to facilitate transfer of care or comanagement in support of a desired TOLAC, and such plans should be initiated early in the course of antenatal care.
- Respect for patient autonomy supports that patients should be allowed to accept increased levels of risk; however, patients should be clearly informed of such a potential increase in risk and management alternatives.
- After counseling, the ultimate decision to undergo TOLAC or repeat cesarean birth should be made by the patient in consultation with her healthcare provider. The potential risks and benefits of both TOLAC and elective repeat cesarean birth should be discussed. Documentation of counseling and the management plan should be included in the medical record.

Rupture of the uterus is an obstetric emergency. Maternal–fetal survival depends on prompt identification and surgical intervention. Rapid volume expanders, blood, and blood products should be readily available. Policies, procedures, and protocols should be written and evaluated to ensure optimum care for women who are having a TOLAC. If the primary care provider is a family practitioner or CNM without privileges or the ability to perform an emergent cesarean birth, clear policies and protocols should be in place to ensure appropriate and timely surgical coverage in case of maternal complications.

Safe care during a trial of labor to attempt VBAC is resource intensive. Many obstetric units do not have the financial and personnel resources to provide in-house anesthesia and a surgical team for the course of VBAC labor. Approximately 37% of U.S. hospitals providing perinatal services have fewer than 500 births per year; 8% have less than 100 births per year (Simpson, 2011a). These hospitals and others without around-the-clock anesthesia and surgical team support may find it challenging to supply the resources to meet the full scope of the ACOG (2019c) recommendations during VBAC labor. Not all obstetricians have the desire or the ability to devote the time to remain in-house during VBAC labor. The decision to offer a trial of labor for women attempting VBAC should be based on a commitment of resources and an agreement of providers to be in-house during labor. If this commitment cannot be made for whatever reason, the hospital should not offer planned VBAC care. Alternatives are repeat cesarean birth or patient referral to another hospital with resources consistent with the ACOG (2019c) recommendations.

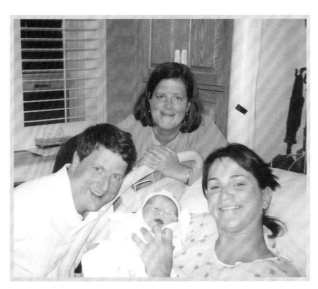

FIGURE 14–23. The nurse and the new family.

SUMMARY

Nurses who care for women during the intrapartum period require knowledge of the labor process and a thorough understanding of techniques and interventions that enhance safe labor and birth. The woman's desires about her labor and birth experience should guide care. We should consider ourselves supportive guests at the woman's momentous life event rather than routine interventionists. A philosophy that labor and birth are normal processes will enable appropriate care and avoid unnecessary interventions that can lead to iatrogenic maternal–fetal injuries. This chapter has presented an overview of nursing considerations for clinical practice during childbirth. Perinatal care based on national standards, current research, and principles of patient safety will enhance quality outcomes for women and newborns. The nurse has an important role in supporting a positive childbirth experience (Fig. 14–23). Attending the birth of a healthy baby and sharing the joy with the new mother is one of the most rewarding experiences in perinatal nursing practice.

REFERENCES

Abalos, E., Oladapo, O. T., Chamillard, M., Díaz, V., Pasquale, J., Bonet, M., . . . Gülmezoglu, A. M. (2018). Duration of spontaneous labour in 'low-risk' women with 'normal' perinatal outcomes: A systematic review. *European Journal of Obstetric, Gynecology, and Reproductive Biology*, 223, 123–132. doi:10.1016/j.ejogrb.2018.02.026

Adams, E. D., Stark, M. A., & Low, L. K. (2016). A nurse's guide to supporting physiologic birth. *Nursing for Women's Health*, 20(1), 76–85. doi:10.1016/j.nwh.2015.12.009

Akhan, S. E., Iyibozkurt, A. C., & Turfanda, A. (2001). Unscarred uterine rupture after induction of labor with misoprostol: A case report. *Clinical and Experimental Obstetrics & Gynecology*, 28(2), 118–120.

Akinsipe, D. C., Villalobos, L. E., & Ridley, R. T. (2012). A systematic review of implementing an elective labor induction policy. *Journal of Obstetric, Gynecologic, and Neonatal Nursing*, 41(1), 5–16. doi:10.1111/j.1552-6909.2011.01320.

Albers, L. L., Anderson, D., Cragin, L., Daniels, S. M., Hunter, C., Sedler, K. D., & Teaf, D. (1997). The relationship of ambulation in labor to operative delivery. *Journal of Nurse-Midwifery*, 42(1), 4–8.

Albers, L. L., Sedler, K. D., Bedrick, E. J., Teaf, D., & Peralta, P. (2006). Factors related to genital tract trauma in normal spontaneous vaginal births. *Birth*, 33(2), 94–100. doi:10.1111/j.0730-7659.2006.00085.x

Aldrich, C. J., D'Antona, D., Spencer, J. A. D., Wyatt, J. S., Peebles, D. M., Delpy, D. T., & Reynolds, E. O. (1995). The effect of maternal pushing on cerebral oxygenation and blood volume during the second stage of labour. *British Journal of Obstetrics and Gynaecology*, 102(6), 448–453.

Alexander, J. M., Sharma, S. K., McIntire, D. D., & Leveno, K. J. (2002). Epidural anesthesia lengthens the Friedman active phase of labor. *Obstetrics & Gynecology*, 100(1), 46–50.

Alfirevic, Z., Aflaifel, N., & Weeks, A. (2014). Oral misoprostol for induction of labour. *Cochrane Database of Systematic Reviews*, (6), CD001338. doi:10.1002/14651858.CD001338.pub3

Alliance for Innovation on Maternal Health. (2017). *Maternal safety bundles*. Washington, DC: Author. Retrieved from http://www.safehealthcareforeverywoman.org/aim.php

American Academy of Pediatrics & American College of Obstetricians and Gynecologists. (2017). *Guidelines for perinatal care* (8th ed.). Elk Grove Village, IL: American Academy of Pediatrics.

American Academy of Pediatrics & American Heart Association. (2016). *Textbook of neonatal resuscitation* (7th ed.). Elk Grove Village, IL: American Academy of Pediatrics.

American College of Nurse-Midwives. (2015a). Intermittent auscultation for intrapartum fetal heart surveillance: American College of Nurse-Midwives. *Journal of Midwifery and Women's Health*, 60(5), 626–632. doi:10.1111/jmwh.12372

American College of Nurse-Midwives. (2015b). *Reducing primary cesareans*. Silver Spring, MD: Author. Retrieved from http://www.birthtools.org/Reducing-Primary-Cesareans

American College of Nurse-Midwives. (2016). Providing oral nutrition to women in labor: American College of Nurse-Midwives. *Journal of Midwifery and Women's Health*, 61(4), 528–534. doi:10.1111/jmwh.12515

American College of Obstetricians and Gynecologists. (2006). *Amnioinfusion does not prevent meconium aspiration syndrome* (Committee Opinion No. 346; Reaffirmed, 2018). Washington, DC: Author.

American College of Obstetricians and Gynecologists. (2009a). *Induction of labor* (Practice Bulletin No. 107; Reaffirmed, 2019). Washington, DC: Author.

American College of Obstetricians and Gynecologists. (2009b). *Intrapartum fetal heart rate monitoring: Nomenclature, interpretation, and general management principles* (Practice Bulletin No. 106; Reaffirmed, 2017). Washington, DC: Author.

American College of Obstetricians and Gynecologists. (2009c). *Oral intake during labor* (Committee Opinion No. 441; Reaffirmed, 2017). Washington, DC: Author.

American College of Obstetricians and Gynecologists. (2010). *Management of intrapartum fetal heart rate tracings* (Practice Bulletin No. 116; Reaffirmed, 2017). Washington, DC: Author.

American College of Obstetricians and Gynecologists. (2011a). *Scheduling induction of labor* (Patient Safety Checklist No. 5). Washington, DC: Author.

American College of Obstetricians and Gynecologists. (2011b). *Scheduling planned cesarean delivery* (Patient Safety Checklist No. 3). Washington, DC: Author.

American College of Obstetricians and Gynecologists. (2012a). *Communication strategies for patient handoffs* (Committee Opinion No. 517; Reaffirmed, 2018). Washington, DC: Author.

American College of Obstetricians and Gynecologists. (2012b). *Documenting shoulder dystocia* (Patient Safety Checklist No. 6). Washington, DC: Author.

American College of Obstetricians and Gynecologists. (2014a). *Preparing for clinical emergencies in obstetrics and gynecology* (Committee Opinion No. 590; Reaffirmed, 2018). Washington, DC: Author.

American College of Obstetricians and Gynecologists. (2014b). *Revitalize: Obstetric data definitions* (Version 1.0). Washington, DC: Author.

American College of Obstetricians and Gynecologists. (2015). *Operative vaginal delivery* (Practice Bulletin No. 154; Reaffirmed, 2018). Washington, DC: Author.

American College of Obstetricians and Gynecologists. (2016a). *Fetal macrosomia* (Practice Bulletin No. 173; Reaffirmed, 2018). Washington, DC: Author.

American College of Obstetricians and Gynecologists. (2016b). *Hospital-based triage of obstetric patients* (Committee Opinion No. 667). Washington, DC: Author.

American College of Obstetricians and Gynecologists. (2017). *Shoulder dystocia* (Practice Bulletin No. 178; Reaffirmed, 2019). Washington, DC: Author.

American College of Obstetricians and Gynecologists. (2018). *Prevention and management of obstetric lacerations at vaginal delivery* (Practice Bulletin No. 198). Washington, DC: Author.

American College of Obstetricians and Gynecologists. (2019a). *Approaches to limit interventions during labor and birth* (Committee Opinion No. 766). Washington, DC: Author.

American College of Obstetricians and Gynecologists. (2019b). *Obstetric analgesia and anesthesia* (Practice Bulletin No. 209). Washington, DC: Author.

American College of Obstetricians and Gynecologists. (2019c). *Vaginal birth after cesarean delivery* (Practice Bulletin No. 205). Washington, DC: Author.

American College of Obstetricians and Gynecologists & Society for Maternal-Fetal Medicine. (2014). Safe prevention of the primary cesarean delivery (Obstetric Care Consensus No. 1). *Obstetrics & Gynecology, 123*(3), 693–711. doi:10.1097/01. AOG.0000444441.04111.1d

American Society of Anesthesiologists. (2016). Practice guidelines for obstetric anesthesia: An updated report by the American Society of Anesthesiologists Task Force on Obstetric Anesthesia and Perinatology. *Anesthesiology, 124*(2), 270–300. doi:10.1097 /ALN.0000000000000935

Andrews, V., Sultan, A. H., Thakar, R., & Jones, P. W. (2006). Risk factors for obstetric anal sphincter injury: A prospective study. *Birth, 33*(2), 117–122. doi:10.1111/j.0730-7659.2006.00088.x

Apfelbaum, J. L., Hagberg, C. A., Caplan, R. A., Blitt, C. D., Connis, R. T., Nickinovich, D. G., . . . Ovassapian, A. (2013). Practice guidelines for management of a difficult airway: An updated report by the American Society of Anesthesiologists task force on management of the difficult airway. *Anesthesiology, 118*(2), 251–270. doi:10.1097/ALN.0b013e31827773b2

Arias, F. (2000). Pharmacology of oxytocin and prostaglandins. *Clinical Obstetrics and Gynecology, 43*(3), 455–468.

Association of Women's Health, Obstetric and Neonatal Nurses. (2006). *High-touch nursing care during labor.* Longmont, CO: Injoy Birth and Parenting Videos.

Association of Women's Health, Obstetric and Neonatal Nurses. (2010). *Guidelines for professional registered nurse staffing for perinatal units.* Washington, DC: Author.

Association of Women's Health, Obstetric and Neonatal Nurses. (2011). *Nursing care of the woman receiving regional analgesia/ anesthesia in labor* (Evidence-Based Clinical Practice Guideline). Washington, DC: Author.

Association of Women's Health, Obstetric and Neonatal Nurses. (2012). *40 Reasons to go the full 40 weeks.* Washington, DC: Author.

Association of Women's Health, Obstetric and Neonatal Nurses. (2015). *Maternal Fetal Triage Index.* Washington, DC: Author. Retrieved from https://www.awhonn.org/general/custom .asp?page=MFTI

Association of Women's Health, Obstetric and Neonatal Nurses. (2016). Immediate and sustained skin-to-skin contact for the healthy term newborn after cesarean birth (Practice Brief No. 5). *Nursing for Women's Health, 20*(6), 614–616. doi:10.1016 /S1751-4851(16)30331-2

Association of Women's Health, Obstetric and Neonatal Nurses. (2017). Advanced cardiac life support in obstetric settings (Position Statement). *Nursing for Women's Health, 21*(1), 67–68. doi:10.1016/S1751-4851(17)30045-4

Association of Women's Health, Obstetric and Neonatal Nurses. (2018a). Continuous labor support for every woman (Position Statement). *Nursing for Women's Health, 22*(1), 93–94. doi:10.1016/S1751-4851(18)30035-7

Association of Women's Health, Obstetric and Neonatal Nurses. (2018b). Fetal heart monitoring (Position Statement). *Journal of Obstetric, Gynecologic and Neonatal Nurses, 47*(6), 874–877. doi:10.1016/j.jogn.2018.09.007

Association of Women's Health, Obstetric and Neonatal Nurses. (2019a). Elective induction of labor (Position Statement). *Nursing for Women's Health, 23*(2), 177–179. doi:10.1016/j.nwh .2019.03.001

Association of Women's Health, Obstetric and Neonatal Nurses. (2019b). *Nursing care and management of the 2nd stage of labor* (Evidence-Based Clinical Practice Guideline, 3rd ed.). Washington, DC: Author.

Association of Women's Health, Obstetric and Neonatal Nurses. (2019c). *Perioperative care of the pregnant woman* (Evidence-Based Clinical Practice Guideline, 2nd ed.). Washington, DC: Author.

Aukee, P., Sundström, H., & Kairaluoma, M. V. (2006). The role of mediolateral episiotomy during labour: Analysis of risk factors for obstetric anal sphincter tears. *Acta Obstetricia et Gynecologica Scandinavica, 85*(7), 856–860. doi:10.1080 /00016340500408283

Bakker, P. C. A. M., Kurver, P. H. J., Kuik, D. J., & Van Geijn, H. P. (2007). Elevated uterine activity increases the risk of fetal acidosis at birth. *American Journal of Obstetrics & Gynecology, 196,* 313.e1–313.e6.

Barnett, M. M., & Humenick, S. S. (1982). Infant outcome in relation to second stage labor pushing method. *Birth, 9*(4), 221–229.

Bassell, G. M., Humayun, S. G., & Marx, G. F. (1980). Maternal bearing down efforts: Another fetal risk? *Obstetrics & Gynecology, 56*(1), 39–41.

Beall, M. H., Spong, C. Y., & Ross, M. G. (2003). A randomized controlled trial of prophylactic maneuvers to reduce head-to-body delivery time in patients at risk for shoulder dystocia. *Obstetrics & Gynecology, 102*(1), 31–35.

Belfort, M. A., White, G. L., & Vermeulen, F. M. (2012). Association of fetal cranial shape with shoulder dystocia. *Ultrasound Obstetrics & Gynecology, 39*(3), 304–309. doi:10.1002/uog.9066

Benavides, L., Wu, J. M., Hundley, A. F., Ivester, T. S., & Visco, A. G. (2005). The impact of occiput posterior fetal head position on the risk of anal sphincter injury in forceps-assisted vaginal deliveries. *American Journal of Obstetrics & Gynecology, 192*(5), 1702–1706. doi:10.1016/j.ajog.2004.11.047

Benedetti, T. J. (1995). Shoulder dystocia. *Contemporary Ob Gyn, 40*(3), 39–43.

Bennett, B. B. (1997). Uterine rupture during induction of labor at term with intravaginal misoprostol. *Obstetrics & Gynecology, 89*(5, Pt. 1), 832–833.

Bernal, A. L. (2003). Mechanisms of labour: Biochemical aspects. *British Journal of Obstetrics and Gynaecology, 110*(20 Suppl.), 39–45.

Bick, D., Briley, A., Brocklehurst, P., Hardy, P., Juszczak, E., Lynch, L., . . . Wilson, M. (2017). A multicentre, randomised controlled trial of position during the late stages of labour in nulliparous women with an epidural: Clinical effectiveness and an economic evaluation (BUMPES). *Health Technology Assessment, 21*(65), 1–176. doi:10.3310/hta21650

Bingham, J., Chauhan, S. P., Hayes, E., Gherman, R., & Lewis, D. (2010). Recurrent shoulder dystocia: A review. *Obstetrical & Gynecological Survey, 65*(3), 183–188. doi:10.1097/OGX .0b013e3181cb8fbc

Bishop, E. H. (1964). Pelvic scoring for elective induction. *Obstetrics & Gynecology, 24,* 266–268.

Blackburn, S. B. (2018). *Maternal, fetal, and neonatal physiology: A clinical perspective* (5th ed.). St. Louis, MO: Elsevier.

Blomquist, J. L., Quiroz, L. H., Macmillan, D., McCullough, A., & Handa, V. L. (2011). Mothers' satisfaction with planned vaginal and planned cesarean birth. *American Journal of Perinatology, 28*(5), 383–388. doi:10.1055/s-0031-1274508

Bloom, S. L., Casey, B. M., Schaffer, J. I., McIntire, D. D., & Leveno, K. J. (2006). A randomized trial of coached versus uncoached maternal pushing during the second stage of labor. *American*

Journal of Obstetrics & Gynecology, 194(1), 10–13. doi:10.1016/j.ajog.2005.06.022

Bloom, S. L., McIntire, D. D., Kelly, M. A., Beimer, H. L., Burpo, R. H., Garcia, M. A., & Leveno, K. J. (1998). Lack of effect of walking on labor and delivery. *The New England Journal of Medicine, 339*(2), 76–79.

Bodner-Adler, B., Bodner, K., Kimberger, O., Lozanov, P., Hussiein, P., & Mayerhofer, K. (2003). Women's position during labour: Influence on maternal and neonatal outcome. *Wiener Klinische Wochenschrift, 115*(19–20), 720–723.

Bofill, J. A., Rust, O. A., Devidas, M., Roberts, W. E., Morrison, J. C., & Martin, J. N., Jr. (1997). Neonatal cephalohematoma from vacuum extraction. *Journal of Reproductive Medicine, 42*(9), 565–569.

Bohren, M. A., Hofmeyr, G. J., Sakala, C., Fukuzawa, R. K., & Cuthbert, A. (2017). Continuous support for women during childbirth. *Cochrane Database of Systematic Reviews,* (7), CD003766. doi:10.1002/14651858.CD003766.pub6

Boie, S., Glavind, J., Velu, A. V., Mol, B. W. J., Uldbjerg, N., de Graaf, I., . . . Bakker, J. J. (2018). Discontinuation of intravenous oxytocin in the active phase of induced labour. *Cochrane Database of Systematic Reviews,* (8), CD012274. doi:10.1002/14651858.CD012274.pub2

Bor, P., Ledertoug, S., Boie, S., Knoblauch, N. O., & Stornes, I. (2016). Continuation versus discontinuation of oxytocin infusion during active phase of labour: A randomized controlled trial. *British Journal of Obstetrics and Gynaecology, 123*(1), 129–135. doi:10.1111/1471-0528.13589

Brancato, R. M., Church, S., & Stone, P. W. (2008). A meta-analysis of passive descent versus immediate pushing in nulliparous women with epidural analgesia in the second stage of labor. *Journal of Obstetric, Gynecologic, and Neonatal Nursing, 37*(1), 4–12. doi:10.1111/j.1552-6909.2007.00205.x

Breedlove, G. (2019). Have we ARRIVEd at a new normal? *MCN: The American Journal of Maternal Child Nursing, 44*(1), 59–60. doi:10.1097/NMC.0000000000000484

Bruner, J. P., Drummond, S. B., Meenan, A. L., & Gaskin, I. M. (1998). All-fours maneuver for reducing shoulder dystocia during labor. *Journal of Reproductive Medicine, 43*(5), 439–443.

Buckley, S. (2015). *Hormonal physiology of childbearing: Evidence and implications for women, babies, and maternity care.* Washington, DC: Childbirth Connection Programs, National Partnership for Women and Families.

Budden, A., Chen, L. J., & Henry, A. (2014). High-dose versus low-dose oxytocin regimens for induction of labour at term. *Cochrane Database of Systematic Reviews,* (10), CD009701. doi:10.1002/14651858.CD009701.pub2

Cahill, A. G., Odibo, A. O., Allsworth, J. E., & Macones, G. A. (2010). Frequent epidural dosing as a marker for impending uterine rupture in patients who attempt vaginal birth after cesarean delivery. *American Journal of Obstetrics & Gynecology, 202*(4), 355.e1–335.e5. doi:10.1016/j.ajog.2010.01.041

Cahill, A. G., Roehl, K. A., Odibo, A. O., Zhao, Q., & Macones, G. A. (2012). Impact of fetal gender on the labor curve. *American Journal of Obstetrics & Gynecology, 206*(4), 335.e1–335.e5. doi:10.1016/j.ajog.2012.01.021

Cahill, A. G., Srinivas, S. K., Tita, A. T. N., Caughey, A. B., Richter, H. E., Gregory, W. T., . . . Tuuli, M. G. (2018). Effect of immediate vs delayed pushing on rates of spontaneous vaginal delivery among nulliparous women receiving neuraxial analgesia: A randomized clinical trial. *JAMA, 320*(14), 1444–1454. doi:10.1001/jama.2018.13986

Cahill, A. G., Stamilio, D. M., Odibo, A. O., Peipert, J. F., Stevens, E. J., & Macones, G. A. (2007). Does a maximum dose of oxytocin affect risk for uterine rupture in candidates for vaginal birth after cesarean delivery? *American Journal of Obstetrics & Gynecology, 197*(5), 495.e1–495.e5. doi:10.1016/j.ajog.2007.04.005

Cahill, A. G., Stamilio, D. M., Odibo, A. O., Peipert, J. F., Stevens, E. J., & Macones, G. A. (2008). Racial disparity in the success and complications of vaginal birth after cesarean delivery. *Obstetrics & Gynecology, 111*(3), 654–658. doi:10.1097/AOG.0b013e318163be22

Cahill, A. G., Tuuli, M., Odibo, A. O., Stamilio, D. M., & Macones, G. A. (2010). Vaginal birth after caesarean for women with three or more prior caesareans: Assessing safety and success. *British Journal of Obstetrics and Gynaecology, 117*(4), 422–427. doi:10.1111/j.1471-0528.2010.02498.x

Caldeyro-Barcia, R. (1979). The influence of maternal bearing-down efforts during second stage on fetal well-being. *Birth and the Family Journal, 6,* 17–21.

Caldeyro-Barcia, R., Giussi, G., Storch, E., Poseiro, J. J., Lafaurie, N., Kettenhuber, K., & Ballejo, G. (1981). The bearing-down efforts and their effects on fetal heart rate, oxygenation, and acid base balance. *Journal of Perinatal Medicine, 9*(1 Suppl.), 63–67.

Caldeyro-Barcia, R., & Poseiro, J. J. (1960). Physiology of the uterine contraction. *Clinical Obstetrics and Gynecology, 3,* 386–408.

Campbell, D. A., Lake, M. F., Falk, M., & Backstrand, J. R. (2006). A randomized control trial of continuous support in labor by a lay doula. *Journal of Obstetric, Gynecologic, and Neonatal Nursing, 35*(4), 456–464. doi:10.1111/j.1552-6909.2006.00067.x

Carbillon, L., Seince, N., & Uzan, M. (2001). Myometrial maturation and labour. *Annals of Medicine, 33,* 571–578.

Carmen, S. (1986). Neonatal hypoglycemia in response to maternal glucose infusion before delivery. *Journal of Obstetric, Gynecologic, and Neonatal Nursing, 15*(4), 319–322.

Castro, M. A., Hoey, S. D., & Towner, D. (2003). Controversies in the use of the vacuum extractor. *Seminars in Perinatology, 27*(1), 46–53.

Catanzarite, V., Cousins, L., Dowling, D., & Daneshmand, S. (2006). Oxytocin-associated rupture of an unscarred uterus in a primagravida. *Obstetrics & Gynecology, 108*(3, Pt. 2), 723–725. doi:10.1097/01.AOG.0000215559.21051.dc

Caughey, A. B. (2017). Evidence-based labor and delivery management: Can we safely reduce the cesarean rate? *Obstetrics and Gynecology Clinics of North America, 44*(4), 523–533. doi:10.1016/j.ogc.2017.08.008

Caughey, A. B., Sandberg, P. L., Zlatnik, M. G., Thiet, M., Parer, J. T., & Laros, R. K. (2005). Forceps compared with vacuum: Rates of neonatal and maternal morbidity. *Obstetrics & Gynecology, 106*(5, Pt. 1), 908–912. doi:10.1097/01.AOG.0000182616.39503.b2

Caughey, A. B., Sundaram, V., Kaimal, A. J., Cheng, Y. W., Gienger, A., Little, S. E., . . . Bravata, D. M. (2009). *Maternal and neonatal outcomes of elective induction of labor* (Evidence Reports/Technology Assessments No. 176). Rockville, MD: Agency for Healthcare Research and Quality. Retrieved from http://www.ahrq.gov/clinic/tp/eiltp.htm

Caughey, A. B., Wood, S. L., Macones, G. A., Wrench, I., Huang, J., Norman, M., . . . Wilson, R. D. (2018). Guidelines for intraoperative care in cesarean delivery: Enhanced Recovery after Surgery Society recommendations (part 2). *American Journal of Obstetrics and Gynecology, 219*(6), 533–544. doi:10.1016/j.ajog.2018.08.006

Chang, S. C., Chou, M. M., Lin, K. C., Lin, L. C., Lin, Y. L., & Kuo, S. C. (2011). Effects of a pushing intervention on pain, fatigue and birthing experiences among Taiwanese women during the second stage of labour. *Midwifery, 27*(6), 825–831. doi:10.1016/j.midw.2010.08.009

Chauhan, S. P., Martin, J. N., Jr., Hendrichs, C. E., Morrison, J. C., & Magann, E. F. (2003). Maternal and perinatal complications with uterine rupture in 142,075 patients who attempted vaginal birth after cesarean delivery: A review of the literature. *American Journal of Obstetrics & Gynecology, 189*(2), 408–417. doi:10.1067/s0002-9378(03)00675-6

Cheng, Y. W., & Caughey, A. B. (2017). Defining and managing normal and abnormal second stage of labor. *Obstetrics and Gynecology Clinics of North America*, 44(4), 547–566. doi:10.1016/j.ogc.2017.08.009

Cheng, Y. W., Hopkins, L. M., & Caughey, A. B. (2004). How long is too long: Does a prolonged second stage of labor in nulliparous women affect maternal and neonatal outcomes? *American Journal of Obstetrics & Gynecology*, 191(3), 933–938. doi:10.1016/j.ajog.2004.05.044

Cheng, Y. W., Hopkins, L. M., Laros, R. K., Jr., & Caughey, A. B. (2007). Duration of the second stage of labor in multiparous women: Maternal and neonatal outcomes. *American Journal of Obstetrics & Gynecology*, 196(6), 585.e1–585.e6. doi:10.1016/j.ajog.2007.03.021

Cheng, Y. W., Shaffer, B. L., & Caughey, A. B. (2006). The association between persistent occiput posterior position and neonatal outcomes. *Obstetrics & Gynecology*, 107(4), 837–844. doi:10.1097/01.AOG.0000206217.07883.a2

Christiaens, W., & Bracke, P. (2007). Assessment of social psychological determinants of satisfaction with childbirth in a cross-national perspective. *BMC Pregnancy Childbirth*, 7, 26. doi:10.1186/1471-2393-7-26

Christianson, L. M., Bovbjerg, V. E., McDavitt, E. C., & Hullfish, K. L. (2003). Risk factors for perineal injury during delivery. *American Journal of Obstetrics & Gynecology*, 189(1), 255–260. doi:10.1067/mob.2003.547

Clark, S. L., Belfort, M. A., Byrum, S. L., Meyers, J. A., & Perlin, J. B. (2008). Improved outcomes, fewer cesarean deliveries, and reduced litigation: Results of a new paradigm in patient safety. *American Journal of Obstetrics & Gynecology*, 199(2), 105.e1–105.e7. doi:10.1016/j.ajog.2008.02.031

Clark, S. L., Belfort, M. A., Dildy, G. A., & Meyers, J. A. (2008). Reducing obstetric litigation through alterations in practice patterns. *Obstetrics & Gynecology*, 112(6), 1279–1283. doi:10.1097/AOG.0b013e31818da2c7

Clark, S. L., Belfort, M. A., Hankins, G. D. V., Meyers, J. A., & Houser, F. M. (2007). Variation in the rates of operative delivery in the United States. *American Journal of Obstetrics & Gynecology*, 196(6), 526.e1–526.e5. doi:10.1016/j.ajog.2007.01.024

Clark, S. L., Simpson, K. R., Knox, G. E., & Garite, T. J. (2009). Oxytocin: New perspectives on an old drug. *American Journal of Obstetrics & Gynecology*, 200(1), 35.e1–35.e6. doi:10.1016/j.ajog.2008.06.010

Cohen, W. R., & Friedman, E. A. (2018). The assessment of labor: A brief history. *Journal of Perinatal Medicine*, 46(1), 1–8. doi:10.1515/jpm-2017-0018

Colachis, S. C., III, Pease, W. S., & Johnson, E. W. (1994). A preventable cause of foot drop during childbirth. *American Journal of Obstetrics & Gynecology*, 171(1), 270–272.

Colombara, D. V., Soh, J. D., Menacho, L. A., Schiff, M. A., & Reed, S. D. (2011). Birth injury in a subsequent vaginal delivery among women with a history of shoulder dystocia. *Journal of Perinatal Medicine*, 39(6), 709–715. doi:10.1515/JPM.2011.074

Cosner, K. R., & deJong, E. (1993). Physiologic second-stage labor. *MCN: The American Journal of Maternal Child Nursing*, 18(1), 38–43.

Crane, J. M. (2006). Factors predicting labor induction success: A critical analysis. *Clinical Obstetrics and Gynecology*, 49(3), 573–584.

Crane, J. M., & Young, D. C. (1998). Meta-analysis of low-dose versus high-dose oxytocin for labour induction. *Journal of the Society of Obstetricians and Gynaecologists of Canada*, 20(13), 1215–1223.

Crane, J. M., Young, D. C., Butt, K. D., Bennett, K. A., & Hutchens, D. (2001). Excessive uterine activity accompanying induced labor. *Obstetrics & Gynecology*, 97(6), 926–931.

Cromi, A., Ghezzi, F., Uccella, S., Agosti, M., Serati, M., Marchitelli, G., & Bolis, P. (2012). A randomized trial of preinduction cervical ripening: Dinoprostone vaginal insert versus double-balloon catheter. *American Journal of Obstetrics & Gynecology*, 207(2), 125.e1–125.e7. doi:10.1016/j.ajog.2012.05.020

Curtin, S. C., Gregory, K. D., Korst, L. M., & Uddin, S. F. G. (2015). Maternal morbidity for vaginal and cesarean deliveries, according to previous cesarean history: New data from the birth certificate, 2013. *National Vital Statistics Reports*, 64(4), 1–14. Hyattsville, MD: National Center for Health Statistics. Retrieved from https://www.cdc.gov/nchs/data/nvsr/nvsr64/nvsr64_04.pdf

Dandolu, V., Chatwani, A., Harmanli, O., Floro, C., Gaaughan, J. P., & Hernandez, E. (2005). Risk factors for obstetrical anal sphincter lacerations. *International Urogynecology Journal and Pelvic Floor Dysfunction*, 16(4), 304–307.

Daniel-Spiegel, E., Weiner, Z., Ben-Shlomo, I., & Shalev, E. (2004). For how long should oxytocin be continued during induction of labour? *British Journal of Obstetrics and Gynaecology*, 111(4), 331–334. doi:10.1111/j.1471-0528.2004.00096.x

da Silva, F. M., de Oliveira, S. M., Bick, D., Osava, R. H., Tuesta, E. F., & Riesco, M. L. (2012). Risk factors for birth-related perineal trauma: A cross-sectional study in a birth centre. *Journal of Clinical Nursing*, 21(15–16), 2209–2218. doi:10.1111/j.1365-2702.2012.04133.x

Davies, J. M., Posner, K. L., Lee, L. A., Cheney, F. W., & Domino, K. B. (2009). Liability associated with obstetric anesthesia: A closed claims analysis. *Anesthesiology*, 110(1), 131–139. doi:10.1097/ALN.0b013e318190e16a

Dawood, M. Y. (1995a). Novel approach to oxytocin induction-augmentation of labor: Application of oxytocin physiology during pregnancy. *Advances in Experimental Medicine and Biology*, 395, 585–594.

Dawood, M. Y. (1995b). Pharmacologic stimulation of uterine contractions. *Seminars in Perinatology*, 19(1), 73–83.

Dawood, M. Y., Wang, C. F., Gupta, R., & Fuchs, F. (1978). Fetal contribution to oxytocin in human labor. *Obstetrics & Gynecology*, 52(2), 205–209.

Dawood, M. Y., Ylikorkala, O., Trivedi, D., & Fuchs, F. (1979). Oxytocin in maternal circulation and amniotic fluid during pregnancy. *Journal of Clinical Endocrinology and Metabolism*, 49(3), 429–434.

Declercq, E. R., Sakala, C., Corry, M. P., Applebaum, S., & Herrlich, A. (2014). Major survey findings of Listening to Mothers[SM] III: New mothers speak out. Report of National Surveys of Women's Childbearing Experiences. Conducted October–December 2012 and January–April 2013. *Journal of Perinatal Education*, 23(1), 17–24. doi:10.1891/1058-1243.23.1.17

Deering, S. H., Tobler, K., & Cypher, R. (2010). Improvement in documentation using an electronic checklist for shoulder dystocia deliveries. *Obstetrics & Gynecology*, 116(1), 63–66. doi:10.1097/AOG.0b013e3181e42220

Deering, S. H., Weeks, L., & Benedetti, T. (2011). Evaluation of force applied during deliveries complicated by shoulder dystocia using simulation. *American Journal of Obstetrics & Gynecology*, 204(3), 234.e1–234.e5. doi:10.1016/j.ajog.2010.10.904

de Jong, P. R., Johanson, R. B., Baxen, P., Adrians, V. D., van der Westhuisen, S., & Jones, P. W. (1997). Randomised trial comparing the upright and supine positions for the second stage of labour. *British Journal of Obstetrics and Gynaecology*, 104(5), 567–571.

De Jonge, A., Teunissen, T. A., & Lagro-Janssen, A. L. (2004). Supine position compared to other positions during the second stage of labor: A meta-analytic review. *Journal of Psychosomatic Obstetrics and Gynaecology*, 25, 35–45.

De Jonge, A., Van Diem, M. T., Scheepers, P. L., Buitendijk, S. E., & Lagro-Janssen, A. L. (2010). Risk of perineal damage is not a reason to discourage a sitting birthing position: A secondary analysis. *International Journal of Clinical Practice*, 64(5), 611–618. doi:10.1111/j.1742-1241.2009.02316.x

Deliktas, A., & Kukulu, K. (2017). A meta-analysis of the effect on maternal health of upright positions during the second stage of labour, without routine epidural analgesia. *Journal of Advanced Nursing, 74*, 263–278. doi:10.1111/jan.13447

DiFranco, J. T., Romano, A. M., & Keen, R. (2007). Care Practice #5: Spontaneous pushing in upright or gravity-neutral positions. *Journal of Perinatal Education, 16*(3), 35–38. doi:10.1624/105812407X217138

Doumouchtsis, S. K., & Arulkumaran, S. (2006). Head injuries after instrumental vaginal deliveries. *Current Opinion in Obstetrics & Gynecology, 18*(2), 129–134. doi:10.1097/01.gco.0000192983.76976.68

Downe, S., Gerrett, D., & Renfrew, M. J. (2004). A prospective randomised trial on the effect of position in the passive second stage of labour on birth outcome in nulliparous women using epidural analgesia. *Midwifery, 20*(2), 157–168.

Draycott, T. J., Crofts, J. F., Ash, J. P., Wilson, L. V., Yard, E., Sibanda, T., & Whitelaw, A. (2008). Improving neonatal outcome through practical shoulder dystocia training. *Obstetrics & Gynecology, 112*(1), 14–20. doi:10.1097/AOG.0b013e31817bbc61

Dupuis, O., Silveira, R., Dupong, C., Mottolese, C., Kahn, P., Dittmar, A., & Rudigoz, R. C. (2005). Comparison of "instrumented-associated" and "spontaneous" obstetric depressed skull fractures in a cohort of 68 neonates. *American Journal of Obstetrics & Gynecology, 192*(1), 165–170. doi:10.1016/j.ajog.2004.06.035

Eason, E., & Feldman, P. (2000). Much ado about a little cut: Is episiotomy worthwhile? *Obstetrics & Gynecology, 95*(4), 616–618.

Eason, E., Labrecque, M., Wells, G., & Feldman, P. (2000). Preventing perineal trauma during childbirth: A systematic review. *Obstetrics & Gynecology, 95*(3), 464–471.

Eslamian, L., Marsoosi, V., & Pakneeyat, Y. (2006). Increased intravenous fluid intake and the course of labor in nulliparous women. *European Journal of Obstetrics and Gynecology, 93*(2), 102–105. doi:10.1016/j.ijgo.2006.01.023

Feldman-Winter, L., & Goldsmith, J. P. (2016). Safe sleep and skin-to-skin care in the neonatal period for healthy term newborns. *Pediatrics, 138*(3), e20161889. doi:10.1542/peds.2016-1889

Ferguson, J. K. W. (1941). Study of motility of intact uterus at term. *Surgery, Gynecology, and Obstetrics, 73*, 359–366.

Ferring Pharmaceuticals. (2017). *Cervidil package insert.* Parsippany, NJ: Author. Retrieved from http://www.ferringusa.com/wp-content/uploads/2018/11/Cervidil-Package-Insert-04.2017.pdf

FitzGerald, M. P., Weber, A. M., Howden, N., Cundiff, G. W., & Brown, M. B. (2007). Risk factors for anal sphincter tear during vaginal delivery. *Obstetrics & Gynecology, 109*(1), 29–34. doi:10.1097/01.AOG.0000242616.56617.ff

Fleming, N., Newton, E. R., & Roberts, J. (2003). Changes in postpartum perineal muscle function in women with and without episiotomies. *Journal of Midwifery & Women's Health, 48*(1), 53–59.

Fox, N. S., Saltzman, D. H., Roman, A. S., Klauser, C. K., Moshier, E., & Rebarber, A. (2011). Intravaginal misoprostol versus Foley catheter for labour induction: A meta-analysis. *British Journal of Obstetrics and Gynaecology, 118*(6), 647–654. doi:10.1111/j.1471-0528.2011.02905.x

Fraser, W. D., Marcoux, S., Krauss, I., Douglas, J., Goulet, C., & Boulvain, M. (2000). Multicenter randomized controlled trial of delayed pushing for nulliparous women in the second stage of labor with continuous epidural analgesia. *American Journal of Obstetrics & Gynecology, 182*(5), 1165–1172.

Freeman, R. K., Garite, T. J., Nageotte, M. P., & Miller, L. A. (2012). *Fetal heart rate monitoring* (4th ed.). Philadelphia, PA: Lippincott Williams & Wilkins.

Friedman, E. A. (1955). Primigravid labor: A graphicostatistical analysis. *Obstetrics & Gynecology, 6*, 567–589.

Friedman, E. A. (1978). *Labor: Clinical evaluation of management* (2nd ed.). New York, NY: Appleton-Century-Crofts.

Friedman, E. A., Niswander, K. R., Bayonet-Rivera, N. P., & Sachtleben, M. R. (1966). Relationship of prelabor evaluation to inducibility and the course of labor. *Obstetrics & Gynecology, 28*, 495–501.

Fuchs, A. R., Fuchs, F., Husslein, P., & Soloff, M. S. (1984). Oxytocin receptors in the human uterus during pregnancy and parturition. *American Journal of Obstetrics & Gynecology, 150*(12), 734–741.

Fuchs, A. R., Husslein, P., & Fuchs, F. (1981). Oxytocin and the initiation of human parturition. II. Stimulation of prostaglandin production in the human decidua by oxytocin. *American Journal of Obstetrics & Gynecology, 141*(6), 694–699.

Fuchs, A. R., Romero, R., Keefe, D., Parra, M., Oyarzun, E., & Behnke, E. (1991). Oxytocin secretion and human parturition: Pulse frequency and duration increase during spontaneous labor in women. *American Journal of Obstetrics & Gynecology, 165*(5, Pt. 1), 1515–1523.

Gannon, J. M. (1992). Delivery on the hands and knees: A case study approach. *Journal of Nurse-Midwifery, 37*(1), 48–52.

Garite, T. J., & Simpson, K. R. (2011). Intrauterine resuscitation during labor. *Clinical Obstetrics and Gynecology, 54*(1), 28–39. doi:10.1097/GRF.0b013e31820a062b

Garite, T. J., Weeks, J., Peters-Phair, K., Pattillo, C., & Brewster, W. R. (2000). A randomized controlled trial of the effect of increased intravenous hydration on the course of labor in nulliparous women. *American Journal of Obstetrics & Gynecology, 183*(6), 1544–1548.

Garpiel, S. J. (2018). Effects of an interdisciplinary practice bundle for second-stage labor on clinical outcomes. *MCN: The American Journal of Maternal Child Nursing, 43*(4), 184–194. doi:10.1097/NMC.0000000000000438

Gherman, R. B. (2002). Shoulder dystocia: An evidence-based evaluation of the obstetric nightmare. *Clinical Obstetrics and Gynecology, 45*(2), 345–362.

Gherman, R. B., Chauhan, S. P., & Lewis, D. F. (2012). A survey of central association members about the definition, management, and complications of shoulder dystocia. *Obstetrics & Gynecology, 119*(4), 830–837. doi:10.1097/AOG.0b013e31824be910

Gherman, R. B., Chauhan, S. P., Ouzounian, J. G., Lerner, H., Gonik, B., & Goodwin, M. (2006). Shoulder dystocia: The unpreventable obstetric emergency with empiric management guidelines. *American Journal of Obstetrics & Gynecology, 195*(3), 657–672. doi:10.1016/j.ajog.2005.09.007

Gherman, R. B., Tramont, J., Muffley, P., & Goodwin, T. M. (2000). Analysis of McRoberts' maneuver by x-ray pelvimetry. *Obstetrics & Gynecology, 95*(1), 43–47.

Gillesby, E., Burns, S., Dempsey, A., Kirby, S., Mogensen, K., Naylor, K., . . . Whelan, B. (2010). Comparison of delayed versus immediate pushing during second stage of labor for nulliparous women with epidural anesthesia. *Journal of Obstetric, Gynecologic, and Neonatal Nursing, 39*(6), 635–644. doi:10.1111/j.1552-6909.2010.01195.x

Golay, J., Vedam, S., & Sorger, L. (1993). The squatting position for the second stage of labor: Effects on labor and on maternal and fetal well-being. *Birth, 20*(2), 73–78.

Goldberg, A. B., Greenberg, M. B., & Darney, P. D. (2001). Misoprostol and pregnancy. *The New England Journal of Medicine, 344*(1), 38–47.

Goodman, P., Mackey, M. C., & Tavakoli, A. S. (2004). Factors related to childbirth satisfaction. *Journal of Advanced Nursing, 46*(2), 212–219. doi:10.1111/j.1365-2648.2003.02981.x

Grobman, W. A., Bailit, J., Lai, Y., Reddy, U. M., Wapner, R. J., Thorp, J. M., Jr., . . . Tolosa, J. E. (2018). Defining failed induction of labor. *American Journal of Obstetrics & Gynecology, 218*(1), 122.e1–122.e8. doi:10.1016/j.ajog.2017.11.556

Grobman, W. A., Bailit, J., Lai, Y., Reddy, U. M., Wapner, R. J., Varner, M. W., . . . Tolosa, J. E. (2016). Association of the duration of active pushing with obstetrics outcomes. *Obstetrics & Gynecology, 127*(4), 667–673. doi:10.1097/AOG.0000000000001354

Grobman, W. A., Hornbogen, A., Burke, C., & Costello, R. (2010). Development and implementation of a team-centered shoulder dystocia protocol. *Simulation in Healthcare*, 5(4), 199–203. doi:10.1097/SIH.0b013e3181da5caa

Grobman, W. A., Miller, D., Burke, C., Hornbogen, A., Tam, K., & Costello, R. (2011). Outcomes associated with introduction of a shoulder dystocia protocol. *American Journal of Obstetrics & Gynecology*, 205(6), 513–517. doi:10.1016/j.ajog.2011.05.002

Grobman, W. A., Rice, M. M., Reddy, U. M., Tita, A. T. N., Silver, R. M., Mallett, G., . . . Macones, G. A. (2018). Labor induction versus expectant management in low-risk nulliparous women. *The New England Journal of Medicine*, 379(6), 513–523. doi:10.1056/NEJMoa1800566

Gross, S. J., Shime, J., & Farine, D. (1987). Shoulder dystocia: Predictors and outcome. A five-year review. *American Journal of Obstetrics & Gynecology*, 156(2), 334–336.

Grylack, L. J., Chu, S. S., & Scanlon, J. W. (1984). Use of intravenous fluids before cesarean section: Effects on perinatal glucose, insulin, and sodium homeostasis. *Obstetrics & Gynecology*, 63(5), 654–658.

Guise, J.-M., Berlin, M., McDonagh, M., Osterwell, P., Chan, B., & Helfand, M. (2004). Safety of vaginal birth after cesarean: A systematic review. *Obstetrics & Gynecology*, 103(3), 420–429.

Guise, J.-M., Eden, K., Emeis, C., Denman, M. A., Marshall, N., Fu, R., . . . McDonagh, M. (2010). *Evidence Report/Technology Assessment Number 191: Vaginal birth after cesarean: New insights* (AHRQ Publication No. 10-E001). Rockville, MD: Agency for Healthcare Research and Quality.

Gupta, J. K., Sood, A., Hofmeyr, G. J., & Vogel, J. P. (2017). Position in the second stage of labour for women without epidural anaesthesia. *Cochrane Database of Systematic Reviews*, (5), CD002006. doi:10.1002/14651858.CD002006.pub4

Gurewitsch, E. D., & Allen, R. H. (2011). Reducing the risk of shoulder dystocia and associated brachial plexus injury. *Obstetrics and Gynecology Clinics of North America*, 38(2), 247–269. doi:10.1016/j.ogc.2011.02.015

Hamilton, B. E., Martin, J. A., & Ventura, S. J. (2011). Births: Preliminary data for 2010. *National Vital Statistics Reports*, 60(2), 1–36.

Hamilton, B. E., Martin, J. A., Osterman, M. J. K., & Rossen, L. M. (2019). *Births: Provisional data for 2018* (Vital Statistics Rapid Release No. 7). Hyattsville, MD: National Center for Health Statistics.

Hamilton, E., Warrick, P., Knox, E., O'Keeffe, D., & Garite, T. (2012). High uterine contraction rates in births with normal and abnormal umbilical artery gases. *Journal of Maternal-Fetal & Neonatal Medicine*, 25(11), 2302–2307.

Handa, V. L., Blomquist, J. L., McDermott, K. C., Friedman, S., & Muñoz, A. (2012). Pelvic floor disorders after vaginal birth: Effect of episiotomy, perineal laceration, and operative birth. *Obstetrics & Gynecology*, 119(2, Pt. 1), 233–239. doi:10.1097/AOG.0b013e318240df4f

Handa, V. L., Harris, T. A., & Ostergard, D. R. (1996). Protecting the pelvic floor: Obstetric management to prevent incontinence and pelvic organ prolapse. *Obstetrics & Gynecology*, 88(3), 470–478.

Hansen, S. L., Clark, S. L., & Foster, J. C. (2002). Active pushing versus passive fetal descent in the second stage of labor: A randomized controlled trial. *Obstetrics & Gynecology*, 99(1), 29–34.

Hanson, L. (2009). Second-stage labor care: Challenges in spontaneous bearing down. *Journal of Perinatal & Neonatal Nursing*, 23(1), 31–39. doi:10.1097/JPN.0b013e318196526b

Harper, L. M., Cahill, A. G., Roehl, K. A., Odibo, A. O., Stamilio, D. M., & Macones, G. A. (2012). The pattern of labor preceding uterine rupture. *American Journal of Obstetrics & Gynecology*, 207(3), 210.e1–210.e6.

Harper, L. M., Caughey, A. B., Odibo, A. O., Roehl, K. A., Zhao, Q., & Cahill, A. G. (2012). Normal progress of induced labor.

Obstetrics & Gynecology, 119(6), 1113–1118. doi:10.1097/AOG.0b013e318253d7aa

Hartmann, K., Viswanathan, M., Palmieri, R., Gartiehner, G., Thorp, J., Jr., & Lohr, K. N. (2005). Outcomes of routine episiotomy: A systematic review. *JAMA*, 293(17), 2141–2148. doi:10.1001/jama.293.17.2141

Hastings-Tolsma, M., Vincent, D., Emeis, C., & Francisco, T. (2007). Getting through birth in one piece: Protecting the perineum. *MCN: The American Journal of Maternal Child Nursing*, 32(3), 158–164. doi:10.1097/01.NMC.0000269565.20111.92

Hawkins, J. L., Chang, J., Palmer, S. K., Gibbs, C. P., & Callaghan, W. M. (2011). Anesthesia-related maternal mortality in the United States: 1979–2002. *Obstetrics & Gynecology*, 117(1), 69–74. doi:10.1097/AOG.0b013e31820093a9

Hellman, L. M., & Prystowsky, H. (1952). The duration of the second stage of labor. *American Journal of Obstetrics & Gynecology*, 63(6), 1223–1233.

Hersh, A. R., Skeith, A. E., Sargent, J. A., & Caughey, A. B. (2019). Induction of labor at 39 weeks of gestation versus expectant management for low-risk nulliparous women: A cost-effectiveness analysis. *American Journal of Obstetrics & Gynecology*, 220(6), 590.e1–590.e10. doi:10.1016/j.ajog.2019.02.017

Heuser, C., Knight, S., Esplin, M. S., Eller, A. G., Holmgren, C. M., Richards, D., . . . Jackson, G. M. (2013). Tachysystole in term labor: Incidence, risk factors, outcomes, and effect on fetal tracings. *American Journal of Obstetrics & Gynecology*, 209, 32.e1–32.e6. doi:10.1016/j.ajog.2013.04.004

Hibbard, J. U., Gilbert, S., Landon, M. B., Hauth, J. C., Leveno, K. J., Spong, C. Y., . . . Gabbe, S. G. (2006). Trial of labor or repeat cesarean delivery in women with morbid obesity and previous cesarean delivery. *Obstetrics & Gynecology*, 108(1), 125–133. doi:10.1097/01.AOG.0000223871.69852.31

Hibbard, J. U., Ismail, M. A., Wang, Y., Te, C., Karrison, T., & Ismail, M. A. (2001). Failed vaginal birth after cesarean section: How risky is it? I. Maternal morbidity. *American Journal of Obstetrics & Gynecology*, 184(7), 1365–1371.

Hilliard, A. M., Chauhan, S. P., Zhao, Y., & Rankins, N. C. (2012). Effect of obesity on length of labor in nulliparous women. *American Journal of Perinatology*, 29(2), 127–132. doi:10.1055/s-0031-1295653

Hirshberg, A., Levine, L. D., & Srinivas, S. (2014). Labor length among overweight and obese women undergoing induction of labor. *Journal of Maternal-Fetal & Neonatal Medicine*, 27(17), 1771–1775. doi:10.3109/14767058.2013.879705

Hodnett, E. D. (2002). Pain and women's satisfaction with the experience of childbirth: A systematic review. *American Journal of Obstetrics & Gynecology*, 186(5 Suppl.), S160–S172.

Hodnett, E. D., Gates, S., Hofmeyr, G., & Sakala, C. (2013). Continuous support for women during childbirth. *Cochrane Database of Systematic Reviews*, (10), CD003766. doi:10.1002/14651858.CD003766.pub4

Hodnett, E. D., Lowe, N. K., Hannah, M. E., Willan, A. R., Stevens, B., Weston, J. A., . . . Stremler, R. (2002). Effectiveness of nurse providers of birth labor support in North American hospitals: A randomized controlled trial. *JAMA*, 288(11), 1373–1381. doi:10.1001/jama.288.11.1373

Hoffman, M. K., Bailit, J. L., Branch, D. W., Burkman, R. T., Van Veldhusien, P., Lu, L., . . . Zhang, J. (2011). A comparison of obstetric maneuvers for the acute management of shoulder dystocia. *Obstetrics & Gynecology*, 117(6), 1272–1278. doi:10.1097/AOG.0b013e31821a12c9

Hoffman, M. K., Vahratian, A., Sciscione, A. C., Troendle, J. F., & Zhang, J. (2006). Comparison of labor progression between induced and noninduced multiparous women. *Obstetrics & Gynecology*, 107(5), 1029–1034. doi:10.1097/01.AOG.0000210528.32940.c6

Hofmeyr, G. J., Gülmezoglu, A. M., & Pileggi, C. (2010). Vaginal misoprostol for cervical ripening and induction of labour.

Cochrane Database of Systematic Reviews, (10), CD000941. doi:10.1002/14651858.CD000941.pub2

Hofmeyr, G. J., & Lawrie, T. A. (2012). Amnioinfusion for potential or suspected umbilical cord compression in labour. *Cochrane Database of Systematic Reviews*, (1), CD000013. doi:10.1002/14651858.CD000013.pub2

Holmgren, C., Scott, J. R., Porter, T. F., Esplin, M. S., & Bardsley, T. (2012). Uterine rupture with attempted vaginal birth after cesarean delivery: Decision-to-delivery time and neonatal outcome. *Obstetrics & Gynecology*, 119(4), 725–731. doi:10.1097/AOG.0b013e318249a1d7

Holvey, N. (2014). Supporting women in the second stage of labour. *British Journal of Midwifery*, 22(3), 182–186. doi:10.12968/bjom.2014.22.3.182

Hudelist, G., Gelle'n, J., Singer, C., Ruecklinger, E., Czerwenka, K., Kandolf, O., & Keckstein, J. (2005). Factors predicting severe perineal trauma during childbirth: Role of forceps delivery routinely combined with mediolateral episiotomy. *American Journal of Obstetrics & Gynecology*, 192(3), 875–881. doi:10.1016/j.ajog.2004.09.035

Hung, K. J., & Berg, O. (2011). Early skin-to-skin after cesarean to improve breastfeeding. *MCN: The American Journal of Maternal Child Nursing*, 36(5), 318–324. doi:10.1097/NMC.0b013e3182266314

Hurd, W. W., Gibbs, S. G., Ventolini, G., Horowitz, G. M., & Guy, S. R. (2005). Shortening increases spontaneous contractility in myometrium from pregnant women at term. *American Journal of Obstetrics & Gynecology*, 192(4), 1295–1301. doi:10.1016/j.ajog.2005.01.030

Husslein, P., Fuchs, A. R., & Fuchs, F. (1981). Oxytocin and the initiation of human parturition. I. Prostaglandin release during induction of labor by oxytocin. *American Journal of Obstetrics & Gynecology*, 141(6), 688–693.

Incerti, M., Locatelli, A., Ghidini, A., Ciriello, E., Consonni, S., & Pezzullo, J. C. (2011). Variability in rate of cervical dilation in nulliparous women at term. *Birth*, 38(1), 30–35. doi:10.1111/j.1523-536X.2010.00443.x

Inglis, S. R., Feier, N., Chetiyaar, J. B., Naylor, M. H., Sumersille, M., Cervellione, K. L., & Predanic, M. (2011). Effects of shoulder dystocia training on the incidence of brachial plexus injury. *American Journal of Obstetrics & Gynecology*, 204(4), 322.e1–322.e6. doi:10.1016/j.ajog.2011.01.027

Institute for Safe Medication Practices. (2007). *High-alert medications*. Huntingdon Valley, PA: Author.

Jackson, J. K., Wickstrom, E., & Anderson, B. (2019). Oxytocin guidelines associated with compliance to national standards. *MCN: The American Journal of Maternal Child Nursing*, 44(3), 128–136. doi:10.1097/NMC.0000000000000520

Jiang, H., Qian, X., Carroli, G., & Garner, P. (2017). Selective versus routine use of episiotomy for vaginal birth. *Cochrane Database of Systematic Reviews*, (2), CD000081. doi:10.1002/14651858.CD000081.pub3

Johnson, J. H., Figueroa, R., Garry, D., Elimian, A., & Maulik, D. (2004). Immediate maternal and neonatal effects of forceps and vacuum-assisted deliveries. *Obstetrics & Gynecology*, 103(3), 513–518.

Jozwiak, M., Bloemenkamp, K. W., Kelly, A. J., Mol, B. W., Irion, O., & Boulvain, M. (2012). Mechanical methods for induction of labour. *Cochrane Database of Systematic Reviews*, (3), CD001233. doi:10.1002/14651858.CD001233.pub2

Kazandi, M., Sendag, R., Akercan, F., Terek, M. C., & Gundem, G. (2003). Different type of variable decelerations and their effects to neonatal outcomes. *Singapore Medical Journal*, 44(5), 243–247.

Keirse, M. J. (2006). Natural prostaglandins for induction of labor and preinduction cervical ripening. *Clinical Obstetrics and Gynecology*, 49(3), 609–626.

Kelly, M., Johnson, E., Lee, V., Massey, L., Purser, D., Ring, K., . . . Wood, D. (2010). Delayed versus immediate pushing in second stage of labor. *MCN: The American Journal of Maternal Child Nursing*, 35(2), 81–88. doi:10.1097/NMC.0b013e3181cae7ad

Keppler, A. B. (1988). The use of intravenous fluids during labor. *Birth*, 15(2), 75–79.

Kettle, C., & Tohill, S. (2011). *Perinatal care*. Retrieved from http://www.ncbi.nlm.nih.gov/pmc/articles/PMC2907946/pdf/2008-1401.pdf

Killion, M. M. (2019). Enhanced recovery after cesarean birth. *MCN: The American Journal of Maternal Child Nursing*, 44(6), 296. doi:10.1097/NMC.0000000000000572

Kilpatrick, S., & Garrison, E. (2017). Normal labor and delivery. In S. G. Gabbe, J. R. Niebyl, J. L. Simpson, M. B. Landon, H. L. Galan, E. R. M. Jauniaux, . . . W. A. Grobman (Eds.). *Obstetrics: Normal and problem pregnancies* (7th ed., pp. 246–270). Philadelphia, PA: Elsevier.

King, T. (2018). Fetal assessment. In S. T. Blackburn (Ed.), *Maternal, fetal, neonatal physiology: A clinical perspective* (5th ed., pp. 162–177). St. Louis, MO: Elsevier.

Kirkendall, C., Jauregui, I., Kim, J. O., & Phelan, J. (2000). Catastrophic uterine rupture: Maternal and fetal characteristics. *Obstetrics & Gynecology*, 95(4 Suppl.), S74.

Knox, G. E., & Simpson, K. R. (2011). Perinatal high reliability. *American Journal of Obstetrics & Gynecology*, 204(5), 373–377. doi:10.1016/j.ajog.2010.10.900

Kominiarek, M. A., Zhang, J., Vanveldhuisen, P., Troendle, J., Beaver, J., & Hibbard, J. U. (2011). Contemporary labor patterns: The impact of maternal body mass index. *American Journal of Obstetrics & Gynecology*, 205(3), 244.e1–244.e8. doi:10.1016/j.ajog.2011.06.014

Korb, D., Goffinet, F., Seco, A., Chevret, S., & Deneux-Tharaux, C. (2019). Risk of severe maternal morbidity associated with cesarean delivery and the role of maternal age: A population-based propensity score analysis. *Canadian Medical Association Journal*, 191(13), E352–E360. doi:10.1503/cmaj.181067

Kozhimannil, K. B., Hardeman, R. R., Attanasio, L. B., Blauer-Peterson, C., & O'Brien, M. (2013). Doula care, birth outcomes, and costs among Medicaid beneficiaries. *American Journal of Public Health*, 103(4), e113–e121. doi:10.2105/AJPH.2012.301201

Krening, C. F., Rehling-Anthony, K., & Garko, C. (2012). Oxytocin administration: The transition to a safer model of care. *Journal of Perinatal & Neonatal Nursing*, 26(1), 15–24. doi:10.1097/JPN.0b013e318240c7d4

Kudish, B., Blackwell, S., Mcneely, S. G., Bujold, E., Kruger, M., Hendrix, S. L., & Sokol, R. (2006). Operative vaginal delivery and midline episiotomy: A bad combination for the perineum. *American Journal of Obstetrics & Gynecology*, 195(3), 749–754. doi:10.1016/j.ajog.2006.06.078

Kwek, K., & Yeo, G. S. H. (2006). Shoulder dystocia and injuries: Prevention and management. *Current Opinion in Obstetrics & Gynecology*, 18(2), 123–128. doi:10.1097/01.gco.0000192976.38858.90

Lagrew, D. C., Kane Low, L., Brennan, R., Corry, M. P., Edmonds, J. K., Gilpin, B. G., . . . Jaffer, S. (2018). National partnership for maternal safety: Consensus bundle on safe reduction of primary cesarean births-supporting intended vaginal births. *Journal of Obstetric, Gynecologic, and Neonatal Nursing*, 47(2), 214–226. doi:10.1016/j.jogn.2018.01.008

Lai, M. L., Lin, K. C., Li, H. Y., Shey, K. S., & Gau, M. L. (2009). Effects of delayed pushing during the second stage of labour on postpartum fatigue and birth outcomes in nulliparous women. *Journal of Nursing Research*, 17(1), 62–72. doi:10.1097/JNR.0b013e3181999e78

Landy, H. J., Laughon, S. K., Bailit, J. L., Kominiarek, M. A., Gonzalez-Quintero, V. H., Ramirez, M., . . . Zhang, J. (2011).

Characteristics associated with severe perineal and cervical lacerations during vaginal delivery. *Obstetrics & Gynecology, 117*(3), 627–635. doi:10.1097/AOG.0b013e31820afaf2

Langer, B., Carbonne, B., Goffinet, F., Le Gouëff, F., Berkane, N., & Laville, M. (1997). Fetal pulse oximetry and fetal heart rate monitoring during stage II of labour. *European Journal of Obstetrics, Gynecology and Reproductive Biology, 72*(Suppl.), S57–S61.

Larkin, P., Begley, C. M., & Devane, D. (2012). 'Not enough people to look after you': An exploration of women's experiences of childbirth in the Republic of Ireland. *Midwifery, 28*(1), 98–105. doi:10.1016/j.midw.2010.11.007

Larson, A., & Mandelbaum, D. E. (2012). Association of head circumference and shoulder dystocia in macrosomic neonates. *Maternal and Child Health Journal, 17*(3), 501–504. doi:10.1007/s10995-012-1013-z

Laughon, S. K., Berghella, V., Reddy, U. M., Sundaram, R., Lu, Z., & Hoffman, M. K. (2014). Neonatal and maternal outcomes with prolonged second stage of labor. *Obstetrics & Gynecology, 124*(1), 57–67. doi:10.1097/AOG.0000000000000278

Laughon, S. K., Branch, D. W., Beaver, J., & Zhang, J. (2012). Changes in labor patterns over 50 years. *American Journal of Obstetrics & Gynecology, 206*(5), 419.e1–419.e9. doi:10.1016/j.ajog.2012.03.003

Lawrence, A., Lewis, L., Hofmeyr, G. J., & Styles, C. (2013). Maternal positions and mobility during first stage labour. *Cochrane Database of Systematic Reviews*, (10), CD003934. doi:10.1002/14651858.CD003934.pub4

Lederman, R. P., Lederman, E., Work, B., Jr., & McCann, D. S. (1985). Anxiety and epinephrine in multiparous women in labor: Relationship to duration of labor and fetal heart rate pattern. *American Journal of Obstetrics & Gynecology, 153*(8), 870–877.

Lemos, A., Amorin, L. A., Dornelas de Andrade, A., de Souza, A. I., Cabral Filho, J. E., & Correia, J. B. (2015). Pushing/bearing down methods for the second stage of labour. *Cochrane Database of Systematic Reviews*, (10), CD009124. doi:10.1002/14651858.CD009124.pub2

Le Ray, C., Audibert, F., Goffinet, F., & Fraser, W. (2009). When to stop pushing: Effects of expulsive efforts on maternal and neonatal outcomes in nulliparous women with epidural analgesia. *American Journal of Obstetrics & Gynecology, 201*(4), 361.e1–361.e7. doi:10.1016/j.ajog.2009.08.002

Lerner, H., Durlacher, K., Smith, S., & Hamilton, E. (2011). Relationship between head-to-body delivery interval in shoulder dystocia and neonatal depression. *Obstetrics & Gynecology, 118*(2, Pt. 1), 318–322. doi:10.1097/AOG.0b013e31822467e9

Leung, A., Farmer, R. M., Leung, E. K., Medearis, A. L., & Paul, R. H. (1993). Risk factors associated with uterine rupture during trial of labor after cesarean birth: A case-control study. *American Journal of Obstetrics & Gynecology, 168*(5), 1358–1363.

Leung, A., Leung, E., & Paul, R. (1993). Uterine rupture after previous cesarean delivery: Maternal and fetal consequences. *American Journal of Obstetrics & Gynecology, 169*(4), 945–950.

Leung, T. Y., Stuart, O., Sahota, D. S., Suen, S. S., Lau, T. K., & Lao, T. T. (2011). Head-to-body delivery interval and risk of fetal acidosis and hypoxic ischaemic encephalopathy in shoulder dystocia: A retrospective review. *British Journal of Obstetrics and Gynaecology, 118*(4), 474–479. doi:10.1111/j.1471-0528.2010.02834.x

Liao, J. B., Buhimschi, C. S., & Norwitz, E. R. (2005). Normal labor: Mechanism and duration. *Obstetrics and Gynecology Clinics of North America, 32*(2), 145–164. doi:10.1016/j.ogc.2005.01.001

Lim, G., Facco, F. L., Nathan, B., Waters, J. H., Wong, C. A., & Eltzschig, H. K. (2018). A review of the impact of obstetric anesthesia on maternal and neonatal outcomes. *Anesthesiology, 129*(1), 192–215. doi:10.1097/ALN.0000000000002182

Liston, R., Sawchuck, D., & Young, D. (2018). No. 197b-fetal health surveillance: Intrapartum consensus guideline. *Journal of Obstetrics and Gynaecology Canada, 40*(4), e298–e322.

Liu, S., Heaman, M., Joseph, K. S., Liston, R. M., Huang, L., Sauve, R., & Kramer, M. S. (2005). Risk of maternal postpartum readmission associated with mode of delivery. *Obstetrics & Gynecology, 105*(4), 836–842. doi:10.1097/01.AOG.0000154153.31193.2c

Liu, Y. C. (1989). The effects of the upright position during childbirth. *Image—The Journal of Nursing Scholarship, 21*(1), 14–18.

Low, L. K., Seng, J. S., Murtland, T. L., & Oakley, D. (2000). Clinician-specific episiotomy rates: Impacts on perineal outcomes. *Journal of Nurse Midwifery & Women's Health, 43*(2), 87–93.

Lydon-Rochelle, M., Holt, V. L., Easterling, T. R., & Martin, D. P. (2001). First-birth cesarean and placental abruption or previa at second birth. *Obstetrics & Gynecology, 97*(5, Pt. 1), 765–769.

Lydon-Rochelle, M., Holt, V. L., Martin, D. P., & Easterling, T. R. (2000). Association between method of delivery and maternal rehospitalization. *JAMA, 283*(18), 2411–2416.

Lyndon, A., Simpson, K. R., & Spetz, J. (2017). Thematic analysis of US stakeholder views on the influence of labour nurses' care on birth outcomes. *BMJ Quality & Safety, 26*(10), 824–831. doi:10.1136/bmjqs-2016-005859

MacKinnon, K., McIntyre, M., & Quance, M. (2005). The meaning of the nurse's presence during childbirth. *Journal of Obstetric, Gynecologic, and Neonatal Nursing, 34*(1), 28–36. doi:10.1177/0884217504272808

Macones, G. A., Caughey, A. B., Wood, S. L, Wrench, I., Huang, J., Norman, M., . . . Wilson, R. D. (2019). Guidelines for postoperative care in cesarean delivery: Enhanced Recovery after Surgery (ERAS) Society recommendations (part 3). *American Journal of Obstetrics and Gynecology, 221*(3), 247.e1–247.e9. doi:10.1016/j.ajog.2019.04.012.

Macones, G. A., Hankins, G. D. V., Spong, C. Y., Hauth, J., & Moore, T. (2008). The 2008 National Institute of Child Health and Human Development workshop report on electronic fetal monitoring: Update on definitions, interpretation, and research guidelines. *Obstetrics & Gynecology, 112*(3), 661–666. doi:10.1097/AOG.0b013e3181841395

Main, E. K., Chang, S.-C., Cape, V., Sakowski, C., Smith, H., & Vasher, J. (2019). Safety assessment of a large-scale improvement collaborative to reduce nulliparous cesarean delivery rates. *Obstetrics & Gynecology, 133*(4), 613–623. doi:10.1097/aog.0000000000003109

Maresh, M., Choong, K. H., & Beard, R. W. (1983). Delayed pushing with lumbar epidural analgesia in labour. *British Journal of Obstetrics and Gynaecology, 90*(7), 623–627.

Martin, J. A., Hamilton, B. E., Osterman, M. J. K., Driscoll, A. K., & Drake, P. (2018). *Births: Final data for 2017*. Hyattsville, MD: National Center for Health Statistics. Retrieved from https://www.cdc.gov/nchs/data/nvsr/nvsr67/nvsr67_08-508.pdf

Martin, J. A., Hamilton, B. E., Ventura, S. J., Osterman, M. J. K., Wilson, E. C., & Mathews, T. J. (2012). Births: Final data for 2010. *National Vital Statistics Reports, 61*(1), 1–72.

Matthews, R., & Callister, L. C. (2004). Childbearing women's perceptions of nursing care that promotes dignity. *Journal of Obstetric, Gynecologic, and Neonatal Nursing, 33*(4), 498–507. doi:10.1177/0884217504266896

Matthews, T. J., & Curtin, S. C. (2015). *When are babies born: Morning, noon, or night? Birth certificate data for 2013* (Data Brief No. 200). Hyattsville, MD: National Center for Health Statistics.

Maul, H., Macray, L., & Garfield, R. E. (2006). Cervical ripening: Biochemical, molecular, and clinical considerations. *Clinical Obstetrics and Gynecology, 49*(3), 551–563.

Mayberry, L. J., Hammer, R., Kelly, C., True-Driver, B., & De, A. (1999). Use of delayed pushing with epidural anesthesia: Findings from a randomized controlled trial. *Journal of Perinatology, 19*(1), 26–30.

Mayerhofer, K., Bodner-Adler, B., Bodner, K., Rabl, M., Kaider, A., Wagenbichler, P., . . . Husslein, P. (2002). Traditional care of the perineum during birth. A prospective, randomized, multicenter study of 1,076 women. *Journal of Reproductive Medicine*, 47(6), 477–482.

Mazouni, C., Porcu, G., Bretelle, F., Loundou, A., Heckenroth, H., & Gamerre, M. (2006). Risk factors for forceps delivery in nulliparous patients. *Acta Obstetricia et Gynecologica Scandinavica*, 85(3), 298–301. doi:10.1080/00016340500500782

McGrath, S. K., & Kennell, J. H. (2008). A randomized controlled trial of continuous labor support for middle-class couples: Effect on cesarean delivery rates. *Birth*, 35(2), 92–97. doi:10.1111/j.1523-536X.2008.00221.x

McKay, S., Barrows, T., & Roberts, J. (1990). Women's views of second-stage labor as assessed by interviews and videotapes. *Birth*, 17(4), 192–198.

McMaster, K., Sanchez-Ramos, L., & Kaunitz, (2015). Balancing the efficacy and safety of misoprostol: A meta-analysis comparing 25 versus 50 micrograms of intravaginal misoprostol for the induction of labor. *British Journal of Obstetrics and Gynaecology*, 122, 468–472. doi:10.1111/1471-0528.12935

Menacker, F., & Martin, J. A. (2008). Expanded health data from the new birth certificate, 2005. *National Vital Statistics Reports*, 56(3), 1–24.

Mendelson, C. L. (1946). The aspiration of stomach contents into the lungs during obstetric anesthesia. *American Journal of Obstetrics & Gynecology*, 52, 191–205.

Mendiola, J., Grylack, L. J., & Scanlon, J. W. (1982). Effects of intrapartum maternal glucose infusion on the normal fetus and newborn. *Anesthesia and Analgesia*, 61(1), 32–35.

Mengert, W., & Murphy, D. (1933). Intra-abdominal pressures created by voluntary muscular effort. *Surgery and Gynecologic Obstetrics*, 57, 745–751.

Merchant, R., Chartrand, D., Dain, S., Dobson, J., Kurrek, M., LeDez, K., . . . Shukla, R. (2012). Guidelines to the practice of anesthesia revised edition 2012. *Canadian Journal of Anesthesia*, 59(1), 1–14. doi:10.1007/s12630-011-9609-0

Miño, M., Puertas, A., Miranda, J. A., & Herruzo, A. J. (1999). Amnioinfusion in term labor with low amniotic fluid due to rupture of membranes: A new indication. *European Journal of Obstetrics, Gynecology, and Reproductive Biology*, 82(1), 29–34.

Miyazaki, F. S., & Nevarez, F. (1985). Saline amnioinfusion for relief of repetitive variable decelerations: A prospective randomized study. *American Journal of Obstetrics & Gynecology*, 153(3), 301–306.

Mollberg, M., Hagberg, H., Bager, B., Lilja, H., & Ladfors, L. (2005). Risk factors for obstetric brachial palsy among neonates delivered by vacuum extraction. *Obstetrics & Gynecology*, 106(5, Pt. 1), 913–918. doi:10.1097/01.AOG.0000183595.32077.83

Moragianni, V. A., Hacker, M. R., & Craparo, F. J. (2011). Improved overall delivery documentation following implementation of a standardized shoulder dystocia delivery form. *Journal of Perinatal Medicine*, 40(1), 97–100. doi:10.1515/JPM.2011.112

Myles, T. D., & Santolaya, J. (2003). Maternal and neonatal outcomes in patients with a prolonged second stage of labor. *Obstetrics & Gynecology*, 102(1), 52–58.

Nathanielsz, P. W. (1998). Comparison studies on the initiation of labor. *European Journal of Obstetrics, Gynecology, and Reproductive Biology*, 78(2), 127–132.

National Institute for Health and Care Excellence. (2014). *Intrapartum care for healthy women and babies*. Retrieved from http://www.nice.org.uk/guidance/cg190

National Institutes of Health. (2010). Vaginal birth after cesarean: New insights. *NIH Consensus and State of the Science Statements*, 27(3), 1–48. Retrieved from http://consensus.nih.gov/2010/vbacstatement.htm

National Quality Forum. (2018). *National quality partners playbook: Shared decision making in healthcare*. Washington, DC: Author.

Neal, J. L., & Lowe, N. K. (2012). Physiologic partograph to improve birth safety and outcomes among low-risk, nulliparous women with spontaneous labor onset. *Medical Hypotheses*, 78(2), 319–326. doi:10.1016/j.mehy.2011.11.012

Neal, J. L., Lowe, N. K., Ahijevych, K. L., Patrick, T. E., Cabbage, L. A., & Corwin, E. J. (2010). "Active labor" duration and dilation rates among low-risk, nulliparous women with spontaneous labor onset: A systematic review. *Journal of Midwifery & Women's Health*, 55(4), 308–318. doi:10.1016/j.jmwh.2009.08.004

Neal, J. L., Lowe, N. K., Patrick, T. E., Cabbage, L. A., & Corwin, E. J. (2010). What is the slowest-yet-normal cervical dilation rate among nulliparous women with spontaneous labor onset? *Journal of Obstetric, Gynecologic, and Neonatal Nursing*, 39(4), 361–369. doi:10.1111/j.1552-6909.2010.01154.x

Neilson, D. R., Freeman, R. K., & Mangan, S. (2008). Signal ambiguity resulting in unexpected outcome with external fetal heart rate monitoring. *American Journal of Obstetrics & Gynecology*, 198(6), 717–724. doi:10.1016/j.ajog.2008.02.030

Nelson, D. B., McIntire, D. D., & Leveno, K. J. (2013). Relationship of the length of the first stage of labor to the length of the second stage. *Obstetrics & Gynecology*, 122(1), 27–32. doi:10.1097/AOG.0b013e3182972907

Ness, A., Goldberg, J., & Berghella, V. (2005). Abnormalities of the first and second stages of labor. *Obstetrics and Gynecology Clinics of North America*, 32(2), 201–220.

Nettina, S. M. (2010). *Lippincott manual of nursing practice* (9th ed.). Philadelphia, PA: Lippincott, Williams & Wilkins.

Newman, R. B. (2005). Uterine contraction assessment. *Obstetrics and Gynecology Clinics of North America*, 32(3), 341–367.

Nguyen, T., Fox, N. S., Friedman, F., Jr., Sandler, R., & Rebarber, A. (2011). The sequential effect of computerized delivery charting and simulation training on shoulder dystocia documentation. *Journal of Maternal-Fetal & Neonatal Medicine*, 24(11), 1357–1361. doi:10.3109/14767058.2010.551151

Nieuwenhuijze, M. J., de Jonge, A., Korstjens, I., Budé, L., & Lagro-Janssen, T. (2013). Influence on birthing positions affects women's sense of control in second stage of labour. *Midwifery*, 29(11), e107–e114. doi:10.1016/j.midw.2012.12.007

Nieuwenhuijze, M. J., Low, L. K., Korstjens, I., & Lagro-Janssen, T. (2014). The role of maternity care providers in promoting shared decision making regarding birthing positions during the second stage of labor. *Journal of Midwifery & Women's Health*, 59, 277–285. doi:10.1111/jmwh.12187

Novikova, N., Hofmeyr, G. J., & Essilfie-Appiah, G. (2010). Prophylactic versus therapeutic amnioinfusion for oligohydramnios in labour. *Cochrane Database of Systematic Reviews*, (9), CD000176. doi:10.1002/14651858.CD000176.pub2

Okby, R., & Sheiner, E. (2012). Risk factors for neonatal brachial plexus paralysis. *Archives of Gynecology and Obstetrics*, 286(2), 333–336. doi:10.1007/s00404-012-2272-z

Oladapo, O. T., Diaz, V., Bonet, M., Abalos, E., Thwin, S. S., Souza, H., . . . Gülmezoglu, A. M. (2018). Cervical dilatation patterns of 'low-risk' women with spontaneous labour and normal perinatal outcomes: A systematic review. *British Journal of Obstetrics and Gynaecology*, 125(8), 944–954. doi:10.1111/1471-0528.14930

Oláh, K. S., & Gee, H. (1996). The active mismanagement of labour. *British Journal of Obstetrics and Gynaecology*, 103(8), 729–731.

O'Rourke, T. P., Girardi, G. J., Balaskas, T. N., Havlisch, R. A., Landstrom, G., Kirby, B., . . . Simpson, K. R. (2011). Implementation of a system-wide policy for labor induction. *MCN: The American Journal of Maternal Child Nursing*, 36(5), 305–311. doi:10.1097/NMC.0b013e3182069e12

Osmundson, S., Ou-Yang, R. J., & Grobman, W. A. (2010). Elective induction compared with expectant management in nulliparous women with a favorable cervix. *Obstetrics & Gynecology*, 116(3), 601–605. doi:10.1097/AOG.0b013e3181eb6e9b

O'Sullivan, G., Liu, B., Hart, D., Seed, P., & Shennan, A. (2009). Effect of food intake during labour on obstetric outcome: Randomized controlled trial. *British Medical Journal, 338,* b784. doi:10.1136/bmj.b784

Ouzounian, J. G., Gherman, R. B., Chauhan, S., Battista, L. R., & Lee, R. H. (2012). Recurrent shoulder dystocia: Analysis of incidence and risk factors. *American Journal of Perinatology, 29*(7), 515–528. doi:10.1055/s-0032-1310522

Ouzounian, J. G., Korst, L. M., Ahn, M. O., & Phelan, J. P. (1998). Shoulder dystocia and neonatal brain injury: Significance of the head–shoulder interval. *American Journal of Obstetrics & Gynecology, 178*(1 Suppl.), S76.

Overland, E. A., Vatten, L. J., & Eskild, A. (2012). Risk of shoulder dystocia: Associations with parity and offspring birthweight. A population study of 1 914 544 deliveries. *Acta Obstetricia et Gynecologica Scandinavica, 91*(4), 483–488. doi:10.1111/j.1600-0412.2012.01354.x

Page, K., McCool, W. F., & Guidera, M. (2017). Examination of the pharmacology of oxytocin and clinical guidelines for use in labor. *Journal of Midwifery & Women's Health, 62*(4), 425–433. doi:10.1111/jmwh.12610

Paré, E., Quiñones, J. N., & Macones, G. A. (2006). Vaginal birth after cesarean section versus elective repeat cesarean section: Assessment of maternal downstream health outcomes. *British Journal of Obstetrics and Gynaecology, 113*(1), 75–85. doi:10.1111/j.1471-0528.2005.00793.x

Parer, J. T., King, T., Flanders, S., Fox, M., & Kilpatrick, S. J. (2006). Fetal acidemia and electronic fetal heart rate patterns: Is there evidence of an association? *Journal of Maternal-Fetal & Neonatal Medicine, 19*(5), 289–294. doi:10.1080/14767050500526172

Paris, A. E., Greenberg, J. A., Ecker, J. L., & McElrath, T. F. (2011). Is an episiotomy necessary with a shoulder dystocia? *American Journal of Obstetrics & Gynecology, 205*(3), 217.e1–217.e3. doi:10.1016/j.ajog.2011.04.006

Parnell, C., Langhoff-Roos, J., Iversen, R., & Damgaard, P. (1993). Pushing method in the expulsive phase of labor. A randomized trial. *Acta Obstetricia et Gynecologica Scandinavica, 72*(1), 31–35.

Penfield, C. A., & Wing, D. A. (2017). Labor induction techniques: Which is best? *Obstetrics and Gynecology Clinics of North America, 44*(4), 567–592. doi:10.1016/j.ogc.2017.08.011

Penney, D. S., & Perlis, D. W. (1992). When to use suprapubic or fundal pressure. *MCN. The American Journal of Maternal Child Nursing, 17,* 34–36.

Phaneuf, S., Asbóth, G., Carrasco, M. P., Liñares, B. R., Kimura, T., Harris, A., & Bernal, A. L. (1998). Desensitization of oxytocin receptors in human myometrium. *Human Reproduction Update, 4*(5), 625–633.

Phaneuf, S., Rodríguez Liñares, B., TambyRaja, R. L., MacKenzie, I. Z., & López Bernal, A. (2000). Loss of myometrial oxytocin receptors during oxytocin-induced and oxytocin-augmented labour. *Journal of Reproduction and Fertility, 120*(1), 91–97.

Phelan, J. P., Ouzounian, J. G., Gherman, R. B., Korst, L. M., & Goodwin, M. (1997). Shoulder dystocia and permanent Erb's palsy: The role of fundal pressure. *American Journal of Obstetrics & Gynecology, 176*(1 Suppl.), S138.

Philipson, E. H., Kalhan, S. C., Riha, M. M., & Pimental, R. (1987). Effects of maternal glucose infusion on fetal acid-base status in human pregnancy. *American Journal of Obstetrics & Gynecology, 157*(4, Pt. 1), 866–873.

Phillips, K. C., & Thomas, T. A. (1983). Second stage of labour with or without extradural analgesia. *Anaesthesia, 38*(10), 972–976.

Plunkett, J., Doniger, S., Orabona, G., Morgan, T., Haataja, R., Hallman, M., . . . Muglia, L. (2011). An evolutionary genomic approach to identify genes involved in human birth timing. *PLoS Genetics, 7*(4), e1001365. doi:10.1371/journal.pgen.1001365

Prins, M., Boxem, J., Lucas, C., & Hutton, E. (2011). Effect of spontaneous pushing versus Valsalva pushing in the second stage of labour on mother and fetus: A systematic review of randomised trials. *British Journal of Obstetrics and Gynaecology, 118*(6), 662–670. doi:10.1111/j.1471-0528.2011.02910.x

Ragnar, I., Altman, D., Tydén, T., & Olsson, S. E. (2006). Comparison of the maternal experience and duration of labour in two upright delivery positions—A randomised controlled trial. *British Journal of Obstetrics and Gynaecology, 113*(2), 165–170. doi:10.1111/j.1471-0528.2005.00824.x

Rayburn, W. F., Tassone, S., & Pearman, C. (2000). Is Cervidil appropriate for outpatient cervical ripening? *Obstetrics & Gynecology, 95*(4 Suppl.), S63.

Rhoades, J. S., & Cahill, A. G. (2017). Defining and managing normal and abnormal first stage of labor. *Obstetrics and Gynecology Clinics of North America, 44*(4), 567–592, 535–545. doi:10.1016/j.ogc.2017.07.001

Ridgeway, J. J., Weyrich, D. L., & Benedetti, T. J. (2004). Fetal heart rate changes associated with uterine rupture. *Obstetrics & Gynecology, 103*(3), 506–512.

Roberts, C. L., Algert, C. S., Cameron, C. A., & Torvaldsen, S. (2005). A meta-analysis of upright positions in the second stage of labor to reduce instrumental deliveries in women with epidural anesthesia. *Acta Obstetricia et Gynecologica Scandinavica, 84*(8), 794–798. doi:10.1111/j.0001-6349.2005.00786.x

Roberts, C. L., Torvaldsen, S., Cameron, C. A., & Olive, E. (2004). Delayed versus early pushing in women with epidural analgesia: A systematic review and meta-analysis. *British Journal of Obstetrics and Gynaecology, 111*(12), 1333–1340. doi:10.1111/j.1471-0528.2004.00282.x

Roberts, J. E. (2002). The "push" for evidence: Management of the second stage. *Journal of Midwifery & Women's Health, 47*(1), 2–15.

Roberts, J. E. (2003). A new understanding of the second stage of labor: Implications for nursing care. *Journal of Obstetric, Gynecologic, and Neonatal Nursing, 32*(6), 794–801. doi:10.1177/0884217503258497

Roberts, J. E., Goldstein, S. A., Gruener, J. S., Maggio, M., & Mendez-Bauer, C. (1987). A descriptive analysis of involuntary bearing-down efforts during the expulsive phase of labor. *Journal of Obstetric, Gynecologic, and Neonatal Nursing, 16*(1), 48–55.

Roberts, J. E., & Hanson, L. (2007). Best practices in second stage labor care: Maternal bearing down and positioning. *Journal of Midwifery & Women's Health, 52*(3), 238–245. doi:10.1016/j.jmwh.2006.12.011

Roberts, J. E., & Woolley, D. (1996). A second look at the second stage of labor. *Journal of Obstetric, Gynecologic, and Neonatal Nursing, 25*(5), 415–423.

Robinson, C., Schumann, R., Zhang, P., & Young, R. C. (2003). Oxytocin-induced desensitization of the oxytocin receptor. *American Journal of Obstetrics & Gynecology, 188*(2), 497–502. doi:10.1067/mob.2003.22

Rouse, D. J., Owen, J., Savage, K. G., & Hauth, J. C. (2001). Active phase labor arrest: Revisiting the 2-hour minimum. *Obstetrics & Gynecology, 98*(4), 550–554.

Rubin, A. (1964). Management of shoulder dystocia. *JAMA, 189,* 835–837.

Ruhl, C., Scheich, B., Onokpise, B., & Bingham, D. (2015a). Content validity testing of the Maternal Fetal Triage Index. *Journal of Obstetric, Gynecologic, and Neonatal Nursing, 44*(6), 701–709. doi:10.1111/1552-6909.12763

Ruhl, C., Scheich, B., Onokpise, B., & Bingham, D. (2015b). Inter-rater reliability testing of the Maternal Fetal Triage Index. *Journal of Obstetric, Gynecologic, and Neonatal Nursing, 44*(6), 710–716. doi:10.1111/1552-6909.12762

Saccone, G., Ciardulli, A., Baxter, J. K., Quiñones, J. N., Diven, L. C., Pinar, B., . . . Berghella, V. (2017). Discontinuing oxytocin in the active phase of labor: A systematic review and meta-analysis. *Obstetrics & Gynecology, 130*(5), 1090–1096. doi:10.1097/AOG.0000000000002325

Sakala, C., Declercq, E. R., Turon, J. M., & Corry, M. P. (2018). *Listening to mothers in California: A population-based survey of women's childbearing experiences.* Washington, DC: National Partnership for Women & Families.

Sampselle, C. M., & Hines, S. (1999). Spontaneous pushing during birth: Relationship to perineal outcomes. *Journal of Nurse Midwifery, 44*(1), 36–39.

Sandberg, E. C. (1999). The Zavanelli maneuver: 12 Years of recorded experience. *Obstetrics & Gynecology, 93*(2), 312–317.

Sargent, J., & Caughey, A. B. (2017). Vaginal birth after cesarean trends: Which way is the pendulum swinging? *Obstetrics and Gynecology Clinics of North America, 44*(4), 655–666. doi:10.1016/j.ogc.2017.08.006

Schaffer, J. I., Bloom, S. L., Casey, B. M., McIntire, D. D., Nihira, M. A., & Leveno, K. J. (2005). A randomized trial of the effects of coached vs uncoached maternal pushing during the second stage of labor on postpartum pelvic floor structure and function. *American Journal of Obstetrics & Gynecology, 192*(5), 1692–1696. doi:10.1016/j.ajog.2004.11.043

Scheich, B., & Bingham, D. (2015). Key findings from the AWHONN perinatal staffing data collaborative. *Journal of Obstetric, Gynecologic, and Neonatal Nursing, 44*(2), 317–328. doi:10.1111/1552-6909.12548

Schiessl, B., Janni, W., Jundt, K., Rammel, G., Peschers, U., & Kainer, F. (2005). Obstetrical procedures influencing the duration of the second stage of labor. *European Journal of Obstetrics, Gynecology, and Reproductive Biology, 118*(1), 17–20.

Schifrin, B. S., & Ater, S. (2006). Fetal hypoxic and ischemic injuries. *Current Opinion in Obstetrics & Gynecology, 18*(2), 112–122. doi:10.1097/01.gco.0000192984.15095.7c

Scholz, H. S., Benedicic, C., Arikan, M. G., Haas, J., & Petru, E. (2001). Spontaneous vaginal delivery in the birth-chair versus in the conventional dorsal position: A matched controlled comparison. *Wiener Klinische Wochenschrift, 113,* 695–697.

Schuit, E., Kwee, A., Westerhuis, M., Van Dessel, H., Graziosi, G., Van Lith, J., . . . Groenwold, R. (2012). A clinical prediction model to assess the risk of operative delivery. *British Journal of Obstetrics and Gynaecology, 119*(8), 915–923. doi:10.1111/j.1471-0528.2012.03334.x

Scifres, C. M., Rohn, A., Odibo, A., Stamilio, D., & Macones, G. A. (2011). Predicting significant maternal morbidity in women attempting vaginal birth after cesarean section. *American Journal of Perinatology, 28*(3), 181–186. doi:10.1055/s-0030-1266159

Scott, J. R. (2005). Episiotomy and vaginal trauma. *Obstetrics and Gynecology Clinics of North America, 32*(2), 307–321.

Scott, J. R. (2011). Vaginal birth after cesarean delivery: A common sense approach. *Obstetrics & Gynecology, 118*(2, Pt. 1), 342–350. doi:10.1097/AOG.0b013e3182245b39

Seitchik, J., Amico, J., Robinson, A. G., & Castillo, M. (1984). Oxytocin augmentation of dysfunctional labor. IV. Oxytocin pharmacokinetics. *American Journal of Obstetrics & Gynecology, 150*(3), 225–228.

Seitchik, J., & Castillo, M. (1982). Oxytocin augmentation of dysfunctional labor. I. Clinical data. *American Journal of Obstetrics & Gynecology, 144*(8), 899–905.

Seitchik, J., & Castillo, M. (1983). Oxytocin augmentation of dysfunctional labor. III. Multiparous patients. *American Journal of Obstetrics & Gynecology, 145*(7), 777–780.

Selin, L., Wennerholm, U. B., Jonsson, M., Dencker, A., Wallin, G., Wiberg-Itzel, E., . . . Berg, M. (2019). High-dose versus low-dose of oxytocin for labour augmentation: A randomized controlled trial. *Women and Birth, 32*(4), 356–363. doi:10.1016/j.wombi.2018.09.002

Shanks, A. L., & Cahill, A. G. (2011). Delivery after prior cesarean: Success rate and factors. *Clinics in Perinatology, 38*(2), 233–245. doi:10.1016/j.clp.2011.03.011

Sharts-Hopko, N. C. (2010). Oral intake in labor: A review of the evidence. *MCN: The American Journal of Maternal Child Nursing, 35*(4), 197–203. doi:10.1097/NMC.0b013e3181db48f5

Sheehan, P. M. (2006). A possible role for progesterone metabolites in human parturition. *Australian and New Zealand Journal of Obstetrics & Gynaecology, 46*(2), 159–163.

Shermer, R. H., & Raines, D. A. (1997). Positioning during the second stage of labor: Moving back to the basics. *Journal of Obstetric, Gynecologic, and Neonatal Nursing, 26*(6), 727–734.

Shilling, T., Romano, A. M., & DiFranco, J. T. (2007). Care Practice #2: Freedom of movement throughout labor. *Journal of Perinatal Education, 16*(3), 21–24. doi:10.1624/105812407X217101

Shrivastava, V. K., Garite, T. J., Jenkins, S. M., Saul, L., Rumney, P., Preslicka, C., & Chan, K. (2009). A randomized, double-blinded, controlled trial comparing parenteral normal saline with and without dextrose on the course of labor in nulliparas. *American Journal of Obstetrics & Gynecology, 200*(4), 379.e1–379.e6. doi:10.1016/j.ajog.2008.11.030

Shyken, J. M., & Petrie, R. H. (1995). Oxytocin to induce labor. *Clinical Obstetrics and Gynecology, 38*(2), 232–245.

Silver, R. M. (2007). Fetal death. *Obstetrics & Gynecology, 109*(1), 153–167. doi:10.1097/01.AOG.0000248537.89739.96

Simon, C. E., & Grobman, W. A. (2005). When has an induction failed? *Obstetrics & Gynecology, 105*(4), 705–709. doi:10.1097/01.AOG.0000157437.10998.e7

Simpson, K. R. (2005). Handling handoffs safely. *MCN: The American Journal of Maternal Child Nursing, 30*(2), 76.

Simpson, K. R. (2010). Reconsideration of the costs of convenience: Quality, operational, and fiscal strategies to minimize elective labor induction. *Journal of Perinatal & Neonatal Nursing, 24*(1), 42–53. doi:10.1097/JPN.0b013e3181c6abe3

Simpson, K. R. (2011a). An overview of distribution of births in United States hospitals in 2008 with implications for small volume perinatal units in rural hospitals. *Journal of Obstetric, Gynecologic, and Neonatal Nursing, 40*(4), 432–439. doi:10.1111/j.1552-6909.2011.01262.x

Simpson, K. R. (2011b). Avoiding confusion of maternal heart rate with fetal heart rate during labor. *MCN: The American Journal of Maternal Child Nursing, 36*(4), 272. doi:10.1097/NMC.0b013e318217a61a

Simpson, K. R. (2015). Physiologic interventions for fetal heart rate patterns. In A. Lyndon & L. U. Ali (Eds.), *AWHONN's fetal heart monitoring principles and practices* (5th ed., pp. 163–189). Dubuque, IA: Kendall Hunt.

Simpson, K. R. (2019a). Immediate vs. delayed pushing. *MCN: The American Journal of Maternal Child Nursing, 44*(2), 124. doi:10.1097/NMC.0000000000000503

Simpson, K. R. (2019b). Partnering with patients and families during childbirth: Confirming knowledge of informed consent. *MCN: The American Journal of Maternal Child Nursing, 443*(3), 124. doi:10.1097/NMC.0000000000000527

Simpson, K. R. (2020). *Cervical ripening, labor induction and labor augmentation* (5th ed.). Washington, DC: Association of Women's Health, Obstetric and Neonatal Nurses.

Simpson, K. R., & James, D. C. (2005a). Effects of immediate versus delayed pushing during second-stage labor on fetal well-being. *Nursing Research, 54*(3), 149–157.

Simpson, K. R., & James, D. C. (2005b). Efficacy of intrauterine resuscitation techniques in improving fetal oxygen status during labor. *Obstetrics & Gynecology, 105*(6), 1362–1368. doi:10.1097/01.AOG.0000164474.03350.7c

Simpson, K. R., & James, D. C. (2008). Effects of oxytocin-induced uterine hyperstimulation during labor on fetal oxygen status and fetal heart rate patterns. *American Journal of Obstetrics & Gynecology, 199*(1), 34.e1–34.e5. doi:10.1016/j.ajog.2007.12.015

Simpson, K. R., James, D. C., & Knox, G. E. (2006). Nurse-physician communication during labor and birth: Implications for patient safety. *Journal of Obstetric, Gynecologic, and Neonatal Nursing, 35*(4), 547–556. doi:10.1111/j.1552-6909.2006.00075.x

Simpson, K. R., & Knox, G. E. (2009). Oxytocin as a high-alert medication: Implications for perinatal patient safety. *MCN: The American Journal of Maternal Child Nursing, 34*(1), 8–15. doi:10.1097/01.NMC.0000343859.62828.ee

Simpson, K. R., Knox, G. E., Martin, M., George, C., & Watson, S. R. (2011). Michigan Health & Hospital Association Keystone Obstetrics: A statewide collaborative for perinatal patient safety in Michigan. *Joint Commission Journal on Quality and Patient Safety, 37*(12), 544–552.

Simpson, K. R., & Lyndon, A. (2009). Clinical disagreements during labor and birth: How does real life compare to best practice? *MCN: The American Journal of Maternal Child Nursing, 34*(1), 31–39. doi:10.1097/01.NMC.0000343863.72237.2b

Simpson, K. R., & Lyndon, A. (2017a). Consequences of delayed, unfinished, or missed nursing care during labor and birth. *Journal of Perinatal & Neonatal Nursing, 31*(1), 32–40. doi:10.1097/JPN.0000000000000203

Simpson, K. R., & Lyndon, A. (2017b). Labor nurses' views of their influence on cesarean birth. *MCN: The American Journal of Maternal Child Nursing, 42*(2), 81–87. doi:10.1097/nmc.0000000000000308

Simpson, K. R., Lyndon, A., Spetz, J., Gay, C. L., & Landstrom, G. L. (2019). Adherence to the AWHONN staffing guidelines as perceived by labor nurses. *Nursing for Women's Health, 23*(3), 217–223. doi:10.1016/j.nwh.2019.03.003

Simpson, K. R., Newman, G., & Chirino, O. R. (2010a). Patient education to reduce elective inductions. *MCN: The American Journal of Maternal Child Nursing, 35*(4), 188–194. doi:10.1097/NMC.0b013e3181d9c6d6

Simpson, K. R., Newman, G., & Chirino, O. R. (2010b). Patients' perspectives on the role of prepared childbirth education in decision-making regarding elective labor induction. *Journal of Perinatal Education, 19*(3), 21–32. doi:10.1624/105812410X514396

Singata, M., Tranmer, J., & Gyte, G. M. (2013). Restricting oral fluid and food intake during labour. *Cochrane Database of Systematic Reviews,* (8), CD003930. doi:10.1002/14651858.CD003930.pub3

Singhi, S. (1988). Effect of maternal intrapartum glucose therapy on neonatal blood glucose levels and neurobehavioral status of hypoglycemic term infants. *Journal of Perinatal Medicine, 16*(3), 217–224.

Slater, D. M., Zervou, S., & Thornton, S. (2002). Prostaglandins and prostanoid receptors in human pregnancy and parturition. *Journal of the Society for Gynecologic Investigation, 9*(3), 118–124.

Smith, G. C. S., Pell, J. P., Cameron, A. D., & Dobbie, R. (2002). Risk of perinatal death associated with labor after previous cesarean delivery in uncomplicated term pregnancies. *JAMA, 287*(20), 2684–2690.

Smith, H., Peterson, N., Lagrew, D., & Main, E. (2016). *Toolkit to support vaginal birth and reduce primary cesareans: a quality improvement toolkit.* Stanford, CA: California Maternal Quality Care Collaborative. Retrieved from https://www.cmqcc.org/VBirthToolkit

Smith, R. (2007). Parturition. *The New England Journal of Medicine, 356*(3), 271–283.

Society for Maternal-Fetal Medicine. (2019). SMFM statement on elective induction of labor in low-risk nulliparous women at term: The ARRIVE trial. *American Journal of Obstetrics & Gynecology, 221*(1), B2–B4. doi:10.1016/j.ajog.2018.08.009

Society of Obstetricians and Gynaecologists of Canada. (2001). *Induction of labour at term* (Clinical Practice Guideline No. 107; Reaffirmed, 2015). Ottawa, Canada: Author.

Society of Obstetricians and Gynaecologists of Canada. (2004). *Guidelines for operative vaginal birth* (Clinical Practice Guideline No. 148; Reaffirmed, 2018). Ottawa, Canada: Author.

Sommer, P. A., Norr, K., & Roberts, J. (2000). Clinical decision-making regarding intravenous hydration in normal labor in a birth center setting. *Journal of Midwifery & Women's Health, 45*(2), 114–121.

Spong, C. Y., Berghella, V., Wenstrom, K. D., Mercer, B. M., & Saade, G. R. (2012). Preventing the first cesarean delivery: Summary of a joint Eunice Kennedy Shriver National Institute of Child Health and Human Development, Society for Maternal-Fetal Medicine, and American College of Obstetricians and Gynecologists Workshop. *Obstetrics & Gynecology, 120*(5), 1181–1193. doi:10.1097/AOG.0b013e3182704880

Spong, C. Y., Mercer, B. M., D'Alton, M., Kilpatrick, S., Blackwell, S., & Saade, G. (2011). Timing of indicated late-preterm and early-term birth. *Obstetrics & Gynecology, 118*(2, Pt. 1), 323–333. doi:10.1097/AOG.0b013e3182255999

Stremler, R., Hodnett, E., Petryshen, P., Stevens, B., Weston, J., & Willan, A. R. (2005). Randomized controlled trial of hands-and-knees positioning for occipitoposterior position in labor. *Birth, 32*(4), 243–251. doi:10.1111/j.0730-7659.2005.00382.x

Stringer, J. L. (1996). *Basic concepts in pharmacology: A student's survival guide.* St. Louis, MO: McGraw-Hill.

Sultatos, L. G. (1997). Mechanisms of drugs that affect uterine motility. *Journal of Nurse Midwifery, 42*(2), 367–370.

Sundin, C., Mazac, L., Ellis, K., & Garbo, C. (2018). Implementation of an oxytocin checklist to improve clinical outcomes. *MCN: The American Journal of Maternal Child Nursing, 43*(3), 133–138. doi:10.1097/NMC.0000000000000428

Terry, R. R., Westcott, J., O'Shea, L., & Kelly, F. (2006). Postpartum outcomes in supine delivery by physicians vs nonsupine delivery by midwives. *Journal of the American Osteopathic Association, 106*(4), 199–202.

The Joint Commission. (2004). *Preventing infant death and injury during delivery* (Sentinel Event Alert No. 30). Oakbrook Terrace, IL: Author.

Thomson, A. M. (1993). Pushing techniques in the second stage of labour. *Journal of Advanced Nursing, 18*(2), 171–177.

Thomson, A. M. (1995). Maternal behaviour during spontaneous and directed pushing in the second stage of labour. *Journal of Advanced Nursing, 22*(6), 1027–1034.

Tilden, E. L., Phillippi, J. C., Ahlberg, M., King, T. L., Dissanayake, M., Lee, C. S., . . . Caughey, A. B. (2019). Describing latent phase duration and associated characteristics among 1281 low-risk women in spontaneous labor. *Birth.* doi:10.1111/birt.12428

Torki, M., Barton, L., Miller, D. A., & Ouzounian, J. G. (2012). Severe brachial plexus palsy in women without shoulder dystocia. *Obstetrics & Gynecology, 120*(3), 539–541. doi:10.1097/AOG.0b013e318264f644

Torvaldsen, S., Roberts, C. L., Bell, J. C., & Raynes-Greenow, C. H. (2004). Discontinuation of epidural analgesia late in labour for reducing the adverse delivery outcomes associated with epidural analgesia. *Cochrane Database of Systematic Reviews,* (4), CD004457. doi:10.1002/14651858.CD004457.pub2

Towner, D., Castro, M. A., Eby-Wilkens, E., & Gilbert, W. M. (1999). Effect of mode of delivery in nulliparous women on neonatal intracranial injury. *The New England Journal of Medicine, 341*(23), 1709–1704.

Treacy, A., Robson, M., & O'Herlihy, C. (2006). Dystocia increases with advancing maternal age. *American Journal of Obstetrics & Gynecology, 195*(3), 760–763. doi:10.1016/j.ajog.2006.05.052

Tsur, A., Sergienko, R., Wiznitzer, A., Zlotnik, A., & Sheiner, E. (2012). Critical analysis of risk factors for shoulder dystocia. *Archives of Gynecology and Obstetrics, 285*(5), 1225–1229. doi:10.1007/s00404-011-2139-8

Tubridy, N., & Redmond, J. M. T. (1996). Neurological symptoms attributed to epidural analgesia in labour: An observational study of seven cases. *British Journal of Obstetrics and Gynaecology, 103*(8), 832–833.

Tumblin, A., & Simkin, P. (2001). Pregnant women's perceptions of their nurse's role during labor and delivery. *Birth*, 28(1), 52–56.

Tuuli, M. G., Frey, H. A., Odibo, A. O., Macones, G. A., & Cahill, A. G. (2012). Immediate compared with delayed pushing in the second stage of labor: A systematic review and meta-analysis. *Obstetrics & Gynecology*, 120(3), 660–668. doi:10.1097/AOG.0b013e3182639fae

Uhing, M. R. (2005). Management of birth injuries. *Clinics in Perinatology*, 32(1), 19–38. doi:10.1016/j.clp.2004.11.007

Ulmsten, U. (1997). Onset and forces of term labor. *Acta Obstetricia et Gynecologica Scandinavica*, 76(6), 499–514.

U.S. Food and Drug Administration. (1998). *Need for caution when using vacuum assisted delivery devices* (FDA Public Health Advisory). Washington, DC: Author.

U.S. Food and Drug Administration. (2002). *FDA approves new labeling information for Cytotec (misoprostol)*. Retrieved from http://www.fda.gov/cder

Vacca, A. (2002). Vacuum-assisted delivery. *Best Practice & Research: Clinical Obstetrics & Gynaecology*, 16(1), 17–30.

Vahratian, A., Hoffman, M. K., Troendle, J. F., & Zhang, J. (2006). The impact of parity on course of labor in a contemporary population. *Birth*, 33(1), 12–17. doi:10.1111/j.0730-7659.2006.00069.x

Vahratian, A., Zhang, J., Troendle, J. F., Savitz, D. A., & Siega-Riz, A. M. (2004). Maternal prepregnancy overweight and obesity and the pattern of labor progression in term nulliparous women. *Obstetrics & Gynecology*, 104(5, Pt. 1), 943–951. doi:10.1097/01.AOG.0000142713.53197.91

Vahratian, A., Zhang, J., Troendle, J. F., Sciscione, A. C., & Hoffman, M. K. (2005). Labor progression and risk of cesarean delivery in electively induced nulliparas. *Obstetrics & Gynecology*, 105(4), 698–704. doi:10.1097/01.AOG.0000157436.68847.3b

Vaughn, K. O. (1937). *Safe childbirth: The three essentials*. London, United Kingdom: Ballière, Tindall, and Cox.

Vause, S., Congdon, H. M., & Thornton, J. G. (1998). Immediate and delayed pushing in the second stage of labour for nulliparous women with epidural analgesia: A randomised controlled trial. *British Journal of Obstetrics and Gynaecology*, 105(2), 186–188.

Wasserstrum, N. (1992). Issues in fluid management during labor: General considerations. *Clinics in Obstetrics and Gynecology*, 35(3), 505–513.

Weeks, A. D., Navaratnam, K., & Alfirevic, Z. (2017). Simplifying oral misoprostol protocols for induction of labour. *British Journal of Obstetrics and Gynaecology*, 124, 1642–1645. doi:10.1111/1471-0528.14657

Werner, E. F., Janevic, T. M., Illuzzi, J., Funai, E .F., Savitz, D. A., & Lipkind, H. S. (2011). Mode of delivery in nulliparous women and neonatal intracranial injury. *Obstetrics & Gynecology*, 118(6), 1239–1246. doi:10.1097/AOG.0b013e31823835d3

Wilson, R. D., Caughey, A. B., Wood, S. L., Macones, G. A., Wrench, I. J., Huang, J., . . . Nelson, G. (2018). Guidelines for antenatal and preoperative care in cesarean delivery: Enhanced Recovery after Surgery Society recommendations (part 1). *American Journal of Obstetrics and Gynecology*, 219(6), 523e.1–532.e15. doi:10.1016/j.ajog.2018.09.015

Wisner, K., & Holschuh, C. (2018). *Fetal heart rate auscultation* (3rd ed.). Washington, DC: Association of Women's Health, Obstetric and Neonatal Nurses. doi:10.1016/j.nwh.2018.10.001

Wong, C. A., Scavone, B. M., Dugan, S., Smith, J. C., Prather, H., Ganchiff, J. N., & McCarthy, R. J. (2003). Incidence of postpartum lumbosacral spine and lower extremity nerve injuries. *Obstetrics & Gynecology*, 101(2), 279–288.

Yap, O. W., Kim, E. S., & Laros, R. K., Jr. (2001). Maternal and neonatal outcomes after uterine rupture in labor. *American Journal of Obstetrics & Gynecology*, 184(7), 1576–1581.

Yildirim, G., & Beji, N. K. (2008). Effects of pushing techniques in birth on mother and fetus: A randomized study. *Birth*, 35(1), 25–30 doi:10.1111/j.1523-536X.2007.00208.x

Zahedi-Spung, L., Stout, M., Wookfolk, C., Litz, T., Macones, G. A., & Cahill, A. G. (2019). Second stage tachysystole is associated with adverse neonatal outcomes. *American Journal of Obstetrics & Gynecology*, 220(Suppl.), S500.

Zaki, M. N., Hibbard, J. U., & Kominiarek, M. A. (2013). Contemporary labor patterns and maternal age. *Obstetrics & Gynecology*, 122(5), 1018–1024. doi:10.1097/AOG.0b013e3182a9c92c

Zeeman, G. G., Khan-Dawood, F. S., & Dawood, M. Y. (1997). Oxytocin and its receptor in pregnancy and parturition: Current concepts and clinical implications. *Obstetrics & Gynecology*, 89(5, Pt. 2), 873–883.

Zeiman, M., Fong, S. K., Benowitz, N. L., Banskter, D., & Darney, P. D. (1997). Absorption kinetics of misoprostol with oral and vaginal administration. *Obstetrics & Gynecology*, 90(1), 88–92.

Zhang, G., Feenstra, B., Bacelis, J., Liu, X., Muglia, L. M., Juodakis, J., . . . Muglia, L. J. (2017). Genetic associations with gestational duration and spontaneous preterm birth. *The New England Journal of Medicine*, 377(12), 1156–1167. doi:10.1056/NEJMoa1612665

Zhang, J., Landy, H. J., Branch, D. W., Burkman, R., Haberman, S., Gregory, K. D., . . . Reddy, U. M. (2010). Contemporary patterns of spontaneous labor with normal neonatal outcomes. *Obstetrics & Gynecology*, 116(6), 1281–1287. doi:10.1097/AOG.0b013e3181fdef6e

Zhang, J., Troendle, J. F., Mikolajczyk, R., Sundaram, R., Beaver, J., & Fraser, W. (2010). The natural history of the normal first stage of labor. *Obstetrics & Gynecology*, 115(4), 705–710. doi:10.1097/AOG.0b013e3181d55925

Zhang, J., Troendle, J. F., Reddy, U. M., Laughon, S. K., Branch, D. W., Burkman, R., . . . van Veldhuisen, P. (2010). Contemporary cesarean delivery practice in the United States. *American Journal of Obstetrics & Gynecology*, 203(4), 326.e1–326.e10. doi:10.1016/j.ajog.2010.06.058

Zhang, J., Troendle, J. F., & Yancey, M. K. (2002). Reassessing the labor curve in multiparous women. *American Journal of Obstetrics & Gynecology*, 187(4), 824–828.

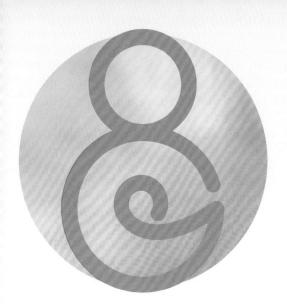

CHAPTER 15

Fetal Assessment during Labor

Nancy O'Brien-Abel • Kathleen Rice Simpson

INTRODUCTION

The introduction of electronic fetal monitoring (EFM) in the late 1960s has had a far-reaching impact on perinatal care and the practice of nursing, midwifery, and medicine. Despite debate about advantages and limitations, effects on perinatal morbidity and mortality, and role in healthcare costs and malpractice litigation, EFM is used in most of the labor and birth units in the United States and Canada today. This chapter discusses the physiologic basis for fetal heart rate (FHR) monitoring, defines FHR patterns, and reviews intrapartum management of FHR patterns.

HISTORICAL PERSPECTIVES

Publication of the discovery of fetal heart tones in 1822 marked the beginning of modern obstetric practice (Goodlin, 1979; Sureau, 1996). Jean Alexandre Le Jumeau Vicomte de Kergaradec used a stethoscope hoping to hear the noise of the water in the uterus. Although M. Maior of Geneva was the first person credited with identifying fetal heart tones, Kergaradec was the first person astute enough to suggest in print potential clinical uses for FHR auscultation (Goodlin, 1979; Kennedy, 1843). In the early 1800s, researchers working independently in Switzerland, Ireland, Germany, France, and the United States described fetal heart tones, and in 1833, the British obstetrician William Kennedy described fetal heart sounds as a "quick double pulsation" with a usual rate of 130 to 140 beats per minute (bpm). Kennedy noted the rate was sometimes slower and sometimes much faster, depending on "inherent vital causes" (Kennedy, 1843, p. 107).

He documented fetal heart variation in labor, including rates as high as 180 to 200 bpm in ill mothers and slowing and cessation of the FHR prior to stillbirth. In 1858, Schwartz of Germany suggested that the FHR be counted often during labor, both between and during contractions, to promote improved outcomes. Schwartz described the association between fetal bradycardia and decreased uteroplacental blood flow during contractions. In 1849, Killian proposed forceps-assisted birth for an FHR of fewer than 100 bpm or greater than 180 bpm (Goodlin, 1979). Soon after, Winckel described specific FHR criteria to be used for the diagnosis of fetal distress via auscultation (Goodlin, 1979). After invention of the fetoscope in the early 1900s, fetal heart sounds were commonly assessed in order to document fetal viability during the prenatal period. Winckel's criteria were used in clinical practice until the 1950s when Hon raised concern about the subjectivity of counting heartbeats during labor.

Although interest in continuous recording of fetal heart tones by various methods dates to the later years of the 19th century, the major development of modern clinical EFM occurred during the 1960s. In 1906, Cramer produced the first electrocardiographic (ECG) recording of the fetal heartbeat. Research using abdominal leads to obtain the fetal ECG continued but remained impractical for clinical use until the mid-1960s, when techniques capable of excluding the maternal ECG from the recording became available. By the 1950s, research on electronic methods of FHR monitoring escalated. In 1958, Hon published the first report of continuous fetal ECG monitoring using a device placed on the maternal abdomen. By the 1960s, Hon, Caldeyro-Barcia, and Hammacher were reporting successful attempts at developing an electronic

413

FHR monitor that could continuously record FHR data (Caldeyro-Barcia et al., 1966; Hammacher, 1969; Hon, 1963). Although many others have contributed to what is known about fetal assessment during labor, EFM, as it is used today, is largely the result of the work of these three investigators working independently on separate continents. In 1968, the first commercially available electronic fetal monitors were introduced.

Coinciding with development of EFM technology was the emergence of data that refuted the effectiveness of intermittent auscultation (IA) with Delee or Pinard fetoscopes. The Benson, Shubeck, Deutschberger, Weiss, and Berendes (1968) study of more than 24,000 births, called the Collaborative Perinatal Project, concluded that FHR auscultation during labor was unreliable in determining fetal distress except in extreme cases of terminal bradycardias. Based on this report and rapid technologic advances, IA of the FHR between contractions was rapidly replaced with continuous EFM during the 1970s. Over the next three decades, EFM became the preferred method of fetal surveillance during the intrapartum period in the United States and Canada.

During the 1980s and 1990s, several randomized trials that compared IA to continuous EFM were conducted (MacDonald, Grant, Sheridan-Pereira, Boylan, & Chalmers, 1985; Thacker, Stroup, & Peterson, 1995; Vintzileos et al., 1993). Continuous EFM did not decrease perinatal mortality or prevent cerebral palsy; however, women in EFM groups experienced a fourfold increase in operative birth (Thacker et al., 1995). Potential reasons why EFM did not demonstrate efficacy in the randomized trials include methodologic flaws, inconsistent criteria and terminology to describe fetal status, and the use of outcome variables for which there were insufficient sample sizes to determine a significant difference between IA and continuous EFM.

The increase in cesarean birth rates fueled reexamination of all aspects of EFM use. In 1997, the National Institute of Child Health and Human Development (NICHD) of the National Institutes of Health convened a panel of FHR monitoring experts. This group proposed quantitative definitions of FHR characteristics to serve as a basis for standardizing research that uses FHR data. Between 1997 and 2004, there was gradual but sporadic adoption of the proposed standardized FHR definitions in clinical practice in the United States. In July 2004, the Joint Commission on Accreditation of Healthcare Organizations (JCAHO, now known as The Joint Commission) recommended use of a standard language for communication and documentation of FHR patterns. In May 2005, the Association of Women's Health, Obstetric and Neonatal Nurses (AWHONN) and the American College

of Obstetricians and Gynecologists (ACOG) formally supported adoption of the NICHD definitions for FHR patterns as the standardized language for communicating fetal status (ACOG, 2005b; AWHONN, 2005). In 2008, the NICHD held an interdisciplinary meeting to consider the status of FHR terminology and whether there was a need for additional guidance regarding interpretation of FHR patterns (Spong, 2008). The 1997 definitions of FHR characteristics were reaffirmed at this meeting (Table 15–1), and a new classification system for interpretation of FHR patterns was proposed (Macones, Hankins, Spong, Hauth, & Moore, 2008) (Table 15–2). These changes were incorporated into ACOG practice bulletins, the AWHONN Fetal Heart Monitoring Program, American College of Nurse-Midwives (ACNM) documents, and National Certification Corporation certification examinations.

Recent research focusing on algorithms for management of category II and category III tracings emphasizing fetal safety versus potential overuse of intervention (Clark et al., 2017; Clark et al., 2013) and electronic visual interpretation of EFM tracings (INFANT Collaborative Group, 2017) is discussed later in this chapter.

Currently, clinical reliance on EFM remains high, despite lack of positive results from published research (Miller, 2016). To date, EFM is the primary screening technique for the clinical determination of the adequacy of fetal oxygenation during labor. This paradox is better understood following a review of the physiology of the fetal heart and its adaptations during labor. The feelings of many clinicians about EFM versus IA were summarized by Cibils in 1996: "It is difficult to understand the premise that the intermittent recording (by a crude method) of a given biologic variable [the FHR] will be better to make a clinical decision affecting the mother and fetus than the continuous, precise recording of the same variable" (p. 1383). Chen, Chauhan, Ananth, Vintzileos, and Abuhamad (2011) conducted a retrospective cohort study of over 4 million U.S. births occurring between 24 and 44 weeks' gestation in 2004, using linked birth certificate and infant death certificate data. They found that EFM was used in 89% of births and EFM use was associated with substantially decreased risk of low Apgar scores (<4), low Apgar score with seizures, and early neonatal death. However, as pointed out by Devoe (2011a), the design of the Chen et al. study cannot address causality or the nature of the relationship between the use of EFM and the observed outcomes because the study did not examine EFM tracings, the labor process, or other myriad circumstances surrounding each birth. A Cochrane review of 13 randomized controlled trials (RCTs) including women with varying risk of fetal acidemia at the onset

TABLE 15–1. Fetal Heart Rate (FHR) Characteristics

Term	Definition
Baseline rate	Approximate mean FHR rounded to increments of 5 bpm during a 10-min window excluding accelerations and decelerations and periods of marked variability. There must be ≥2 min of identifiable baseline segments (not necessarily contiguous) in any 10-min window, or the baseline for that period is indeterminate. In such cases, one may need to refer to the previous 10-min window for determination of the baseline.
Bradycardia	Baseline rate of <110 bpm.
Tachycardia	Baseline rate of >160 bpm.
Baseline variability	Determined in a 10-min window, excluding accelerations and decelerations. Fluctuations in the baseline FHR that are irregular in amplitude and frequency and are visually quantified as the amplitude of the peak-to-trough in bpm.
- Absent variability	Amplitude range undetectable.
- Minimal variability	Amplitude range visually detectable but ≤5 bpm. (Greater than undetectable but ≤5 bpm.)
- Moderate variability	Amplitude range 6 to 25 bpm.
- Marked variability	Amplitude range >25 bpm.
Acceleration	Visually apparent *abrupt* increase in FHR. *Abrupt* increase is defined as an increase from onset of acceleration to peak in <30 sec. Peak must be ≥15 bpm and must last ≥15 sec from the onset to return. Acceleration lasting ≥10 min is defined as a baseline change. Before 32 weeks of gestation, accelerations are defined as having a peak ≥10 bpm and duration of ≥10 sec.
Prolonged acceleration	Acceleration ≥2 min but <10 min in duration.
Early deceleration	Visually apparent, usually symmetrical, *gradual* decrease and return of FHR associated with a uterine contraction. The *gradual* FHR decrease is defined as one from the onset to FHR nadir of ≥30 sec. The decrease in FHR is calculated from onset to nadir of deceleration. The nadir of the deceleration occurs at the same time as the peak of the contraction. In most cases, the onset, nadir, and recovery of the deceleration are coincident with the beginning, peak, and ending of the contraction, respectively.
Late deceleration	Visually apparent, usually symmetrical, *gradual* decrease and return of FHR associated with a uterine contraction. The *gradual* FHR decrease is defined as from the onset to FHR nadir of ≥30 sec. The decrease in FHR is calculated from onset to the nadir of deceleration. The deceleration is delayed in timing, with nadir of the deceleration occurring after the peak of the contraction. In most cases, the onset, nadir, and recovery of the deceleration occur after the beginning, peak, and ending of the contraction, respectively.
Variable deceleration	Visually apparent *abrupt* decrease in FHR. An *abrupt* FHR decrease is defined as from the onset of the deceleration to beginning of FHR nadir of <30 sec. The decrease in FHR is calculated from the onset to the nadir of deceleration. The decrease in FHR is ≥15 bpm, lasting ≥15 sec, and <2 min in duration. When variable decelerations are associated with uterine contractions, their onset, depth, and duration commonly vary with successive uterine contractions.
Prolonged deceleration	Visually apparent decrease in FHR from baseline that is ≥15 bpm, lasting ≥2 min, but <10 min. A deceleration that lasts ≥10 min is baseline change.
Recurrent	Occurring with ≥50% of contractions in any 20-min window.
Intermittent	Occurring with <50% of contractions in any 20-min window.
Sinusoidal pattern	Visually apparent, smooth, sine wave–like undulating pattern in FHR baseline with cycle frequency of three to five per minute that persists for ≥20 min.

Adapted from Macones, G. A., Hankins, G. D., Spong, C. Y., Hauth, J. D., & Moore, T. (2008). The 2008 National Institute of Child Health Human Development Workshop report on electronic fetal monitoring: Update on definitions, interpretations, and research guidelines. *Journal of Obstetric, Gynecologic, and Neonatal Nursing, 37*(5), 510–515, and *Obstetrics & Gynecology, 112*(3), 661–666.

of labor found continuous EFM was associated with a slight increase in cesarean births and instrumental vaginal births when compared to IA. However, continuous EFM was associated with halving the rate of early neonatal seizures, but no differences were found in the rates of perinatal death or cerebral palsy when compared to IA (Alfirevic, Devane, & Gyte, 2013). Nevertheless, most clinicians in the United States prefer continuous EFM as the intrapartum method of fetal assessment (Miller, 2016), and it is recommended by ACOG (2009b) for high-risk maternal–fetal conditions during labor.

DEFINITIONS AND APPROPRIATE USE OF TERMS DESCRIBING FETAL HEART RATE PATTERNS

Appropriate clinical management of variant FHR patterns and effective clinical communication are both enhanced by use of standardized definitions that convey agreed-upon meanings among the members of the healthcare team. Adoption of a common language for FHR characteristics and pattern definitions, as well as medical record documentation that is mutually agreed upon and routinely used by all providers, enhances

TABLE 15–2. Three-Tiered System for Fetal Heart Rate Interpretation

Classification	Definition	Interpretation
Category I	Includes **all** of the following characteristics: Baseline rate 110 to 160 bpm Moderate baseline variability Accelerations present or absent Late or variable decelerations absent Early decelerations present or absent	Normal: Predictive of normal fetal acid–base balance at the time of observation May be followed in a routine manner
Category II	All tracings that do not meet criteria for category I or category III Represents an "appreciable fraction" of tracings encountered in clinical care	Indeterminate: Not predictive of abnormal fetal acid–base status, yet we do not have adequate evidence to classify these as category I or III Require evaluation, continued surveillance, and reevaluation, assessing the entire clinical situation
Category III	Either: Absent baseline variability and any of the following: Recurrent late deceleration Recurrent variable decelerations Bradycardia or Sinusoidal pattern	Abnormal: Associated with abnormal fetal acid–base status at the time of observation Require prompt evaluation and efforts to expeditiously resolve the abnormal fetal heart rate pattern

Adapted from Macones, G. A., Hankins, G. D., Spong, C. Y., Hauth, J., & Moore, T. (2008). The 2008 National Institute of Child Health and Human Development Workshop report on electronic fetal monitoring: Update on definitions, interpretation, and research guidelines. *Journal of Obstetric, Gynecologic, and Neonatal Nursing, 37*(5), 510–515. doi:10.1111/j.1552-6909.2008.00284.x and *Obstetrics and Gynecology, 112*(3), 661–666. doi:10.1097/AOG.0b013e3181841395

interdisciplinary communication and, therefore, maternal–fetal safety (JCAHO, 2004). Both oral communication and written documentation must accurately convey the clinician's level of concern and/or record the presumed diagnosis. The chances of miscommunication between care providers, especially during telephone conversations about fetal status, are decreased when everyone is speaking the same language (Simpson & Knox, 2006, 2009). Timely intervention is dependent on clear communication between providers sharing care of an individual patient (Fox, Kilpatrick, King, & Parer, 2000; Miller, 2005; Simpson & Knox, 2009). The NICHD (Macones et al., 2008) nomenclature is the basis for the pattern descriptions in this chapter.

The three-tiered classification system for FHR pattern interpretation put forth by the NICHD reflects both the presence and absence of scientific consensus on FHR interpretation (Macones et al., 2008) (see Table 15-2). There is little controversy concerning what constitutes a normal (category I) FHR tracing: baseline rate within 110 to 160 bpm, moderate FHR variability, and absence of late or variable decelerations; accelerations (spontaneous or elicited by digital scalp or vibroacoustic stimulation [VAS]) and early decelerations may both be present or absent in a normal tracing. Category I tracings are not associated with fetal acidemia and confer an extremely high predictability of a normally oxygenated fetus at the time of observation (ACOG, 2009b; 2010; Clark et al., 2013; Dellinger, Boehm, & Crane, 2000; Macones et al., 2008; Parer, 1997; Parer, King, Flanders, Fox, & Kilpatrick, 2006).

At the other end of the spectrum from normality, several patterns are likely predictive of current or impending fetal asphyxia so severe that the fetus is at risk for neurologic and other fetal damage or death (Macones et al., 2008). These patterns are classified as abnormal (category III) FHR tracings and include absent baseline FHR variability with recurrent late or variable decelerations or bradycardia, or a sinusoidal FHR pattern. Category III tracings convey an increased risk for fetal acidemia at the time of observation requiring evaluation and interventions, and if unresolved, most often prompt birth (ACOG, 2010).

Many fetuses have FHR tracings that are intermediate between these two extremes, and there is no consensus on their presumed condition or clinical management because there is inconsistent evidence in the literature regarding their predictive value in relation to fetal acid–base status. These tracings are classified as indeterminate (category II). Category II tracings include all tracings that are not categorized as category I or III. This includes tracings with alterations in baseline (e.g., bradycardia with minimal or moderate variability) and tracings with recurrent late or variable decelerations and moderate variability, among others. Category II tracings are not considered predictive of abnormal acid–base status at the time they are observed, but they also cannot reliably be placed in category I based on current evidence (Macones et al., 2008). These tracings can be conceptualized as representing some level of fetal physiologic stress. Thus, evaluation, attempts to ameliorate or reduce any identified stressors, reevaluation, and close surveillance of these tracings are appropriate (ACOG, 2010). Most clinicians do not wait until the FHR pattern is at the extreme end of abnormality before intervening to attempt to improve fetal status via one or more intrauterine resuscitation techniques (Garite & Simpson, 2011; Simpson, 2007).

A review of the literature on the association between FHR patterns and fetal acidemia found moderate FHR variability was strongly associated with an umbilical cord pH >7.15 or newborn vigor (5-minute Apgar score ≥7). Absent or minimal FHR variability with recurrent late or variable decelerations was the strongest predictor of newborn acidemia. The correlation between diminished variability and acidemia was 23%, which the investigators suggest was low because studies reviewed did not always differentiate between decreased and absent variability and the association with absent variability is likely stronger. The investigators found increasing depth of decelerations was correlated with low pH (<7.15). Acidemia took time to develop except in situations of sudden profound bradycardia. In the context of decreasing variability with recurrent decelerations, newborn acidemia developed over a period approaching 1 hour (Parer et al., 2006).

Further data suggest normal fetal status (category I) is associated with normal short-term neonatal outcomes. Based on an analysis of 48,444 EFM tracings of women in term labor in 10 hospitals, babies whose tracings during last 2 hours prior to birth were exclusively normal (category I) did well, with only 0.6% having Apgar scores <7 at 5 minutes of life and 0.2% having low Apgar scores with neonatal intensive care unit (NICU) admission. However, when more than 75% of the EFM tracing in last 2 hours prior to birth was indeterminate (category II), low Apgar scores at 5 minutes increased to 1.3% of babies and low Apgar score at 5 minutes with NICU admission increased to 0.7% (Jackson, Holmgren, Esplin, Henry, & Varner, 2011). Analysis of this large database of women in term labor allowed estimation of the frequency of types of EFM tracings based on the NICHD-defined FHR categories. When all of labor was included, most tracings (77.9%) were normal (category I), 22.1% were indeterminate (category II), and 0.004% were abnormal (category III). During the last 2 hours of labor prior to birth, normal (category I) decreased to 60.9% of the duration, indeterminate (category II) increased to 39.1%, and abnormal (category III) increased to 0.006% (Jackson et al., 2011). These last 2 hours included women in second-stage labor who had a vaginal or cesarean birth and women who had a cesarean birth without second-stage labor. The strength of the association between time in an indeterminate (category II) tracing and the risk of Apgar score less than 7 with a NICU admission did not increase until more than 50% of the last

2 hours of labor were spent in category II. This is consistent with the findings of Parer et al. (2006) that, in the absence of catastrophic events, acidemia develops over a period of time approximating 1 hour. Thus, there is supportive evidence for the classification system developed by the NICHD in relation to presumed fetal acid–base status across a continuum of FHR findings. Ideally, members of the perinatal team have a shared method of interpreting FHR patterns and an agreed-upon management guideline for specific FHR patterns (Fox et al., 2000; Knox & Simpson, 2011).

Terms such as *stress* and *distress* lack the precise meaning needed to discriminate levels of concern. In 1998, ACOG recommended that *nonreassuring fetal status* replace the term *fetal distress* in its committee opinion *Inappropriate Use of the Terms Fetal Distress and Birth Asphyxia*. This committee opinion was reaffirmed in 2005 (ACOG, 2005a). The three-tiered interpretation system developed by the NICHD EFM expert group was introduced in 2008 (Macones et al., 2008). The term *fetal distress* has a low positive predictive value, even in high-risk populations, and is often associated with an infant who is in good condition at birth as determined by the Apgar score or umbilical cord blood gas analysis or both. Communication between clinicians caring for the woman and those caring for her baby is best served by categorization of the FHR as normal, indeterminate, or abnormal, followed by a further description of findings when the tracing is indeterminate (category II) or abnormal (category III). Further description should include baseline variability, recurrent variable or late decelerations, prolonged decelerations, fetal tachycardia or bradycardia, maternal risk factors, proximity to birth, and identification of the level of urgency for intervention. It is important that team members explicitly reach and confirm agreement on the necessity of intervention or the parameters for continued close surveillance (Lyndon, Zlatnik, & Wachter, 2011).

Whereas in the past, the term *fetal distress* generally referred to an ill fetus, categorization of the FHR pattern describes the clinician's interpretation of data on fetal status (i.e., the presumptive relationship between the FHR pattern and fetal acid–base status). The three-tiered categorization system acknowledges the imprecision inherent in interpretation of the data, as well as the dynamic nature of the fetal response to labor (Macones et al., 2008). Therefore, the diagnosis of category II or III tracing can be consistent with the birth of a vigorous baby as the predictive value of even category III tracings for neurologic outcome in infants is poor despite an indication of increased risk for fetal acidemia (ACOG, 2010).

Another problematic issue is use of *asphyxia* and or *acidosis* when making a presumptive diagnosis of intrapartum hypoxia. *Asphyxia* means insufficiency or absence of exchange of respiratory gases. The pathologic consequence of asphyxia is injury to the fetal tissues, primarily the brain, with subsequent neurologic impairment. However, asphyxia is a continuum of oxygen deficit that moves from hypoxemia (decreased oxygen content in blood) to acidemia (increased hydrogen ion concentration in blood) and then acidosis (increased hydrogen ion concentration in the tissue) (King, 2018; King & Parer, 2000). Hypoxemia and acidemia are detectable via pH measurements of fetal scalp blood or umbilical cord blood at birth. These values reveal the acid–base balance within blood but not within tissue and therefore cannot directly reveal the extent or duration of metabolic acidosis or level of asphyxia in tissue. Thus, the use of terms like *asphyxia* and *acidosis* in communication and medical record documentation about characteristics of the FHR and fetal and/or newborn status is both inappropriate and confusing (Fahey & King, 2005) and should be avoided.

TECHNIQUES OF FETAL HEART RATE MONITORING

Assessment of Uterine Activity

During the intrapartum period, the FHR is interpreted relative to uterine activity. Therefore, interpretation of FHR patterns includes a complete assessment of four components of the uterine contractions: (1) frequency, (2) duration, (3) intensity, and (4) the uterine resting tone between contractions. These assessments can be made by either palpation, external tocodynamometer (*tokos* is Greek for *childbirth*), or the use of an intrauterine pressure catheter (IUPC). See Table 15-3 for definitions of the four uterine contraction components and assessment techniques.

Assessment of uterine activity begins with palpation. Contraction frequency is measured from the beginning of one contraction to the beginning of the next and is described in minutes. Duration is the length of the contraction and is described in seconds. Intensity refers to the strength of the contraction and is described as mild, moderate, or strong by palpation or in millimeters of mercury (mm Hg) or Montevideo Units (MVUs) if an IUPC is used. Uterine resting tone is assessed in the absence of contractions or between contractions. By direct palpation, resting tone is described as soft or hard and via IUPC in terms of mm Hg or MVUs. As with any procedure, the least invasive approach is preferred unless maternal–fetal status indicates need for more precise data.

Each technique has some limitation. Intensity cannot be determined with a tocodynamometer. The tocodynamometer detects pressure changes from the tightening of the fundus during contractions through the maternal abdomen. This technique gives a relatively accurate reading of the duration and frequency of contractions but is unable to assess intensity or resting tone. Thus, manual palpation is an essential component of external uterine activity monitoring (Killion, 2015). With an IUPC, the peak of the contraction as indicated on the fetal monitor tracing depicts the actual strength of the contraction measured in mm Hg pressure within the amniotic fluid. The IUPC is most accurate because direct measurement of intraamniotic pressure is recorded, but it requires ruptured membranes for insertion and technical difficulties requiring troubleshooting are not uncommon. An IUPC may be inserted by a physician, midwife, or registered nurse; however, state guidelines and hospital policies vary regarding registered nurses placing IUPCs.

Normal contraction characteristics in the active phase of labor include frequency every 2 to 3 minutes, duration of 80 to 90 seconds, and strong to palpation (Clark, Simpson, Knox, & Garite, 2009). Both contraction characteristics and labor progress are evaluated to determine the adequacy of uterine activity (Miller, 2018). Clinical goals are labor contractions that result in progressive cervical change and fetal descent within a reasonable time frame to maintain maternal–fetal well-being and to avoid unnecessary interventions (i.e., oxytocin, cesarean birth) that have a small, yet real risk patient harm (Simpson & Miller, 2011). If oxytocin is used, additional goals are to avoid excessive uterine contractions by titrating the oxytocin dose to maternal–fetal response and, if excessive contractions occur, timely identification and management based on the clinical situation (Simpson & Miller, 2011).

Some uterine activity patterns are dysfunctional or inadequate for generating progress in labor (Fig. 15–1 A–C). Normal uterine activity is defined as five or less contractions in 10 minutes, averaged over 30

TABLE 15–3. Assessment of Uterine Contractions

Uterine assessment	Definition and assessment techniques
Frequency	Time, in minutes, from beginning of one contraction to the beginning of next contraction
	Assessed by palpation, tocodynamometer (TOCO), or intrauterine pressure catheter (IUPC)
Duration	Time, in seconds, of the duration of the contraction, onset to offset
	Assessed by palpation, TOCO, or IUPC
Intensity	Strength of uterine contraction
	If assessed by palpation, described as mild, moderate, or strong
	If measured by IUPC, described in millimeters of mercury (mm Hg)
Resting tone	Uterine tone between contractions or in absence of contractions
Normal uterine activity	If assessed by palpation, described as soft or hard
	If measured by IUPC, the peak of the contraction is described in mm Hg.
	In the active phase of labor, every 2 to 3 min

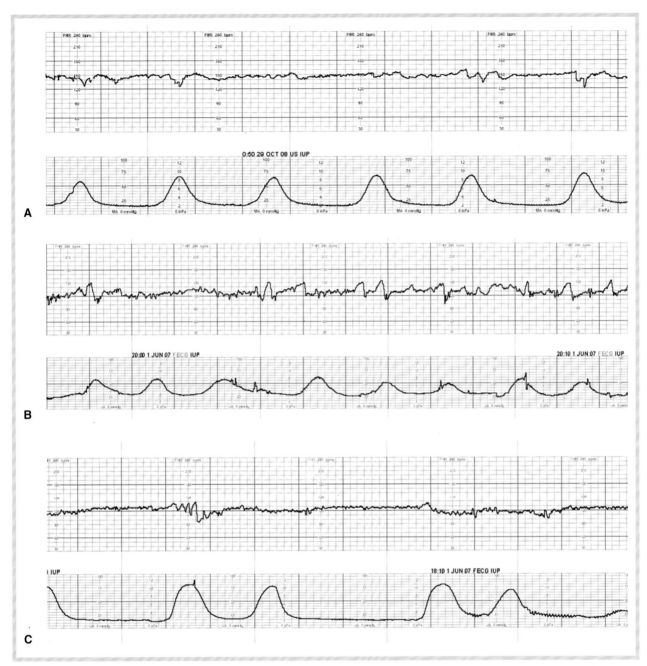

FIGURE 15-1. Three types of uterine contractions. **A**, Normal contraction frequency, duration, and intensity and uterine resting tone. **B**, Tachysystole. **C**, Coupling of contractions.

minutes; tachysystole is defined as more than five contractions in 10 minutes, averaged over 30 minutes (ACOG, 2009a, 2010; Macones et al., 2008). Clark et al. (2009) propose consistent achievement of 200 to 220 MVUs as an indication of adequate labor forces in women receiving oxytocin; however, excessive uterine activity should be avoided to minimize risk of fetal harm. There is an association between higher MVUs and risk of neonatal acidemia at birth. In a study of 1,433 FHR and uterine activity patterns, babies of women with MVUs averaging 236 during first-stage labor were not acidemic at birth, whereas babies of

mothers with MVUs averaging 261 had an umbilical artery pH of 7.11 or less (Bakker, Kurver, Kuik, & Van Geijn, 2007). Tachysystole can be spontaneous as a result of endogenous maternal oxytocin or prostaglandins; however, it is more often seen during exogenous stimulation with agents used in cervical ripening and induction and augmentation of labor (Simpson, 2015).

Coupling or *tripling* refers to a pattern of two or three contractions with little or no interval followed by a regular interval of approximately 2 to 5 minutes. This pattern may be indicative of a dysfunctional labor process and saturation or down-regulation

TABLE 15–4. Assessment of Fetal Status Using Electronic Fetal Monitoring*

	Latent phase (<4 cm)	Latent phase (4 to 5 cm)	Active phase (≥6 cm)	Second stage (passive fetal descent)	Second stage (active pushing)
Low risk without oxytocin	Insufficient evidence to make a recommendation. Frequency at the discretion of the midwife or physician	Every 30 min	Every 30 min	Every 30 min	Every 15 min
With oxytocin or risk factors	Every 15 min with oxytocin; every 30 min without	Every 15 min	Every 15 min	Every 15 min	Every 5 min

*Frequency of assessment should always be determined based on the status of the mother and fetus and at times will need to occur more often based on their clinical needs (e.g., in response to a temporary or ongoing change). Summary documentation is acceptable, and individual hospital policy should be followed.
From Association of Women's Health, Obstetric and Neonatal Nurses. (2018). *Fetal heart monitoring*. Washington, DC: Author. Used with permission from Elsevier.

of uterine oxytocin receptor sites (Dawood, 1995; Phaneuf, Rodriguez Linares, TambyRaja, MacKenzie, & Lopez Bernal, 2000; Zeeman, Khan-Dawood, & Dawood, 1997). If coupling or tripling occurs, a suggested intervention to promote normal uterine activity is temporary discontinuation of oxytocin, maternal repositioning, and an intravenous (IV) fluid bolus of lactated Ringer's solution with resumption of oxytocin after 30 to 60 minutes.

External Doppler versus Fetal Scalp Electrode

The FHR can be detected via a Doppler ultrasound transducer or a fetal scalp electrode (FSE). Frequency of FHR assessment is determined by identified maternal and/or fetal risk factors and the phase and stage of labor (AWHONN, 2019) (Table 15–4). The Doppler transducer is applied to the maternal abdomen over the fetal back or chest and transmits a high-frequency ultrasound. Leopold maneuvers are used to determine the fetal position prior to applying the Doppler transducer (see Chapter 14). The transducer detects the ultrasound wave that is bounced back off the fetal heart and then counts the FHR by measuring the shift in ultrasound wave frequency between the generated wave and the returning wave reflected off the moving heart (Fig. 15–2). The resulting "Doppler shift" waveform goes through "autocorrelation," where it is digitized, smoothed, compared with adjacent wave forms, and averaged over three consecutive heartbeats to produce the FHR. This signal is amplified and converted by the monitor to both visual and auditory output of the FHR. The ultrasound wave will not conduct to the fetus if there is air between the emission of the wave and the object it is reflecting off. Gel applied to the transducer helps eliminate air between the transducer and maternal abdomen.

In the United States, the monitor plots the calculated FHR on paper that is moving at 3 cm/min or on a graphic computer representation of monitor paper moving at the same speed. Because there is variability

in the time interval between heartbeats in a normally oxygenated fetus, the line produced over time has a jagged, irregular appearance resulting from the different rates of consecutively recorded heartbeats. Early Doppler technology tended to exaggerate the FHR variability, but improvements in technology have resulted in a Doppler recording that sufficiently reflects the true variability in the FHR under observation. In some other countries, the recording speed may be set at 1 cm/min, changing the appearance of the FHR patterns observed. Although the Doppler is easy to apply, maternal or fetal movement, uterine contractions, or maternal positions can interrupt a continuous recording. In cases where the mother is significantly overweight, a continuous recording via external monitoring may be challenging.

The direct FSE is the most accurate way to assess the FHR but is invasive and should not be used unless the cervix is at least 2 to 3 cm dilated and the membranes

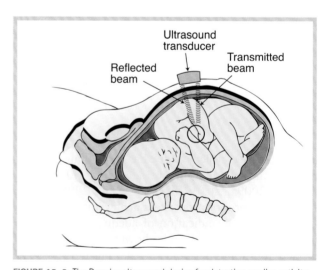

FIGURE 15–2. The Doppler ultrasound device for detecting cardiac activity. The frequency of the reflected beam is changed when it is reflected from a moving structure. (Adapted from Parer, J. T. [1997]. *Handbook of fetal heart rate monitoring* [2nd ed., p. 104]. Philadelphia, PA: W. B. Saunders. Used with permission from Elsevier.)

have ruptured. The electrode has three leads, which detect the PQRST complex. The filter within the electronics of the machine removes all components except the R wave. The R wave then triggers the machine to count; it waits for a second complex, filters all but the R wave, and then calculates how much time elapsed from the first to the second R wave in a fashion similar to the technique used with Doppler ultrasound. The elapsed time between R intervals is converted into beats per minute (bpm), and the pen records that rate on the paper. Both Doppler ultrasound and FSE are appropriate methods for electronic detection and interpretation of FHR patterns (Macones et al., 2008).

It is important to avoid confusing the maternal heart rate with the FHR. Clinical conditions that increase risk of confusion include low FHR baseline, maternal pushing efforts during second-stage labor, maternal repositioning, maternal obesity, and maternal tachycardia, which may be associated with an elevated temperature, anxiety, or medications (Neilson, Freeman, & Mangan, 2008; Simpson, 2011). An abrupt change in the characteristics of the FHR tracing or FHR accelerations consistently coincident with uterine contractions or coincident with maternal pushing efforts should be evaluated to confirm that the tracing is of fetal origin. In the case of fetal demise, a recording may be produced of the maternal heart rate either via the external ultrasound transducer detecting maternal aortic pulsations or via the FSE detecting the maternal ECG. When there are two sources of data (e.g., maternal heart rate via pulse oximetry and fetal or maternal heart rate via external ultrasound or via FSE), the fetal monitor may display coincident alerts to suggest that both data sources are detecting the same heart rate. When these alerts are displayed, confirmation of two distinct heart rates, one from the fetus and one from the mother, should be undertaken. Potential strategies to minimize risk of confusing maternal heart rate with FHR include confirming maternal heart rate by palpation of maternal pulse during initiation of EFM and comparing it with FHR, repeating this confirmation periodically during first- and second-stage labor, playing close attention to distinguishing between maternal heart rate and FHR during second-stage pushing efforts, and recognizing other clinical situations that could result in maternal heart rate being recorded as FHR such as extremes of maternal weight (Simpson, 2011). Coincidence alerts generated from the electronic fetal monitor warrant confirmation that the signal being recorded is fetal rather than maternal.

Both Doppler ultrasound and FSEs can produce FHR recordings that are inadequate for interpretation. Use of EFM during labor requires knowledge of sources of artifact and solutions for resolution. Often, the problem is secondary to equipment malfunction and can be remedied easily. The most common reasons why FHR tracings do not record accurately, the FHR tracing that is produced, and the solution to the problem are listed in Table 15–5. In November 2009, the U.S. Food and Drug Administration (FDA) issued a recall of specific models of fetal monitors and sent a letter to healthcare providers outlining potential problems. The FDA (2009) noted that the following technical issues had been reported: switching between the FHR and

TABLE 15–5. Sources of Artifact or Error in Fetal Heart Rate (FHR) Recordings

	Recording produced	Solution
Signal errors		
Faulty leg plate, electrode, or monitor	No recording	Replace equipment.
Transducer does not detect fetal heart	Intermittent recording consistently	Move transducer.
• Maternal muscle movements		
• Uterine contractions		
• Maternal positioning		
• Maternal obesity		
Interference by maternal signal	Recording will be maternal heart rate.	Recognize maternal heartbeat and use alternative method or adjust placement of transducer.
Limitation of machinery		
Counting process omits FHR that is >30 bpm different from preceding beat.	Arrhythmia will be audible but does not appear on record.	Use fetal ECG if improved recording needed. Arrhythmias tend to be regular, and artifact tends to be irregular.
Halving or doubling of audible FHR	Very slow rates may be doubled and very fast rates (>240 bpm) may be halved.	Auscultate to determine correct rate.
Interpretive errors		
Maternal heart rate recorded	Rate recorded will equal maternal pulse. EFM may provide electronic cues that recording is maternal in nature.	Compare with maternal pulse. Palpate maternal pulse.
• Fetal death		
• Electrode on cervix		

ECG, electrocardiogram; EFM, electronic fetal monitoring.
Adapted with permission from Parer, J. T. (1997). *Handbook of fetal heart rate monitoring* (2nd ed.). Philadelphia, PA: W. B. Saunders.

maternal heart rate, halving of the FHR, a mismatch between the audible and printed FHR, false decelerations, and noisy or erratic signals. The concern was that clinical decisions based on unrecognized inaccuracies in the FHR tracing could lead healthcare professionals to perform unnecessary interventions such as cesarean birth, fail to identify the need for interventions, and/or fail to identify and treat fetal compromise (FDA, 2009).

Application of the FSE is invasive and increases risk of maternal–fetal infection. Therefore, it should be used only when continuous recordings are indicated and are unable to be obtained with external monitoring. If the recording obtained via external EFM is continuous, there is no need for an FSE as there is no clinical difference in data interpretation. The FSE should not be applied to the fetal face, fontanels, or genitalia (CardinalHealth, n.d.). Relative contraindications to the FSE include maternal HIV infection and other high-risk factors for fetal infection, including herpes simplex virus, hepatitis B virus, or hepatitis C virus (American Academy of Pediatrics [AAP] & ACOG, 2017). Conditions in which the fetus is at moderate to severe risk of bleeding based on inherited conditions (e.g., von Willebrand disease or hemophilia) are also contraindicated (AAP & ACOG, 2017).

Intermittent Auscultation

Continuous EFM was introduced as an alternative to IA to decrease the incidence of perinatal death and cerebral palsy. However, because widespread use of continuous EFM has not been able to demonstrate improved outcomes for women with low-risk pregnancies (ACOG, 2019), IA remains an option for women preferring this method. Either a handheld Doppler ultrasound unit, a fetoscope, or Pinard-type stethoscope may be used by the clinician. With Doppler ultrasound, the transducer detects the ultrasound wave that is bounced back off the fetal heart and then counts the FHR by measuring the shift in ultrasound wave frequency between the generated wave and the returning wave reflected off the moving heart (see Fig. 15–2). The nonelectric devices use bone conduction to allow the clinician to hear the actual sound emitted from the opening and closing of the ventricular valves. Table 15–6 compares the abilities of IA techniques versus EFM in assessing FHR characteristics.

ACNM (2015) recommends IA as the preferred method for monitoring the FHR during labor in women at term who are at the onset of labor and are at low risk for developing fetal acidemia. ACOG (2010, 2019) recommends for low-risk women desiring IA during labor that obstetric care providers and facilities consider adopting protocols and training staff to use a handheld Doppler device. Low risk includes healthy women without complications, generally women who have no meconium staining, intrapartum bleeding, and undetermined or abnormal fetal test results; no known factors that could increase risk of fetal acidemia during labor (e.g., congenital anomalies, intrauterine growth restriction); no maternal condition that may affect fetal well-being (e.g., prior cesarean scar, diabetes, hypertensive disease); and no requirement for either oxytocin induction or augmentation of labor (ACOG, 2019). Likewise, AWHONN (Wisner & Holschuh, 2018) supports the use of IA in low-risk women and urges facilities to establish and/or ensure the availability of educational programs for guided clinical experience, skills validation, and ongoing competency assessment. In both Canada (Liston, Sawchuck, & Young, 2018) and the United Kingdom (National Institute for Health and Care Excellence, 2014), IA is the preferred fetal surveillance method for healthy women at term in

TABLE 15–6. Fetal Heart Rate (FHR) Characteristics Determined via Auscultation versus Electronic Monitor

FHR characteristic*	Fetoscope	Doppler device without paper printout	Electronic FHR monitor
Variability	No	No	Yes
Baseline rate	Yes	Yes	Yes
Accelerations	Detects increases[†]	Detects increases[†]	Yes
Decelerations	Detects decreases	Detects decreases	Differentiates types of decelerations
Rhythm[‡]	Yes	Yes	Yes
Double counting or half counting FHR	Can clarify	May double count or half count	May double count or half count
Differentiation of maternal and FHR	Yes	May detect maternal heart rate	May detect and record maternal heart rate

*Definitions of each FHR characteristic based on those reported in Macones et al.
[†]Per method described by Paine et al.[12] and Paine et al.[13]
[‡]Determined as regular or irregular. None of these devices can diagnose the type of fetal arrhythmia.
From Association of Women's Health, Obstetric and Neonatal Nurses. (2018). *Fetal heart monitoring*. Washington, DC: Author. Used with permission from Elsevier; "Intermittent Auscultation for intrapartum Fetal Heart Rate Surveillance," by American College of Nurse Midwives. *Journal of Midwifery & Women's Health, 60*, p. 627. Copyright 2015 by the American College of Nurse Midwives. Used with permission; and Macones, G. A., Hankins, G. D., Spong, C. Y., Hauth, J., & Moore, T. (2008). The 2008 National Institute of Child Health and Human Development Workshop report on electronic fetal monitoring: Update on definitions, interpretation, and research guidelines. *Journal of Obstetric, Gynecologic, and Neonatal Nursing, 37*(5), 510–515. doi:10.1111/j.1552-6909.2008.00284.x and *Obstetrics & Gynecology, 112*(3), 661–666. doi:10.1097/AOG.0b013e3181841395

TABLE 15–7. Auscultation Procedure

Procedure	Rationale
1. Explain the procedure to the woman and her support person(s).	1. Allays fears and anxiety; offers opportunity for emotional and informational support
2. Assist the woman to a semi-Fowler's or wedged lateral position.	2. Prevents supine hypotension syndrome and promotes comfort
3. Palpate the maternal abdomen and perform Leopold's maneuvers.	3. Locates the fetal vertex, buttocks, and back and determines the best location for auscultation (fetal heart sounds are best heard through the fetal back)
4. Assess uterine contractions (frequency, duration, intensity) and uterine resting tone by palpation.	4. Determines uterine activity
5. Apply conduction gel to underside of the Doppler device, if used.	5. Provides an airtight seal and aids in the transmission of ultrasound waves
6. Position the bell of fetoscope or Doppler device on the area of maximum intensity of the fetal heart sounds (usually over the fetal back). Use firm pressure if using the fetoscope.	6. Obtains the strongest FHR signal
7. Place a finger on woman's radial pulse if using a Doppler device or ultrasound transducer.	7. Differentiates maternal heart rate from FHR
8. Determine FHR baseline by listening between contractions for at least 30 sec.	8. Identifies the baseline FHR (in bpm), the rhythm (regular or irregular), and the presence or absence of FHR accelerations or decelerations
9. Assess the FHR for the latter part of a contraction and after uterine contractions for at least 15 to 30 sec to detect periodic changes.	9. Clarifies the presence of FHR changes. Clarifies the nature of FHR changes, such as abrupt versus gradual changes, and amplitude.
10. A multicount strategy may be used to detect FHR accelerations. This method has not been validated for detecting decelerations.	10. May be used as an adjunctive technique to assess for FHR accelerations.

FHR, fetal heart rate.
From Killion, M. M. (2015). Techniques for fetal heart and uterine activity assessment. In A. Lyndon & L. U. Ali (Eds.), *Fetal heart monitoring: Principles and practices* (5th ed., p. 90). Washington, DC: Association of Women's Health, Obstetric and Neonatal Nurses. Copyright 2015 by Association of Women's Health, Obstetric and Neonatal Nurses. Used with permission from Elsevier.

spontaneous labor in the absence of risk factors for adverse perinatal outcomes. An IA procedure is offered in Table 15–7.

Current recommendations for using IA during labor are outlined by AWHONN (2018), ACNM (2015), Society of Obstetricians and Gynaecologists of Canada (SOGC) (Liston et al., 2018), and by AAP and ACOG in the *Guidelines for Perinatal Care* (AAP & ACOG, 2017). However, there are inconsistencies in the recommendations from AAP, ACOG, AWHONN, ACNM, and SOGC regarding patients for whom IA is appropriate, and the frequency of assessment when using IA. In the most recent AWHONN (2018) practice position statement on fetal heart monitoring, AWHONN recommends IA assessments for low-risk women, without oxytocin, every 15 to 30 minutes starting from

cervical dilation of 4 cm in the first stage of labor, every 15 minutes in the second stage of labor (passive fetal descent phase), and every 5 to 15 minutes in the second stage (active pushing phase) as described in Table 15–8. In the *Guidelines for Perinatal Care*, AAP and ACOG (2017) recommend an IA assessment of every 30 minutes in the active phase of the first stage of labor and every 15 minutes in the second stage for women without identified risk factors; however, for women with identified risk factors, at least every 15 minutes in the active phase of first-stage labor and at least every 5 minutes during second-stage labor. In Canada, SOGC (Liston et al., 2018) recommends hourly assessments in the latent phase of labor, every 15 to 30 minutes in the active phase of first-stage labor, and every 5 minutes during active second stage. The ACNM recommends

TABLE 15–8. Assessment and Documentation of Fetal Status Using Intermittent Auscultation*

	Latent phase (<4 cm)	Latent phase (4 to 5 cm)	Active phase (≥6 cm)	Second stage (passive fetal descent)	Second stage (active pushing)
Low risk without oxytocin	Insufficient evidence to make a recommendation. Frequency at the discretion of the midwife or physician	Every 15 to 30 min	Every 15 to 30 min	Every 15 min	Every 5 to 15 min

*Frequency of assessment should always be determined based on the status of the mother and fetus and at times will need to occur more often based on their clinical needs (e.g., in response to a temporary or ongoing change). Summary documentation is acceptable, and individual hospital policy should be followed. From Association of Women's Health, Obstetric and Neonatal Nurses. (2018). *Fetal heart monitoring.* Washington, DC: Author. Used with permission from Elsevier.

TABLE 15–9. Classification and Interpretation of Auscultated Fetal Heart Rate (FHR)

	Characteristics	Interpretation
Category I	**All** of the following: Normal FHR baseline between 110 and 160 bpm Regular rhythm Presence of FHR increases or accelerations from the baseline Absence of FHR decreases of decelerations from the baseline	Normal: Normal FHR characteristics are predictive of fetal well-being at the time of auscultation. Presence of FHR increases, or accelerations, may or may not be present in an FHR auscultated to be normal.
Category II	**Any** of the following: Irregular rhythm Presence of FHR decreases or decelerations from the baseline Tachycardia (baseline >160 bpm >10 min in duration) Bradycardia (baseline <110 bpm >10 min in duration)	Indeterminate: Findings cannot be classified as abnormal as variability cannot be determined by auscultation. These findings require evaluation, ongoing surveillance, and reevaluation consistent with overall clinical circumstances. If recurrent decelerations, bradycardia, or tachycardia are detected, a transfer to continuous electronic fetal monitoring is indicated to evaluate the FHR pattern, to determine a diagnostic category II or III, and to provide appropriate clinical interventions.

auscultation every 15 to 30 minutes in the active phase of the first stage of labor, every 15 minutes in second stage prior to pushing, and every 5 minutes while pushing (ACNM, 2010). No clinical trials have examined methods of fetal assessment during the latent phase of labor. The variation in recommendations among professional societies reflects the variation in protocols used for clinical trials and the mix of both low- and high-risk patients in most trials. Therefore, clinical judgment and unit policy should guide decisions when deciding the method and frequency of fetal assessment. When auscultation is used as the primary method of fetal surveillance during labor, 1 to 1 nursing care is recommended (AAP & ACOG, 2017; ACNM, 2010; AWHONN, 2010, 2018; Liston et al., 2018; Wisner & Holschuh, 2018). Categories for interpretation of IA findings are listed in Table 15–9.

The decision to use IA or EFM is made in collaboration with the laboring woman because there remains a lack of consistent, high-quality evidence to definitively recommend one approach over the other (Devoe, 2011a). The decision is based on many factors, including patient history, fetal condition, risk classification, and hospital policies and procedures. As with continuous EFM, there are benefits and limitations to the use of IA. Both IA and EFM are effective in fetal evaluation when used appropriately (AAP & ACOG, 2017; ACNM, 2015; ACOG, 2010, 2019; AWHONN, 2018; Liston et al., 2018; Martis, Emilia, Nurdiati, & Brown, 2017; Miller, Miller, & Cypher, 2017; Wisner & Holschuh, 2018).

PHYSIOLOGIC BASIS FOR FETAL HEART RATE MONITORING

EFM is a technique for assessing the adequacy of fetal oxygenation. However, while a normal FHR tracing (category I) is a good predictor of a normoxic fetus, the reverse is not true. Because the high rate of false-positive indeterminate (category II) and abnormal (category III) FHR tracings has many origins and several clinical implications, a working knowledge of FHR physiology can aid clinical interpretation of FHR patterns during labor. The following section reviews the importance of maternal oxygenation, uteroplacental exchange, umbilical blood flow, and factors influencing FHR regulation. Subsequently, we review the characteristics of the normal FHR, interventions for managing alterations in FHR, and FHR pattern evolution.

Maternal Oxygen Status

Fetal oxygenation depends on well-oxygenated maternal blood flow to the placenta. Adequate maternal hemoglobin levels, adequate maternal oxygen saturation, and adequate oxygen tension in maternal arterial blood are needed for fetal oxygenation. While most pregnant women are healthy and well oxygenated, maternal conditions that may impair oxygen delivery to the fetus include severe anemia, asthma, congenital cardiac defects, congestive heart failure, lung disease, or seizures.

Uterine, Placental, and Umbilical Blood Flow

Adequate uterine blood flow is required for the passage of respiratory gases and substances across the placenta. Uterine blood flow increases throughout pregnancy and in a singleton pregnancy at term is approximately 700 mL/min, or 10% to 15% of maternal cardiac output (King, 2018; Parer, 1997). While uterine blood also supplies the myometrium and endometrium, the intervillous space within the placenta receives 70% to 90% of the total uterine blood flow near term (King, 2018; Parer, 1997). In the intervillous space, well-oxygenated maternal blood propelled by maternal arterial blood pressure surrounds the fetal chorionic villi, allowing exchange of oxygen, carbon

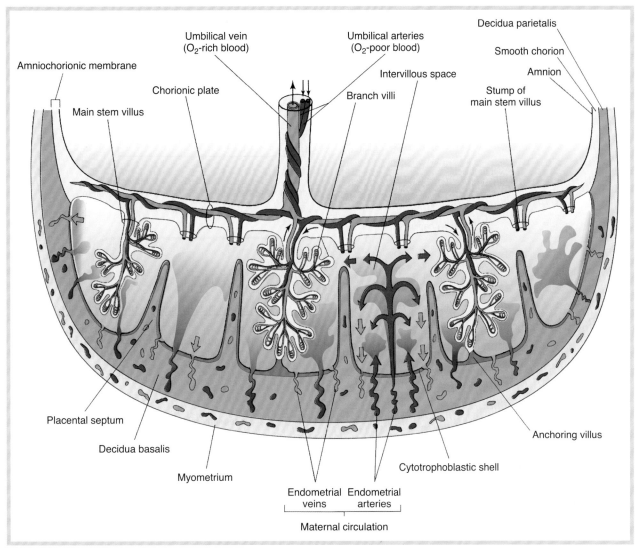

FIGURE 15–3. Schematic drawing of a transverse section through a full-term placenta showing maternal uteroplacental circulation and fetal–placental circulation. (From Moore, K. L., Persaud, T. V. N., & Torchia, M. G. [2016]. *The developing human: Clinically oriented embryology* [10th ed.]. Philadelphia, PA: Elsevier. Used with permission from Elsevier.)

dioxide, and other substances between the maternal and fetal circulations (Fig. 15–3). The newly oxygenated fetal blood within the fetal villi flows into veins that converge into a single umbilical vein, which carries the oxygenated blood and nutrients to the fetus. Deoxygenated blood and waste products return from the fetus to the placenta via two umbilical arteries, which divide successively into smaller vessels, eventually creating an arteriovenous system within each chorionic villus.

Maternal–fetal exchange of oxygen, carbon dioxide, nutrients, waste products, water, and other substances is facilitated by the large surface area of the placental membrane separating the maternal and fetal blood (Fig. 15–4). Mechanisms by which these substances transfer across the placental membrane include passive diffusion, facilitated diffusion, active transport, pinocytosis, bulk flow, capillary leaks or breaks,

independent movement, and infections (Blackburn, 2018; Moore, Persaud, & Torchia, 2016). Oxygen and carbon dioxide exchange rapidly by passive diffusion, which allows movement of a substance down the concentration gradient from an area of high concentration, across a membrane, to an area of lower concentration. The concentration gradients and characteristics of fetal hemoglobin favor transfer of oxygen from mother to fetus and transfer of carbon dioxide from fetus to mother.

Clinical factors that can potentially decrease uteroplacental perfusion and fetal oxygenation include excessive uterine contractions, tachysystole, or hypertonus; maternal hypotension or hypertension; placental changes due to decreased surface area, degenerative changes, infarcts, calcification, infection, or edema; and vasoconstriction. In addition, umbilical cord entanglement, compression, or occlusion may impede

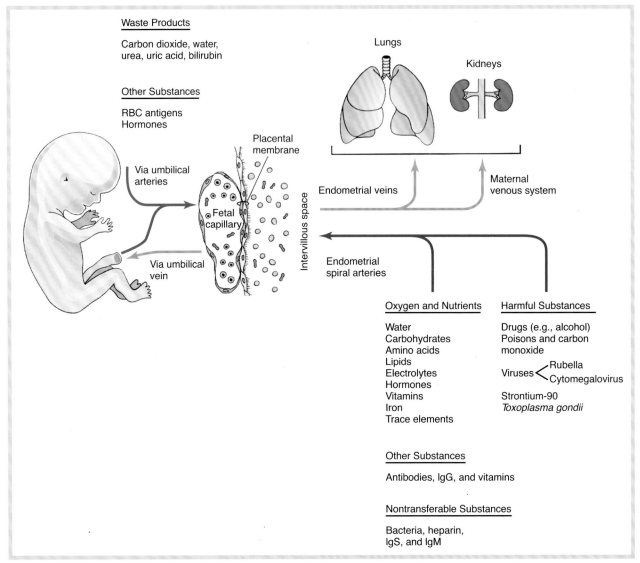

FIGURE 15–4. Transfer of substances between the mother and the fetus across the placental membrane.
Ig, immunoglobulin; RBC, red blood cell. (From Moore, K. L., Persaud, T. V. N., & Torchia, M. G. [2016]. *The developing human: Clinically oriented embryology* [10th ed.]. Philadelphia, PA: Elsevier. Used with permission from Elsevier.)

fetal oxygenation. Therefore, a primary goal in intrapartum care is to maximize uterine blood flow, uteroplacental exchange, and umbilical blood flow, thereby minimizing risk to the fetus.

Fetal Heart Rate Regulation

The cardioregulatory center in the medulla oblongata interacts with the parasympathetic and sympathetic branches of the autonomic nervous systems, baroreceptors, chemoreceptors, fetal hormones, sleep/wake cycles, breathing movements, painful stimuli, sound vibrations, and temperature to influence FHR (O'Brien-Abel, 2015). Major factors believed to influence the integration of FHR control are outlined in Table 15–10. Interplay between the two components of the autonomic nervous system (sympathetic

and parasympathetic), higher cortical functions in the brain, and chemoreceptors and baroreceptors are all reflected in the baseline rate and, in part, make up the FHR variability seen on the recording from an FHR monitor (King, 2018).

Sympathetic nervous system fibers are widely distributed throughout the fetal myocardium at term. Stimulation of these nerve fibers releases norepinephrine, causing increased heart rate, strength of cardiac contractions, and cardiac output (Parer, 1997). The average baseline FHR in the normal fetus at 20 weeks' gestation is 155 bpm; at 30 weeks, 144 bpm; and at term before labor, 140 bpm (normal range, 110 to 160 bpm) (Parer, 1997). This slow, gradual decrease in FHR seen with advancing gestational age is due to an increased dominance of the parasympathetic over the sympathetic branch of the autonomic nervous system.

TABLE 15–10. Factors Influencing Fetal Heart Rate (FHR) Control

Influence	Action	FHR effect
Cardioregulatory center • Collection of neurons in ventral and lateral surface of medulla oblongata	• Integrating source for control of FHR • Interacts with parasympathetic and sympathetic nervous systems, baroreceptors, chemoreceptors, fetal hormones, sleep/wake cycles, breathing movements, painful stimuli, sound, vibrations, and temperature to influence FHR	• Baseline rate, variability, and various FHR patterns provide indirect insights into functioning of CNS. • Presence of FHR variability represents an intact nervous pathway through cerebral cortex, midbrain, vagus nerve, and normal cardiac conduction system.
Parasympathetic branch of the autonomic nervous system • Originates in medulla oblongata • Vagus nerve (10th cranial) innervates SA and AV nodes.	• Stimulation releases acetylcholine. • Pathway for transmission of variability	• ↓ FHR • Slow, gradual ↓ FHR with ↑ gestational age (approximately 10 bpm difference in baseline FHR between 28 weeks and term) • Maintains transmission of beat-to-beat variability • Moderate variability indicates absence of severe hypoxia or metabolic acidemia. • Modulates baseline FHR with sympathetic branch
Sympathetic branch of the autonomic nervous system • At term, nerve fibers widely distributed throughout myocardium	• Stimulation releases catecholamines (e.g., norepinephrine, epinephrine) • Reserve mechanism to improve the heart's pumping ability during intermittent stress • Catecholamines can also cause fetal vasoconstriction and hypertension.	• ↑ FHR • Blocking with propranolol results in ↓ FHR of approximately 10 bpm. • Modulates baseline FHR with parasympathetic branch
Baroreceptors • Protective, stretch receptors • Located in aortic arch and carotid sinuses at bifurcation of external and internal carotid arteries	• When ↑ arterial BP, the baroreceptors quickly detect amount of stretch, sending impulses via vagus nerve to midbrain. • Impulses return via vagus nerve, causing sudden ↓ FHR, ↓ CO, and ↓ blood pressure, thereby protecting fetus.	• Abrupt ↓ FHR • Abrupt ↓ CO • Abrupt ↓ BP • Variable decelerations with moderate variability are baroreceptor influenced
Chemoreceptors • Central—located in medulla oblongata • Peripheral—in aortic arch and carotid sinuses	In the adult: • When arterial blood perfusing chemoreceptors contains ↑ PCO_2 or ↓ PO_2: • Central chemoreceptors respond with reflex tachycardia and hypertension, most likely in an attempt to circulate blood and ↓ PCO_2. • Peripheral chemoreceptors respond with bradycardia.	In the fetus: • Interaction of central and peripheral chemoreceptors poorly understood • Combined effect is slowing of FHR. • Described in mechanism of late decelerations and variable decelerations resulting from umbilical arterial occlusion coupled with hypoxemia • When blood flow is below threshold for normal respiratory gas exchange, ↑ PCO_2 stimulates chemoreceptors to slow FHR
Hormonal regulation • Epinephrine and norepinephrine secreted from the adrenal medulla • Arginine vasopressin secreted from posterior pituitary • Renin-angiotensin-aldosterone secreted from kidneys	• In response to stressful situations, compensatory response shunts blood away from less vital organs and toward brain, heart, and adrenal glands. • In adult, responds to ↓ plasma volume, ↑ plasma osmolarity • In fetal sheep, hypoxemia most potent stimulus; distributes blood flow • Responds to ↓ plasma volume or ↓ BP; protects fetus from hemorrhagic stress by stimulating vasoconstriction	• ↓ FHR, ↑ strength of cardiac contractions, ↑ CO, ↑ arterial BP • ↑ FHR, ↑ CO, ↑ arterial BP • Sinusoidal heart rate pattern in experimental studies • ↑ FHR, ↑ CO, ↑ arterial BP
Cardiac output • In the adult, CO = HR × SV. • The Frank-Starling mechanism dictates ↑ inflow of blood into heart stretches cardiac muscle, thereby resulting in ↑ force of contraction and ↑ SV.	• In the fetus, this mechanism has not been found to apply on the basis of studies involving fetal and adult lambs. • Compared with adult, fetal SV does not fluctuate significantly; fetal heart appears to operate near the top of its cardiac function curve.	• Therefore, fetal CO ≈ HR. • Modest variations in baseline FHR probably have little effect on fetal CO. • At extreme rates (e.g., tachycardia >240 bpm or bradycardia <60 bpm), fetal CO can be significantly decreased.

AV, atrioventricular; BP, blood pressure; bpm, beats per minute; CNS, central nervous system; CO, cardiac output; HR, heart rate; PCO_2, partial pressure of carbon dioxide; PO_2, partial pressure of oxygen; SA, sinoatrial; SV, stroke volume.
From O'Brien-Abel, N. (2015). Physiologic basis for fetal monitoring. In A. Lyndon & L. U. Ali (Eds.), *Fetal heart monitoring: Principles and practices* (5th ed., pp. 23–47). Washington, DC: Association of Women's Health, Obstetric and Neonatal Nurses/Kendall Hunt. Used with permission from Elsevier.

While the sympathetic branch is dominant in an extremely premature fetus, a baseline FHR greater than 160 bpm should be further evaluated to rule out fetal compromise rather than assuming the tachycardia is secondary to prematurity (Freeman, Garite, Nageotte, Miller, 2012).

The parasympathetic nervous system influences the fetal heart via the vagus nerve, which innervates the sinoatrial (SA) and atrioventricular (AV) nodes within the heart. Stimulation of the vagus nerve releases acetylcholine, which decreases firing of the SA node, resulting in a slower heart rate in a normal fetus (Dalton, Phill, Dawes, & Patrick, 1983; Parer, 1997). With advancing gestational age, this vagal influence results in approximately 10 bpm difference in baseline FHR between 28 to 30 weeks' gestation and term. The second important function of the parasympathetic system is the transmission of FHR variability. Vagal stimulation of the SA node is the primary influence in the transmission of impulses causing FHR variability. Because severe hypoxia and metabolic acidosis will decrease central nervous system (CNS) function, the presence of moderate FHR variability reliably indicates a well-oxygenated fetus without metabolic acidosis at the time of observation (Freeman et al., 2012; Parer, 1997).

Chemoreceptors, located centrally in the medulla oblongata and peripherally in the aortic arch and carotid sinuses, have their greatest effect on the regulation of respiration and in the control of circulation (Parer, 1997). When chemoreceptors detect a decrease in circulating oxygenation and an increase in carbon dioxide (PCO_2) (e.g., uteroplacental blood flow falls below a threshold needed for normal respiratory gas exchange), chemoreceptors stimulate a vagally mediated reflex fetal bradycardia and increase in blood pressure (King, 2018; Parer, 1997). The influence of chemoreceptors may be seen in the mechanism of late decelerations and in variable decelerations with hypoxemia.

Baroreceptors, located in the aortic arch and carotid sinuses, are small protective stretch receptors that quickly detect increases in fetal arterial blood pressure (Parer, 1997). When umbilical blood flow is occluded, fetal arterial blood pressure quickly increases and stretches the artery walls, triggering the baroreceptors to send impulses via the vagus nerve to the midbrain to abruptly decrease the FHR, cardiac output, and blood pressure, thereby protecting the fetus. The influence of baroreceptors may be seen in the mechanism of variable decelerations.

Fetal monitoring is an ongoing indirect assessment of physiologic factors affecting fetal oxygenation and thereby fetal acid–base status. Uteroplacental blood flow, intervillous space perfusion, umbilical blood flow, and intrinsic influences of parasympathetic and sympathetic nervous system, baroreceptors and chemoreceptors, are reflected in the characteristics of the observed FHR. Ongoing assessment and interpretation of FHR characteristics are used to determine fetal oxygenation and rule out fetal acidemia.

CHARACTERISTICS OF THE NORMAL FETAL HEART RATE

The FHR pattern interpretation involves assessment of five components of the FHR as well as the relationship of FHR characteristics to both uterine activity and the overall clinical situation. Characteristics of the FHR to be evaluated include (1) baseline rate, (2) FHR variability, (3) presence or absence of accelerations, (4) other periodic and/or episodic changes, and (5) evolution over time (Macones et al., 2008). Periodic and episodic changes refer to accelerations and decelerations. Periodic changes in FHR occur in response to uterine activity. Episodic changes are not associated with uterine activity and may occur randomly. This section reviews characteristics of the normal FHR (category I tracings), and the next section reviews etiology and management of the most common periodic and episodic changes seen in category II and III tracings as well as some other less common alterations in FHR.

Baseline Rate

The baseline FHR is the approximate mean FHR rounded to increments of 5 bpm during a 10-minute segment, excluding accelerations and decelerations, and periods of marked FHR variability (Macones et al., 2008). In determining the baseline rate, at least 2 minutes of identifiable baseline are required, although they do not need to be contiguous. If during a 10-minute segment, there are not at least 2 minutes of identifiable baseline; the baseline for that period is indeterminate. In this case, one may need to refer to the previous 10-minute segment(s) for determination of the baseline. The normal baseline FHR range is 110 to 160 bpm (Macones et al., 2008). Bradycardia is a baseline FHR <110 bpm; tachycardia is a baseline FHR >160 bpm (Macones et al., 2008). Since the baseline is determined over a 10-minute period, a baseline change has occurred once the change in FHR has been sustained for at least 10 minutes. In the absence of tachycardia or bradycardia, the FHR baseline changes frequently during labor in term, singleton fetuses, often reaching amplitudes ≥20 and ≥30 bpm, and does not require clinical interventions (Yang et al., 2017).

Variability

Baseline FHR variability is defined as fluctuations in the baseline FHR that occur with irregular amplitude and frequency during a 10-minute window, excluding accelerations and decelerations (Macones et al., 2008). The FHR of the healthy fetus is displayed as an irregular line on the monitor tracing. The irregular fluctuations reflect the slight difference in time interval between successive heartbeats (short-term component) and cyclic fluctuations over time (long-term component). Clinically, variability is visually determined as a unit without separating short- and long-term components (Macones et al., 2008; NICHD Research Planning Workshop, 1997). These irregular FHR fluctuations are visually quantitated as the amplitude of the peak to trough in bpm as follows (see Fig. 15–8):

> *Absent variability*: amplitude range undetectable
> *Minimal variability*: amplitude range detectable, but less than or equal to 5 bpm
> *Moderate variability*: amplitude range of 6 to 25 bpm
> *Marked variability*: amplitude range greater than 25 bpm

Presence of variability represents an intact nervous pathway from the cerebral cortex, through the midbrain, the vagus nerve, and the normal cardiac conduction system (King, 2018; Parer, 1997). Moderate variability, therefore, reliably indicates a well-oxygenated fetus without metabolic acidemia at the time of observation (ACOG, 2009b; Freeman et al., 2012; King, 2018; Macones et al., 2008; Parer, 1997; Parer et al., 2006). A discussion of minimal, absent, and marked FHR variability following in the section discussing alterations in variability.

Accelerations

An acceleration is a visually apparent abrupt increase (defined as onset of acceleration to peak in <30 seconds) in FHR above the baseline (Fig. 15–5). The peak of the acceleration is at least 15 bpm above the baseline, and the acceleration must last at least 15 seconds but less than 2 minutes from the onset to return to baseline (Macones et al., 2008). The FHR only needs to reach a peak ≥15 bpm above baseline; it does not need to be sustained at ≥15 bpm above baseline. Before 32 weeks of gestation, accelerations are defined as having a peak of at least 10 bpm above the baseline and duration of at least 10 seconds (Macones et al., 2008). Accelerations may be present or absent in a normal (category I) FHR tracing (Macones et al., 2008). Similar to moderate variability, while the presence of FHR accelerations indicates the absence of fetal metabolic acidemia (ACOG, 2009b; Clark, Gimovsky, & Miller, 1984; Macones et al., 2008), the absence of FHR accelerations is not a reliable predictor of fetal metabolic acidemia (Macones et al., 2008).

Early Decelerations

Early decelerations may or may not be present in a normal (category I) FHR tracing (Macones et al., 2008). Early decelerations are characterized by a visually apparent, *gradual* (defined as onset of deceleration to nadir ≥30 seconds) decrease and return to baseline FHR associated with a uterine contraction. Early decelerations are typically symmetrical with the nadir of the contraction occurring at the same time as the peak of the uterine contraction. In most cases, the onset, nadir, and recovery of the deceleration occur at the same time as the beginning, peak, and ending of the contraction, respectively (Macones et al., 2008).

Early decelerations are presumed to be a response to fetal head compression. Altered cerebral blood flow causes the decrease in FHR through a vagal reflex. The FHR begins to gradually slow at the onset of the contraction with head compression and then gradually returns to the baseline rate at the end of the contraction, when the head is no longer compressed. Early decelerations tend to "mirror" the contraction, rarely decreasing more than 20 to 30 bpm below baseline, and are not common. Early decelerations are associated with moderate variability and are not associated with fetal hypoxia, acidosis, or low Apgar scores (Freeman et al., 2012; King, 2018; Parer, 1997).

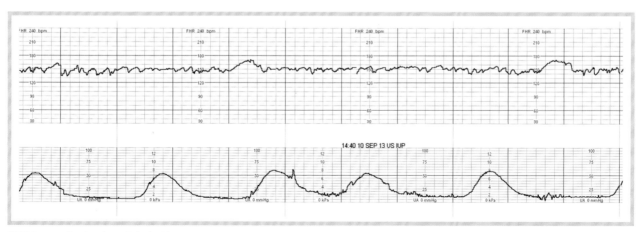

FIGURE 15–5. Accelerations of the fetal heart rate.

The key to assessment of early decelerations is to make sure to distinguish them from late decelerations. The presence of variability is a key clinical factor.

Uterine Activity

Uterine activity is a key characteristic for interpretation of the overall clinical picture and the FHR pattern. Uterine activity is quantified by determining the number of contractions present in a 10-minute window, averaged over 30 minutes (Macones et al., 2008). Uterine activity should be further characterized in terms of contraction duration and intensity and the quality and duration of resting tone (Lyndon, O'Brien-Abel, & Simpson, 2015; Macones et al., 2008). See Table 15–3 for definitions of the four uterine contraction components and assessment techniques.

Frequency of uterine activity is further classified as either normal or tachysystole (Macones et al., 2008). *Normal uterine activity* is five or less contractions in 10 minutes, averaged over 30 minutes. *Tachysystole* occurs when there are more than five contractions in 10 minutes, averaged over 30 minutes, and is further characterized by the presence or absence of associated FHR decelerations. Tachysystole applies to contractions that are either spontaneous or as a result of agents used in cervical ripening and/or induction and augmentation of labor. Although the definition for tachysystole includes an averaging of contractions over a 30-minute period, this is not meant to imply that 30 minutes is required before tachysystole can be determined or that interventions to decrease uterine activity should be delayed until tachysystole has been occurring for 30 minutes. One or two 10-minute segments of more than five contractions are sufficient to identify excessive uterine activity and initiate appropriate interventions. Interventions for reducing uterine activity are discussed in the next section.

INTERVENTIONS FOR INDETERMINATE OR ABNORMAL FETAL HEART RATE PATTERNS

Before discussing the etiology and individual management of periodic or episodic changes in the FHR, a general review of the initial assessment and interventions used to maximize fetal oxygenation in the presence of variant FHR patterns is warranted. When an indeterminate (category II) or abnormal (category III) FHR pattern is identified, initial assessment may include a cervical exam to rule out umbilical cord prolapse, rapid cervical dilation, or rapid descent of the fetal head; a review of uterine activity to rule out tachysystole; and an evaluation of maternal vital signs, in particular temperature and blood pressure, to rule out maternal fever or maternal hypotension (ACOG, 2010). These assessment data can guide appropriate treatment to attempt to resolve the pattern. *Intrauterine resuscitation* refers to one or more of a series of interventions to improve fetal oxygen delivery when a category II or III FHR tracing is observed. Potential interventions include initiate maternal lateral maternal positioning (either right or left), reduce uterine contraction frequency, discontinue oxytocin or cervical ripening agents, administer IV fluids, administer maternal oxygen, modify second-stage pushing efforts, and, sometimes, administer tocolytic medications (e.g., terbutaline sulfate) or initiate amnioinfusion (ACOG, 2010; ACOG & AAP, 2014; Garite & Simpson, 2011; Simpson, 2015). The type of resuscitative technique is based on the specific characteristics of the observed FHR pattern and maternal condition. See Figure 15–6 for an algorithm suggested by ACOG (2010), and reaffirmed in 2017, to manage FHR patterns. In some cases, a combination of techniques will be required. A summary of the goals and techniques for intrauterine resuscitation are presented in Table 15–11. These interventions are directed at improving maternal blood flow to the placenta and oxygen delivery to the fetus. Data suggest that these techniques can improve fetal oxygen status, but there is no evidence that these techniques will reverse asphyxia. If the clinical characteristics of the FHR patterns are thought to represent a serious risk for metabolic acidemia, these measures should be initiated only if doing so does not delay the move toward expeditious birth (Lyndon et al., 2015; Simpson, 2007, 2015).

Position Change

Changing maternal position alters the relationship between the umbilical cord and fetal parts or the uterine wall and alters maternal cardiac output. It is usually done to minimize or correct cord compression and improve uterine blood flow (increased uterine blood flow may also decrease the frequency of uterine contractions) (Simpson, 2015). Position change can resolve or decrease the severity of prolonged decelerations and/or variable decelerations. Position change may also modify late decelerations if the etiology of this pattern is decreased uterine blood flow (usually secondary to supine positioning with inferior vena caval compression), as venous return and cardiac output are increased in the lateral position (Clark et al., 1991). Generally, it is best to avoid supine positioning to prevent compression of the vena cava, reduced cardiac output, and supine hypotensive syndrome. Several studies comparing the effects of right lateral, left lateral, and supine maternal positions on fetal oxygen status suggest that lateral positioning on either the left or the right is more favorable for enhancing fetus oxygenation when compared to a supine position (Aldrich et al., 1995; ACOG & AAP, 2014; Carbonne, Benachi, Leveque, Cabrol, & Papiernik, 1996; Simpson & James, 2005b).

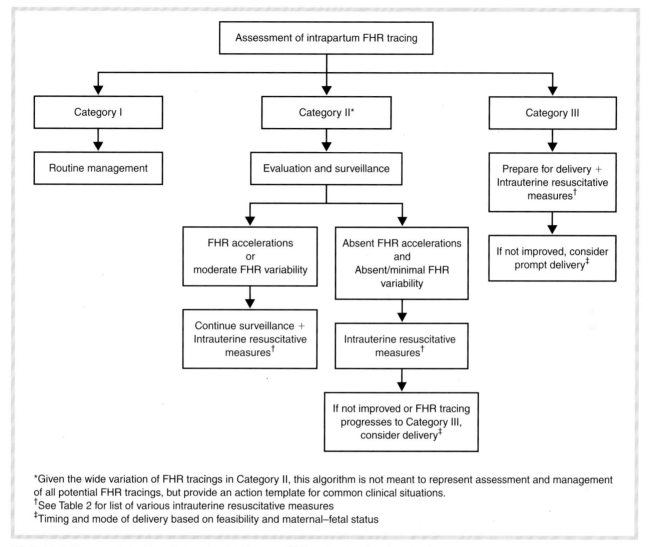

*Given the wide variation of FHR tracings in Category II, this algorithm is not meant to represent assessment and management of all potential FHR tracings, but provide an action template for common clinical situations.
†See Table 2 for list of various intrauterine resuscitative measures
‡Timing and mode of delivery based on feasibility and maternal–fetal status

FIGURE 15–6. Management algorithm of intrapartum fetal heart rate (FHR) tracings based on three-tiered category system. (From American College of Obstetricians and Gynecologists. [2010]. *Management of intrapartum fetal heart rate tracings* [Practice Bulletin No. 116; Reaffirmed, 2017]. Washington, DC: Author. Used with permission.)

TABLE 15–11. Intrauterine Resuscitation

Goal	Techniques/methods
Promote fetal oxygenation	Lateral positioning (either left or right)
	Oxygen administration at 10 L/min via nonrebreather facemask
	IV fluid bolus of at least 500 mL of lactated Ringer's solution
	Discontinuation of oxytocin/removal of Cervidil/withholding next dose of misoprostol (Cytotec)
	Stopping pushing temporarily or pushing with every other, or every third, contraction (during second-stage labor)
Reduce uterine activity	Discontinuation of oxytocin/removal of Cervidil/withhold next dose of Cytotec
	IV fluid bolus of at least 500 mL of lactated Ringer's solution
	Lateral positioning (either left or right)
	If no response, consider terbutaline 0.25 mg subcutaneously.
Alleviate umbilical cord compression	Repositioning
	Amnioinfusion (during first-stage labor)
	Stopping pushing temporarily or pushing with every other, or every third, contraction (during second-stage labor)
Correct maternal hypotension	Lateral positioning (either left or right)
	IV fluid bolus of at least 500 mL of lactated Ringer's solution
	If no response, consider ephedrine 5 to 10 mg IV push.

IV, intravenous.

Reduction of Uterine Activity

Uterine contractions produce an intermittent decrease in uteroplacental blood flow and oxygen exchange within the intervillous space of the placenta. When uterine contractions are too frequent, as with tachysystole, the interruption in blood flow and oxygen exchange decrease to an abnormal level, resulting in a fetus at risk for hypoxemia (ACOG & AAP, 2014). If FHR decelerations occur with tachysystole, reduction of contraction activity will improve fetal oxygenation (Simpson, 2015; Simpson & James, 2008). Reduction of uterine activity can occur by reducing oxytocin dosage or discontinuing oxytocin administration, if in use. Lateral positioning of the mother and a crystalloid IV fluid bolus may also reduce uterine activity (Simpson & James, 2008). If oxytocin is in use, tachysystole is present, and the FHR is abnormal (category III), oxytocin should be discontinued (Simpson, 2020). Oxytocin should be decreased when tachysystole occurs in the context of a normal (category I) FHR tracing (Simpson, 2020). Clinical judgment is required to determine whether to decrease or discontinue oxytocin for category II tracings, depending on their specific presentation (ACOG, 2010). For example, oxytocin may need to be discontinued in the context of category II tracings with minimal variability and recurrent decelerations, but it may be appropriate to continue oxytocin at a decreased rate in a tracing with moderate variability and intermittent variable decelerations. A suggested protocol for management of oxytocin-induced tachysystole is present in Table 15–12. Similarly, the next dose of pharmacologic agents used to ripen the cervix or stimulate

contractions should be delayed until uterine activity returns to normal and the FHR improves. Administration of tocolytics is another option occasionally used as a temporary measure to provide intrauterine resuscitation for a prolonged deceleration or other variant FHR patterns secondary to tachysystole, by reducing uterine activity (ACOG, 2010). A subcutaneous dose of terbutaline 0.25 mg is often used for this purpose.

Intravenous Fluid Administration

IV fluid administration is thought to improve uteroplacental perfusion through expansion of maternal intravascular volume. Reductions in uterine blood flow may occur as a result of hypovolemia, hypotension, and sympathetic nervous system blockade following regional analgesia/anesthesia and other conditions. Data suggest that increasing IV fluids will positively affect uterine blood flow and, thus, fetal oxygenation, even in women who are normotensive and well-hydrated. Fetal oxygen saturation ($FSpO_2$) was significantly increased after at least a 500-mL bolus of lactated Ringer's solution over 20 minutes in normotensive women who were otherwise receiving lactated Ringer's solution at 125 mL/hr (Simpson & James, 2005b). The increase in $FSpO_2$ was greatest with a 1,000-mL IV fluid bolus. The positive effects on fetal oxygen status continued for more than 30 minutes after the IV fluid bolus (Simpson & James, 2005b). Thus, an IV fluid bolus of approximately 500 to 1,000 mL may be useful as an intrauterine resuscitation technique. However, caution is indicated when increasing IV fluids or giving repeated IV fluid boluses. Some clinical situations, such as preeclampsia, preterm labor treated with

---

TABLE 15–12. Suggested Clinical Protocol for Oxytocin-Induced Uterine Tachysystole

Oxytocin-induced tachysystole (normal FHR)

- Assist the mother to a lateral position.
- Give IV fluid bolus of at least 500 mL lactated Ringer's solution as indicated.
- If uterine activity has not returned to normal after 10 to 15 min, decrease oxytocin rate by at least half; if uterine activity has not returned to normal after 10 to 15 more min, discontinue oxytocin until uterine activity less than five contractions in 10 min.
- Resume oxytocin after resolution of tachysystole: If oxytocin has been discontinued for less than 20 to 30 min; the FHR is normal; and contraction frequency, intensity, and duration are normal, resume oxytocin at no more than half the rate that caused the tachysystole and gradually increase the rate as appropriate based on unit protocol and maternal–fetal status. If the oxytocin is discontinued for more than 30 to 40 min, resume oxytocin at the initial dose ordered.

Oxytocin-induced tachysystole (indeterminate or abnormal FHR)

- Discontinue oxytocin.
- Assist the mother to a lateral position.
- Give IV fluid bolus of at least 500 mL of lactated Ringer's solution as indicated.
- Consider oxygen at 10 L/min via nonrebreather face mask (discontinue as soon as possible based on the FHR pattern).
- If no response, consider 0.25 mg terbutaline SQ.
- To resume oxytocin after resolution of tachysystole: If oxytocin has been discontinued for less than 20 to 30 min; the FHR is normal; and contraction frequency, intensity, and duration are normal, resume oxytocin at no more than half the rate that caused the tachysystole and gradually increase the rate as appropriate based on unit protocol and maternal–fetal status. If the oxytocin is discontinued for more than 30 to 40 min, resume oxytocin at the initial dose ordered.

FHR, fetal heart rate; IV, intravenous; SQ, subcutaneous.

magnesium sulfate, or preterm labor treated with corticosteroids and beta-sympathomimetic medications, carry an increased risk for pulmonary edema that might necessitate fluid restriction. Oxytocin has an antidiuretic effect, so prolonged use of oxytocin can also lead to fluid overload if IV fluids are used too liberally. An extreme effect of fluid overload related to excessive use of oxytocin is water intoxication. Glucose-containing IV fluids should not be used for volume expansion (Simpson, 2015).

Oxygen Administration

Intrauterine resuscitation frequently includes maternal oxygen administration. Although this therapy appears to be beneficial in improving fetal oxygen status during labor, recent concern for potential adverse effects of oxygen therapy suggests adoption of a judicious approach to the use of oxygen in laboring women. In a classic study about the effects of maternal oxygen administration on the fetus, 100% oxygen via facemask corrected "nonreassuring" FHR patterns by decreasing the baseline FHR during fetal tachycardia and reducing or eliminating late decelerations (Althabe, Schwarcz, Pose, Escarcena, & Caldeyro-Barcia, 1967). There is evidence that $FSpO_2$ will increase as a result of maternal oxygen administration of at least 10 L/min via nonrebreather facemask (Haydon et al., 2006; McNamara, Johnson, & Lilford, 1993; Simpson & James, 2005b) and some evidence that maternal oxygen administration increases fetal cerebral oxygenation (Aldrich, Wyatt, Spencer, Reynolds, & Delpy, 1994). Fetuses with lower oxygen saturation appear to benefit most from maternal oxygen administration (Haydon et al., 2006; Simpson & James, 2005b).

Even though healthy women in labor have nearly 100% SpO_2 (usually between 96% and 99%), increasing inspired oxygen increases blood oxygen tension and results in more oxygen delivered to the fetus and the fetal cerebral tissues (Aldrich et al., 1994; McNamara et al., 1993; Simon, Fong, & Nageotte, 2018). There is a more rapid increase in $FSpO_2$ when oxygen is given as compared to the decrease in $FSpO_2$ when it is discontinued, suggesting that the fetus responds to the change in oxygen concentration gradient by accepting oxygen more rapidly than it releases it (McNamara et al., 1993). In one study, increased $FSpO_2$ persisted 30 minutes after discontinuation of maternal oxygen (Simpson & James, 2005b). Fetal hemoglobin has a higher affinity for oxygen than adult hemoglobin, and fetal hematocrit is higher than adults. These physiologic factors allow for a steeper increase in fetal oxygen concentration and $FSpO_2$ during maternal oxygen therapy.

When administering oxygen to the mother, the nonrebreather facemask works best because the fraction of inspired oxygen (FIO_2) at 10 L/min is approximately 80% to 100%, as compared to a simple facemask (FIO_2 27% to 40%) or nasal cannula (FIO_2 31%) (Simpson & James, 2005b). There is inconsistent evidence concerning how long maternal oxygen therapy should be continued and its effects on fetal acid–base status. One study found a deterioration in umbilical cord blood values when maternal oxygen was administered for more than 10 minutes during second-stage labor (Thorp, Trobough, Evans, Hedrick, & Yeast, 1995), while others found no change in acid–base status as measured by umbilical cord gases when maternal oxygen was administered from 15 to 60 minutes during second-stage labor or prior to cesarean birth (Haruta, Funato, Sumida, & Shinkai, 1984; Jozwik et al., 2000; Simon et al., 2018). Of note, much of the research on maternal oxygen administration was conducted with very small samples of women and their fetuses, the interventions were not randomized, and there was often no control group. A Cochrane Review concluded there is not enough evidence to support prophylactic oxygen administration and there were no randomized trials of oxygen administration for "fetal distress" (Fawole & Hofmeyr, 2012). Questions have also been raised regarding the production potentially deleterious of oxygen-free radicals in both the mother and fetus under conditions of increased oxygen tension (Simpson, 2008). However, fetal hypoxia also produces oxygen-free radicals. Thus, based on the available evidence, maternal oxygen therapy as an intrauterine resuscitation technique for 15 to 30 minutes appears to be reasonable, based on the fetal response as noted by the FHR pattern (Haydon et al., 2006; Jozwik et al., 2000; Simpson, 2008). Prolonged oxygen administration should be avoided because there are not enough data on beneficial versus potentially negative effects of prolonged administration.

Treatment for Anesthesia–Related Hypotension

Regional anesthetics/analgesics produce a sympathetic blockade, increasing the risk of decreased uteroplacental blood flow with or without overt maternal hypotension (Dado, 2011). Correction of maternal hypotension and any late or prolonged decelerations or fetal bradycardia that occur may be attempted with maternal lateral positioning and an IV fluid bolus of non–glucose-containing fluids (ACOG, 2010; ACOG & AAP, 2014; Garite & Simpson, 2011). If maternal repositioning and IV fluid bolus are not successful in resolving maternal hypotension and FHR decelerations or bradycardia, IV administration of either ephedrine or phenylephrine may be ordered by the anesthesia provider to increase maternal blood pressure (ACOG & AAP, 2014; American Society of Anesthesiologists [ASA], 2016). In the absence of maternal bradycardia, ASA (2016) suggests considering phenylephrine because of improved fetal acid–base status in uncomplicated pregnancies.

Amnioinfusion

Amnioinfusion may be helpful in the treatment of recurrent variable decelerations during first-stage labor that have not resolved with maternal position changes (ACOG, 2010; ACOG & AAP, 2014). During amnioinfusion, normal saline or lactated Ringer's solution is introduced transcervically via a double-lumen IUPC into the uterus either by gravity flow or through an infusion pump. Amnioinfusion may significantly resolve patterns of "moderate to severe" variable decelerations but may not affect late decelerations or patterns with absent variability (Mino, Puertas, Miranda, & Herruzo, 1999; Miyazaki & Nevarez, 1985; Garite & Simpson, 2011). Amnioinfusion is no longer recommended as a treatment for meconium-stained fluid (ACOG, 2006) because it did not reduce the risk of moderate or severe meconium aspiration syndrome or perinatal death in a multinational study of 1,998 women in labor at term (Fraser et al., 2005). When recurrent variable decelerations are observed in women attempting a vaginal birth after cesarean and are not relieved by maternal position change, consideration must be given to uterine rupture rather than attempting amnioinfusion. FHR abnormalities are the most common sign of uterine rupture, occurring in 70% of cases (ACOG, 2017), and variable decelerations are the most frequent FHR change observed during uterine rupture (Holmgren, Scott, Porter, Esplin, & Bardaley, 2012). In addition, the increase in intrauterine pressure from the amnioinfusion may further disruption of the scar. See Chapter 14 for a comprehensive discussion of the technique for amnioinfusion.

Modification of Maternal Pushing Efforts

When the FHR demonstrates recurrent decelerations during second-stage pushing, stopping pushing temporarily or pushing with every other or every third contraction based on the fetal response can be effective in allowing the fetus to recover and maintain adequate physiologic reserves (AWHONN, 2019). As a potential preventive measure, delaying active pushing until the woman feels the urge to push can minimize fetal stress (AWHONN, 2019; Simpson & James, 2005a). See Chapter 14 for a comprehensive discussion of nursing care during second-stage labor.

FETAL HEART RATE PATTERNS

Alterations in Baseline Rate

Changes in baseline rate that can occur are tachycardia (sustained FHR greater than 160 bpm for at least 10 minutes) and bradycardia (sustained FHR below 110 bpm for at least 10 minutes) (Macones et al., 2008).

Tachycardia

Fetal tachycardia (FHR >160 bpm for at least 10 minutes) should be evaluated for underlying maternal conditions such as fever, dehydration, infection (e.g., chorioamnionitis, pyelonephritis), medications and drugs (e.g., terbutaline, atropine, cocaine, other stimulants), and medical problems (e.g., hyperthyroidism) (ACOG, 2010; Freeman et al., 2012). Fetal conditions that may cause sustained fetal tachycardia include fetal bleeding (e.g., placental abruption), fetal anemia, fetal sepsis, fetal heart failure, fetal cardiac arrhythmia (e.g., supraventricular tachycardia [SVT] greater than 200 bpm), and fetal hypoxia (ACOG, 2010; Freeman et al., 2012). The most common cause of fetal tachycardia is maternal fever. Maternal fever increases maternal core temperature, thereby also increasing the fetus's metabolic rate. The baseline rate of premature fetuses should be in the upper range of the normal baseline range. When tachycardia is assessed in preterm fetuses, a bedside evaluation by a physician may be indicated (Freeman et al., 2012).

Tachycardia represents increased sympathetic and/or decreased parasympathetic autonomic tone. When observed in isolation, fetal tachycardia is a poor predictor of fetal hypoxemia or acidemia, unless accompanied by minimal or absent variability or recurrent decelerations or both (ACOG, 2010; Parer, 1997).

In term fetuses, brief periods of tachycardia sometimes occur as a normal compensatory response following a transient hypoxemic event such as a prolonged deceleration. These brief periods of tachycardia are most likely a recovery response caused by a transient rise in catecholamine levels following sympathetic nervous or adrenal medullary activity (King, 2018; Parer, 1997). When observed in isolation, fetal tachycardia is a poor predictor of fetal hypoxemia or acidemia, unless accompanied by minimal or absent variability or recurrent decelerations or both (ACOG, 2010; Parer, 1997).

Management of tachycardia should be directed at the underlying etiology and include the concurrent assessment of FHR variability and the presence or absence of accelerations and decelerations maternal temperature, hydration status, medication history, and uterine activity. Nursing interventions include notifying the physician or midwife and maximizing uteroplacental perfusion (e.g., assisting the woman to a lateral position, administering IV fluids, avoiding excessive uterine activity and administration of oxygen at 10 L/min via nonrebreather facemask). If the fetal tachycardia is associated with absent variability, or recurrent late or variable decelerations, bedside evaluation by a physician or midwife is necessary.

Bradycardia

Fetal bradycardia is defined as a sustained FHR of less than 110 bpm for at least 10 minutes, whereas a prolonged deceleration is defined as decrease in FHR from baseline of at least 15 bpm, lasting at least 2 minutes in duration, but less than 10 minutes (Macones et al., 2008). Because it is often difficult to initially distinguish between fetal bradycardia and prolonged deceleration, immediate clinical management may be similar (ACOG, 2010). Bradycardia may be due to normal physiologic variation, hypoxemia secondary to an acute decrease in uteroplacental blood flow or gas exchange (e.g., maternal hypotension, umbilical cord prolapse, tachysystole, uterine rupture, placental abruption, eclamptic seizure), medications, vagal stimulation (e.g., rapid fetal descent), hypothermia, and fetal cardiac arrhythmia (e.g., complete heart block [CHB], with FHR baseline less than 70 bpm).

Bradycardia within the range of 80 to 110 bpm with moderate variability is associated with an oxygenated, nonacidemic fetus and is most likely a response to increased vagal tone (Freeman et al., 2012; Gull et al., 1996; Parer, 1997). Likewise, end-stage bradycardias at the end of the second stage of labor, in which the FHR remains greater than 80 bpm with variability, are not associated with newborn acidemia (King, 2018). However, efforts should be made to modify maternal pushing efforts to allow the fetus to recover because prolonged deceleration or bradycardia may reflect a progressive decrease in fetal oxygenation. A sudden drop of a normal FHR to a rate below 110 bpm, especially less than 80 bpm, represents the fetus's initial response to an acute asphyxia event (Parer, 1997). If the FHR falls less than 80 bpm, the FHR variability will diminish, resulting in a pattern associated with neonatal metabolic acidemia (King, 2018). Because the

fetus has minimal ability to increase stroke volume, an extremely low heart rate provides inadequate cardiac output to sustain oxygenation. Bradycardias with rates of less than 60 bpm, those associated with late or variable decelerations, and those with minimal or absent variability are most often associated with adverse outcome (Beard, Filshie, Knight, & Roberts, 1971; Berkus, Langer, Samueloff, Xenakis, & Field, 1999; Dellinger et al., 2000; Low, Victory, & Derrick, 1999; Parer, 1997). The presence of thick meconium may also be a factor in the relationship of bradycardia to fetal outcomes (Xu, Mas-Calvet, Wei, Luo, & Fraser, 2009).

A sudden, profound bradycardia is an obstetric emergency that may signal conditions such as uterine rupture, prolapsed umbilical cord, rupture of a vasa previa, or placental abruption (Fig. 15–7). This pattern, sometimes called "terminal" bradycardia, may precede death in utero if birth does not occur rapidly. Because it is often difficult to initially distinguish between fetal bradycardia and prolonged deceleration, immediate management may be similar (ACOG, 2010). The clinical picture at the onset of the bradycardia and the depth, duration, and variability are essential factors to assess fetal condition and need for emergent cesarean birth. When a woman is laboring after a prior cesarean birth, the onset of recurrent variable or late decelerations, prolonged deceleration, or fetal bradycardia should cause concern for the onset of uterine rupture, prompt provider evaluation at the bedside and preparation for an emergent cesarean birth. FHR abnormalities are the most common sign of uterine rupture, occurring in 70% of cases (ACOG, 2017).

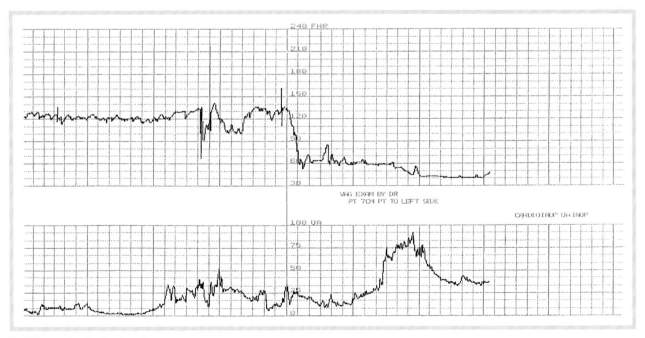

FIGURE 15–7. Terminal bradycardia.

Leung, Leung, and Paul (1993) evaluated the fetal consequences of catastrophic uterine rupture when the diagnosis was made at the onset of a prolonged deceleration. All newborns with a previously normal FHR pattern born within 17 minutes following the onset of a prolonged deceleration that progressed to bradycardia survived without significant perinatal morbidity. However, when "severe" late and variable decelerations precede the onset of a prolonged deceleration associated with uterine rupture, perinatal asphyxia can occur as early as 10 minutes after the onset of a prolonged deceleration (Leung et al., 1993). Similarly, in a study of 36 cases of uterine rupture, which occurred during 11,195 cases of labor after cesarean birth in nine hospitals, signs of uterine rupture were fetal (n = 24), maternal (n = 8), or combination of the two (n = 3), and occult (n = 1) (Holmgren et al., 2012). The FHR characteristics associated with uterine rupture included variable decelerations in 30.5% of the cases and prolonged deceleration/bradycardia in 19.4%. Of the 17 babies born in less than 18 minutes after suspicion of the uterine rupture, none had an umbilical cord pH less than 7.0 or neurologic injury. Of the 18 babies born in greater than 18 minutes after the uterine rupture was suspected, 11 had either an umbilical pH of less than 7.0 or 5-minute Apgar score of less than 7. See Chapter 14 for a discussion of uterine rupture associated with women attempting a trial of labor after a previous cesarean birth.

When bradycardia is assessed upon admission, differentiation of maternal heart rate and FHR is needed to rule out the possibility of a fetal demise, with the maternal heart rate being transmitted through dead fetal tissue. Either the external ultrasound transducer or the direct FSE can record maternal heart rate, which will appear the same as a bradycardic FHR. The external transducer can record maternal heart rate from the aorta, and the direct lead will record maternal heart rate conducted through the dead fetal tissue. Likewise, the external transducer can record maternal heart rate with a live fetus if incorrectly positioned. Therefore, one of the initial nursing interventions when bradycardia is assessed upon admission is to palpate maternal pulse to differentiate it from FHR. When the monitor is recording the maternal heart rate, maternal pulse is synchronous with the monitor signal. As previously mentioned, some fetal monitors provide cues or alerts that the heart rate being detected may be maternal rather than fetal. If these cues are displayed, confirmation that FHR is the source of the tracing is warranted.

Nursing interventions for bradycardia include notifying the physician or midwife with a request for bedside evaluation and directing interventions at the underlying cause. For example, if prolapse umbilical cord is determined, elevate the presenting part while preparations are being made for operative delivery. If bradycardia is caused by uterine tachysystole, discontinue oxytocin and notify the provider. In addition, promote fetal oxygenation and improve uteroplacental blood flow by maternal lateral positioning, IV fluid bolus, oxygen at 10L/min via nonrebreather facemask, and, if ordered, a tocolytic medication. If the bradycardia persists, preparations for an operative birth, including moving the patient to the location where birth can be accomplished most expeditiously, may be warranted.

Alterations in Baseline Variability

FHR baseline variability is described as either absent, minimal, moderate, or marked (Fig. 15–8). While moderate FHR variability reliably predicts the absence of fetal acidemia at the time of observation, minimal or absent baseline variability alone does not reliably predict the presence of abnormal acid–base balance, fetal hypoxemia, or metabolic acidemia (Macones et al., 2008). Therefore, the FHR tracing should be evaluated in the context of the whole clinical picture.

When minimal baseline variability is observed, it is essential to carefully evaluate the FHR tracing for concurrent late, variable, or prolonged decelerations, which may indicate ongoing hypoxemia.

Minimal variability can be seen with maternal medications (e.g., administration of opioids for labor pain, general anesthesia, magnesium sulfate, meperidine, methadone, heroin), fetal sleep cycles, extreme prematurity, congenital anomalies, preexisting neurologic abnormality, or fetal metabolic acidemia (ACOG, 2010; Freeman et al., 2012; Parer, 1997). Careful evaluation of the whole clinical picture is essential to identify the potential cause and determine appropriate interventions. If a mother presents to the labor and birth unit with minimal to absent baseline FHR variability and there is no prior FHR tracing to review, prompt assessment of fetal well-being is indicated because it is not known whether the decreased variability was preceded by other FHR changes indicative of fetal hypoxemia. Asking the mother about perceived fetal movement over the past few hours and days and performing VAS per unit protocol may help distinguish between fetal sleep cycles (20 to 60 minutes) and fetal hypoxemia. An FHR tracing with persistent minimal to absent baseline variability, absent accelerations, without significant decelerations, may represent a fetus with preexisting CNS injury and marked metabolic acidemia or a fetus who has recovered metabolically but not neurologically (Clark et al., 2013). Because this group of fetuses may be less likely to tolerate the additional hypoxia and acidemia of even normal labor without intrapartum demise, close

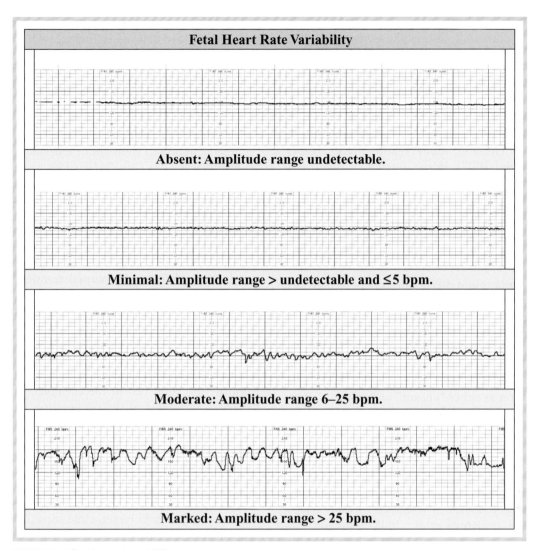

FIGURE 15–8. Fetal heart rate variability.

observation for 1 hour while providing intrauterine resuscitation and preparing for delivery may be appropriate (Clark et al., 2013).

Absent baseline variability observed in conjunction with recurrent late or variable decelerations or bradycardia is presumed to reflect significant fetal risk for metabolic acidemia (ACOG, 2010; Clark et al., 2013; King, 2018; Parer et al., 2006; Paul, Suidan, Yeh, Schifrin, & Hon, 1975). This abnormal (category III) tracing requires prompt evaluation, intrauterine resuscitation measures, and, if unresolved, operative delivery as expeditiously as possible (ACOG, 2010; Clark et al., 2013). Nursing interventions for absent variability include promptly notifying the physician or midwife with a request for bedside evaluation, repositioning the woman to a lateral position, and administering IV fluids and oxygen at 10 L/min via nonrebreather facemask. Oxytocin infusion should be discontinued if infusing or the next dose of pharmacologic agents used

to ripen the cervix or stimulate contractions should be delayed until the FHR improves. Fetal stimulation may be used to attempt to elicit an acceleration.

Marked variability (previously termed *saltatory pattern*) is less common, occurring in approximately 2% of FHR tracings, and is usually benign (O'Brien-Abel & Benedetti, 1992). Marked variability is presumed to result from an increase in alpha-adrenergic activity, which causes selective vasoconstriction of certain vascular beds. In fetal sheep and monkeys, marked variability has been observed with episodes of acute hypoxemia or hypoxia (Dalton, Dawes, & Patrick, 1977; Martin, 1978; Parer et al., 1980). Other studies of human fetuses have associated marked variability with prolonged pregnancies (Cibils, 1976; O'Brien-Abel & Benedetti, 1992), maternal ephedrine administration (O'Brien-Abel & Benedetti, 1992; R. G. Wright, Shnider, Levinson, Rolbin, & Parer, 1981), fetal breathing (Dawes, Visser, Goodman, &

Levine, 1981), and decreased uteroplacental perfusion or umbilical cord compression (Leveno et al., 1984; O'Brien-Abel & Benedetti, 1992).

Interventions to eliminate marked variability aim to promote uteroplacental blood flow and fetal oxygenation. Strategies may include maternal lateral positioning, correcting maternal hypotension or uterine tachysystole, IV fluid bolus, or administration of oxygen at 10 L/min via nonrebreather mask (ACOG, 2010; Simpson, 2007). In the absence of other variant FHR changes, marked variability is not associated with fetal acidemia (O'Brien-Abel & Benedetti, 1992; R. G. Wright et al., 1981).

Periodic and Episodic Changes in Fetal Heart Rate

FHR accelerations and decelerations may be classified as either periodic (occurring in association with a uterine contractions) or episodic (not associated with uterine contractions). Variable decelerations and accelerations may be periodic or episodic; however, late and early decelerations are periodic. Accelerations and decelerations are further characterized by the onset of their waveform as either "abrupt" or "gradual." If the onset to either peak or nadir of the FHR change occurs in less than 30 seconds, it is described as "abrupt" (e.g., accelerations, variable decelerations), whereas if it takes 30 seconds or longer, it is described as "gradual" (e.g., late and early decelerations) (Macones et al., 2008). In addition, accelerations and decelerations are determined in reference to the adjacent baseline FHR (Macones et al., 2008). Baseline variability cannot be determined during accelerations or decelerations as FHR accelerations and decelerations are excluded from the definition of FHR variability (Macones et al., 2008).

The four types of FHR decelerations are described as early, late, variable, and prolonged decelerations (Fig. 15–9 A–D and Table 15–1). Differentiation is based on the shape of their onset and their relationship to the timing of the uterine contractions. Decelerations are defined as either recurrent (occurring with ≥50% of the uterine contractions in a 20-minute segment) or intermittent (occurring with <50% of the contractions in a 20-minute segment). For further discussion of early decelerations and accelerations, see the prior discussion of characteristics of the normal FHR.

Late Decelerations

A late deceleration is defined as a visually apparent, usually symmetrical, *gradual* (defined as onset of deceleration to nadir ≥30 seconds) decrease and return to baseline FHR associated with a uterine contraction (Macones et al., 2008). The decrease in FHR is calculated from onset to nadir of the deceleration. Late decelerations are delayed in timing, with the nadir of the deceleration occurring after the peak of the contraction. In most cases, the onset, nadir, and recovery of the deceleration occur after the beginning, peak, and ending of the contraction, respectively (Macones et al., 2008).

Recurrent late decelerations are thought to reflect the fetal response to transient or chronic uteroplacental insufficiency (ACOG, 2010; Freeman et al., 2012; King, 2018; Martin, 1978). Late decelerations, therefore, must be evaluated in the context of FHR variability and the overall clinical picture.

When a previously well-oxygenated fetus with a normal (category I) tracing experiences an acute reduction in uterine blood flow, the resulting decreased oxygen supply is overlaid on the normal transient reduction in oxygenation that occurs during each contraction. In this situation, chemoreceptors detect the hypoxemia and initiate the vagal bradycardic response. Once the contraction recedes, the fetus resumes normal metabolism and the heart rate recovers. There is a brief delay in the detection of hypoxemia as the fetal blood travels from the placental bed to the chemoreceptors. Thus, the onset and nadir of the deceleration are late relative to the peak of the contraction because there is a lag in time between the hypoxemic event and the FHR response. These late decelerations observed with concurrent moderate baseline variability suggests the fetus does not have significant metabolic acidemia at the time such a pattern is observed (ACOG, 2009b; Parer et al., 2006); however, close surveillance is warranted, and intrauterine resuscitation measures are appropriate (ACOG, 2010). If recurrent late decelerations persist for more than 1 hour despite intrauterine resuscitation measures, additional considerations include assessment of the stages and phases of labor and whether normal labor progress is being made (Clark et al., 2013).

Late decelerations with concomitant minimal or absent baseline variability and no accelerations are associated with abnormal fetal acid–base status (Beard et al., 1971; Berkus et al., 1999; Clark, Gimovsky, & Miller, 1984; Clark et al., 2013; King, 2018; Parer et al., 2006). This type of periodic change occurs when there is insufficient oxygen for myocardial metabolism and/or normal cerebral function. These FHR patterns are likely to occur when there is chronic placental insufficiency that cannot support the transient hypoxemia that occurs with contractions during normal labor. Late decelerations with minimal variability may be associated with significant acidemia (Parer et al., 2006). This type of category II pattern warrants intrauterine resuscitation, reevaluation, and consideration for expediting birth if no improvement with intrauterine resuscitation (ACOG, 2010). If recurrent

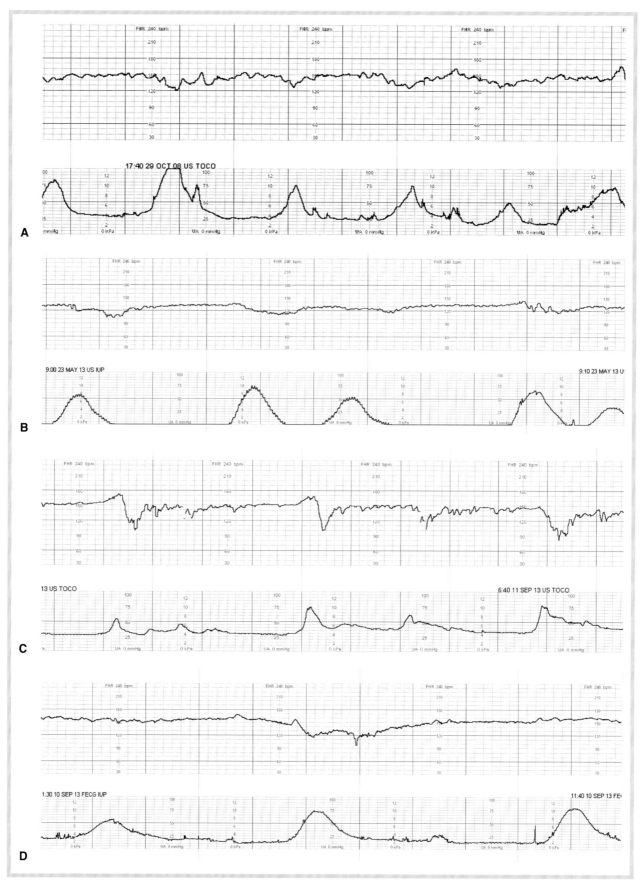

FIGURE 15–9. Four types of fetal heart rate decelerations. **A,** Early. **B,** Late. **C,** Variable. **D,** Prolonged.

late decelerations with minimal or absent variability and no accelerations persist for more than 30 minutes despite intrauterine resuscitation measures, expeditious delivery is recommended (Clark et al., 2013). Recurrent late decelerations with absent variability (category III) are associated with abnormal fetal acid–base status (ACOG, 2010; Macones et al., 2008) and warrant preparation for expeditious birth while simultaneously implementing intrauterine resuscitation measures (ACOG, 2010; Clark et al., 2013; Fox et al., 2000; Parer & Ikeda, 2007).

It follows from the above discussion that late decelerations are evaluated in the context of baseline FHR variability as well as other factors in the overall clinical picture. Intermittent late decelerations seen with moderate variability, normal baseline rate, and accelerations are less concerning and usually easier to correct than recurrent late decelerations seen with minimal to absent baseline variability, abnormal baseline rate, and absence of accelerations. Bedside evaluation and management of clinical events (e.g., maternal hypotension from regional analgesia or supine positioning, placental abruption), excessive uterine activity, and maternal–fetal history and risk factors for uteroplacental insufficiency (e.g., pregnancy-induced hypertension/preeclampsia, postmaturity, intrauterine growth restriction) are essential.

Nursing interventions for late decelerations focus on maximizing placental function, thus improving uteroplacental exchange by maintaining a lateral maternal position, increasing IV fluids to correct dehydration or volume depletion, discontinuing oxytocin, and administering oxygen at 10 L/min via nonrebreather facemask (Garite & Simpson, 2011). The next dose of pharmacologic agents used to ripen the cervix or stimulate contractions should be delayed until uterine activity returns to normal and the FHR improves. The physician or midwife should be notified. If the late decelerations do not resolve after these interventions, bedside evaluation by the physician or midwife is warranted. In addition, iatrogenic insults that may further compromise maternal–fetal exchange such as oxytocin-induced tachysystole or maternal hypotension secondary to maternal supine position should be avoided. If there are late decelerations during second-stage labor, pushing efforts should be modified based on the fetal response.

Variable Decelerations

A variable deceleration is defined as a visually apparent *abrupt* (defined as onset of deceleration to beginning of nadir <30 seconds) decrease in FHR below the baseline (Macones et al., 2008). The decrease is calculated from the onset to the nadir of the contraction and is ≥15 bpm, lasting ≥15 seconds, and <2 minutes from onset to return to baseline. Variable decelerations typically vary in their shape, depth, and duration and the timing relative to uterine contractions. Intermittent variable decelerations (occurring with <50% of contractions) are the most common FHR abnormality seen during labor (Macones et al., 2008).

Most commonly, the abrupt FHR change characteristic of variable decelerations is caused by occlusion of umbilical blood flow. Any circumstance that allows compression of the umbilical cord can result in umbilical cord occlusion and variable decelerations (e.g., cord prolapse or impingement, nuchal cord, knots in the cord, oligohydramnios). When the umbilical arteries are occluded, the low-resistance placental circuit is abruptly withdrawn, resulting in increased peripheral vascular resistance and sudden fetal hypertension. Hypertension immediately stimulates fetal baroreceptors, producing a vagal reflex response and rapid slowing of the FHR. When the umbilical cord is released, the FHR typically returns rapidly to pre-deceleration values (Freeman et al., 2012; Lee, Di Loreto, & O'Lane, 1975; Parer, 1997). When variable decelerations occur during the second stage of labor, they may also be caused by the marked head compression and resultant intense vagal stimulation that occurs during rapid descent (Ball & Parer, 1992; King, 2018). Variable decelerations have multiple appearances in all aspects except one: The initial FHR drop is abrupt.

Interpretation of FHR tracings with recurrent variable decelerations requires assessment of the depth and duration of the decelerations, accompanying baseline variability, baseline rate, presence of accelerations, and evolution of the pattern over time. The presence of moderate variability or a spontaneous or induced acceleration suggests a fetus who not currently acidemic (ACOG, 2010; Clark et al., 2013). Considering recurrent variable decelerations represent a physiologic response to intermittent fetal stress, it may be reasonable to follow this pattern with close observation as long as moderate variability and a baseline FHR in the normal range is maintained (Freeman et al., 2012; Parer & Ikeda, 2007; Parer et al., 2006), labor is progressing (Clark et al., 2013), and there exists adequate time between uterine contractions for fetal oxygenation recovery (Bakker, 2007), and resources are available to rapidly respond the fetal deterioration (Freeman et al., 2012). However, recurrent variable decelerations with minimal to absent baseline variability in which the nadir become increasingly deeper and the decelerations last longer are more likely associated with fetal acidemia requiring prompt evaluation and management (ACOG, 2010; Parer et al., 2006). In the context of significant variable decelerations (lasting longer than 60 seconds and reaching a nadir more than 60 bpm below baseline or lasting longer than 60 seconds and reaching a nadir less than 60 bpm regardless of baseline), that are recurrent, with either minimal or absent baseline variability, persist for more than 30 minutes despite intrauterine resuscitation measures, expeditious birth is recommended (Clark et al., 2013). Recurrent variable decelerations in the context of absent variability, not improved by intrauterine resuscitation measures, are abnormal (category III) and associated with abnormal acid–base status (Macones et al., 2008) requiring expeditious birth (ACOG, 2010; Clark et al., 2013).

It follows from the above discussion that variable decelerations are evaluated in the context of baseline FHR variability, depth, duration, whether they are intermittent or recurrent, as well as other factors in the overall clinical picture. Intermittent variable decelerations seen with moderate variability, normal baseline rate, and accelerations are less concerning and usually easier to correct as compared to recurrent, deep variable decelerations, seen with minimal to absent baseline variability, abnormal baseline rate, and absence of accelerations, which would necessitate bedside evaluation and management of clinical events (e.g., prolapsed umbilical cord), excessive uterine activity, and maternal–fetal history and risk factors (e.g., oligohydramnios). Nursing interventions for variable decelerations focus on modifying or eliminating the stressors causing the umbilical cord occlusion and include measures such as maternal position change, decreasing or discontinuing oxytocin infusion, checking for an umbilical cord prolapse, modified pushing, and preparing for amnioinfusion. If maternal position changes do not result in resolution of the variable decelerations, notification of the physician or midwife is warranted and a request for bedside evaluation may be indicated based on the clinical situation

Prolonged Decelerations

A prolonged deceleration of the FHR is a visually apparent decrease in FHR below the baseline that is ≥15 bpm, lasting ≥2 minutes, but <10 minutes from onset to return to baseline (Macones et al., 2008). The decrease is calculated from the adjacent baseline. Prolonged decelerations may occur in the presence or absence of contractions and may have either an abrupt or slow return to the baseline rate.

Prolonged decelerations are often caused by more sustained incidences of any of the previously discussed FHR deceleration mechanisms. Potential causes of prolonged deceleration include interruption of uteroplacental perfusion or exchange (e.g., uterine tachysystole, acute maternal hypotension, maternal seizure respiratory or cardiac arrest, placental abruption, uterine rupture), interruption of umbilical blood flow (cord compression, cord prolapse, ruptured vasa previa), and vagal stimulation (profound head compression, rapid fetal descent).

When prolonged deceleration occurs, assessment includes baseline variability immediately prior and following the deceleration, frequency of occurrence, duration of the deceleration, and the overall clinical picture including the unit's ability to expedite birth should variably become absent or the deceleration progress to bradycardia. In clinical practice, clinicians do not wait to differentiate between prolonged deceleration and bradycardia before initiating intrauterine resuscitation measures and mobilizing a team response. See management considerations for bradycardia previously discussed. Nonrecurrent prolonged decelerations that are preceded and followed by an FHR that has a normal baseline and moderate variability are not associated with fetal hypoxemia of clinical significance. However, ACOG (2010) recommends prompt birth in cases of prolonged deceleration with minimal or absent variability. A decision tree with suggested general guidelines for the management of selected FHR tracings is provided in Figure 15–10.

Unusual Fetal Heart Rate Patterns

Whenever an unusual FHR tracing is observed from the beginning of EFM, the possibility of a prior unobserved hypoxic insult or a fetal congenital anomaly should be considered. An initial tracing with minimal or absent baseline variability without accelerations or with other unusual characteristics should prompt an urgent assessment of fetal well-being. This may include fetal vibroacoustic or scalp stimulation, an ultrasound evaluation, or other assessments as indicated by the overall clinical picture. In anencephalic fetuses, FHR evidence of CNS dysfunction varies with the level of the defect ranging from a normal FHR to an FHR pattern with absent variability (Freeman et al., 2012). Additional, rarely seen FHR patterns associated with fetal CNS dysfunction include flat FHR, blunted variable decelerations, an unstable baseline, acceleration with absent variability following a variable deceleration (overshoot), sinusoidal pattern, or the check mark pattern (Freeman et al., 2012).

Sinusoidal Heart Rate Pattern

The sinusoidal FHR pattern is a visually apparent, undulating, smooth sine wave–like pattern in FHR baseline with a cycle frequency of three to five per minute that persists for at least 20 minutes (Macones et al., 2008) (Fig. 15–11). First identified in 1972, the sinusoidal FHR pattern was associated with severely affected, Rh-sensitized, and dying fetuses (Manseau, Vaquier, Chavinie, & Sureau, 1972). The FHR pattern was named "sinusoidal" due to its sine waveform.

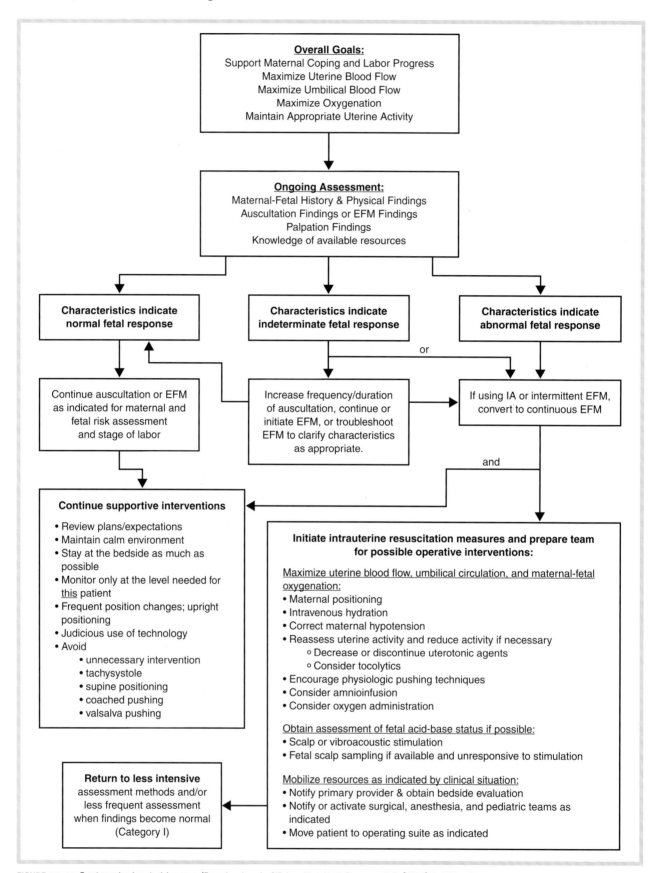

FIGURE 15–10. Fetal monitoring decision tree. (From Lyndon, A., O'Brien-Abel, N., & Simpson, K. R. [2015]. Fetal heart rate interpretation. In A. Lyndon & L. U. Ali [Eds.], *Fetal heart monitoring: Principles and practices* [5th ed., p. 139]. Used with permission.)

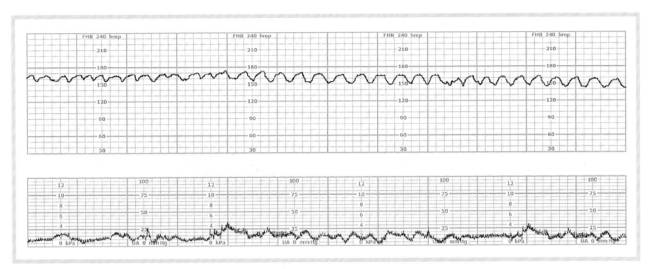

FIGURE 15–11. Sinusoidal fetal heart rate pattern.

A true sinusoidal FHR pattern is a visually apparent, smooth, sine wave–like undulating pattern in the FHR baseline with cycle frequency of three to five per minute that persists for 20 minutes or longer and classified as a category III pattern (Macones et al., 2008). The sinusoidal pattern is rare; however, when identified, it has been associated with severe fetal anemia as a result of Rh isoimmunization, massive fetomaternal hemorrhage, twin-to-twin transfusion syndrome, ruptured vasa previa, traumatic fetal bleeding with severe anemia, or fetal intracranial hemorrhage (Modanlou & Murata, 2004). Other conditions associated with a sinusoidal FHR include fetal infection, fetal cardiac anomalies, neonatal hypoxia, congenital hydrocephalus, gastroschisis, and maternal cardiopulmonary bypass (Modanlou & Murata, 2004). Research suggests that the sinusoidal pattern is related to a change in the CNS control of FHR and implies cerebral ischemia (Freeman et al., 2012). Because the sinusoidal pattern is associated with abnormal fetal acid–base status at the time of observation, it is labeled a category III pattern and, as such, requires prompt evaluation and intrauterine resuscitation measures (ACOG, 2010; Macones et al., 2008).

A sinusoidal-appearing FHR pattern (pseudosinusoidal) has been noted to follow the maternal administration of some analgesic medications (e.g., butorphanol fentanyl, meperidine), fetal sleep cycles, thumb sucking, or rhythmic movements of the fetal mouth (Modanlou & Murata, 2004). In contrast to the true sinusoidal FHR pattern, this undulating pattern is of short duration and preceded and followed by a normal FHR (Modanlou & Murata, 2004). No treatment is indicated.

Fetal Arrhythmias

Fetal cardiac arrhythmias occur in approximately 1% to 2% of all pregnancies and are usually benign (Kleinman, Nehgme, Copel, 2004). Of those, approximately 90% are due to irregular rhythm and less than 10% are due to sustained brady- or tachyarrhythmias with clinical significance to the fetus (Kleinman & Nehgme, 2004).

Arrhythmias due to irregular rhythm have been recognized with increasing frequency at routine prenatal visits (Fig. 15–12). Most of these arrhythmias are ectopic premature atrial contractions (PACs) detected by listening to the fetal heart. The most common finding is the impression that the fetal heart is intermittently "skipping" beats. In most cases, the skipping represents either a pause following an extrasystole that has not reset the sinus node pacemaker or an extrasystole occurring early in the cardiac cycle with a stroke volume that is inadequate to produce a detectable Doppler signal (Kleinman & Nehgme, 2004). PACs may be exacerbated by maternal caffeine ingestion, decongestant medications, or tobacco (Sklansky, 2009). While the extrasystoles may be a source of anxiety for the parents, they usually resolve spontaneously later in pregnancy or in the first few days after birth, and only rarely, do PVC develop into a persistent tachyarrhythmias requiring further evaluation.

The most common fetal tachyarrhythmia is SVT, which typically occurs in the range of 240 to 260 bpm with minimal or absent FHR variability. SVT is most commonly diagnosed in fetuses with structurally normal hearts and frequently is a result of electrical reentry arising from a circus movement of electrical energy between the atrial and ventricular myocardium (Kleinman & Nehgme, 2004). Initially, SVT may manifest as an intermittent, nonsustained tachyarrhythmia; however, sustained SVT may develop. In utero pharmacologic treatment of sustained fetal SVT has used single drugs or combinations of digoxin, calcium-channel blockers, beta-blockers, procainamide, and quinidine (Freeman et al., 2012). Because these drugs are not benign, a

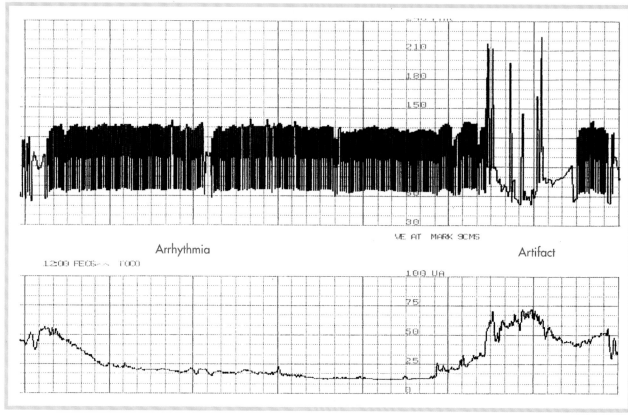

FIGURE 15–12. Arrhythmia. This tracing demonstrates fetal arrhythmia and artifact. Notice the randomness of the artifactual information compared with the organization of the arrhythmia.

careful risk/benefit analysis is needed with focus on the development of hydrops fetalis, gestational age, lung maturity, provider experience with in utero cardioversion, neonatal intensive care experience with varying gestational ages for fetuses with and without hydrops, and parental wishes (Kleinman & Nehgme, 2004).

The most common bradyarrhythmia is complete or third-degree AV heart block in which the atrial electrical impulses are unable to pass through the conduction system to activate the ventricles. This results in the ventricles depolarizing at their own intrinsic rate of approximately 40 to 80 bpm. Approximately 50% of fetuses with CHB have structurally normal hearts in early development; however, typically after 18 to 20 weeks' gestation, transplacental passage of maternal antibodies (e.g., maternal anti-Rho immunoglobulin) can damage the cardiac conduction system after it was normally formed (Copel, Friedman, & Kleinman, 1997; Freeman et al., 2012; Sklansky, 2009). Often, mothers of these fetuses have symptoms consistent with Sjögren's syndrome, systemic lupus erythematosus, or related connective tissue disorders (Sklansky, 2009). In the absence of any significant underlying congenital heart disease, these fetuses are generally hemodynamically compensated if they are able to maintain a ventricular rate greater than 55 bpm and often do well, although some may require a pacemaker soon

after birth (Kleinman & Nehgme, 2004). The other 50% of fetuses with CHB have underlying congenital heart disease, often appearing as a complex lesion in the central portion of the heart involving the AV junction. The prognosis for fetuses with structural cardiac defects or nonimmune hydrops from heart failure in utero is quite poor (Freeman et al., 2012; Kleinman & Nehgme, 2004).

Assessment of the FHR with external ultrasound component of the EFM may be difficult in the presence of extrasystoles due to the inability to see a consistent baseline or evaluate variability. These arrhythmias may be verified by auscultating the FHR for irregular rhythm or, if appropriate, applying the FSE to accurately record the extrasystoles as brief upward or downward excursions. Tachyarrhythmias and bradyarrhythmias may appear as halved or doubled the actual heart rate when monitored electronically. Auscultating and counting the actual FHR or ultrasound imaging may verify the arrhythmia. If the FHR is regular to auscultation, yet there are unusual excursions on the EFM tracing, the most likely explanation is that it is artifactual information. Artifact may be caused by the FSE having a poor attachment to the fetal presenting part or equipment problems. Attempts to correct the problem include changing the cable or fetal monitor and/or replacing the direct electrode (see Table 15–5).

CLINICAL IMPLICATIONS FOR MONITORING THE FETUS LESS THAN 32 WEEKS' GESTATION DURING LABOR

While the principles of EFM are the same for the preterm fetus as for the term fetus, there are differences in FHR patterns of preterm fetuses when compared to those in term labor, and there are unique clinical implications for obtaining and interpreting EFM data during preterm labor. Perinatal complications such as preeclampsia, intraamniotic infection, oligohydramnios, umbilical cord compression, placental abruption, intrauterine growth restriction, uteroplacental insufficiency, and multiple gestation are more common during preterm labor and often associated with indeterminate or abnormal FHR patterns.

An abnormal FHR pattern and some types of indeterminate FHR patterns (e.g., minimal to absent variability, late decelerations, recurrent variable decelerations, tachycardia) may be predictive of perinatal asphyxia and long-term neurologic outcome for the preterm fetus (Braithwaite, Milligan, & Shennan, 1986; Douvas, Meeks, Graves, Walsh, & Morrison, 1984; Low et al., 1992; Matsuda, Maeda, & Kouno, 2003; Shy et al., 1990; Westgren, Malcus, & Svenningsen, 1986).

In fetuses less than 28 weeks' gestation, approximately 60% will have an indeterminate or abnormal FHR tracing during the 24 hours prior to birth (Ayoubi et al., 2002). Decelerations (five or more per hour, in which FHR amplitude decreased at least 60 bpm for greater than 30 seconds) and "bradycardia" (less than 120 bpm for greater than 10 minutes) were most common (56%), followed by tachycardia greater than 160 bpm (25%) and minimal or absent variability (20%). Of these findings, minimal or absent variability was most significantly correlated with neonatal death at 2 months of age, with only 38% of these infants surviving. Neither decelerations or bradycardia nor fetal tachycardia appeared to affect neonatal mortality rates, with 65% and 74%, respectively, surviving. If FHR abnormalities are persistent, intrauterine resuscitation measures, ancillary tests to ensure fetal well-being, and possibly birth should occur (ACOG, 2009b). Compared to the term fetus, the progression from a normal to an indeterminate or abnormal FHR tracing occurs more often and more quickly in the premature fetus (Freeman et al., 2012; Matsuda et al., 2003; Parer, 1997). Thus, timeliness of identification and initiation of interventions for variant FHR patterns may be more critical and of more lasting consequences when the fetus is preterm.

Baseline Rate

With advancing gestational age, average baseline FHR at term decreases to approximately 140 bpm before labor. In the preterm fetus, baseline FHR is often in the upper end of the normal range, closer to 160 bpm. In one study, 78% of fetuses less than 33 weeks' gestation had periods of tachycardia (greater than 160 bpm) as compared to only 20% of fetuses greater than 33 weeks' gestation (Westgren et al., 1986). An FHR greater than 160 bpm may indicate evolving fetal hypoxemia, maternal fever, intraamniotic infection, or the side effects of terbutaline administration. The presence of fetal tachycardia is more predictive of acidemia, low Apgar scores, and adverse neonatal outcomes in the preterm fetus compared to the term fetus (Burrus, O'Shea, Veille, & Mueller-Heubach, 1994; Freeman et al., 2012; Westgren, Holmquist, Svenningsen, & Ingemarsson, 1982). Another potential cause of fetal tachycardia, however unrelated to acidemia, is beta-sympathomimetic drugs, such as terbutaline, given to the mother in preterm labor.

Variability

Minimal variability may be seen more often in the preterm fetus than in the term fetus (Freeman et al., 2012; To & Leung, 1998; Westgren et al., 1982). Loss of variability in the preterm fetus is more predictive of low Apgar scores and acidemia compared to when observed in the fetus at term (Douvas et al., 1984; Freeman et al., 2012; Westgren, Hormquist, Ingemarsson, & Svenningsen, 1984). At term, approximately 20% of fetuses with abnormal FHR patterns will be depressed, whereas when abnormal FHR patterns are observed in preterm fetuses <33 weeks' gestation, approximately 70% to 80% will be depressed and/or have acidemia (Freeman et al., 2012). When compared with FHR decelerations, bradycardia, or tachycardia, the finding of minimal or absent variability is most strongly associated with neonatal death in fetuses less than 28 weeks' gestation (Ayoubi et al., 2002). The combination of loss of variability and fetal tachycardia is more often associated with low Apgar scores and acidemia in the preterm fetus (Freeman et al., 2012). While minimal variability is observed more frequently in preterm fetus ≤30 weeks' gestation that develop interventricular hemorrhage (IVH), EFM patterns do not discriminate in identifying very preterm fetuses at risk for developing IVH (Hannaford, Stout, Smyser, Mathur, & Cahill, 2016).

Medications may also influence FHR variability in the preterm fetus. IV magnesium sulfate may be used for prevention and treatment of seizures in women with preeclampsia or eclampsia and fetal neuroprotection before anticipated early preterm (less than 32 weeks' gestation) delivery (ACOG, 2016). Magnesium sulfate may also be used for the short-term prolongation of pregnancy (up to 48 hours) to allow for administration of antenatal corticosteroids (ACOG, 2016). While studies vary regarding the effect of magnesium sulfate on FHR variability, decreased variability should always be assessed with caution taking into consideration additional factors (e.g., early gestational age, preeclampsia) that may be causing the decreased variability (ACOG, 2009b; J. W. Wright, Ridgway, Wright, Covington, & Bobitt, 1996). Antenatal corticosteroids may be given to the women in preterm labor to enhance fetal lung maturity. Betamethasone (not dexamethasone) may cause a transient decrease in baseline FHR variability, which returns to pretreatment variability by the fourth to the seventh day (ACOG, 2009b). This transient decrease in FHR variability is not indicative of deterioration in fetal status (ACOG, 2009b; Lunshof et al., 2005; Senat et al., 1998; Subtil et al., 2003). IV or intramuscular (IM) opioids may result in minimal variability. It is important to know the duration of the effects of any pain medication given to be able to accurately distinguish between expected FHR side effects and evolving fetal hypoxemia.

Accelerations

Accelerations of the preterm FHR are generally lower in amplitude and less frequent than those of the term fetus, although most preterm fetuses, even at 24 to 26 weeks' gestation and beyond, will have accelerations of at least 15 bpm lasting 15 seconds (Freeman et al., 2012). The number and amplitude of accelerations increase over the course of gestation as the fetus matures (Kisilevsky, Hains, & Low, 2001). Before 32 weeks of gestation, accelerations are defined as having an acme of at least 10 bpm above baseline with a duration of at least 10 seconds above the baseline (ACOG, 2009b, 2010; Macones et al., 2008). Similar to moderate variability, the presence of FHR accelerations is highly predictive of normal acid–base status at the time of assessment (ACOG, 2010).

Antenatal corticosteroid administration may cause a transient increase in fetal movement and FHR accelerations within 12 hours of the first injection and within 6 hours of a second dose (Lunshof et al., 2005; Subtil et al., 2003). The increase in fetal movement and FHR accelerations may be more common in 29- to 33-week-gestation fetuses compared to 25- to 28-week-gestation fetuses (Lunshof et al., 2005). As with variability, IV or IM opioid medication may temporarily depress the fetal neurologic system, resulting in fewer FHR accelerations and/or FHR accelerations of lower amplitude.

Decelerations

During labor of a preterm fetus, variable decelerations are more common, occurring 55% (34 to 36 weeks' gestation) and 70% (28 to 33 weeks' gestation) of the time compared with 20% to 30% in normal term fetuses (Westgren et al., 1982). Variable decelerations may progress rapidly from indeterminate (category II) to abnormal (category III) with loss of variability (Freeman et al., 2012). Variable decelerations during preterm labor

are associated with a higher rate of fetal hypoxemia, acidemia, neurologic abnormalities, and adverse long-term outcomes (Douvas et al., 1984; Freeman et al., 2012; Holmes, Oppenheimer, Gravelle, Walker, & Blayney, 2001; Westgren et al., 1984). There is evidence to suggest variable decelerations in the premature fetus may also be associated with intraventricular hemorrhage in a manner unrelated to fetal acidemia (Holmes et al., 2001).

Although there does not appear to be an increased incidence of late decelerations during preterm labor, conditions more likely to result in late decelerations are more common (Freeman et al., 2012). These include uteroplacental insufficiency, intraamniotic infection, preeclampsia, intrauterine growth restriction, and placenta abruption. Late decelerations during preterm labor are associated with adverse outcomes such as fetal hypoxemia, acidemia, and long-term neurologic abnormalities (Westgren et al., 1984; Zanini, Paul, & Huey, 1980). Prolonged decelerations occur at a similar frequency for the preterm and term fetus (Freeman et al., 2012).

Monitoring Preterm Multiple Gestations

When monitoring more than one fetus, it is important to maintain two distinct FHRs. Some newer generation monitors designed to accommodate multiple gestations have features to distinguish the two fetuses being monitored. Independent volume controls aid transducer placement by allowing both FHRs to be heard simultaneously. FHRs recorded on the tracing may be offset to facilitate interpretation. Some monitors even provide visual and audible indications when synchronous fetal or maternal heart rate signals are detected. These system cues can be helpful but do not replace careful nursing assessment of each FHR pattern. The mother may be able to provide assistance in determining the position of each baby by indicating where she feels fetal movement, or ultrasound guidance may be needed to accurately locate and identify individual FHRs for placement of transducers. Despite attempts to continuously monitor multiples for prolonged periods of time, an interpretable tracing may be difficult to obtain. In a study of monoamniotic twins, successful monitoring occurred in only half of the fetuses 27 to 30 weeks' gestation. At earlier gestations (<27 weeks), successful monitoring of both fetuses was accomplished only 37% of the time (Quinn, Cao, Lacoursiere, & Schrimmer, 2011).

Although some fetal twin pairs may have synchronous FHR patterns at times, most fetuses in multiple gestations will not have completely synchronous FHR patterns during labor (Fig. 15–13 A–B). Tactile communication occurs between twins in utero, and these movements often result in simultaneous accelerations of the FHR during nonstress testing (Sherer, Nawrocki, Peco, Metlay, & Woods, 1990). Periods of reactivity and nonreactivity of the FHR also are similar during nonstress testing (Sherer, D'Amico, Cox, Metlay,

& Woods, 1994). The assumption can be made that these conditions and FHR reactions would apply to the intrapartum period, but there have been no confirmatory studies. The published data are limited to FHR patterns of twins during antepartum testing, although authors mentioned incidental data. Some twin fetuses will have asynchronous FHR patterns over the course of labor, especially if there are differences in fetal well-being. Accelerations and decelerations usually occur within the same time frame but will not be identical in duration or excursion from the baseline (Gallagher, Costigan, & Johnson, 1992). There were no studies found about intrapartum FHR patterns of triplets and higher order multiples, presumably because these pregnancies almost always result in cesarean birth without labor. However, in selected cases when fetal status is normal and fetal presentation is favorable, women with triplets can labor and give birth vaginally.

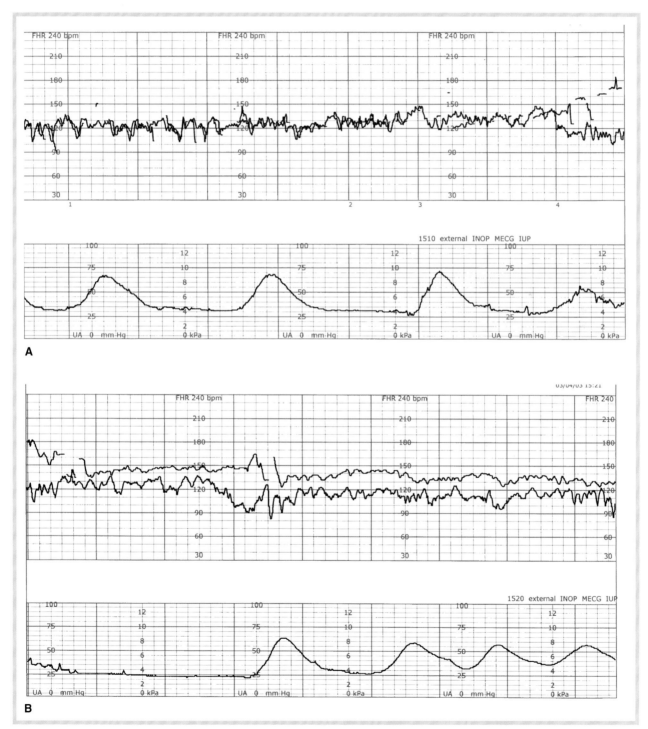

FIGURE 15–13. **A**, Synchronous fetal heart rate patterns of twins. **B**, Asynchronous fetal heart rate patterns of twins.

ASSESSMENT OF PATTERN EVOLUTION

In clinical practice, interpretation of the FHR is an ongoing assessment that includes multiple perinatal factors, specific FHR characteristics, and, most important, the evolution of the FHR pattern as labor progresses (Fig. 15–14). An abnormal FHR can suddenly develop spontaneously, but usually, the evolution from normal follows a typical pattern over time. FHR patterns that result from an acute event such as umbilical cord prolapse, uterine rupture, or placental abruption are typically noted immediately and acted on quickly by the perinatal team. However, when fetal deterioration occurs progressively over a long period, the clinical symptoms may not be fully appreciated by all members of the perinatal team. A loss of situational awareness can occur, and as a result, timely interventions may be delayed. When the FHR evolves from a baseline within normal limits, moderate variability, and accelerations to variant patterns with minimal to absent variability and recurrent late, variable or prolonged decelerations, the risk of fetal deterioration toward metabolic acidemia is significant, despite the low predictive value of abnormal (category III) tracings for abnormal neurologic outcomes in the neonate (ACOG, 2010; Freeman et al., 2012). Oxytocin-induced tachysystole can exacerbate the situation, so it is essential to carefully titrate the oxytocin infusion based on contraction frequency and the fetal response (Simpson, 2015). If the usual intrauterine resuscitation techniques do not result in pattern resolution, consider

expeditious birth. A request for bedside evaluation by the primary provider is warranted so that plans can be made and implemented for fetal rescue in a timely manner (Simpson, 2005b).

The significance of evolving FHR patterns during second stage labor that suggest fetal deterioration can be missed when clinicians become focused on imminent birth at the expense of careful assessment of the FHR tracing. The active pushing phase of the second stage often involves increased physiologic fetal stress with maternal bearing down efforts (Roberts, 2002), and care should be taken to avoid iatrogenic stress and allow recovery between uterine contractions. If the etiology of this pattern is cord occlusion that is worsening as the fetus descends, the decelerations may become more severe and develop a concomitant loss of variability as the fetus develops hypoxemia. One way to minimize fetal risk during the second stage is to allow the fetus to descend passively and to delay pushing until the woman feels the urge to push. Shortening the active pushing phase by allowing passive fetal descent can minimize the decrease in fetal oxygen status that is associated with maternal pushing efforts (Simpson & James, 2005a).

When oxytocin is continued during second-stage pushing, it is especially important to avoid tachysystole. Normally during the second stage, contractions tend to become slightly less frequent, which may allow the fetus to tolerate the stress of maternal pushing efforts, umbilical cord compression, and vagal stimulation. When contractions are too frequent over a

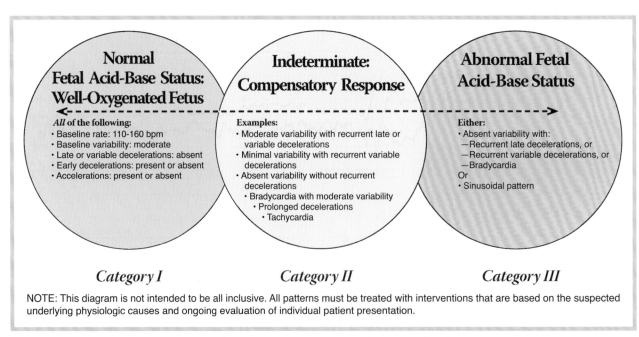

FIGURE 15–14. Dynamic physiologic response model. (From Lyndon, A., O'Brien-Abel, N., & Simpson, K. R. [2015]. Fetal heart rate interpretation. In A. Lyndon & L. U. Ali [Eds.], *Fetal heart monitoring: Principles and practices* [5th ed., p. 139]. Used with permission.)

prolonged period, the fetus may not be able to tolerate this physiologic stress (Bakker et al., 2007).

Interventions for variable decelerations during the second stage should also include assessment of the pushing technique used. When recurrent variable decelerations during the second stage are associated with closed-glottis pushing, the most appropriate approach is to encourage the woman to push with every other, or every third, contraction and to discourage prolonged breath holding (AWHONN, 2019) (Fig. 15–15). In some cases, it is best to temporarily discontinue pushing to allow the fetus to recover. These techniques can be attempted for all women but are most effective for women who have regional analgesia/anesthesia. Open-glottis pushing with the woman bearing down for no more than 6 to 8 seconds per pushing effort will have less negative effect on fetal status than repetitive closed-glottis pushing (AWHONN, 2019; Simpson & James, 2005a) (Fig. 15–16). Encouraging the woman to bear down as long as she can is more favorable for fetal well-being than telling the woman to take a deep breath and hold it for 10 seconds without making a sound (Simpson & James, 2005a). Counting to 10 with each pushing effort to encourage pushing efforts lasting 10 seconds or more is no longer considered the most appropriate method of second-stage labor coaching (AWHONN, 2019; Roberts, 2002). Three to four

pushing efforts per contraction will minimize risk of fetal compromise and promote adequate fetal descent (AWHONN, 2019). The provider should assess variable decelerations that evolve into longer or deeper decelerations or are associated with tachycardia or decreasing variability and should intervene to minimize additional stress via intrauterine resuscitation, discontinuation of oxytocin, and potentially emergent birth (ACOG, 2009b, 2010). Appropriate care during the second stage of labor can prevent iatrogenic fetal stress and the birth of a depressed baby.

The end-stage bradycardia that retains mild to moderate variability is another expression of head compression during rapid descent. If moderate variability is retained and the rate remains above 80 to 90 bpm, this pattern should be watched but considered as a benign variant. Conversely, a bradycardia that slopes down over several minutes and loses variability within the first 4 minutes of descent is a pattern evolution that signals fetal decompensation and warrants rapid intervention (Gull et al., 1996).

It is extremely important to recognize FHR patterns that precedes death. In any stage of labor, bradycardias that are preceded by a period of late or variable decelerations or minimal variability and bradycardias that are associated with absent variability are associated with metabolic acidosis in the fetus (Beard et al., 1971;

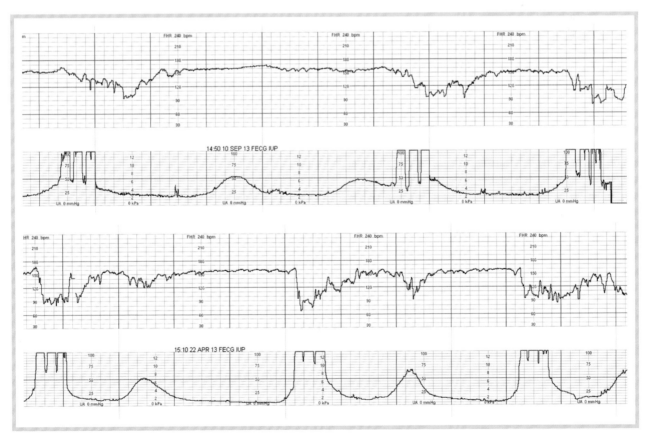

FIGURE 15–15. Modification of Maternal Pushing Efforts Based on Fetal Response.

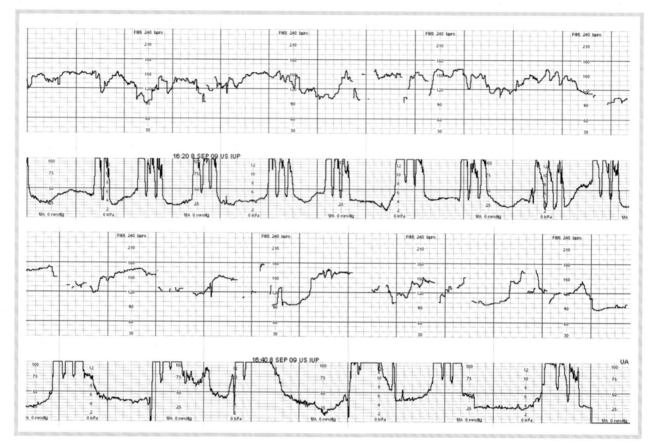

FIGURE 15–16. Iatrogenic category II fetal heart rate pattern as a result of coached closed-glottis pushing during the second stage of labor.

Berkus et al., 1999; Clark et al., 1984; Dellinger et al., 2000; Low et al., 1999; Macones et al., 2008), and birth is recommended if the pattern cannot be resolved (ACOG, 2010) (see Fig. 15–6). In either situation, if the problem causing fetal hypoxia is not corrected, the FHR eventually becomes a flat, fixed pattern with absent variability prior to death. Scalp stimulation elicits no response. Multiple authors have reviewed the relationship between FHR patterns and neonatal outcomes. The presence of accelerations most reliably indicates adequate oxygenation to the brain, and moderate baseline variability is highly suggestive of the same. A normal baseline rate with moderate variability, with or without accelerations, conveys a high level of security that the fetus is well oxygenated at the time of observation (ACOG, 2009b, 2010; Macones et al., 2008). Many FHR tracings obtained during labor include some type of variant pattern, and most of these fetuses are also well oxygenated. In a study examining the frequency of categories of FHR patterns during term labor, most tracings (77.9%) were normal (category I), 22.1% were indeterminate (category II), and 0.004% were abnormal (category III) (Jackson et al., 2011). Because the range of tracings in category II is quite wide, clinical judgment and knowledge of the underlying physiology are required to determine the appropriate level of concern and level of intervention needed. Nurses caring for women during labor should be able to promptly recognize abnormal (category III) patterns and request immediate medical consultation, as these abnormal tracings do convey a risk for fetal metabolic acidemia.

ANCILLARY METHODS FOR ASSESSING FETAL ACID–BASE STATUS

Because most variant FHR tracings are not associated with an underlying fetal hypoxemia, it is occasionally helpful to use ancillary testing that can discriminate between the fetus with hypoxemia and the fetus that is centrally well oxygenated. This discrimination can potentially avoid unnecessary interventions if the results of the test are normal. Preferred ancillary methods for evaluating fetal status are fetal scalp stimulation and VAS. Umbilical cord blood gas and pH values are used to determine fetal acid–base status at the time of birth.

Fetal Scalp and Vibroacoustic Stimulation

Accelerations of the FHR of at least 15 bpm above the baseline with a duration of at least 15 seconds correlate highly with a fetal blood pH ≥7.19 (Clark et al., 1984; Freeman at al., 2012). These FHR accelerations, either spontaneous or elicited by digital scalp or VAS, are highly predictive of normal fetal acid–base status and may help guide clinical management during labor and birth (ACOG, 2010). FHR stimulation should be performed during a time when the FHR is at its baseline rate and the acceleration evoked is above the FHR baseline (Clark et al., 1984). Performing scalp stimulation or VAS during a deceleration is inappropriate (Freeman et al., 2012). The absence of an acceleration response to scalp or VAS is not diagnostic of fetal acidemia; rather, it is an indeterminate finding (Freeman et al., 2012; Macones et al., 2008; Porter & Clark, 1999; Skupski, Rosenberg, & Eglinton, 2002) and should be managed accordingly (ACOG, 2010).

Digital scalp stimulation is performed by placing firm, digital pressure on the fetal scalp during a vaginal examination. However, excessive pressure or pressure applied directly over a fetal fontanelle may result in vagal stimulation and a transient decrease in the FHR. To perform VAS, a commercially distributed vibroacoustic stimulator or a battery-powered artificial larynx is positioned over the fetal vertex or breech and a stimulus of 1 to 2 seconds is applied (ACOG, 2014). This may be repeated up to three times for progressively longer durations up to 3 seconds to elicit FHR accelerations (ACOG, 2014; Druzin, Smith, Gabbe, & Reed, 2007). While some evidence supports the use of VAS during labor (ACOG, 2010), no RCTs to date have addressed the safety and efficacy of VAS during labor and birth. Because digital scalp stimulation and VAS are less invasive and easier to perform than fetal scalp pH sampling, while providing similar information about the likelihood of fetal acidemia, scalp pH sampling is used rarely in the United States (ACOG, 2009b; Freeman et al., 2012). ACOG (2010) recommends that when an FHR tracing has minimal or absent variability and no accelerations and does not respond to intrauterine resuscitation measures, additional assessment such as digital scalp stimulation or VAS should be done.

Umbilical Cord Blood Gas and Acid–Base Analysis

At birth, newborn metabolic status is most accurately determined by assessing the acid–base parameters of the umbilical cord blood. While all newborns have a small degree of metabolic acidosis, a severe accumulation of metabolic acids in response to hypoxia-ischemia and anaerobic metabolism correlates with the risk of permanent neurologic abnormalities in some newborns (ACOG & AAP, 2014). However, most severely acidotic newborns do not develop cerebral palsy, as the majority of cases of cerebral palsy are unrelated to events during labor and birth (ACOG & AAP, 2014). Newborns who are depressed at birth or at risk for acidemia due to maternal–fetal indications or complications during labor and birth often have umbilical cord blood sampling performed immediately after birth. Indications for umbilical cord pH include nonelective cesarean, instrumented vaginal birth, abnormal or indeterminate FHR pattern within 1 hour of birth, Apgar score <7 at 1 and/or 5 minutes, shoulder dystocia, breech or other malpresentation at birth, intrapartum vaginal bleeding more than "bloody show," maternal fever ≥100.4°F, maternal thyroid disease, severe intrauterine growth restriction, premature birth less than 34 weeks, moderate to thick meconium, and suspected fetal anomaly (Freeman et al., 2012).

To obtain umbilical cord gases, efforts should be made by the obstetric care provider to double clamp the umbilical cord promptly after birth. Depending on perinatal unit resources, physicians, midwives, nurses, or respiratory therapists may draw the umbilical cord gases and send them expeditiously for analysis. Both umbilical artery and venous samples should be obtained separately and analyzed for pH and PCO_2, and the base excess or base deficit calculated. Samples taken either from unclamped vessels in continuity with placental vessels or with a delay of more than 20 minutes to blood gas analysis showed significant increases in base deficit and lactate values and therefore should be interpreted with caution (ACOG & AAP, 2014).

The umbilical artery provides the most accurate information for determining neonatal acid–base status at birth. Drawing a separate sample from the umbilical vein will help verify that a true arterial specimen was obtained. While normal cord blood values are usually described in ranges, Table 15–13 provides single-digit values to serve as an initial reference of normal and abnormal umbilical artery cord blood acid–base values. Table 15–14 provides a quick reference for each type of acidemia (respiratory, metabolic, mixed) and corresponding increases or decreases in acid–base measurements (pH, PCO_2, bicarbonate [HCO_3^-], base deficit, base excess). Respiratory acidemia may occur when the flow of gases in the umbilical cord is interrupted, resulting in an elevated fetal PCO_2. Metabolic acidemia may occur with prolonged disruption of fetal oxygenation, resulting in anaerobic metabolism and the buildup of lactic acid in excess of fetal capacity to buffer acids. Decreased bicarbonate and increased base deficit or decreased base excess are reflective of this process. While metabolic acidemia is more serious than respiratory acidemia, most infants born with metabolic acidemia will develop normally as metabolic acidemia has a relatively weak predictive value for longer term complications such as neonatal encephalopathy or cerebral palsy (ACOG & AAP, 2014).

TABLE 15–13. Single-Digit Value Guideline for Initial Assessment of Normal and Abnormal Umbilical Artery Cord Blood Acid–Base Values

	Normal values	Respiratory acidemia	Metabolic acidemia
pH	≥7.10	<7.10	<7.10
PO₂ (mm Hg)	≥20	Variable	<20
PCO₂ (mm Hg)	<60	>60	<60
Bicarbonate (mEq/L)	>22	≥22	<22
Base deficit (mEq/L)	≤12	<12	>12
Base excess (mEq/L)	≥−12	>−12	<−12

The values presented are suggested as a guide for evaluating acid–base status. All umbilical cord blood values should be evaluated in relation to the specific clinical findings and situation for a given patient. Note that greater absolute values of base deficit or excess are associated with acidemia.
PCO₂, partial pressure of carbon dioxide; PO₂, partial pressure of oxygen.
Adapted from Andres, R. L., Saade, G., Gilstrap, L. C., Wilkins, I., Witlin, A., Zlatnik, F., & Hankins, G. V. (1999). Association between umbilical blood gas parameters and neonatal morbidity and death in neonates with pathologic fetal acidemia. *American Journal of Obstetrics and Gynecology, 181*(4), 867–871 and Low, J. A., Lindsay, B. G., & Derrick, E. J. (1997). Threshold of metabolic acidosis associated with newborn complications. *American Journal of Obstetrics and Gynecology, 177*(6), 1391–1394.

ST Segment Analysis

Ongoing efforts to improve the predictive value of FHR data for differentiating the compromised fetus from the uncompromised fetus when variant FHR patterns are present have included fetal pulse oximetry and ST segment analysis (STAN). While fetal pulse oximetry initially appeared promising, it did not gain widespread clinical use in the United States because it did not reduce the overall cesarean rate in a large multicenter trial (Garite et al., 2000), and it was eventually withdrawn from the market in the United States, although still is in use in Europe. STAN uses select components of the fetal ECG signal to determine whether fetal myocardial ischemia is present. The system includes a fetal ECG electrode, a maternal skin reference electrode, and a microprocessor-based fetal monitor that continuously identifies the fetal ST segment and T-wave changes from the fetal cardiac cycle (Belfort & Saade, 2011). When the STAN monitor detects significant changes in the ST interval compared to the baseline T/QRS ratio, it flags an ST event on the monitor and in the event log (Devoe, 2011b). The fetal STAN system is manufactured by Neoventa Medical in Mölndal, Sweden.

While fetal STAN has been used and studied in Europe, enthusiasm for this practice in the United States has been somewhat lacking. Study results in Europe are difficult to extrapolate to the U.S. population due to differences in obstetric practice and patient case mix as well as differences in definitions of key terms such as *metabolic acidosis* and *neonatal encephalopathy* (Belfort & Saade, 2011). Additionally, as STAN is not a stand-alone component that can be used with current fetal monitors, the cost of replacing fetal monitors with those that can provide STAN data is a concern and a significant barrier to widespread adoption in the United States. The Maternal-Fetal Medicine Units Networks of NICHD conducted an RCT of over 11,000 women in labor comparing use of the STAN technology as an adjunct to EFM versus FHR monitoring alone. No reduction in the composite outcome of intrapartum fetal death, neonatal death, Apgar score <3 at 5 minutes, neonatal seizure, umbilical artery pH <7.05 with base deficit >12 mmol/L, neonatal intubation, or neonatal encephalopathy was found. There was also no difference in cesarean birth or operative vaginal birth rates between groups (Belfort et al., 2015). A Cochrane systematic review and meta-analysis of six trials concluded that use of STAN made no difference in cesarean birth rates, severe neonatal metabolic acidosis, or neonatal encephalopathy (Neilson, 2015).

Computerized Interpretation of Electronic Fetal Monitoring Data

For many years, researches have made efforts to develop and use computer algorithms to interpret EFM and generate alarms for FHR tachycardia and bradycardia. Some systems accurately identified rate and variability; however, they had difficulty with decelerations

TABLE 15–14. Significance of Deviation from Normal Values

Type of acidemia	pH	PO₂	PCO₂	HCO₃⁻	Base deficit	Base excess
Respiratory	Decreased	Variable	Increased	Normal	Normal	Normal
Metabolic	Decreased	Decreased	Normal	Decreased	Increased	Decreased
Mixed	Decreased	Decreased	Increased	Decreased	Increased	Decreased

HCO₃⁻, bicarbonate; PCO₂, partial pressure of carbon dioxide; PO₂, partial pressure of oxygen.

and accelerations. In the last few years, computer systems using artificial intelligence technology have demonstrated increased accuracy in identifying types of FHR deceleration and accelerations, similar to the level of agreement between clinicians. However, not until two recent RCTs in United Kingdom and Ireland has a computerized interpretation system been combined with a decision support software system (INFANT) to make an assessment of the overall FHR pattern and issue real-time alerts (INFANT Collaborative Group, 2017; Nunes et al., 2017).

In the first RCT, 47,062 women in United Kingdom and Ireland were randomly assigned (23,515 in the decision-support group [INFANT]; 23,547 in the no-decision-support group) and 46,042 were analyzed (22,987 in the decision-support group [INFANT]; 23,055 in the no-decision-support group) (INFANT Collaborative Group, 2017). This RCT was designed to evaluate whether intrapartum fetal monitoring with computer analysis and real-time alerts (INFANT system) compared to visual analysis without alerts decreases the rate of poor neonatal outcome (intrapartum stillbirth or early neonatal death excluding lethal congenital anomalies, or neonatal encephalopathy, admission to NICU within 24 hours for ≥48 hours with evidence of feeding difficulties, respiratory illness, or encephalopathy with evidence of compromise at birth) and developmental assessment at 2 years in a subset of surviving children. No differences were noted in the incidence of poor neonatal outcome between groups (adjusted odds ratio, 1.01; 95% confidence interval [CI], 0.82 to 1.25). Nor were significant differences found in terms of developmental assessment at 2 years.

In the second RCT, which also recruited in the United Kingdom, evaluated whether intrapartum EFM with computer analysis and real-time alerts (INFANT) decreases the rate of newborn metabolic acidosis or obstetric intervention when compared with visual analysis of the FHR tracing alone (Nunes et al., 2017). Continuous central EFM by computer analysis and online alerts (experimental group) was compared with visual analysis (control group). There were 32,306 women who were assessed for eligibility, and 7,730 were randomized: 3,961 to computer analysis and online alerts and 3,769 to visual analysis. Baseline characteristics were similar in both groups. Metabolic acidosis occurred in 16 participants (0.40%) in the experimental group compared with 22 participants (0.58%) in the control group (relative risk, 0.69; 95% CI, 0.36 to 1.31). No significant differences were found in the incidence of secondary outcomes (operative delivery, use of fetal blood sampling, low 5-minute Apgar score, NICU admission, hypoxic-ischemic encephalopathy, and perinatal death). Compared with visual analysis, computer analysis of fetal monitoring signals with real-time alerts did not significantly reduce the rate of metabolic acidosis or obstetric intervention. These two recent studies demonstrate the continued importance of nurses, midwives, and physicians visually assessing the EFM tracing, accurately interpreting the FHR patterns, and providing timely interventions.

NURSING ASSESSMENT AND MANAGEMENT STRATEGIES

Patient Education about Fetal Heart Rate Monitoring

Preparation for fetal monitoring includes a discussion of risks and benefits of methods of fetal assessment in the context of the woman's values, preferences, obstetric history, and treatment plan so that the woman may make an informed decision about monitoring (Carter et al., 2010). While continuous EFM may be recommended for many women (i.e., those with obstetric risk factors and those receiving induction or augmentation of labor), EFM is not without risk and may often be used simply out of routine and convenience. In *Listening to Mothers in California*, a statewide, population-based survey in 2016, 84% of women who experienced labor had EFM, either exclusively (68%) or used in conjunction with either a handheld device such as an electronic Doppler or fetal stethoscope (Sakala, Declercq, Turon, & Corry, 2018). Only 3% of women reported being exclusively monitored with a handheld device.

An assessment of the woman's preferences, knowledge, and prior discussions with providers about monitoring methods is a good starting point for discussion. Monitoring methods appropriate to the woman's individual situation should be described and offered, with adequate time provided for answering the woman's questions (ACOG, 2019). Ideally, concerns about fetal assessment and monitoring during labor would have been discussed between the woman and her perinatal healthcare provider prior to admission to the hospital for labor. It is important to keep in mind that options for ongoing fetal assessment may include intermittent EFM and IA for many women, in addition to continuous EFM (ACOG, 2009b, 2010, 2017; AWHONN, 2018; Wisner & Holschuh, 2018).

Nursing Assessment of the Fetal Heart Rate

A systematic, organized approach to interpreting FHR patterns prevents misinterpretation and confusion. The deceleration in the middle of the tracing can sometimes draw immediate attention, but it may not be the most important aspect of the tracing. Assessment of the entire FHR tracing, including previous fetal status, uterine contractions, and all procedures that transpired prior to the deceleration, is required. Integration of maternal obstetric and medical history is of critical importance for appropriate interpretation of FHR findings. Assessment should include but are not limited to the following: (1) maternal–fetal risk for uteroplacental insufficiency, (2) administration of regional analgesia/anesthesia, (3) administration of medications or maternal substance use, (4) pharmacologic agents used for cervical ripening and labor induction/augmentation, and (5) trends or changes in FHR characteristics over time.

Physical assessment should include maternal vital signs, hydration status, and position as these factors can have an influence on fetal status. For example, maternal fever can cause fetal tachycardia, whereas supine positioning or hypotension can cause fetal bradycardia.

Experienced perinatal nurses assess FHR patterns for evidence of fetal well-being very quickly. They use a mental checklist that includes the following questions (Simpson, 1997):

- What is the baseline FHR?
- Is it within normal limits for this fetus?
- If not, what clinical factors could be contributing to this baseline rate?
- Is there evidence of moderate baseline variability?
- Are accelerations present?
- If accelerations are not present and variability is minimal or absent, does external or fetal scalp stimulation elicit an acceleration of the FHR appropriate for gestational age?
- What clinical factors could be contributing to this baseline variability?
- Are there periodic or episodic FHR patterns?
- If so, what are they and what are the appropriate interventions (if any)?
- Does the FHR pattern suggest a chronic or acute maternal–fetal condition?
- Is uterine activity normal in frequency, duration, intensity, and resting tone?
- What is the relationship between the FHR and uterine activity?
- How has the FHR changed over time?
- If the FHR pattern is indeterminate (category II) or abnormal (category III), do the appropriate interventions resolve the situation?
- If not, are further interventions needed based on the overall clinical picture?
- Is the FHR pattern such that notification of the physician or midwife is warranted?
- How close or far is the woman from birth?
- What team members need to be aware of current maternal–fetal status?
- Are there complications team members should prepare for?

Nurses who are learning the principles of EFM may require more time to complete an assessment of fetal status; however, the essential components of a comprehensive assessment remain the same. It is helpful to devise a systematic method for FHR assessment and related appropriate interventions and consistently use that method in clinical practice to enhance optimal maternal–fetal outcomes.

After collecting all pertinent data, the following characteristics of the FHR tracing are interpreted and documented in the medical record: (1) uterine activity: frequency, duration, intensity, and resting tone; (2) baseline FHR and variability; (3) presence or absence of accelerations; and (4) presence or absence of decelerations (Display 15–1). There is no need to provide detailed descriptions of FHR decelerations in medical record documentation: Simply identify them by name. In the past, some clinicians were taught to descriptively document decelerations by depth, duration, and return to baseline rate (i.e., deceleration down to 60 bpm for 90 seconds with a slow return to baseline). However, this advice was based on concern for loss of the tracing in systems where paper tracings were microfilmed separately from the rest of the medical record. In the current environment, this type of description is time-consuming and unnecessary when the electronic tracing is recorded and integrated in the labor record as it is with most obstetric surveillance systems. Additional detailed descriptions of the tracing reduces time available for nursing care and may increase professional liability if the case should be reviewed after an adverse outcome, and the medical record documentation concerning the decelerations does not match exactly with the decelerations as noted on the FHR tracing. Identification of the deceleration as early, late, variable, or prolonged implies that the deceleration meets criteria for these types of decelerations as defined by NICHD (Macones et al., 2008), and this is sufficient for the medical record. During interdisciplinary communication about FHR patterns,

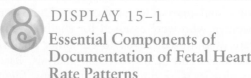

DISPLAY 15–1

Essential Components of Documentation of Fetal Heart Rate Patterns

1. Baseline rate
2. Baseline variability
3. Presence or absence of accelerations
4. Periodic or episodic decelerations
5. Changes of trends of fetal heart rate patterns over time

Adapted from National Institute of Child Health and Human Development Research Planning Workshop. (1997). Electronic fetal heart rate monitoring: Research guidelines for interpretation. *American Journal of Obstetrics & Gynecology, 177*(6), 1385–1390, and *Journal of Obstetric Gynecology and Neonatal Nursing, 26*(6), 635–640. doi:10.1016/S0002-9378(97)70079-6 detailed descriptions may be necessary and appropriate for clarification and appreciation of the need for immediacy of intervention.

If the FHR pattern is indeterminate or abnormal, nursing intervention is based first on identification of the precipitating event, when possible, and then prioritized based on the level of concern. Eliminating the cause (e.g., uterine tachysystole or maternal hypotension) and/or instituting interventions that provide intrauterine resuscitation may be all that is necessary for the resumption of a normal FHR pattern (see Table 15–11). Conversely, the presence of any category III tracing and some category II tracings warrants immediate bedside evaluation by a physician who can initiate a cesarean birth. A decision tree for FHR management is presented in Figure 15–10. Depending on the clinical situation, there may be a decision for operative birth.

Clinical Algorithms for Standardization of Response to and Management of Indeterminant (Category II) Fetal Heart Rate Patterns

In 2013, a group of fetal monitoring researchers and clinicians offered suggestions for standard management of indeterminant (category II) FHR patterns (Clark et al., 2013) (Fig. 15–17). The goal was to provide guidance for FHR patterns that are included in category II and to avoid situations in which fetal resuscitative efforts or expeditious birth were delayed until the FHR pattern evolved to category III or metabolic acidemia. Application of the algorithm in clinical practice has potential to avoid preventable fetal harm during labor; however, there are significant limitations of the ability of EFM to accurately predict neonatal metabolic acidemia (Clark et al., 2017). The Clark et al. (2013) standard FHR management algorithm was modified by Shields, Wiesner, Klein, Pelletreau, and Hedriana (2018) with more details and specific time frames for clinical intervention and applied to practice in six birthing hospitals. Results were compared with data from 23 hospitals in the same health system that did not use the standard management of FHR algorithm. Use of the algorithm was associated with a shorter time that labor was allowed to continue in the context of "significant" decelerations, a goal of the original version of the Clark et al. algorithm, along with a reduction in low 5-minute Apgar scores and severe unexpected newborn complications (Shields et al., 2018). Significant decelerations were defined as per Clark et al. The algorithm was found to be feasible to apply to clinical practice as physicians followed the standardized approach in over 97% of patients. More data are needed on application of standardized algorithms for management of category II FHR tracings; however, the Shields et al. results are promising.

Interdisciplinary Communication

It is not unusual for disagreements in the interpretation of FHR patterns to exist between different members of the perinatal healthcare team (ACOG, 2009b; Beckmann, Van Mullem, Beckmann, & Broekhuizen, 1997; Lyndon et al., 2011; Simpson, James, & Knox, 2006; Simpson & Lyndon, 2009). Intrapartum fetal assessment is one of the most important clinical situations in which nurses, physicians, and midwives need to work together and trust each other's judgment (Clark et al., 2009; Fox et al., 2000; Miller & Miller, 2013; Simpson et al., 2006; Simpson & Knox, 2009). Much of the communication about ongoing maternal–fetal status during labor occurs while the nurse is at the bedside and the provider is in the office or at home (Simpson, 2005a; Simpson et al., 2006). If the nurse determines that the FHR pattern is indeterminate or abnormal, the physician or midwife should be notified. Effective clinical communication is timely, direct, respectful, and explicitly identifies the level of concern and urgency (Lyndon et al., 2011). Nurses should describe their concerns and observations so that a clear plan of management can collaboratively be determined. Requests for orders for interventions and a bedside evaluation, if necessary, should be clearly stated. "Please come in to review the FHR pattern" is more effective in obtaining a bedside evaluation than "I'm worried about the fetus." If the situation is acute, "I need you to come now" is a clear, concise request for immediate action. Communication about indeterminate or abnormal FHR patterns should include characteristics of the pattern (baseline rate, variability, and presence or absence of accelerations and decelerations), pattern evolution (i.e., how long this FHR pattern has been developing and changing over time), the clinical context (e.g., bleeding, tachysystole, hypotension), intrauterine resuscitation techniques implemented and the fetal response, and request for further interventions and evaluation (e.g., amnioinfusion, ephedrine or phenylephrine, terbutaline, bedside evaluation as soon as possible, immediate bedside evaluation, preparations for emergent cesarean birth) (Fox et al., 2000; Simpson & Knox, 2009). The general content of this conversation, including the provider's response, should be documented in the medical record. If the discussion results in a clinical disagreement that cannot be resolved by the direct care providers, nurses should follow institutional policy about resolution of clinical disagreements. This type of policy is usually known as the chain of consultation or chain of command.

Physicians, midwives, and nurses are responsible for maintaining competence in FHR pattern interpretation and appropriate use of interventions. One way to both maintain competence and promote interdisciplinary collaboration is participation in EFM

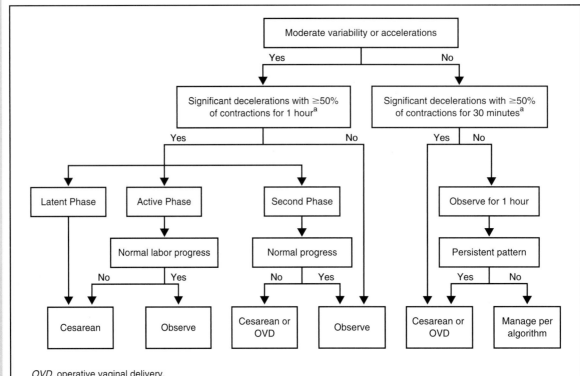

OVD, operative vaginal delivery.

[a]That have not resolved with appropriate conservative corrective measures, which may include supplemental oxygen, maternal position changes, intravenous fluid administration, correction of hypotension, reduction or discontinuation of uterine stimulation, administration of uterine relaxant, amnioinfusion, and/or changes in second stage breathing and pushing techniques.

Clark. Category II FHRT. Am J Obstet Gynecol 2013.

Management of category II fetal heart rate patterns: clarifications for use in algorithm

1. Variability refers to predominant baseline FHR pattern (marked, moderate, minimal, absent) during a 30-minute evaluation period, as defined by NICHD.
2. Marked variability is considered same as moderate variability for purposes of this algorithm.
3. Significant decelerations are defined as any of the following:
   • Variable decelerations lasting longer than 60 seconds and reaching a nadir more than 60 bpm below baseline.
   • Variable decelerations lasting longer than 60 seconds and reaching a nadir less than 60 bpm regardless of the baseline.
   • Any late decelerations of any depth.
   • Any prolonged deceleration, as defined by the NICHD. Due to the broad heterogeneity inherent in this definition, identification of a prolonged deceleration should prompt discontinuation of the algorithm until the deceleration is resolved.
4. Application of algorithm may be initially delayed for up to 30 minutes while attempts are made to alleviate category II pattern with conservative therapeutic interventions (eg, correction of hypotension, position change, amnioinfusion, tocolysis, reduction or discontinuation of oxytocin).
5. Once a category II FHR pattern is identified, FHR is evaluated and algorithm applied every 30 minutes.
6. Any significant change in FHR parameters should result in reapplication of algorithm.
7. For category II FHR patterns in which algorithm suggests delivery is indicated, such delivery should ideally be initiated within 30 minutes of decision for cesarean.
8. If at any time tracing reverts to category I status, or deteriorates for even a short time to category III status, the algorithm no longer applies. However, algorithm should be reinstituted if category I pattern again reverts to category II.
9. In fetus with extreme prematurity, neither significance of certain FHR patterns of concern in more mature fetus (eg, minimal variability) or ability of such fetuses to tolerate intrapartum events leading to certain types of category II patterns are well defined. This algorithm is not intended as guide to management of fetus with extreme prematurity.
10. Algorithm may be overridden at any time if, after evaluation of patient, physician believes it is in best interest of the fetus to intervene sooner.

FHR, fetal heart rate; NICHD, Eunice Kennedy Shriver National Institute of Child Health and Human Development.
Clark. Category II FHRT. Am J Obstet Gynecol 2013.

FIGURE 15-17. Algorithm for management of category II fetal heart rate tracings. (From Clark, S. L., Nageotte, M. P., Garite, T. J., Freeman, R. K., Miller, D. A., Simpson, K. R., . . . Hankins, G. D. V. [2013]. Intrapartum management of category II fetal heart tracings: Towards standardization of care. *American Journal of Obstetrics & Gynecology, 209*[2], 89-97. doi:10.1016/j.ajog.2013.04.030. Used with permission.)

education programs that include physicians, midwives, and nurses (Miller & Miller, 2013). A group process can be used to review EFM strips, expected responses, appropriate interpretations, and related interventions. Interdisciplinary team discussions can lead to an increased knowledge of EFM principles for everyone involved and can be a mechanism for decreasing hierarchy and improving interdisciplinary understanding and teamwork. Developing case studies containing clinical ambiguity is an ideal avenue for clarifying ongoing clinical issues where interpretation and expectations of all provider groups are not in sync (Miller, 2005). Educational collaboration between nurses, midwives, and physicians who are jointly responsible for FHR pattern interpretation and clinical interventions enhances collaboration in everyday clinical interactions and thus promotes maternal–fetal safety (JCAHO, 2004).

Certification in EFM is another option to promote interdisciplinary knowledge related to fetal assessment (Miller, 2017). When all members of the team hold certification in EFM, there is recognition that everyone has the same level of EFM knowledge and skill and that this knowledge and these skills are not discipline specific. Preparing for the certification exam as a group can enhance interdisciplinary team collegiality and effective communication when there is a question concerning fetal status based on the FHR pattern.

ISSUES IN THE USE OF FETAL HEART RATE MONITORING DURING LABOR

Efficacy of Electronic Fetal Heart Rate Monitoring

When EFM was developed and introduced into clinical practice, the hope was that this technique for fetal assessment would lead to a reduction in the overall incidence of cerebral palsy and intrapartum stillbirth (ACOG, 2009b; ACOG & AAP, 2014). This expectation was due in part to the opinion of experts in the 1960s and 1970s that most cases of cerebral palsy and other neurologic morbidity were the result of asphyxia during labor and birth. The randomized trials conducted during the 1980s failed to show a decrease in the incidence of cerebral palsy among infants who were monitored during labor (Shy et al., 1990). Yet the incidence of cesarean birth and assisted operative birth in the cohorts monitored increased fourfold (Thacker et al., 1995). These results have led many to the conclusion that EFM is not efficacious (Freeman, 1990). More recent reviews of the methodology used in the randomized trials in combination with newer information on the genesis of cerebral palsy have brought to light some of the reasons why FHR monitoring did poorly in the randomized trials that were conducted

(Parer & King, 2000). Because this controversy remains unresolved, it is worth reviewing in the context of this text.

Fetal Heart Rate Monitoring and Cerebral Palsy

EFM has been in wide use for more than 40 years with no change in the incidence of cerebral palsy (2 per 1,000 live births) (ACOG, 2009b; ACOG & AAP, 2014). Thus, the original hope that EFM would predict and therefore prevent fetal asphyxia, which would in turn prevent cerebral palsy, has not been realized. The majority of cases of infant and childhood cerebral palsy are related to prenatal events rather than the labor and birth process. Most cases of cerebral palsy are associated with prematurity, disorders of coagulation, and intrauterine exposure to maternal infections (Grether & Nelson, 1997). Interruption of the oxygen supply to the fetus contributes to approximately 6% of cases of cerebral palsy (Nelson & Grether, 1999), and most experts believe that no more than 2% to 20% of cases of cerebral palsy are due to intrapartum events of any cause (MacDonald, 1996; Nelson, 1988). These wide-ranging estimates are the result of imprecise interpretation of EFM data during labor as well as variations in diagnostic classification of the severity and type of cerebral palsy (Lent, 1999). No more than 4% of encephalopathy cases can be attributed to intrapartum events in isolation (ACOG, 2009b). The dramatically improved survival rates of extremely preterm infants have the potential to increase the incidence of cerebral palsy, and advances in neonatal care may also improve the survival rate of asphyxiated infants of any gestational age. These factors may obscure any effect that EFM has had on the incidence of cerebral palsy. Suggestions for assessment of an acute peripartum or intrapartum event sufficient to cause neonatal encephalopathy are offered by ACOG and AAP (2014) (Display 15–2).

Sensitivity, Specificity, and Reliability of Electronic Fetal Monitoring

EFM sensitivity (the ability to detect a healthy fetus when it is indeed healthy) is high, while specificity (the ability to detect a compromised fetus when it is compromised and not include healthy fetuses in the criteria) is low (Simpson & Knox, 2000). When the FHR is normal, there is a very high probability that the fetus is adequately oxygenated and not acidemic at the time of observation (Macones et al., 2008). Thus, EFM is a sensitive screening tool as it is very good at ruling out fetal compromise. Conversely, it is estimated that even the most ominous FHR patterns are associated with at most a 50% to 65% incidence of neonatal depression (Martin, 1998). EFM can have up to a 99.8%

DISPLAY 15-2

Assessment of Acute Peripartum or Intrapartum Event Sufficient to Cause Neonatal Encephalopathy

I. Neonatal Signs Consistent with an Acute Peripartum or Intrapartum Event

A. Apgar score of less than 5 at 5 and 10 min
- Low Apgar scores at 5 and 10 min clearly confer an increased relative risk of cerebral palsy. The degree of Apgar abnormality at 5 and 10 min correlates with the risk of cerebral palsy. However, most infants with low Apgar scores will not develop cerebral palsy. There are many potential causes for low Apgar scores.

B. Fetal umbilical artery acidemia
- Fetal umbilical artery pH less than 7.0, base deficit greater than or equal to 12 mmol/L, or both increases the probability that neonatal encephalopathy, if present, had an intrapartum hypoxic component; lesser degrees of acidemia decrease that likelihood. Even in the presence of significant acidemia, most newborns will be neurologically normal.

C. Neuroimaging evidence of acute brain injury seen on brain magnetic resonance imaging or magnetic resonance spectroscopy consistent with hypoxic-ischemia

D. Presence of multisystem organ failure consistent with hypoxic-ischemic encephalopathy

II. Type and Timing of Contributing Factors that Are Consistent with an Acute Peripartum or Intrapartum Event

A. A sentinel hypoxic or ischemic event occurring immediately before or during labor and delivery
- Examples include ruptured uterus, severe abruptio placenta, umbilical cord prolapse, amniotic fluid embolism with coincident severe and prolonged maternal hypotension and hypoxemia, maternal cardiovascular collapse, fetal exsanguination from ruptured either vasa previa, or massive fetomaternal hemorrhage.

B. Fetal heart rate (FHR) monitor patterns consistent with acute peripartum or intrapartum event
- A category I or category II FHR tracing when associated with Apgar scores of 7 or higher at 5 min, normal umbilical cord arterial blood (±1 standard deviation), or both is not consistent with an acute hypoxic-ischemic event.
- A category II FHR pattern lasting 60 min or more that was identified on initial presentation with persistently minimal or absent variability and lacking accelerations, even in the absence of decelerations, is suggestive of a previously compromised or injured fetus. If fetal well-being cannot be established by appropriate response to scalp stimulation or biophysical testing, the patient should be evaluated for the method and timing of delivery. An emergency cesarean delivery may not benefit a fetus with previous severe compromise.
- The patient who presents with a category I FHR pattern that converts to a category III as defined by the *Eunice Kennedy Shriver* National Institute of Child Health and Human Development guidelines is suggestive of intrapartum timing of a hypoxic-ischemic event.
- Additional FHR patterns that develop after a category I FHR pattern on presentation, which may suggest intrapartum timing of a hypoxic-ischemic event, include tachycardia with recurrent decelerations and persistent minimal variability with recurrent decelerations.

C. Timing and type of brain injury patterns based on imaging studies consistent with an etiology of an acute peripartum or intrapartum event

D. No evidence of other proximal or distal factors that could be contributing factors
- In the presence of other significant risk factors (e.g., abnormal fetal growth, maternal infection, fetomaternal hemorrhage, neonatal sepsis, and chronic placental lesions), an acute intrapartum event as the sole underlying pathogenesis of neonatal encephalopathy becomes less likely.

III. Developmental Outcome Is Spastic Quadriplegia or Dyskinetic Cerebral Palsy
- Other subtypes of cerebral palsy are less likely to be associated with acute intrapartum hypoxic-ischemic events.

Adapted from American College of Obstetricians and Gynecologists & American Academy of Pediatrics. (2014). *Neonatal encephalopathy and neurologic outcome* (2nd ed.). Washington, DC: American College of Obstetricians and Gynecologists.

false-positive rate for predicting cerebral palsy in term fetuses (Nelson, Dambrosia, Ting, & Grether, 1996). Therefore, EFM is not very specific or highly accurate for definitively identifying fetal compromise. The sensitivity and specificity limitations of EFM are related to its inability to directly evaluate fetal oxygen status.

Further complicating the issue is the fact that both inter- and intraobserver reliability in interpreting EFM data is inconsistent (Martin, 1998; Paneth, Bommarito, & Stricker, 1993). Not only do experienced clinicians continue to differ in interpretations when evaluating a specific FHR pattern (Wolfberg et al., 2008), they

also disagree with their own interpretation when asked to review the same FHR tracing, and their interpretations of the tracing may be influenced by knowledge of the outcome (Di Lieto et al., 2003; Figueras et al., 2005). This phenomenon particularly affects interpretations suggesting fetal compromise (Simpson & Knox, 2000). By contrast, diagnosis of fetal well-being (adequate fetal oxygenation) has much higher inter- and intraobserver reliability: Agreement is highest on identification of normal baseline, "normal" variability, and presence of accelerations (Di Lieto et al., 2003; Figueras et al., 2005; Wolfberg et al., 2008).

Therefore, communication issues and professional disagreements about EFM interpretation are much more likely to occur when attempting to assign a diagnosis of fetal compromise than that of fetal well-being.

The differential predictability between sensitivity and specificity and lack of reliability between different providers is the basis of the fundamental issue confounding the use of EFM (Simpson & Knox, 2000). The lack of common understanding by all involved professionals about how FHR monitoring can be relied on when determining fetal status undermines the ability of this technique to guide clinical management (Fox et al., 2000). If the FHR pattern has a normal baseline rate and moderate variability and no late, variable, or prolonged decelerations (i.e., a category I tracing), there is little disagreement about the prediction of fetal well-being. Similarly, category III patterns, those with absent variability and either bradycardia, variable, or late decelerations, or a sinusoidal FHR, generate significant agreement. These patterns clearly suggest the fetus is at risk for acidemia. However, many FHR patterns are between these two extremes, falling into category II. When different members of the care team simultaneously make different assumptions concerning EFM data, communication between the involved professionals is compromised (Fox et al., 2000). Therefore, interdisciplinary processes that promote common understanding of EFM principles are highly recommended to promote the safest care possible for the mother and fetus (JCAHO, 2004).

Artificial Intelligence and Electronic Fetal Monitoring

In the future, it is likely that computerized interpretation of the FHR and clinical decision support systems will be integrated into nursing care during labor and birth; however, research studies to date have suggested that clinicians are not yet prepared to rely on computer-generated data for EFM interpretation (Belfort & Clark, 2017; Clark et al., 2017; INFANT Collaborative Group, 2017; Simpson & Lyndon, 2019). In a recent randomized clinical trial of over 47,000 women in England and Ireland a decision support system analyzed features of the FHR pattern and uterine activity and, if necessary, generated a color-coded warning to the user ranging from blue (least severe), yellow (moderate severity), to red (most severe) (INFANT Collaborative Group, 2017). The system did not offer advice or suggestions about what types of clinical interventions were required based on the features of the FHR pattern and uterine activity. Results indicated no differences in incidence of poor neonatal outcomes between groups, and at the 2-year follow-up, there were no differences noted in infant development. Accuracy issues may have played a role in the results as only 58% of tracings designated in the red category by the system were judged by expert reviewers to be of valid concern and 70% of the remaining cases were noted to be recording maternal heart rate (INFANT Collaborative Group, 2017).

Some clinicians have found computer-generated interpretation data and clinical alerts less than helpful (INFANT Collaborative Group, 2017; Simpson & Lyndon, 2019). In other areas of clinical practice such as intensive care units, nurses have indicated that experience with repeated episodes of false alarms can cause them to tune out the sounds or respond more slowly, even when some of the alarms are accurately notifying potential patient risk (Bonafide et al., 2017; Paine et al., 2016; Simpson & Lyndon, 2019). Nurses using EFM have reported similar responses (Simpson & Lyndon, 2019). False alarms and alerts are common when using EFM surveillance systems and mainly involve loss of signal (Simpson & Lyndon, 2019; Simpson, Lyndon, & Davidson, 2016). Nurses are more reliant on the visual assessment of the FHR pattern rather than system-generated alerts and alarms (Simpson & Lyndon, 2019). Greater sophistication in system design and better accuracy will be needed before artificial intelligence in EFM interpretation and decision support can be useful.

SUMMARY

Monitoring and interpretation of the FHR and uterine activity are critical elements of intrapartum care that promote safe care for the woman and fetus (see Fig. 15–10). Standardized terms and definitions must be routinely used by all members of the perinatal healthcare team (Miller & Miller, 2013). Knowledge of the physiology underlying specific FHR patterns has increased over time. Nurses, midwives, and physicians must keep abreast of evolving knowledge to provide the best care for mothers and babies during labor. An appreciation of FHR pattern evolution and use of variability in determining the risk for fetal acidemia is critical. Clinicians caring for women in labor should be able to rapidly identify FHR patterns that reflect the absence of fetal acidemia and those that consistently indicate a significant risk for fetal acidemia (Parer et al., 2006). An interdisciplinary team approach in which there is mutual respect and true collaboration between nurses, midwives, and physicians will create a clinical environment that enhances safe and effective intrapartum care. Involving the woman in labor as a partner in her care must be the expected standard. Providing accurate information to the woman and her family at the appropriate literacy level and in understandable terms is vital to make sure the woman is able to be an informed participant in shared decision making.

REFERENCES

Aldrich, C. J., D'Antona, D., Spencer, J. A., Wyatt, J. S., Peebles, D. M., Delpy, D. T., & Reynolds, E. O. (1995). The effect of maternal posture on fetal cerebral oxygenation during labour. *British Journal of Obstetrics and Gynaecology, 102*(1), 14–19.

Aldrich, C. J., Wyatt, J. S., Spencer, J. A., Reynolds, E. O., & Delpy, D. T. (1994). The effect of maternal oxygen administration on human fetal cerebral oxygenation measured during labour by near infrared spectroscopy. *British Journal of Obstetrics and Gynaecology, 101*(6), 509–513.

Alfirevic, Z., Devane, D., & Gyte, G. M. (2013). Continuous cardiotocography (CTG) as a form of electronic fetal monitoring (EFM) for fetal assessment during labour. *Cochrane Database of Systematic Reviews,* (5), CD006066. doi:10.1002/14651858.CD006066.pub2

Althabe, O., Jr., Schwarcz, R. L., Pose, S. V., Escarcena, L., & Caldeyro-Barcia, R. (1967). Effects on fetal heart rate and fetal pO2 of oxygen administration to the mother. *American Journal of Obstetrics & Gynecology, 98*(6), 858–870.

American Academy of Pediatrics & American College of Obstetricians and Gynecologists. (2017). *Guidelines for perinatal care* (8th ed.). Elk Grove Village, IL: American Academy of Pediatrics.

American College of Nurse-Midwives. (2010). *Standardized nomenclature for electronic fetal monitoring* (Position Statement). Silver Spring, MD: Author.

American College of Nurse-Midwives. (2015). Intermittent auscultation for intrapartum fetal heart rate surveillance. *Journal of Midwifery & Women's Health, 60,* 626–632. doi:10.1111/jmwh.12372

American College of Obstetricians and Gynecologists. (1998). *Inappropriate use of the terms fetal distress and birth asphyxia* (Committee Opinion No. 197). Washington, DC: Author.

American College of Obstetricians and Gynecologists. (2005a). *Inappropriate use of the terms fetal distress and birth asphyxia* (Committee Opinion No. 326). Washington, DC: Author.

American College of Obstetricians and Gynecologists. (2005b). *Intrapartum fetal heart rate monitoring* (Practice Bulletin No. 70). Washington, DC: Author.

American College of Obstetricians and Gynecologists. (2006). *Amnioinfusion does not prevent meconium aspiration syndrome* (Committee Opinion No. 346; Reaffirmed, 2018). Washington, DC: Author.

American College of Obstetricians and Gynecologists. (2009a). *Induction of labor* (Practice Bulletin No. 107; Reaffirmed, 2016). Washington, DC: Author.

American College of Obstetricians and Gynecologists. (2009b). *Intrapartum fetal heart rate monitoring: Nomenclature, interpretation, and general management principles* (Practice Bulletin No. 106; Reaffirmed, 2017). Washington, DC: Author.

American College of Obstetricians and Gynecologists. (2010). *Management of intrapartum fetal heart rate tracings* (Practice Bulletin No. 116; Reaffirmed, 2017). Washington, DC: Author.

American College of Obstetricians and Gynecologists. (2014). *Antepartum fetal surveillance* (Practice Bulletin No. 145; Reaffirmed, 2016). Washington, DC: Author.

American College of Obstetricians and Gynecologists. (2016). *Magnesium sulfate use in obstetrics* (Committee Opinion No. 652). Washington, DC: Author.

American College of Obstetricians and Gynecologists. (2017). *Vaginal birth after cesarean delivery* (Practice Bulletin No. 184). Washington, DC: Author.

American College of Obstetricians and Gynecologists. (2019). *Approaches to limit interventions during labor and birth* (Committee Opinion No. 776). Washington, DC: Author.

American College of Obstetricians and Gynecologists & American Academy of Pediatrics. (2014). *Neonatal encephalopathy and neurologic outcome* (2nd ed.). Washington, DC: American College of Obstetricians and Gynecologists.

American Society of Anesthesiologists. (2016). Practice guidelines for obstetric anesthesia: An updated report by the American Society of Anesthesiologists Task Force on Obstetric Anesthesia and Perinatology. *Anesthesiology, 124*(2), 270–300. doi:10.1097/ALN.0000000000000935

Andres, R. L., Saade, G., Gilstrap, L. C., Wilkins, I., Witlin, A., Zlatnik, F., & Hankins, G. V. (1999). Association between umbilical blood gas parameters and neonatal morbidity and death in neonates with pathologic fetal acidemia. *American Journal of Obstetrics and Gynecology, 181*(4), 867–871.

Association of Women's Health, Obstetric and Neonatal Nurses. (2005). *NICHD transitional teaching guide.* Washington, DC: Author.

Association of Women's Health, Obstetric and Neonatal Nurses. (2010). *Guidelines for professional registered nurse staffing for perinatal units.* Washington, DC: Author.

Association of Women's Health, Obstetric and Neonatal Nurses. (2018). *Fetal heart monitoring* (Position Statement). Washington, DC: Author. doi:10.1016/j.jogn.2018.09.007

Association of Women's Health, Obstetric and Neonatal Nurses. (2019). *Nursing care and management of the second stage of labor* (Evidence-Based Clinical Practice Guideline, 3rd ed.). Washington, DC: Author.

Ayoubi, J. M., Audibert, F., Vial, M., Pons, J. C., Taylor, S., & Frydman, R. (2002). Fetal heart rate and survival of the very premature newborn. *American Journal of Obstetrics & Gynecology, 187*(4), 1026–1030.

Bakker, P. C., Kurver, P. H., Kuik, D. J., & Van Geijn, H. P. (2007). Elevated uterine activity increases the risk of fetal acidosis at birth. *American Journal of Obstetrics & Gynecology, 196*(4), 313.e1–e313.e6. doi:10.1016/j.ajog.2006.11.035

Ball, R. H., & Parer, J. T. (1992). The physiologic mechanism of variable decelerations. *American Journal of Obstetrics & Gynecology, 166*(6, Pt. 1), 1683–1688.

Beard, R. W., Filshie, G. M., Knight, C. A., & Roberts, G. M. (1971). The significance of the changes in the continuous fetal heart rate in the first stage of labour. *Journal of Obstetrics and Gynaecology of the British Commonwealth, 78*(10), 865–881.

Beckmann, C. A., Van Mullem, C., Beckmann, C. R., & Broekhuizen, F. F. (1997). Interpreting fetal heart rate tracings. Is there a difference between labor and delivery nurses and obstetricians? *Journal of Reproductive Medicine, 42*(10), 647–650.

Belfort, M. A., & Clark, S. L. (2017). Computerised cardiotocography—Study design hampers findings. *Lancet, 389*(10080), 1674–1676. doi:10.1016/S0140-6736(17)30762-6

Belfort, M. A., & Saade, G. R. (2011). ST segment analysis (STAN) as an adjunct to electronic fetal monitoring, part II: Clinical studies and future directions. *Clinics in Perinatology, 38*(1), 159–167, vii. doi:10.1016/j.clp.2010.12.010

Belfort, M. A., Saade, G. R., Thom, E., Blackwell, S. C., Reddy, U. M., Thorp, J. M., Jr., . . . VanDorsten, J. P. (2015). A randomized trial of intrapartum fetal ECG ST-segment analysis. *The New England Journal of Medicine, 13*(7), 632–641. doi:10.1056/NEJMoa1500600

Benson, R. C., Shubeck, F., Deutschberger, J., Weiss, W., & Berendes, H. (1968). Fetal heart rate as a predictor of fetal distress. A report from the collaborative project. *Obstetrics & Gynecology, 32*(2), 259–266.

Berkus, M. D., Langer, O., Samueloff, A., Xenakis, E. M., & Field, N. T. (1999). Electronic fetal monitoring: What's reassuring? *Acta Obstetricia et Gynecologica Scandinavica, 78*(1), 15–21.

Blackburn, S. T. (2018). Prenatal period and placental physiology. In S. T. Blackburn (Ed.), *Maternal, fetal, and neonatal physiology: A clinical perspective* (5th ed., pp. 61–114). St. Louis, MO: Elsevier.

Bonafide, C. P., Localio, A. R., Holmes, J. H., Nadkarni, V. M., Stemler, S., MacMurchy, M., . . . Keren, R. (2017). Video analysis of factors associated with response time to physiologic monitor alarms in a children's hospital. *JAMA Pediatrics, 171*(6), 524–531. doi:10.1001/jamapediatrics.2016.5123

Braithwaite, N. D., Milligan, J. E., & Shennan, A. T. (1986). Fetal heart rate monitoring and neonatal mortality in the very preterm infant. *American Journal of Obstetrics & Gynecology, 154*(2), 250–254.

Burrus, D. R., O'Shea, T. M., Jr., Veille, J. C., & Mueller-Heubach, E. (1994). The predictive value of intrapartum fetal heart rate abnormalities in the extremely premature infant. *American Journal of Obstetrics & Gynecology, 171*(4), 1128–1132.

Caldeyro-Barcia, R., Mendez-Bauer, C., Poseiro, J. J., Escarcena, B. S., Pose, S. V., Bieniarz, J., . . . Althabe, O. (1966). Control of human fetal heart rate during labor. In D. E. Cassels (Ed.), *The heart and circulation in the newborn and infant* (pp. 7–36). New York, NY: The Chicago Heart Association/ Grune & Stratton.

Carbonne, B., Benachi, A., Leveque, M. L., Cabrol, D., & Papiernik, E. (1996). Maternal position during labor: Effects on fetal oxygen saturation measured by pulse oximetry. *Obstetrics & Gynecology, 88*(5), 797–800. doi:10.1016/0029 -7844(96)00298-0

CardinalHealth. (n.d.). *Kendall™ fetal spiral electrode system*. Retrieved from https://www.cardinalhealth.com/en/product-solutions /medical/woman-and-baby/labor-and-delivery-essentials/kendall -fetal-spiral-electrode-system.html

Carter, M. C., Corry, M., Delbanco, S., Foster, T. C., Friedland, R., Gabel, R., . . . Simpson, K. R. (2010). 2020 Vision for a high-quality, high-value maternity care system. *Women's Health Issues, 20*(1 Suppl.), S7–S17. doi:10.1016/j.whi.2009.11.006

Chen, H. Y., Chauhan, S. P., Ananth, C. V., Vintzileos, A. M., & Abuhamad, A. Z. (2011). Electronic fetal heart rate monitoring and its relationship to neonatal and infant mortality in the United States. *American Journal of Obstetrics & Gynecology, 204*(6), 491.e1–491.e10. doi:10.1016/j.ajog.2011.04.024

Cibils, L. A. (1976). Clinical significance of fetal heart rate patterns during labor. I. Baseline patterns. *American Journal of Obstetrics & Gynecology, 125*(3), 290–305.

Cibils, L. A. (1996). On intrapartum fetal monitoring. *American Journal of Obstetrics and Gynecology, 174*(4), 1382–1389.

Clark, S. L., Cotton, D. B., Pivarnik, J. M., Lee, W., Hankins, G. D., Benedetti, T. J., & Phelan, J. P. (1991). Position change and central hemodynamic profile during normal third-trimester pregnancy and post partum. *American Journal of Obstetrics & Gynecology, 164*(3), 883–887.

Clark, S. L., Gimovsky, M. L., & Miller, F. C. (1984). The scalp stimulation test: A clinical alternative to fetal scalp blood sampling. *American Journal of Obstetrics & Gynecology, 148*(3), 274–277.

Clark, S. L., Hamilton, E. F., Garite, T. J., Timmons, A., Warrick, P. A., & Smith, S. (2017). The limits of electronic fetal heart rate monitoring in the prevention of neonatal metabolic acidemia. *American Journal of Obstetrics & Gynecology, 216*, 163.e1–163.e6. doi:10.1016/j.ajog.2016.10.009

Clark, S. L., Nageotte, M. P., Garite, T. J., Freeman, R. K., Miller, D. A., Simpson, K. R., . . . Hankins, G. D. V. (2013). Intrapartum management of category II fetal heart tracings: Towards standardization of care. *American Journal of Obstetrics & Gynecology, 209*(2), 89–97. doi:10.1016/j.ajog.2013.04.030

Clark, S. L., Simpson, K. R., Knox, G. E., & Garite, T. J. (2009). Oxytocin: New perspectives on an old drug. *American Journal of Obstetrics & Gynecology, 200*(1), 35.e1–35.e6. doi:10.1016 /j.ajog.2008.06.010

Copel, J. A., Friedman, A. H., & Kleinman, C. S. (1997). Management of fetal cardiac arrhythmias. *Fetal Diagnosis and Therapy, 24*(1), 201–221.

Cramer, M. V. (1906). Ueber die dierkte ableitung der akionsstrome des menschlchen hersens vom oesophagus und uber das elektrokardiogramm des fotus []. *Muenchener Medizinische Wochenschrift, 53*, 811–813.

Dado, L. A. (2011). Anesthesia for the complicated obstetric patient. In M. L. Foley, T. H. Strong, Jr., & T. J. Garite (Eds.), *Obstetric intensive care manual* (3rd ed., pp. 231–246). New York, NY: McGraw-Hill.

Dalton, K. J., Dawes, G. S., & Patrick, J. E. (1977). Diurnal, respiratory, and other rhythms of fetal heart rate in lambs. *American Journal of Obstetrics & Gynecology, 127*(4), 414–424.

Dalton, K. J., Phill, D., Dawes, G. S., & Patrick, J. E. (1983). The autonomic nervous system and fetal heart rate variability. *American Journal of Obstetrics & Gynecology, 146*(4), 456–462.

Dawes, G. S., Visser, G. H., Goodman, J. D., & Levine, D. H. (1981). Numerical analysis of the human fetal heart rate: Modulation by breathing and movement. *American Journal of Obstetrics & Gynecology, 140*(5), 535–544.

Dawood, M. Y. (1995). Pharmacologic stimulation of uterine contraction. *Seminars in Perinatology, 19*(1), 73–83.

Dellinger, E. H., Boehm, F. H., & Crane, M. M. (2000). Electronic fetal heart rate monitoring: Early neonatal outcomes associated with normal rate, fetal stress, and fetal distress. *American Journal of Obstetrics & Gynecology, 182*(1, Pt. 1), 214–220.

Devoe, L. D. (2011a). Electronic fetal monitoring: Does it really lead to better outcomes? *American Journal of Obstetrics & Gynecology, 204*(6), 455–456. doi:10.1016/j.ajog.2011.04.023

Devoe, L. D. (2011b). Fetal ECG analysis for intrapartum electronic fetal monitoring: A review. *Clinical Obstetrics and Gynecology, 54*(1), 56–65. doi:10.1097/GRF.0b013e31820a0ee7

Di Lieto, A., Giani, U., Campanile, M., De Falco, M., Scaramellino, M., & Papa, R. (2003). Conventional and computerized antepartum telecardiotocography. Experienced and inexperienced observers versus computerized analysis. *Gynecologic and Obstetric Investigation, 55*(1), 37–40. doi:10.1159/000068955

Douvas, S. G., Meeks, G. R., Graves, G., Walsh, D. A., & Morrison, J. C. (1984). Intrapartum fetal heart rate monitoring as a predictor of fetal distress and immediate neonatal condition in low-birth weight (less than or equal to 1,800 grams) infants. *American Journal of Obstetrics & Gynecology, 148*(3), 300–302.

Druzin, M. L., Smith, J. F., Gabbe, S. G., & Reed, K. L. (2007). Antepartum fetal evaluation. In S. G. Gabbe, J. R. Niebyl, & J. L. Simpson (Eds.), *Obstetrics: Normal and problem pregnancies* (5th ed., pp. 267–300). Philadelphia, PA: Churchill Livingstone.

Fahey, J., & King, T. L. (2005). Intrauterine asphyxia: Clinical implications for providers of intrapartum care. *Journal of Midwifery & Womens Health, 50*(6), 498–506. doi:10.1016 /j.jmwh.2005.08.007

Fawole, B., & Hofmeyr, G. J. (2012). Maternal oxygen administration for fetal distress. *Cochrane Database of Systematic Reviews,* (12), CD000136. doi:10.1002/14651858.CD000136.pub2

Figueras, F., Albela, S., Bonino, S., Palacio, M., Barrau, E., Hernandez, S., . . . Cararach, V. (2005). Visual analysis of antepartum fetal heart rate tracings: Inter- and intra-observer agreement and impact of knowledge of neonatal outcome. *Journal of Perinatal Medicine, 33*(3), 241–245. doi:10.1515/JPM.2005.044

Fox, M., Kilpatrick, S., King, T., & Parer, J. T. (2000). Fetal heart rate monitoring: Interpretation and collaborative management. *Journal of Midwifery & Women's Health, 45*(6), 498–507.

Fraser, W. D., Hofmeyr, J., Lede, R., Faron, G., Alexander, S., Goffinet, F., . . . Wei, B. (2005). Amnioinfusion for the prevention of the meconium aspiration syndrome. *The New England Journal of Medicine, 353*(9), 909–917. doi:10.1056/NEJMoa050223

Freeman, R. (1990). Intrapartum fetal monitoring: A disappointing story. *The New England Journal of Medicine, 322*(9), 624–626.

Freeman, R. K., Garite, T. J., Nageotte, M. P., & Miller, L. (2012). *Fetal heart rate monitoring* (4th ed.). Philadelphia, PA: Lippincott Williams & Wilkins.

Gallagher, M. W., Costigan, K., & Johnson, T. R. (1992). Fetal heart rate accelerations, fetal movement, and fetal behavior patterns in twin gestations. *American Journal of Obstetrics & Gynecology, 167*(4, Pt. 1), 1140–1144.

Garite, T. J., Dildy, G. A., McNamara, H., Nageotte, M. P., Boehm, F. H., Dellinger, E. H., . . . Swedlow, D. B. (2000). A multicenter controlled trial of fetal pulse oximetry in the intrapartum management of nonreassuring fetal heart rate patterns. *American*

Journal of Obstetrics & Gynecology, 183(5), 1049–1058. doi:10.1067/mob.2000.110632

Garite, T. J., & Simpson, K. R. (2011). Intrauterine resuscitation during labor. *Clinical Obstetrics and Gynecology, 54*(1), 28–39. doi:10.1097/GRF.0b013e31820a062b

Goodlin, R. C. (1979). History of fetal monitoring. *American Journal of Obstetrics & Gynecology, 133*(3), 323–352.

Grether, J. K., & Nelson, K. B. (1997). Maternal infection and cerebral palsy in infants of normal birth weight. *JAMA, 278*(3), 207–211.

Gull, I., Jaffa, A. J., Oren, M., Grisaru, D., Peyser, M. R., & Lessing, J. B. (1996). Acid accumulation during end-stage bradycardia in term fetuses: How long is too long? *British Journal of Obstetrics and Gynaecology, 103*(11), 1096–1101.

Hammacher, K. (1969). The clinical significance of cardiotocography. In P. Huntingford, K. Huter, & E. Salez (Eds.), *Perinatal medicine: 1st European Congress, Berlin* (p. 81). New York, NY: Academic Press.

Hannaford, K. E., Stout, M. J., Smyser, C. D., Mathur, A., & Cahill, A. G. (2016). Evaluating the sensitivity of electronic fetal monitoring patterns for the prediction of intraventricular hemorrhage. *American Journal of Perinatology, 33*(14), 1420–1425. doi:10.1055/s-0036-1584140

Haruta, M., Funato, T., Sumida, T., & Shinkai, T. (1984). The influence of maternal oxygen inhalation for 30 to 60 minutes on fetal oxygenation. *Nippon Sanka Fujinka Gakkai Zasshi. Acta Obstetrica et Gynaecologica Japonica, 36*(10), 1921–1929.

Haydon, M. L., Gorenberg, D. M., Nageotte, M. P., Ghamsary, M., Rumney, P. J., Patillo, C., & Garite, T. J. (2006). The effect of maternal oxygen administration on fetal pulse oximetry during labor in fetuses with nonreassuring fetal heart rate patterns. *American Journal of Obstetrics & Gynecology, 195*(3), 735–738. doi:10.1016/j.ajog.2006.06.084

Holmes, P., Oppenheimer, L. W., Gravelle, A., Walker, M., & Blayney, M. (2001). The effect of variable heart rate decelerations on intraventricular hemorrhage and other perinatal outcomes in preterm infants. *Journal of Maternal-Fetal Medicine, 10*(4), 264–268.

Holmgren, C., Scott, J. R., Porter, T. F., Esplin, M. S., & Bardaley, T. (2012). Uterine rupture with attempted vaginal birth after cesarean delivery: Decision-to-delivery time and neonatal outcome. *Obstetrics & Gynecology, 119*(4), 725–731. doi:10.1097/AOG .0b013e318249a1d7

Hon, E. H. (1958). The electronic evaluation of the fetal heart rate: Preliminary report. *American Journal of Obstetrics & Gynecology, 75*(6), 1215–1230.

Hon, E. (1963). The classification of fetal heart rate. I. A revised working classification. *Obstetrics & Gynecology, 22*(2), 137–146.

INFANT Collaborative Group. (2017). Computerised interpretation of fetal heart rate during labour (INFANT): A randomized controlled trial. *Lancet, 389*(10080), 1719–1729. doi:10.1016 /S0140-6736(17)30568-8

Jackson, M., Holmgren, C. M., Esplin, M. S., Henry, E., & Varner, M. W. (2011). Frequency of fetal heart rate categories and short-term neonatal outcome. *Obstetrics & Gynecology, 118*(4), 803–808. doi:10.1097/AOG.0b013e31822f1b50

Joint Commission on Accreditation of Healthcare Organizations. (2004). *Preventing infant death and injury during delivery* (Sentinel Event Alert No. 30). Oakbrook Terrace, IL: Author.

Jozwik, M., Sledziewski, A., Klubowicz, Z., Zak, J., Sajewska, G., & Pietrzycki, B. (2000). Use of oxygen therapy during labour and acid-base status in the newborn. *Medycyna Wieku Rozwojowego, 4*(4), 403–411.

Kennedy, E. (1843). Audible evidences of pregnancy. In *Observations on obstetric auscultation: With an analysis of the evidences of pregnancy and an inquiry into the proofs of the life and death of the foetus in utero* (pp. 71–146). New York, NY: J. & H. G. Langley. (Original work published 1833)

Killion, M. M. (2015). Techniques for fetal heart and uterine activity assessment. In A. Lyndon & L. U. Ali (Eds.), *Fetal heart monitoring: Principles and practices* (5th ed., pp. 85–121). Washington,

DC: Association of Women's Health, Obstetric and Neonatal Nurses/Kendall Hunt.

King, T. L. (2018). Fetal assessment. In S. T. Blackburn (Ed.), *Maternal, fetal, and neonatal physiology: A clinical perspective* (5th ed., pp. 162–179). St. Louis, MO: Elsevier.

King, T., & Parer, J. (2000). The physiology of fetal heart rate patterns and perinatal asphyxia. *Journal of Perinatal & Neonatal Nursing, 14*(3), 19–39, 102–103.

Kisilevsky, B. S., Hains, S. M., & Low, J. A. (2001). Maturation of fetal heart rate and body movement in 24-33-week-old fetuses threatening to deliver prematurely. *Developmental Psychobiology, 38*(1), 78–86. doi:10.1002/1098-2302(2001)38:1<78::AID -DEV7>3.0.CO

Kleinman, C. S., & Nehgme, R. A. (2004). Cardiac arrhythmias in the human fetus. *Pediatric Cardiology, 25*(3), 234–251. doi:10.1007/s00246-003-0589-x

Kleinman, C. S., Nehgme, R., & Copel, J. A. (2004). Fetal cardiac arrhythmias. In R. K. Creasy & R. Resnick (Eds.), *Maternal-fetal medicine* (5th ed., pp. 465–482). Philadelphia, PA: W. B. Saunders.

Knox, G. E., & Simpson, K. R. (2011). Perinatal high reliability. *American Journal of Obstetrics & Gynecology, 204*(5), 373–377. doi:10.1016/j.ajog.2010.10.900

Lee, C. Y., Di Loreto, P. C., & O'Lane, J. M. (1975). A study of fetal heart rate acceleration patterns. *Obstetrics & Gynecology, 45*(2), 142–146.

Lent, M. (1999). The medical and legal risks of the electronic fetal monitor. *Stanford Law Review, 51*(4), 807–837.

Leung, A. S., Leung, E. K., & Paul, R. H. (1993). Uterine rupture after previous cesarean delivery: Maternal and fetal consequences. *American Journal of Obstetrics & Gynecology, 169*(4), 945–950.

Leveno, K. J., Quirk, J. G., Jr., Cunningham, F. G., Nelson, S. D., Santos-Ramos, R., Toofanian, A., & DePalma, R. T. (1984). Prolonged pregnancy. I. Observations concerning the causes of fetal distress. *American Journal of Obstetrics & Gynecology, 150*(5), 465–473.

Liston, R., Sawchuck, D., & Young, D. (2018). No. 197b-Fetal Health Surveillance: Intrapartum consensus guideline. *Journal of Obstetrics and Gynaecology Canada, 40*(4), e298–e322.

Low, J. A., Galbraith, R. S., Muir, D. W., Killen, H. L., Pater, E. A., & Karchmar, E. J. (1992). Mortality and morbidity after intrapartum asphyxia in the preterm fetus. *Obstetrics & Gynecology, 80*(1), 57–61.

Low, J. A., Lindsay, B. G., & Derrick, E. J. (1997). Threshold of metabolic acidosis associated with newborn complications. *American Journal of Obstetrics and Gynecology, 177*(6), 1391–1394.

Low, J. A., Victory, R., & Derrick, E. J. (1999). Predictive value of electronic fetal monitoring for intrapartum fetal asphyxia with metabolic acidosis. *Obstetrics & Gynecology, 93*(2), 285–291.

Lunshof, M. S., Boer, K., Wolf, H., Koppen, S., Velderman, J. K., & Mulder, E. J. (2005). Short-term (0-48 h) effects of maternal betamethasone administration on fetal heart rate and its variability. *Pediatric Research, 57*(4), 545–549. doi:10.1203 /01.PDR.0000155948.83570.EB

Lyndon, A., & Ali, L. U. (Eds.). (2015). *Fetal heart monitoring: Principles and practices* (5th ed.). Washington, DC: Association of Women's Health, Obstetric and Neonatal Nursing/Kendall Hunt.

Lyndon, A., O'Brien-Abel, N., & Simpson, K. R. (2015). Fetal heart rate interpretation. In A. Lyndon & L. U. Ali (Eds.), *Fetal heart monitoring: Principles and practices* (5th ed., pp. 125–162). Washington, DC: Association of Women's Health, Obstetric and Neonatal Nurses/Kendall Hunt.

Lyndon, A., Zlatnik, M. G., & Wachter, R. M. (2011). Effective physician-nurse communication: A patient safety essential for labor and delivery. *American Journal of Obstetrics & Gynecology, 205*(2), 91–96. doi:10.1016/j.ajog.2011.04.021

MacDonald, D. (1996). Cerebral palsy and intrapartum fetal monitoring. *The New England Journal of Medicine, 334*(10), 659–660. doi:10.1056/NEJM199603073341011

MacDonald, D., Grant, A., Sheridan-Pereira, M., Boylan, P., & Chalmers, I. (1985). The Dublin randomized controlled trial of intrapartum fetal heart rate monitoring. *American Journal of Obstetrics & Gynecology, 152*(5), 524–539.

Macones, G. A., Hankins, G. D., Spong, C. Y., Hauth, J., & Moore, T. (2008). The 2008 National Institute of Child Health and Human Development Workshop report on electronic fetal monitoring: Update on definitions, interpretation, and research guidelines. *Journal of Obstetric, Gynecologic, and Neonatal Nursing, 37*(5), 510–515. doi:10.1111/j.1552-6909.2008.00284.x and *Obstetrics & Gynecology, 112*(3), 661–666. doi:10.1097/AOG.0b013e3181841395

Manseau, P., Vaquier, J., Chavinie, J., & Sureau, C. (1972). Sinusoidal fetal cardiac rhythm. An aspect evocative of fetal distress during pregnancy. *Journal de Gynecologie, Obstetrique et Biologie de la Reproduction, 1*(4), 343–352.

Martin, C. B., Jr. (1978). Regulation of the fetal heart rate and genesis of FHR patterns. *Seminars in Perinatology, 2*(2), 131–146.

Martin, C. B., Jr. (1998). Electronic fetal monitoring: A brief summary of its development, problems and prospects. *European Journal of Obstetrics, Gynecology, and Reproductive Biology, 78*(2), 133–140.

Martis, R., Emilia, O., Nurdiati, D. S., & Brown, J. (2017). Intermitent auscultataion (IA) of the fetal heart rate in labour for fetal well-being. *Cochrane Database of Systematic Reviews*, (2), CD008680. doi:10.1002/14651858.CD008680.pub2

Matsuda, Y., Maeda, T., & Kouno, S. (2003). The critical period of non-reassuring fetal heart rate patterns in preterm gestation. *European Journal of Obstetrics, Gynecology, and Reproductive Biology, 106*(1), 36–39.

McNamara, H., Johnson, N., & Lilford, R. (1993). The effect on fetal arteriolar oxygen saturation resulting from giving oxygen to the mother measured by pulse oximetry. *British Journal of Obstetrics and Gynaecology, 100*(5), 446–449.

Miller, L. A. (2005). System errors in intrapartum electronic fetal monitoring: A case review. *Journal of Midwifery & Women's Health, 50*(6), 507–516. doi:10.1016/j.jmwh.2004.09.012

Miller, L. A. (2016). The more things change, the more they stay the same: Thirty years of fetal monitoring in perspective. *Journal of Perinatal and Neonatal Nursing, 30*(2), 255–258. doi:10.1097/JPN.0000000000000180

Miller, L. A. (2017). Education, competency, certification, credentialing: What's the difference? *Journal of Perinatal & Neonatal Nursing, 31*(2), 101–103. doi:10.1097/JPN.0000000000000249

Miller, L. A. (2018). Uterine activity: What you don't know can hurt you. *MCN: The American Journal of Maternal Child Nursing, 43*(3), 180. doi:10.1097/NMC.0000000000000431

Miller, L. A., & Miller, D. A. (2013). A collaborative interdisciplinary approach to electronic fetal monitoring: Report of a statewide initiative. *Journal of Perinatal & Neonatal Nursing, 27*(2), 126–133. doi:10.1097/JPN.0b013e31828ee7fe

Miller, L. A., Miller, D. A., & Cypher, R. L. (2017). *Mosby's pocket guide to fetal monitoring: A disciplinary approach* (8th ed.). St. Louis: Elsevier.

Mino, M., Puertas, A., Miranda, J. A., & Herruzo, A. J. (1999). Amnioinfusion in term labor with low amniotic fluid due to rupture of membranes: A new indication. *European Journal of Obstetrics, Gynecology, and Reproductive Biology, 82*(1), 29–34.

Miyazaki, F. S., & Nevarez, F. (1985). Saline amnioinfusion for relief of repetitive variable decelerations: A prospective randomized study. *American Journal of Obstetrics & Gynecology, 153*(3), 301–306.

Modanlou, H. D., & Murata, Y. (2004). Sinusoidal heart rate pattern: Reappraisal of its definition and clinical significance. *Journal of Obstetrics and Gynaecology Research, 30*(3), 169–180. doi:10.1111/j.1447-0756.2004.00186.x

Moore, K. L., Persaud, T. V. N., & Torchia, M. G. (2016). *The developing human: Clinically oriented embryology* (10th ed.). Philadelphia, PA: Elsevier.

National Institute for Health and Care Excellence. (2014). *Intrapartum care for healthy women and babies*. London, UK: Author.

National Institute of Child Health and Human Development Research Planning Workshop. (1997). Electronic fetal heart rate monitoring: Research guidelines for interpretation. *American Journal of Obstetrics & Gynecology, 177*(6), 1385–1390, and *Journal of Obstetric Gynecology and Neonatal Nursing, 26*(6), 635–640. doi:10.1016/S0002-9378(97)70079-6

Neilson, D. R., Jr., Freeman, R. K., & Mangan, S. (2008). Signal ambiguity resulting in unexpected outcome with external fetal heart rate monitoring. *American Journal of Obstetrics & Gynecology, 198*(6), 717–724. doi:10.1016/j.ajog.2008.02.030

Neilson, J. P. (2015). Fetal electrocardiogram (ECG) for fetal monitoring during labour. *Cochrane Database of Systematic Reviews*, (12), CD000116. doi:10.1002/14651858.CD000116.pub5

Nelson, K. B. (1988). What proportion of cerebral palsy is related to birth asphyxia? *Journal of Pediatrics, 112*(4), 572–574.

Nelson, K. B., Dambrosia, J. M., Ting, T. Y., & Grether, J. K. (1996). Uncertain value of electronic fetal monitoring in predicting cerebral palsy. *The New England Journal of Medicine, 334*(10), 613–618. doi:10.1056/NEJM199603073341001

Nelson, K. B., & Grether, J. K. (1999). Causes of cerebral palsy. *Current Opinion in Pediatrics, 11*(6), 487–491.

Nunes, I., Ayres-de-Campos, D., Ugwumadu, A., Amin, P., Banfield, P., Nicoll, A., . . . Bernardes, J. (2017). Central fetal monitoring with and without computer analysis: A randomized controlled trial. *Obstetrics & Gynecology, 129*(1), 83–90. doi:10.1097/AOG.0000000000001799

O'Brien-Abel, N. (2015). Physiologic basis for fetal monitoring. In A. Lyndon & L. U. Ali (Eds.), *Fetal heart monitoring: Principles and practices* (5th ed., pp. 23–47). Washington, DC: Association of Women's Health, Obstetric and Neonatal Nurses/Kendall Hunt.

O'Brien-Abel, N. E., & Benedetti, T. J. (1992). Saltatory fetal heart rate pattern. *Journal of Perinatology, 12*(1), 13–17.

Paine, C. W., Goel, V. V., Ely, E., Stave, C. D., Stemler, S., Zander, M., & Bonafide, C. P. (2016). Systematic review of physiologic monitor alarm characteristics and pragmatic interventions to reduce alarm frequency. *Journal of Hospital Medicine, 11*(2), 136–144. doi:10.1002/jhm.2520

Paneth, N., Bommarito, M., & Stricker, J. (1993). Electronic fetal monitoring and later outcome. *Clinical and Investigative Medicine. Medecine Clinique et Experimentale, 16*(2), 159–165.

Parer, J. T. (1997). *Handbook of fetal heart rate monitoring* (2nd ed.). Philadelphia, PA: W. B. Saunders.

Parer, J. T., Dijkstra, H. R., Vredebregt, P. P., Harris, J. L., Krueger, T. R., & Reuss, M. L. (1980). Increased fetal heart rate variability with acute hypoxia in chronically instrumented sheep. *European Journal of Obstetrics, Gynecology, and Reproductive Biology, 10*(6), 393–399.

Parer, J. T., & Ikeda, T. (2007). A framework for standardized management of intrapartum fetal heart rate patterns. *American Journal of Obstetrics & Gynecology, 197*(1), 26.e1–26.e6. doi:10.1016/j.ajog.2007.03.037

Parer, J. T., & King, T. (2000). Fetal heart rate monitoring: Is it salvageable? *American Journal of Obstetrics & Gynecology, 182*(4), 982–987.

Parer, J. T., King, T., Flanders, S., Fox, M., & Kilpatrick, S. J. (2006). Fetal acidemia and electronic fetal heart rate patterns: Is there evidence of an association? *Journal of Maternal Fetal and Neonatal Medicine, 19*(5), 289–294. doi:10.1080/14767050500526172

Paul, R. H., Suidan, A. K., Yeh, S., Schifrin, B. S., & Hon, E. H. (1975). Clinical fetal monitoring. VII: The evaluation and significance of intrapartum baseline FHR variability. *American Journal of Obstetrics & Gynecology, 123*(2), 206–210.

Phaneuf, S., Rodriguez Linares, B., TambyRaja, R. L., MacKenzie, I. Z., & Lopez Bernal, A. (2000). Loss of myometrial oxytocin receptors during oxytocin-induced and oxytocin-augmented labour. *Journal of Reproduction and Fertility, 120*(1), 91–97.

Porter, T. F., & Clark, S. L. (1999). Vibroacoustic and scalp stimulation. *Obstetrics and Gynecology Clinics of North America, 26*(4), 657–669.

Quinn, K. H., Cao, C. T., Lacoursiere, D. Y., & Schrimmer, D. (2011). Monoamniotic twin pregnancy: Continuous inpatient electronic fetal monitoring—An impossible goal? *American Journal of Obstetrics & Gynecology, 204*(2), 161.e1–161.e6. doi:10.1016/j.ajog.2010.08.044

Roberts, J. E. (2002). The "push" for evidence: Management of the second stage. *Journal of Midwifery and Women's Health, 47*(1), 2–15.

Sakala, C., Declercq, E. R., Turon, J. M., & Corry, M. P. (2018). *Listening to mothers in California: A population-based survey of women's childbearing experiences, full survey report.* Washington, DC: National Partnership for Women & Families.

Senat, M. V., Minoui, S., Multon, O., Fernandez, H., Frydman, R., & Ville, Y. (1998). Effect of dexamethasone and betamethasone on fetal heart rate variability in preterm labour: A randomised study. *British Journal of Obstetrics and Gynaecology, 105*(7), 749–755.

Sherer, D. M., D'Amico, M. L., Cox, C., Metlay, L. A., & Woods, J. R., Jr. (1994). Association of in utero behavioral patterns of twins with each other as indicated by fetal heart rate reactivity and nonreactivity. *American Journal of Perinatology, 11*(3), 208–212. doi:10.1055/s-2008-1040747

Sherer, D. M., Nawrocki, M. N., Peco, N. E., Metlay, L. A., & Woods, J. R., Jr. (1990). The occurrence of simultaneous fetal heart rate accelerations in twins during nonstress testing. *Obstetrics & Gynecology, 76*(5, Pt. 1), 817–821.

Shields, L. E., Wiesner, S., Klein, C., Pelletreau, B., & Hedriana, H. L. (2018). A standardized approach for category II fetal heart rate with significant decelerations: Maternal and neonatal outcomes. *American Journal of Perinatology, 35*(14), 1405–1410. doi:10.1055/s-0038-1660459

Shy, K. K., Luthy, D. A., Bennett, F. C., Whitfield, M., Larson, E. B., van Belle, G., . . . Stenchever, M. A. (1990). Effects of electronic fetal-heart-rate monitoring, as compared with periodic auscultation, on the neurologic development of premature infants. *The New England Journal of Medicine, 322*(9), 588–593. doi:10.1056/NEJM199003013220904

Simon, V. B., Fong, A., & Nageotte, M. P. (2018). Supplemental oxygen study: A randomized controlled study on the effect of maternal oxygen supplementation during planned cesarean delivery on umbilical cord gases. *American Journal of Perinatology, 35*(1), 84–89. doi:10.1055/s-0037-1606184

Simpson, K. R. (1997). Electronic fetal heart rate monitoring: A primer for the critical care nurse. *AACN Clinical Issues, 8*(4), 516–523.

Simpson, K. R. (2005a). The context and clinical evidence for common nursing practices during labor. *MCN: The American Journal of Maternal Child Nursing, 30*(6), 356–363.

Simpson, K. R. (2005b). Failure to rescue: Implications for evaluating quality of care during labor and birth. *Journal of Perinatal and Neonatal Nursing, 19*(1), 24–34.

Simpson, K. R. (2007). Intrauterine resuscitation during labor: Review of current methods and supportive evidence. *Journal of Midwifery & Women's Health, 52*(3), 229–237. doi:10.1016/j.jmwh.2006.12.010

Simpson, K. R. (2008). Intrauterine resuscitation during labor: Should maternal oxygen administration be a first-line measure? *Seminars in Fetal and Neonatal Medicine, 13*(6), 362–367. doi:10.1016/j.siny.2008.04.016

Simpson, K. R. (2011). Avoiding confusion of maternal heart rate with fetal heart rate during labor. *MCN: The American Journal of Maternal Child Nursing, 36*(4), 272. doi:10.1097/NMC.0b013e318217a61a

Simpson, K. R. (2020). *Cervical ripening & induction & augmentation of labor* (5th ed.). Washington, DC: Association of Women's Health, Obstetric and Neonatal Nurses.

Simpson, K. R. (2015). Physiologic interventions for fetal heart rate patterns. In A. Lyndon & L. U. Ali (Eds.), *Fetal heart monitoring: Principles and practices* (5th ed., pp. 163–189). Washington, DC: Association of Women's Health, Obstetric and Neonatal Nurses/Kendall Hunt.

Simpson, K. R., & James, D. C. (2005a). Effects of immediate versus delayed pushing during second-stage labor on fetal well-being: A randomized clinical trial. *Nursing Research, 54*(3),149–157.

Simpson, K. R., & James, D. C. (2005b). Efficacy of intrauterine resuscitation techniques in improving fetal oxygen status during labor. *Obstetrics & Gynecology, 105*(6), 1362–1368. doi:10.1097/01.AOG.0000164474.03350.7c

Simpson, K. R., & James, D. C. (2008). Effects of oxytocin-induced uterine hyperstimulation during labor on fetal oxygen status and fetal heart rate patterns. *American Journal of Obstetrics & Gynecology,199*(1), 34.e1–34.5. doi:10.1016/j.ajog.2007.12.015

Simpson, K. R., James, D. C., & Knox, G. E. (2006). Nurse-physician communication during labor and birth: Implications for patient safety. *Journal of Obstetric, Gynecologic & Neonatal Nursing, 35*(4), 547–556. doi:10.1111/j.1552-6909.2006.00075.x

Simpson, K. R., & Knox, G. E. (2000). Risk management and electronic fetal monitoring: Decreasing risk of adverse outcomes and liability exposure. *Journal of Perinatal and Neonatal Nursing, 14*(3), 40–52.

Simpson, K. R., & Knox, G. E. (2006). Essential criteria to promote safe care during labor and birth. *AWHONN Lifelines, 9*(6), 478–483.

Simpson, K. R., & Knox, G. E. (2009). Communication of fetal heart monitoring information. In A. Lyndon & L. U. Ali (Eds.), *Fetal heart monitoring: Principles and practices* (4th ed., pp. 177–209). Washington, DC: Association of Women's Health, Obstetric and Neonatal Nurses/Kendall Hunt.

Simpson, K. R., & Lyndon, A. (2009). Clinical disagreements during labor and birth: How does real life compare to best practice? *MCN: The American Journal of Maternal Child Nursing, 34*(1), 31–39. doi:10.1097/01.NMC.0000343863.72237.2b

Simpson, K. R., & Lyndon, A. (2019). False alarms and overmonitoring: Major factors in alarm fatigue among labor nurses. *Journal of Nursing Care Quality, 34*(1), 66–72. doi:10.1097/NCQ.0000000000000335

Simpson, K. R., Lyndon, A., & Davidson, L. A. (2016). Patient safety implications of electronic alerts and alarms of maternal–fetal status during labor. *Nursing for Women's Health, 20*(4), 358–366. doi:10.1016/j.nwh.2016.07.004

Simpson, K. R., & Miller, L. (2011). Assessment and optimization of uterine activity during labor. *Clinical Obstetrics and Gynecology, 54*(1), 40–49.

Sklansky, M. (2009). Fetal cardiac malformations and arrhythmias. In R. K. Creasy & R. Resnick (Eds.), *Maternal-fetal medicine* (6th ed., pp. 305–345). Philadelphia, PA: Saunders.

Skupski, D. W., Rosenberg, C. R., & Eglinton, G. S. (2002). Intrapartum fetal stimulation tests: A meta-analysis. *Obstetrics & Gynecology, 99*(1), 129–134.

Spong, C. Y. (2008). Electronic fetal heart rate monitoring: another look. *Obstetrics & Gynecology, 112*(3), 506–507. doi:10.1097/AOG.0b013e318185f872

Subtil, D., Tiberghien, P., Devos, P., Therby, D., Leclerc, G., Vaast, P., & Puech, F. (2003). Immediate and delayed effects of antenatal corticosteroids on fetal heart rate: A randomized trial that compares betamethasone acetate and phosphate, betamethasone phosphate, and dexamethasone. *American Journal of Obstetrics & Gynecology, 188*(2), 524–531.

Sureau, C. (1996). Historical perspectives: Forgotten past, unpredictable future. *Baillieres Clinical Obstetrics and Gynaecology, 10*(2), 167–184.

Thacker, S. B., Stroup, D. F., & Peterson, H. B. (1995). Efficacy and safety of intrapartum electronic fetal monitoring: An update. *Obstetrics & Gynecology, 86*(4, Pt. 1), 613–620.

Thorp, J. A., Trobough, T., Evans, R., Hedrick, J., & Yeast, J. D. (1995). The effect of maternal oxygen administration during the second stage of labor on umbilical cord blood gas values: A randomized controlled prospective trial. *American Journal of Obstetrics & Gynecology, 172*(2, Pt. 1), 465–474.

To, W. W., & Leung, W. C. (1998). The incidence of abnormal findings from intrapartum cardiotocogram monitoring in term and preterm labours. *Australian and New Zealand Journal of Obstetrics and Gynaecology, 38*(3), 258–261.

U.S. Food and Drug Administration. (2009). *Safety alert: Phillips avalon fetal monitors (Safety alerts for human medical products). MedWatch: The FDA Safety Information and Adverse Event Reporting Program* Washington, DC; Author.

Vintzileos, A. M., Antsaklis, A., Varvarigos, I., Papas, C., Sofatzis, I., & Montgomery, J. T. (1993). A randomized trial of intrapartum electronic fetal heart rate monitoring versus intermittent auscultation. *Obstetrics & Gynecology, 81*(6), 899–907.

Westgren, M., Holmquist, P., Svenningsen, N. W., & Ingemarsson, I. (1982). Intrapartum fetal monitoring in preterm deliveries: Prospective study. *Obstetrics & Gynecology, 60*(1), 99–106.

Westgren, M., Hormquist, P., Ingemarsson, I., & Svenningsen, N. (1984). Intrapartum fetal acidosis in preterm infants: Fetal monitoring and long-term morbidity. *Obstetrics & Gynecology, 63*(3), 355–359.

Westgren, M., Malcus, P., & Svenningsen, N. W. (1986). Intrauterine asphyxia and long-term outcome in preterm fetuses. *Obstetrics & Gynecology, 67*(4), 512–516.

Wisner, K., & Holschuh, C. (2018). *Fetal heart rate auscultation* (3rd ed.). Washington, DC: Association of Women's Health, Obstetric and Neonatal Nurses.

Wolfberg, A. J., Derosier, D. J., Roberts, T., Syed, Z., Clifford, G. D., Acker, D., & Plessis, A. D. (2008). A comparison of subjective and mathematical estimations of fetal heart rate variability. *Journal of Maternal Fetal and Neonatal Medicine, 21*(2), 101–104. doi:10.1080/14767050701836792

Wright, J. W., Ridgway, L. E., Wright, B. D., Covington, D. L., & Bobitt, J. R. (1996). Effect of MgSO4 on heart rate monitoring in the preterm fetus. *Journal of Reproductive Medicine, 41*(8), 605–608.

Wright, R. G., Shnider, S. M., Levinson, G., Rolbin, S. H., & Parer, J. T. (1981). The effect of maternal administration of ephedrine on fetal heart rate and variability. *Obstetrics & Gynecology, 57*(6), 734–738.

Xu, H., Mas-Calvet, M., Wei, S. Q., Luo, Z. C., & Fraser, W. D. (2009). Abnormal fetal heart rate tracing patterns in patients with thick meconium staining of the amniotic fluid: Association with perinatal outcomes. *American Journal of Obstetrics & Gynecology, 200*(3), 283.e1–283.e7. doi:10.1016/j.ajog.2008.08.043

Yang, M., Stout, M. J., López, J. D., Colvin, R., Macones, G. A., & Cahill, A. G. (2017). Association of fetal heart rate baseline changes and neonatal outcomes. *American Journal of Perinatology, 34*(9), 879–886. doi:10.1055/s-0037-1600911

Zanini, B., Paul, R. H., & Huey, J. R. (1980). Intrapartum fetal heart rate: Correlation with scalp pH in the preterm fetus. *American Journal of Obstetrics & Gynecology, 136*(1), 43–47. doi:10.1016/0002-9378(80)90562-1

Zeeman, G. G., Khan-Dawood, F. S., & Dawood, M. Y. (1997). Oxytocin and its receptor in pregnancy and parturition: Current concepts and clinical implications. *Obstetrics & Gynecology, 89*(5, Pt. 2), 873–883.

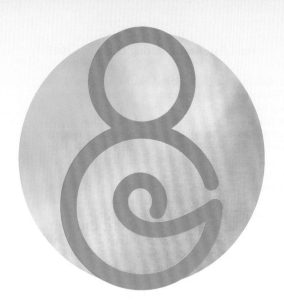

CHAPTER 16

Pain in Labor: Nonpharmacologic and Pharmacologic Management

Carol Burke

INTRODUCTION

A woman's experience of pain in labor and satisfaction with the birth process is multifaceted, multidimensional, individualistic, and unique (Bossano, Townsend, Walton, Blomquist, & Handa, 2017). Labor is a normal, physiologic process that causes a paradoxical experience of severe pain for most women. For most women in all societies and cultures, natural childbirth is likely to be one of the most painful events in their lifetime (Lowe, 2002). This severe pain may lead to emotional distress and suffering mediated by fear and anxiety. Numerous variables influence whether or not suffering occurs including supportive presence of significant others and prior traumatic experiences. An appreciation of each woman's unique experience of pain is possible when the nurse understands the physiologic, psychological, emotional, social, and cultural factors influencing pain perception (Johnson, 2016). This chapter focuses on the physiologic basis for pain, psychosocial factors influencing pain perception, recent trends in labor pain assessment, management, and nursing care using both nonpharmacologic and pharmacologic methods. Nursing care is focused on acute assessment and enabling optimal comfort tailored to the woman's needs throughout the labor and recovery process. Pain in labor is a symptom not easily defined or simple to assess (Roberts, Gulliver, Fisher, & Cloyes, 2010). During labor, responsibility for managing pain and providing comfort is shared by the laboring woman, nurses, physicians, certified nurse midwives (CNMs), and labor support persons. A continuum of interventions from nonpharmacologic to pharmacologic exist, with an increasing potential for complications and side effects with progression. A variety of nonpharmacologic and pharmacologic methods can be used to help women cope with the pain of labor (American College of Obstetricians and Gynecologists [ACOG], 2019a; Association of Women's Health, Obstetric and Neonatal Nurses [AWHONN], 2018).

The goal of pain management during labor is to assist the woman in managing her pain without interrupting labor or doing harm to the woman, her fetus, or her newborn. Approaches to pain management in childbirth are multidimensional; addressing the sensory, affective, cognitive, and behavioral dimensions of pain (Lowe, 2002; Wesselmann, 2008). A systematic review of low-risk women in labor found that four factors were critical to women's experience of childbirth: (1) personal expectations, (2) the amount of support from caregivers, (3) the quality of the caregiver–woman relationship, and (4) personal involvement in decision making (Hodnett, Gates, Hofmeyr, & Sakala, 2013). The birth experience leaves a long-lasting impression on women (Bossano et al., 2017).

PHYSIOLOGIC BASIS FOR PAIN

Most pain during childbirth results from normal physiologic events. During the first stage of labor, visceral pain results from uterine contractions leading to uterine muscle hypoxia; lactic acid accumulation; cervical and lower uterine segment stretching; traction on ovaries, fallopian tubes, and uterine ligaments; and pressure on the bony pelvis. Afferent pain impulses are carried along sympathetic nerve fibers entering the neuraxis between the 10th and 12th thoracic and first lumbar spinal segments. An additional somatic component arises from perineal stretching and pressure on the urethra, bladder, and rectum causing afferent pain impulses to fire late in the first stage and persist throughout the second stage. Contraction pain is mediated by mechanical distension of the lower uterine segment and cervix. In addition to pain associated with uterine contractions, descent of the fetal head may cause pressure on the roots of the lumbosacral plexus and other structures to cause pain in the thighs, legs, vagina, perineum, and rectum. This pain is transmitted along the pudendal nerve carried along sympathetic nerve fibers entering the neuraxis between the second and fourth sacral spinal segments (El-Wahab & Robinson, 2011). Some women in labor experience continuous low-back pain that is distinct from uterine contractions. This pain may be related to pressure from the fetal occipital bone on the neural plexus and bony structures of the maternal spine and pelvis. In comparison, the third stage is usually not particularly painful.

Physiologic Responses to Pain

Pain during labor may result in anxiety and a stress response. Pain induces a sympathetic stress response that can precipitate widespread physiologic and potentially adverse effects on the progress of labor and the well-being of the mother and fetus. Unrelieved anxiety and stress cause increased production of cortisol, glucagon, and catecholamines, which increase metabolism and oxygen consumption (Hawkins, 2010; Reynolds, 2011). Labor pain has an indirect effect on the fetus due to the reduction in uteroplacental perfusion. Increased levels of catecholamines have been shown to cause uterine hypoperfusion and decreased blood flow to the placenta, resulting in uterine irritability, preterm labor, dystocia, and decreased fetal oxygenation (Gonzalez, Gaurav, & Ihab, 2016; Wesselmann, 2008). The release of epinephrine from the stress response leads to uterine artery vasoconstriction, which may prolong labor through beta-receptor–mediated uterine relaxation leading to a tocolytic effect (Wesselmann, 2008). Increased maternal heart rate and blood pressure is partly in response to pain and partly due to uterine contractions causing an increase

in central volume. Both will cause a rise in cardiac output increasing myocardial workload and oxygen demand. During labor, painful stress causes an increase in minute ventilation resulting in maternal hypocapnia. While these responses may be innocuous during the course of an uncomplicated labor, they can compromise uteroplacental circulation or precipitate heart failure and even ischemia in women with poor cardiorespiratory reserve (El-Wahab & Robinson, 2011). Cortisol output is activated by mental negative stress such as fear, anxiety, depression, and lack of control. Table 16–1 lists the physiologic and psychosocial responses to pain. It has been suggested that postnatal depression may be less common among women who receive effective analgesia in labor (Flink, Mroczek, Sullivan, & Linton, 2009). Communication, shared understanding of the labor plan, empowerment, and greater patient knowledge may influence health outcome and modulate the physiologic response.

The Experience of Pain

Unique circumstances of every labor influence the experience of pain. Responsiveness of the cervix to uterine contractions is influenced by prior surgical or diagnostic procedures that compromise the integrity of the cervix. Prior surgical procedures may result in cervical injury and shorter labor or cause scarring and adhesions, resulting in failure to dilate and protract labor. Many medical and nursing procedures are uncomfortable. Interventions such as placement of an intravenous (IV) catheter, continuous application of an automatic blood pressure cuff, pharmacologic agents used for cervical ripening, induction and augmentation of labor, vaginal examinations, bed rest, amniotomy, and external electronic fetal monitor (EFM) belts may change the character of labor contractions and increase discomfort. Length of labor does not necessarily correlate directly with a woman's perception of pain. Women with precipitous labor may experience very intense pain due to frequent uterine contractions. Women with a fetus in

TABLE 16–1. Physiologic and Psychosocial Response to Labor Pain

Maternal organ	Response to pain in labor	Effect on mother/fetus
Heart and vasculature	Increase in systemic vascular resistance and increased cardiac output	Decreased uteroplacental perfusion
Lung	Increase in minute ventilation, hyperventilation leads to increased oxygen consumption → maternal hypocarbia and transient hypoxemia → respiratory alkalosis	Decreased O_2 offloading to the fetus leading to fetal hypoxemia and fetal acidemia
Uterus	Uncoordinated uterine contraction pattern and tocolytic effect; uterine artery vasoconstriction	Prolonged labor
Endocrine	Increased cortisol levels	Inhibits lactation
Gastrointestinal	Increased gastrin secretion and decrease gastrointestinal motility	Increased risk of aspiration
Psychosocial effect	Fear, anxiety, depression	Anxiety with future pregnancies

O_2, oxygen.

a persistent posterior position report severe back pain during and between uterine contractions.

As duration of intense pain increases, discouragement and fatigue increase, decreasing the woman's ability to cope effectively with contractions. Fatigue may occur with a prolonged latent phase, as reported by the woman on admission that she has not slept well for days. Differences in use of pain medication during labor are based in part on cultural variances with labor pain, acceptance, and personal control in pain relief. Use of pain medication is lowest if women have a positive attitude toward labor pain and experience control over the reception of pain medication (Christiaens, Verhaeghe, & Bracke, 2010). Catastrophizing (where a person may think only in terms of negative thoughts about the pain and outcome) is associated with increased pain reports, even when coping strategies are being used (Escott, Slade, & Spiby, 2009). Pain in labor may be associated with suffering. Suffering is influenced by other emotional factors such as anxiety, fear, and depression and is expressed by moaning, crying, grimacing, hyperventilating, writhing, and shaking.

Labor pain is an example of acute pain that can come on quickly but lasts a relatively short time. It has a high degree of variability among individuals and at different points during labor. In a study of primiparous women during the first stage of labor, 60% described the pain during first stage of labor as unbearable, intolerable, extremely severe, and excruciating (Melzack, 1984). Descriptions of pain during the first and second stage of labor are described in Table 16–2. Some women describe a decrease in intensity during the second stage, perhaps because of maternal focus on pushing. Others experience more painful sensations, possibly because of the position of the fetus descending through the birth canal.

Many women experience intense pain in labor that may increase in severity and duration over time. Childbirth pain is one of the most severe types of pain a woman will experience in her lifetime (Camann, 2005). When the McGill Pain Questionnaire was used to compare reports of intensity of pain for a variety of clinical experiences (e.g., chronic back pain, nonterminal cancer pain, phantom limb pain, sprains, fractures), only the pain associated with accidental amputation of a digit and causalgia pain caused more pain than labor (Niven & Gijsbers, 1989). A woman's expectation of

her labor helps shape her experience and that the level of pain for many women is different than anticipated (Lally, Murtagh, Macphail, & Thomson, 2008).

While pain is unique to the individual, clinicians assisting with pain management can impose preconceived notions on the pain management process when discerning a woman's needs. The woman's involvement in planning pain management involves collaboration with all healthcare providers to arrive at realistic expectations and clear goals.

Pain Assessment

Achieving a satisfactory level of pain for the laboring woman is a shared goal for all healthcare providers. Pain is a culturally bound phenomenon. When a woman expresses pain, the form that expression takes is related to what her culture has taught her is appropriate. Nurses play a critical role in the assessment, relief, and evaluation of pain. The Joint Commission (TJC) released updated standards on pain assessment and management effective January 1, 2019 (TJC, 2018). They recommended women develop a personal treatment plan and set realistic expectations and measurable goals (TJC, 2018). The modification in pain assessment standards is reflective of the unintended consequence of overprescribing opioids. Evaluating a woman's response to the labor experience is crucial. A traditional method to quantify pain used a rating scale from 0 to 10 with 10 being excruciating pain and that a pain scale of 4 or greater required intervention. Simplistic rating scales are ineffective for use with the laboring woman because pain with contractions ebb and flow and the subjective experience of coping with labor is not assessed (Howard, 2017; Roberts et al., 2010). Although pain may be quantified, it is only one component of a woman's overall experience of labor and birth. Personal satisfaction does not always correlate with the level of pain and should be included in the evaluation of pain (Tournaire & Theau-Yonneau, 2007).

Roberts et al. (2010) developed and implemented an alternative tool to the 0 to 10 rating scale, the Coping with Labor Algorithm, which qualifies the woman's ability and internal consciousness as coping or not coping with her labor. Signs of coping and not coping with labor are presented in Table 16–3. The algorithm

TABLE 16–2. Descriptions of Pain Experience during Labor and Birth

Stage	Sensory	Affective
Stage 1	Cramping, pulling, aching, heavy, sharp, stabbing, cutting, intermittent, localized, global, sore, heavy, throbbing	Exciting, intense, tiring, exhausting, scary, frightening, bearable or unbearable, distressing, horrible, agonizing, indescribable, overwhelming, engulfing
Stage 2	Painful pressure, burning, ripping, tearing, piercing, explosive, localized	Exhausting, overwhelming, out-of-body feeling, inner focused or tunnel vision, exciting, horrible, excruciating, terrifying, less intense

TABLE 16–3. Signs of Coping/Not Coping in Labor

Signs of coping	Signs of not coping
• States she is coping	• States she is not coping
• Rhythmic activity during contraction (rocking, swaying)	• Crying (may see with self-hypnosis)
• Focused inward	• Sweaty
• Rhythmic breathing	• Tremulous voice
• Able to relax in between contractions	• Thrashing, wincing, writhing
• Vocalization: moaning, chanting, counting	• Inability to focus or concentrate
	• Clawing, biting
	• Panicked activity during contractions
	• Tense

features both coping and not coping pathways and incorporates nursing and supportive actions such as providing physical, emotional, and psychosocial interventions to increase coping ability. This algorithm has been implemented in hospital settings with success (Fairchild, Roberts, Zelman, Michelli, & Hastings-Tolsma, 2017). More research is needed to find a suitable assessment instrument for the evaluation of labor pain (Bergh, Stener-Victorin, Wallin, & Mårtensson, 2011).

Pain tolerance may be defined as the level of stimuli at which the laboring woman asks to have the stimulation stopped. In labor, it is the point at which a woman requests pharmacologic pain relief or increased comfort measures. Descriptive words such as mild, moderate, and severe do not provide a measure of pain tolerance because laboring women may describe pain as severe but not request pain medication. A woman's pain tolerance or the length of time she is able to go without medication may be increased by the use of nonpharmacologic pain management techniques (O'Sullivan, 2009). Helping women cope with labor through methods to impact the affective component and decrease the sensory component may be viewed as ineffective by clinicians supportive of the pharmacologic model (Lowe, 2002).

Suffering and pain are not equal concepts in childbirth. Suffering incorporates numerous variables such as prior experience, social support, and unique circumstances of a particular pregnancy (Hensley, Collins, & Leezer, 2017). Women can feel intense pain during labor, and the ability to cope is mediated by non-pharmacologic approaches. Research has shown that alternative coping techniques may improve a woman's sense of control and satisfaction with childbirth (Kimber, McNabb, Mc Court, Haines, & Brocklehurst, 2008). However, those approaches may become insufficient, leading to suffering thereby increasing maternal anxiety. A meta-analysis found that pharmacologic pain-relieving interventions, used in addition to nonpharmacologic approaches, can contribute to reducing medical interventions (Chaillet et al., 2014).

Healthcare Environment

Generally, in the United States, maternity care is intervention intensive. As reported in the *Listening to Mothers III* survey, labor care is technology intensive with most mothers reporting continuous fetal monitoring, and IV line, epidural or spinal anesthesia, having their labor augmented or induced with oxytocin, artificial rupture of membranes, and an episiotomy (Declercq, Sakala, Corry, Applebaum, & Herrlich, 2013).

Care givers in every perinatal unit take a unique approach to caring for laboring women. A culture develops over time and is accepted by most of those working within the department as a reflection of their values and beliefs. Cultural differences may be as significant as the separation of the mother and baby after birth or as subtle as the routine initiation of IV fluids on admission. These practices reflect the evolution of intrapartum care within a particular institution. Display 16–1 lists suggestions to create a relaxed environment. Unit culture extends to treatment of pain and influences the woman's perception of pain. In any birth setting, nurses can influence use of facilities and equipment that support physiologic birth (ACOG, 2019b; Stark, Remynse, & Zwelling, 2016). Nurses who value nonpharmacologic approaches to pain management use these techniques in clinical practice. Guidelines and clinical practices should accommodate and elicit women's preferences for birth (Kukla et al., 2009).

The Birth Plan

Birth plans are popular, widely available, and prepared as an instrument for women to use to communicate goals and choices in their birth process. Many interactive birth plans offering hundreds of choice points

---

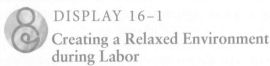

DISPLAY 16–1

Creating a Relaxed Environment during Labor

• Control the amount of light, noise, and interruptions.
• Maintain an unhurried demeanor.
• Use a calm, soft, slow voice.
• Recognize the signs of tension:
  ○ Changes in voice
  ○ Frowning
  ○ Clenched fists
  ○ Stiff, straight posture
  ○ Tense arms or legs
  ○ Stiff, raised shoulders
• Maintain eye contact.
• Use touch or massage if this is acceptable to the woman.
• Sit, rather than stand, next to the woman.
• Introduce caregivers to the woman and her support partner(s).
• Respect the birth plan.

can be found on-line. Nurses have a responsibility whenever possible to facilitate an experience for each couple that matches their expectations. Asking about their plans and goals validates their efforts to prepare for labor and birth. Nurses should assure the woman and her support persons that the couple's goals are understood and that achievement is a shared objective. Labor admission assessment should include questions related to the type and amount of childbirth preparation and birth choices. The nurse should ask about the couple's plans for pain management during labor and whether this subject was discussed with their maternity provider. Knowledge and skills learned in childbirth preparation classes are enhanced when the nurse present during labor and birth believes in and actively supports the couple as they apply these principles.

Templates are available in pregnancy books and Web sites and, however, may include inconsistent, outdated, and unrealistic choices leading to a breakdown in communication instead of partnership. Hostility may develop between the woman and healthcare team, and distrust can build on both sides (DeBaets, 2017). Even when birth plans are discussed during an antepartum visit, communication breakdowns may occur during labor when an unfamiliar hospitalist or on-call provider assumes care and the woman is challenged with advocating for individual choices. Women may express a religious need for female-only staff or limitation on blood products, and these values should be shared proactively and respected. Economic and logistic realities and cultural understandings of birth and safety influence a woman's choice and satisfaction with their birth process (Miller & Shriver, 2012).

NONPHARMACOLOGIC APPROACHES

The nonpharmacologic approach to labor pain management views childbirth as a unique individual experience and a normal physiologic process. The nonpharmacologic approach includes a wide variety of techniques to address both physical sensations of pain and eliminate the suffering, helplessness, distress, and loss of control by addressing the emotional and spiritual components of care (Simkin & Bolding, 2004). Interventions will not provide complete pain relief but rather use techniques that allow a woman to cope with her labor pain. Therefore, it is inaccurate to use terms such as *pain relief* when referring to these interventions. Alternatively, the complete removal of pain does not always convert to a more satisfying experience. A woman's ability to actively participate in her labor can transform the experience from suffering to active participation and confidence in her ability to cope, with the aid of her support system. Nonpharmacologic interventions are appealing to women and caregivers who are interested in reducing labor pain without creating

potentially serious side effects and high costs. Increasing women's access to nonmedical approaches during labor, such as continuous labor support, has been shown to reduce cesarean birth rates (Adams, Stark, & Low, 2016). The 2018 pain management standards of TJC require that nonpharmacologic pain treatment modalities should be provided by the hospital in addition to pharmacologic strategies (TJC, 2017).

Women choose pain management strategies based on their previous experience with pain, what they learned from reading and in prenatal classes, primary healthcare providers' recommendations, and listening to what worked for family members and friends. The advantage of nonpharmacologic pain management strategies is their simplicity and relative ease to initiate, the sense of control women achieve when they actively manage their pain, the lack of serious side effects, and that they do not generally add more cost to the birth process (Simkin & O'Hara, 2002). Nonpharmacologic techniques do not require additional medical interventions and provide the opportunity for the woman's support team to be involved in the birth experience. The 2013 *Listening to Mothers III* survey noted that 73% of women used at least one nonpharmacologic method of pain relief, an increase from 69% reported 5 years earlier. None of the techniques were used by a majority of mothers and 17% reported using no pain medication. Figure 16–1 provides results comparing the second to the third *Listening to Mother's* survey with little change noted overall (Declercq et al., 2013).

There are three classifications of nonpharmacologic methods or comfort measures that can be used to decrease or alter painful sensations associated with labor and birth: (1) cognitive processes to control the degree to which a sensation is interpreted as painful, (2) addition of painful stimulation at any site of the body, and (3) cutaneous measures to reduce painful stimuli (gate control theory). Table 16–4 lists the classifications and methods used for nonpharmacologic pain management. Few randomized, controlled clinical trials exist validating all these techniques.

Cognitive Processes

The cognitive process focuses on auditory or visual stimulation and pain is modulated by conditioning the areas which are responsible for memory, emotions, and reaction to pain. Many forms of distraction are used during labor to decrease pain perception. Interventions such as continuous support, relaxation, imagery, focusing, breathing techniques, meditation, yoga, hypnosis, aromatherapy, and music are likely to benefit a woman by decreasing anxiety, improving overall mood, and increasing the individual's sense of control in a painful situation by conditioning the areas, which are responsible for memory, emotions, and reaction to pain (Challiet et al., 2014; McCaffery & Pasero, 1999).

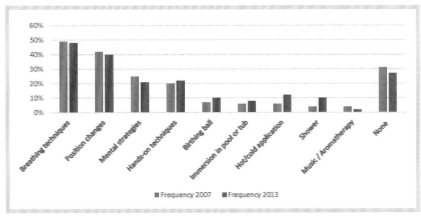

FIGURE 16–1. Comparison between 2007 and 2013 of use of nonpharmacologic techniques during labor. (Adapted from Declercq, E. R., Sakala, C., Corry, M. P., & Applebaum, S. [2007]. Listening to mothers II: Report of the second national U.S. survey of women's childbearing experiences: Conducted January–February 2006 for Childbirth Connection by Harris Interactive® in partnership with Lamaze International. *The Journal of Perinatal Education, 16*(4), 15–17. doi:10.1624/105812407X244778; Declercq, E. R., Sakala, C., Corry, M. P., Applebaum, S., & Herrlich, A. [2013]. *Listening to mothers III pregnancy and birth: Report of the third national U.S. survey of women's childbearing experiences.* Retrieved from http://transform.childbirthconnection.org/wp-content/uploads/2013/06/LTM-III_Pregnancy-and-Birth.pdf)

Prenatal education and labor support are effective pain management strategies because they enhance maternal confidence and a sense of control.

These approaches allow the brain to modulate the pain stimulus and are associated with a reduction in epidural use, significant reduction in cesarean and operative birth, use of oxytocin, and duration of labor while contributing to improved maternal satisfaction with childbirth and neonatal outcomes (Challiet et al., 2014).

In addition to the physiologic factors that influence the perception of pain, psychosocial and emotional factors influence a woman's feelings of accomplishment and satisfaction with the birth experience (Richardson, Lopez, Baysinger, Shotwell, & Chestnut, 2017). These factors include pain relief, labor support, childbirth preparation, and the healthcare environment. Promotion of support begins with an overall philosophy that the mother–baby dyad is the true center of care, and her ability to birth is respected and encouraged.

Labor Support

Women identify labor support as continuous presence by another, emotional support, physical comforting, or information and guidance for the woman and her partner. Supportive care may enhance the physiologic labor progress and provide a sense of control and confidence in the woman's ability to achieve spontaneous vaginal birth and improved outcomes (ACOG, 2019b; Bohren, Hofmeyr, Sakala, Fukuzawa, & Cuthbert, 2017; Caughey, Cahill, Guise, & Rouse, 2014). Stress hormones lower and oxytocin rises, promoting progressive contractions when a woman receives supportive care. Emotional support includes behaviors such as giving praise, encouragement, and reassurance; being positive; appearing calm and confident; assisting with breathing and relaxation; providing explanations about labor progress; identifying ways to include family members in the experience; and treating women with respect (Bryanton, Fraser-Davey, & Sullivan, 1994; Hodnett et al., 2013; Sleutel, 2000). Continuous emotional support is crucial for an easier, safer birth (Green & Hotelling, 2014). Providing for physical comfort includes comforting touch, massage, encouraging mobility, promoting adequate fluid intake, and offering a variety of nonpharmacologic and

TABLE 16–4. Nonpharmacologic Methods to Control Pain	
Technique	Examples
Cognitive processes to control the degree to which a sensation is interpreted as painful (attention deviation)	Continuous labor support Hypnotherapy Music Aromatherapy Meditation/yoga Relaxation/breathing techniques Guided imagery/focal point Distraction Patterned breathing Childbirth preparation
Painful stimulation at any site of the body	Acupressure Acupuncture Intradermal injections of sterile water
Cutaneous measures to reduce painful stimuli (gate control theory)	Movement and positioning Birth ball Touch, massage, back rub Counterpressure Hydrotherapy, water immersion Warm packs Ice/cold compress

pharmacologic interventions. Information regarding decision making, labor progress, anticipatory guidance, explanations of procedures, and advocating on behalf of the woman facilitate communication between the woman, her family, and the healthcare providers (Bohren et al., 2017). Methods of labor support are found in Display 16–2. In a meta-analysis of 15 clinical trials, continuous support from a nurse, CNM, certified doula, or companions of the mother's choice from her network (partner, mother, and friend) resulted in a more satisfying birth experience. This continuous support led to decreased operative vaginal births and cesarean births and resulted in significantly shorter labors, decreased use of analgesia and oxytocin, and 5-minute Apgar scores <7 (Association of Women's Health, Obstetric and Neonatal Nurses [AWHONN], 2018; Hodnett et al., 2013). These findings are supported by another meta-analysis on nonpharmacologic approaches validating a reduction in obstetric interventions (Challiet et al., 2014). Programs and policies to include support personnel providing continuous one-on-one emotional support should be considered given the evidence of benefits (ACOG, 2019b).

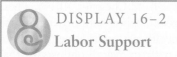

DISPLAY 16–2
Labor Support

Emotional Support
Continuous presence, companionship
Eye contact
Encouragement, praise
Distraction
Reassurance

Physical Comfort
Comforting touch
Promoting adequate fluid intake and output
Personal hygiene
Applications of heat or cold
Massage
Hydrotherapy: warm baths/showers
Position change, encouraging mobility

Advocacy
Providing information
Offering advice
Coaching in breathing, relaxation techniques
Interpreting medical jargon
Supporting the woman's decisions
Translating the woman's wishes to others

Support for Family Members
Role model labor support
Providing opportunity for breaks
Encouragement

Registered Nurse

Ultimately, it is a nurse's role to support the laboring woman to make informed choices that achieve a woman's vision of birth while ensuring the safety of both the mother and infant. It is the position of AWHONN (2018) that supporting and caring for women during labor is best performed by a registered nurse (RN) (Display 16–3). The labor nurse is a constant care provider during labor and birth in the hospital and may partner with a variety of individuals chosen by the woman (e.g., a family member or friend, trained doula), helping to create a supportive environment promoting healthy birth outcomes. Comprehensive nursing education, clinical patient management skills, and previous experience make the RN uniquely qualified to provide the professional care and complex emotional care that women and families need during labor and birth (AWHONN, 2018). The perinatal nurse must be able to support the laboring woman and assist her in maximizing the potential of a woman's birth experience. Multiple strategies may be necessary during the course of labor, and the nurse may encourage activities and positions in labor that are known to be beneficial to the progress of labor (Hodnett et al., 2013). Perinatal nurses should develop expertise in both nonpharmacologic and pharmacologic pain management and coping strategies through enhanced training. Length of the nurses' intrapartum experience, personal attitudes, and own birth experiences are positively correlated with intent to provide labor support (Sleutel, 2000; Sleutel, Schultz, & Wyble, 2007; Stark et al., 2016). Nurses allocate from 12% (Gale, Fothergill-Bourbonnais, & Chamberlain, 2001) to 58% (Miltner, 2002) of their time providing supportive care to women in labor, usually doing so in conjunction with some technical activity. Factors that have contributed to nurses spending less direct time with women include increased documentation requirements, technology, fetal heart rate (FHR) surveillance, physician assistance with epidural anesthesia, and institutional staffing patterns. As use of technology has expanded in obstetrics, the perinatal nurse added monitoring the equipment, imputing data into the electronic health record, and relying on pharmacologic interventions to the basic provision of hands-on comfort. Technology, especially when coupled with epidural analgesia, requires nurses to have coexisting responsibilities that divide their focus between the laboring woman and machines. If pharmacologic methods have been used, the woman's pain may be lessened and the nurse may feel that her presence is no longer needed. The nurse may perceive that caring for a woman with an epidural is less physically and emotionally draining for the nurse than caring for a woman who is planning nonpharmacologic management. If the culture of the perinatal unit allows ease of access to neuraxial analgesia, nurses

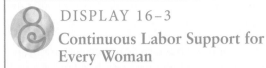

DISPLAY 16–3

Continuous Labor Support for Every Woman

The Association of Women's Health, Obstetric and Neonatal Nurses (AWHONN) asserts that continuous labor support from a registered nurse (RN) is critical to achieve improved birth outcomes. In partnership with the woman, the RN conducts an assessment and then implements and evaluates an individualized plan of care based on the woman's physical, psychological, and sociocultural needs. This plan incorporates the woman's desires for and expectations of the process of labor. The RN coordinates the woman's support team, which may include a partner, family, friends, and/or a doula, to assist the woman to achieve her childbirth goals. Care and support during labor are powerful nursing functions, and it is incumbent on healthcare facilities to provide a level of staffing that facilitates the unique patient–RN relationship during childbirth. Childbirth education and doula services contribute to the woman's preparation for and support during childbirth and supports consideration of these services as a covered benefit in public and private health insurance plans.

The childbirth experience is an intensely dynamic, physical, and emotional event with lifelong implications. Women who receive continuous support during labor from hospital clinicians, nonhospital professionals such as doulas (Kozhimannil, Hardeman, Attanasio, Blauer-Peterson, & O'Brien, 2013), and family or friends may have improved outcomes compared with women who do not have such support. Improved maternal and newborn outcomes include the following:

- Increased spontaneous vaginal birth
- Shorter duration of labor
- Decreased cesarean birth
- Decreased instrumental vaginal birth
- Decreased use of any analgesia
- Decreased use of regional analgesia
- Improved 5-min Apgar score
- Fewer negative feelings about childbirth experiences

The American College of Obstetricians and Gynecologists (ACOG, 2019a) recommended continuous support as one strategy to limit intervention during labor and birth. Despite the many benefits of continuous support in labor, RNs are challenged by competing priorities for their time and attention. Increasingly, RNs care for women with higher acuity levels, and the care of these women often demands increased attention to technology and documentation. Adequate staffing is essential for the RN to support the woman in labor and her family and to provide safe care that meets the accepted standards for maternal and fetal assessment. However, perinatal nurses indicated that inadequate staffing was a barrier to the provision of all aspects of labor support: physical and emotional support, information, and advocacy (Simpson & Lyndon, 2017). The *Guidelines for Professional Registered Nurse Staffing for Perinatal Units* (AWHONN, 2010) indicate that a one-to-one RN-to-patient ratio is needed to ensure the safety of women in labor who have medical or obstetric complications, receive oxytocin, choose minimal intervention in labor, or are in second-stage labor.

The RN integrates nursing theory with knowledge and clinical expertise to provide individualized, patient-centered care for each woman in labor and coordinates the woman's support team in accordance with institutional policies to ensure a safe birth.

The support provided by the RN should include the following (Adams et al., 2016):

- Assessment of the physiologic and psychological processes of labor
- Facilitation of normal physiologic processes, for example, allow movement in labor
- Provision of physical comfort measures, emotional support, information, and advocacy
- Evaluation of maternal and fetal status, including uterine activity and fetal oxygenation
- Instruction regarding the labor process and comfort and coping measures
- Role modeling to facilitate the participation of the family and companions during labor and birth
- Direct collaboration with other members of the healthcare team to coordinate patient care

The RN should help the woman to cope with labor (Roberts et al., 2010). Support during early labor builds the woman's confidence and helps her establish realistic expectations. When regional anesthesia is used, the nurse should encourage frequent position changes, use labor progress tools to help the fetus rotate and descend, allow labor to progress naturally and wait for passive descent until the woman has the urge to push, and monitor for fever associated with the use of epidural anesthesia.

- Nurse leaders, including unit managers, nurse educators, and clinical nurse specialists, can be instrumental in advocating for staffing levels that ensure the provision of continuous labor support based on national guidelines. They can help to create cultures of care in which continuous labor support is prioritized. They can also ensure that women are educated about reasons to delay admission until active labor, strategies to deal with early labor at home, and how they will be supported in active labor by the nursing staff. Nurse leaders can review and revise policies to facilitate the ability of the nurse to directly provide labor support and coordinate the labor support team. These policies may include the following:
  - Comprehensive and ongoing education on labor support techniques and tools for nurses
  - Policies and education on intermittent fetal monitoring and auscultation, including the identification of appropriate patients and procedures
  - Early labor support and therapeutic rest policies
  - Nurse staffing policies, including policies about contingency and on-call staffing, which plan for appropriate numbers of nurses to provide direct labor support consistent with national guidelines as well as RN coordination of the support team (American Academy of Pediatrics [AAP] & ACOG, 2017; AWHONN, 2010)
  - Liberal visitor policies permitting and encouraging a woman to have the support persons she desires to provide her effective support, in accordance with maintaining a safe physical environment.

Providing coverage and reimbursement for childbirth education and doula services that improve birth outcomes and save healthcare dollars should be a priority. As covered benefits for all pregnant women, these services could enhance goals to reduce racial and ethnic disparities in birth outcomes. Continued research about the effect of nursing support on maternal–newborn outcomes and the potential financial benefits of such support for healthcare systems is vital.

Adapted from Association of Women's Health, Obstetric and Neonatal Nurses. (2018). *Continuous labor support for every woman* (Position Statement). Washington, DC: Author.

new to the specialty will have limited opportunity to learn about or use nonpharmacologic measures.

It is essential that nurses recognize the value of caregiver presence and not be distracted by the technology. The RN, who understands the physiologic events of labor and has been educated about supportive care in labor, should take the lead in providing labor support and positively model labor support behaviors for others present during labor and birth. Perinatal nurses should remain at the bedside when women are experiencing severe pain (AWHONN, 2010). Women who are laboring with minimal to no pain relief require 1 to 1 nursing care (AWHONN, 2010). This allows the nurse to assess the underlying etiology for the pain and provide support to the laboring woman and her partner. According to Chapman (2000), nurses who remained at the bedside, explained what was occurring with the labor, and included the support person were viewed as providing the most support. The woman may change her mind about choice of pain relief and comfort options at any time during labor. Some labors last longer than anticipated and are more painful than expected. In some cases, unplanned interventions such as augmentation of labor with oxytocin can occur, which have the potential to exacerbate labor pain due to an increase in contraction frequency, duration, and intensity. The nurse should facilitate pain relief measures when and if requested by the woman during labor.

Husband, Partner, and Support Person(s)

Labor support is ideally provided by a variety of individuals (Table 16–5). On admission, the laboring woman should identify the husband or partner, family members or friends who will act as labor support persons. It should be up to the woman as to how many support persons she desires. According to *Listening to Mothers III*, a husband or partner provided labor support 77% of the time (Declercq et al., 2013). Fathers have an important role in providing physical and emotional support during childbirth. Being in a hospital and seeing the woman in labor may be very stressful for some fathers, and although their presence is important, the partner may not be the best coach (Klaus, Kennell, & Klaus, 2002). In a classic study, Chapman (1992) described three roles assumed by expectant fathers during labor without epidural analgesia or anesthesia. These roles were identified by organizing behaviors that partners were observed performing during labor or behaviors women described in interviews after birth. Most men in the study adopted the role of witness rather than teammate or coach (Chapman, 1992).

- Coaches actively assisted their partners during and after labor contractions with breathing and relaxation techniques. Coaches led or directed their partners through labor and birth and viewed themselves as managers or directors of the experience.
- Teammates assisted their partners throughout the experience of labor and birth by responding to requests for physical or emotional support or both. They sometimes led their partners, but their usual role was that of follower or helper.
- Witnesses viewed themselves primarily as companions who were there to provide emotional and moral support. They were present during labor and birth to observe the process and to witness the birth of their child. Chandler and Field (1997) report that witnessing their partners in severe pain caused men to feel helpless and fearful. They became discouraged when the comfort measures they tried did not help their partners. Ultimately, they felt they had failed in their role. These results contrast with the intentions of childbirth educators, who perceive themselves as preparing coaches and teammates for laboring women, and with perinatal nurses, who expect fathers and other family members to take a more active role in labor support.

TABLE 16–5. Providing Labor Support

Clinical practice	Referenced rationale
1. Labor support ideally is continuous and provided by a variety of individuals.	A Cochrane review of 26 studies that provided data from 17 countries, involving more than 15,000 women, concluded that women who had continuous 1:1 support were (1) more likely to have a spontaneous vaginal birth and have shorter labors, (2) less likely to require analgesia, (3) less likely to report dissatisfaction with their childbirth, (4) postpartum depression could be lower, (5) Apgar scores are less likely to be 6 or lower at 5 min (Hodnett et al., 2013).
2. Trained lay doulas are effective in providing labor support.	Pain was reduced by continuous labor support, particularly those in which doulas provided the support (Simkin & Bolding, 2004).
3. Labor support should begin in early labor and continued through birth.	Support in early labor and continued throughout seems to have provided greatest benefit (American College of Obstetricians and Gynecologists, 2019b).
4. Fathers and other support persons may require assistance and suggestions with support measures.	As pain intensifies, women become frustrated, irritable, exhausted, and panicky. These personality changes may be totally unfamiliar qualities that the partner had never seen the woman demonstrate.
5. Content related to changing emotions should be presented in prenatal classes.	Childbirth educators should present content related to coping and not coping, discuss the transition, and teach support partners in their classes about the emotions they can expect to witness and experience themselves during labor.

DISPLAY 16-4

Grounded Theory of the Expectant Father's Epidural Labor Experience

Holding-out phase: during labor, when couples are planning to avoid an epidural or seeing how far they can get in labor without needing an epidural

Surrendering phase: the point at which the decision is made to receive an epidural, which is described as yielding to the need for an epidural, giving up, feeling they have experienced all the pain they can handle and done everything they can to avoid an epidural

Waiting phase: period after making the decision to receive an epidural until the anesthesia care provider arrives

Getting phase: period when the anesthesia provider is present, making assessments, preparing equipment, and placing the epidural

Cruising phase: the time after the epidural has provided pain relief. Couples' focus changes to rest and relaxation. Labor has gone from a stressful process to a calm experience. Both may fall asleep, due to exhaustion from the stress of coping with the pain of labor.

From Chapman, L. L. (2000). Expectant fathers and labor epidurals. *MCN: The American Journal of Maternal Child Nursing, 25*(3), 133–138.

The theoretical experience of expectant fathers when their partners received epidural analgesia or anesthesia is outlined in Display 16–4 (Chapman, 2000). During labor, critical experiences for men occurred at two points. In the holding-out phase of labor, before making the decision to receive an epidural, men experienced a sense of "losing her." As pain became more severe, women underwent personality changes, becoming frustrated, irritable, exhausted, and panicky. These personality changes may be totally unfamiliar qualities that the men had never seen their partners demonstrate or demonstrate to the degree that they do while in labor. Women also gradually turn inward as they attempt to cope with the pain. Withdrawing into themselves causes women to be unable to communicate their needs and to become unresponsive to their partners' attempts at labor support. Men feel increased levels of anxiety, helplessness, frustration, and emotional pain (Chapman, 2000). These findings are consistent with the work of Somers-Smith (1999), who found that fathers experience childbirth as a stressful event.

The second and most dramatic phase for men sharing the experience of labor is during the cruising phase. After the epidural has provided relief from the pain of labor, men describe a sensation of "she's back." The laboring woman again is aware of her surroundings and interacting with those around her. From a man's perspective, labor has gone from a stressful event to a calm experience. Rather than describing their experience in terms of the role they assumed during labor and the frustration and disconnected feelings they had as labor intensified and the woman's behavior changed (Chapman, 1991, 1992), these men described their experience by the degree of frustration they felt before the epidural and the degree of enjoyment after the epidural (Chapman, 2000). It is important that childbirth educators present this content, discuss this process, and teach men in their classes about the emotions they can expect to witness and experience during labor.

Doula

Doulas (also known as labor assistant, birth companion, labor support specialist, professional labor assistant, and monitrice), may be volunteers or paid and are available through a variety of programs, either hospital based, community based, or as a private, contracted service. Hospital- and community-based programs may be available to underserved populations, women who may be newly emigrating, or women who might be alone during childbirth, for example, adolescents or incarcerated women. Individual hospitals or community-based healthcare agencies may be involved in training doulas, and national organizations offer specialized education and certification (Display 16–5). In 1992, Doulas of North America (now DONA International) was founded and the name "doula" was coined. Doulas have a variety of credentials and education (Ahlemeyer & Mahon, 2015). They assist women and their partners by providing physical, emotional, and informational support during pregnancy, birth, and the postpartum period (Green & Hotelling, 2014). There is increased interest in the role of the professional or lay labor support doula. The doula can advocate for the woman and assist with communication of needs. The movement toward professional or lay labor support may be a result of the inability of perinatal nurses or husband/significant others to provide women with the support they want during labor.

DISPLAY 16-5

Associations that Educate and Certify Doulas

BirthWorks International: https://birthworks.org

CAPPA (Childbirth and Postpartum Professional Association): https://www.cappa.net

DONA International (formerly Doulas of North America): https://www.dona.org

Childbirth International: https://childbirthinternational.com

ICEA (International Childbirth Education Association): https://icea.org

Each member of the mother's care team should respect each other's skills and contributions to ensure coordinated, optimal safe care. The role of the doula is different from that of the provider, the father, and the nurse. The husband or significant other, family members and friends, and/or a doula should be welcomed and encouraged to provide labor support. The presence of one or all of these additional individuals does not decrease the ultimate responsibility of the perinatal nurse but instead may add to a positive birth experience (Ballen & Fulcher, 2006). While not provided by all programs, a unique aspect of the doula role occurs during postpartum, usually after discharge from the hospital. During a home visit, the doula is able to make time to review the labor and birth experience with the goal of creating a satisfying birth experience for the new mother. "The doula allows the woman to reflect on her experience, fills in gaps in her memory, praises her, and sometimes helps reframe upsetting or difficult aspects of the birth" (Ballen & Fulcher, 2006, p. 305). Table 16–6 compares the role of a doula with the perinatal nurse. Women who had the benefit of a doula during labor expressed significantly less emotional distress and had higher self-esteem at 4 months postpartum than women who had attended a traditional Lamaze class (Manning-Orenstein, 1998). When low-income pregnant women were randomized to be accompanied in labor by their family and a trained doula or just family members, those in the doula group had significantly shorter labors and greater cervical dilation at

the time of epidural anesthesia (Campbell, Lake, Falk, & Backstrand, 2006).

Qualitative research has demonstrated that one of the most effective aspects of the experience of labor for women is strong and prolonged continuous support provided by caregivers who are not employees of the institution (Hodnett et al., 2013). Women place a high value on their partners' presence and support in labor, leading to reduced anxiety, less perceived pain, greater satisfaction with the birth experience, lower rates of postnatal depression, and improved outcomes in the child (Dellman, 2004). In a culture in which women experience traditional labor without their partner, those accompanied by a female support person had significantly shorter labors, less use of analgesia and oxytocin, and fewer admissions to the neonatal intensive care unit (NICU) (Mosallam, Rizk, Thomas, & Ezimokhai, 2004).

Hypnotherapy

Hypnotherapy or clinical hypnosis is an integrative mind–body technique using entrancing suggestions communicated between the therapist and the participant (Cyna, McAuliffe, & Andrew, 2004). Three components of hypnosis are used in labor: reframing the birth process to a satisfying event through positive messaging, altering perception of sensations, and advocacy by a prepared partner (Beebe, 2014). Positive affirmations such as renaming uterine contractions to

TABLE 16–6. Differentiating the Roles of the Registered Nurse and the Doula

Registered nurse	Doula
Professional education and license to practice nursing; follows evidence-based standards and guidelines from professional organizations	Often educated, though not required; may be prepared through a formal education program; may be certified
Meets the woman for the first time during labor	Usually meets and begins to form a relationship with the woman during her pregnancy to try to understand her expectations, needs, fears, and concerns
Performs clinical tasks within the scope of practice of the registered nurse	Supportive role; performs no clinical nursing tasks
Consults with the perinatal care provider	Advocates for communication with the perinatal care team
Provides intermittent labor support; presence in the bedside or in the labor room is not continuous; may be caring for more than one woman; depending on the length of labor, more than one nurse may care for the woman	Provides continuous labor support; leaves the bedside/labor room only for intermittent breaks; stays with the woman throughout her labor and birth and into the early recovery period
Keeps woman informed of labor progress: what is normal and what to expect	Keeps woman informed of labor progress in lay terms: what is normal and what to expect
Advocates for the woman by communicating her needs and desires to the perinatal care provider	Assists the woman to formulate and articulate her questions and concerns to the nurse and the perinatal care provider
Responsible for documenting assessments in the woman's record	May document events of the labor and birth in a private journal to share and review with the woman later to ensure positive memories
Has a legal accountability and responsibility for his or her actions	Responsibilities determined between doula and the family
May have minimal or no contact with the woman after the birth	Some type of follow-up visit or visits with the woman is usually part of the program.

Adapted from Roberts, L., Gulliver, B., Fisher, J., & Cloyes, K. G. (2010). The Coping with Labor Algorithm: An alternate pain assessment tool for the laboring woman. *Journal of Midwifery & Women's Health, 55*(2), 107–116. doi:10.1016/j.jmwh.2009.11.002

uterine surges or waves are means to support visualizations to relax the body, guide thoughts, and control breathing. A recorded voice on tape may be played to help the woman enter a calm state of self-hypnosis. One method of altering perception of sensation is "glove anesthesia" in which the woman imagines that her hand is numb and that it can spread numbness to other areas by placing her hand on painful areas. The effectiveness of self-hypnosis for childbirth is subject to the amount and consistency of conditioning and practice. Use of hypnotherapy may not be accepted or understood by the healthcare team, which could undermine its use, leading to power struggles between the mother, her partner, and the healthcare team. It is crucial to balance institutional standards while attempting to accommodate the woman's birthing preferences.

Research on self-hypnosis for birthing is limited due to lack of standardized metrics and problems evaluating overall effectiveness (Beebe, 2014). A systematic review found hypnosis may reduce the overall use of analgesia during labor but not epidural use. Satisfaction with pain relief or sense of coping was similar in control groups and those using hypnosis (Madden, Middleton, Cyna, Matthewson, & Jones, 2016).

Music

Music can be used during labor as a distraction and to provide focus. The perception and response to pain and music travel through the same neural pathways in the limbic system and that use of particular types of music perceived as relaxing may decrease anxiety associated with the perception of pain (Browning, 2000). Familiar music associated with restful or pleasant recollections may be an adjunct to relaxation and imagery to manage the pain of labor (Nayak, Rastogi, & Kathuria, 2014).

Music creates an atmosphere in the birthing room that also may change the approach of healthcare professionals to laboring women. Perinatal nurses and physicians become more relaxed, slow their activities, and respond with increased respect for the unique personal event in progress (DiFranco, 2000). When women use earphones or headsets to listen to music, the music provides a distraction and the woman is in constant control of the volume. Ultimately, choosing music that helps her relax or improve her mood will give the woman a greater sense of control.

Music can be effective in increasing pain tolerance or a cue to the mother to move or breathe rhythmically. Most studies, however, lack significance or validate benefits (DiFranco, 2000).

Aromatherapy

Aromatherapy with lavender is reported to decrease anxiety during labor in nulliparous women and decrease cortisol secretion from the adrenal gland while increasing serotonin secretion from the gastrointestinal tract (Mirzaei, Keshtgar, Kaviana, Rajaeifard, 2015). Lavender is also used to help with pain relief, to lighten mood, and to calm contractions if rest is needed in early labor. Peppermint oil is found to ease nausea and vomiting. Avoidance of clary sage is recommended due to increased uterine contractions. Overall, there is insufficient evidence from randomized controlled trials about the benefits of aromatherapy on pain management in labor. More research is needed (Smith, Collins, & Crowther, 2011; Smith, Levett, Collins, & Crowther, 2011).

Yoga

Yoga, a method of Indian origin, proposes control of the body and mind. Energy yoga uses special training of breathing and achieves changes in levels of consciousness, relaxation, and inner peace. Yoga during pregnancy may contribute with reducing labor pain, increasing satisfaction, and reducing the rate of assisted vaginal birth (Jahdi et al., 2017).

Relaxation

Achieving a state of relaxation is the basis of all nonpharmacologic interventions during labor. Women benefit from a state of relaxation because it conserves energy rather than creating fatigue from the prolonged tension of voluntary muscles. Relaxation enhances the effectiveness of nonpharmacologic and pharmacologic pain management strategies. Relaxation is a skill and a physical state. The degree of relaxation a woman can achieve will influence the amount of anxiety she feels. Women may be first introduced to relaxation techniques during childbirth classes. How well they learn and are able to use these skills depends on quality of instruction, the amount of time they practice, and their belief that this technique can be beneficial. Relaxation is as contagious as panic, tension, and feelings of being overwhelmed. Relaxation skills cannot be taught during active labor, but an environment that promotes relaxation can be created by the perinatal nurse (see Display 16–1). When faced with the forces of labor, women who learned relaxation techniques will need the presence of an informed perinatal nurse to reinforce and encourage the use of these techniques during labor.

Guided Imagery

Guided imagery is a relaxation technique using visualization to purposefully direct thoughts to relieve stress and provide a sense of relief. Childbirth educators teach imagery as a skill, encouraging expectant women to focus on pleasant scenes or experiences to increase their level of relaxation. Nurses encourage women to use imagery by making statements such as "think of the baby moving through the birth canal," "think of the baby moving down and out," and "think about the cervix gently opening like a flower one petal at a time." Imagery is used to keep women focused and to encourage the use of the contraction as a stimulus for strength and power.

Attention Focusing and Distraction

During early labor, distraction is an effective strategy. Distraction is the process by which stimuli from the environment draw a woman's attention away from her pain. Walking in the hallway, sitting in a chair, talking with visitors, watching television, playing cards, and using the telephone or Internet keep laboring women occupied. Most women reach a point during labor when they no longer are able to talk comfortably through contractions. Labor is hard work that requires intense concentration to maintain a sense of control. Women are helped to concentrate by focusing on an object in the room or a support person's face or eyes. Attention focusing involves deliberate, intentional activities on the part of the laboring woman. These activities include patterned breathing and visualization or imagery.

Patterned Breathing

Breathing techniques may be taught in prenatal classes and are used as a distraction during labor to decrease pain and promote relaxation. On admission, the perinatal nurse reviews with the woman and her support person the specific techniques they were taught in prenatal class. If a woman has not attended class, early labor is the time to discuss and practice a slow, controlled breathing pattern. Most women are taught to take a deep breath at the beginning of a contraction. This breath ensures oxygen to the mother and baby, signals to people in the room that a contraction is beginning and stretches and tenses respiratory muscles. Exhaling this breath relaxes respiratory muscles and voluntary muscles. At some point during labor, perinatal nurses may find it necessary to breathe synchronously with a couple through several contractions. Women are encouraged to breathe slowly. However, as labor pain increases, women may need to use a lighter, more accelerated breathing (i.e., no more than 2 times their normal rate). Alternatively, a pant-blow method of breathing, in which a woman takes three to four light panting breaths, followed by an exhale (i.e., blow), may be used. When attempting to control the urge to push, a rapid and shallow breathing pattern may be helpful.

Childbirth Preparation

An awareness of the childbirth preparation and skills that the woman and her partner are prepared to use is helpful when planning nursing support strategies during labor. The desire for pain relief during labor varies in women with a spectrum from natural childbirth to neuraxial analgesia. Nonpharmacologic and pharmacologic pain management strategies provide women with specific techniques they can use to cope with the discomfort of labor, thereby increasing their feelings of control. Prenatal education should provide information on an assortment of pain management, support, and coping skills to hopefully meet the expectations of the woman. Most pregnant women have concerns about labor process and their ability to handle painful contractions. Childbirth classes provide an opportunity to help women understand the normal process of labor and begin to develop confidence in their ability to give birth. Antenatal education in preparation for childbirth is available in a number of formats including classroom, online, and video display. Content and bias vary dependent on the author and presenter of the material. *Listening to Mother's III* survey noted that content focused on the labor and birth process and what to expect in the hospital (Declercq et al., 2013). They reported that overall, 53% of mothers took a childbirth class or a series of classes either with the current pregnancy or a prior pregnancy.

Both pharmacologic and nonpharmacologic pain relief methods may be presented as alternatives or complementary to each other, which may influence the woman's coping ability and choice. The common goal of all birthing classes is to provide the knowledge and confidence to give birth and make informed decisions. Anxiety-reducing strategies and a variety of coping techniques integrated into the physiology of the birth process will provide an aid to pain management. Knowledge regarding pregnancy, birth, and parenting is increased following attendance of antenatal classes. The desire to receive this information is a strong motivator for attending classes. Classes need to include information about decision making, including both informed consent and women's right to informed refusal. For the woman, it takes courage and confidence to communicate effectively with the healthcare team and her provider in making clear her expectations of labor and birth (Lothian, 2005). A broad range of nonpharmacologic behavioral strategies including controlled breathing, relaxation, positioning, and massage are usually presented in both the Lamaze and Bradley courses. The Lamaze® philosophy teaches that birth is a normal, natural, and healthy process. The Bradley Method® (also called "Husband-Coached Birth") places an emphasis on a natural approach to birth and on the active participation and teamwork with the baby's father as the birth coach. Hospital-based prenatal class presents content usually particular to specific institutional practices and may focus primarily on the medical model. Table 16–7 provides a detailed comparison of the potential content covered in classes.

TABLE 16–7. Comparison of Prenatal Education Classes

Type	Objective	Class content
Lamaze® International https://www.lamaze.org	Supports birth as normal, natural, safe, and healthy and empowers expectant women and their partners to make informed decisions about what to expect and what choices are available	4- to 6-week class, newsletter, free app and online courses Labor rehearsals, normal labor, birth, and early postpartum Positioning for labor and birth Relaxation and massage techniques to ease pain Labor support Communication skills Information about interventions, including risks and benefits Breastfeeding Healthy lifestyle
The Bradley Method® http://www.bradleybirth.com	Helps women and her partner to prepare for a natural labor and birth and take the responsibility needed for preparation	12-week series to promote natural birth Importance of nutrition and exercise Relaxation techniques to manage pain Labor rehearsals How to avoid a cesarean birth Postpartum care Breastfeeding Guidance for coach/doula about supporting and advocating for the mother
Hospital based	Provides information about procedures available at the particular hospital; usually taught by RN from the hospital	1- or 2-day class May include elements of Lamaze® and Bradley Method® Physical/emotional changes in pregnancy Information on cesarean birth, induction, augmentation and common labor and birth interventions, medication options specific to the facility May include postpartum and newborn care

RN, registered nurse.

Carlton, Callister, and Stoneman (2005) question whether some hospital-based education serves to socialize women about the "appropriate" ways of giving birth rather than educating them. Women who wish to avoid medications can be successful with the help of educational preparation, their support system, and perinatal nurses who respect that plan.

Addition of Stimulation at Any Site of the Body

Acupressure

Acupressure is a directed form of massage in which the support person or healthcare provider applies pressure to specific acupuncture points using fingers, elbows, or special devices. Acupressure may relieve back pain, headache, anxiety, stress, tension, nausea, and vomiting. Pericardium 6 (PC6) acupressure can reduce nausea in pregnancy using elasticated wristbands with a pressure dome applied to the site. PC6 is located on the palm side of the wrist in the midline between the two tendons (palmaris longus and flexor carpi radialis). To accurately locate the PC6 point, have the woman lay one hand palm up with the other hand placed palm down at right angles to the upturned arm. The first three fingers of the palm down hand are held close together and the edge of the ring finger is placed at the crease of the wrist closest to the palm. The acupressure point is now readily palpable under the tip of the index finger of the examining hand. Other acupressure points affect uterine contractions or duration of labor by stimulating the secretion of oxytocin from the hypophysis (Beal, 1999). Acupressure can also facilitate the progress of labor by reducing the neuroendocrine response to pain. In a randomized control trial that included 88 pregnant women, acupressure applied to point LI4, and the SP6 was found to decreased perception of labor pains and shortened labor (Calik & Komurcu, 2014). More research is needed on the effects of acupressure on labor.

Acupuncture

Acupuncture is the insertion of fine needles into specific areas of the body. It has been used for centuries in China and is gaining popularity in Western countries. One proposed theory is that acupuncture blocks pain stimuli from reaching the spinal cord. Acupuncture might have benefit as an alternative or complement to women who seek another method of pain relief in labor (Florence & Palmer, 2003); however, another study found that acupuncture did not reduce the need for epidural anesthesia (MacKenzie et al., 2011). More research is needed on the effects of acupuncture on labor.

Intradermal Injections of Sterile Water

Intradermal injections of sterile water (IISW) to control the pain of labor was first introduced in midwifery and obstetric literature in the late 1980s and uses counter-irritation to offset localized pain in the same dermatome distribution. Four subdermal injections are placed over the sacrum of a woman's back. The placement of IISW causes a brief intense, stinging, significant degree of additional pain, which could be viewed as counterintuitive (N. Lee, Kildea, & Stapleton, 2017). The National Institute for Health and Care Excellence (2017) guideline from the United Kingdom no longer recommends this painful procedure.

Transcutaneous Electrical Nerve Stimulation

Transcutaneous electrical nerve stimulation (TENS) is a pain management approach that places electrodes on the skin, conducting electrical stimuli, causing analgesia. There is limited evidence that TENS reduces pain in labor, and it does not seem to have any impact on other outcomes for mothers or infants (Bedwell, Dowswell, Neilson, & Lavender, 2011). In a controlled study, the application of TENS affected pain relief in the first and second stages of labor and 4 hours after labor (Shahoei, Shahghebi, Rezaei, & Nagshbandi, 2017). Given the absence of adverse effects and the limited evidence base, more robust studies of effectiveness are needed.

Cutaneous Measures to Reduce Painful Stimuli (Gate Control Theory)

Melzack and Wall's (1965) early work on the gate control theory modulates the sensory intensity component of pain. Gate control is explained by the structure of the central nervous system, which is composed of large and small sensory nerve fibers. Impulses are carried by the spinal cord from the site of the stimuli to the cerebral cortex, where impulses are interpreted. Small, thinly myelinated or unmyelinated fibers transport impulses such as pressure and pain from the uterus, cervix, and pelvic joints. Large myelinated fibers transport impulses from the skin. Because passage along large fibers occurs more quickly, it is possible for cutaneous stimulation to block or alter painful impulses. Based on this premise, tactile stimulation in the form of touch or massage is often used effectively during labor. The second process modulates the intensity of pain by triggering an endorphinergic system, which reduces pain everywhere except in the stimulated area. Melzack (1999) has reevaluated the gate control theory, adding to it the possibility of multiple influences within the brain; a neuromatrix that is responsible ultimately for how each individual perceives pain. These other influences include past experiences, cultural conditioning, emotional state, level of anxiety, understanding of the labor process, and the meaning that the current situation has for the individual are used by the cerebral cortex to interpret a sensation as painful. Just as thoughts and emotions can increase pain, they can also increase feelings of confidence and control, thereby decreasing painful sensations. Positioning/movement, light massage, counterpressure, water immersion, use of a birth ball, and warm or cold packs may decrease pain by the gate control theory (Challiet et al., 2014).

Maternal Position and Movement

Mobility in labor should be viewed as supporting the national physiologic process for optimal birth. Women who use upright positions and are mobile during labor have shorter, more efficient labors due to more intense and frequent contractions leading to progressive cervical dilation, receive fewer interventions, report less severe pain, and describe more satisfaction with their childbirth experience than women in recumbent positions (AWHONN, 2019; Cluett, Burns, & Cuthbert, 2018; Ondeck, 2014). Women naturally choose positions of comfort and are more likely to change position during early labor. Changing position alters the relationship between the fetus and pelvis and the efficiency of uterine contractions (Zwelling, 2010). Positioning and movements in labor are recommended for purposes other than comfort, such as rotating an asynclitic fetus and correcting slow progress in dilation or descent. Women who labor with the baby's head in an occipitoposterior position report significantly less back pain when using hands-and-knees positioning (Zwelling, 2010). Table 16–8 lists a variety of positions available to women in labor along with the benefits of each.

Women should be encouraged to change their position frequently during labor. *Listening to Mothers III* reported that only 40% of mothers changed positions in labor and only 43% walked after admission to the hospital (Declercq et al., 2013). Modern technology (e.g., internal EFM, IV tubing, catheters, automatic blood pressure monitors, neuraxial anesthesia, and pharmacologic use) may interfere with a woman's ability to change positions or safely ambulate and frequently restricts her to bed. Nurses and physicians may encourage bed rest for labor because it helps them feel more in control of the situation, and they believe it may be safer for the woman and fetus. Nevertheless, it is possible to use most of the technology available in maternity care without maintaining continuous bed rest. Frequent position changes during labor to enhance maternal comfort and promote optimal fetal positioning are recommended by ACOG (2019a) as long as appropriate monitoring can be achieved and the positioning is not contraindicated by maternal medical or obstetrical complications.

An upright position can be accomplished in a chair, recliner, rocking chair, or birthing bed adjusted to a chair position. Telemetry units for EFM, transducers that can be submerged in water or intermittent auscultation of the FHR can be used to evaluate fetal response to labor

TABLE 16–8. Labor Positions

Positions	Effect of positions
Standing or any upright position	Takes advantage of gravity during and between contractions Contractions less painful and more productive Fetus well aligned with angle of pelvis May speed labor if woman has been recumbent May increase urge to push in second stage
Walking	Movement causes changes in pelvic joints, encouraging rotation and descent
Standing and leaning forward on person or object (e.g., partner/support team, bed, or birth ball)	May relieve backache; good position for back rub More restful than standing Can maintain continuous electronic fetal monitor
Slow dancing (mother embraces significant other around neck, rests head on his or her chest or shoulder; with dancing partner's arms around mother's trunk, interlocking fingers at her low back, she can drop her arms and rests against the other person to increase relaxation)	Swaying movements to music may causes changes in pelvic joints, encouraging rotation and descent Rhythm and music add comfort Being embraced by loved one increases sense of well-being Position permits partner to give back pressure to relieve back pain.
Sitting upright	Resting position More gravity advantage than supine
Rocking in chair	Rocking movement is relaxing and increases comfort. Using foot stool decreases tension in lower extremities.
Sitting on toilet or commode	May help relax perineum for effective bearing down
Hands and knees (can achieve this position by kneeling on bed with head raised, kneeling on floor while leaning on a chair or birthing ball)	Helps relieve backache from occipitoposterior Allows freedom of movement for pelvic rocking Vaginal examinations possible Takes pressure off hemorrhoids
Side lying	Helps lower elevated blood pressure; increases perfusion of blood to the placenta and fetus Takes pressure off hemorrhoids Easier to relax between pushing efforts Effective position for pushing during second stage
Squatting while supporting herself on object like side of the bed or chair	Takes advantage of gravity Widens pelvic outlet; may enhance rotation and descent of the fetus Makes bearing down efforts more spontaneous
Supported squat: mother leans with back against standing partner who holds her under the arms and takes all her weight during contraction	Helpful if mother does not feel an urge to push
Supported squat: significant other sits on high bed or counter with feet supported on chairs or foot stool; with thighs spread, mother backs between legs and places flexed arms over thighs; significant other grips woman's sides with his or her thighs; she lowers herself, allowing other person to support her full weight	Mechanical advantage during second stage as upper trunk presses on uterine fundus Lengthens mother's trunk, allowing more room for asynclitic fetus to maneuver into position Eliminates restriction of pelvic joint mobility that can be caused by external pressure from bed or chair

Adapted from Simkin, P. (1995). Reducing pain and enhancing progress in labor: A guide to nonpharmacologic methods for maternity caregivers. *Birth, 22*(3), 161–171. doi:10.1111/j.1523-536X.1995.tb00693.x

while the woman is ambulating or using hydrotherapy. Maintaining a horizontal position during labor is associated with decreased blood flow and may increase uterine muscle hypoxia, resulting in the increased perception of pain associated with uterine contractions. Mayberry et al. (2000) and Molina, Solá, López, and Pires (1997) noted decreased pain in vertical as compared with horizontal positions before 6 cm of dilation.

Women may initially resist suggestions to change position or may find new positions uncomfortable. When encouraging a woman to change position, the nurse should provide extra support and encouragement and suggest that she remain in the new position through several contractions before deciding whether it will be sustained. Pillows, blanket wedges, and birthing balls should be generously used to maintain positions and

support extremities. When a side-lying position is used, supportive devices can be placed behind the back and between the knees. In a semi-Fowler's position, pillows can be placed under knees or arms. Shorter women sitting in a chair may find that a pillow or stool under their feet decreases stretching of leg muscles. While position changes during labor may be challenging due to resistance, unit culture, maternal obesity, and use of technology, encouraging, and using different positions will have a positive impact on the labor progress.

Birthing Ball

Standard physiotherapy balls routinely used in physical therapy and exercise programs are used in the labor setting. The woman can maintain an upright position by sitting on the ball or kneeling on the bed with her arms and chest draped over the ball. The rotation of the ball helps the mother to sway her hips side to side or in a circle. The birthing ball can facilitate position changes and be used as a comfort tool for women in labor. A woman can sit on it and rock or lightly bounce to decrease perineal pressure. She can also lean over the ball, decreasing back pain with an occiput posterior position. The peanut-shaped ball may be used to lift the upper leg resting around the narrow part of the ball opening the pelvic outlet. This position has been used to help rotate a fetal posterior position, decrease the length of labor, and increase the likelihood of spontaneous vaginal birth for women laboring under epidural analgesia (Roth, Dent, Parfitt, Hering, & Bay, 2016; Tussey et al., 2015). Birthing balls are one of the best tools for facilitating labor and can also be used for women with an epidural but only with assistance and support.

Touch and Massage

Touch in the form of hand holding, stroking, embracing, or patting communicates caring and reassurance. Cultural influences and personal factors may affect individual responses to touch; however, touch is universal and may soothe and reassure the laboring woman.

In hospitals, nurses have varying comfort levels with touch, and some may be more likely to advise support persons to provide the intervention. Usual touch by the nurse (only as necessary to perform clinical procedures) is different than comforting (nonclinical) touch. Perinatal nurses and others who provide support during labor use touch consciously and unconsciously throughout labor to communicate their support and presence, to relieve muscle tension, and to decrease the pain of labor. Most women appreciate touch in labor, and it may relieve pain and anxiety.

Massage is the manipulation of the soft tissues of the body to enhance health and healing. Massage has been used to decrease fatigue, tension, emotional distress, chronic, and acute pain. Purposeful use of back and shoulder massage is employed during labor as a relaxation and stress-reduction technique. This technique is effective for reducing pain because it functions as a distraction, may stimulate cutaneous nerve fibers that block painful impulses, and stimulates the local release of endorphins (Gentz, 2001; Huntley, Coon, & Ernst, 2004). Massage is accomplished with moderate pressure, activating large myelinated nerve fibers. Because habituation can occur, decreasing the beneficial effects of massage, the type of stroke and location should vary during labor. Effleurage is a technique moving the fingertips in a light circular stroke applied to the lower abdomen, usually performed in rhythm with breathing during a uterine contraction. The reaction of each woman should guide the nurse in the acceptability and value of this soothing measure (Declercq et al., 2013). Massage has been shown to promote labor progress, decrease pain perception, and increase the woman's ability to cope with labor (Zwelling, Johnson, & Allen, 2006). In a randomized controlled trial during which partners provided massage during labor, women reported significantly less pain and anxiety (Field, Hernandez-Reif, Taylor, Quintino, & Burman, 1997). In two randomized controlled trials, where the experimental group received several massages during labor, self-reports of anxiety levels were the same in both groups, but nurses reported observing significantly less behavioral manifestation of pain (Chang, Wang, & Chen, 2002), and pain scores were significantly less during early and active labor (Chang, Chen, & Huang, 2006).

Counterpressure

Back labor can be relieved by interventions used by the perinatal nurse or other labor support people. These techniques include counterpressure, bilateral hip pressure (e.g., double-hip squeeze), and the knee press (Simkin, 1995). These maneuvers are performed by applying localized pressure to reduce sacroiliac pain resulting from strain on sacroiliac ligaments caused by mechanisms of labor. Counterpressure requires application of enough force to meet the intensity of pressure from the fetal occipital bone against the sacrum (Fig. 16–2). Sacral pressure may help when a woman has back pain, usually most intense when the fetus is in a posterior position. Sacral pressure may be applied using the palm or fist of a hand or a firm object such as a tennis ball rotating in the hand. A variation of sacral pressure is the double hip squeeze in which the attendant's palms are placed on the woman's hips while she is in a standing or in a hands-and-knees position. Pressure is applied to both hips and pressed downward and inward toward the symphysis. When counterpressure is used, the woman should guide the support person as to the amount and exact location as to where to apply the pressure.

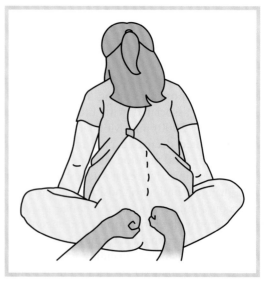

FIGURE 16–2. Firm counterpressure of the fists on the lower back.

Hydrotherapy

Hydrotherapy, or the use of warm water as a complementary nonpharmacologic pain relief technique, is an effective method of pain management in labor (Vanderlaan, 2017). It is capable of promoting relaxation, decreased anxiety, and pain. Positive benefits of water immersion include ease of positioning, buoyancy, hydrostatic pressure, and thermal relaxation. Hydrotherapy allows freedom of movement and helps facilitate maternal participation leading to a more normal labor process. Buoyancy in the tub allows for an almost weightless feeling, and women may have more opportunity to move during labor, which enhances progress due to the ease of movement. Using water immersion and covering the abdomen with warm water, the hydrostatic pressure of the water provides stability and relieves some of the pain associated with uterine contractions. Hydrostatic pressure moves fluid from the extravascular to the intravascular spaces reducing blood pressure and edema and promoting diuresis (Florence & Palmer, 2003). Warm water provides soothing stimulation of nerves in the skin, promoting vasodilation, reversal of sympathetic nervous system response, and a reduction in catecholamine production (Florence & Palmer, 2003). Hydrotherapy is thought to provide pain relief through the perception of warmth by nerve receptors in the skin. These nerve impulses travel to the cerebral cortex, and initiate the gate mechanism, thereby decreasing pain perception. Potential combined effects of these changes are proposed to result in increased intravascular volume, improved uterine perfusion, decreased pain, decreased blood pressure due to vasodilatation, increased relaxation, and shortened labor (Simkin & O'Hara, 2002). The water temperature should be maintained between 36° and 37.5°C to promote relaxation and maintain warmth (American College of Nurse-Midwives [ACNM], 2014).

Warmer water may raise both maternal and fetal temperature and lead to fetal tachycardia and elevated neonatal temperature (Simkin & O'Hara, 2002). Maternal effects of hydrotherapy include weakness, dizziness, nausea, tachycardia, or hypotension. These effects are usually related to an increase in body temperature or dehydration. Cool liquids should be provided to the mother to maintain her comfort and hourly monitoring of the water temperature will help to maintain optimal temperature. A repeated concern regarding the safety to the fetus is whether hydrotherapy can be used with ruptured membranes. Water does not enter the vagina during tub bathing. Additional safety concerns include planning for rapid draining of the water and movement to the birthing bed due to an indeterminate or abnormal FHR pattern, imminent birth, or maternal concern. A safety huddle including the woman and her support person and nursing and provider staff should occur prior to entry to the tub, which includes expectations of duration of hydrotherapy, need for emergent exit, and avoidance of injury from falls.

Tubs may be ordinary bathtubs, water-saving reclining tubs, or portable tubs. The manufacturer's recommendations and the hospital's infection control department are sources for appropriate cleaning and safety requirements.

If water immersion is not an option, a warm shower spray using a flexible handheld unit guided by the mother, her support person, or the nurse may provide comfort. Aiming at the lower uterine segment, the warm stream of water may help to relieve the stretching sensations of the ligaments and promote local vasodilatation that facilitates muscle relaxation and reduces pain of tense muscles (Mackey, 2001). Individuals supporting the woman in labor can assist her by holding the shower wand and adjusting the temperature as needed. The mother may stand or sit in the shower on a supportive bench or chair as tolerated and desired, even for long periods of time. Whether in a tub or a shower, hydrotherapy can provide relaxation and temporary pain relief in labor (Simkin & O'Hara, 2002). Hospital policies and culture may influence the use of hydrotherapy and other alternative methods of pain relief (Stark, Rudell, & Haus, 2008).

Water immersion is supported by ACOG (2019a) as a beneficial nonpharmacologic pain management technique for women in latent labor. Benfield, Herman, Katz, Wilson, and Davis (2001) published a small study of laboring women at 4-cm cervical dilation, noting a therapeutic effect of decreased anxiety at 15 minutes of warm water immersion with an added benefit of decreased pain and anxiety at 60 minutes compared to nonbathers. A randomized controlled study of 108 women found the pain index scores among women who used the immersion bath were significantly lower than those women without immersion (da Silva, de Oliveira, & Nobre, 2009). Kiani, Shahpourian, Sedighian, and Hosseini (2009) concluded that a warm water pool can be an effective way to decrease labor pain and alleviate suffering especially during the first and second stages of labor. Numerous positive benefits have been shown by use of hydrotherapy during labor (Cluett et al., 2018) and are listed in Display 16–6. See Table 16–9 for suggestions on use of hydrotherapy.

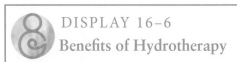

DISPLAY 16–6

Benefits of Hydrotherapy

- Pain and anxiety relief
- Increased diuresis
- Decreased edema
- Decreased blood pressure
- Enhanced fetal rotation due to increased buoyancy
- Less use of intramuscular and intravenous medication
- Less use of epidural anesthesia
- Fewer operative births (vacuum and forceps)
- Less perineal trauma
- Fewer episiotomies

TABLE 16–9. Hydrotherapy in Labor

Clinical practice	Referenced rationale
1. Warm water immersion using a tub may be considered as a complementary therapy for pain relief of the laboring women meeting the following eligibility criteria: • 37 weeks or greater gestation • Cephalic presentation, singleton • 30-min category I FHR tracing prior to tub entry • Active labor	The use of hydrotherapy during labor, whether in a shower or a tub, is a proven means of relaxation and pain relief (Cluett et al., 2018; Royal College of Obstetricians and Gynaecologists, 2012). The warm water stimulates the release of endorphins, relaxes muscles to decrease tension, stimulates large-diameter nerve fibers to close the gate on pain, and promotes better circulation and oxygenation (Garland & Jones, 1997).
2. If baseline FHR >160 or maternal temperature >100.4°F develops during water immersion, the water should be cooled or the mother assisted out of the tub to cool. If fetal tachycardia or elevated temperature persists despite these measures, the mother should not return to the tub, and the physician/midwife should be notified.	Fetal tachycardia may be a result of maternal hyperthermia because there were no differences for Apgar score less than 7 at 5 min, neonatal unit admissions, or neonatal infection rates when immersion was used (Cluett et al., 2018).
3. FHR may be auscultated or telemetry used according to the institution's fetal monitoring protocol while in the tub or shower.	Changes in water temperature by as little as 2°F have been noted to be associated with impact on maternal heart rate, cardiac output, diastolic blood pressure, and core body temperature. Recommended temperature to avoid potentially harmful effects is 96° to 98.6°F (36° to 37°C) (Eriksson, Ladfors, Mattsson, & Fall, 1996; Florence & Palmer, 2003).
4. Water temperature should remain between 96° and 98.6°F (36° and 37°C). The water temperature is documented every hour while the patient is in the tub. Water in the tub should cover the maternal abdomen.	With relaxation and comfort, stress hormone production may decrease. Increased comfort with submersion and decreased stress hormone production may improve uterine contractility. In a study of nulliparous women with dystocia, immersion in water reduced the rate of labor augmentation without resulting in longer labors (Cluett, Pickering, Getliffe, & St. George Saunders, 2004).
5. Vital signs are assessed and documented according to hospital protocol.	Cervical dilation at the onset of the bath may indirectly influence the duration of labor. Early labor use of the tub may result in a longer duration of the bath and suppression of the posterior gland's production of oxytocin (Cluett et al., 2018; Nikodem, 2004).
6. Ambulation and other nonpharmacologic measures are recommended until cervical dilation is 4 to 5 cm and contraction pattern is well established. Earlier entry into the tub may slow the progress of labor.	Frequency of fetal monitoring should be consistent with recognized standards of care and institutional policies and based on the stage of labor. When cervical dilation was 5 cm or greater upon entry to the tub, a decreased use of oxytocin, epidural analgesia, and shorter labor resulted (Eriksson et al., 1996).
7. Provide hydration for the mother with cold/cool drinks, for example, water, juice, sport drinks, or any clear liquid.	Several physiologic changes occur with immersion in warm water. Buoyancy allows for support of extremities, while hydrostatic pressure gives equal resistance to all muscle groups, providing stability. This support and stability allow for freedom of movement and a sense of weightlessness that may encourage movement (Simkin & O'Hara, 2002). Women with a normal, uncomplicated active labor may drink modest amounts of clear liquids such as water, fruit juice without pulp, carbonated beverages, clear tea, black coffee, and sports drinks (American College of Obstetricians and Gynecologists, 2009).
8. If an IV is started, protect the site with plastic covering.	The data on IV fluids type and infusion rate is insufficient for a strong recommendation (Berghella, Baxter, & Chauhan, 2008).
9. Water is changed or the woman leaves the tub if excessive feces or debris accumulates during labor that cannot be easily removed with a tropical fish net.	Contraindications include thick meconium, oxytocin infusion, bleeding or large bloody show, epidural analgesia or anesthesia, and concern about fetal status.
10. Use of water immersion for labor is documented in the woman's record.	Documentation and record keeping are a fundamental part of clinical practice (Williams, Davies, & Ross, 2009). Warm water may cause dizziness and a decrease in catecholamine release will decrease blood pressure.
11. Support person or member of the nursing staff should be present at all times. Shower seat should be available in the shower for the laboring woman as well as a seat outside of the shower or tub for their support person.	Labor support is essential, especially for the woman with an unmedicated labor.

FHR, fetal heart rate; IV, intravenous.

Warm Packs

Hospital resources may not accommodate immersion tubs or allow women to bring inflatable devices for use in labor or provide the opportunity to shower during labor. An alternative source of heat may be provided by the use of a hot water bottle, warm moist towel, heating pad, and chemical warm packs. Warmth increases local blood flow, relaxes muscles, and raises the pain threshold. Caution must be used when using external devices so that scalding of the skin does not occur.

Hospital-established protocols may prohibit use of external heating devices. The advantages of using thermal interventions as a nonpharmacologic method of pain relief may include a reduction and/or delay in the use of pharmacotherapy, allowing the laboring woman to have a more active role in the labor process.

Ice/Cold Compress

Cold compresses may provide relief of musculoskeletal pain and may be an appropriate intervention to suggest if heat is not an option or not desired. An ice pack, frozen gel pack, cold towels, or chemical cool pack applied to the lower back may provide pain relief for the laboring woman. A cool cloth to the forehead, neck, wrist areas may provide comfort.

PHARMACOLOGIC APPROACHES

The pharmacologic approach to labor pain management views pain as a potential physical threat, which should be eased to an acceptable pain threshold or eliminated. Unlike acute pain, labor pain is considered by some women as tolerable and an empowering natural sign of labor progression, while others suffer with excruciating pain depriving them of a positive experience and sometimes resulting in psychological harm (Flink et al., 2009). The woman's autonomy should be respected, allowing for flexibility to change the birth plan regarding analgesia as labor progresses. Maternal request for pain relief in labor is a sufficient indication in the absence of a medical contraindication (ACOG, 2019b) (Display 16–7). Alleviation and control of pain are of major importance for the laboring woman and her caregivers. Pain management options should be offered to the laboring woman and the decision for pain

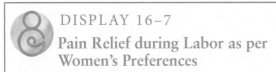

DISPLAY 16–7

Pain Relief during Labor as per Women's Preferences

Labor causes severe pain for many women. There is no other circumstance where it is considered acceptable for an individual to experience untreated severe pain, amenable to safe intervention, while under a physician's care. Many women desire pain management during labor and birth. In the absence of a medical contraindication, maternal request is a sufficient medical indication for pain relief during labor. A woman who requests epidural analgesia during labor should not be denied this service based on the status of her health insurance or her ability to pay.

Adapted from American College of Obstetricians and Gynecologists. (2019b). *Obstetric analgesia and anesthesia* (Practice Bulletin No. 209). Washington, DC: Author.

management should be based on the woman's preference in collaboration with her maternity care provider rather than insurance status or ability to pay (ACOG, 2019b; American Society of Anesthesiologists [ASA], 2016a; AWHONN, 2011; Collins, 2018). The ASA (2016a) optimal goals for anesthesia care in obstetrics are listed in (Display 16–8).

The use of pain-relieving drugs during labor is now part of standard care in many countries throughout the world (Ullman, Smith, Burns, Mori, & Dowswell, 2010). Neuraxial use has tripled between 1981 and 2001 with approximately 75% of women in the United States using this technique in labor (Briggs & Wan, 2006; Declercq et al., 2013; Martin, Hamilton, Osterman, Driscoll, & Drake, 2018; Oesterman & Martin, 2011). Figure 16–3 reflects maternal recall from the *Listening to Mothers II* and *III* report revealing a slight change from 2007 to 2013 in pharmacologic methods used in labor. The patterns of pain may vary during the day, with peak and trough times reported at different times of the day. Therapeutic effects of opioids and local anesthetics also demonstrate circadian variations (Touitou, Dispersyn, & Pain, 2010).

The woman should clearly understand benefits and potential maternal–fetal side effects of pharmacologic methods. This information is best discussed during the prenatal period with her prenatal provider. During labor, the woman may be exhausted, distressed, and not coping. She may feel remorseful following the birth if pharmacologic methods were not in her birth plan or suffer from posttraumatic stress disorder if the pain was unrelenting (Flink et al., 2009). Women who plan to avoid the use of medication for pain control should not be pressured into using medication but neither should they have such medication withheld if they change their minds during labor. The neuraxial procedure and potential complications must be discussed between the anesthesiologist, maternity care provider, and the woman with sufficient time for her questions to be answered. Some institutions provide the opportunity for women to meet with an anesthesia provider before admission. The perinatal nurse assesses preferences for pain management on admission and conducts ongoing assessments of factors influencing pain perception throughout labor.

Pharmacologic pain management strategies used during labor include sedatives and hypnotics, parenteral opioids, neuraxial analgesia, and local anesthesia. Pharmacologic use during labor brings unique concerns that are not faced in other clinical areas. These include concerns about the effect medications may have on the course and outcome of labor and the fetus or newborn. In some situations, women experiencing prolonged latent labor may benefit from the brief period of therapeutic rest or sleep.

DISPLAY 16–8

Optimal Goals for Anesthesia Care in Obstetrics

Good obstetric care requires the availability of qualified personnel and equipment to administer general or neuraxial anesthesia. The extent and degree to which anesthesia services are available varies widely among hospitals. For any hospital providing obstetric care, certain optimal anesthesia goals should be sought. These include the following:

I. Availability of a licensed practitioner who is credentialed to administer an appropriate anesthetic whenever necessary. For many childbearing women, neuraxial anesthesia (epidural, spinal, or combined spinal epidural) will be the most appropriate anesthetic.

II. Availability of a licensed practitioner who is credentialed to maintain support of vital functions during any obstetric emergency

III. Availability of anesthesia and surgical personnel to permit the start of a cesarean birth in a timely manner in accordance with clinical needs and local resources.

IV. Because the risks associated with trial of labor after cesarean birth (TOLAC) and uterine rupture may be unpredictable, the immediate availability of appropriate facilities and personnel (including obstetric anesthesia; nursing personnel; and a physician capable of monitoring labor and performing cesarean birth, including an emergency cesarean birth) is optimal. When resources for immediate cesarean birth are not available, patients considering TOLAC should discuss the hospital's resources and availability of obstetric, anesthetic, pediatric, and nursing staff with their obstetric provider and patients should be clearly informed of the potential increase in risk and the management alternatives. The definition of immediately available personnel and facilities remains a local decision based on each institution's available resources and geographic location.

V. Appointment of a qualified anesthesiologist to be responsible for all anesthetics administered. There are many obstetric units where physicians or physician-supervised nurse anesthetists administer labor anesthetics. The administration of general or neuraxial anesthesia requires both medical judgment and technical skills. Thus, a physician with privileges in anesthesiology should be readily available.

Persons administering or supervising obstetric anesthesia should be qualified to manage the infrequent but occasionally life-threatening complications of neuraxial anesthesia, such as respiratory and cardiovascular failure, toxic local anesthetic convulsions, or vomiting and aspiration. Mastering and retaining the skills and knowledge necessary to manage these complications requires adequate training and frequent application.

To ensure the safest and most effective anesthesia for obstetric patients, the physician director of anesthesia services, with the approval of the medical staff, should develop and enforce written policies regarding provision of obstetric anesthesia. These include the following:

I. A qualified physician with obstetric privileges to perform operative vaginal or cesarean birth who concurs with the patient's management and has knowledge of the maternal and fetal status and progress of labor should be readily available during administration of anesthesia. Readily available should be defined by each institution within the context of its resources and geographic location. Neuraxial and/or general anesthesia should not be administered until the patient has been examined and the fetal status and progress of labor evaluated by a qualified individual.

II. Availability of equipment, facilities, and support personnel equal to that provided in the surgical suite. This should include the availability of a properly equipped and staffed recovery room capable of receiving and caring for all patients recovering from neuraxial or general anesthesia. Birthing facilities, when used for labor anesthesia services or surgical anesthesia, must be appropriately equipped to provide safe anesthetic care during labor and birth or post-anesthesia recovery care.

III. Personnel other than the surgical team should be immediately available to assume care of the newborn. The obstetric provider and anesthesiologist are responsible for the mother and may not be able to leave her care for the newborn.

In larger maternity units and those functioning as high-risk centers, 24-hour in-house anesthesia, obstetric, and neonatal specialists are usually available. Preferably, the obstetric anesthesia services should be directed by an anesthesiologist with special training or experience in obstetric anesthesia. These units will also frequently require the availability of more sophisticated monitoring equipment and specially trained nursing personnel.

Good interpersonal relations between obstetric providers, anesthesiologists, and certified registered nurse anesthetists are important. Joint meetings between the two departments should be encouraged. Anesthesiologists should recognize the special needs and concerns of obstetric providers, who in turn should recognize the anesthesiologist as a consultant in the management of pain and life-support measures. Both should recognize the need to provide high-quality care for all patients.

Adapted from American Society of Anesthesiologists. (2016a). *Optimal goals for anesthesia care in obstetrics.* Washington, DC: Author.

Sedatives and Hypnotics

The term *sedative–hypnotic* describes the effect this group of medications has on the individual; it is not a classification of drugs. The effect of these drugs is dose related. In low doses, they cause sedation and higher doses cause a hypnotic effect. Two classifications of drugs used in labor to provide sedative–hypnotic effects are barbiturates and H_1-receptor antagonists (i.e., antihistamines).

Historically, women experiencing prolonged latent labor were thought to benefit from the brief period of therapeutic rest or sleep following administration

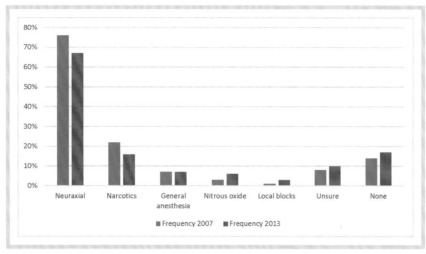

FIGURE 16–3. Comparison between 2007 and 2013 of pharmacologic use during labor. (Adapted from Declercq, E. R., Sakala, C., Corry, M. P., & Applebaum, S. [2007]. Listening to mothers II: Report of the second national U.S. survey of women's childbearing experiences: Conducted January-February 2006 for Childbirth Connection by Harris Interactive® in partnership with Lamaze International. *The Journal of Perinatal Education, 16*[4], 15–17. doi:10.1624/105812407X244778; Declercq, E. R., Sakala, C., Corry, M. P., Applebaum, S., & Herrlich, A. [2013]. *Listening to mothers III pregnancy and birth: Report of the third national U.S. survey of women's childbearing experiences.* Retrieved from http://transform.childbirth connection.org/wp-content/uploads/2013/06/LTM-III_Pregnancy-and-Birth.pdf)

of barbiturates. Barbiturates such as secobarbital sodium (Seconal) and pentobarbital (Nembutal) given orally or as an intramuscular injection have little analgesic action, depress the central nervous system, and decrease anxiety and can potentiate respiratory depression (Faucher & Brucker, 2000). Barbiturates are lipid soluble, easily cross the placenta, and have a long half-life. Seconal has been found in maternal and fetal blood samples for up to 40 hours after administration and therefore is rarely used in modern-day obstetrics (Florence & Palmer, 2003).

Zolpidem tartrate (Ambien) is unrelated to barbiturates but possesses the sedative and hypnotic properties of benzodiazepines. The usual dosage of 5 to 10 mg has a mean peak blood concentration of 1.6 hours and half-life of 1.4 to 4.5 hours. This drug may enable the exhausted woman to rest and recover from hypertonic uterine dysfunction or prolonged latent phase so that she is better able to cope with active labor (Florence & Palmer, 2003).

H_1-receptor antagonists include promethazine hydrochloride (Phenergan), hydroxyzine hydrochloride (Vistaril), and propiomazine (Largon). These medications may be administered with opioids during labor to relieve anxiety, increase sedation, and decrease nausea and vomiting. Promethazine hydrochloride can cause respiratory depression and if combined with an opioid may cause hypotension and sedation leading to a fall risk, should the woman ambulate (Poole, 2003). H_1-receptor antagonists traditionally have been thought to potentiate the effects of opioids;

however, there is no objective evidence to support this belief (Wakefield, 1999). Although all H_1-receptor antagonists have a sedative effect on the woman in labor, they cross the placenta, and when administered close to birth, neonatal respiratory depression may occur, and resuscitation may be required (McKenzie & Pulley, 2016).

Inhalational Analgesia

Nitrous oxide is a colorless, almost odorless, and tasteless gas provided in a 50:50 ratio of nitrous oxide to oxygen and inhaled to provide analgesia during labor. In addition to labor use, nitrous oxide has been used for initiation of regional anesthesia, external cephalic version, and other procedures during intrapartum including placement of an inflatable bulb for cervical ripening, laceration repair, and manual removal of the placenta (Collins, 2017). The analgesic effect is thought to be via the stimulation of an endogenous endorphin release creating a euphoric effect that decreases pain perception (Sanders, Weimann, & Maze, 2008; Stewart & Collins, 2012). Nitrous oxide is self-administered with a demand valve connected to a facemask or mouthpiece. The aim being that the mother should remain conscious with preservation of her laryngeal reflexes (O'Sullivan, 2010). This form of analgesia is widely used in the United Kingdom, Australia, Finland, and Canada. Collins (2017) reports this method is gaining acceptance in the United States with more than 300 hospitals and 70 birth centers offering nitrous oxide as an option for laboring women. According to ACNM (2010), all women in the United States should have universal access to nitrous for labor pain relief. Likewise, per AWHONN, nitrous oxide should be a vital component in the provision of quality maternity care and may be initiated by the bedside nurse (Collins, 2018).

Due to the rapid onset and offset of action, timing of use is central to effectiveness and satisfaction. The peak-onset analgesic effect of nitrous oxide is 30 to 50 seconds and will require patient education and coaching as to timing of inhalation in relation to uterine activity. Nitrous oxide is rapidly cleared from the maternal system within 30 to 60 seconds allowing the woman options to change to another form of pain management or utilize nonpharmacologic methods such as water immersion, hypnosis, and acupressure. The laboring woman can remain ambulatory, IV access is not necessary, and intermittent fetal monitoring can be used (Stewart & Collins, 2012). Nitrous oxide administration does not affect uterine activity and thus would not be expected to affect the course of the first and second stage of labor or rate of cesarean birth. Nitrous oxide readily passes across the placenta; however, there is little apparent effect on Apgar score, acid–base balance, neurologic, and adaptive capacity scores (Reynolds, 2010). Adverse maternal effects of vertigo, nausea, and vomiting are reported; however, it is unclear if this is due to the normal progress of labor or use of nitrous oxide (Jones et al., 2012; Volmanen, Palomäki, & Ahonen, 2011). Contraindications to the use of nitrous oxide are included in Display 16–9 (Collins, 2017).

Results on efficacy are mixed. A Cochrane review noted this modality appeared to be effective as a labor analgesic without increasing risk or adverse neonatal outcomes (Klomp et al., 2012). Current published data does not provide clear quantitative objective evidence of sufficient pain management; thus, more robust studies are needed (Likis et al., 2014; Richardson et al., 2017).

DISPLAY 16–9

Contraindications to Nitrous Oxide Use

- Inability to hold or self-administer the mask or inability to cooperate
- Recent collapsed lung, bowel, or gastric surgery (recent history of gastric bypass)
- Increased intraocular or intracranial pressure
- Very low vitamin B_{12} levels associated with celiac sprue disease, Crohn disease, and pernicious anemia

---

Parenteral Opioids

Opioids are agents for relief of severe pain. An opioid is a chemical that binds to opioid receptors, which are widely distributed in the central and peripheral nervous system and gastrointestinal tract. The pain-killing effect of opioids is induced by the synergy of the two events, namely, reduction of pain threshold and emotional detachment from pain. The opioid effects transcending analgesia include sedation, constipation, and a strong sense of euphoria with respiratory depression being the greatest hazard. Repeated use can lead to tolerance, physical dependence, and addiction (Phillips, Fernando, & Girard, 2017). The use of opiates in labor is approximately 40% to 56%, both in the United States and in the United Kingdom (Ullman et al., 2010). Women not desirous of or not able to use neuraxial technique may choose parenteral opioids. Advantages include cost, ease of availability, and administration.

There are three main types of opioid receptors found in the central and peripheral nervous system: the mu, delta, and kappa receptors. Additional receptor types were proposed (e.g., sigma, epsilon, orphanin) but are no longer considered "classical" opioid receptors (Stein, 2016). Once bound, opioids lead to a reduction in nerve transmission and therefore pain impulses. Table 16–10 highlights the most commonly used opioids and their receptor-binding patterns. Individual drugs have an affinity for one or more receptor sites, which accounts for differences in pharmacodynamics, variable degree of analgesia, and side effects. There are three types of drugs, which may be administered parenteral during labor: opioids (morphine), synthetic opioids (fentanyl and remifentanil), and opioid agonist-antagonists (butorphanol and nalbuphine). Parenteral opioids can be administered intramuscularly, as IV intermittent boluses, or through a woman-controlled IV administration system.

Depending on the dose, route of administration, and stage of labor, parenteral analgesia does not eliminate pain but instead causes a blunting effect, inducing somnolence and decreasing the perception of pain allowing women to relax and rest between contractions.

Table 16–11 lists parenteral opioid analgesics used in labor including dose, route of administration, onset of action, time of peak effect, and duration of action. The opioid choice for analgesia in labor is dependent on what is available and customary in each facility. There is insufficient evidence to support the choice of one opioid over another (Ullman et al., 2010).

Morphine has a strong affinity for mu receptors, resulting in effective analgesia and dose-dependent respiratory depression. While parenteral opioids may provide sedation and comfort, there is strong evidence to suggest that morphine does not decrease pain intensity (Silva & Halpern, 2010). Morphine sulfate may cause allergic reactions in sulfite-sensitive people,

TABLE 16–10. Parenteral Opioid Agents Used in Labor and Their Receptor-Binding Relationships

Receptor	Receptor properties	Medication
Mu	Supraspinal analgesia Respiratory depression Euphoria Physical dependence Constipation	Morphine Meperidine—no longer recommended Butorphanol (weak) Fentanyl Sufentanil Remifentanil Alfentanil
Kappa	Spinal analgesia Dysphoria Sedation Diuresis Slight respiratory depression	Morphine (weak) Butorphanol Nalbuphine
Delta	Spinal analgesia and smooth muscle relaxation Constipation	Morphine (weak) Codeine (weak)

Adapted from Faucher, M. A., & Brucker, M. C. (2000). Intrapartum pain: Pharmacologic management. *Journal of Obstetric, Gynecologic, and Neonatal Nursing, 29*(2), 169–180.

more common in women with asthma. Morphine may be used during a prolonged period of early labor to rest prior to active labor. The use of meperidine is no longer recommended for peripartum analgesia due to the active metabolite normeperidine's half-life of up to 72 hours in the neonate and may lead to respiratory depression (ACOG, 2019b).

The synthetic opioids, fentanyl and remifentanil, have advantages of short duration of action, IV pharmacologic action, and are suited for systemic labor analgesia. Fentanyl may be administered via several routes, most commonly via epidural or IV injection. The time to peak effect of fentanyl is 3 to 4 minutes; it is well tolerated and administered using a patient-controlled analgesia pump. One study found that intranasal use was also effective (Kerr, Taylor, & Evans, 2015). Remifentanil rapidly transfers across the placenta and is metabolized rapidly in the fetus; therefore, neonatal depression is minimized. These synthetic opioids do not cause as much sedation, nausea, and emesis

as women experienced with opioids (Reynolds, 2010). Remifentanil is a more expensive, novel mu receptor agonist that has been used in obstetric anesthesia and analgesia for almost 10 years. It is preferred for the rapid onset of effect (approximately 1 minute), rapid degradation, and elimination in the fetus. It does not accumulate even after prolonged administration. Efficacy and safety in labor are well established; however, fetal and maternal monitoring is recommended with this drug (Evron & Ezri, 2007; Hinova & Fernando, 2009; Volmanen et al., 2011). Remifentanil regimen requires close maternal monitoring (suggested 1:1 nursing ratio), continuous oxygen saturation monitoring due to the potential for maternal respiratory depression, and a dedicated IV cannula for this particular drug administration (Hinova & Fernando, 2009; Volmanen et al., 2011). No study has identified an increased incidence of indeterminate or abnormal FHR recording after remifentanil has been used for labor analgesia and no neonate has required naloxone

TABLE 16–11. Parenteral Opioid Dosing

Drug	Dose	Route	Onset of action (min)	Duration of action (hr)
Morphine	2 to 5 mg	IV	10	1 to 3
	5 to 10 mg	IM	30	
Butorphanol (Stadol)		IV	5 to 10	3 to 4
	1 to 2 mg	IM	30 to 60	4 to 6
Nalbuphine (Nubain)		IV	2 to 3	2 to 4
	10 to 20 mg	IM, SQ	10 to 15	
Fentanyl (Sublimaze)	50 to 100 mcg	IV	2 to 4	0.5 to 1
	50 mcg load	PCA		
	10 to 25 mcg Q 10 to 12 min			
Remifentanil	20 mcg	IV (PCA)	1	15 min

IM, intramuscular; IV, intravenous; PCA, patient-controlled analgesia; Q, every; SQ, subcutaneous.
Adapted from American College of Obstetricians and Gynecologists. (2017). *Obstetric analgesia and anesthesia* (Practice Bulletin No. 177). Washington, DC: Author.

after birth (D'Onofrio, Novelli, Mecacci, & Scarselli, 2009; Hinova & Fernando, 2009).

Butorphanol (Stadol) and nalbuphine (Nubain), with affinity for the kappa receptors, provide effective analgesia with less respiratory depression than synthetic opioids. Agonist-antagonists have limited effect on maternal respiratory depression, regardless of the number of doses (Althaus & Wax, 2005). IV butorphanol and nalbuphine during labor have been associated with transient sinusoidal-like FHR patterns during labor (ACOG, 2009). This nonpathologic sinusoidal pattern may be noted for 10 to 90 minutes but without any adverse neonatal outcomes (Florence & Palmer, 2003). Because it can increase blood pressure, butorphanol should be avoided if the woman has hypertension or preeclampsia (ACOG, 2009).

All opioids can cause unwanted maternal side effects such as nausea, vomiting, constipation, sedation, and respiratory depression (Phillips et al., 2017). After administration of these medications, the frequency and duration of contractions may decrease and may be the result of decreased anxiety and serum concentrations of catecholamines (Althaus & Wax, 2005; Mussell, 1998). For this reason, parenteral analgesia is usually not administered until a labor pattern is well established. When given during labor, these medications often cause women to doze between contractions. If medication administration does result in dozing, coaching by a support person or nurse is important to help the woman anticipate and recognize the beginning of a contraction rather than have her startled awake at the peak of a contraction.

Any drug present in maternal blood and transferred to the central nervous system must readily cross the blood–brain barrier and therefore also the placenta and can have a cumulative effect, increasing the potential for neonatal respiratory depression as the woman receives more medication (Florence & Palmer, 2003; Reynolds, 2010). The greatest risk of harm is to the fetus related to placental transfer and longer half-life due to reduced neonatal metabolism leading to respiratory depression, lower Apgar, and neurobehavioral scores, with the potential for decreased suckling, leading to impaired breastfeeding (Ullman et al., 2010). Neonatal effects may be apparent for the first few hours and include reduced oxygen saturation, increased carbon dioxide levels, acidosis, and diminished thermoregulation (Reynolds, 2010). Because of the potential for adverse neonatal effects, the timing of administration relative to birth of the newborn is important. The greatest risk is if an opioid is administered 2 to 3 hours prior to birth; therefore, ideally, birth should occur within 1 hour or after 4 hours following administration (Althaus & Wax, 2005). Naloxone hydrochloride (Narcan), an opioid antagonist, reverses the respiratory depression caused by parenteral opioids received by the mother within the past 4 hours.

This agent is administered directly to the newborn who continues to experience respiratory depression after positive pressure ventilation has restored a normal heart rate (American Heart Association & American Academy of Pediatrics [AAP], 2016). Naloxone should not be given to infants of mothers who are addicted or suspected of being addicted to narcotics or who are in a methadone treatment program. In these infants, naloxone can cause withdrawal signs and symptoms including seizures.

Opioid-dependent women present with special needs and nonpharmacologic or neuraxial labor pain management methods may be a better choice (Reddy, Davis, Zhaoxia, & Greene, 2017). Currently, the prescription drug abuse milieu increases the possibility that a laboring woman has a history of opioid abuse (Saia et al., 2016). Opioid-dependent women have an 80% to 90% unintended pregnancy rate, almost double the overall unintended pregnancy rate: 40% globally and 51% in North America (Saia et al., 2016). Providing adequate pain relief to opioid-dependent women during labor is challenging; however, the efficacy of local anesthetics is not affected. It is important to avoid treating opioid-dependent women with antagonists and agonists (e.g., nalbuphine or butorphanol) because these can precipitate drug withdrawal because of its strong antagonist effect at the mu receptor site. Women on a methadone or buprenorphine treatment program should be continued at the usual dose throughout the peripartum period to avoid withdrawal (Reddy et al., 2017). Of note, opioid-naive women after cesarean birth are at risk to become persistent users, therefore limiting prescription dosing for discharge is essential (Reddy et al., 2017).

Neuraxial Analgesia

Neuraxial analgesia in labor refers to the epidural or spinal administration of opioids combined with a local anesthetic. Methods of administration include single injection, continuous or intermittent infusion, combined spinal and epidural (CSE) technique, or patient-controlled epidural analgesia (PCEA) (Apfelbaum et al., 2016; Wong, 2014). The goal of neuraxial analgesia techniques during labor is to provide sufficient analgesia effect with as little motor block as possible. Lower concentrations of local anesthetic, in combination with opioids such as fentanyl (Sublimaze), sufentanil (Sufenta), alfentanil (Alfenta), and remifentanil (Ultiva), result in increased pain relief without major motor block (Apfelbaum et al., 2016). The anesthesia care provider may have preferences regarding type of local anesthetic agent in a variety of concentrations combined with an opioid choice. When a local anesthetic is combined with an opioid, there is less motor blockade, no difference in rate of spontaneous versus operative vaginal birth or perineal pain during second-stage labor and increased maternal satisfaction with pain management (Hong, 2010; Russell & Reynolds, 1996; Wong, McCarthy, & Hewlett, 2011). As cervical dilatation progresses, some women require an increase in the rate of the continuous infusion or a second bolus with a higher concentration of medication. Of the various pharmacologic methods available for use during labor, neuraxial analgesia techniques are the most effective, widely used by laboring women and results in the least central nervous system depression of the mother and neonate (ACOG, 2019b; Declercq et al., 2013; Oesterman & Martin, 2011). In 2017 (the most recent year for which data are available), in the United States, approximately 75% of women had epidural or spinal anesthesia during labor (Martin et al., 2018). The benefits and limitations of neuraxial analgesia are outlined in Display 16–10. Successful epidural analgesia produces a segmental sympathetic and sensory nerve block and a decrease in endogenous catecholamines with the onset of pain relief. The anesthesiologist or certified registered nurse anesthetist (CRNA) is responsible for identifying women with contraindications to the procedure (Display 16–11). Medications commonly used for neuraxial analgesia including adverse effects are described in Table 16–12.

DISPLAY 16–11

Contraindications to Neuraxial Analgesia

- Coagulation disorders
- Local infection at the site of injection
- Maternal hypotension and shock
- Abnormal fetal heart rate pattern requiring immediate birth
- Maternal inability to cooperate or nondesirous of neuraxial analgesia
- Allergy to local anesthetics
- Progressive neurologic diseases, raised intracranial pressure
- Last dose of low-dose low molecular weight heparin within 12 hr or high dose <24 hr

The neuraxial block may be performed for a woman who is in a seated or sitting or lateral position that maximizes the distance between the spinous processes. The decision for position is usually based on anesthesia provider preference or the woman's choice. In some women, the sitting position may result in orthostatic hypotension and syncope. Maternal cardiac output may be reduced in the left lateral position (Silva & Halpern, 2010). It is important to align the vertebrae so that the spinous processes can be palpated and the needle correctly inserted into the epidural space. Excess adipose tissue or well-developed paraspinous muscles create difficulty for the provider to palpate the spinous processes, and therefore, the sitting position may be preferred. In some cases, ultrasound identification of the midline may be useful in determining approximate depth to the epidural space and level of puncture (Silva & Halpern, 2010). It is critical for a healthcare assistant to provide continuous support to the woman during the procedure.

Anesthesia guidelines and systematic reviews support epidural administration in early labor (less than 5 cm dilation) and not withholding neuraxial analgesia on the basis of achieving an arbitrary cervical dilation (ASA, 2016b; O'Hana et al., 2008; Sng et al., 2014; Wong et al., 2005). Use of neuraxial analgesia techniques and the timing of catheter placement does not influence cesarean birth rate (ACOG, 2019b; Caughey et al., 2014). Use of epidural or spinal anesthesia is more common in vaginal births assisted by forceps (84%) or vacuum extraction (77%) than in spontaneous vaginal births (60%) (Oesterman & Martin, 2011). There is no evidence that discontinuing the epidural infusion during the second stage of labor may improve the woman's ability to push. Efforts to sustain adequate epidural analgesia in the second stage should always be made (Abenhaim & Fraser, 2008).

Pregnancy conditions such as twin gestation, maternal hypertension, difficult airway, or obesity validates the practice of prophylactic placement of an

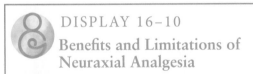

DISPLAY 16–10

Benefits and Limitations of Neuraxial Analgesia

Benefits	Limitations
• Generally provides superior pain relief, and position changes are less uncomfortable • Usually provides sufficient anesthesia for episiotomy and/or repair of lacerations • Placement of an epidural catheter in labor means that an emergent cesarean section can occur more quickly, should this become necessary • Women for whom general anesthesia is a risk (e.g., marked obesity, history of difficult/failed intubation, abnormalities of face, neck, spine, severe medical complications such as cardiac pulmonary or neurologic disease) may benefit from having an epidural catheter placed and functioning in early labor.	• Decreases ambulation and movement potential • Increases probability for operative vaginal birth (forceps and vacuum) • Increased risk of maternal adverse events leading to potential fetal compromise (hypotension, fever, systemic toxicity, etc.) • American Society of Anesthesiologists (2016b) Practice Guidelines suggest that an anesthesia care provider must be in-house during the conduct of a labor epidural. Availability may be limited or increased wait times for pain relief.

TABLE 16–12. Medications Commonly Used for Regional Analgesia/Anesthesia during Labor

Anesthesia agents

Drug	Route	Concentration (%)	Volume (mL)	Dose (mg)	Side effects/adverse reactions*	Nursing implications
Bupivacaine	Epidural block	0.25	10 to 20	25 to 50	Hypotension† FHR changes† Dysrhythmias† Bronchospasm† Seizures† Respiratory arrest† Cardiovascular collapse†	Monitor maternal vital signs. Monitor FHR. Ensure resuscitation equipment available.
		0.50	10 to 20	50 to 100		
	Intermittent infusion	0.125 to 0.375	5 to 10			
	Continuous infusion	0.0625 to 0.25	8 to 15			
	Caudal block	0.25	15 to 30	37.5 to 75		
		0.5	15 to 30	75 to 150		
	Surgical spinal	0.75 in 8.25% dextrose				
Lidocaine	Epidural block	1	25 to 30	250 to 300	Hypotension† FHR changes† Muscular twitching† Light-headedness† Edema† CNS depression† Tinnitus† Coma† Seizures† Respiratory arrest† Cardiovascular collapse†	Monitor maternal vital signs. Monitor FHR. Ensure resuscitation equipment available.
		1.5	15 to 20	225 to 300		
	Intermittent injection	2	10 to 15	200 to 300		
	Continuous infusion	0.75 to 1.5	5 to 10			
	Caudal block	0.5–1.0	8–15			
		1	20 to 30	200 to 300		
	Spinal surgical	5 in 7.5% dextrose	1.5 to 2.0	75 to 100		
Ropivacaine	Intermittent injection	0.125 to 0.25	5 to 10	20 to 30	Hypotension† FHR changes† Neonatal jaundice†	Monitor maternal vital signs. Monitor FHR. Ensure resuscitation equipment available.
	Continuous infusion	0.125 to 0.25	6 to 12	12 to 28		

Narcotic agents

Drug	Route	Concentration (mcg/mL)	Rate (mL/hr)	Side effects/adverse reactions*	Nursing implications
Fentanyl	PCEA	1 to 3	8 to 20	FHR changes† Hypotension† Nausea† Pruritus† Sedation† Vomiting† Urinary retention† Dysrhythmias† Respiratory depression†	Prolonged administration may ↑ risk of maternal/fetal/neonatal respiratory/CNS depression. Crosses placenta rapidly. Monitor for maternal/neonatal respiratory depression. Determine allergy status. Ensure naloxone and resuscitation equipment available.
	CSE	10 to 25			
Sufentanil	PCEA	0.75 to 1	5 to 15	FHR changes† Hypotension† Nausea† Vomiting† Pruritus† Sedation† Respiratory depression†	May improve and prolong anesthesia. Monitor for maternal/neonatal respiratory depression. Ensure naloxone and resuscitation equipment available.
	CSE	5 to 11.5			

CNS, central nervous system; CSE, combined spinal epidural; FHR, fetal heart rate; PCEA, patient-controlled epidural analgesia.

*Adverse reactions are rare.

†Potential side effect.

†Potential adverse reaction.

epidural catheter early in labor and may make the process easier and more controlled due to her ability to cooperate. This access catheter permits rapid administration and/or extension of the block for emergent cesarean birth and lessens the risks associated with urgent use of general anesthesia (ASA, 2016b). Women who are obese, defined as a body mass index (BMI) of 30 kg/m² or greater, present unique challenges for the anesthesia care provider in terms of positioning, identification of anatomic landmarks, and the midline and location of the epidural space (Roofthooft, 2009; Saravanakumar, Rao, & Cooper, 2006). Significant physiologic changes with the woman who is obese include the airway and respiratory and cardiovascular systems, which lead to increased anesthetic and obstetric risk. Difficult or failed tracheal intubation rate is higher in women whose BMI is 33 kg/m² and greater (Roofthooft, 2009). Obesity also increases the need for cesarean birth due to fetal macrosomia and labor dystocia. Not only are perinatal risks increased with obesity, but the anesthetic complications are more frequent. Therefore, careful anticipatory planning and consult with the anesthesia provider is paramount to coordinate care for the woman with obesity. See Chapter 12 for a detailed review of the implications of obesity in pregnancy.

Risks and Complications

Adverse events are known to occur with neuraxial analgesia. Unintended maternal, fetal, and neonatal effects associated with epidural analgesia include a lower rate of spontaneous vaginal birth, a higher rate of instrumental vaginal birth, longer labors, particularly in nulliparous women, and an increase in the likelihood of admittance of the newborn to a higher level of care. Other, more common adverse effects are reported with varying degrees of frequency and include maternal hypotension, FHR changes, reduced success in breastfeeding initiation, headache, epidural failure, and maternal fever (Adams, Frawley, Steel, Broom, & Sibbritt, 2015; Brancato, Church, & Stone, 2008; Gillesby et al., 2010; Lieberman & O'donoghue, 2002; Thangamuthu, Russell, & Purya, 2013). Rare, life-threatening and life-altering major complications occur in approximately 1:3,000 obstetric cases and include high neuraxial block, respiratory arrest with accidental intravascular injection, epidural hematoma, and meningitis (Gruzman, Shelef, Weintraub, Zlotnik, & Erez, 2017).

Hypotension

Maternal hypotension is thought to be due to an anesthetic-induced sympathectomy and vasodilatation. The sympathetic nerve blockade and the decrease in circulating catecholamines may lead to hypotension, which may result in a reduction in venous return and cardiac output, resulting in a decrease in uteroplacental blood flow. For some women, the reduction in vascular resistance results in a statistically significant improvement in uteroplacental blood flow (Hong, 2010). Hypotension is defined as a systolic reading less than 100 mm Hg or a 20% decrease in systolic blood pressure compared with baseline (Poole, 2003). The incidence of hypotension after the initiation of neuraxial analgesia during labor is estimated to be about 10% (ACOG, 2019b). Pre-epidural hydration with a crystalloid IV infusion such as lactated Ringer's solution of 500 to 1,000 mL increases vascular volume and may blunt the hypotension. Because uterine blood flow and fetal oxygenation is directly related to maternal arterial pressure, hypotension is a serious adverse effect that must be treated rapidly especially if there is an abnormal FHR pattern or if the mother is symptomatic. If it persists, despite adequate IV hydration, lateral positioning with complete uterine displacement, IV ephedrine can be given in 5- to 10-mg incremental injections for a total dosage of 30 mg (Poole, 2003).

Fetal and Neonatal Risks

Fetal and neonatal effects to neuraxial analgesia are related to maternal hypotension or to transplacental passage of analgesic or anesthetic drugs (ACOG, 2019b). Opioids used in both CSE and epidural anesthesia do pass into maternal blood, cross the placenta, and produce fetal and neonatal depression when given in large doses (Reynolds, 2010). Low-dose local anesthetic and opioid solutions may cause minimal variability of the FHR (O'Sullivan, 2009). Late and prolonged decelerations and fetal bradycardia are more common with CSE but are not associated with an increased cesarean birth rate (Reynolds, 2010). Agents may also be found in breast milk. Neonatal depression or drowsiness can interfere with suckling. The effect of epidural analgesia on breastfeeding continues to be controversial and suggests a relationship with breastfeeding rates (ACOG, 2019b; Beilin et al., 2005; Henderson, Dickinson, Evans, McDonald, & Paech, 2003; Montgomery & Hale, 2012). Epidural analgesia decreases oxytocin levels during labor and affects oxytocin and prolactin levels on day 2 postpartum (ACOG, 2019b). More studies are needed to determine the long-term effects of labor analgesia or birth anesthesia on infant development (Sun, 2011).

Headache

A postdural puncture headache may occur after a spinal anesthetic or after inadvertent dural puncture during epidural catheter placement also known as a *wet tap*. The incidence of a wet tap is about 1:100 with approximately 70% of women complaining of a severe headache (El-Wahab & Robinson, 2011; Hawkins, 2010). The pain that results from accidental dural puncture can severely limit a new mother's ability to care for her newborn. The headache is caused by leakage of cerebrospinal fluid through the dural hole, leading to relative intracranial hypotension and traction of the meninges and meningeal vessels (Pages-Arroyo & Plan-Smith, 2013). An epidural blood patch, using 15 to 25 mL of the woman's own blood aseptically drawn and injected into the epidural space will provide immediate relief to 65% to 90% of women (Hawkins, 2010).

Hyperthermia

The precise etiology of the maternal hyperthermia related to epidural analgesia remains unknown. It is likely that the rise is due to an alteration in maternal thermoregulatory physiology due to an imbalance between heat production and heat loss. However, an infectious etiology can never be completely discounted. Women with intrapartum fever are more likely to deliver by cesarean birth or operative vaginal birth. As a result of maternal fever, the infant may undergo an evaluation for neonatal sepsis including antibiotic therapy, which may result in maternal/neonatal separation and prolonged hospital stay for the newborn (Osborne et al., 2008; Verani, McGee, & Schrag, 2010; Yancey, Zhang, Schwarz, Dietrich, & Klebanoff, 2001). Epidurals associated with maternal hyperthermia are more common in nulliparous women and the risk appears to increase with duration of labor (El-Wahab & Robinson, 2011; Kuczkowski & Reisner, 2003; Yancey et al., 2001). The maternal–fetal temperature affects uteroplacental blood flow and fetal oxygen delivery due to higher maternal oxygen consumption and is associated with an increased risk of neonatal encephalopathy (Kuczkowski & Reisner, 2003).

Pruritus

Pruritus is a common side effect of neuraxial opioid administration, which for most women will last approximately 45 to 60 minutes after the initial loading dose (Wong, 2014). Fentanyl and sufentanil causes pruritus on maternal legs, abdomen, and thorax. Morphine and hydromorphone may cause pruritus in the neck and head. The cause of pruritus is not well understood. Opioid antagonists (naloxone) or partial agonist-antagonists (nalbuphine) are somewhat effective in relieving pruritus.

Systemic Toxicity

Inadvertent placement of the catheter and infusion into the intrathecal space can cause a high spinal block resulting in immediate upper thoracic sensory loss and severe lower extremity motor blockade. The anesthetic agent may ascend intrathecally to the brainstem leading to respiratory paralysis, total autonomic blockage, and loss of consciousness. An accidental IV injection of epinephrine and a local anesthetic agent into an epidural vein may lead to systemic toxicity causing almost immediate increased maternal heart rate, palpitations, increased blood pressure, numbness of the tongue or around the mouth, metallic taste, tinnitus, slurred speech, jitteriness, or agitation, which may culminate in seizures and cardiac arrest.

As a safety measure, a test dose of a local anesthetic mixed with epinephrine may be injected to determine that the catheter is not in the epidural vein (Fig. 16–4). In some women, a test dose may not determine intravascular injection because there is existing maternal tachycardia or because the effects occur too quickly to be observed. For this reason, some practitioners prefer to place a 10-mL anesthetic dose combining bupivacaine, fentanyl, and epinephrine in 5-mL increments through the catheter. When the anesthesiologist or CRNA is satisfied that the catheter is properly placed, a bolus of anesthetic medication is injected. The nurse must be prepared to always have emergency equipment immediately available, recognize these complications, and anticipate the need for cardiopulmonary support. IV lipid emulsion has emerged as an effective therapy for cardiotoxic effects of lipid soluble local anesthetics such as bupivacaine or ropivacaine (Hawkins & Bucklin, 2017).

Catheter Migration/Inadequate Analgesia

Placement of catheter is associated with problems like kinking, knotting, breakage and dislodgment, or migration. Change of posture, type of epidural catheter or needle may influence the potential of migration. Catheter migration carries potential risks of inadequate analgesia, subdural, spinal, or intravascular injection (Farooq, Tagi, & Khawaj, 2016). A potential effect is that women may experience what is called "windows," areas or even whole sides of their body where pain relief is not obtained. The failure to obtain complete pain relief despite proper placement of the catheter may be due to the presence of connective tissue bands in the epidural space that limit areas that can be reached by the medication infused into the epidural space (Althaus & Wax, 2005). In circumstances where the woman is not satisfied with her pain relief, a bolus might be given or the catheter removed and replaced.

Spinal Epidural Hematoma

Laboring women with altered coagulation due to prophylactic anticoagulants or preexisting coagulation disorders create a need for multidisciplinary planning and health education.

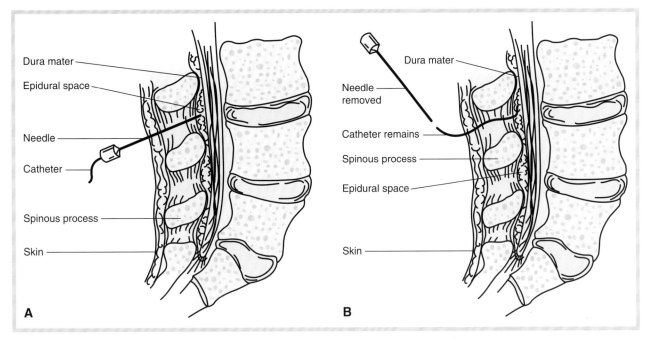

FIGURE 16–4. **A,** A needle is inserted into the epidural space. **B,** A catheter is threaded into the epidural space; the needle is then removed. The catheter allows medication to be administered intermittently or continuously to relieve pain during labor and childbirth.

Bleeding within the spinal neuraxis can lead to a very rare spinal or epidural hematoma (Horlocker et al., 2010; Ruppen, Derry, McQuay, & Moore, 2006). Early signs of a hematoma include severe back pain, progressive sensory or motor blockade following initial signs of regression, deteriorating function of the lower extremities and the bowel and bladder (Horlocker et al., 2010). Once a hematoma is suspected, spinal imaging followed by emergency neurosurgery maximizes neurologic recovery (Horlocker et al., 2010).

Anticoagulant drugs can increase the risk of the rare spinal hematoma after neuraxial anesthesia, and evidence-based management utilizing the pharmacokinetics and pharmacodynamics of anticoagulants has led to greater appreciation for withholding anticoagulation before and after neuraxial anesthesia (L. O. Lee, Bateman, Kheterpal, Klumpner, & Housey, 2017; Leffert et al., 2018). Tables 16–13 and 16–14 outline the timing and recommendations for administration or withholding neuraxial analgesia for the woman using unfractionated heparin and low molecular weight heparin. A retrospective cohort study found the risk of epidural hematoma correlated with a platelet count of 0 to 49,000 mm^{-3} is 11%, for 50,000 to 69,000 mm^{-3} is 3%, and for 70,000 to 100,000 mm^{-3} is 0.2% (L. O. Lee et al., 2017).

Meningitis

Infectious complications of neuraxial analgesia include epidural, spinal, or subdural abscess, meningitis, encephalitis, sepsis, and bacteremia among others. Infection leading to meningitis has been reported to be approximately 1 in 39,000 neuraxial blocks (Pages-Arroyo & Plan-Smith, 2013). The most common organisms not only come from the oral and nasal passages of healthcare providers but also can originate from contaminated equipment, poor aseptic technique, and the woman's skin and blood. The ASA (2017) indicates no clear preference for chlorhexidine with or without alcohol or povidone-iodine with or without alcohol as skin preparation solution prior to performing a neuraxial technique. Sterile occlusive dressings should be used at the catheter insertion site and disconnection and reconnection of neuraxial delivery systems should be limited. Women should be evaluated following neuraxial placement for labor or cesarean birth for signs and symptoms of infection: for example, fever, backache, unrelenting headache, erythema, and tenderness at the insertion site. Additional signs and symptoms of meningitis may occur within 12 hours to a few days following birth and include signs of infection and neck stiffness, sensitivity to light, nausea, and vomiting. Drowsiness, confusion, and seizure are advanced signs. Bacterial meningitis is serious and requires prompt antibiotic treatment to improve the chances of a recovery without serious complications. Meningitis can lead to serious long-term consequences such as deafness, epilepsy, hydrocephalus, and cognitive deficits, especially if not treated quickly. Cerebral spinal fluid obtained through a lumbar puncture will reveal an increased leukocytosis and protein level and a lowered glucose level. Vancomycin and

TABLE 16–13. Anesthesia Plan for Women on Unfractionated Heparin Anticoagulation Therapy

Medication	Time since last dose	Coagulation status	Anesthesia plan
UFH SQ low dose (5,000 U twice or three times daily)	>4 to 6 hr		Proceed with neuraxial.
	<4 to 6 hr	aPTT within normal range or anti-factor Xa level is undetectable.	
		aPTT outside normal range or anti-factor Xa level is present.	Assess difficult airway and balance relative risks of GA compared to SEH.
UFH SQ intermediate dose (7,500 U or 10,000 U twice daily) *Total daily dose ≤ 20,000 U*	>12 hr	aPTT within normal range or anti-factor Xa level is undetectable.	Proceed with neuraxial.
	<12 hr	aPTT within normal range or anti-factor Xa level is undetectable.	Assess difficult airway and balance relative risks of GA compared to SEH.
		aPTT outside normal range or anti-factor Xa level is present.	Consider not proceeding with neuraxial.
UFH SQ high dose (individual dose >10,000 U per dose) *Total daily dose >20,000 U*	≥24 hr	aPTT within normal range or anti-factor Xa level is undetectable.	Proceed with neuraxial.
	<24 hr	Minimal data to guide risk	Consider not proceeding with neuraxial.

aPTT, activated partial thromboplastin time; GA, general anesthesia; SEH, spinal epidural hematoma; SQ, subcutaneous; UFH, unfractionated heparin.
Adapted from Figure 3. Decision aid for urgent or emergent neuraxial procedures in the obstetric patient receiving UFH in Leffert, L., Butwick, A., Carvalho, B., Arendt, K., Bates, S. M., Friedman, A., . . . Toledo, P. (2018). The Society for Obstetric Anesthesia and Perinatology consensus statement on the anesthetic management of pregnant and postpartum women receiving thromboprophylaxis or higher dose anticoagulants. *Anesthesia and Analgesia, 126*(3), 928–944.

third-generation cephalosporin are the recommended first-line antibiotic therapy (Horlocker et al., 2010).

Methods of Neuraxial Anesthesia

Single-Injection Spinal Anesthesia

Spinal anesthesia is commonly used for cesarean birth and given as a single injection needle puncture of the dura mater and medication administration into the cerebrospinal fluid. Its rapid onset provides dense sensory time limited blockade due to the coadministration of opioid and local anesthetic agents injected into the subarachnoid space. Adverse events of spinal anesthesia for cesarean include perioperative hypothermia with the incidence reported as high as 91% (Allen & Habib, 2018). Hypothermia is associated with increased blood loss, higher surgical site infection rates, dysrhythmias, and prolonged hospitalization.

TABLE 16–14. Anesthesia Plan for Women on Low Molecular Weight Heparin Anticoagulation Therapy

Medication	Time since last dose	Anesthesia plan
Low-dose LMWH Enoxaparin <40 mg SQ once daily or 30 mg SQ twice daily or dalteparin 5,000 U SQ once daily	>12 hr	Proceed with neuraxial.
	<12 hr	Consider not proceeding with neuraxial. Balance potential increased risk for SEH with risk of GA.
Intermediate-dose LMWH Enoxaparin >40 mg SQ once daily or 30 mg SQ twice daily and <1 mg/kg SQ twice daily or 1.5 mg/kg SQ once daily or dalteparin >5,000 U SQ once daily and <120 U/kg SQ twice daily or 200 U/kg SQ once daily		Insufficient published data to recommend a specific interval between 12 and 24 hr to delay neuraxial anesthesia
High-dose LMWH Enoxaparin 1 mg/kg SQ twice daily or 1.5 mg/kg SQ once daily or dalteparin 120 U/kg SQ twice daily or 200 U/kg SQ once daily	>24 hr	Proceed with neuraxial.
	<24 hr	Consider not proceeding with neuraxial. Balance potential increased risk for SEH with risk of GA.

GA, general anesthesia; LMWH, low molecular weight heparin; SEH, spinal epidural hematoma; SQ, subcutaneous.
Adapted from Figure 4: Decision aid for urgent or emergent neuraxial procedures in the obstetric patient receiving UFH in Leffert, L., Butwick, A., Carvalho, B., Arendt, K., Bates, S. M., Friedman, A., . . . Toledo, P. (2018). The Society for Obstetric Anesthesia and Perinatology consensus statement on the anesthetic management of pregnant and postpartum women receiving thromboprophylaxis or higher dose anticoagulants. *Anesthesia and Analgesia, 126*(3), 928–944.

Attempts to prevent hypothermia include active warming with either forced air or warmed IV fluids, which increases maternal thermal comfort and reduces shivering (Allen & Habib, 2018). Hypotension with spinal anesthesia is reported in 10% to 24% of cases (Rollins & Lucero, 2012).

Standard Epidural

Epidural anesthesia is noted as "the gold standard" pain relief for labor and birth (Hawkins, 2010; O'Sullivan, 2009). It involves the injection of a local anesthetic agent (e.g., lidocaine or bupivacaine) and an opioid analgesic agent (e.g., morphine or fentanyl) into the lumbar epidural space between the fourth and fifth lumbar vertebrae (see Fig. 16–4). The injected agent gradually diffuses across the dura into the subarachnoid space, where it acts primarily on the spinal nerve roots binding to opiate receptors in the dorsal horn of the spinal cord and paravertebral nerves. Depending on the specific medications used, women begin to feel relief in 5 to 10 minutes. A complete block usually occurs in 15 to 20 minutes (Wong, 2014). The epidural block requires more medication than a spinal block for similar clinical effects. Adding a narcotic to the local anesthetic lessens the risk of toxicity by decreasing the amount of local anesthetic needed, reducing the motor blockade, increasing the duration of pain relief, and improving the quality of pain relief (ASA, 2016b).

Continuous epidural infusion or intermittent boluses given by licensed anesthesia providers or the midwife can provide satisfactory analgesia for labor. Professional guidelines restrict nurses from manipulation of dosing or restarting an infusion (AWHONN, 2015). Advantages of a continuous infusion include a consistent level of pain relief and prevention of hemodynamic changes associated with the repeated occurrence of pain. Continuous flow through the catheter also stabilizes the catheter, decreasing the risk of migration into an epidural vein or through the dura into the subarachnoid space. The continuous infusion may be a local anesthetic alone (bupivacaine, lidocaine, or ropivacaine) or a combination of a local and an opioid (fentanyl or sufentanil). Intermittent boluses are given for breakthrough pain. Boluses can also be programmed at prescribed intervals. A randomized study compared women who received programmed intermittent boluses to continuous infusion and found the women who received programmed intermittent epidural boluses received less drug dose than those with continuous epidural infusion with no difference in pain control or side effects (Ferrer, Romero, Vásquez, Matute, Van de Velde, 2017).

PCEA is a reliable and effective method of maintaining epidural labor analgesia (Halpern & Carvalho, 2009). A basal infusion is suitable for most women because it reduces the need for unscheduled clinician interventions and may provide better analgesia compared with when a basal infusion is omitted. Basal infusion rates between 2 and 10 mL/hr have been used effectively (Halpern & Carvalho, 2009). Table 16–15 compares patient-controlled neuraxial to parenteral analgesia (Gillesby et al., 2010; Halpern et al., 2004; Liu & Sia, 2004; Wong et al., 2005). A systematic review of randomized controlled trials on PCEA for labor revealed a reduction of unscheduled clinician interventions, total dose of local anesthetic, and lower extremity motor block. Settings and drug combinations used for PCEA are varied and no ideal bolus dose or lockout interval setting has been established (Halpern & Carvalho, 2009).

Combined Spinal Epidural

CSE offers the advantages of both the epidural and spinal techniques as it provides rapid-onset pain relief

TABLE 16–15. Patient-Controlled Options: Comparison of Neuraxial to Parenteral Opioid Analgesia

PCEA	IV opioid analgesia
Higher maternal satisfaction scores	Higher level of maternal control and choice
Maternal hypotension, some nausea	More nausea
Maternal pain relief	Maternal sedation
Can be given early in labor	Not recommended until active labor; may prolong latent phase
Labor duration longer and second stage longer	
Potential increase need for oxytocin administration	
Increased births by vacuum and forceps	No increase in operative vaginal birth
Maternal fever, which may lead to fetal tachycardia and neonatal septic workup	Newborns required more resuscitation, required naloxone, and lower 1-min Apgar score
Larger doses of fentanyl may be associated with slightly impaired breastfeeding.	No documented problems in breastfeeding
Rare, life-threatening complications	Maternal respiratory depression
No difference in cesarean birth rate	

IV, intravenous; PCEA, patient-controlled epidural analgesia.

and minimal motor blockade to the laboring woman. It is performed by first placing a 17- or 18-gauge Tuohy needle in the epidural space using the loss-of-resistance technique. After the needle is positioned in the epidural space, the smaller gauge spinal needle is placed through the epidural needle into the adjacent dural sac ("needle-through-needle" technique) (Hong, 2010). Within the dural sac are the contents of the intrathecal space including cerebrospinal fluid, the spinal cord, and the spinal nerve roots. Intrathecal analgesia is achieved faster and with a very low dose of local and opioid analgesia (combination of bupivacaine and fentanyl) necessary to produce epidural analgesia (Atiénzar et al., 2008). The spinal needle is removed, and an epidural catheter is then threaded through the epidural needle. The epidural needle is removed and the catheter is taped in place. The epidural catheter allows for continuation of neuraxial analgesia after the initial spinal dose wears off. Maternal hypotension, pruritus, and motor nerve block are a few of the more prevalent problems. Women who receive CSE analgesia report significantly more pruritus than women receiving standard epidural (Hong, 2010). Fetal bradycardia can occur with reported rates exceeding the risk with epidural analgesia alone (Wong, 2014).

Sustained or Extended-release Epidural Morphine

Following cesarean birth, administration of preservative-free morphine given by the intrathecal or epidural route is commonly used to achieve 12 to 24 hours of postoperative analgesia. Adverse effects include pruritus, nausea, and respiratory depression (ACOG, 2019b). Some women are at increased risk for respiratory depression including those with an unstable medical condition, obesity, obstructive sleep apnea, or concomitant administration of opioid analgesics. The ASA recommends monitoring for adequacy of ventilation (e.g., respiratory rate, depth of respiration [assessed without disturbing a sleeping woman]), oxygenation (e.g., pulse oximetry when appropriate), and level of consciousness at least once every hour should be performed during the first 12 hours after administration and at least once every 2 hours for the next 12 hours. After 24 hours, the monitoring frequency should be dictated by the woman's overall condition and concurrent medications (ASA, 2016c).

Nursing Care with Neuraxial Analgesia

In 2015, AWHONN updated the position statement: *Role of the Registered Nurse in the Care of the Pregnant Woman Receiving Analgesia and Anesthesia by Catheter Techniques.*

The position statement states that RNs in communication with the obstetric and anesthesia care providers, may:

- Monitor the woman's vital signs, level of mobility, level of consciousness, and perception of pain and level of pain relief
- Monitor fetal status
- Pause the infusion to replace empty infusion syringes or infusion bags with new, pre-prepared solutions containing the same medication and concentration, according to orders provided by the anesthesia care provider and restart the infusion
- Stop the continuous infusion if there is a safety concern or the woman has given birth
- Remove the catheter if the RN has had appropriate educational training, criteria have been met, and institutional policy and law allow. Removal of the catheter by an RN is contingent upon receipt of a specific order from a qualified anesthesia or physician provider.
- Initiate emergency therapeutic measures if complications arise according to institutional policy, protocol, and RN scope of practice
- Communicate clinical assessments and changes in maternal status to the obstetric and anesthesia care providers as indicated by institutional policy

RNs who are not licensed anesthesia providers should not:

- Bolus or rebolus regional/intrathecal analgesia or anesthesia doses by injecting medication into the catheter
- Manipulate doses of regional/intrathecal analgesia and anesthesia delivered by continuous infusion
- Manipulate doses of regional/intrathecal analgesia and anesthesia or dosage intervals for PCEA
- Increase or decrease the rate of a continuous infusion
- Reinitiate an infusion once it has been stopped
- Be responsible for obtaining informed consent for analgesia and anesthesia procedures; however, the nurse may witness the woman's signature for informed consent prior to analgesia and anesthesia administration

Perinatal nurses must be comfortable with the operation of additional technology, familiar with nursing care during all phases of the procedure, and able to recognize potential complications when a laboring woman receives neuraxial analgesia. Continuous epidural anesthesia is always delivered through an infusion pump, and continuous EFM is required following placement. Depending on institutional practice, women may also be monitored using a cardiac monitor, pulse oximeter, and automatic blood pressure devices. *Guidelines for Perinatal Care* (AAP & ACOG, 2017) and AWHONN (2010) nurse staffing guidelines suggest one nurse to one woman in labor staffing for initiating epidural anesthesia including, specifically, continuous bedside attendance during the initiation of regional anesthesia until the mother's condition is stable (at least for the first 30 minutes).

Published statements from professional organizations, individual state nursing practice acts, and facilities are inconsistent about the role of the nurse in caring for women in labor, who receive anesthesia or analgesia. Controversy exists in the literature and in clinical practice about the frequency of maternal–fetal assessments during epidural anesthesia or analgesia for laboring women. Many perinatal units have policies that require completion of specific aspects of maternal–fetal assessment every 15 to 30 minutes for women with epidurals. There are, however, no published standards of care or practice guidelines from the ASA, American Association of Nurse Anesthetists, ACOG, or AWHONN that prescribe what the maternal–fetal assessment includes or the specific frequencies for making assessments during epidural infusion for labor and birth because there are no research-based data to demonstrate optimal time intervals for maternal–fetal assessments during epidural infusion. Existing published standards are general and outlined in Display 16–12.

Close monitoring of the blood pressure and pulse oximetry is critical during placement and initiation. Suggestions from AWHONN (2011) for maternal vital sign assessment during the initiation and rebolusing process include the following: Assess maternal blood pressure after the initiation or rebolus of a regional block, including PCEA. Blood pressure may be assessed every 5 minutes for the first 15 minutes and then repeated at 30 minutes and at 1 hour after the procedure. More or less frequent monitoring may be indicated based on consideration of factors such as the type of analgesia/anesthesia, route and dose of medication used, the maternal–fetal response to medication, maternal–fetal condition, the stage of labor, and facility protocol. Use of continuous or intermittent oxygen saturation monitoring (pulse oximetry) should be reserved for select women at highest risk for respiratory depression, hypoventilation, or apnea, such as those with obstructive sleep apnea or cardiovascular disease (Wong, 2014). The nurse observes for meticulous adherence to aseptic technique during epidural placement and provides continuous emotional and positional support to the woman during the procedure. Nursing and medical textbooks may contain suggested protocols and valuable clinical information, but they do not alone define standards of care. Perinatal nurses, in collaboration with other providers in each institution, must develop protocols that delineate responsibilities and care for women receiving epidural anesthesia or analgesia during labor and birth.

Table 16–16 presents an overview of the nursing care to consider as policies and procedures are developed for care of the woman in labor receiving neuraxial analgesia.

Local Anesthetic

During the second stage of labor, a local anesthetic agent may be injected into the perineum and posterior vaginal wall before performing an episiotomy. The duration of action is approximately 20 to 40 minutes for these medications (Briggs & Wan, 2006). This area may be reinjected after delivery of the placenta in preparation for perineal repair.

Pudendal Block

A pudendal nerve block is a minor regional block that is safe and usually effective. A pudendal block is performed during the second stage of labor by injecting a local anesthetic just below the ischial spines through the lateral vaginal walls into the area of the pudendal nerve. Aspiration of the needle before injection is important to verify appropriate placement. This application anesthetizes the lower vagina, vulva, and perineum. This block provides satisfactory anesthesia for spontaneous vaginal birth, application of outlet forceps or vacuum, and perineal repair. The potential risks for pudendal block are hematoma, infection, and nerve damage as well as local anesthetic toxicity and extension of the nerve block, but the complications are unusual (Volmanen et al., 2011).

SUMMARY

The perinatal nurse is an essential member of the healthcare team and as such, works collaboratively with the perinatal and anesthesia healthcare providers to meet women's needs for pain management during labor and birth. Labor causes intense pain, which leads to a physiologic stress response. A woman should be given options regarding both nonpharmacologic and pharmacologic choices for pain management, which maintains her sense of control and allows participation of her birthing partner. None of the methods described constitute the ideal analgesic for labor; all have pros and cons and risks and benefits. A combination of techniques is often more effective than reliance on a single plan of action. Nurses should encourage women in labor to use a variety of techniques to decrease pain perception and sustain her ability to cope. Pharmacologic pain management strategies represent one aspect of intrapartum pain management and may be used to augment, not substitute for nonpharmacologic strategies. The nurse must remember that a woman who has been given IV pain medication or

Professional Organizations' Guidelines for Maternal–Fetal Assessment Frequency During Neuraxial Analgesia

	Association of Women's Health, Obstetric and Neonatal Nurses (2011, 2015)	American Society of Anesthesiologists (2016b)	American College of Obstetricians and Gynecologists (2019b)
Maternal assessments	Blood pressure assessment after the initiation or rebolus of a regional block, including PCEA Blood pressure, pulse, and respirations are assessed every 5 min for the first 15 min and then repeated at 30 min and at 1 hr after the procedure. Monitor the woman's vital signs, level of mobility, level of consciousness, and perception of pain and level of pain relief. Communicate clinical assessments and changes in patient status to the obstetric and anesthesia care providers as indicated by institutional policy. More or less frequent monitoring may be indicated based on consideration of factors such as the type of analgesia/anesthesia, route and dose of medication used, the maternal–fetal response to medication, maternal–fetal condition, and the stage of labor or facility protocol.	Requires that the laboring woman's vital signs and the FHR be monitored and documented by a qualified individual. Additional monitoring appropriate to the clinical condition of the laboring woman and the fetus should be used when indicated.	When regional anesthesia is administered during labor, the woman's vital signs should be monitored at regular intervals by a qualified member of the healthcare team.
Fetal assessments	The RN is responsible for monitoring fetal well-being either electronically or via frequent auscultation of the FHR. Assess the FHR tracing before initiating regional analgesia, if a category II or III FHR pattern is identified, initiate corrective measures as needed and notify the anesthesia/obstetric care provider. Assess FHR after the initiation or rebolus of a regional block, including PCEA. FHR may be assessed every 5 min for the first 15 min. More or less frequent monitoring may be indicated based on consideration of factors such as the type of analgesia/anesthesia, route and dose of medication used, the maternal–fetal response to medication, maternal–fetal condition, and the stage of labor or facility protocol. The frequency of subsequent assessment should be based on consideration of the variables listed above.	FHR should be monitored by a qualified individual before and after administration of regional analgesia for labor. Continuous electronic recording of the FHR may not be possible during placement of a neuraxial catheter.	

FHR, fetal heart rate; PCEA, patient-controlled epidural analgesia; RN, registered nurse.

American Academy of Pediatrics & American College of Obstetricians and Gynecologists (2017). *Guidelines for perinatal care* (8th ed.). Elk Grove Village, IL: American Academy of Pediatrics; American Society of Anesthesiologists. (2016b). Practice guidelines for obstetric anesthesia: An updated report by the American Society of Anesthesiologists Task Force on Obstetric Anesthesia and the Society for Obstetric Anesthesia and Perinatology. *Anesthesiology, 124*(2), 270–300; Association of Women's Health, Obstetric and Neonatal Nurses. (2011). *Nursing care of the woman receiving regional analgesia/anesthesia in labor.* Washington, DC: Author; Association of Women's Health, Obstetric and Neonatal Nurses. (2015). *Role of the registered nurse in the care of the pregnant woman receiving analgesia and anesthesia by catheter techniques* (Position Statement). Washington, DC: Author.

TABLE 16–16. Care of Women Receiving Neuraxial Analgesia

Nursing care	Referenced rationale
1. Review understanding of neuraxial analgesia and clarify concerns and information as needed. Include support systems as available.	Women are encouraged and supported to take an active role in decision making about pregnancy, labor, and birth (Adams et al., 2016; Lally et al., 2008).
2. Notify the perinatal and anesthesia care providers of the woman's desire for or against for neuraxial analgesia.	The woman has a right to request pain relief during labor. A focused history and physical should be completed prior to initiation of anesthesia/analgesia (American Society of Anesthesiologists [ASA], 2016b). Labor progress and fetal status must be evaluated prior to initiation of neuraxial analgesia by a qualified perinatal provider (ASA, 2016a).
3. Assess for any contraindications to the procedure prior to initiation, including the following: • Coagulopathy and/or thrombocytopenia • Local or systemic infection • Inadequate staffing	A specific platelet count predictive of neuraxial anesthetic complications has not been determined. A platelet count is clinically useful for laboring women with suspected preeclampsia or HELLP syndrome and for other disorders associated with coagulopathy (Leffert et al., 2018). The recommendation from ASA (2016b) is that a blood type and screen or cross-match should be based on maternal history, anticipated hemorrhage complications, and the institution's policies. Significant anesthetic or obstetric risk factors should encourage consultation between the anesthesia and obstetric healthcare providers (ASA, 2016b). Continuous bedside nursing attendance should be provided during the initiation of regional anesthesia until the woman's condition is stable (at least for the first 30 min following the initial dose of medication (Association of Women's Health, Obstetric and Neonatal Nurses [AWHONN], 2010).
4. The FHR should be monitored 20 to 30 min before and continuously after administration of neuraxial analgesia. Continuous EFM may not be possible during placement of the epidural catheter.	Anesthetic and analgesia agents may influence the FHR pattern. Recording the FHR reduces fetal and neonatal complications (ASA, 2017). Administration of regional analgesia during labor has resulted in decreased uteroplacental blood flow, and alterations in the FHR, such as late decelerations, variable decelerations, bradycardia, tachycardia, and increased and decreased variability, have been reported (Wong, 2014).
5. Initiate large-bore IV access and provide a bolus of 500 to 1,000 mL Hartmann's solution (Ringer's lactate) 15 to 30 min before the procedure.	Avoid rapidly infusing IV fluids into women with cardiac disease or severe preeclampsia without direct measurement of hemodynamic status.
6. Conduct a preprocedural verification process (time-out) prior to initiation of the neuraxial procedure and document completion of this verification.	The purpose of the time-out is to conduct a final validation that the correct patient, site, and procedure are identified (TJC, 2019).
7. Emergency preparedness: Verify the immediate availability of emergency response and equipment. Advise colleagues that the procedure will soon begin. An emergency cesarean birth may become necessary due to a prolonged deceleration, or bradycardia occurs that does not respond the intrauterine resuscitation techniques.	Regional anesthesia should be initiated and maintained only in areas in which resuscitation equipment and drugs are immediately available (ASA, 2016a; AWHONN, 2015).
8. Assist the woman to maintain a sitting or side-lying position with feet supported on a chair or stool; head flexed forward supported by herself with elbows resting on knees or leaning against the shoulder of a support person. Stress the importance of remaining motionless during insertion of the catheter. Encourage the use of breathing and relaxation techniques during the procedure.	Avoid severe spinal flexion because it can decrease the epidural space and increase the possibility of puncturing the dura. The respiratory effect of obesity in pregnancy is minimal when placed in the sitting position (Roofthooft, 2009).
9. Maintain aseptic technique.	Use of sterile gloves is required by the anesthesia provider; however, a sterile gown is not necessary. Wearing a mask will decrease potential for droplet contamination of the sterile field.
10. Provide anticipatory guidance for the woman to normal sensations felt with skin preparation, taping, local injection stinging, and needle placement.	No clear preference for chlorhexidine with or without alcohol or povidone-iodine with or without alcohol as skin preparation solution prior to performing a neuraxial technique (ASA, 2017)

(continued)

TABLE 16–16. Care of Women Receiving Neuraxial Analgesia *(Continued)*

Nursing care	Referenced rationale
11. Monitor for intravascular injection of local anesthetic during the test dose.	Signs of intravascular injection include the following: • Maternal tachycardia or bradycardia • Hypertension • Seizures • Dizziness • Restlessness • Tinnitus • Metallic taste in mouth • Perioral paresthesia • Difficulty speaking • Loss of consciousness
12. Monitor for signs of infusion of medication into the intrathecal space.	Signs of infusion into the intrathecal space leading to a high spinal block include the following: • Immediate upper thoracic sensory loss • Severe lower extremity motor blockade • Respiratory paralysis • Total autonomic blockage • Loss of consciousness
13. Monitor BP, pulse, respiration, and FHR every 5 min during the first 15 min following initiation or rebolus of regional analgesia to identify and manage side/adverse effects and then repeated at 30 min and at 1 hr after the procedure.	Women who have received neuraxial opioids should be observed for adequate ventilation by assessing respiratory rate, depth of respiration, level of consciousness, and pulse oximetry when appropriate (ASA, 2016b; AWHONN, 2011).
14. Temperature should be assessed according to hospital protocol and based on risk factors with ruptured membranes.	Use of labor epidural analgesia is associated with a clinically significant increase in the incidence of intrapartum fever (Yancey et al., 2001).
15. If maternal hypotension occurs (systolic <100 or a 20 mmHg decrease from prior readings), initiate IV bolus, place in lateral position, administer oxygen at 10 L per nonrebreather facemask, stop oxytocin administration, notify perinatal and anesthesia providers, and prepare for IV administration of ephedrine to improve maternal hypotension.	An indeterminate or abnormal FHR pattern associated with regional analgesia/anesthesia may respond to maternal position change, an IV fluid bolus and/or oxygen supplementation (Simpson, 2007; Simpson & James, 2005). Maternal hypotension has been treated successfully with maternal position change, IV administration of 5 to 10 mg of ephedrine or 50 to 100 mcg of phenylephrine, and an IV fluid bolus of non–glucose-containing solution (Skupski, Abramovitz, Samuels, Pressimone, & Kjaer, 2009).
16. Assess uterine activity following neuraxial placement and infusion or rebolus of a regional block, including PCEA. Uterine activity may be assessed every 5 min for the first 15 min. More or less frequent monitoring may be indicated based on consideration of factors such as the type of analgesia/anesthesia, route and dose of medication used, the maternal–fetal response to medication, maternal–fetal condition, the stage of labor, and facility protocol. Tachysystole or a decrease in uterine activity may occur requiring an oxytocin infusion to be initiated for augmentation of labor.	Tachysystole and uterine hypertonus may be noted after combined spinal epidural analgesia, epidural analgesia, or intrathecal opioids (Reynolds, 2011; Skupski et al., 2009). Uterine activity may slow in the first 30 to 60 min after regional block administration secondary to rapid preload of 500 mL or more of IV fluid. There is an increase in oxytocin use in the first stage of labor among women who receive epidural analgesia when compared to women who received parenteral opioids. The use of epidural analgesia was associated with a statistically significant longer duration of both first and second stages of labor among nulliparous (nearly 4 hr) and multiparous women (Cheng, Nicholson, Shaffer, Lyell, & Caughey, 2009).
17. Evaluate pain and coping using a visual or verbal analogue scale according to institutional policy. If pain continues to be felt on one side of the body, lying on that side will potentially achieve increased relief. Request that the anesthesia care provider reevaluate the woman as needed for further pain management.	Of women with labor epidurals, 93% reported a pain score of >3 using a 0 to 10 numeric rating scale and desired additional medication (Beilin, Hossain, & Bodian, 2003). Coping with labor scale may provide a better assessment of maternal response than scales used outside of intrapartum (Roberts et al., 2010).
18. Encourage the woman to void frequently during labor. If the bladder is distended and the woman experiences decreased bladder sensation or is unable to use a bed pan to void, placement of an indwelling catheter eliminates the need for repeated catheterizations.	Inability to void and need for catheterization have been reported in up to two thirds of women after epidural analgesia during labor (Mayberry, Clemmens, & De, 2002).
19. Women who experience pruritus should be assured that this is usually a transitory symptom and should decrease within an hour on onset.	The most common side effect of intrathecal opioid administration is pruritus and is more frequently observed with intrathecal opioid administration compared to epidural administration (Wong, 2014).

TABLE 16–16. Care of Women Receiving Neuraxial Analgesia *(Continued)*

Nursing care	Referenced rationale
20. Oral intake of modest amounts of clear liquids should be encouraged for uncomplicated laboring women.	Oral liquid intake of clear liquids during labor does not increase maternal complications. Clear liquids include but are not limited to water, fruit juices without pulp, carbonated beverages, clear team, black coffee, and sports drinks. Women with additional risk factors for aspiration (morbid obesity, diabetes, difficult airway) may have restricted intake based on the decision of the anesthesiologist (ASA, 2016b).
21. Assist with second-stage management and prepare for possibility of operative vaginal birth.	Regional anesthesia/analgesia diminishes the sensation of the urge to push in varying degrees, depending on the type of agents used and route of administration. Research has demonstrated that delaying pushing for various time intervals after complete cervical dilation vs. pushing immediately has been accomplished without lengthening the second stage of labor or negatively affecting birth outcomes in women who received epidural analgesia (Beilin, Mungall, Hossain, & Bodian, 2009; Brancato et al., 2008; Mayberry et al., 2002; Wong, 2014). There may be an increased risk for vacuum-assisted birth and labor dystocia with epidural analgesia (O'Hana et al., 2008).

BP, blood pressure; EFM, electronic fetal monitoring; FHR, fetal heart rate; HELLP, hemolysis, elevated liver enzymes, low platelet count; IV, intravenous; PCEA, patient-controlled epidural analgesia.

From Association of Women's Health, Obstetric and Neonatal Nurses. (2011). *Nursing care of the woman receiving regional analgesia/anesthesia in labor* (Evidence-Based Clinical Practice Guideline). Washington, DC: Author; Association of Women's Health, Obstetric and Neonatal Nurses. (2015). *Role of the registered nurse in the care of the pregnant woman receiving analgesia and anesthesia by catheter techniques* (Position Statement). Washington, DC: Author.

received neuraxial anesthesia may still need, and can benefit from, all the available nonpharmacologic nursing interventions. Labor pain is a unique, individual, and multifaceted phenomenon compounded by various contributing physiologic, emotional, social, and cultural components.

REFERENCES

Abenhaim, H. A., & Fraser, W. D. (2008). Impact of pain level on second-stage delivery outcomes among women with epidural analgesia: Results from the PEOPLE study. *American Journal of Obstetrics & Gynecology, 199*(5), 500.e1–500.e6. doi:10.1016/j.ajog.2008.04.052

Adams, E. D., Stark, M. A., & Low, L. K. (2016). A nurse's guide to supporting physiologic birth. *Nursing for Women's Health, 20*(1), 76–86. doi:10.1016/j.nwh.2015.12.009

Adams, J., Frawley, J., Steel, A., Broom, A., & Sibbritt, D. (2015). Use of pharmacological and non-pharmacological labour pain management techniques and their relationship to maternal and infant birth outcomes: Examination of a nationally representative sample of 1835 pregnant women. *Midwifery, 31,* 458–463.

Ahlemeyer, J., & Mahon, S. (2015). Doulas for childbearing women. *MCN: The American Journal of Maternal Child Nursing, 40*(2), 122–127. doi:10.1097/NMC.0000000000000111

Allen, T. K., & Habib, A. S. (2018). Inadvertent perioperative hypothermia induced by spinal anesthesia for cesarean delivery might be more significant than we think: Are we doing enough to warm our parturients? *Anesthesia and Analgesia, 126*(1), 7–9. doi:10.1213/ANE.0000000000002604

Althaus, J., & Wax, J. (2005). Analgesia and anesthesia in labor. *Obstetrics and Gynecology Clinics of North America, 32*(2), 231–244. doi:10.1016/j.ogc.2005.01.002

American Academy of Pediatrics & American Heart Association. (2016). *Textbook of neonatal resuscitation (NRP)* (7th ed.). Dallas, TX: American Heart Association.

American Academy of Pediatrics & American College of Obstetricians and Gynecologists. (2017). *Guidelines for perinatal care* (8th ed.). Elk Grove Village, IL: American Academy of Pediatrics.

American College of Nurse-Midwives. (2010). From the American College of Nurse-Midwives. Nitrous oxide for labor analgesia. *Journal of Midwifery & Women's Health, 55*(3), 292–296.

American College of Nurse-Midwives. (2014). *Hydrotherapy during labor and birth* (Position Statement). Silver Spring, MD: Author.

American College of Obstetricians and Gynecologists. (2009). *Intrapartum fetal heart rate monitoring: Nomenclature, interpretation, and general management principles* (Practice Bulletin No. 106). Washington, DC: Author.

American College of Obstetricians and Gynecologists. (2019a). *Approaches to limit intervention during labor and birth.* (Committee Opinion No. 766). Washington, DC: Author.

American College of Obstetricians and Gynecologists. (2019b). *Obstetric analgesia and anesthesia* (Practice Bulletin No. 209). Washington, DC: Author.

American Society of Anesthesiologists. (2016a). *Optimal goals for anesthesia care in obstetrics.* Washington, DC: Author.

American Society of Anesthesiologists. (2016b). Practice guidelines for obstetric anesthesia: An updated report by the American Society of Anesthesiologists Task Force on Obstetric Anesthesia and the Society for Obstetric Anesthesia and Perinatology. *Anesthesiology, 124*(2), 270–300. doi:10.1097/ALN.0000000000000935

American Society of Anesthesiologists. (2016c). Practice guidelines for the prevention, detection, and management of respiratory depression associated with neuraxial opioid administration: An updated report by the American Society of Anesthesiologists Task Force on Neuraxial Opioids and the American Society of Regional Anesthesia and Pain Medicine. *Anesthesiology, 124*(3), 535–552. doi:10.1097/ALN.0000000000000975

American Society of Anesthesiologists. (2017). Practice advisory for the prevention, diagnosis, and management of infectious complications associated with neuraxial techniques: An updated report by the American Society of Anesthesiologists Task Force on Infectious Complication Associated with Neuraxial Techniques and the American Society of Regional and Pain Medicine. *Anesthesiology*, 126(4), 585–601. doi:10.1097/ALN.0000000000001521

Apfelbaum, J. L., Hawkins, J. L., Agarkar, M., Bucklin, B. A., Connis, R. T., Gambling, D. R., & Yaghmour, E. T. A. (2016). Practice guidelines for obstetric anesthesia: An updated report by the American Society of Anesthesiologists Task Force on Obstetric Anesthesia and the Society for Obstetric Anesthesia and Perinatology. *Anesthesiology*, 124(2), 270–300. doi:10.1097/ALN.0000000000000935

Association of Women's Health, Obstetric and Neonatal Nurses. (2010). *Guidelines for professional nurse staffing for perinatal units*. Washington, DC: Author.

Association of Women's Health, Obstetric and Neonatal Nurses. (2011). *Nursing care of the woman receiving regional analgesia/anesthesia in labor* (Evidence-Based Clinical Practice Guideline). Washington, DC: Author.

Association of Women's Health, Obstetric and Neonatal Nurses. (2015). *Role of the registered nurse in the care of the pregnant woman receiving analgesia and anesthesia by catheter techniques* (Position Statement). Washington, DC: Author.

Association of Women's Health, Obstetric and Neonatal Nurses. (2018). *Continuous labor support for every woman* (Position Statement). Washington, DC: Author.

Association of Women's Health, Obstetric and Neonatal Nurses. (2019). *Nursing care and management of the second stage of labor* (Evidence-Based Clinical Practice Guideline, 3rd ed.). Washington, DC: Author.

Atiénzar, M, C., Palanca, J. M., Torres, F., Borrás, R., Gil, S., & Esteve, I. (2008). A randomized comparison of levobupivacaine, bupivacaine and ropivacaine with fentanyl, for labor analgesia. *International Journal of Obstetric Anesthesia*, 17(2), 106–111.

Ballen, L. E., & Fulcher, A. J. (2006). Nurses and doulas: Complementary roles to provide optimal maternity care. *Journal of Obstetrics, Gynecologic, and Neonatal Nursing*, 35(2), 304–311. doi:10.1111/j.1552-6909.2006.00041.x

Beal, M. W. (1999). Acupuncture and acupressure. Applications to women's reproductive health care. *Journal of Nurse-Midwifery*, 44(3), 217–230.

Bedwell, C., Dowswell, T., Neilson, J. P., & Lavender, T. (2011). The use of transcutaneous electrical nerve stimulation (TENS) for pain relief in labour: A review of the evidence. *Midwifery*, 27(5), e141–e148.

Beebe, K. R. (2014). Hypnotherapy for labor and birth. *Nursing for Women's Health*, 18(1), 48–59. doi:10.1111/1751-486X.12093

Beilin, Y., Bodian, C. A., Weiser, J., Hossain, S., Arnold, I., Feierman, D. E., . . . Holzman, I. (2005). Effect of labor epidural analgesia with and without fentanyl on infant breast-feeding: A prospective, randomized, double-blind study. *Anesthesiology*, 103(6), 1211–1217.

Beilin, Y., Hossain, S., & Bodian, A. A. (2003). The numeric rating scale and labor epidural analgesia. *Anesthesia and Analgesia*, 96(6), 1794–1798.

Beilin, Y., Mungall, D., Hossain, S., & Bodian, C. A. (2009). Labor pain at the time of epidural analgesia and mode of delivery in nulliparous women presenting for an induction of labor. *Obstetrics & Gynecology*, 114(4), 764–769. doi:10.1097/AOG.0b013e3181b6beee

Benfield, R., Herman, J., Katz, V. L., Wison, S. P., & Davis, J. M. (2001). Hydrotherapy in labor. *Research in Nursing & Health*, 24(1), 57–67. doi:10.1002/1098-240X(200102)24:1<57::AID-NUR1007>3.0.CO;2-J

Bergh, I., Stener-Victorin, E., Wallin, G., & Mårtensson, L. (2011). Comparison of the PainMatcher and the visual analogue scale for assessment of labour pain following administered pain relief treatment. *Midwifery*, 27, e134–e139. doi:10.1016/j.midw.2009.03.004

Berghella, V., Baxter, J. K., & Chauhan, S. P. (2008). Evidence-based labor and delivery management. *American Journal of Obstetrics & Gynecology*, 199(5), 445–454. doi:10.1016/j.ajog.2008.06.093

Bohren, M. A., Hofmeyr, G., Sakala, C., Fukuzawa, R. K., & Cuthbert, A. (2017). Continuous support for women during childbirth. *Cochrane Database of Systematic Reviews*, (7), CD003766. doi:10.1002/1465/858

Bossano, C. M., Townsend, K. M., Walton, A. C., Blomquist, J. L., & Handa, V. L. (2017). The maternal childbirth experience more than a decade after delivery. *American Journal of Obstetrics & Gynecology*, 217(3), 342.e1–342.e8.

Brancato, R. M., Church, S., & Stone, P. W. (2008). A meta-analysis of passive descent versus immediate pushing in nulliparous women with epidural analgesia in the second stage of labor. *Journal of Obstetric, Gynecologic, and Neonatal Nursing*, 37(1), 4–12. doi:10.1111/j.1552-6909.2007.00205.x

Briggs, G. G., & Wan, S. R. (2006). Drug therapy during labor and delivery, part 2. *American Journal of Health-System Pharmacy*, 63(12), 1131–1139. doi:10.2146/ajhp050265.p2

Browning, C. A. (2000). Using music during childbirth. *Birth*, 27(4), 272–276. doi:10.1046/j.1523-536x.2000.00272.x

Bryanton, J., Fraser-Davey, H., & Sullivan, P. (1994). Women's perceptions of nursing support during labor. *Journal of Obstetric, Gynecologic, and Neonatal Nursing*, 23(8), 638–644.

Calik, K. Y., & Komurcu, N. (2014). Effects of SP6 acupuncture point stimulation on labor pain and duration of labor. *Iranian Red Crescent Medical Journal*, 16(10), e16461. doi:10.5812/ircmj.16461

Camann, W. (2005). Pain relief during labor. *The New England Journal of Medicine*, 352(7), 718–720.

Campbell, D. A., Lake, M. F., Falk, M., & Backstrand, J. R. (2006). A randomized control trial of continuous support in labor by a lay doula. *Journal of Obstetric, Gynecologic, and Neonatal Nursing*, 35(4), 456–464. doi:10.1111/j.1552-6909.2006.00067.x

Carlton, T., Callister, L. C., & Stoneman, E. (2005). Decision making in laboring women: Ethical issues for perinatal nurses. *The Journal of Perinatal & Neonatal Nursing*, 19(2), 145–154.

Caughey, A. B., Cahill, A. G., Guise, J. M., & Rouse, D. J. (2014). Safe prevention of the primary cesarean delivery. *American Journal of Obstetrics & Gynecology*, 210(3), 179–193.

Challiet, N., Belaid, L., Crochetière, C., Roy, L., Gagne, G., Mautquin, J. M., . . . Bonapace, J. (2014). Nonpharmacologic approaches for pain management during labor compared with usual care: A meta-analysis. *Birth*, 41(2), 122–137.

Chandler, S., & Field, P. (1997). Becoming a father: First-time fathers' experience of labor and delivery. *Journal of Nurse-Midwifery*, 42(1), 17–24. doi:10.1016/s0091-2(96)00067-5

Chang, M. Y., Chen, C. H., & Huang, K. F. (2006). A comparison of massage effects on labor pain using the McGill Pain Questionnaire. *Journal of Nursing Research*, 14(3), 190–197. doi:10.1097/01.JNR.0000387577.51350.5f

Chang, M. Y., Wang, S. Y., & Chen, C. H. (2002). Effects of massage on pain and anxiety during labour: A randomized controlled trial in Taiwan. *Journal of Advanced Nursing*, 38(1), 68–73. doi:10.1046/j.1365-2648.2002.02147.x

Chapman, L. L. (1991). Searching: Expectant fathers' experience during labor and birth. *The Journal of Perinatal & Neonatal Nursing*, 4(4), 21–29.

Chapman, L. L. (1992). Expectant fathers' roles during labor and birth. *Journal of Obstetric, Gynecologic, and Neonatal Nursing*, 21(2), 114–120. doi:10.1111/j.1552-6909.1992.tb01729.x

Chapman, L. L. (2000). Expectant fathers and labor epidurals. *MCN: The American Journal of Maternal Child Nursing*, 25(3), 133–138.

Cheng, Y., Nicholson, J., Shaffer, B., Lyell, D., & Caughey, A. (2009). The second stage of labor and epidural use: A larger effect than previously suggested. *American Journal of Obstetrics & Gynecology*, 201(6), S46. doi:10.1016/j.ajog.2009.10.097

Christiaens, W., Verhaeghe, M., & Bracke, P. (2010). Pain acceptance and personal control in pain relief in two maternity care models: A cross-national comparison of Belgium and the Netherlands. *BMC Health Services Research*, 10, 268.

Cluett, E. R., Burns, E., & Cuthbert, A. (2018). Immersion in water during labour and birth. *Cochrane Database of Systematic Reviews*, (2), CD000111. doi:10.1002/14651858.CD000111.pub4

Cluett, E. R., Pickering, R., Getliffe, K., & St. George Saunders, N. J. (2004). Randomised controlled trial of labouring in water compared with standard of augmentation for management of dystocia in first stage of labour. *BMJ*, 328(7435), 314–320.

Collins, M. (2017). Nitrous oxide utility in labor and birth: A multipurpose modality. *The Journal of Perinatal & Neonatal Nursing*, 31(2), 137–144. doi: 10.1097/JPN.0000000000000248

Collins, M. (2018). Use of nitrous oxide in maternity care (AWHONN Practice Brief No. 6). *Journal of Obstetric, Gynecologic, and Neonatal Nursing*, 47(2), 239–242. DOI: https://doi.org/10.1016/j.jogn.2018.01.009

Cyna, A. M., McAuliffe, G. I., & Andrew, M. I. (2004). Hypnosis for pain relief in labour and childbirth: A systematic review. *British Journal of Anaesthesia*, 93, 505–511. doi:10.1093/bja/aeh225

da Silva, F. M., de Oliveira, S. M., & Nobre, M. R. (2009). A randomised controlled trial evaluating the effect of immersion bath on labour pain. *Midwifery*, 25(3), 286–294. doi:10.1016/j.midw.2007.04.006

DeBaets, A. M. (2017). From birth plan to birth partnership: Enhancing communication in childbirth. *American Journal of Obstetrics & Gynecology*, 216(1), 31.e1–31.e4. doi: 10.1016/j.ajog.2016.09.087

Declercq, E. R., Sakala, C., Corry, M. P., & Applebaum, S. (2007). Listening to mothers II: Report of the second national U.S. survey of women's childbearing experiences: Conducted January-February 2006 for Childbirth Connection by Harris Interactive® in partnership with Lamaze International. *The Journal of Perinatal Education*, 16(4), 15–17. doi:10.1624/105812407X244778

Declercq, E. R., Sakala, C., Corry, M. P., Applebaum, S., & Herrlich, A. (2013). *Listening to mothers III pregnancy and birth: Report of the third national U.S. survey of women's childbearing experiences* New York: Childbirth Connection.

Dellman, T. (2004). "The best moment of my life": A literature review of fathers' experience of childbirth. *Australian Midwifery*, 17(3), 20–26. doi:10.1016/S1448-8272(04)80014-2

DiFranco, J. (2000). Relaxation: Music. In F. Nichols & S. Humernick (Eds.), *Childbirth education: Practice, research and theory* (2nd ed.). Philadelphia, PA: WB Saunders.

D'Onofrio, P., Novelli, A. M., Mecacci, F., & Scarselli, G. (2009). The efficacy and safety of continuous intravenous administration of remifentanil for birth pain relief: An open study of 205 parturients. *Anesthesia and Analgesia*, 109(6), 1922–1924. doi:10.1213/ane.0b013e3181acc6fc

El-Wahab, N., & Robinson, N. (2011). Analgesia and anaesthesia in labour. *Obstetrics, Gynaecology & Reproductive Medicine*, 21, 137–141.

Eriksson, M., Ladfors, L., Mattsson, L. A., & Fall, O. (1996). Warm tub bath during labor: A study of 1385 women with prelabor rupture of the membranes after 34 weeks of gestation. *Acta Obstetricia et Gynecologica Scandinavica*, 75(7), 642–644. doi:10.3109/00016349609054689

Escott, D., Slade, P., & Spiby, H. (2009). Preparation for pain management during childbirth: The psychological aspects of coping strategy development in antenatal education. *Clinical Psychology Review*, 29(7), 617–622.

Evron, S., & Ezri, T. (2007). Options for systemic labor analgesia. *Current Opinion in Anaesthesiology*, 20(3), 181–185. doi:10.1097/ACO.0b013e328136c1d1

Fairchild, E., Roberts, L., Zelman, K., Michelli, S., & Hastings-Tolsma, M. (2017). Implementation of Robert's Coping with Labor Algorithm© in a large tertiary care facility. *Midwifery*, 50, 208–218. doi:10.1016/j.midw.2017.03.008

Farooq, A., Tagi, A., & Khawaj, S. (2016). The frequency of epidural catheter migration in patients receiving epidural analgesia during labor increases with time. *Pakistan Armed Forces Medical Journal*, 66(3), 351–353.

Faucher, M. A., & Brucker, M. C. (2000). Intrapartum pain: Pharmacologic management. *Journal of Obstetric, Gynecologic, and Neonatal Nursing*, 29(2), 169–180. doi:10.1111/j.1552-6909.2000.tb02037.x

Ferrer, L. E., Romero, D. J., Vásquez, O. I., Matute, E. C., & Van de Velde, M. (2017). Effect of programmed intermittent epidural boluses and continuous epidural infusion on labor analgesia and obstetric outcomes: A randomized controlled trial. *Archives of Gynecology and Obstetrics*, 296, 915–922. doi:10.1007/s00404-017-4510-x

Field, T., Hernandez-Reif, M., Taylor, S., Quintino, O., & Burman, I. (1997). Labor pain is reduced by massage therapy. *Journal of Psychosomatic Obstetrics and Gynaecology*, 18(4), 286–291. doi:10.3109/01674829709080701

Flink, I. K., Mroczek, M., Sullivan, M., & Linton, S. J. (2009). Pain in childbirth and postpartum recovery: The role of catastrophizing. *European Journal of Pain*, 13(3), 312–316. doi:10.1016/j.ejpain.2008.04.010

Florence, D. J., & Palmer, D. G. (2003). Therapeutic choices for the discomforts of labor. *The Journal of Perinatal & Neonatal Nursing*, 17(4), 238–251.

Gale, J., Fothergill-Bourbonnais, F., & Chamberlain, M. (2001). Measuring nursing support during childbirth. *MCN: The American Journal of Maternal Child Nursing*, 26(5), 264–271.

Garland, D., & Jones, K. (1997). Waterbirth: Updating the evidence. *British Journal of Midwifery*, 5, 6.

Gentz, B. A. (2001). Alternative therapies for the management of pain in labor and delivery. *Clinical Obstetrics & Gynaecology*, 44(4), 704–732.

Gillesby, E., Burns, S., Dempsey, A., Kirby, S., Mogensen, K., Naylor, K., . . . Whelan, B. (2010). Comparison of delayed versus immediate pushing during second stage of labor for nulliparous women with epidural anesthesia. *Journal of Obstetrics, Gynecologic, and Neonatal Nursing*, 39(6), 635–644. doi:10.1111/j.1552-6909.2010.01195.x

Gonzalez, M., Gaurav, T., & Ihab, K. (2016). Pain management during labor part 1: Pathophysiology of labor pain and maternal evaluation for labor analgesia. *Topics in Obstetrics & Gynecology*, 36(11), 1–7. doi:10.1097/01.PGO.0000488508.99543.41

Green, J., & Hotelling, B. A. (2014). Healthy Birth Practice #3: Bring a loved one, friend, or doula for continuous support. *The Journal of Perinatal Education*, 23(4), 194–197. doi:10.1891/1058-1243.23.4.194

Gruzman, I., Shelef, I., Weintraub, A. Y., Zlotnik, A., & Erez, O. (2017). Puerperal ventral epidural hematoma after epidural labor analgesia. *International Journal of Obstetric Anesthesia*, 31, 100–104.

Halpern, S. H., & Carvalho, B. (2009). Patient-controlled epidural analgesia for labor. *Anesthesia and Analgesia*, 108(3), 921–928.

Halpern, S., Muir, H., Breen, T. W., Campbell, D. C., Barrett, J., Liston, R., & Blanchard, J. W. (2004). A multicenter randomized controlled trial comparing patient-controlled epidural with intravenous analgesia for pain relief in labor. *Anesthesia and Analgesia*, 99(5), 1532–1538. doi:10.1213/01.ANE.0000136850.08972.07

Hawkins, J. L. (2010). Epidural analgesia for labor and delivery. *The New England Journal of Medicine*, 362(16), 1503–1510.

Hawkins, J. L., & Bucklin, B. A. (2017). Obstetric anesthesia. In S. G. Gabbe, J. R. Niebyl, R. J. Weber, & G. G. Briggs (Eds.), *Obstetrics: Normal and problem pregnancies* (7th ed., pp. 344–367). Philadelphia, PA: Elsevier.

Henderson, J. J., Dickinson, J. E., Evans, S. F., McDonald, S. J., & Paech, M. J. (2003). Impact of intrapartum epidural analgesia on breast-feeding duration. *The Australian & New Zealand Journal of Obstetrics & Gynecology*, 43(5), 372–377.

Hensley, J. G., Collins, M. R., & Leezer, C. L. (2017). Pain management in obstetrics. *Critical Care Nursing Clinics of North America*, 29, 471–485. doi:10.1016/j.cnc.2017.08.007

Hinova, A., & Fernando, R. (2009). Systemic remifentanil for labor analgesia. *Anesthesia and Analgesia, 109*(6), 1925–1929. doi:10.1213/ANE.0b013e3181c03e0c

Hodnett, E. D., Gates, S., Hofmeyr, G., & Sakala, C. (2013). Continuous support for women during childbirth. *Cochrane Database of Systematic Reviews*, (10), CD003766. doi:10.1002/14651858.CD003766.pub5

Hong, R. W. (2010). Less is more: The recent history of neuraxial labor analgesia. *American Journal of Therapeutics, 17*(5), 492–497. doi:10.1097/MJT.0b013e3181ea7838

Horlocker, T. T., Wedel, D. J., Rowlinson, J. C., Enneking, F. K., Kopp, S. L., Benzon, H. T., . . . Yuan, C. S. (2010). Regional anesthesia in the patient receiving antithrombotic or thrombolytic therapy: American Society of Regional Anesthesia and Pain Medicine Evidence-Based Guidelines (Third Edition). *Regional Anesthesia and Pain Medicine, 35*(1), 64–101

Howard, E. D. (2017). An innovation in the assessment of labor pain. *The Journal of Perinatal & Neonatal Nursing, 31*(2), 96–98. doi:10.1097/JPN.0000000000000246

Huntley, A. L., Coon, J. T., & Ernst, E. (2004). Complementary and alternative medicine for labor pain: A systematic review. *American Journal of Obstetrics & Gynecology, 191*(1), 36–44. doi:10.1016/j.ajog.2003.12.008

Jahdi, F., Sheikhan, F., Haghani, H., Sharifi, B., Ghaseminejad, A., Khodarahmian, M., & Rouhana, N. (2017). Yoga during pregnancy: The effects on labor pain and delivery outcomes (A randomized controlled trial). *Complementary Therapies in Clinical Practice, 27*, 1–4. doi:10.1016/j.ctcp.2016.12.002

Johnson, N. (2016). *The use of hydrotherapy in labor to promote physiologic labor.* Retrieved from http://scholarworks.wmich.edu/honors_theses/2759

Jones, L., Othman, M., Dowswell, T., Alfirevic, Z., Gates, S., Newburn, M., . . . Neilson, J. P. (2012). Pain management for women in labour: An overview of systematic reviews. *Cochrane Database of Systematic Reviews*, (3), CD009234. doi:10.1002/14651858.CD009234.pub2.

Kerr, D., Taylor, D., & Evans, B. (2015). Patient-controlled intranasal fentanyl analgesia: A pilot study to assess practicality and tolerability during childbirth. *International Journal of Obstetric Anesthesia, 24*(2), 117–123.

Kiani, K., Shahpourian, F., Sedighian, H., & Hosseini, A. F. (2009). O472 effect of water birth on labor pain during active phase of labor. *International Journal of Gynecology & Obstetrics, 107*(Suppl. 2), S93–S96.

Kimber, L., McNabb, M., Mc Court, C., Haines, A., & Brocklehurst, P. (2008). Massage or music for pain relief in labour: A pilot randomised placebo controlled trial. *European Journal of Pain (London, England), 12*(8), 961–969. doi:10.1016/j.ejpain.2008.01.004

Klaus, M. H., Kennell, J. H., & Klaus, P. H. (2002). *The doula book: How a trained labor companion can help you have a shorter, easier, and healthier birth.* Cambridge, MA: Perseus.

Klomp, T., van Poppel, M., Jones, L., Lazet, J., Di Nisio, M., & Lagro-Janssen, A. L. (2012). Inhaled analgesia for pain management in labour. *Cochrane Database of Systematic Reviews*, (9), CD009351.

Kozhimannil, K. B., Hardeman, R. R., Attanasio, L. B., Blauer-Peterson, C., & O'Brien, M. (2013). Doula care, birth outcomes, and costs among Medicaid beneficiaries. *American Journal of Public Health, 103*(4), e113–e121. doi:10.2105/AJPH.2012.301201

Kuczkowski, K. M., & Reisner, L. S. (2003). Anesthetic management of the parturient with fever and infection. *Journal of Clinical Anesthesia, 15*, 478–488. doi:10.1016/S0952-8180(03)00081-3

Kukla, R., Kuppermann, M., Little, M., Lyerly, A. D., Mitchell, L. M., Armstrong, E. M., & Harris, L. (2009). Finding autonomy in birth. *Bioethics, 23*(1), 1–8. doi:10.1111/j.1467-8519.2008.00677.x

Lally, J. E., Murtagh, M. J., Macphail, S., & Thomson, R. (2008). More in hope than expectations: A systematic review of women's expectations and experience of pain relief in labour. *BMC Medicine, 6*, 7. doi:10.1186/1741-7015-6-7

Lee, L. O., Bateman, B. T., Kheterpal, L., Klumpner, T. T., & Housey, M. (2017). Risk of epidural hematoma after neuraxial techniques in thrombocytopenic parturients: A report from the multicenter perioperative outcomes group. *Anesthesiology, 126*(6), 1053–1063. doi:10.1097/ALN.0000000000001630

Lee, N., Kildea, S., & Stapleton, H. (2017). "Tough love": The experiences of midwives giving women sterile water injections for the relief of back pain in labour. *Midwifery, 53*, 80–86.

Leffert, L., Butwick, A., Carvalho, B., Arendt, K., Bates, S. M., Friedman, A., . . . Toledo, P. (2018). The Society for Obstetric Anesthesia and Perinatology consensus statement on the anesthetic management of pregnant and postpartum women receiving thromboprophylaxis or higher dose anticoagulants. *Anesthesia and Analgesia, 126*(3), 928–944.

Lieberman, E., & O'donoghue, C. (2002). Unintended effects of epidural analgesia during labor: A systematic review. *American Journal of Obstetrics & Gynecology, 186*(5 Suppl.), S31–S68.

Likis, F. E., Andrews, J. C., Collins, M. R., Lewis, R. M., Seroogy, J. J., Starr, S. A., . . . McPheeters, M. L. (2014). Nitrous oxide for the management of labor pain: A systematic review. *Anesthesia and Analgesia, 118*(1), 153–167.

Liu, E. H., & Sia, A. T. (2004). Rates of cesarean section and instrumental vaginal delivery in nulliparous women after low concentration epidural infusions or opioid analgesia: Systematic review. *BMJ, 328*(7453), 410–415. doi:10.1136/bmj.38097.590810.7C

Lothian, J. (2005). Birth plans: The good, the bad, and the future. *Journal of Obstetric, Gynecologic, and Neonatal Nursing, 35*, 295–303. doi:10.1111/J.1552-6909.2006.00042.x

Lowe, N. (2002). The nature of labor pain. *American Journal of Obstetrics & Gynecology, 186*, S16–S24. doi:10.1067/mob.2002.121427

MacKenzie, I. Z., Xu, J., Cusick, C., Midwinter-Morten, H., Meacher, H., Mollison, J., & Brock, M. (2011). Acupuncture for pain relief during induced labor in nulliparae: A randomised controlled study. *BJOG, 118*(4), 440–447. doi:10.1111/j.1471-0528.2010.02825.x

Mackey, M. M. (2001). Use of water in labor and birth. *Clinical Obstetrics and Gynecology, 44*(4), 733–749.

Madden, K., Middleton, P., Cyna, A. M., Matthewson, M., & Jones, L. (2016). Hypnosis for pain management during labour and childbirth. *Cochrane Database of Systematic Reviews*, (5), CD009356. doi:10.1002/14651858.CD009356.pub3

Manning-Orenstein, G. (1998). A birth intervention: The therapeutic effects of doula support versus Lamaze preparation on first-time mother's working models of caregiving. *Alternative Therapies in Health and Medicine, 4*(4), 73–81.

Martin, J. A., Hamilton, B. E., Osterman, M. J. K., Driscoll, A. K., & Drake, P. (2018). Births: Final data for 2017. *National Vital Statistics Reports, 67*(8), 1–50.

Mayberry, L. J., Clemmens, D., & De, A. (2002). Epidural analgesia side effects, co-interventions, and care of women during childbirth: A systematic review. *American Journal of Obstetrics & Gynecology, 186*(5 Suppl.), S81–S94.

Mayberry, L. J., Wood, S. H., Strange, L. B., Lee, L., Heisler, D. R., & Nielsen-Smith, K. (2000). *Second stage labor management: Promotion of evidence-based practice and a collaborative approach to patient care.* Washington, DC: Author.

McCaffery, M., & Pasero, C. (1999). Practical nondrug approaches to pain. In M. McCaffery & C. Pasero (Eds.), *Pain: Clinical manual for nursing practice* (2nd ed., pp. 399–427). St. Louis, MO: Mosby.

McKenzie, H., & Pulley, D. (2016). The pregnant patient: Assessment and perioperative management. *Anesthesiology Clinics, 34*(1), 213–222. doi:10.1016/j.anclin.2015.10.016

Melzack, R. (1984). The myth of painless childbirth (the John J. Bonica lecture). *Pain, 19*(4), 321–327. doi:10.1016/0304-3959(84)90079-4

Melzack, R. (1999). From the gate to the neuromatrix. *Pain, 82*(Suppl. 1), S121–S126. doi:10.1016/s0304-3959(99)00145-1

Melzack, R., & Wall, P. D. (1965). Pain mechanisms: A new theory. *Science, 150,* 971–979.

Miller, A. C., & Shriver, T. E. (2012). Women's childbirth preferences and practices in the United States. *Social Science & Medicine, 75*(4), 709–716.

Miltner, R. S. (2002). More than support: Nursing interventions provided to women in labor. *Journal of Obstetric, Gynecologic, and Neonatal Nursing, 31*(6), 753–761. doi:10.1177/0884217502239214

Mirzaei, F., Keshtgar, S., Kaviana, M., & Rajaeifard, A. R. (2015). The effect of lavender essence smelling during labor on cortisol and serotonin plasma levels and anxiety reduction in nulliparous women. *Journal of Kerman University of Medical Sciences, 16,* 245–254.

Molina, F. J., Solá, P. A., López, E., & Pires, C. (1997). Pain in the first stage of labor: Relationship with the patient's position. *Journal of Pain and Symptom Management, 13*(2), 98–103. doi:10.1016/S0885-3924(96)00270-9

Montgomery, A., & Hale, T. W. (2012). ABM Clinical Protocol #15: Analgesia and anesthesia for the breastfeeding mother, revised 2012. *Breastfeeding Medicine, 7*(6), 547–553. doi:10.1089/bfm.2012.9977

Mosallam, M., Rizk, D. E., Thomas, L., & Ezimokhai, M. (2004). Women's attitudes towards psychosocial support in labour in United Arab Emirates. *Archives of Gynecology and Obstetrics, 269*(3), 181–187. doi:10.1007/s00404-002-0448-7

Mussell, S. (1998). Narcotic analgesia during labor and birth: Maternal and newborn effects. *Mother-Baby Journal, 3*(6), 19–23.

National Institute for Health and Care Excellence. (2017). *Intrapartum care for healthy women and their babies* (Clinical Guideline No. 190). London, UK: Author.

Nayak, D., Rastogi, S., & Kathuria, K. (2014). Effectiveness of music therapy on anxiety level, and pain perception in primipara mothers during first stage of labor in selected hospitals of Odisha. *Journal of Nursing and Health Science, 3*(2), 7–14.

Nikodem, V. C. (2004). Immersion in water in pregnancy, labour and birth. *Cochrane Database of Systematic Reviews,* (2), CD000111.

Niven, C. A., & Gijsbers, K. J. (1989). Do low levels of labour pain reflect low sensitivity to noxious stimulation? *Social Science & Medicine (1982), 29*(4), 585–588. doi:10.1016/0277-9536(89)90204-9

Oesterman, M. J., & Martin, J. A. (2011). Epidural and spinal anesthesia use during labor: 27-State reporting area, 2008. *National Vital Statistics Reports, 59*(5), 1–13, 16.

O'Hana, H. P., Levy, A., Rozen, A., Greemberg, L., Shapira, Y., & Sheiner, E. (2008). The effect of epidural analgesia on labor progress and outcome in nulliparous women. *The Journal of Maternal-Fetal & Neonatal Medicine, 21*(8), 517–521. doi:10.1080/14767050802040864

Ondeck, M. (2014). Healthy Birth Practice #2: Walk, move around, and change positions throughout labor. *The Journal of Perinatal Education, 23*(4), 188–193.

Osborne, L., Snyder, M., Villecco, D., Jacob, A., Pyle, S., & Crum-Cianflone, N. (2008). Evidence-based anesthesia: Fever of unknown origin in parturients and neuraxial anesthesia. *AANA Journal, 76*(3), 221–226.

O'Sullivan, G. (2009). Epidural analgesia and labor. *European Journal of Pain Supplements, 3,* 65–70. doi:10.1016/j.eujps.2009.08.006

O'Sullivan, G. (2010). Non-neuraxial analgesia during labour. *Anaesthesia and Intensive Care Medicine, 11*(7), 270–273. doi:10.1016/j.mpaic.2010.04.009

Pages-Arroyo, E., & Plan-Smith, M. C. (2013). Neurologic complications of neuraxial anesthesia. *Anesthesiology Clinics, 31*(3), 571–594.

Phillips, S. N., Fernando, R., & Girard, T. (2017). Parenteral opioid analgesia: Does it still have a role? *Best Practice & Research. Clinical Anaesthesiology, 31,* 3–14.

Poole, J. (2003). Analgesia and anesthesia during labor and birth: Implications for mother and fetus. *Journal of Obstetrics, Gynecology, and Neonatal Nursing, 32*(6), 780–793. doi:10.1177/0884217503258498

Reddy, U. M., Davis, J. M., Zhaoxia, R., & Greene, M. F. (2017). Opioid use in pregnancy, neonatal abstinence syndrome, and childhood outcomes: Executive summary of a joint workshop by the Eunice Kennedy Shriver National Institute of Child Health and Human Development, American College of Obstetricians and Gynecologists, American Academy of Pediatrics, Society for Maternal-Fetal Medicine, Centers for Disease Control and Prevention, and the March of Dimes Foundation. *Obstetrics & Gynecology, 130*(1), 10–28.

Reynolds, F. (2010). The effects of maternal labour analgesia on the fetus. *Best Practice & Research. Clinical Obstetrics & Gynaecology, 24*(3), 289–302. doi:10.1016/j.bpobgyn.2009.11.003

Reynolds, F. (2011). Labour analgesia and the baby: Good news is no news. *International Journal of Obstetric Anesthesia, 20*(1), 38–50. doi:10.1016/j.ijoa.2010.08.004

Richardson, M. G., Lopez, B. M., Baysinger, C. L., Shotwell, M. S., & Chestnut, D. H. (2017). Nitrous oxide during labor: Maternal satisfaction does not depend exclusively on analgesic effectiveness. *Anesthesia and Analgesia, 124*(2), 548–553.

Roberts, L., Gulliver, B., Fisher, J., & Cloyes, K. G. (2010). The Coping with Labor Algorithm: An alternate pain assessment tool for the laboring woman. *Journal of Midwifery & Women's Health, 55*(2), 107–116. doi:10.1016/j.jmwh.2009.11.002

Rollins, M., & Lucero, J. (2012). Overview of anesthetic considerations for cesarean delivery. *British Medical Bulletin, 101,* 105–125.

Roofthooft, E. (2009). Anesthesia for the morbidly obese parturient. *Current Opinion in Anaesthesiology, 22*(3), 341–346. doi:10.1097/ACO.0b013e328329a5b8

Roth, C., Dent, S. A., Parfitt, S. E., Hering, S. L., & Bay, R. C. (2016). Randomized controlled trial of use of the peanut ball during labor. *MCN: The American Journal of Maternal Child Nursing, 41*(3), 140–146. doi:10.1097/NMC.0000000000000232

Royal College of Obstetricians and Gynaecologists. (2012). *Immersion in water during labor and birth.* London, UK: Author.

Ruppen, W., Derry, S., McQuay, H., & Moore, R. A. (2006). Incidence of epidural hematoma, infection, and neurologic injury in obstetric patients with epidural analgesia/anesthesia. *Anesthesiology, 105*(2), 394–399.

Russell, R., & Reynolds, F. (1996). Epidural infusion of low-dose bupivacaine and opioid in labour. Does reducing motor block increase the spontaneous delivery date? *Anaesthesia, 51*(3), 266–273. doi:10.1111/j.1365-2044.1996.tb13645.x

Saia, K., Schiff, D., Wachman, E. M., Mehta, P., Vilkins, A., Sia, M., . . . Bagley, S. (2016). Caring for pregnant women with opioid use disorder in the USA: Expanding and improving treatment. *Current Obstetrics & Gynecology Reports, 5,* 257–263. doi:10.1007/s13669-016-0168-9

Sanders, R. D., Weimann, J., & Maze, M. (2008). Biologic effects of nitrous oxide. *Anesthesiology, 109*(4), 707–722. doi:10.1097/ALN.0b013e3181870a17

Saravanakumar, K., Rao, S. G., & Cooper, G. M. (2006). The challenges of obesity and obstetric anaesthesia. *Current Opinion in Obstetrics & Gynecology, 18*(6), 631–635.

Shahoei, R., Shahghebi, S., Rezaei, M., & Nagshbandi, S. (2017). The effect of transcutaneous electrical nerve stimulation on the severity of labor pain among nulliparous women: A clinical trial. *Complementary Therapies in Clinical Practice, 28,* 176–180.

Silva, M., & Halpern, S. H. (2010). Epidural analgesia for labor: Current techniques. *Local and Regional Anesthesia, 3,* 143–153. doi:10.2147/LRA.S10237

Simkin, P. (1995). Reducing pain and enhancing progress in labor: A guide to nonpharmacologic methods for maternity caregivers. *Birth, 22*(3), 161–171. doi:10.1111/j.1523-536X.1995.tb00693.x

Simkin, P., & Bolding, A. (2004). Update on nonpharmacologic approaches to relieve labor pain and prevent suffering. *Journal of Midwifery & Women's Health*, 49(6), 489–504. doi:10.1016/j/jmwh.2004.07.007

Simkin, P., & O'Hara, M. A. (2002). Nonpharmacologic relief of pain during labor: Systematic reviews of five methods. *American Journal of Obstetrics & Gynecology*, 186(5 Suppl.), S131–S159. doi:10.1067/mob.2002.122382

Simpson, K. R. (2007). Intrauterine resuscitation during labor: Review of current methods and supportive evidence. *Journal of Midwifery & Women's Health*, 52(3), 229–237. doi:10.1016/j.jmwh.2006.12.010

Simpson, K. R., & James, D. C. (2005). Efficacy of intrauterine resuscitation techniques in improving fetal oxygen status during labor. *Obstetrics & Gynecology*, 105(6), 1362–1368. doi:10.1097/01.AOG.0000164474.03350.7c

Simpson, K. R., & Lyndon, A. (2017). Consequences of delayed, unfinished, or missed nursing care during labor and birth. *The Journal of Perinatal & Neonatal Nursing*, 31(1), 32–40. doi:10.1097/JPN.0000000000000203

Skupski, D. W., Abramovitz, S., Samuels, J., Pressimone, V., & Kjaer, K. (2009). Adverse effects of combined spinal-epidural versus traditional epidural analgesia. *International Journal of Gynecology and Obstetrics*, 106(3), 242–245. doi:10/1016/j.ijgo.2009.04/019

Sleutel, M. R. (2000). Climate, culture, context, or work environment? Organizational factors that influence nursing practice. *The Journal of Nursing Administration*, 30(2), 53–58.

Sleutel, M. R., Schultz, S., & Wyble, K. (2007). Nurses' views of factors that help and hinder their intrapartum care. *Journal of Obstetric, Gynecologic, and Neonatal Nursing*, 36(3), 203–211.

Smith, C. A., Collins, C. T., & Crowther, C. A. (2011). Aromatherapy for pain management in labour. *Cochrane Database of Systematic Reviews*, (7), CD009215. doi:10.1002/14651858.CD009215

Smith, C. A., Levett, K. M., Collins, C. T., & Crowther, C. A. (2011). Relaxation techniques for pain management in labour. *Cochrane Database of Systematic Reviews*, (12), CD009514. doi:10.1002/14651858.CD009514

Sng, B. L., Leong, W. L., Zeng, Y., Siddiqui, F. J., Assam, P. N., Lim, Y., . . . Sia, A. T. (2014). Early versus late initiation of epidural analgesia for labour. *Cochrane Database of Systematic Reviews*, (10), CD007238. doi:10.1002/14651858.CD007238.pub2

Somers-Smith, M. J. (1999). A place for the partner? Expectations and experiences of support during childbirth. *Midwifery*, 15(2), 101–108. doi:10.1016/S0266-6138(99)90006-2

Stark, M. A., Remynse, M., & Zwelling, E. (2016). Importance of the birth environment to support physiologic birth. *Journal of Obstetric, Gynecologic, and Neonatal Nursing*, 45(2), 285–294.

Stark, M. A., Rudell, B., & Haus, G. (2008). Observing position and movements in hydrotherapy: A pilot study. *Journal of Obstetric, Gynecologic, and Neonatal Nursing*, 37(1), 116–122. doi:10.1111/j.1552-6909.2007.00212.x

Stein, C. (2016). Opioid receptors. *Annual Review of Medicine*, 67, 433–451.

Stewart, L. S., & Collins, M. (2012). Nitrous oxide as labor analgesia: Clinical implications for nurses. *Nursing for Women's Health*, 16(5), 400–409.

Sun, L. S. (2011). Labor analgesia and the developing human brain. *Anesthesia and Analgesia*, 112(6), 1265–1267. doi:10.1213/ANE.0b013e3182135a4d

Thangamuthu, A., Russell, I. F., & Purya, M. (2013). Epidural failure rate using a standardized definition. *International Journal of Obstetric Anesthesia*, 22(4), 310–315.

The Joint Commission. (2017). Joint Commission enhances pain assessment and management requirements for accredited hospitals. *Perspectives*, 37(2), 1–4.

The Joint Commission. (2018). *Approved: New and revised pain assessment and management standards*. Oakbrook Terrace, IL: Author.

The Joint Commission. (2019). *Hospital: 2019 national patient safety*. Oakbrook Terrace, IL: Author.

Touitou, Y., Dispersyn, G., & Pain, L. (2010). Labor pain, analgesia, and chronobiology: What factor matters? *Anesthesia and Analgesia*, 111(4), 838–840. doi:10:1213/ANE.0b013e3181ee85d9

Tournaire, M., & Theau-Yonneau, A. (2007). Complementary and alternative approaches to pain relief during labor. *Evidence-Based Complementary and Alternative Medicine*, 4(4), 409–417.

Tussey, C. M., Botsios, E., Gerkin, R. D., Kelly, L. A., Gamez, J., & Mensik, J. (2015). Reducing length of labor and cesarean surgery rate using a peanut ball for women laboring with an epidural. *The Journal of Perinatal Education*, 24(1), 16–24. doi:10.1891/1058-1243.24.1.16

Ullman, R., Smith, L. A., Burns, E., Mori, R., & Dowswell, T. (2010). Parenteral opioids for maternal pain relief in labour. *Cochrane Database of Systematic Reviews*, (9), CD007396. doi:10.1002/14651858.CD007396.pub2

Vanderlaan, J. (2017). Retrospective cohort study of hydrotherapy in labor. *Journal of Obstetric, Gynecologic, and Neonatal Nursing*, 46, 403–410.

Verani, J. R., McGee, L., & Schrag, S. J. (2010). Prevention of perinatal group B streptococcal disease—Revised guidelines from CDC, 2010. *MMWR Morbidity and Mortality Weekly Report*, 59(RR-10), 1–36.

Volmanen, P., Palomäki, O., & Ahonen, J. (2011). Alternatives to neuraxial analgesia for labor. *Current Opinion in Anaesthesiology*, 24(3), 235–241. doi:10.1097/ACO.0b013e328345ad18

Wakefield, M. L. (1999). Systemic analgesia: Opioids, ketamine, and inhalational agents. In D. H. Chestnut (Ed.), *Obstetric anesthesia: Principles and practice* (pp. 340–353). St. Louis, MO: Mosby.

Wesselmann, U. (2008). Pain in childbirth. In M. C. Bushnell, D. V. Smith, G. K. Beauchamp, S. J. Firestein, P. Dallos, D. Oertel, . . . A. I. Basbaum (Eds.), *The senses: A comprehensive reference* (pp. 579–583). St. Louis, MO: Elsevier.

Williams, M. S., Davies, J. M., & Ross, B. K. (2009). Medicolegal issues in obstetric anesthesia. In D. H. Chestnut, L. S. Polley, L. C. Tsen, & C. A. Wong (Eds.), *Chestnut's obstetric anesthesia: Principles and practice* (4th ed., pp. 727–746). Philadelphia, PA: Elsevier.

Wong, C. A. (2014). Epidural and spinal analgesia/anesthesia for labor and vaginal delivery. In D. H. Chestnut, L. S. Polley, L. C. Tsen, & C. A. Wong (Eds.), *Chestnut's obstetric anesthesia: Principles and practice* (5th ed., pp. 429–492). St. Louis, MO: Mosby.

Wong, C. A., McCarthy, R. J., & Hewlett, B. (2011). The effect of manipulation of the programmed intermittent bolus time interval and injection volume on total drug use for labor epidural analgesia: A randomized controlled trial. *Anesthesia and Analgesia*, 112(4), 904–911. doi:10.1213/ANE.0b013e31820e7c2f

Wong, C. A., Scavone, B. M., Peaceman, A. M., McCarthy, R. J., Sullivan, J. T., Diaz, N. T., . . . Grouper, S. (2005). The risk of cesarean delivery with neuraxial analgesia given early versus late in labor. *The New England Journal of Medicine*, 352(7), 655–665.

Yancey, M. K., Zhang, J., Schwarz, J., Dietrich, C. S., III, & Klebanoff, M. (2001). Labor epidural analgesia and intrapartum maternal hyperthermia. *Obstetrics & Gynecology*, 98(5, Pt. 1), 763–770.

Zwelling, E. (2010). Overcoming the challenges: Maternal movement and positioning to facilitate labor progress. *MCN: The American Journal of Maternal Child Nursing*, 35(2), 72–80. doi:10.1097/NMC.0b013e3181caeab3

Zwelling, E., Johnson, K., & Allen, J. (2006). How to implement complimentary therapies for laboring women. *MCN: The American Journal of Maternal Child Nursing*, 31(6), 364–370.

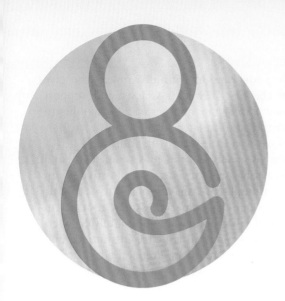

CHAPTER 17

Postpartum Care

Dotti C. James • Patricia D. Suplee

INTRODUCTION

A woman experiences significant alterations in physical and psychosocial status after childbirth. The postpartum period is a time of transition involving physiologic changes, adaptation to the maternal role, and modification of the family system with the addition of the baby. Nurses have a unique opportunity to promote and support maternal and family adaptation. Inpatient postpartum care routines are ideally focused on the needs of the mother, baby, and family rather than on arbitrary rules and unit traditions. Postpartum nursing care should be as individualized and flexible as needed. The perinatal nurse recognizes women and their families as integral members of the healthcare team and encourages them to be partners in decision-making processes and planning of care (Association of Women's Health, Obstetric and Neonatal Nurses [AWHONN], 2019b). Open visiting and family interaction with the new mother and newborn are encouraged and supported. The woman's partner and other support persons should be encouraged to be present, according to the desires of the woman, and actively involved in postpartum and newborn care. Family-centered maternity care is based on the philosophy that the physical, social, psychological, and spiritual needs of the family are included in all aspects of the nursing care provided (AWHONN, 2019b).

Implementation of family-centered maternity care requires collaboration among childbearing women, families, and healthcare providers. The family is defined by the woman and frequently extends beyond traditional definitions. Cultural beliefs and values of the woman and her family should be respected and accommodated. Chapter 2 provides a comprehensive review and discussion of various cultural and religious perspectives and can be helpful in developing nursing care for specific women.

PLANNING FOR THE TRANSITION TO PARENTHOOD

According to current trends, length of stay (LOS) for childbirth is now more realistically in line with the physical and psychosocial needs of the new mother and her family rather than with the previous arbitrary mandates from health insurance companies in an effort to control costs. However, although LOS has slightly increased over the past several years, it is still relatively short in hospital settings. A shortened hospital stay (less than 48 hours after birth) for all term newborns may not be appropriate for every mother and newborn, especially for those mothers who have preexisting medical conditions or complications postbirth (American Academy of Pediatrics [AAP] and American College of Obstetricians and Gynecologists [ACOG], 2017). Newborn infants discharged before 48 hours of age should be examined by a provider within 3 to 4 days of life (AAP & ACOG, 2017). The most frequent causes of newborn readmission are jaundice, dehydration, feeding difficulties, and infection (Gracia et al., 2016).

Rubin's (1961a) classic research suggests that during the immediate postpartum period, the new mother is not physically or emotionally ready to listen to extensive presentations of how to care for herself and her newborn. Postpartum women have transient deficits in cognition, particularly in memory function, the first day after giving birth. According to Henry and Sherwin (2012), pregnant women can temporarily develop mild cognitive defects, especially related to tasks of verbal recall and processing speed, during labor and after birth when compared with nonpregnant women. In their study, cortisol levels were significantly associated with verbal recall scores at both the pregnancy and at postpartum periods and with spatial abilities at postpartum only. This decline was not attributed to depression, anxiety, sleep deprivation, or other physical changes associated with pregnancy. Based on available evidence, traditional discharge education that includes verbal transmission of information or instruction in child care techniques provided immediately after birth or on the first postpartum day may be poorly remembered. These findings underscore the importance of providing the family with appropriate written material they can review after discharge. Priorities for most women in the first 24 hours postpartum are rest; time to touch, hold, and get to know their baby; and an opportunity to review and discuss their labor and birth (Rubin, 1961a).

The childbearing experience is very different today than it was over 50 years ago when Rubin (1961a, 1961b) began her research. Major changes include the availability of prenatal classes; women and families as active participants in all aspects of perinatal care; fathers, siblings, and other support persons present for labor and birth; the use of epidural anesthesia/analgesia for pain management; open visiting and single-room maternity care; couplet care models; and shorter hospitalizations. However, despite the progress made toward a healthcare environment where childbearing women have more participation and control, much of Rubin's work about the taking-in and taking-hold phases of the postpartum period is still valid today.

Childbirth education discharge planning process should be ongoing from preconception counseling, pregnancy, labor, and the postpartum period. Although education about maternal and infant care can occur during the inpatient stay, information should be offered during pregnancy and reinforced after discharge in many different settings using a variety of teaching methods. The prenatal period provides a window of opportunity to prepare families not only about pregnancy and birth but also about the postpartum and infant periods. Prenatal visits to the primary healthcare provider are an ideal time for the perinatal nurse to assess family learning needs and concerns and to offer information, support, and resources in a personalized way. Prenatal classes should provide education about pregnancy, health promotion, labor and birth, postpartum, interconception, maternal and infant care, and the transition to parenthood. During the postpartum period, critical concepts can then be reviewed and reinforced again prior to discharge.

Postpartum home care visits offer the perinatal nurse another opportunity to assess knowledge, skills, and learning needs as well as to provide individualized education, support, and referrals to new mothers (Ladewig, London, & Davidson, 2017). If home visits are not possible, follow-up phone calls after discharge provide the perinatal nurse an opportunity to clarify information and answer additional questions. ACOG (2018a) recommends a touch point with all women who give birth within the first 3 weeks. Classes and support groups for new parents are another way for families to continue learning about maternal and infant care, parenting, and how to nurture family relationships.

Healthcare providers continue to struggle to find innovative ways to provide safe, cost-effective, comprehensive perinatal care in response to economic pressures. Although consumer pressures resulted in state and federal laws mandating minimal LOS coverage, costs remain a very real issue for institutions and individual healthcare providers. Prenatal education in healthcare provider offices and in the classroom combined with written materials and/or videos are some methods that prepare women and their families for discharge. Women feel more in control and express greater feelings of maternal confidence and competence when they have adequate knowledge about how to care for themselves and their newborns after discharge.

Prenatal Patient Database

Early identification and entry into the system can facilitate prenatal preparation for hospitalization and postpartum discharge. Successful programs require communication among primary healthcare providers, prenatal care sites, prenatal educators, community resources, and the birthing facility. A simple, user-friendly system that incorporates demographic data, estimated date of birth, significant clinical history, family assessment and learning needs, participation in prenatal education programs, and a mechanism to communicate all pertinent information to the inpatient unit is critical. Healthcare providers at each institution can develop a prenatal patient database to meet specific needs. For example, when a woman registers her intent to give birth at the institution early in pregnancy, demographic and insurance data can be entered into the system. Primary healthcare providers and those in community prenatal clinics that refer women for inpatient care can be encouraged to send notification about women who have selected the institution for childbirth. Lack of interoperability between software systems used in the birthing hospital, other hospitals where the woman may have received care, prenatal clinics, and physician and midwife offices is major factor in the inability to share important information about prenatal care with the clinicians at the hospital. There is risk of critical data being missed as well as testing being repeated unnecessarily. Women may seek prenatal care at multiple sites. Until electronic health records (EHRs) are able to be used between health systems, hospitals, clinics, and providers' offices, birthing hospitals will be challenged to have processes to make sure they have all prenatal care and testing data available when women present for care in the hospital.

Some hospitals have developed Internet Web sites where women can register for childbirth classes, seek prenatal care information, download patient education materials, and take a virtual tour of the facilities or schedule a live tour. Summaries of the educational and clinical backgrounds, services, office hours, and insurance plan participation of healthcare providers that have privileges at the institutions can offer valuable information to women who are in the process of selecting a healthcare provider and an institution for birth. Links to offices of obstetricians, family practice physicians, and nurse midwives on staff can be helpful as well. Information about financial criteria for eligibility to participate in programs such as Medicaid and the Special Supplemental Nutrition Program for Women, Infants, and Children's are useful for selected families. As most families of childbearing age have access to the Internet, these Web sites can meet the needs of patients and healthcare institutions.

Brochures describing all perinatal services available at the institution including telephone numbers are especially helpful and ideally should be available in the offices of all healthcare providers affiliated with the institution and online. Written materials should be available in the languages of the population served. Families should be informed about prenatal classes and encouraged to attend. Ideally, these classes are low cost and affordable or at no cost. Selected women and their families can be referred for case management, especially when the pregnancy and the social or economic situation are complex.

By the 36th week of pregnancy, a record of prenatal care should be sent by the primary healthcare provider to the birthing facility to be available when the woman is admitted for labor and birth (AAP & ACOG, 2017). Specific individualized care plans or guides developed by the case manager, social worker, or perinatal nurse in collaboration with the pregnant woman should also be added to the patient database. With this type of system, when the woman is admitted for childbirth, the perinatal nurse has valuable information about current maternal–fetal health status, family learning needs, and the education programs the family attended. The quality and quantity of prenatal data about the childbearing family enhance the perinatal nurse's ability to provide individualized care and teaching.

Prenatal Education and Shared Decision Making

In the past, most prenatal education was offered in a series of weekly classes lasting 6 to 8 weeks during the last trimester of pregnancy. The focus of the education was on preparation for labor and birth and to a lesser extent on pregnancy, infant care, and the transition to parenthood. For many working couples, making the time commitment to attend a series of six classes was

difficult. Multiple factors such as perceived knowledge, support systems, transportation issues, work schedules, childcare availability, and previous newborn and childbirth experience now influence the decision to attend prenatal classes. Many institutions and perinatal educators have responded to consumer needs by streamlining content to decrease program length and offering alternatives such as weekend programs, flexible hours, informative Web sites and webinars, and antepartum home visits.

Information about health promotion should be presented to women early in pregnancy to have the opportunity to potentially make a difference in pregnancy outcomes. Topics in early pregnancy classes may include the following:

- Fetal growth and development
- Expected physical changes during pregnancy
- Normal discomforts of pregnancy
- Lifestyle modifications
- Nutrition
- Activity and exercise
- Effects of smoking cigarettes, drinking alcohol, and using illegal drugs
- Use of over-the-counter medications, herbal supplements, and medications prescribed by other healthcare providers
- Warning signs of pregnancy complications and when to call the provider if these signs and symptoms should occur

Traditionally, prepared childbirth classes are usually offered during the third trimester when the mother and her partner are intent on learning about what to expect during labor and birth. Although the process of labor and birth is valuable content, information about maternal postpartum self-care, parenthood, and infant care is also important for expectant parents.

There is a significant need for information to assist in preparing couples for labor and birth, thus pregnant women and their partners can benefit from a comprehensive educational program that includes preconception health promotion, healthy behaviors during the prenatal period, breastfeeding, the postpartum period, and infant care content. Prenatal education should be designed to meet the needs of the population served and based on the knowledge of what information and skills are useful and relevant to expectant parents, at various stages of pregnancy. The education should be presented in a manner that supports women's ability to have the information they need to make informed decisions about based on their personal reproductive goals and values. Shared decision making should be the norm, not the exception. Classes focusing on parenting, breastfeeding, sibling preparation, grandparents, car seat safety, exercise during pregnancy, the benefits and risks of a trial of labor after a cesarean birth, the benefits of spontaneous labor, the risks of nonmedically indicated interventions, labor preparation for women who desire a vaginal birth after cesarean birth (VBAC), and families expecting more than one baby complement the core curriculum. All prenatal information should be discussed in a manner that empowers and supports shared decision making.

Parent and birth educators play a significant role in preparing families for the postpartum period. It is important that their work is valued and that there is ongoing communication between the educators and the perinatal unit staff, especially if the educators are not formally affiliated with the institution. Disappointments and unmet expectations for the labor, birth, and postpartum experience can be avoided if childbirth educators are fully familiar with the policies of the perinatal unit.

Educational Methods and Materials

Whether education is provided at the bedside or in a classroom, the teaching method must complement the information presented and must be appropriate for the learner. Feelings and beliefs are best addressed individually or in a small group setting. Consideration should be given to personal learning styles and basic education level and knowledge. Parents should be allowed to bring up their own topics of interest along with the traditional topics being proposed so their concerns can be addressed. Some institutions periodically hold new parent focus groups or use telephone or mailed surveys to validate the content of their educational materials and classes and to make sure they are consistent with the needs of their patients.

Written materials support and reinforce interactive learning. Books, pamphlets, brochures, and other handouts must have a consistent message and support the philosophy of the perinatal institution. There are a number of excellent resources in print, or the prenatal educators may develop their own education materials. Women and their families can be referred to online resources such as those provided by AWHONN (https://www.health4mom.org/). The Centers for Disease Control and Prevention (CDC) offers accurate and timely education on a number of pregnancy and parenting topics (English, Alden, Zomorodi, Travers, & Ross, 2018). Thus, referrals to these sites for online education can be made with confidence that the information is accurate and up to date: pregnancy (https://www.cdc.gov/pregnancy/index.html), breastfeeding (https://www.cdc.gov/breastfeeding/), and parenting (https://www.cdc.gov/parents/).

Selection or development of written materials should be based on the education level of the population served and the financial resources available. The healthcare provider, educator, and representatives from the perinatal institution should collectively choose written materials and be familiar with the contents. Parents should be asked to evaluate the usefulness and helpfulness of the written materials. Providing families with standardized written materials can be a time-saving and cost-effective strategy. If the institution chooses to use materials purchased from companies that specialize in developing childbirth and parenting educational materials, it is important to thoroughly review the content for accuracy before distributing to patients. Standardized materials (either purchased or developed by the institution) provide a ready resource for parents at any time and potentially decrease the volume of calls to the perinatal center and to the primary healthcare provider. Written materials should be developed or chosen with consideration to the basic language level of the family and to the language they speak. Families who do not speak English should be supplied with language-appropriate materials.

Some institutions use in-hospital television channels with programs on newborn bath, cord and circumcision care, and breast-feeding and formula feeding. Purchased videos or those produced by the institution are another method of providing important information. The videos can be given as gifts, loaned to families, or purchased in the hospital gift shop. As with written materials, television instruction, links to online resources, and videos need to be evaluated for consistent, correct information that is learner appropriate and reflects the philosophy of the perinatal institution.

Family Preference Plan

Involving women and their families in decisions about their perinatal care increases satisfaction and promotes a collaborative relationship between healthcare providers and families. A birth preference plan contains written suggestions of what a woman would prefer to happen during her childbirth stay. A preference plan helps to individualize the family's care (Display 17–1). The preference plan can be given to all pregnant women registered for birth or given to families during prenatal classes. The preference plan provides the healthcare provider with information about the family's special needs, concerns, and requests and allows the healthcare provider to have a meaningful discussion with the family about their expectations. This discussion should occur during the pregnancy with the primary healthcare provider and with the perinatal nurse on admission to the unit for labor and birth.

Reviewing preference plans with the woman prior to presenting in labor can be helpful in clarifying unit protocols and avoiding unmet expectations when women have plans for techniques or procedures that are not available on the unit. For example, a woman may have read about the benefits of hydrotherapy in labor,

DISPLAY 17–1

Family Preference Plan

My name: _____   My midwife or physician's name: _____

1. My main support person is: _____

   Relationship: _____

2. I would like to have these persons visit during labor:

   _____   _____

   _____   _____

3. For pain control/positioning during labor and birth, I would like to:

   _____ walk in room/halls   _____ listen to special music

   _____ sit in recliner   _____ use special focal point

   _____ use shower   _____ use my own pillows

   _____ use Jacuzzi   _____ use squat bar

   _____ use heat/cold/massage   _____ use foot pads on bed

4. I would like to have these persons present during birth:

   _____   _____

5. I have these religious requests:

   _____ birth blessing by chaplain

   _____ Eucharist or communion

   _____ have visit by my own clergy

   _____ other: _____

   _____ none

6. After birth, I would like to:

   _____ place baby skin-to-skin   _____ have doctor circumcise my son

   _____ wrap baby in blanket before holding   _____ have pictures taken of my baby

   _____ breastfeed my baby   _____ keep baby in my room as long as he or she is stable

   _____ bathe my baby

7. During my hospital stay, I would like to have my support person:

   _____ put baby skin-to-skin to him or her

   _____ assist with baby care

   _____ give the baby's first bath

   _____ spend the night in my room

   _____ take pictures of birth experience

8. I plan to attend, or have already attended, these classes/services during this pregnancy:

   _____ prenatal class

   _____ hospital OB tour

   _____ sibling class

   _____ exercise sessions

   _____ Lamaze

9. Child care has been arranged for other dependent children:

   _____ during the hospital stay

   _____ after mom and baby go home

   _____ not applicable

   _____ other: _____

10. I plan to have my other child(ren) come to visit:

    _____ during birth

    _____ in the first 2-hour recovery time

    _____ after I arrive in my postpartum room

    _____ not at all

    _____ not applicable

11. After going home, these persons will help out for the first 2 days:

    _____

    _____

12. Additional ideas:

    _____

    _____

    _____

    _____

    _____

    _____

but the unit does not have a Jacuzzi tub available; wants to use candles for aromatherapy, however the unit may not allow burning candles for safety reasons; or may plan to use a birthing ball during labor, and the unit doesn't have birthing balls. If the woman is aware of these limitations in advance of admission, she can make alternative plans. In the examples described here, there are other methods that could meet the woman's expectations. Hydrotherapy can be provided in the shower, use of scented lotions can be used for aromatherapy, and a birthing ball can be obtained on loan from a childbirth educator or purchased before admission. The preference plan can be sent to the birthing facility along with the prenatal care records and a hard copy brought to the labor and delivery unit by the woman on admission for childbirth. It is important that any record-keeping process about childbirth preferences includes a system to ensure that it is available to all healthcare providers when the woman is admitted for labor and birth.

Ideally, the amount of childbirth preparation and type of pain management anticipated during labor are covered prior to or during the admission assessment. A review of preferences for childbirth, including reinforcement of options that are available at the institution, works best to facilitate a positive experience. Although some nurses and physicians have negative feelings about written birth plans, a birth plan helps the nurse meet the couple's expectations and indicates that the woman has given considerable thought to how she would like labor and birth to proceed. Every effort should be made to meet the expectations and wishes of the woman. The woman's desires for positioning, ambulation, and method of fetal assessment should be honored in ways that are consistent with safe care. If maternal and/or fetal status is such that the woman's wishes cannot be met within reason, a thorough discussion with adequate explanation of the rationale for the decision should occur. The woman should be allowed and encouraged to ask any questions and be given appropriate answers to those questions. It may be necessary for the primary healthcare provider to talk to the woman in person or by telephone about her concerns. The nurse should acknowledge the woman's disappointment and assure her that every attempt to meet her expectations will be made if the clinical situation changes.

Arbitrary rules prohibiting more than one support person during labor and birth are contrary to the philosophy that the birth experience belongs to the woman and her family rather to those providing clinical care. Although healthcare providers are sometimes inclined to attempt to control this aspect of the birth process using various arguments for safety and convenience, when examined critically, these arguments have little scientific merit. Women should be able to choose who will be with them during this very special and unique life experience. Family-centered care supports the concept that the "family" is defined by childbearing women. Families should be free to take still pictures and record video and/or audio tapes during labor and birth. If there are specific policies in place at the woman's selected birthing facility, these should be shared with the woman and her partner early in pregnancy so they can make an informed decision on where to give birth.

Learning Needs Assessment

Needs assessment tools, care paths, or teaching lists can assist nurses and families in identifying learning needs and in documentation of the type and timing of prenatal and postpartum education. A learning needs assessment can be initiated at various times during the perinatal period depending on when a woman has first contact with the hospital system. Opportunities include prenatal classes, prenatal visits, hospital tours, and telephone contact with a case manager, during admission to the hospital, following birth, and at the mother–infant follow-up visit or contact. Many families attending prenatal classes are first-time parents. A detailed assessment of individual learning needs discussed during the first prenatal class alerts prospective parents to information and skills they need to acquire by the time they are discharged from the hospital. The learning needs assessment tool and supporting written materials should include the information, instruction provided, and the skills taught.

For women who have not attended prenatal classes or completed a learning needs assessment during a prenatal visit, the process begins on admission to the hospital. With the help of the labor nurse, families identify specific learning needs they want to address during the inpatient stay. Whether the needs assessment is completed prior to admission, during early labor, or after birth, the education process begins as soon as possible for each woman and family.

Primary responsibility for patient and family education varies with the institution. Patient education may be coordinated by the case manager, clinical nurse specialist, or perinatal educator; however, in any practice model, the perinatal staff nurse plays a key role. Critical concepts and essential information that families need have been identified. They are presented regardless of the family's past experience or self-assessment. Critical concepts include the following:

Maternal care
- Activity and rest
- Pain relief and comfort measures
- Care of the perineum and care of lacerations or episiotomy
- Breast care for breastfeeding women and lactation suppression for women who are formula feeding
- Postbirth instructions
- Expected emotional adaptations

- Signs of urgent and emergency postpartum complications to report to the nurse in the hospital or to the healthcare provider after discharge
- Importance of and scheduled postpartum follow-up visit

Newborn care

- Newborn adaptation to extrauterine life: need to be held, need for thermoregulation, need for comfort
- Newborn feeding cues
- Breastfeeding basics
- Formula feeding basics
- Care of an infant who is spitting up or choking
- Use of the bulb syringe
- Umbilical cord care
- Circumcision care and care of the uncircumcised penis
- Position for sleep: Safe to Sleep campaign to reduce the risk of sudden infant death syndrome
- Information about immunizations and newborn screening tests
- Signs of newborn complications to report to the nurse in the hospital or to the healthcare provider after discharge and contact telephone numbers
- Safe use of infant and child car seats
- Appointment made for follow-up clinic or home visit offered by the hospital or community nursing agency

Written materials provided to the woman and her family should contain information about all critical concepts related to her self-care as well as care of the infant. Some institutions use interactive documentation forms signed by the mother and the nurse providing the education. Before discharge, knowledge and skills about self-care and infant care are validated. Validation can be accomplished by discussion with the new mother during which understanding is verbalized or by demonstration of critical skills such as feeding, sleeping position, or umbilical cord care. No one method of validation is superior; rather, nurses in each institution can develop a system with enough flexibility to meet the needs of the population served. Validation ensures that women who indicate they need no additional information are, in reality, prepared and knowledgeable. The goal is for all women to verbalize understanding or demonstrate skills related to all critical concepts. Women with special needs, who have not demonstrated knowledge of critical concepts or have not acquired the skills to care for themselves or their infants, are referred for follow-up support and care. Referrals are made to the clinical nurse specialist, lactation consultant, social worker, dietitian, and/or home care agency. Follow-up contacts to ensure that the critical concepts have been learned and to verify the woman can safely care for her infant and herself can occur at a clinic or home visit, during a phone assessment, through involvement in support groups and community programs, or at healthcare provider office visits. Assessment of maternal knowledge and skills is documented on the discharge teaching record or other appropriate medical record form.

ANATOMIC AND PHYSIOLOGIC CHANGES DURING THE POSTPARTUM PERIOD

Perinatal nurses should have knowledge of normal anatomical and physiologic changes that occur during the postpartum period in order to perform comprehensive assessments, plan comprehensive care, and carry out appropriate interventions for new mothers. The postpartum period does not end at the 6-week checkup but extends over the first year postbirth.

Uterus

Involution results from a decrease in myometrial cell size not in the number of myometrial cells. This decrease is the result of ischemia, autolysis, and phagocytosis. Ischemia occurs when the retraction of uterine musculature necessary for hemostasis after placental separation results in decreased blood flow to the uterus. Proteolytic enzymes are released, and macrophages migrate to the uterus, resulting in autolysis or self-digestion and subsequent reduction in myometrial cell size. Within 24 hours of giving birth, the uterus is approximately the size it was at 20 weeks' gestation (Cunningham et al., 2018). Immediately after birth, the uterus weighs approximately 1,000 g. As involution occurs, the uterine weight continues to decrease to 500 g (1 week); 300 g (2 weeks); and by 6 weeks postpartum, it weighs 100 g or less. Immediately after birth, the uterine fundus can be palpated midway between the umbilicus and symphysis pubis. During the first 12 hours after birth, the muscles relax slightly, and the fundus returns to the level of the umbilicus. Beginning on postpartum day 2 or 3, the usual progression of uterine descent into the pelvis is 1 cm/day (Display 17–2).

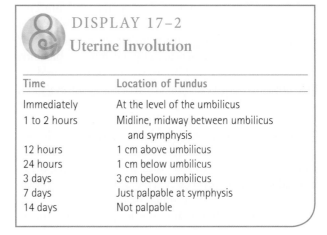

DISPLAY 17–2

Uterine Involution

Time	Location of Fundus
Immediately	At the level of the umbilicus
1 to 2 hours	Midline, midway between umbilicus and symphysis
12 hours	1 cm above umbilicus
24 hours	1 cm below umbilicus
3 days	3 cm below umbilicus
7 days	Just palpable at symphysis
14 days	Not palpable

TABLE 17–1. Types of Lochia

	Rubra	Serosa	Alba
Normal color	Red	Pink, brown tinged	Yellowish-white
Normal duration	1 to 3 days	3 to 10 days	10 to 14 days, but not abnormal to last longer
Normal discharge	Bloody with clots; fleshing odor; increased flow on standing or breast-feeding, or during physical activity	Serosanguineous (blood and mucus) consistency; fleshy odor	Mostly mucus, no strong odor
Abnormal discharge	Foul smell; numerous and/or large clots; quickly saturates perineal pad	Foul smell; quickly saturates perineal pad	Foul smell; saturates perineal pad; reappearance of pink or red lochia; discharge lasts far too long (past 4 weeks)

During the first few days after birth, oxytocin secretion from the posterior pituitary gland causes strong uterine contractions and a further reduction in size, especially after breastfeeding and in multiparas. Multiparity, multiple gestation, polyhydramnios, and bladder distention can influence uterine size and the progression of uterine involution.

Placental Site and Lochia

The placenta separates spontaneously from the uterus within 15 minutes of birth in 90% of women and within 30 minutes after birth in 95% of women. Separation of the placenta and membranes includes the spongy layer of the endometrium, leaving the decidua basalis in the uterus. This remaining layer reorganizes into basal and superficial layers. The superficial layer becomes necrotic and is sloughed in the lochia, and the basal layer becomes the source of new endometrium. The endometrium is regenerated by 2 to 3 weeks after birth, except at the site of placental attachment (Blackburn, 2017; Cunningham et al., 2018). Immediately after delivery of the placenta, the placental site is approximately 8 to 10 cm, and by end of the second week, it is about 3 to 4 cm. Exfoliation, the process of placental site healing, occurs over the first 6 weeks after birth by necrotic sloughing of the infarcted superficial tissues. A reparative process follows in which the endometrium regenerates from the margins and base. This process prevents the formation of a fibrous scar in the decidua. At 7 to 14 days postpartum, the infarcted superficial tissue over the placental site sloughs. At this time, the woman may notice an episode of increased vaginal bleeding, which is usually self-limited. Bleeding lasting more than 1 to 2 hours should be evaluated for late postpartum hemorrhage. Ultrasonography can be useful in determining the presence of retained placental tissue (Thorpe & Laughon, 2014).

Lochia is the postpartum uterine discharge. Although lochia varies in amount, the total volume lost usually is 150 to 400 mL. Initially, lochia rubra is reddish and continues 3 to 4 days. Lochia serosa, a pinkish discharge, continues from day 4 to day 10. Lochia alba, a yellow-white discharge, follows lochia serosa (Table 17–1). There is a slight musty odor to lochia; however, it should not be foul smelling. The choice of feeding method for the baby and the use of oral contraceptives do not affect duration of lochia (Cunningham et al., 2018).

Cervix, Vagina, and Pelvic Floor

The cervix and lower uterine segment are thin and flaccid immediately postpartum. Cervical lacerations can occur during any birth; however, women with precipitous labor and operative procedures are at increased risk for lacerations. At 2 to 3 days, the cervix has resumed its customary appearance but remains dilated 2 to 3 cm. By the end of the first week, the cervical os narrows to a diameter of 1 cm. The external cervical os remains wider than its pregravid state, and bilateral depressions are typically seen at the site of lacerations. Cervical edema may persist for several months (Cunningham et al., 2018). The vagina and vaginal outlet are smooth walled and may appear bruised early in the puerperium. The apparent bruising, caused by pelvic congestion, disappears quickly after birth. Rugae reappear in the distended vagina by the third week. The voluntary muscles and supports of the pelvic floor gradually regain tone during the first 6 weeks postpartum. These changes occur in response to the reduced amount of circulating progesterone. For some women, vaginal tone may be improved by perineal tightening exercises, such as Kegel exercises (Ladewig et al., 2017). In the lactating woman, the hypoestrogenic state resulting from ovarian suppression may cause the vagina to appear pale and without rugae. This may result in dyspareunia.

Ovarian Function and Return of Menses

Although the return of menses and ovulation vary, the first menstrual period usually occurs within 7 to 9 weeks postpartum in nonnursing mothers. There are great variations in the return of menses for women who are nursing because of depressed estrogen levels. In nursing mothers, menstruation usually returns between months 2 and 18.

Estrogen and progesterone levels decrease suddenly after placental delivery. For the first 2 to 3 weeks after birth, there is minimal gonadotropin activity, possibly because of a transient pituitary insensitivity to luteinizing hormone–releasing factor. As sensitivity returns, hormonal function returns to normal levels. The first menstrual cycle is usually anovulatory, but 25% of women may ovulate before menstruation. The mean for the return of ovulation is 10 weeks postpartum for women who are not lactating and approximately 17 weeks postpartum for women who are breastfeeding. The delay in the resumption of menses in lactating women in part may result from elevated prolactin levels (Cunningham et al., 2018).

Metabolic Changes

Prolactin, a pituitary hormone, is responsible for stimulating and sustaining lactation. Like estrogen and progesterone, prolactin levels decrease with placental delivery, although they remain elevated over nonpregnant levels. The decrease in estrogen and progesterone stimulates the anterior pituitary to produce prolactin. Between the third and fourth week postpartum, the prolactin level returns to normal in women who formula-feed their infants. For those who breast-feed, prolactin levels increase with each nursing episode (Cunningham et al., 2018).

Thyroid function returns to prepregnant levels within 4 to 6 weeks after birth. Because immunosuppression is a normal physiologic consequence of pregnancy, there is an increased risk of developing transient autoimmune thyroiditis, followed by hypothyroidism. This depression of thyroid function may cause depression, carelessness, and impairment of memory and concentration. There is a slightly increased risk of recurrence of autoimmune hypothyroidism or hyperthyroidism postpartum (Cunningham et al., 2018; Nader, 2014).

Low levels of placental lactogen, estrogen, cortisol, growth hormone, and the placental enzyme insulinase reduce their anti-insulin effect in the early puerperium. This results in lower glucose levels for women during this period and a reduction in insulin requirements for insulin-dependent diabetic women (Cunningham et al., 2018). Breastfeeding may precipitate hypoglycemic episodes in women with insulin-dependent diabetes. Women with gestational diabetes often have normal glucose levels immediately postpartum. Nutritional needs must be reassessed during this period. The basal metabolic rate (BMR) increases 20% to 25% during pregnancy because of fetal metabolic activity. The BMR remains elevated for 7 to 14 days after giving birth.

During the first 2 hours postpartum, plasma renin and angiotensin II levels (involved in blood pressure maintenance) fall to normal, nonpregnant levels and then rise again and remain elevated for up to 14 days (Markham & Funai, 2014). Blood pressure should remain stable during the postpartum period but lowered vascular resistance in the pelvis may result in orthostatic hypotension when a woman moves from a supine to a sitting position. An increase in blood pressure, especially if accompanied by headaches or visual changes, may indicate postpartum preeclampsia and should be evaluated.

Kidneys and Bladder

Mild proteinuria (1+) may exist for 1 to 2 days after birth in 40% to 50% of women. Nonpathology can be assumed only in the absence of the symptoms of infection or preeclampsia (Blackburn, 2017). If one of these diagnoses is suspected, a urine specimen should be obtained through catheterization or as a clean-catch technique. These methods avoid contamination by protein-laden lochia. Glycosuria of pregnancy disappears, and creatinine clearance is usually normal by 1 week postpartum. Pregnancy-induced hypotonia and dilation of the ureters and renal pelves return to the prepregnant state by 8 weeks postpartum. The catabolic process of involution causes an increase of the blood urea nitrogen (BUN). By the end of the first week postpartum, the BUN level rises to values of 20 mg/dL, compared with 15 mg/dL in the late third trimester (Cunningham et al., 2018). Glomerular filtration rate, renal blood flow, and plasma creatinine return to normal levels by 6 weeks postpartum.

Labor may result in displacement of the urinary bladder and stretching of the urethra. Other factors that interfere with normal micturition include the numbing effect of anesthesia and the temporary neural dysfunction of the traumatized bladder. These may cause decreased sensitivity. As a result, overdistention and incomplete emptying may occur. Signs of bladder distention include uterine atony reflected in increased lochia, displacement of the uterus to the right and significantly above the umbilicus, decreased urine output compared with oral and intravenous intake, and a "soft fullness" sometimes with a palpable margin in the suprapubic area. Normal postpartum diuresis combined with the often large amount of intravenous fluids administered during labor can result in bladder filling in a relatively short time. The woman should be encouraged to void as soon as possible after birth to avoid bladder filling, which can inhibit uterine contraction, thus predisposing the woman to postpartum hemorrhage. Assistance to the bathroom or on a bedpan may be helpful in facilitating bladder emptying. Women may report an urge but inability to urinate. Spontaneous voiding, however, should resume by 6 to 8 hours after birth, and bladder tone usually returns to normal levels 5 to 7 days later. Each voiding should be at least 150 mL. Edema, hyperemia, and submucous extravasation of blood are frequently evident in the bladder postpartum (Cunningham et al., 2018). The effects of trauma from labor on the bladder and urethra diminish during the first 24 hours, unless a urinary tract infection (UTI) is present. Some women may require in-and-out catheterization to empty their bladder in the immediate postpartum period. There is no maximum amount of urine that should be removed by catheterization at one time; however, it is important that the woman be assessed on an individual basis during the procedure.

Stress Incontinence

Impairment of muscle function near and surrounding the urethra underlies stress incontinence. Prompt catheterization for urinary retention during the postpartum can prevent urinary difficulties (Cunningham et al., 2018). Many women report transient stress incontinence during the first 6 weeks postpartum. There are conflicting data on the effect of vaginal birth on future urinary status. A meta-analysis of 16 studies suggested that vaginal delivery is associated with almost double the odds of long-term stress urinary incontinence, an absolute increase of approximately 8% when compared with cesarean section. The effect is largest in younger women but diminishes with age (Tähtinen et al., 2016). Other researchers have suggested that pregnancy itself may be a predisposing factor for urinary incontinence and pelvic organ prolapse, thus cesarean birth may not be protective against these conditions but this benefit, if true, has not been quantified (Tähtinen et al., 2016). The risks for the mother and infant must also be considered. Persistent stress incontinence may result from pregnancy, labor, operative birth, giving birth to a large baby, and perineal tissue damage. The influences of obstetric factors diminish over 3 months. The length of the second stage of labor, infant head size, birth weight, and episiotomy can correlate with the development of postpartum stress incontinence and levator ani injury (Hoyte, Wyman, & Hahn, 2015). Schaffer et al. (2005) suggest that the pelvic floor is exposed to compression and extreme pressures during vaginal delivery and maternal expulsive efforts. Uncoached (non-Valsalva) pushing, a response to the urge to push, is characterized by several short bearing-down efforts per contraction with breath holding for 6 to 8 seconds. In contrast, coached pushing begins as soon as a contraction is noted by the coach, and the mother is urged to push for 10 seconds, take a deep breath, and push again, repeating this cycle for the duration of the contraction. Coached pushing may potentially increase the pressure on the pelvic floor with subsequent deleterious effects. See Chapter 14 for a comprehensive discussion of second-stage pushing techniques that can minimize risk of injuries to the perineum and pelvic floor. Knowledge about clinical factors implicated in stress incontinence allows anticipatory guidance and interventions for women at risk.

Fluid Balance and Electrolytes

The physiologic reversal of the extracellular or interstitial fluid accumulated during a normal pregnancy begins during the immediate postpartum period. Diuresis begins within 12 hours after birth and continues up to 5 days. Diuresis occurs in response to the decrease in estrogen that stimulated fluid retention during pregnancy, the reduction of venous pressure in the lower half of the body, and the decrease in residual hypervolemia (Cunningham et al., 2018). Urine output may be 3,000 mL or more each day. Additional fluid is lost through increased perspiration. Diuresis results in a decrease in body weight of 2 to 3 kg. Electrolyte levels return to nonpregnant homeostasis by 21 days or earlier. Fluid loss is greater in women who have experienced preeclampsia or eclampsia. By the third postpartum day, resolution of the vasoconstriction and additional extracellular fluid of gestational hypertension contribute to significant expansion of the vascular volume (Cunningham et al., 2018).

Neurologic Changes

Discomfort and fatigue are common concerns after birth. Afterpains or painful uterine contractions during the first 2 to 3 days after birth; discomfort associated with episiotomy, incisions, lacerations, or tears; muscle aches; and breast engorgement may contribute to a woman's discomfort during the postpartum period. Neurologic changes related to anesthesia and analgesia are transient and, if present, require attention to ensure the woman's safety. Deep tendon reflexes remain normal. Sleep disturbances contributing to fatigue are related to discomfort and the demands of newborn care. The presence of children or a lack of social support may limit the time available for rest. Natural or pharmacologic comfort measures should be offered. Psychosocial support is necessary, and referral to home-care nursing may be appropriate.

Some women may develop carpal tunnel syndrome while pregnant resulting from compression of the median nerve by the physiologic edema of pregnancy. This syndrome will be relieved by postpartum diuresis. Headaches may result from fluid shifts in the first week after birth, leakage of cerebrospinal fluid into the extradural space during spinal anesthesia, fluid and electrolyte imbalance, hypertensive disorders, and/or stress. A thorough assessment of the timing, quality, and location of the headache is necessary. Interventions such as environmental control of lighting, noise levels, and visitors and administration of analgesic medications may be effective for nonpathologic headaches. Postpartum preeclampsia should be ruled especially because a headache is often one of the first signs that a woman complains of. Women can develop preeclampsia or eclampsia in the postpartum period without having a prenatal diagnosis of hypertensive disorders. Because women may experience prodromal signs and symptoms after discharge from the hospital, information should be provided about these subjective signs and symptoms, which include a severe and persistent headache, scotomata (i.e., spots before the eyes), blurred vision, photophobia, and epigastric or right upper-quadrant pain. Women should be encouraged to notify their primary healthcare provider if any of these symptoms develop to facilitate immediate evaluation.

Hemodynamic Changes

Changes in the cardiovascular system occur early in the postpartum period, with a variable rate of return to baseline levels that ranges from 6 to 12 weeks. Blood volume changes occur rapidly. Autotransfusion occurs as a result of elimination of blood flow to the placenta. The blood flow of 500 to 750 mL/min, formerly flowing to the uteroplacental unit, is diverted to maternal systemic venous circulation immediately after birth. Women usually lose less than 500 mL of blood during a vaginal birth and 1,000 mL following a cesarean birth (March of Dimes, 2018). Plasma volume is diminished by approximately 1,000 mL as a result of blood loss and diuresis. By the third day postpartum, blood volume has decreased 16% from peak pregnancy levels and returns to nearly prepregnant levels by 1 to 2 weeks postpartum.

Cardiac output after birth depends on use and choice of anesthesia or analgesia, mode of birth, blood loss, and maternal position. Cardiac output peaks immediately after birth to approximately 80% above the pre-labor value in women who have received only local anesthesia. After reaching a maximum value at 10 to 15 minutes after birth, cardiac output begins to decline, reaching pre-labor values approximately 1 hour postpartum, although it remains elevated for 48 hours after birth (Blackburn, 2017). It returns to prepregnant levels by 2 to 3 weeks after birth. Because the heart rate is stable or slightly decreased, the cardiac output is most likely caused by an increased stroke volume from venous return. Cesarean birth before labor onset avoids the hemodynamic effect of contractions but not the rise in cardiac output immediately postpartum. It is thought that epidural anesthesia during labor moderates the increase in cardiac output after birth by decreasing pain and anxiety (Cunningham et al., 2018).

The pulse rate remains stable or decreases slightly after birth. If the pulse rate is above 100 beats per minute (bpm), the woman should be assessed for potential complications such as infection or delayed postpartum hemorrhage. Some women may exhibit puerperal bradycardia, with a pulse rate of 40 to 50 bpm. No conclusive proof has been given for this phenomenon. Orthostatic hypotension may occur when a woman sits up from a reclining position. During the postpartum period, blood pressure remains within the woman's normal range. Any elevation in blood pressure requires additional assessment. Preeclampsia should be suspected if blood pressure values are 140/90 mm Hg on two or more occasions at least 6 hours apart or begin to trend upward.

Hematologic and Liver Changes

The decrease in plasma volume is greater than the loss of red blood cells after birth, causing an increase in the hematocrit between day 3 and day 7. The hematocrit returns to normal levels 4 to 8 weeks later as red blood cells reach the end of their normal life span (Cunningham et al., 2018; Kilpatrick, 2014; Monga & Matrobattista, 2014). In assessing postpartum laboratory values, a 1 to 1.5 g decrease in hemoglobin levels or 2 to 3-point decrease in the hematocrit value reflects a 500 mL blood loss. During the first 48 hours after birth, the physiologic reversal of the extracellular fluid accumulated during a normal pregnancy and intravenous fluids given during labor makes accurate blood loss assessment difficult because hemodilution occurs as this fluid enters the vascular system. This phenomenon is seen even in women who have lost 20% of their circulating blood volume during birth. Hemoconcentration may occur with minimal blood loss if a woman has preexisting polycythemia (Cunningham et al., 2018; Monga & Matrobattista, 2014).

Normal serum iron levels are regained by the second week postpartum. A relative erythrocytosis is seen in women who have received iron supplementation during pregnancy and had an average blood loss during the birth process. In the absence of iron supplementation, iron deficiency develops in most women (Cunningham et al., 2018; Stotland, Boonar, & Abrams, 2014). The serum ferritin level correlates closely with the body's iron stores and is predictive of iron deficiency anemia (Cunningham et al., 2018; Stotland et al., 2014). Changes in blood coagulation factors remain for variable periods postpartum. Plasma fibrinogen levels and sedimentation rate levels remain elevated for at least the first week.

Leukocytosis from the stress of labor and birth is seen in the postpartum period. A nonpathologic white blood cell (WBC) count may reach 25,000 to 30,000/μL, with the increase predominantly granulocytes. Relative lymphopenia (i.e., lymphocyte deficiency) and absolute eosinopenia (i.e., decreased eosinophils) may also be seen. This phenomenon, coupled with the increase in the sedimentation rate, may confuse the interpretation or assessment of infections during this period. Pathology should be suspected, and further evaluation is indicated when the WBCs increase 30% over a 6-hour period (Cunningham et al., 2018; Kilpatrick, 2014).

The alterations in liver enzymes and lipids that occurred in response to increased estrogen levels and hemodilution during pregnancy are reversed and returned to normal levels within 3 weeks postpartum. Elevated levels of free fatty acids, cholesterol, triglycerides, and lipoproteins seen during pregnancy return to normal levels within 10 days. Alkaline phosphatase, derived from the placenta, liver, and bone during pregnancy, may remain elevated for 6 weeks. The previously atonic gallbladder demonstrates increased contractility as progesterone levels decrease (Cunningham et al., 2018; Williamson, Mackillop, & Heneghan, 2014).

Respiratory and Acid–Base Changes

The respiratory system quickly returns to its prepregnant state after the birth of the baby. These changes result from the decrease in progesterone levels, the decrease in intraabdominal pressure that accompanies emptying of the uterus, and the increased excursion of the diaphragm. This reduction of diaphragmatic pressure results in the immediate return of chest wall compliance to normal levels and partially relieves the dyspnea experienced during pregnancy. Residual volume (i.e., amount of air remaining in the lung after maximum expiration) and tidal volume (i.e., volume of air inhaled and exhaled during each breath) normalize soon after birth; the expiratory reserve volume (i.e., maximum amount of air that can be exhaled), however, may remain in the abnormal range for several months. Vital capacity, inspiratory capacity, and maximum breathing capacity decrease after birth. The response to exercise may therefore be affected in the early postpartum weeks (Cunningham et al., 2018; Whitty & Dombrowski, 2014).

Length and severity of the second stage of labor appear to contribute to an "oxygen debt" (i.e., extra oxygen required after strenuous exercise) that extends into the immediate postpartum period (Cunningham et al., 2018; Whitty & Dombrowski, 2014). The BMR remains elevated for 7 to 14 days into the postpartum period and is attributable to mild anemia, lactation, and psychological factors.

As progesterone levels fall, the P_aCO_2 rises to the normal prepregnant values (35 to 40 mm Hg) within the first 2 days after birth. During the postpartum period, the P_aO_2 should be normal at 95% or higher. Normal levels of pH and base excess gradually return by approximately 3 weeks postpartum.

Skin, Muscle, and Weight Changes

Overdistention of the abdominal wall as a result of pregnancy can rupture collagen fibers of the dermis, resulting in striae, which can occur also on the breasts, buttocks, and thighs. Striae eventually become irregular white lines. Diastasis (i.e., separation) of the rectus muscles is common and usually is reapproximated by the late postpartum period. Evidence of diastasis can be assessed by asking the woman to lift her head while lying in a supine position. If diastasis has occurred, a tentlike protrusion in the lower abdomen is noticeable. Abdominal binders are not recommended; however, mild exercise to restore tone may be started after 1 to 2 weeks. The joint instability that occurred during pregnancy may not resolve until 6 to 8 weeks postpartum.

A woman loses an average of 12 lb (5.5 kg) at birth. Additional weight is lost between 2 weeks and 6 months postpartum, especially if the woman is breastfeeding (Cunningham et al., 2018). Women who choose formula feeding can expect a 0.5 to 1 kg/week loss when eating a balanced diet containing slightly fewer calories than their usual daily expenditure. Weight loss occurs more rapidly in women of lower parity, age, and prepregnancy weight.

Gastrointestinal Changes

After birth, there is a decrease in gastrointestinal muscle tone and motility. When these changes are coupled with relaxation of abdominal muscles, gaseous distention can occur during the first 2 to 3 days postpartum. Decreased motility can result in postpartum ileus. Constipation may result from hemorrhoids, perineal trauma, dehydration, pain, fear of having a bowel movement, immobility, and medication (i.e., magnesium sulfate antenatally for tocolysis, iron supplementation, codeine for pain, and anesthetics during labor or surgery). Constipation can be minimized by encouraging the woman to drink adequate fluids and eat foods high in fiber. Hemorrhoids that develop during pregnancy may increase in size during labor and result in significant discomfort during the postpartum period. If the woman has hemorrhoids, suggesting warm or cold sitz baths and applying topical anesthetics can decrease discomfort. Stool softeners and laxatives are sometimes given. Bowel movements typically resume 2 to 3 days after birth, and normal bowel elimination patterns resume by 2 weeks postpartum.

Hernias and Perineal, Pelvic Floor, and Anal Sphincter Damage

The prevalence of urinary incontinence among women, regardless of type of delivery, ranges from 2.8% to 30.8% (Tähtinen et al., 2016). Approximately one-fifth to one-third of U.S. women have symptoms of urinary incontinence or pelvic organ prolapse (Tähtinen et al., 2016). Genital hernias (i.e., cystocele, rectocele, uterine prolapse, enterocele) may occur because of overstretching or tearing of the muscles or fascia during birth. Meta-analysis suggests that digital perineal massage from 34 weeks and more of gestation was associated with a modest reduction in perineal trauma requiring repair with suture and decreased episiotomy in women with no previous vaginal birth (ACOG, 2016b). Controversy exists regarding the use of episiotomy. Some practitioners suggest using mediolateral episiotomy when the risk for extension is increased (i.e., macrosomia, shallow perineal body, operative vaginal birth), but there is little supportive evidence for that practice (Hoyte et al., 2015). Episiotomy does not always prevent third- or fourth-degree lacerations. Risk factors for lacerations include nulliparity, increased gestational age, second-stage labor arrest, macrosomia, persistent occiput posterior positions, episiotomy, forceps assistance, and use of vacuum extractors. Routine episiotomy is not recommended by ACOG (2016b; see Chapter 14 more details on episiotomy).

Obstetric trauma such as injury to the sphincter muscle or damage to the innervation of the pelvic floor is a leading cause of anal incontinence in healthy women (ACOG, 2016b). Other associations with anal incontinence include prolonged second-stage labor, macrosomia, labor augmentation, and episiotomy. One-half of women with third-degree tears experience anal incontinence. Disturbances in bowel function (i.e., fecal urgency and anal incontinence of stool and flatus) from mechanical or neurologic injury to the anal sphincter during vaginal birth may also be the result of damage from the large size of the baby's head in relation to the vaginal opening. Women who experience a third- or fourth-degree perineal laceration report a greater incidence of incontinence of flatus than those without anal sphincter rupture. Women with a history of anal sphincter injury have an increased risk of developing anal incontinence (ACOG, 2016b). Women with a long second-stage of labor, a large newborn, or both have the greatest risk of nerve damage (ACOG, 2016b; Cunningham et al., 2018). Warm compresses applied to the perineum during pushing reduces the incidence of third- and fourth-degree lacerations (ACOG, 2016b).

Parity is associated with an increased risk for urinary incontinence. Vaginal delivery increases the risk for urinary incontinence, but labor and pushing alone, without subsequent vaginal birth, do not appear to increase risk (Tähtinen et al., 2016). Pelvic floor exercises have shown to reduce urinary incontinence and increase pelvic floor strength and pregnant women should be encouraged to perform them during the antepartum period (Hoyte et al., 2015).

Embarrassment may prevent women from reporting symptoms of anal sphincter damage. The prevalence of fecal incontinence (FI) varies considerably depending on the studied population and the definition of FI with rates of 2.2% to 25% (Meyer & Richter, 2015). Symptoms may disappear or worsen with time. An accurate history is helpful so that women with major sphincter defects can be offered a cesarean birth when appropriate. Aging, menopause, progression of neuropathy, and effects of subsequent births may contribute

to long-term sphincter weakness. In addition, women report that anal incontinence results in negative emotional health and a decrease in their quality of life (Meyer & Richter, 2015).

Fluid and Nutritional Needs

After vaginal birth, there are no dietary restrictions for women without underlying medical conditions or pregnancy-induced complications. Oral fluids or intravenous fluid administration helps restore the balance altered by fluid loss during the labor and birth process. Women should be encouraged to drink approximately 2,000 mL of water and other liquids every 24 hours. Nurses should encourage healthy food choices with respect for ethnic and cultural preferences. Snack trays should be available for women who give birth when regular food service is unavailable. After cesarean birth, women usually receive clear liquids until bowel sounds are present and then advance to solid foods. For each 20 mL of breast milk produced, the woman must consume an additional 30 calories. This results in a dietary increase of 500 to 1,000 calories each day for women who are maintaining body weight (Lawrence & Lawrence, 2014). By 6 weeks postpartum, decreased pressure and distortion of the stomach from the gravid uterus and the normalization of lower esophageal sphincter pressure and tone resolves the heartburn experienced by many pregnant women.

NURSING ASSESSMENT AND CARE DURING POSTPARTUM

Immediate Postpartum Period

During the immediate postpartum period, the perinatal nurse focuses on maternal and newborn stabilization and recovery from the birth process. There should be a registered nurse in continuous attendance with the new mother and baby during the 2-hour recovery period. The nurse should have no other patient assignment beyond the mother–baby couplet (AWHONN, 2010). A separate nurse is needed for the baby at birth and during transition until the critical elements of care have been met. These critical elements during postpartum recovery before the mother's nurse accepts the baby as part of the care assignment have been defined by AWHONN (2010):

- Critical elements for the mother's care after vaginal birth before the mother's nurse accepts the baby as part of the patient care assignment are defined as: (a) initial assessment is completed and documented; (b) repair of episiotomy or perineal laceration(s) is completed; and (c) the woman is hemodynamically stable.
- Critical elements for the mother's post-anesthesia care after cesarean birth before the mother's nurse

accepts the baby as part of the patient care assignment are defined as: (a) report has been received from the anesthesia provider, questions answered, and the transfer of care has taken place; (b) woman is conscious, with adequate respiratory status; (c) initial assessment is completed and documented; (d) woman is hemodynamically stable.

• Critical elements for the baby's care before the mother's nurse accepts the baby as part of the patient care assignment are defined as: (a) report has been received from the baby nurse, questions answered, and the transfer of care has taken place; (b) initial assessment and care are completed and documented; (c) identification bracelets have been applied; and (d) baby's condition is stable.

These critical elements for both the mother and the baby should be completed by each nurse assigned to the mother and each nurse assigned to the baby before care can be transitioned to one nurse caring for the mother and baby simultaneously.

When mother and baby are stable and critical elements of care are met, one nurse can care for both the mother and the baby. Critical elements are usually accomplished within 30 to 45 minutes. Nurses who care for mothers and babies during recovery and those in leadership positions that determine nurse staffing should be aware of these definitions and use them to guide their care and assignment (Simpson, 2015).

Healthy mothers and babies should stay together as much as possible, based on their condition and the desires of the mother. Maternal–newborn attachment and breastfeeding (if the woman desires) should be promoted and encouraged (Figs. 17–1 and 17–2). Nursing assessments and interventions should occur concurrently with activities celebrating the joy of childbirth and welcoming the new baby into the family. Family and visitor interactions, including holding the new baby and taking video and still pictures of the first hours of life, should be supported as much as possible based on the condition of the mother and

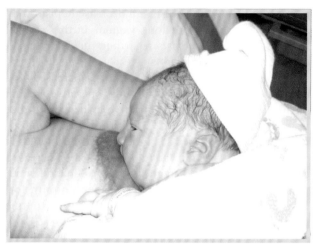
FIGURE 17–2. Promoting breastfeeding immediately after birth.

newborn. Every effort should be made to accommodate the wishes of the woman and her family.

If the baby is stable, immediate and sustained skin-to-skin contact (SSC) between the mother and the baby should be encouraged (AAP & ACOG, 2017; AWHONN, 2016). A blanket covering the baby up to the neck during SSC helps maintain warmth while allowing ongoing nursing assessment, including the baby's color and respiratory efforts (AAP, 2016). The baby's head should be turned to the side when not breastfeeding so the baby can breathe without obstruction and the nurse can make sure the baby's nose and mouth are easily assessed. Some mothers may not be fully awake or may fall asleep during recovery, so maternal status is a major factor in SSC (AAP, 2016). Breastfeeding should be initiated within 1 hour after birth for breastfeeding mothers. Some babies may lack ability to move their head to maintain normal breathing during SSC and attempts at breastfeeding processes, so all babies being held by their mothers during the 2-hour transition and recovery process require frequent assessment to assure safety. The mother and her support person(s) should be instructed about maintaining the baby's airway (AAP, 2016). Continued nursing bedside attendance during this 2-hour period is recommended since the nurse caring for the mother and baby (after the critical elements are met [AWHONN, 2010]) should have no other responsibilities.

When regional analgesia or anesthesia or general anesthesia has been used for vaginal or cesarean birth, the woman should be observed in an appropriately staffed and equipped labor–delivery–recovery room or post-anesthesia care unit until she has recovered from the anesthetic (AAP & ACOG, 2017; American Society of Anesthesiologists [ASA], 2016). The patient's desires for support persons to be with her during the post-anesthesia care period should be honored as much as possible. At a minimum, at least one support person should be encouraged and allowed (Fig. 17–3). The woman should be discharged from post-anesthesia

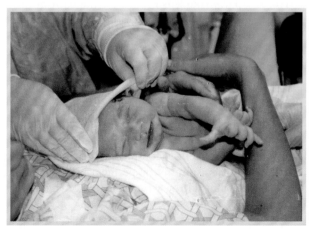
FIGURE 17–1. Promoting mother–baby attachment at birth.

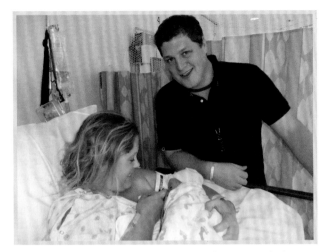

FIGURE 17–3. Support person with mother in the OB post-anesthesia care unit.

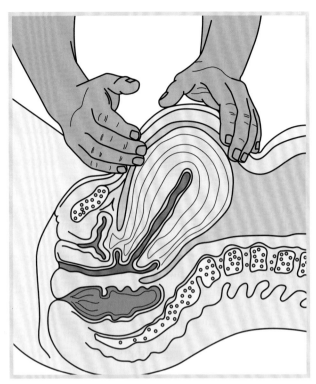

FIGURE 17–4. Fundal massage. The nurse uses two hands for fundal massage. One hand anchors the lower uterine segment just above the symphysis. The other gently massages the fundal area.

care only at the discretion of and after communication among the attending physician or a certified nurse midwife, anesthesiologist, and certified registered nurse anesthetist (AAP & ACOG, 2017; ASA, 2016). See Chapter 14 for an in-depth discussion of post-anesthesia care.

During the immediate postpartum period, maternal blood pressure and pulse should be monitored and recorded at least every 15 minutes for 2 hours or more often as indicated (AAP & ACOG, 2017). The newborn's temperature, heart rate, skin color, peripheral circulation, respiration, level of consciousness, tone, and activity should be monitored and recorded at least once every 30 minutes until the infant's condition has remained stable for 2 hours (AAP & ACOG, 2017).

Most institutions have protocols that include comprehensive maternal assessments after the first 2 hours of the immediate recovery period that are every 1 to 2 hours and then every 4 hours (or more frequently if complications are present) for 12 to 24 hours. If the mother is stable, some institutions defer the 4-hour assessments after the first 12 hours when the mother is sleeping. Assessment of maternal status every 8 to 12 hours in the second postpartum day and thereafter is common. There are no data from prospective clinical trials to determine how often maternal status should be assessed during the postpartum period to promote safety and optimal outcomes. Each institution should develop protocols that are reasonable and based on the condition of the mother and type of birth. The following clinical parameters are included in a comprehensive assessment during the immediate postpartum period:

- Assess blood pressure and pulse every 15 minutes for the first 2 hours (AAP & ACOG, 2017).
- Assess the uterine fundus for tone and position. Uterine massage is indicated if the uterus is not firmly contracted.

- Support the lower uterine segment during massage to prevent uterine prolapse or inversion (Fig. 17–4). Uterine inversion is an obstetric emergency associated with hemorrhage and shock.
- Assess the amount of lochia on perineal pad and under buttocks.
- Assess the condition of the perineum.
- Assess the condition of episiotomy after assisting the woman into lateral position with upper leg flexed; use the acronym REEDA (redness, edema, ecchymosis, discharge, approximation of edges of episiotomy) to guide assessment.
- Assess pain status.
- Assess the temperature hourly during the first 2 hours (AWHONN, 2019a), then at least every 4 hours for the first 8 hours after birth, and at least every 8 hours subsequently (AAP & ACOG, 2017).
- Decisions about post-anesthesia status and readiness for discharge from the recovery area are made at the discretion of the attending physician, nurse midwife, anesthesiologist, or certified registered nurse anesthetist (AAP & ACOG, 2017; ASA, 2016).

Ongoing Postpartum Care

According to the wishes and condition of the woman, she and the newborn should be kept together as much as possible during the inpatient stay. Most maternity units have models of care that support maternal–newborn attachment. Mother–baby or couplet care in which one nurse is responsible for both patients facilitates optimal interaction between the mother and baby and coordination of appropriate nursing assessments and interventions. If the mother is tired, in pain, medicated such that she cannot unable to safely care for her baby, or requests nursing care for the baby in the nursery, accommodations must be available for nursing care of the baby outside of the mother's room in the nursery (Simpson, 2017b). Nurse staffing for care of newborns should be flexible to adjust to these situations. The World Health Organization and United Nations Children's Fund (2018) have recently published updated *Baby-Friendly Hospital Initiative Guidance and 10 Steps to Successful Breastfeeding*. They recommend *enabling* mothers and babies to remain together and to practice rooming-in 24 hours a day. Baby-Friendly USA (2019) has not yet adopted the updated guidelines; however, their language about rooming-in is similar, *allow* mothers and babies to remain together 24 hours a day. Healthy mothers and babies should be enabled and encouraged (but not forced) to remain together as much as possible based on individual clinical situations. Partnering with women and their families to meet their needs and requests during the postpartum hospitalization is essential.

Guidelines for nurse staffing during the postpartum period as per AWHONN (2010) include the following:

- The nurse-to-patient ratio for normal healthy mother–baby couplets should be no more than 1 to 3. This means actual care assignments and responsible nurses, not averaged based on a charge nurse (or lactation consultant) without a patient assignment.
- Patient assignment should consider acuity and type of birth.
- Nurses caring for women receiving magnesium sulfate during the postpartum period should not have more than 1 other mother–baby couplet or one other patient (if not providing couplet care) as part of their patient care assignment because assessment of maternal status for women receiving magnesium sulfate is required at least hourly.
- For couplet care assignments, nurses should not have more than two women recovering from cesarean birth on the immediate postoperative day as part of the nurse to patient ratio of 1 nurse to 3 mother–baby couplets.
- For assignments that include only new mothers, nurses should not have more than 5 to 6 postpartum women without complications, with no more than 2 to 3 women on the immediate postoperative day who are recovering from cesarean birth, as part of the nurse-to-patient ratio of 1 nurse to 5 to 6 postpartum women without complications (when the babies are cared for by other nursing staff).
- For assignments that include only new mothers, nurses should not have more than three postpartum patients with complications who are stable (when the babies are cared for by other nursing staff).
- For assignments that include only babies, the ratio should not exceed 1 nurse physically present in the nursery to 5 to 6 newborns requiring routine care (when the mothers are cared for by other nursing staff).
- After cesarean birth, patients need assistance with newborn care, especially in the immediate recovery period. They should not be required to keep their babies in their rooms if they do not feel up to it and/or a support person is not available to stay with them. Until the new mother recovering from cesarean birth is no longer receiving pain relief via patient-controlled analgesia pumps or epidural catheters, babies should not be left alone in mothers' arms without nursing personnel or support people in attendance to reduce risk of a baby falling from the mother's arms and to reduce risk of a mother falling asleep with the baby in the bed. This recommendation also applies to mothers who have been given medication for sleep.
- Availability of lactation consultants 7 days a week is recommended to assist with complex breastfeeding issues. 1.9 full-time equivalent lactation consultants are recommended for every 1,000 births based on annual birth volume in level III perinatal centers; 1.6 full-time equivalent lactation consultants are recommended for every 1,000 births based on annual birth volume in level II perinatal centers, and 1.3 full-time equivalent lactation consultants are recommended for every 1,000 births based on annual birth volume in level I perinatal centers.
- One nurse to 1 baby newborn boy undergoing circumcision or other surgical procedures during the immediate preoperative, intraoperative, and immediate postoperative periods. The steps involved in the process of a surgical procedure require the presence of a nurse.

Guidelines on newborn safety for SSC between new mothers and their newborn babies, rooming-in, and supporting breastfeeding from AAP (2016) should be followed for newborn safety. Analyze skin-to-skin and rooming practices to make sure they are consistent with AAP (2016) guidelines. A key aspect of the AAP recommendations is frequent checking on the mother and baby during rooming-in.

- For high-risk women, AAP (2016) recommends every 30-minute rounding during nighttime and early morning hours.
- The advisory on safety and quality issues from The Joint Commission (2018) *Preventing Newborn Falls and Drops* recommends at least hourly rounding on mother–baby couplets and more often as needed based on individual clinical situations.

Opportunities for rest for the new mother should be promoted, although this may be challenging for the nurse because of the number of congratulatory telephone calls and visitors and because of the unit routines that interrupt sleep. Nursing care should be planned so that necessary interventions and medication administration (if needed) can be grouped together, minimizing the need to wake the woman during daytime naps or during the night. A plan for rest designed collaboratively with the new mother and her family works well. Ambulation as soon as the mother feels able should be encouraged, but the woman should be instructed not to get out of bed on her own without assistance the first time after birth (AAP & ACOG, 2017). In the absence of complications or surgical recovery, a regular diet should be resumed as soon as the woman desires. Education for the new mother and her family about maternal postpartum care and newborn care should focus on easing the transition from hospital to home.

Pain Management

Pain during the postpartum period may be caused by the episiotomy, lacerations, perineal trauma, incisions, uterine contractions after birth, hemorrhoids, breast engorgement, and nipple tenderness. Nursing assessments, such as fundal assessment, may also result in discomfort. Some strategies can reduce the level of discomfort. After cesarean birth, pain may be related to the incision and intestinal gas. Pain causes stress and interferes with the woman's ability to interact with and care for her infant. Evidence for the effectiveness of topically applied local anesthetics for treating perineal pain is not compelling (Rhodes, 2017). While manufactured ice packs may provide increased comfort, ice-filled gloves or zip locked bags are considerably less expensive. Petersen (2011) recommends that if a community ice machine is used to fill these, consideration should be given to conducting cultures to determine the presence of harmful bacteria.

The following interventions are included in a comprehensive assessment during the immediate postpartum period:

- Ask about type and severity of pain.
- Explain rationale for uterine massage and periodic assessments. Encourage slow, deep breathing during the assessment.
- Gentle palpation with warm hands can enhance comfort and encourage participation in the procedure.
- Apply ice pack to perineum during first 24 hours to reduce edema (some women may prefer an ice pack to the perineum intermittently after the first 24 hours). Ice packs are most beneficial when they are applied for 10- to 20-minute intervals rather than leaving them in place continually (Petersen, 2011).
- Apply moist heat (i.e., sitz bath) after 24 hours to increase circulation and promote healing.

- Administer analgesic medication as ordered.
- Women who have cesarean birth may or may not require uterine massage to stimulate uterine contraction. If the amount of lochia indicates excessive bleeding, combine palpation and pain management measures. If pain management is inadequate, additional pain medication, reassurance, and comfort measures may be helpful after necessary procedures.
- Abdominal binders may be offered to women after cesarean birth.
- Gas pains can be relieved by ambulation, rocking in a rocking chair, gum chewing, and avoiding gas-forming foods and carbonated beverages.

The opioid crisis in the United States has resulted in changes in how pain is treated and managed for all patients, including women during the postpartum period. Pain can interfere with a woman's ability to care for herself and her infant; however, caution is needed in prescribing opioids postpartum because 1 in 300 opioid-naive patients exposed to opioids after cesarean birth will become persistent users of opioids (ACOG, 2018b). Nonpharmacologic and pharmacologic therapies are important components of postpartum pain management. Recommendations from ACOG (2018b) include the following:

- Using a multimodal combination of agents
- Standard oral and parenteral analgesics should include acetaminophen, nonsteroidal anti-inflammatory drugs, opioids, and opioids in combination formulations with either acetaminophen or an nonsteroidal anti-inflammatory drug for women after cesarean birth.
- Reserving parenteral or oral opioids for treating breakthrough pain when analgesia from the combination of neuraxial opioids and nonopioid adjuncts is inadequate
- Shared decision making for postpartum discharge opioid prescription to allow for optimal pain control while reducing amount of unused opioid tablets
- If a codeine-containing medication is the selected choice for postpartum pain management, medication risks and benefits, including education on newborn signs of toxicity, should be shared with the family.
- Advise women who are prescribed opioid analgesics about risk of central nervous system depression in the woman and the breastfed infant. Duration of use of opiate prescriptions should be limited to the shortest reasonable time expected for treating acute pain.

Psychosocial Status

Ongoing assessment of the psychosocial status should be personalized during the postpartum period to promote the development of healthy mother–infant relationships and maternal confidence (AAP & ACOG, 2017).

The following interventions are included in a comprehensive assessment during the immediate postpartum period:

- Determine the level of emotional lability and level of social support.
- Identify actual and potential sources of support.
- Assess the fatigue level.
- Ascertain educational needs and the level of confidence.
- Assess the teaching needs based on interview and observation.
- Use interactions with mothers as potential teaching moments.
- Use assessment of the fundus as an opportunity to provide information about involution.
- During perineal care, explain cleansing the vulva from front to back to avoid contamination, changing the pad at least four times each day or after each voiding or bowel movement, and washing hands before and after changing pads.
- Use bathing of the newborn at mother's bedside as an opportunity to discuss basic techniques of newborn care such as feeding, clothing, holding, and safety.
- Assess the interaction with the newborn and attachment behaviors.
  - Note whether the mother looks directly at the infant and maintains eye contact (i.e., en face position).
  - Note whether the mother touches and talks to the infant.
  - Note whether the mother interprets the infant's behaviors positively.
- Provide an early opportunity to hold infant after birth and keep the infant with the parents as much as possible.
- Ensure flexibility in visiting policies and opportunities for privacy.
- Demonstrate acceptance of expression of maternal feelings and reinforce parenting behaviors.
- Be a role model for infant-care activities.
- Assist parents in interpreting infant cues.
- Offer appropriate educational materials (i.e., consider age, educational level, and resources).
- Identify risk factors for parenting (i.e., lack of economic or psychosocial resources) and assist in obtaining appropriate referrals and assistance.
- Conduct hourly rounding on mother–baby couplets (The Joint Commission, 2018) and every 30-minute rounding during nighttime and early morning hours for high-risk mother–baby couplets (AAP, 2016).

Physical Status

Physical assessment is an essential part of comprehensive nursing care during the postpartum period. Changes in the breasts, uterus, lochia, bladder, abdomen, perineum, legs, and feet should be assessed periodically and appropriate nursing interventions initiated as needed. The nurse should include all of the following assessments during the immediate postpartum period:

- Assess breasts for redness, pain, engorgement, and if nursing, correct latch-on and removal of the newborn from the breast.
- Assess the uterus and lochia as described previously.
- Note any foul-smelling lochia.
- Assess the bladder for fullness before and after voiding.
- Measure amount of the first void (repeat if an insufficient amount).
- Assess for burning and/or frequency on urination and flank tenderness.
- Assess the abdomen for muscle tone and check the incision site if applicable.
- Assess bowel sounds in all four quadrants.
- Assess the perineum, labia, and anus for edema, redness, pain, bruising, and hematoma.
- Assess the episiotomy or abdominal incision for approximation and drainage.
- Assess for the presence, size, and condition of hemorrhoids.
- Assess dietary intake and elimination patterns.
- Assess legs and feet for edema and varicosities.
- Assess for signs or symptoms of a deep vein thrombosis (DVT) such as swelling or pain/tenderness in the affected leg (usually in the calf area), red or discolored skin on the leg, or a feeling of warmth in the affected leg. Of note, the Homan's sign has not been found to be consistently predictive of the presence of deep vein thrombosis.
- Assess activity tolerance.
- Assess the comfort level and response to pain medication.
- Assess breath sounds if the woman has received magnesium sulfate, other tocolytics, or oxytocin; has been on bed rest; has an infection; or had a multiple birth (i.e., greater risk for pulmonary edema, especially if the patient received large amounts of intravenous therapy).
- Use the acronym BUBBLERS (*b*reasts, *u*terus, *b*ladder, *b*owel, *l*ochia, *e*pisiotomy or incision, emotional *r*esponse) to guide this assessment.

COMPLICATIONS DURING POSTPARTUM

Postpartum Hemorrhage

Postpartum hemorrhage is the leading cause of maternal mortality worldwide, followed by infections and hypertensive disorders (World Health Organization & United Nations Children's Fund, 2018). See Chapter 1 for a detailed discussion of maternal morbidity and mortality. *Healthy People 2020* includes an objective to reduce maternal illness and complications due to pregnancy during hospitalized labor and delivery (U.S. Department of Health and Human Services, 2018). The baseline of pregnant females who suffered complications during hospitalized labor and birth in 2007 was 31.1%. The target for 2020 is 28.0%. The physiologic changes that occur during pregnancy are in anticipation of natural blood loss at birth. These changes include a plasma volume increase of approximately 40% and a red cell mass increase of approximately 25% (ACOG, 2017). Uterine bleeding after birth is controlled by the contraction of the myometrium, which constricts blood vessels supplying the placenta, and local decidual hemostatic factors such as tissue factor, type-1 plasminogen activator inhibitor, and systemic coagulation from platelets and circulating clotting factors. Some women experience a greater than normal blood loss evolving into postpartum hemorrhage. The acute anemia resulting from postpartum hemorrhage interferes with oxygen delivery to tissue. Acute blood loss leads to tissue hypoxia with subsequent vasodilation of vascular beds in an attempt to bring more blood to the area. Tissue hypoxia then results in anaerobic metabolism and production of lactate with resultant lactic acidosis. The effects of hypovolemia are outlined in Figure 17–5.

Postpartum hemorrhage occurs in about 2% to 6% of women who have a vaginal birth (Cunningham et al., 2018). It can occur early (first 24 hours) or secondary (>24 hours and <6 weeks after birth). Early or primary postpartum hemorrhage is caused by uterine atony in 80% or more of cases (ACOG, 2017). Display 17–3 lists factors associated with postpartum

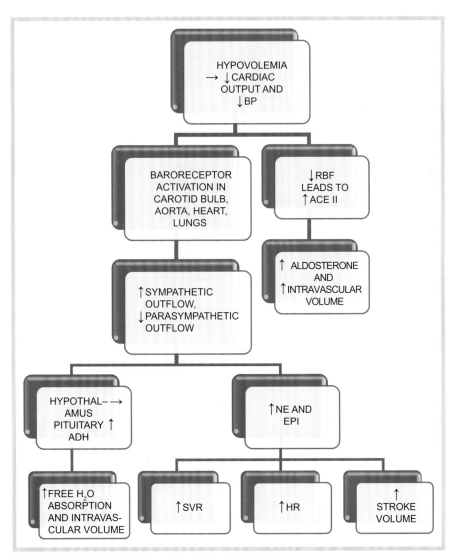

FIGURE 17–5. Physiology of blood loss. Note that changes in maternal vital signs are late signs of decompensation. ACE, angiotensin-converting enzyme; ADH, antidiuretic hormone; BP, blood pressure; EPI, epinephrine; HR, heart rate; H_2O, water; NE, norepinephrine; RBF, renal blood flow; SVR, systemic vascular resistance. (Used with permission of Mercy Hospital St. Louis, Perinatal Service, 2011.)

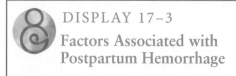

DISPLAY 17–3

Factors Associated with Postpartum Hemorrhage

Etiology

Early or primary postpartum hemorrhage

    Uterine atony (most common)

    Retained placenta

    Placenta accreta

    Defects in coagulation

    Uterine inversion

    Genital tract hematomas

Late or secondary postpartum hemorrhage

    Infection

    Subinvolution of placental site

    Retained placenta

    Inherited coagulation defects

Risk Factors

History of uterine atony or postpartum hemorrhage

Family history of postpartum hemorrhage in first-degree relatives (possible coagulopathy undiagnosed)

Trauma, lacerations, or hematoma of cervix and/or birth canal

Large uterine fibroids

Precipitous labor and birth

Prolonged labor

Induced or augmented labor

Chorioamnionitis

Difficult third stage (i.e., use of aggressive fundal manipulation or cord traction)

Operative vaginal birth (e.g., use of forceps or vacuum)

Cesarean birth

Uterine overdistention (e.g., large infant, multiple gestation, polyhydramnios)

Multiparity

Sepsis

Coagulopathies

Uterine rupture

Fetal demise

Low platelets (<100,000/mm^3)

Drugs (large dosages of oxytocin, magnesium sulfate, beta-adrenergic tocolytic agents; diazoxide [potent antihypertensive agent]; calcium channel blockers, such as nifedipine; and halothane [anesthetic agent])

---

hemorrhage etiology and clinical factors predisposing women to risk. Some hospitals have found use of a risk assessment tool for postpartum hemorrhage to be successful in reducing maternal morbidity and mortality related to postpartum hemorrhage (Lyndon, Lagrew, Shields, Main, & Cape, 2015). See Table 17–2 for a risk assessment tool (AWHONN, 2018). It is

important to consider that more than half of women who have postpartum hemorrhage due to uterine atony have no known risk factors (Bateman, Berman, Riley, & Leffert, 2010).

The term *postpartum hemorrhage* is a description of an event, not a diagnosis. Estimates of blood loss after birth are notoriously inaccurate with significant under-reporting most common (ACOG, 2017; Cunningham et al., 2018). Postpartum hemorrhage has traditionally been defined as blood loss of greater than 500 mL after vaginal birth and greater than 1,000 mL after a cesarean birth. However, these numbers reflect estimates and more likely represent average blood loss after vaginal and cesarean birth (Màin et al., 2015). Per ACOG (2014), postpartum hemorrhage is defined as cumulative blood loss of ≥1,000 mL *or* blood loss accompanied by signs and symptoms of hypovolemia within 24 hours following the birth process" (p. 1). Cumulative blood loss of 500 to 999 mL alone should trigger increased supervision and potential interventions as clinically indicated (ACOG, 2014). Signs and symptoms of maternal hypovolemia may include tachycardia, hypotension, tachypnea, low oxygen saturation (<95%), oliguria, pallor, dizziness, or altered mental status (ACOG, 2014). Excessive bleeding immediately postpartum can cause a number of symptoms beyond hypovolemia such as, pallor, light-headedness, weakness, palpitations, diaphoresis, restlessness, confusion, air hunger, syncope. Clinical signs and symptoms such as hypotension, dizziness, pallor, and oliguria do not occur until blood loss is substantial; approximately 10% or more of total blood volume (ACOG, 2017).

During birth, a normal, healthy woman tolerates blood loss equal to the volume of blood added during pregnancy without any significant decrease in the postpartum hematocrit. Hematocrit and hemoglobin levels are often used to estimate blood loss after birth; however, laboratory values may not always reflect current hematologic status, especially when blood is drawn soon after the event before equilibrium has occurred and large amounts of rapid volume expanders have been administered intravenously (ACOG, 2017). Within the clinical context of these limitations, blood loss is often estimated at 500 mL for every 3% drop in hematocrit values when comparing the admission hematocrit with the postpartum hematocrit (Cunningham et al., 2018). For example, a decrease in hematocrit from 38% on admission to 32% postpartum would represent an approximate blood loss of 1,000 mL. Hemoglobin values can be used similarly. The hemoglobin value can be assumed to decrease 1 to 1.5 g/dL for each 500 mL of blood loss (ACOG, 2017; Cunningham et al., 2018). Acute blood loss can be classified as mild, moderate, or severe (Table 17–3).

The greatest risk for early postpartum hemorrhage is during the first hour after birth because large venous

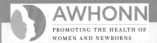

TABLE 17–2. Postpartum Hemorrhage Risk Assessment

CLINICIAN GUIDELINES:

- Each box ❑ represents ONE risk factor. Treat patients with 2 or more medium risk factors as high risk.
- Prenatal risk assessment is beyond the scope of this document, however performing a prenatal hemorrhage risk assessment and planning is highly recommended. Early identification and management preparation for patients with special considerations such as placental previa/accreta, bleeding disorder, or those who decline blood products will assist in better outcomes.

- Adjust blood bank orders based on the patient's most recent risk category. When a patient is identified to be at high risk for hemorrhage verify that the blood can be available on the unit within 30 minutes of a medical order.
- Plan appropriately for patient and facility factors that may affect how quickly the blood is delivered to the patient. For example,
  - Patient issues: Pre-existing red cell antibody
  - Facility issues: Any problems at your facility related to the blood supply and obtaining blood

	RISK CATEGORY: ADMISSION		
	Low risk	Medium risk (two or more medium-risk factors, advance patient to high-risk status)	High risk
	❑ No previous uterine incision	❑ Induction of labor (with oxytocin) or cervical ripening	❑ Has two or more medium risk factors
	❑ Singleton pregnancy	❑ Multiple gestation	❑ Active bleeding more than "bloody show"
	❑ ≤4 previous vaginal births	❑ >4 previous vaginal births	❑ Suspected placenta accreta or percreta
		❑ Prior cesarean birth or prior uterine incision	❑ Placenta previa, low lying placenta
	❑ No known bleeding disorder	❑ Large uterine fibroids	❑ Known coagulopathy
	❑ No history of PPH	❑ History of one previous PPH	❑ History of more than one previous PPH
		❑ Family history in first-degree relatives who experienced PPH (known or unknown etiology with possible coagulopathy)	❑ Hematocrit <30 *and* other risk factors
		❑ Chorioamnionitis	❑ Platelets <100,000/mm^3
		❑ Fetal demise	
		❑ Polyhydramnios	
	Anticipatory interventions: Monitor patient for a change in risk factors at admission and implement anticipatory interventions as indicated.		
❑ **Blood bank order:** Change blood bank orders as needed if risk category changes.	❑ Clot only (type and hold)	❑ Obtain type and screen.	❑ Obtain type and cross (see Clinical Guidelines).
		❑ Notify appropriate personnel such as the provider (physician/CNM), anesthesia, blood bank, charge nurse, clinical nurse specialist.	❑ Notify appropriate personnel such as the provider (physician/CNM), anesthesia, blood bank, charge nurse, clinical nurse specialist.
			❑ Consider delivering at a facility with the appropriate level of care capable of managing a high-risk mother.

(continued)

AWHONN PROMOTING THE HEALTH OF WOMEN AND NEWBORNS | TABLE 17–2. Postpartum Hemorrhage Risk Assessment *(Continued)*

		RISK CATEGORY: PREBIRTH	
		(Approximately 30 to 60 minutes prior to giving birth)	
	Low risk	Medium risk (two or more medium-risk factors, advance patient to high-risk status)	High risk
	INCLUDE ADMISSION LOW-RISK FACTORS.	INCLUDE ADMISSION MEDIUM-RISK FACTORS.	INCLUDE ADMISSION HIGH-RISK FACTORS.
		❑ Labor greater than 18 hours	❑ Has two or more medium risk factors
		❑ Temperature greater than 100.4°F (38°C)	❑ Active bleeding more than "bloody show"
		❑ Augmentation of labor (with oxytocin)	❑ Suspected abruption
		❑ Magnesium sulfate	
		❑ Prolonged second stage (>2 hours)	
		Anticipatory interventions:	
		Monitor patient for any change risk factors during labor and implement anticipatory interventions as indicated.	
❑ Blood bank order: Change blood bank orders as needed if risk category changes.	❑ Clot only (type and hold)	❑ Confirm type and screen	❑ Confirm type and cross (see Clinical Guidelines).
	❑ Ensures the availability of calibrated drapes, scales to weigh, and measure blood loss for every birth	❑ Review the hemorrhage protocol.	❑ Review the hemorrhage protocol.
		❑ Review lab work, for example, platelets (PLTs), hemoglobin (Hgb).	❑ Review lab work, for example, PLTs, Hgb.
		❑ Notify the provider and charge nurse.	❑ Notify the provider and charge nurse.
		❑ Initiate and/or maintain IV access.	❑ Insertion of a second large bore IV is optional.
		❑ Confirm availability of anesthesia provider.	❑ Notify anesthesia provider to come to the unit.
		❑ Ensure uterotonics (oxytocin, methylergonovine [Methergine], carboprost tromethamine [Hemabate], misoprostol) and supplies for administrations (such as syringes, needles, alcohol swabs) are immediately available.	❑ Check and ensure uterotonics (oxytocin, Methergine, Hemabate, misoprostol) and supplies for administration (such as syringes, needles, alcohol swabs) are immediately available.
		❑ Ensure that the hemorrhage supplies are near the patient's room.	❑ Bring the hemorrhage supplies to the bedside.
		❑ Transfer from a birthing center to an intrapartum unit.	❑ Ensure operating room (OR) and staff available.
		❑ Ensure the availability of calibrated drapes, scales to weigh, and measure blood loss with every birth.	❑ Ensure the availability of calibrated drapes, scales, and other equipment to measure and weigh blood loss with every birth.

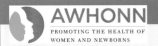

TABLE 17–2. Postpartum Hemorrhage Risk Assessment *(Continued)*

	RISK CATEGORY: POSTBIRTH (Within 60 minutes after birth)		
	Low risk	Medium risk (two or more medium-risk factors, advance patient to high-risk status)	High risk
	INCLUDE ADMISSION LOW-RISK FACTORS.	INCLUDE ADMISSION AND PREBIRTH MEDIUM-RISK FACTORS.	INCLUDE ADMISSION AND PREBIRTH HIGH-RISK FACTORS.
	❏ No known bleeding disorder	❏ Large uterine fibroids	❏ Has two or more medium-risk factors
	❏ No previous uterine incision	❏ Operative vaginal delivery	❏ Active bleeding
	❏ No history of PPH	❏ Third- or fourth-degree perineal laceration	❏ Difficult placental extraction
		❏ Vaginal or cervical laceration and/or mediolateral episiotomy	❏ Concealed abruption
		❏ Cesarean birth	❏ Uterine inversion
		❏ Precipitous delivery	
		❏ Shoulder dystocia	

Anticipatory interventions:			
Continue to monitor patient for any change in risk factors after birth and implement anticipatory interventions as indicated.			
❏ **Blood bank order:** Change blood bank orders as needed if risk category changes.	❏ **Clot only (type and hold)**	❏ **Confirm type and screen.**	❏ **Confirm type and cross (see Clinical Guidelines).** ❏ **Notify the blood bank.**
	❏ Utilize scales and calibrated equipment to weigh and measure maternal blood loss for every birth.	❏ Review your hemorrhage protocol.	❏ Review you hemorrhage protocol.
		❏ Notify the provider and the charge nurse.	❏ Notify the provider, charge nurse, and obtain additional nursing personnel.
		❏ Heightened postpartum assessment surveillance	❏ Heightened postpartum assessment surveillance
		❏ Utilize scales and calibrated equipment to quantify cumulative maternal blood loss for every birth.	❏ Utilize scales and calibrated equipment to quantify cumulative maternal blood loss for every birth.
		❏ Maintain IV access.	❏ Insertion of a second large bore IV is optional.
		❏ Confirm availability of anesthesia provider.	❏ Notify anesthesia provider to come to the unit.
		❏ Ensure immediate availability of uterotonics (oxytocin, methylergonovine [Methergine], carboprost tromethamine [Hemabate], misoprostol).	❏ Check and ensure immediate availability of uterotonics (oxytocin, Methergine, Hemabate, misoprostol,) and supplies for administration (such as syringes, needles, alcohol swabs).
		❏ Ensure the hemorrhage cart with supplies is near the patient's room.	❏ Bring hemorrhage cart with supplies to the bedside
		❏ Ensure OR and staff available.	❏ Consider notifying team to prepare the OR.
			❏ Consider notifying interventional radiology if available in facility.

IV, intravenous; CNM, certified nurse midwife; PPH, postpartum hemorrhage.
From Association of Women's Health, Obstetric and Neonatal Nurses. (2018). *Obstetric patient safety classroom course for postpartum hemorrhage* (pp. 225–227). Washington, DC: Author.

TABLE 17–3. Hemorrhage and Physical Findings				
	Mild	Moderate	Severe	
Volume	900 to 1,000 mL	1,200 to 1,500 mL 20% to 25% blood volume	2,000 mL 30% to 35% blood volume	>2,400 mL 40% blood volume
Vital signs	Class 1 Normal or ↑ diastolic BP	Class 2 Mild tachycardia Narrowed pulse pressure Orthostatic hypotension	Class 3 Tachycardia—120 ↓ BP/systolic 90 to 100 Tachypnea ↓ urine output	Class 4 Shock
Exam	Normal	Delayed capillary refill Anxiety	Restless Cool, pale skin	Oliguria Anuria

BP, blood pressure.

areas are exposed after placental separation. According to ASA (2016), the following resources should be available in the event of an obstetric hemorrhagic emergency: large-bore intravenous catheters; intravenous fluid warmer; forced-air body warmer; an available blood blank; and equipment for infusing intravenous fluids or blood products rapidly, such as hand-squeezed fluid chambers, hand-inflated pressure bags, and automatic infusion devices. The frontline treatment for the management of postpartum hemorrhage is uterotonic agents (oxytocin, methylergonovine, 15-methylprostaglandin F$_{2\alpha}$, dinoprostone, misoprostol) when atony is the cause of the bleeding (ACOG, 2017). If these medications fail, an exploratory laparotomy is the next step. Maintaining uterine contraction by using fundal massage (see Fig. 17–4) and intravenous oxytocin administration (20 U/L) reduces the incidence of hemorrhage from uterine atony (AAP & ACOG, 2017; ACOG, 2017; Cunningham et al., 2018; Thorpe & Laughon, 2014). Late or secondary postpartum hemorrhage occurs between 24 hours up to 6 weeks postpartum.

Preexisting risk factors for postpartum hemorrhage include the following:

- High parity
- Previous postpartum hemorrhage
- Previous uterine surgery
- Coagulation defects or medical disorders of clotting

Current pregnancy risk factors for postpartum hemorrhage include the following:

- Antepartal hemorrhage
- Uterine overdistention (macrosomia, multiple gestation, or polyhydramnios)
- Chorioamnionitis/intraamniotic infection
- Placental abnormality (succenturiate lobe, placenta previa, placenta accreta, abruptio placentae, hydatidiform mole)
- Fetal death

Risk factors for postpartum hemorrhage associated with labor and birth include the following:

- Rapid or prolonged labor
- Use of tocolytic or halogenated anesthetic agents
- Large episiotomy
- Operative vaginal birth
- Cesarean birth
- Abnormally located or attached placenta
- Inversion of uterus

When postpartum hemorrhage occurs, the perinatal team must work together to treat the underlying condition, manage the blood loss, and minimize the risk to the mother (Fig. 17–6). Timely identification and quick coordinated evidence-based actions are essential to minimize maternal morbidity and mortality.

The California Maternal Quality Care Collaborative (CMQCC) developed a toolkit to improve healthcare providers' response to maternal hemorrhage (Lyndon et al., 2015). Their recommendations include the following:

- Every hospital has a protocol outlining the steps for activation and response to maternal hemorrhage. Charge nurses triage and designate staff to respond to specific protocol steps, and all phone numbers of potentially needed personnel are included.
- Either physicians and nursing staff can activate an emergency maternal hemorrhage protocol.
- Develop a collaborative policy/procedure with the blood bank for issue of a specified "OB Emergency Hemorrhage Pack" that includes red blood cells, fresh frozen plasma (FFP), cryoprecipitate, and platelets.
- Identify a local expert with experience in hemorrhage and disseminated intravascular coagulation treatment for contact as needed.
- Post medicine doses and suture techniques in labor and delivery and operating room suites for reference.
- Perform scheduled hemorrhage protocol drills and assessments for both physicians and registered nurses.

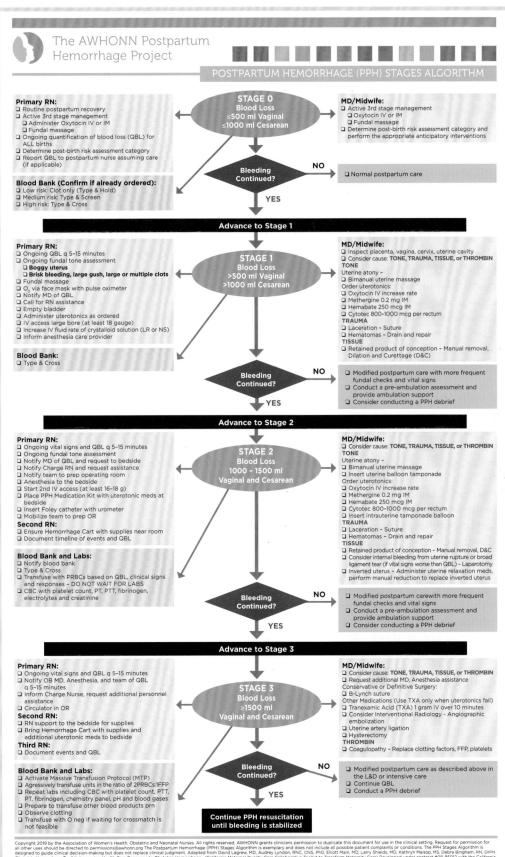

FIGURE 17–6. Postpartum hemorrhage stages algorithm.

The following assessments and interventions are included in comprehensive care during postpartum hemorrhage based on the individual clinical situation:

- Plan for care and assessment to ensure early recognition of hemorrhage.
- Packed red blood cells should be typed and cross-matched if excessive blood loss is anticipated (AAP & ACOG, 2017).
- Assess blood loss. Tips include assessing spill on floor:
  - 24 inches is about 500 mL.
  - 34 inches is about 1,000 mL.
  - 45 inches is about 1,500 mL.
- Weigh Peri-Pads or Chux dressing (1 g = 1 mL) (keep a gram scale on unit). Quantification of blood loss assessment is superior to estimated blood loss. See AWHONN (2015) practice brief on quantification of blood loss for more details. A calibrated under-buttocks drape can be useful as part of accurate measurement of blood loss.
- Assess excessive bleeding, which is defined as one perineal pad saturated within 15 minutes.
- Look for severe loss that may occur with steady, slow seepage.
- Assess vital signs at least every 15 minutes or more often if indicated.
- Mean arterial pressure (MAP), which is the mean blood pressure (BP) in arterial circulation, should be assessed because the first blood pressure response to hypovolemia may be a pulse pressure decreased to 30 mm Hg or less (Cunningham et al., 2018). MAP in nonpregnant women is normally 86.4 ± 7.5 mm Hg, with a slightly higher value for pregnant women, 90.3 ± 6 (Cunningham et al., 2018). MAP can be calculated with this formula:
  MAP = systolic BP + 2 (diastolic BP) / 3.
- Assess for tachypnea and tachycardia, which may occur while the BP is constant or slightly lowered.
- Assess for shock. Normal vital signs do not mean that the woman is not in shock. Traditional signs of hypovolemic shock are not evident until 10% to 30% of the total blood volume is lost due to the pregnancy-induced hypervolemia that accounts for the 30% to 70% increase in blood volume (an additional 1 to 2 L) that prevents symptoms with the typical 500 mL blood loss (ACOG, 2017; Robbins, Martin, & Wilson, 2014). The initial response of vasoconstriction shunts blood to vital organs to maintain their function and viability.
- Maintain accurate measurements of intake and output.
- Ensure large-bore (14, 16, or 18 gauge) needle intravenous access (two sites preferably).
- Replace volume with crystalloid (normal saline or lactated Ringer's) 1:3 or colloid (Hespan or albumin) 1:1 while waiting for blood or deciding on transfusion.

Goal is to produce at least 30 mL/hour of urine output and hematocrit values of 30% (Cunningham et al., 2018).

- Draw blood for hemoglobin and hematocrit (compare with prenatal or admission values), type and cross-match, coagulation studies (i.e., fibrinogen, prothrombin time, partial thromboplastin time, fibrin split products, and fibrin degradation products), and blood chemistry. The blood bank should be notified that transfusion may be necessary.
- The clot observation test provides a simple measure of fibrinogen. A volume of 5 mL of the patient's blood can be placed into a clean, red-topped tube and observed frequently. Normally, blood will clot within 8 to 10 minutes and will remain intact. If the fibrinogen concentration is low, generally less than 150 mg/dL, the blood in the tube will not clot, or if it does, it will undergo partial or complete dissolution in 30 to 60 minutes (ACOG, 2017).
- Arterial blood may be drawn for blood gas determinations.
- If blood transfusion is necessary, each unit of packed red blood cells (240 mL is the usual volume of 1 U) can be expected to increase hematocrit 3 percentage points and hemoglobin by 1 g/dL. Packed red blood cells contain red blood cells, WBCs, and plasma (ACOG, 2017).
- Transfusion can be withheld with adequate urine output and no appreciable postural hypotension or tachycardia (AAP & ACOG, 2017).
- Deficits in clotting factors may necessitate cryoprecipitate (i.e., for fibrinogen deficiency), recombinant activated factor VII, or FFP (i.e., for decreased levels of clotting factors) (AAP & ACOG, 2017; ACOG, 2017; Park, Yeom, Han, Jo, & Kim, 2017). Each unit of 50 mL of platelets can be expected to increase platelet count 5,000 to 10,000/mm³. Platelets contain platelets, red blood cells, WBCs, and plasma. Each unit of 250 mL of FFP can be expected to increase fibrinogen by 10 mg/dL. FFP contains fibrinogen, antithrombin III, and factors V and VIII. Each unit of cryoprecipitate can be expected to increase fibrinogen by 10 mg/dL. Cryoprecipitate contains fibrinogen, factors VII and XIII, and von Willebrand factor (ACOG, 2017).
- Use correct uterine massage to avoid ligament damage and potential uterine inversion (see Fig. 17–4). Place one hand pointing toward the woman's head with thumb resting on one side of the uterus and fingers along the other side. Use other hand to massage with *only the force needed to effect contraction or expulsion of clots.* Overaggressive uterine massage may tire muscle fibers and contribute to further atony.
- Early recognition minimizes blood loss and potential sequelae such as anemia, puerperal infection, thromboembolism, and necrosis of the anterior pituitary (i.e., Sheehan's syndrome).

- Anticipate pain management needs for fundal massage and uterotonic medications for treatment of hemorrhage.
- Urine should be sent to the laboratory as indicated.
- Insert a Foley catheter to empty the bladder and allow accurate measurement of output. A full bladder can impede complete uterine contraction.
- Administer prescribed medication. Labor and birth units should have the following pharmacologic agents available: oxytocin, methylergonovine, ergot alkaloids, 15-methyl-prostaglandin $F_{2\alpha}$, prostaglandin $F_{2\alpha}$, misoprostol, and dinoprostone (AAP & ACOG, 2017; ACOG, 2017).
  - See Table 17–4 for pharmacologic management of postpartum hemorrhage.
- Apply pulse oximeter and administer oxygen according to unit protocol. This is usually accomplished with a nonrebreather facemask at 10 to 12 L/min.
- Continuous electrocardiographic monitoring may be indicated for hypotension, continuous bleeding, tachycardia, or shock.
- Elevate the legs to a 20- to 30-degree angle to increase venous return.
- Prepare for additional interventions if the situation does not resolve. These include packing the uterus with gauze or using a balloon tamponade, dilatation and curettage, exploratory laparotomy, bilateral uterine artery ligation, arterial embolization, and other surgical techniques. In some cases, postpartum hemorrhage may require a transfer or return to the surgical suite. The surgical team should be notified that they may be needed.
- Provide emotional support and explanations for the woman and her family.

Based on interdisciplinary collaboration, the CMQCC (Lyndon et al., 2015) suggests a methodology for blood and fluid replacement following a postpartum hemorrhage.

- Use a ratio of packed red blood cells to FFP to platelets that is 4 to 6 units packed red blood cell:4 units FFP:1 unit pheresis platelets.
- Stat labs
  - If bleeding exceeds expected volume for routine delivery and there is no response to initial therapy, request stat laboratory analysis for the following:
    - Complete blood count with platelets
    - Prothrombin time/partial thromboplastin time
    - Fibrinogen
    - Repeat labs one to three times every 30 minutes until patient is stable.
- Packed red blood cells
  - Initial request: 3 to 6 units of red blood cells
  - O-negative or type-specific blood initially until cross-match units are released

TABLE 17–4. Pharmacologic Management of Postpartum Hemorrhage

Medication (Brand name)	Dose	Route	Frequency	Adverse effects	Contraindications
Oxytocin* (Pitocin)	10 to 40 units in 500 to 1,000 mL NS or LR 10 U	IV IM	Continuous infusion	Water intoxication With prolonged administration, nausea, vomiting, and hyponatremia	Hypersensitivity to drug High-dose IV push—hypotension; IV push associated with myocardial ischemia
Methylergonovine* (Methergine)	0.2 mg	IM	Every 2 to 4 hours	Hypertension Hypotension Nausea and vomiting	Hypertension Heart disease
Carboprost tromethamine* (Hemabate)	0.25 mg Total dose should not exceed 2 mg (8 doses of 0.25 mg).	IM or intramyometrial	Every 15 to 90 minutes	Nausea and vomiting Diarrhea Flushing	Asthma Hypersensitivity to drug Acute pelvic inflammatory disease
Misoprostol* (Cytotec)	800 to 1,000 mcg 200 to 400 mcg	Rectal Sublingual or oral	Single dose	Fever Chills Shivering	Hypersensitivity to drug Known allergy to prostaglandin
Tranexamic acid (TXA) (Administer TXA when uterotonics fail to control bleeding.)	1 g slow IV injection or diluted in 50 or 100 mL IV infusion	IV over 10 minutes	Administer first dose within 3 hours after birth When bleeding persists, repeat only once after 30 minutes.	Visual abnormalities Hypotension (with rapid injection) Nausea Vomiting Diarrhea Anaphylaxis	History or risk of thrombosis or active thromboembolic disease (DVT, PE) Use cautiously with renal impairment, renal failure, active vascular disease, thromboembolic history.

DVT, deep vein thrombosis; IM, intramuscular; IV, intravenous; LR, lactated Ringers; NS, normal saline; PE, pulmonary embolism.
*Uterotonics.
From Association of Women's Health, Obstetric and Neonatal Nurses. (2018). *Obstetric patient safety classroom course for postpartum hemorrhage* (pp. 231–232). Washington, DC: Author.

- FFP
  - Red blood cells-to-FFP ratio not to exceed 3:2
  - Infuse FFP to maintain international normalized ratio <1.5 to 1.7.
- Platelets
  - Single donor apheresis platelet pack
  - Infuse to maintain platelet count >50,000 to 100,000/μL in the face of ongoing hemorrhage.
- Cryoprecipitate
  - Initial request: 6 to 10 units cryoprecipitate if fibrinogen is less than 100 mg/dL
  - Additional units to maintain fibrinogen concentration ≥100 to 125 mg/dL
- Recombinant activated factor VII
  - Not universally recommend

Once the woman is stable, replacement of red blood cell mass is an important clinical intervention. She should be instructed to continue prenatal vitamins that contain about 60 mg of elemental iron and 1 mg of folate during the hospitalization and at least until the first postpartum office visit. Additional iron should be encouraged (two tablets of 300 mg ferrous sulfate) to maximize red cell production and restoration (ACOG, 2017).

In 2004 and 2010, The Joint Commission recommended conducting periodic drills for obstetric emergencies such as postpartum hemorrhage. Although there are few data supporting improved outcomes in units where postpartum hemorrhage birth drills are routine, it would seem likely that when all members of the perinatal team know their roles and responsibilities, the location of key medications and equipment and whom to call, and the chances of the chaotic environment often associated with a significant postpartum hemorrhage would be minimized. During postpartum hemorrhage, immediate access to required medications can be challenging. Common medications used to treat postpartum hemorrhage such as oxytocin, Methergine, Prostin, and misoprostol are kept in locked drug-dispensing systems often remote from the labor room. Intravenous fluids required for rapid volume expansion also may be not be available in the labor room. Development of a clinical algorithm for interventions during postpartum hemorrhage in addition to drills to evaluate the feasibility of getting necessary medications and intravenous fluids quickly may be helpful. Documenting interventions is important to keep both the drill and actual response organized.

To prepare for a drill, develop a list of roles and responsibilities for each team member. Some have found it helpful to use a scribe or video recording of the drill so that the organization of events and interventions can be analyzed retrospectively. Using a volunteer staff member as a surrogate for the patient can make the drill seem more realistic. See Display 17–4 for a form to use for debriefing after a postpartum hemorrhage. See AWHONN's resources for postpartum hemorrhage (https://www.awhonn.org/general/custom.asp?page=PPH, https://cdn.ymaws.com/www.awhonn.org/resource/resmgr/PDFs/PPH/PPHPoster.pdf, https://www.jognn.org/article/S0884-2175(15)31768-8/fulltext, https://onlinelibrary.wiley.com/doi/full/10.1111/j.1552-6909.2012.01371.x).

Postpartum Infections

A puerperal infection should be suspected when a woman has an oral temperature higher than 38°C (100.4°F) on two occasions that are 6 hours apart during the first 10 days postpartum, exclusive of the first 24 hours. Interventions may begin prior to waiting 6 hours between temperature assessments. The cardinal symptoms of a postpartum infection are elevated temperature, tachycardia, and pain. The nursery should be notified of these findings, although the newborn need not be separated from the mother (AAP & ACOG, 2017; Cunningham et al., 2018; Duff, 2014).

Endometritis

Postpartum endometritis occurs in 1% to 3% of vaginal births and is 10 times more common in cesarean births (Cunningham et al., 2018; Duff, 2014). Postpartum uterine infections, called *endometritis* (i.e., inflammation of endometrium), *endomyometritis* (i.e., inflammation of endometrium and myometrium), or endomyoparametritis (i.e., inflammation of endometrium and parametrial tissue), are the most commonly identified causes of puerperal morbidity. One of the most effective methods of prevention of infection is handwashing.

The most common cause of uterine infection tends to be polymicrobial, including aerobic and anaerobic organisms that have ascended to the uterus from the lower genital tract. Isolated organisms include streptococci A and B, enterococci, *Staphylococcus aureus*, *Gardnerella vaginalis*, *Escherichia coli*, *Enterobacter*, *Proteus mirabilis*, *Klebsiella pneumoniae*, *Bacteroides* species, *Peptostreptococcus* species, *Ureaplasma urealyticum*, *Mycoplasma hominis*, and *Chlamydia trachomatis*. *C. trachomatis* has been specifically associated with late-onset postpartum endometritis (Cunningham et al., 2018; Duff, 2014). Blood cultures are positive in about 10% of women. Endometrial cultures may have limited value because of cervicovaginal contamination of the specimen, yet they may provide useful information if the woman does not respond to initial antibiotic therapy (Cunningham et al., 2018; Duff, 2014). If the infection does not respond to antibiotic therapy, an antiviral regimen should be considered for pathogens such as herpes simplex virus or cytomegalovirus (Giraldo-Isaza, Jaspan, & Cohen, 2011; Moldenhauer, 2018).

DISPLAY 17–4
Immediate Focused Postpartum Hemorrhage Debrief Form

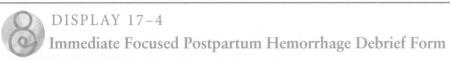

AWHONN
PROMOTING THE HEALTH OF
WOMEN AND NEWBORNS

IMMEDIATE FOCUSED POSTPARTUM HEMORRHAGE (PPH) DEBRIEF FORM

> **For quality improvement (QI) processes only.**
> Follow hospital QI policies regarding recording the patient's name and medical record number.

Date of the event: _____

Form completed by: _____

Type of event: Please check one.
Postpartum Hemorrhage ❑ Stage 2   ❑ Stage 3

Description: A quick focused debrief immediately after an event helps capture important lessons learned and identify areas for needed improvement.

> **Facilitator Guidelines:**
> 1. RN and MD partner as facilitators. (Primary RN is responsible for calling the debrief. Ensure that the family is debriefed and debrief is recorded).
> 2. Blame-free and shame-free session
> 3. No interruptions or side conversations

Clinical Debrief Guidelines:
- Conduct a team debrief for ALL stage 2 or 3 postpartum hemorrhages and other emergencies as indicated.
- Empower all team members who cared for the patient to participate.
- Keep the debrief short, maximum of 15 minutes. Be as specific as possible.
- Conduct the debrief as soon possible once the patient is stabilized.
- The RN debrief leader should follow up with the family.
- Learn from debriefs by sharing what went well and any concerns.

Debrief Attendees: Indicate the number (#) of team members that attended the debriefing.

#	RN debrief attendees	#	Provider debrief attendees	#	Anesthesia and Pediatric debrief attendees (MDs and RNs)	#	Support staff debrief attendees
	Primary RN		Primary MD (MFM, OB, FP)		Neonatology/Pediatrics MD		Unit Secretary/Clerk
	Nurse Manager or Supervisor		OB Resident(s)		Anesthesia Provider		OB Scrub/Surgical Tech
	Charge RN		Certified Nurse Midwife		NICU RN		Other Departments
	Other RN		Other		Other		Clergy or Social Worker

Overall Team Management: Check all that apply.

RECOGNITION				READINESS			
Risk and Hemorrhage Identification	Performed Well	Needs Improvement	Comments	**Resources and Equipment**	Performed Well	Needs Improvement	Comments
1. Were ongoing PPH risk assessments performed on admission, pre- and post-birth?	❑	❑		1. Was there adequate staffing on the unit?	❑	❑	
2. Was there prompt recognition of the emergency?	❑	❑		2. Were necessary supplies and/or equipment available?	❑	❑	
				3. Were additional supplies and/or equipment easily accessible?	❑	❑	

RESPONSE							
Teamwork and Clinical Management	Performed Well	Needs Improvement	Comments	**Medications, Blood Loss, and Blood Administration**	Performed Well	Needs Improvement	Comments
1. Was the team mobilized in a timely manner?	❑	❑		1. Were the appropriate uterotonic medications given?	❑	❑	
2. Were appropriate clinical decisions followed as per the hemorrhage policy?	❑	❑		2. Was blood loss quantified by direct measurement?	❑	❑	
3. Were other interventions, e.g., tamponade balloons, B-Lynch suture utilized in a timely manner?	❑	❑		3. Were blood products administered in a timely manner?	❑	❑	
4. Was additional support requested and obtained in a timely manner?	❑	❑		4. Was blood readily available?	❑	❑	

Team and Family Communication	Performed Well	Needs Improvement	Comments	**Additional Comments**	Performed Well	Needs Improvement	Comments
1. Did team members communicate important or critical information in a timely manner?	❑	❑		1.	❑	❑	
2. Were the patient and family informed and the team's plan of care communicated?	❑	❑		2.	❑	❑	
3. Did the team meet the patient's and family's spiritual and emotional needs?	❑	❑		3.	❑	❑	

(continued)

DISPLAY 17–4

Immediate Focused Postpartum Hemorrhage Debrief Form *(Continued)*

Issue Identified	Action Needed	Person(s) Responsible for Follow Up

From Association of Women's Health, Obstetric and Neonatal Nurses. (2018). *Obstetric patient safety classroom course for postpartum hemorrhage* (pp. 233). Washington, DC: Author.

Parenteral broad-spectrum antibiotic therapy is promptly initiated when postpartum endometritis is diagnosed. Treatment continues until the woman has been afebrile for 48 hours. A common treatment regimen is a combination of clindamycin and gentamicin, with ampicillin in refractory cases. Women usually respond rapidly (48 to 72 hours) to antibiotic therapy. Occasional complications include pelvic abscesses, infected hematoma, septic pelvic thrombophlebitis, persistent fever, and retained infected placenta (AAP & ACOG, 2017; Shepherd & Pizzarello, 2017).

Other causes of postpartum infection include wound and UTI; pneumonia (usually related to general anesthesia); mastitis; pelvic thrombophlebitis; and necrotizing fasciitis, an uncommon but serious localized infection of the deep soft tissues.

Risk factors for endometritis are:

- Operative birth
- Prolonged labor or rupture of membranes
- Use of invasive procedures (i.e., internal monitoring, amnioinfusion, fetal scalp sampling, lacerations)
- Multiple pelvic examinations
- Excessive blood loss
- Pyelonephritis or diabetes
- Socioeconomic and nutritional factors compromising host defense mechanisms
- Anemia and systemic illness
- Smoking
- Diabetes

The following assessments and interventions are included in comprehensive nursing care for postpartum infections:

- Fever occurring about the third postnatal day is the most important finding.
- Observe for tachycardia (rise of 10 bpm for every degree Celsius).
- Determine possible causes of malaise.
- Assess lower abdominal pain.
- Assess uterine tenderness on palpation (extending laterally) and slight abdominal distention.
- Determine cause of foul-smelling lochia (if organism is anaerobic).
- Obtain urinalysis to rule out UTIs.
- Assess leukocytosis (WBC count >20,000/mm^3 with increased neutrophils or polymorphonuclear leukocytes).
- Blood cultures are positive in about 10% of women.
- Endometrial cultures may have limited value because of cervicovaginal contamination of the specimen, but they may provide useful information if the woman does not respond to initial antibiotic therapy (Cunningham et al., 2018; Duff, 2014).
- Parenteral broad-spectrum antibiotic therapy is promptly initiated when postpartum endometritis is diagnosed. Treatment continues until the woman has been afebrile for 48 hours. A common treatment regimen is a combination of clindamycin and an aminoglycoside such as gentamicin, with ampicillin added in refractory cases. A protocol including activity against the Bacteroides fragilis group and other penicillin-resistant anaerobic bacteria is better than one without. No one regimen is associated with fewer side effects, with the exception of cephalosporins, which are associated with less diarrhea.
- Women usually respond rapidly (48 to 72 hours) to antibiotic therapy. Occasional complications include pelvic abscesses, septic pelvic thrombophlebitis, persistent fever, and retained infected placenta (AAP & ACOG, 2017).
- Increase fluid intake and encourage adequate nutrition.
- Encourage intake of a minimum of six to eight glasses (1,500 to 2,000 mL) of water, milk, or juices; 2,000 mL is the preferred amount.
- Encourage intake of at least 1,800 to 2,000 calories daily if lactating and 1,500 calories if not lactating.
- Encourage the woman to eat a varied diet, with representation of foods from all food groups, that is high in protein and vitamin C to promote wound healing.
- Ensure adequate output (30 mL/hour) because renal toxicity can occur with antibiotic therapy.
- Provide comfort through meeting the woman's personal hygiene needs. Cool compresses, linen changes, massage, and positioning may enhance comfort.
- Assess maternal vital signs every 4 hours or every 2 hours if her temperature is elevated.
- Use a semi-Fowler position, ambulation, or both to promote uterine drainage.
- Administer oxytocics as ordered to promote uterine contraction and drainage.
- Observe for signs of septic shock: tachycardia (>120 bpm), hypotension, tachypnea, changes in sensorium, and decreased urine output (i.e., oliguria) (Cunningham et al., 2018). If septic shock develops, increase the frequency of obtaining vital signs and other assessments, depending on the clinical situation.

Wound Infections

Wound infections can be classified as early onset (within 48 hours) or late onset (within 6 to 8 days). Early-onset wound infections are usually treated with antibiotic therapy and excision of necrotic tissue. Late-onset infections are treated with incision and drainage, and they may not require antibiotics unless there is extensive cellulitis (Cunningham et al., 2018; Duff, 2014). The following are risk factors for wound infections:

- History of chorioamnionitis or intraamniotic infection
- Hemorrhage or anemia
- Obesity
- Underlying medical problems such as diabetes and malnutrition

- Multiple vaginal examinations
- Corticosteroid therapy
- Immunosuppression
- Advancing age
- Malnutrition

The following assessments and interventions are included in comprehensive nursing care for wound infections:

- Observe for wound erythema, swelling, tenderness, and purulent discharge.
- Assess for localized pain and dysuria.
- Assess vital signs.
  - Low-grade temperature (101°F or 38.3°C).
  - Temperature of 40°C (104°F) may be exhibited by sudden onset of chills
  - Pulse usually is <100 bpm.
- Perform cultures as ordered.
- Assist with drainage, irrigation, and occasionally, débridement procedures.
- Sitz baths are used for cleaning and promotion of increased circulation to the affected area.
- Wound may be packed. Treatment is directed toward cleaning the wound and promoting granulation.
- Change dressings and dispose appropriately of soiled dressings.
- Dressings may be continued after discharge. The patient and family will need instruction for dressing and wound care.
- Ensure frequent changes of Peri-Pads.
- Ensure pain management and appropriate administration of analgesia.
- Ensure adequate room ventilation prior to dressing changes.
- Continued hospitalization or readmission may be required.
- Provide explanations during this stressful period.
- Offer reassurance and encouragement.
- Encourage frequent visits by the family to help reduce anxiety.
- Assist breastfeeding women with pumping or lactation suppression.
- Administer antibiotic therapy as ordered (may be continued after discharge).
- Provide referrals for postpartum follow-up visits by home care nurses.
- Reduce anxiety and the incidence of rehospitalization by early identification and treatment of infections.

Necrotizing Fasciitis

Necrotizing fasciitis is a severe infection (polymicrobial more common) that is characterized by severe tissue necrosis, erythema, discharge, and severe pain. Partial liquefaction of fascia adjacent to the incision may also occur. Secondary healing may take 6 to 12 weeks (Cunningham et al., 2018; Duff, 2014).

Risk factors for necrotizing fasciitis include the following:

- Diabetes
- Obesity
- Hypertension

The following assessments and interventions are included in comprehensive nursing care for necrotizing fasciitis:

- Wound status (i.e., erythema, discharge)
- Pain
- Administration of broad-spectrum antibiotics, as ordered
- Surgical debridement

Mastitis

Both congestive and infectious mastitis are more commonly seen in primigravidas and nursing mothers. Symptoms usually appear between the third and fourth week after birth and are typically unilateral. Symptoms of mastitis may include fever; chills; localized tenderness; and a palpable, hard, reddened mass. Nipple trauma has been implicated in the development of mastitis. Trauma from incorrect latch-on or removal of the newborn from the breast permits the introduction of organisms from the newborn into the mother's breast. *S. aureus* is the most common causative organism. Administration of penicillinase-resistant antibiotics such as dicloxacillin for 7 to 10 days is recommended.

If a breast abscess develops, incision and drainage may be indicated. The decision to continue breastfeeding should be made jointly by the woman and the healthcare provider. If breastfeeding is delayed while purulent drainage continues, the woman may need assistance with breast pumping to reestablish lactation. If advised to discontinue breastfeeding, emotional support, reassurance, and comfort measures are important. Lactation consultant referral is indicated as a preventive or treatment measure when these services are available.

Risk factors for mastitis include the following:

- Infrequent breastfeeding
- Incomplete breast emptying
- Plugged milk duct
- Cracked and bleeding nipples (may be secondary to improper latch-on and removal)

The following assessments and interventions are included in comprehensive nursing care for mastitis:

- Assess fever and chills.
- Assess localized tenderness and a palpable, hard, reddened mass.
- Assess for tachycardia.
- Assess for purulent discharge.
- Offer education about preventive measures (i.e., hand washing, breast cleanliness, frequent breast-pad

changes, exposure of the nipples to air, and correct infant latch-on and removal from the breast).
- Obtain a culture of the breast milk before initiating antibiotic therapy, if ordered.
- The infection usually resolves within 24 to 48 hours of antibiotic therapy.
- Suggest comfort measures, including warm or cold compresses, wearing a supportive bra, and analgesia as ordered.
- Offer education about completing the full regimen of antibiotic therapy.
- Encourage an increase in fluid intake from 2 to 2.5 L/day.
- Massage, positioning the newborn in the direction of the site, and frequent breastfeeding promote milk flow.
- Assist with the use of a breast pump or manual expression if indicated (Cunningham et al., 2018; Duff, 2014).

Urinary Tract Infections

UTIs are the most common medical complication occurring during pregnancy. They may be asymptomatic (i.e., bacteriuria) or symptomatic (i.e., cystitis, acute pyelonephritis). Asymptomatic UTIs occur in 4% to 7% of pregnant women. Diagnosis and treatment of bacteriuria can prevent the development of pyelonephritis, which places the fetus at increased risk for preterm birth or low birth weight. Women who develop UTIs during pregnancy are at increased risk for a UTI during the postpartum period (Cunningham et al., 2018; Duff, 2014).

Risk factors for UTIs include the following:

- A shorter urethra in women than men
- Contamination of the urethra with pathogenic bacteria from vagina and rectum
- High probability that women do not completely empty bladders
- Movement of bacteria into bladder during sexual intercourse
- Pregnancy-related changes (i.e., decreased ureteric muscle tone and activity from progesterone and pressure of gravid uterus, resulting in lower rate of urine passing through urinary collecting system)
- Urinary catheterization, frequent pelvic examinations, epidural anesthesia, genital tract injury, and cesarean birth

Asymptomatic Bacteriuria

The following assessments and interventions are included in comprehensive nursing care of asymptomatic bacteriuria:

- Evaluate urinalysis for bacteriuria (presence of 10^5 or more bacterial colonies per milliliter of urine on two consecutive clean-catch, midstream voided specimens).

- *E. coli* is cultured in 60% to 90% of cases. (Other pathogens include *P. mirabilis*, *K. pneumoniae*, group B hemolytic streptococci, and *Staphylococcus saprophyticus*)
- Educate women about the importance of repeat urinalysis to determine the effectiveness of antibiotics.
- Risk is associated with sickle cell trait, lower socioeconomic status, increased parity, and reduced availability of medical care.
- Administer or educate the woman to take antibiotics as ordered to eliminate bacteria in urine.
- Ampicillin and cephalosporins are used (no significant risk to the fetus); antibiotics are administered for 7 days.
- If continuous antimicrobial therapy is required, typically use a single daily dose of nitrofurantoin (100 mg), preferably after the evening meal (Duff, 2014).

Pyelonephritis and Cystitis

The following assessments and interventions are included in comprehensive nursing care for pyelonephritis and cystitis:

- Assess urinalysis for presence of untreated, asymptomatic bacteriuria.
  - High risk for pyelonephritis with untreated bacteriuria
  - Bacterial growth more than 100,000 colonies/mL
  - May have increased WBCs, protein, or blood in specimen
  - Most common bacteria: *E. coli* (80%), *Klebsiella*, *Enterobacter*, *Proteus*
  - First choice of therapy: cephalosporins for single-agent therapy
- Assess for symptoms of cystitis.
  - Urinary urgency, frequency, dysuria
  - Suprapubic pain without fever or tenderness at the costovertebral angle
  - Gross hematuria
- Assess for symptoms of pyelonephritis.
  - Shaking chills, fever, tachycardia, flank pain, nausea, vomiting
  - Urinary frequency, urgency, dysuria, and costovertebral angle tenderness
  - Possible endotoxin-mediated tissue damage (Duff, 2014)
- Administer antibiotics as ordered.
  - Short courses (1 to 3 weeks) of sulfonamides, ampicillin, or nitrofurantoin recommended for pyelonephritis
  - Recommended 7-day course of antibiotics for acute cystitis in pregnant women
- Monitor intake and output.
  - Maintain adequate hydration (at least 2,000 mL/day) mainly water.
  - Measure urinary output for adequacy (at least 30 mL/hour).

- Administer antipyretics, antispasmodics, or urinary analgesics (phenazopyridine [Pyridium]) and antiemetics as ordered.
- Encourage rest.
- Monitor vital signs every 4 hours.
- Educate the woman about monitoring temperature, bladder function, appearance of urine, importance of completing antibiotic therapy, proper perineal care (i.e., wiping front to back), wearing cotton underwear, adequate hydration, and balanced nutrition.

If readmission for treatment of a UTI is necessary, reassurance and family support are essential. Separation from the newborn is distressing to the mother and child. If the woman has been breastfeeding, interventions such as pumping and newborn visits can help to maintain lactation after antibiotic therapy has been initiated. If breastfeeding is temporarily contraindicated, the nurse can provide emotional support and offer strategies to maintain lactation (i.e., breast pump) until breastfeeding can be resumed (Cunningham et al., 2018; Duff, 2014).

Thrombophlebitis and Thromboembolism

Thrombophlebitis (inflammation of a vein after formation of a thrombus) is classified as superficial or deep. Superficial thrombophlebitis involves the superficial veins of the saphenous system. Deep vein thrombophlebitis affects the veins of the calf, thigh, or pelvis and can lead to a pulmonary embolism (PE), which is among the leading causes of maternal mortality in the United States.

During pregnancy, risk is increased because

- Venous capacitance and venous pressure in the legs are increased, resulting in stasis.
- Pregnancy causes a degree of hypercoagulability.

However, most thromboemboli develop postpartum and result from vascular trauma during birth (Douketis, 2018; Tapson, 2018). Cesarean birth can also increase the risk. Stasis is a significant predisposing event to the development of deep vein thrombosis, thus early ambulation after birth is encouraged as the new mother is able. Symptoms of thrombophlebitis or their absence does not accurately predict the diagnosis, disease severity, or risk of embolization. Thromboembolic disorders can occur without symptoms, with only minimal symptoms, or with significant symptoms. Numerous studies have questioned the accuracy and utility of Homans' sign. Accuracy estimates range from a positive result in 8% to 56% of documented cases of deep vein thrombosis (DVT) to a positive result in more than 50% of patients without DVT. Most authors conclude that Homans' sign is unreliable, insensitive, and nonspecific in the diagnosis of DVT.

When a clot becomes friable, and the pieces detach from the vessel wall and travel through the heart into the pulmonary circulation, it is known as a pulmonary emboli. PE should be treated as a life-threatening event; interruption of blood flow to the pulmonary bed can result in cardiovascular collapse and death (Cunningham et al., 2018; Leung & Lockwood, 2014).

Risk Factors for Thrombophlebitis and Thromboembolism

- Normal changes in coagulation status during pregnancy
  - Increasing concentrations of coagulation factors and fibrinogen
  - Decreasing natural anticoagulants protein S and activated protein C
  - Shift of coagulation and fibrinolytic systems to hypercoagulability (Douketis, 2018; Friel, 2018; Tapson, 2018)
- History of thromboembolic disease or varicosities
- Increased parity
- Obesity
- Advanced maternal age (≥30 years)
- Immobility associated with extended antepartum bed rest
- Use of forceps
- Cesarean birth
- Blood vessel and tissue trauma
- Prolonged labor with multiple pelvic examinations
- Sepsis/trauma
- Dehydration

Prevention of Thrombus Formation

- Early ambulation or leg exercises for women on bed rest
- Education about correct posture
- Avoiding crossing legs
- Avoiding extreme flexion of legs at the groin
- Positioning without pressure on the backs of knees
- Use of support hose by women with a history of thrombophlebitis
- Padding of pressure points during birth while in the lithotomy position

Diagnosis

Diagnosis of DVT is usually by Doppler ultrasonography. In the postpartum period, if Doppler ultrasonography and plethysmography are normal but iliac, ovarian, or other pelvic venous thrombosis is suspected, computed tomography (CT) with contrast is used. Diagnosis of PE is increasingly being made by helical CT rather than ventilation/perfusion scanning because CT involves less radiation and is equally sensitive. If the diagnosis of PE is uncertain, pulmonary angiography is required.

If DVT or PE is detected during pregnancy, the anticoagulant of choice is a low molecular weight heparin. Low molecular weight heparin, because of its molecular size, does not cross the placenta. It does not cause maternal osteoporosis and may be less likely to cause thrombocytopenia, which can result from prolonged (≥ 6 months) use of unfractionated heparin. Warfarin crosses the placenta and may cause fetal abnormalities or death (Douketis, 2018; Friel, 2018; Tapson, 2018).

The following assessments and interventions are included in comprehensive nursing care of thrombophlebitis:

- Evaluate the woman's physical status.
- Apply a supportive bandage or antiembolic support stockings.
- Apply a soothing agent (i.e., glycerin and Ichthyol).
- Apply warm packs to the affected area.
- Slightly elevate the involved leg.
- Perform serial measurements of the circumferences of the calves; a circumference difference of more than 2 cm is classified as leg swelling.
- Monitor vital signs every 4 hours; there may be a slight increase in temperature.
- Compare pulses in both extremities, which may reveal decreased venous flow to the affected area.
- Heparin anticoagulation therapy may be ordered.
- Bed rest with elevation of involved extremity until swelling is reduced and anticoagulation therapy are effective (promote venous return and decreases edema).
- As soon as symptoms allow, ambulation is encouraged as bed rest can increase venous stasis.
- Anticoagulation therapy with intravenous heparin, followed by oral warfarin
  - Maintenance of activated partial thromboplastin time that is prolonged by 1.5 to 2 times laboratory control value (Cunningham et al., 2018)
  - Dosing regimens (Cunningham et al., 2018):
    - 5,000 U bolus of heparin and then continuous infusion to a total 24,000 to 32,000 U/day
    - Intermittent intravenous injections of 5,000 U every 4 hours or 7,500 U every 6 hours
    - Subcutaneous heparin at dose of 10,000 U every 8 hours or 20,000 U every 12 hours
  - Monitor coagulation laboratory values.
- Carefully assess unusual bleeding. Heavy vaginal bleeding, generalized petechiae, bleeding from the mucous membranes, hematuria, or oozing from venipuncture sites should be reported to the physician. The heparin antidote protamine sulfate should be readily available.
- Educate and prepare women for diagnostic testing:
  - Physical assessments look for muscle pain, palpable deep linear cord, tenderness, swelling, and dilated superficial veins.
  - Doppler ultrasonography provides more sensitivity and is more specific for the diagnosis of popliteal and femoral vein thrombosis than for calf vein thrombosis. It can evaluate venous flow and possible occlusion.
  - Venography is a more specific test, but it is invasive, expensive, and difficult to interpret. Contrast material may cause chemical phlebitis.
  - Impedance plethysmography has had little research to support its efficacy during pregnancy, but coupled with ultrasound, the reliability increases. A thigh cuff is inflated, resulting in temporary occlusion of venous return. Release results in a rapid decrease in volume as blood drains proximally. Volume changes are detected by measurement of electrical resistance in the calf.
  - Blood studies can determine the formation of intravascular fibrin; results are positive in cases of thrombosis. Results are also positive in presence of hematomas or inflammatory exudates containing fibrin.

Septic Pelvic Thrombophlebitis

Septic pelvic thrombophlebitis is a condition more common in women after a cesarean birth and occurs with infections of the reproductive tract. Ascending infection within the venous system results in thrombophlebitis. This condition should be suspected when the infection does not respond to antibiotics and is accompanied by abdominal or flank pain and guarding on the second or third postpartum day. A more serious complication occurs when a thrombus forms in any of the dilated pelvic veins. The following assessments and interventions are included in comprehensive nursing care of septic pelvic thrombophlebitis:

- Assess the woman for physical symptoms:
  - Fever and tachycardia
  - Spiking fever persisting despite antibiotic therapy
  - Abdominal and flank pain (paralytic ileus may develop)
  - Prepare and support the woman during examination (i.e., parametrial mass found on bimanual examination).
- Obtain appropriate laboratory testing:
  - Complete blood count
  - Blood chemistry
  - Coagulation profile
  - Chest radiography, CT, magnetic resonance imaging
- Administer medications as ordered:
  - Heparin regimen initiated with diagnosis
  - Coumarin agent substituted and continued for total course of anticoagulation of 3 to 6 weeks

Pulmonary Embolism

The following assessments and interventions are included in comprehensive nursing care of PE:

- The most common signs are dyspnea, chest pain, hemoptysis, and abdominal pain.
- The most serious signs are sudden collapse, cyanosis, and hypotension.

- Prepare the woman for diagnostic testing:
  - Ventilation/perfusion (V/Q) scan
  - Blood gas studies
  - Radiography
  - Pulmonary angiography
- Elevate the head of the bed to facilitate breathing.
- Administer oxygen 10 L/min using a nonrebreather facemask; use pulse oximetry.
- Maintain the $P_aO_2 \geq 70$ mm Hg.
- Monitor arterial blood gases.
- Frequently assess vital signs.
- Provide for intravenous fluids (i.e., pulmonary artery catheter may be placed).
- Administer salt-poor or hypertonic intravenous fluids, as ordered.
- Administer medications as ordered to counteract symptoms:
  - Medium dose of intravenous heparin (continued subcutaneous heparin or oral anticoagulant therapy for 6 months)
  - Total daily heparin dose of 30,000 to 40,000 U (Cunningham et al., 2018)
  - Dopamine to maintain blood pressure
  - Morphine for analgesia
- Maintain adequate staffing:
  - Personnel who have completed an Advanced Cardiac Life Support course should be available for full resuscitation support, if needed. Because ongoing care may occur in an intensive care unit (ICU) setting, collaboration between the ICU staff and perinatal staff is essential. Maternal transport should be considered if the level of care and supportive staff necessary are unavailable.

Although most women have a normal postpartum course, complications can occur. Comprehensive, frequent nursing assessments contribute to early identification and prompt treatment. Collaboration between the perinatal nurse and the primary healthcare provider is essential.

INDIVIDUALIZING CARE FOR WOMEN WITH SPECIAL NEEDS

Cesarean Birth

In the United States, the cesarean birth rate is 32% (CDC, 2018), higher than most industrialized countries. The VBAC rate, vaginal births among women with a previous cesarean birth, was 12.8% in 2017, a 3% increase from 2016 when the VBAC rate was 12.4% (Martin, Hamilton, Osterman, Driscoll, & Drake, 2018). In 2017, the primary cesarean birth rate (cesareans among women who have not had a previous cesarean) was 21.9%, up from 21.8% in 2016 (Martin et al., 2018). Elective labor induction for nulliparous women is one factor that has long been thought to have

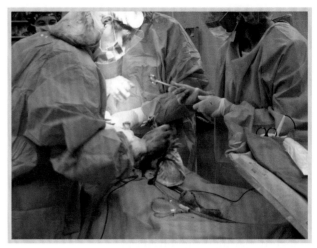

FIGURE 17–7. Emergent cesarean birth.

an impact on the rise in primary cesarean births; however, this may not always be a factor when labor induction is conducted in the context of established labor guidelines (Grobman et al., 2018). When labor ends in cesarean birth, there is risk of lowered self-esteem related to failure to achieve the planned vaginal birth. The desired outcome of birth is for each couple to verbalize a positive birth experience and to feel happiness and excitement about a healthy baby, even if labor and birth do not go as planned. Nurses can assist in achieving this outcome for women experiencing a cesarean birth by involving the couple as much as possible in the decision-making process, keeping the couple informed, supporting the coach and family, encouraging verbalization, and providing reassurance that a cesarean birth is not a failure. If the cesarean birth was unexpected and/or emergent (Fig. 17–7) with minimal time to prepare the couple, time should be allocated as soon as possible after birth to discuss what occurred and why the provider felt cesarean birth was the safest option at that time for the mother and baby. Efforts should be made to allow mother's partner to see the baby as soon as possible if the emergent birth resulted in the baby's admission to the special care nursery or neonatal intensive care unit (NICU); thus, the baby has been separated from the couple during post-anesthesia care (Fig. 17–8).

Nurses caring for women after a cesarean birth should stress that the woman is a new mother with the same needs as other new mothers; however, she also requires supportive postoperative care. It is important to provide that extra level of care and include consideration of women in the postoperative period when planning nurse staffing. The woman who has experienced a cesarean birth usually has increased levels of fatigue, activity intolerance, and incisional pain. Women who have cesarean birth after a long labor may be especially fatigued. Women who are in the postoperative recovery period and during the first day or two postoperatively

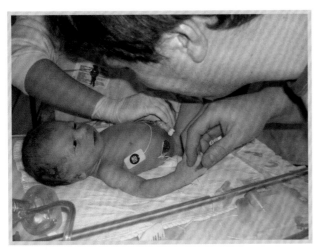

FIGURE 17–8. Promoting partner visiting baby in the neonatal intensive care unit after emergent cesarean birth.

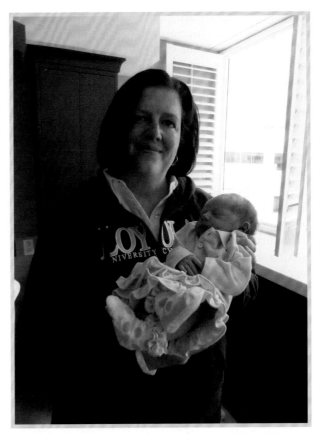

FIGURE 17–10. Support person in attendance to help mother care for baby during rooming in.

should have a support person with them to help care for the baby while rooming-in (Fig. 17–9). Policies that require rooming-in for these patients are not appropriate if the mother does not have a support person available to stay with her continuously until she can assume newborn care on her own (Fig. 17–10). The Newborns' and Mothers' Health Protection Act prohibits the restriction of mothers' and newborns' benefits for hospitals length-of-stay in connection with childbirth to less than 48 hours for a vaginal birth or 96 hours for a cesarean section (National Conference of State Legislatures, 2018). Chapter 14 provides a full discussion of cesarean birth and the immediate postoperative recovery period.

Antepartum Bed Rest and Postpartum Recovery

Approximately 18% of pregnant women will be on bed rest at some point during their pregnancy (Van Eerden, 2017). Bed rest has not been supported as an effective

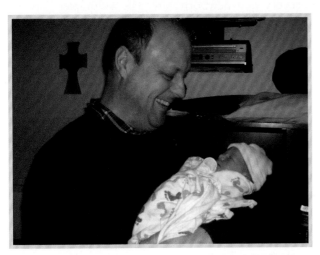

FIGURE 17–9. Support person in attendance to help mother care for baby after cesarean birth.

treatment for preterm labor or prolonging multifetal pregnancy and is not recommended by ACOG (2016a). Despite lack of evidence to support bed rest therapy as contributing to positive outcomes, it has been prescribed routinely for women with high-risk pregnancies. Women with bleeding, preterm labor, and pregnancy-induced hypertension are frequently encouraged to maintain modified or strict bed rest in the hope of prolonging the pregnancy. Some research suggests that modified rest or some level of activity restriction at home, rather than strict bed rest, is an acceptable form of treatment for women with pregnancy-induced hypertension remote from term and women at risk for preterm labor and birth (ACOG, 2016a, 2019).

Extended periods of activity restriction result in deconditioning or loss of muscle and bone. Pregnancy is associated with an increased risk of developing blood clots in the legs (deep venous thrombosis, or DVT) and movement of clots to the lungs (pulmonary embolism, or PE).

Bed rest increases the risk of DVT and PE among pregnant women placed on bed rest compared to pregnant women who were not placed on bed rest as well as an increased risk of blood clots (Van Eerden, 2017). During pregnancy, physical inactivity is recognized as an independent risk factor for maternal obesity and related pregnancy complications. Normally, blood volume, heart rate, stroke volume, and cardiac output normally increase during pregnancy, while systemic vascular resistance decreases.

These hemodynamic changes establish the circulatory reserve necessary to sustain the pregnant woman and fetus at rest and during exercise. Motionless postures, such as the supine position, may cause decreased venous return and hypotension. Patients prescribed prolonged bed rest or restricted physical activity are at risk of venous thromboembolism, bone demineralization, and deconditioning (ACOG, 2015). Isometric and isotonic conditioning exercises, Kegel exercises, pelvic tilts, and range-of-motion exercises can be used during hospitalization for the woman on bed rest. Deep breathing and coughing are added to exercise abdominal muscles and promote venous return.

After birth, the woman requires additional time, support, and education to prepare for safe and progressive levels of activity. Postpartum recovery may be prolonged. Ambulation after prolonged bed rest requires the continued presence of the perinatal nurse. Women should be alerted to the possibility of weakness, dizziness, shortness of breath, and muscle soreness and be reassured that these are normal physiologic consequences of prolonged bed rest that will reverse over time after resumption of normal activity (Maloni, 2010).

Preterm Birth

The March of Dimes (2016) has established goals to reduce preterm birth rates in the United States to 8.1% by 2020 and 5.5% by 2030. The U.S. preterm birth rate (birth at less than 37 completed weeks of gestation) increased to 9.93% in 2017, a 1% increase from 9.85% in 2016. This represents the third year in a row that the preterm birth rate has risen in the United States. The preterm birth rate has risen 10.44% since 2007. The low-birth-weight rate (babies weighing less than 2,500 g) remained relatively stable at 8.17% in 2016, compared with 8.1% in 2015 (March of Dimes, 2016; Martin et al., 2018). Women who have experienced a preterm birth may have special needs related to a long period of antepartum bed rest and/or a cesarean birth as previous described. In addition, based on the gestational age and condition of the baby, they may be worried about their baby's survival. The day-to-day fluctuations in the baby's status can be emotionally draining for the woman and her family. Even if the preterm baby is healthy with no apparent life-threatening conditions, the woman and her family will likely be spending time visiting the baby in the NICU. Travel to and from the hospital and NICU observation can be physically exhausting. The mother is likely not to get adequate rest and nutrition for recovery. Nursing education prior to the mother's discharge should include an explanation of the importance of rest and proper diet to promote postpartum recovery. Some hospitals provide hospitality rooms for mothers and their families after discharge when the baby has to remain in the NICU. These accommodations can be helpful in avoiding maternal exhaustion and offer easy access to the baby. For a more in-depth review of nursing care for women who experience preterm birth and the implications for postpartum recovery, see Chapter 7.

Multiple Birth

A rise in the rate of multiple births, associated with older age at childbearing and greater use of assisted reproductive technologies and fertility drugs, has occurred (March of Dimes, 2017). Multiple births trend upward with a women's age, an increased tendency to delay childbirth has played a major part in rising rates. Women who have a multiple birth have special needs during the postpartum period for multiple reasons. They may have experienced antepartum bed rest and/or a cesarean birth and are likely to have preterm babies admitted to the NICU. As compared to singleton births (10%), in 2014, multiple birth babies were much more likely to be born preterm (twins: 59%, triplets and higher order births: 98%) and are more likely to need NICU care (March of Dimes, 2016). After the babies are discharged, mothers of multiples have additional responsibilities related to the condition and number of babies. Although often there are many offers of help for some families, as time goes on, the burden of ongoing care falls to the mother.

A recent meta-analysis of qualitative research about mothers of multiples revealed five themes that can help increase understanding of what the mother experiences caring for multiples during the first year of life. These themes include "bearing the burden," "riding an emotional roller coaster," "lifesaving support," "striving for maternal justice," and "acknowledging individuality" (Beck, 2002). The mother's experiences are helpful for nurses when reviewing realistic expectations with patients with multiple births for postpartum recovery and newborn care. For a complete discussion of the nursing care of women with multiple birth, see Chapter 11.

Perinatal Loss

Not all pregnancies end with birth of a healthy baby. Some women experience a pregnancy loss, stillbirth, or a neonatal death. Postpartum nursing care for these women can be a challenging and humbling experience. Nurses must examine their own thoughts, feelings, and assumptions about the death of a baby and the bereaved family. This self-examination covers preconceived ideas, judgments, and experiences of loss (Côté-Arsenault, 2011). To provide effective nursing care, the nurse must display an open and caring attitude expressed through appreciation and acceptance of validation of the experiences of the mother and her family (Côté-Arsenault, 2011). Sensitivity to the mother's wishes is critical. Some women who experience a perinatal loss may prefer a room on another unit away from the nursery and postpartum area. Other women prefer to be with nurses in labor and delivery or postpartum who are more comfortable with this type of loss. Ideally, the nursing unit is situated so these families do not have to come in contact with newborn infants. It is important to allow the woman and her family as much time as they need to be with their baby. The woman and her family's desires should guide postpartum nursing care. A comprehensive guide to caring for women who experience a perinatal loss is the March of Dimes nursing module *Loss and Grief in the Childbearing Period* (Côté-Arsenault, 2011).

POSTPARTUM LEARNING NEEDS

Planning for education during the postpartum period begins as soon as possible after inpatient admission. Ideally, women have had opportunities during the prenatal period to learn about postpartum and baby care by attending classes and reading appropriate materials. However, this may not be true for all pregnant women because of access to care issues, complications of pregnancy, unavailability of resources, language barriers, literacy issues, or lack of knowledge about existing programs. During the hospital stay, nurses need to take advantage of all of the potential opportunities for assessment and education of new mothers. Access, availability, and acceptability must be considered when providing postpartum education. All available resources may not be able to be integrated within the hospital stay. Closed-circuit educational television and printed materials collaboratively developed by obstetric and pediatric professionals are helpful to new parents. Individual and group educational sessions held regularly during the postpartum period are beneficial. Baby care and normal infant behaviors and expected maternal physical and psychological changes should be included in the educational plans for each mother. New mothers should be aware of available community and healthcare resources (AAP & ACOG, 2017).

Discharge processes that meet patient needs are not based on arbitrary discharge times rather when the woman can arrange for safe transportation. Nurses need enough time to make sure discharge teaching is comprehensive and individualized. A nurse-to-mother–baby couplet ratio of 1:3 should allow for adequate discharge teaching. Scheduling follow-up appointments before discharge can be invaluable. Some parents may not have transportation, so ability to get to the clinic should be assessed. If English is not the primary language, efforts should be made to make sure the information that is conveyed is understood. Translation services should be offered as needed. A list of local resources for breastfeeding assistance is useful if the hospital does not offer this service, as is a list of maternal and newborn signs and symptoms that should warrant a call to the provider along with their telephone numbers. With EHR use more widespread, transitions in care from inpatient to outpatient should be easier and more accurate; however, many EHRs in the outpatient setting still do not "talk" to hospitals' EHRs. Recommendations from Agency for Healthcare Research and Quality (2014) about hospital discharges for other populations apply to mothers and babies: Use whole-person transitional care for all patients; adapt processes as needed; identify patients at risk for readmission; communicate simply and effectively; link patients to follow-up and posthospital services; and give accurate, real-time information to receiving providers. A high-quality discharge process for new mothers and babies is a vital part of excellent maternity nursing care (Simpson, 2017a).

Selected Postpartum Teaching Topics

Pelvic Floor Exercises

Patient education should include instruction on pelvic muscle exercises. Kegel exercises help the woman to regain muscle tone lost as pelvic tissues are stretched. Each contraction should be held at least 10 seconds, with a 10-second or longer rest between contractions for muscular recovery. Women with third- or fourth-degree lacerations, a long second stage of labor, a large newborn, or a combination of these factors should be taught to report potential anal sphincter symptoms, such as incontinence of flatus or stool, to the primary healthcare provider.

Postpartum Exercise

A thorough clinical evaluation should be conducted before recommending an exercise program to ensure that a patient does not have a medical reason to avoid exercise. Exercise may begin soon after birth with simple exercises such as arm raises, leg rolls, and buttock lifts. Walking works well to get back to prepregnancy shape. After cesarean birth, abdominal exercises should be postponed for 4 weeks. Exercise benefits the mood, self-image, and energy level and improves or maintains muscular endurance, strength, and tone but only if the exercise is stress relieving rather than stress provoking (ACOG, 2015). Women who exercise demonstrate better scores on measures of postpartum adaptation and are more likely to engage in social activities, hobbies, and entertainment.

Regular physical activity during pregnancy improves or maintains physical fitness, helps with weight management, and enhances psychologic well-being. An exercise program that leads to an eventual goal of moderate-intensity exercise for at least 20 to 30 min/day on most or all days of the week should be developed with the patient and adjusted as medically indicated.

Studies have shown that exercise during pregnancy can contribute to controlling glucose levels in women with gestational diabetes (Padayachee & Coombes, 2015). Exercise has shown only a modest decrease in overall weight gain (1 to 2 kg) in normal weight, overweight, and obese women (ACOG, 2015). Discharge instructions should include written information regarding activity, rest, and exercise for women who have given birth vaginally or by cesarean. Women should be instructed to listen to their bodies and avoid fatigue and pain.

Sexuality

Sexuality is one of the least understood and most superficially discussed topics by healthcare providers during a woman's postpartum experience. Sexuality encompasses physical capacity for sexual arousal and pleasure (i.e., libido), personalized and shared social meanings attached to sexual behavior, and formation of sexual and gender identities. Sexuality and gender attitudes and behaviors carry profound significance for women and men in every society. Sexuality is a vital component of physical and emotional well-being for men and women. Display 17–5 lists factors contributing to decline in sexual interest during the postpartum period.

Nurses must assume responsibility for anticipatory guidance, reassurance, and counseling or referral. Research about dyspareunia (i.e., painful intercourse) suggests some nontraditional forms of therapy, such as counseling, physiotherapy, acupuncture, and ultrasound, may be helpful. Information about sexuality can be provided to the couple prenatally and after birth. Knowledge about normal physiologic and emotional changes allows the couple to discuss coping mechanisms and alternate means of maintaining intimacy during this challenging period. Education about sexuality during the postpartum period should include the following information:

- Although it is recommended for the woman to wait a few weeks postbirth to resume sexual intercourse to aid in the healing process (some providers still recommend waiting until the 6-week postpartum visit), it is ultimately the woman's decision.
- Sexual intercourse should be avoided until vaginal bleeding has stopped.
- A water-soluble gel may be necessary for additional lubrication.
- It is vital to include a discussion about birth control during this discussion since women can get pregnant prior to regaining her menstrual cycle.

Contraception

The infant feeding method and the involution process influence the woman's choice and use of postpartum contraception. Ideally, the primary healthcare provider has discussed the choice, use, advantages, and disadvantages of a variety of contraceptive methods with both partners during prenatal care. The nurse should encourage the woman to ask questions regarding contraception prior to discharge from the hospital. Although many couples wait 4 to 6 weeks after birth to resume sexual relations, some couples choose earlier resumption; thus, it is important to have this discussion while still in the hospital and not wait until the first postpartum office or clinic visit. Consideration of the couple's needs and preferences is important when selecting a contraceptive method that is acceptable and effective for their unique situation. This approach allows sharing of responsibility, an opportunity to discuss advantages and disadvantages of methods, clarification of misconceptions, and discussion of prevention of sexually transmitted infections (STIs). Information about contraception should include effectiveness, acceptability, and safety. Some of the available options for women and their partners are described in the following sections. This list is not all-inclusive. Although it is not the responsibility of the postpartum nurse to provide in-depth counseling to women regarding contraception, some basic knowledge is necessary if women have questions and if these types of discussions are not discouraged because of the institution's religious affiliation.

The CDC (2011) recommends that women do not begin combined hormonal contraceptives for at least 21 days postpartum due to the high risk of developing a venous thromboembolism. There are methods of birth control that can be initiated in the immediate postpartum period such as progestin-only pills, depot medroxyprogesterone acetate injections (aka Depo), or implants and intrauterine devices (IUDs) (CDC, 2018). Each have various levels of effectiveness (CDC, 2011, 2018; Peragallo Urrutia et al., 2018).

DISPLAY 17–5

Factors Contributing to a Decline in Sexual Interest or Activity during the Postpartum Period

- Fatigue
- Fear of not hearing the infant
- Emotional distress on a continuum from baby blues to postpartum depression
- Adjustments to role change
- Hormonal changes
- Physical discomfort related to changes of vulva, vagina, perineum, and breasts
- Breastfeeding
- Decreased sense of attractiveness

Depo-Provera

- Injections are given four times each year (150 mg given intramuscularly in the deltoid or gluteus maximus).
- The effectiveness rate is 96%.
- Advantages include long-lasting action, unimpaired lactation, and independence from coitus.
- Disadvantages include prolonged amenorrhea or uterine bleeding, weight gain, increased risk of venous thrombosis and thromboembolism, no STI protection, need for continued injections, fluid retention or edema, abdominal discomfort, decrease in bone density, and glucose intolerance.

Implanon

- The subdermal implant is inserted surgically and provides up to 3 years of contraception.
- The effectiveness rate is 99%.
- Advantages include long-lasting and reversible action.
- Disadvantages include menstrual irregularities, need for surgical removal, headaches, weight gain, breast pain, nervousness, nausea, skin changes, vertigo, no STI protection, and raised area on the arm.

Oral Contraceptives—Combined Estrogen–Progestin

- Dosage is one pill each day.
- The effectiveness rate is 93%.
- Advantages include coitus independent; decreased menstrual blood loss; decreased incidence of dysmenorrhea and premenstrual syndrome; reduction in endometrial adenocarcinoma, ovarian cancer, and benign breast disease; improvement in acne; protection against development of functional ovarian cysts; and decreased risk of ectopic pregnancy (Ladewig et al., 2017).
- Disadvantages include contraindications for women with a history of thromboembolic disorders; cerebrovascular or coronary artery disease; breast cancer; estrogen-dependent tumors; pregnancy; impaired liver function or tumors; hypertension; or diabetes of 20 years' duration; and for women who smoke (if older than 35 years), are lactating, or have had a period of immobilization (Ladewig et al., 2017). The drug can cause libido changes, breast tenderness, weight gain, nausea, and a delay in return of fertility.

Oral Contraceptives—Progestin-Only

- Dosage is one pill each day.
- The effectiveness rate is 93%.
- In addition to the advantages of oral contraceptives listed previously, lactation is not impaired by this formulation, which is less likely to cause cardiovascular complications, headaches, or hypertension.
- In addition to the disadvantages of oral contraceptives listed previously, drug interactions are more likely, and irregular bleeding, amenorrhea, and functional ovarian cysts can occur. The pill must be taken at same time each day.

Barrier Methods

- Device must be used at the time of sexual act.
- The effectiveness rate is 73% to 87%, depending on the device.
- Advantages include prevention of pregnancy, STIs, or both (used in combination with spermicides to achieve maximal protection); newer male condoms have various lengths, shapes, and adhesives.
- Female condom has two rings connected by a polyurethane sheath. The inner ring is fitted like a diaphragm; the outer ring protects the vulva and prevents slipping. It has a 21% failure rate.
- A diaphragm covers the cervix and requires fitting by healthcare professional. Its effectiveness is increased with the use of spermicide. It must be refitted after weight loss or gain greater than 22 kg and after birth. It has a 17% failure rate.
- A male condom is a latex or synthetic sheath placed over the erect penis before coitus. It must be applied before penile–vulvar contact and removed before the penis becomes flaccid to prevent sperm leakage at withdrawal. It has a 13% failure rate.

Chemical Methods (Spermicidal Creams, Jellies, Foams, Suppositories, and Vaginal Film Containing Nonoxynol-9)

- Agent must be used at the time of the sex act.
- The effectiveness rate is 50% to 95%.
- Advantages include ease of application, safety, low cost, no prescription required, and help in lubrication.
- Disadvantages include a maximum effect that lasts no longer than 1 hour, required reapplication for repeat intercourse, possibility of an allergic response or irritation, and messiness.

Intrauterine Devices

- No action is required at time of intercourse.
- Two types are approved for use in United States:
  Copper IUDs—can be placed in the uterus and can last up to 10 years
  Hormonal IUDs—can be placed in the uterus and can last from 3 to 7 years depending on the brand.
- The effectiveness rate is 99%.
- Advantages include use for postpartum and breastfeeding women, long-term and continuous use requiring minimal effort, and no continual expense.
- Disadvantages include contraindications for women with a history of pelvic inflammatory disease or STIs; need for professional insertion; and generation of cramping, pain, and bleeding, which should be evaluated.

Postpartum Tubal Ligation/Vasectomy (Sterilization)

- It requires no additional effort after surgical procedure.
- The effectiveness rate is 99.5% (female) to 99.9% (male).

- Advantages include no need for additional contraception (should be considered permanent although reversal is technically possible).
- Its disadvantage is no STI protection.
- Before surgery, appropriate counseling is necessary regarding risks of failure, surgical risks, and potential psychosocial reactions to the procedure. A signed consent form according to institutional protocol is required.

Natural Family Planning

- It relies on fertility awareness, observations, and abstinence during the fertile portion of a woman's menstrual cycle.
- It requires an understanding of the changes occurring in a woman's ovulatory cycle.
- The fertile period is calculated with a set formula, basal body temperature, cervical mucus assessment, symptothermal techniques (i.e., combines body temperature and cervical mucus assessment), or over-the-counter ovulation test kit (i.e., Creighton Model, Billings Method, or Sympto Thermal).
- Advantages include a couple-centered method, low cost, lack of harm to fertility, no side effects, usefulness in diagnosing gynecologic disorders and infertility, and use in achieving pregnancy when desired.
- Disadvantages include no STI protection, difficult application during irregular cycles postpartum, need to begin charting 3 weeks after birth, and ovulation possibly occurring before the first postpartum menses (Ladewig et al., 2017).

PSYCHOLOGICAL ADAPTATION TO THE POSTPARTUM PERIOD

Postpartum Mood and Anxiety Disorders

Women with postpartum depression report feeling very alone and helpless. Although family members notice abnormal changes in the woman's mood and behavior, they frequently underestimate the extent of the illness. Women are told by well-meaning others that they just have the "baby blues" and they should snap out of it and take care of their beautiful baby. Women suffering from postpartum depression wish it could be that easy. Prompt diagnosis and treatment is needed for postpartum depression. Nurses can be helpful in identifying women who could benefit from referral and treatment.

During the postpartum hospital stay, the new mother has to move quickly from self-concern to other-concern: her baby. It is important that her physical and psychological needs be met so that she will be better able to focus on her newborn's care. She may become intensely focused on the cognitive learning needs related to newborn feeding and physical care. The new mother may verbalize anxiety and concern. If so, she needs to be heard, and her concerns must be validated. The newly evolving relationship between the mother and her newborn is based on connection and care. If the woman has difficulty with these beginning skills, it may alter her self-esteem and maternal development. Postpartum depression can negatively affect the mother–infant interaction during the first 12 months after birth (Beck, 2008). The nurse can assist the mother in this attachment process by establishing a responsive, nurturing environment; maximizing mother–infant contact; and assisting the mother to understand the newborn's behaviors (Ghadery-Sefat, Abdeyazdan, Badiee, & Zargham-Boroujeni, 2016).

The woman brings with her many performance expectations that need to be discussed and clarified. Mercer (1986) described maternal role attainment as a process that takes a period of about 10 months to develop. During this postpartum phase, the new mother attaches to her newborn, gains competence as a mother, and should express gratification in the mother–baby interaction. This adaptation can be delayed or altered if the woman's health and mental status is less than optimal. The reality of the current healthcare delivery system is that much of the work of the postpartum maternal adjustment and role attainment is done after discharge. Referral to community resources and discharge planning are thus imperative in the total care plan.

Emotionally, the early days after giving birth can be disconcerting. It is supposed to be such an exciting time, but in reality, the new mother may be experiencing alternating periods of crying and joy, irritability, anxiety, headaches, confusion, forgetfulness, depersonalization, and fatigue. These are characteristics of the "baby blues." About 4 in 5 new moms (80%) of new mothers experience this transitory mood disorder (March of Dimes, 2017). Unfortunately, this phenomenon occurs so frequently that it is often considered normal and therefore does not get the attention that it deserves.

Postpartum depression may be biologic, psychologic, situational, or multifactorial (Beck, 2002; Beck & Indman, 2005). It is felt that this disorder is related to the normal physiologic and psychosocial changes that occur in the process of becoming a new mother. The rapid decrease in the levels of female reproductive hormones after birth may dysregulate the complex balance of neurotransmitters, stress hormones, and reproductive hormones (Driscoll, 2006b). Having the "baby blues" can greatly affect the new mother and her family, especially if they are unaware of the possibility or what to do about it.

Women and their families need information about normal mood changes after childbirth. They should be aware that with a lot of support, reassurance, rest, and good nutrition, these labile moods usually balance out, and the woman will begin to feel better and feel more organized and confident. However, if the moods do not stabilize, referral should be made to the psychiatric/mental health team specialists in postpartum mood and anxiety disorders (Driscoll, 2006a). Inpatient perinatal nurses interact with women during the first days after birth and are in the position to make initial assessments of mother–baby interactions and mood alterations. An important aspect of this nursing assessment is determining when the mother's behaviors are beyond normal "baby blues" and pathologic such as postpartum depression (Beck, 2006). This is challenging because alterations in mood are common during the immediate hours after labor and birth. An awareness of the risk factors for postpartum depression facilitates prompt diagnosis, treatment, and early recovery (Display 17–6). Because most postpartum LOSs are 1 to 4 days, there is a greater likelihood of mood disorders occurring at home rather than in the hospital environment. If a follow-up appointment with a healthcare provider occurs at 4 to 6 weeks after birth, the woman experiences these conditions alone, without medical or nursing support. Thus, women and their families need anticipatory information about postpartum mood disorders so that prompt identification and early treatment can be initiated. A heightened awareness among perinatal healthcare providers about the incidence of postpartum mood and anxiety disorders, knowledge of common signs and symptoms, and the prospects for recovery can contribute to successful outcomes for affected women and their families.

Each woman should be routinely assessed for maternal mental status and adjustment and mood disorders as a standard part of postpartum clinical nursing assessments (Driscoll, 2006a, 2006b). This assessment is facilitated by a professional nurse who is willing to listen to the woman's birth experience, observant of mother–baby interactions, and knowledgeable about the normal physiologic adaptations that are similar to symptoms of depression such as appetite fluctuations, fatigue, and decreased libido. Prior to discharge from the hospital, the woman should be given a list of telephone numbers of her care providers as well as any emergency services that she may need. It is important to go over the key support people with the new mother and her partner during discharge teaching. When home visits by skilled perinatal nurses are available, the nurse should include a thorough assessment of the psychological adaptation of the new mother.

Psychiatric professionals have several instruments available for assessing women for postpartum depression (Display 17–7). These assessments require careful planning and knowledge about the instruments themselves and appropriate referral options. If perinatal care providers are knowledgeable about the woman's psychological well-being, appropriate referral and early identification of these disorders can be made, thus potentially preventing a crisis. Preparation for appropriate assessments and interventions can result from interdisciplinary efforts involving physicians, nurse practitioners, nurse midwives, nurses, perinatal educators, lactation consultants, and support services such as social services and counselors. Educational programs sponsored by experts in postpartum mood disorders can be helpful to increase awareness and lead to appropriate, timely referral. Educational programs should also be offered within the community to increase public awareness and knowledge of available resources.

DISPLAY 17–6

Risk Factors for Postpartum Depression

- Prenatal depression
- Low self-esteem
- Stress of child care
- Prenatal anxiety
- Life stress
- Lack of social support
- Marital relationship problems
- History of depression
- "Difficult" infant temperament
- Postpartum blues
- Single status
- Low socioeconomic status
- Unplanned or unwanted pregnancy
- Young maternal age

Adapted from Beck, C. (2001). Predictors of postpartum depression: An update. *Nursing Research, 50*(5), 275–285; Beck, C. (2002). Revision of the Postpartum Depression Predictors Inventory. *Journal of Obstetric, Gynecologic, and Neonatal Nursing, 31*(4), 394–402; Breese McCoy, S., J. (2011). Postpartum depression: An essential overview for the practitioner. *Southern Medical Journal, 104*(2), 128–132; Records, K., Rice, M. J., & Beck, C. T. (2007). Psychometric assessment of the Postpartum Depression Predictors Inventory-Revised. *Journal of Nursing Measurement, 15*(3), 189–202.

DISPLAY 17–7

Instruments for Assessing Postpartum Depression, Mood Disorders, and Psychosis

- Edinburgh Postnatal Depression Scale (EPDS) (Cox, Holden, & Sagovsky, 1987)
- Postpartum Depression Predictors Inventory (PDPI)-Revised (Beck, 2001, 2002; Records, Rice, & Beck, 2007)
- Postpartum Depression Checklist (PDC) (Beck, 2001, 2002; Beck, Records, & Rice, 2006)
- Brisbane Postnatal Depression Index (Webster, Pritchard, Creedy, & East, 2003)
- Schedule for Affective Disorders and Schizophrenia (SADS) (Beck & Gable, 2005)
- Postpartum Depression Screening Scale (PDSS) (Beck & Gable, 2005)

Validating the woman's experience as normal may provide needed reassurance. Talking with the woman in a familiar, comfortable environment about the stresses and challenges of new motherhood provides opportunities for early interventions, such as counseling, referrals to support services, and pharmacologic assistance. Help with infant and self-care, coupled with support from family members, promotes recovery. Providing appropriate interventions and therapy has far-reaching effects—improving the health of the women, their infants, and the family itself. These interventions become an investment in the future.

Psychosocial adaptation to pregnancy and postpartum is a dynamic process. The nurse plays a significant role in the promotion and facilitation of this experience in a healthy way. It is a time when the woman is open to great psychological growth and relies on the healthcare team for information and support. The nurse needs to be aware of the normal process in order to identify those that are abnormal. It is helpful in the assessment of mood, anxiety, and emotional states to remember three words: *frequency, duration, and intensity*. If the woman describes that she is having difficulty functioning in her activities of daily living and having a tough time coping due to emotional, mood, and/or anxiety changes, referral is necessary. The referral process needs to be managed in an empowering, supportive way. Letting her know that she is valued and her concerns and feelings are important is a way for the perinatal nurse to give the woman the message that she deserves good care. Appropriate healthcare provider attitudes support the referral process. Due to the rapid changes in the healthcare delivery system and decreasing lengths of stay, it is imperative for the perinatal nurse to actively pursue, nurture, and promote collaborative relationships with colleagues in the community. It is this active communication and relational approach to the care of this new mother and her family that will promote, facilitate, and encourage healthy maternal and paternal psychosocial adaptation and adjustment.

FATIGUE

The first 6 weeks after giving birth are a time of change and adjustment for the woman and the family. Fatigue, stress, depression, and infection are interrelated in postpartum mothers. These variables change over time, possibly placing mothers and infants in a psychoneuroimmunologically vulnerable group (Groër et al., 2005). The variables reinforce one another and make it difficult to determine which occurs first, fatigue causing depression and stress or the reverse. Their alteration of immune function in new mothers may result in increased vulnerability to infection. In the breastfeeding woman, fatigue is associated with increased levels of melatonin in the mother's milk, which is transferred to the infant and influence the sleep–wake cycle. Fatigue affects emotional adjustment and adaptation to the maternal role, and it may cause feelings of inadequacy in meeting the needs of other family members and in assuming household responsibilities. Anticipatory guidance in identifying rest opportunities and organizing new responsibilities and tasks is important for the new mother. Education about the causes of fatigue and possible community and family resources enables the new mother to assume control and promotes problem-solving behaviors. Together, the nurse and woman can develop strategies for requesting help with newborn care, household chores, and sibling care. Listing daily and weekly tasks provides an organizational framework and may serve as a readily available wish list that can be used when family and friends offer to help. Identification of family members and friends available to help provides an initial supportive structure for the new family.

FAMILY TRANSITION TO PARENTHOOD

After birth, the woman experiences psychological changes as well as physiologic reversal of the physical changes of pregnancy. For the woman, adoption of a maternal role begins during pregnancy as she develops an attachment to the fetus. This role evolution continues postpartum with the birth separation of the mother–infant pair, or polarization (Rubin, 1977). As the mother develops her style of parenting, she considers her behavior in relation to the infant and notices familial characteristics in the infant. These changes in the mother are referred to as maternal role attainment (Mercer, 1995). Mercer (1995) identified four stages in this process: anticipatory, formal, informal, and personal. The anticipatory stage, occurring during pregnancy, involves the observation of role models for mothering behaviors. During the formal stage, the new mother tries to perform infant care tasks as expected by others. The mother begins to make personal choices about mothering during the informal stage and attains comfort with the role during the personal stage. The final stages, informal and formal, correspond to the taking-in and taking-hold stages identified by Rubin (1961a). During the taking-in phase (first 24 hours or longer), the woman relives the birth experience, clarifies her understanding of the experience, and focuses on food and sleep. The taking-hold phase (second to fourth day) centers on concern with bodily functions, and the woman focuses on regaining control over her life and succeeding in infant-care responsibilities. Rubin (1961b) includes the letting-go phase to describe the new mother's letting go of who she was and full participation in the mothering role. Nurses can foster success in these processes by meeting the woman's needs during each stage and providing a supportive environment for listening and educating the new mother.

Paternal satisfaction with the birth experience and its associated stresses influences marital happiness and family life. For most women, being comfortable as a mother occurs during the first 3 to 10 months after birth. Nursing assessments about the quality of parenting behaviors during the postpartum period can guide the educational plan for the new couple. Display 17–8 lists adaptive and maladaptive parenting behaviors. Evidence of maladaptive parenting behaviors should prompt nursing communication with the primary healthcare provider and appropriate referral.

Nurses caring for women and families during the postpartum period must consider their cultural expectations and norms when planning care. This requires an open-minded, sensitive, and creative approach. Knowledge about various traditions and services within ethnic groups and a willingness to give up control demonstrate respect and encourage a collaborative approach to providing these women with a positive and satisfying birth experience. We must accept that maternity care system has a culture that may class with the cultures of our clients (Lewallen, 2011).

The changes that occur within the family are not limited to the woman. The family, however it is defined, experiences changes in structure and process. Parents adapt to these changes more easily when they are involved with a support network. This network may include family, friends, and institutional components. New parents often report a change in their immediate

DISPLAY 17–8
Adaptive and Maladaptive Parenting Behaviors

	Adaptive	Maladaptive
Feeding	Provides an appropriate amount and type of food	Makes inappropriate types or inadequate amounts of food available
	Burps the child both during and after feeding	Does not burp the baby, although she or he knows it is necessary to do so
	Prepares the meal appropriately	Prepares the meal inappropriately
	Feeds the infant regularly and as frequently as necessary	Rushes or delays feeding the child
Rest	Provides a quiet and relaxed environment for the resting baby	Does not provide a quiet and relaxed environment
	Schedules rest periods	Does not schedule rest periods
Stimulating caring for infant	Speaks to the child and makes other appropriate sounds	Speaks aggressively or not at all to the infant
	Provides tactile stimulation at a variety of times and not only when the baby is hungry or in danger	Plays aggressively with the baby or does not touch her or him
	Provides age-appropriate toys	Provides inappropriate toys
	Positions infant comfortably while holding the child	Does not hold the baby or ignores child's discomfort when being held
	The baby seems satisfied with the way it is being handled	The baby seems frustrated with the way it is handled
	Sees that the baby is dry, warm, and not hungry	Does not care for the baby who is hungry, cold, or soiled
	Exhibits initiative in trying to find how to deal with the baby's problems	Lacks initiative and does not try to meet the baby's needs
Self-perception/ emotional state of parent	Usually maintains a realistic perception of and realistic expectations for the baby	Develops distorted perceptions of and unrealistic expectations for the baby
	Exhibits a realistic perception of her or his own mothering and fathering abilities	Holds unrealistic expectations of her or his own parenting abilities
	Shows some interest in understanding and/or discussing the childbirth	Is unable or unwilling to discuss the childbirth
	Exhibits friendly or neutral behavior with other children	Exhibits hostility/aggression toward other children
	Appears generally satisfied to be a parent	Appears dissatisfied to be a parent
	Is able or willing to turn to other people for social support when necessary	Is unable to provide adequately for relaxation and own emotional needs
		Is isolated and without adequate social support
		Is depressed

social network. This change typically involves increased contact with other new parents or with families facing similar challenges. For new parents living without immediate access to family, referral to support groups sponsored by hospitals or community centers may provide an opening into a circle of new parents and friends. New parents may place increased importance on family and the traditions they include. For other couples, increased familial contacts may result in an increased level of stress as the new family attempts to meet the external demands placed on them by enthusiastic or demanding family members. If the new mother decides not to return to a work environment outside the home, she may face the challenge of redefining herself. Individuals respond differently to life changes, other areas that may prove stressful to certain individuals include physical changes and complications, role-adaptation conflicts, newborn needs, relationship changes, returning to the work, and/or selecting a child care setting.

Nurses caring for families during this time can provide anticipatory guidance about possible areas of stress and options for stress reduction. Providing this information in a written format enables the couple to review the information as situations develop.

POSTPARTUM DISCHARGE FOLLOW-UP

In response to the current LOS, many perinatal centers now offer postdischarge follow-up home visits, clinic visits, or telephone calls. The AAP (2015) Committee on the Fetus and Newborn recommends that newborns discharged less than 48 hours after birth, be examined by a licensed healthcare professional, preferably within 48 hours of discharge based on risk factors but no later than 72 hours in most cases so that infections, poor infant feeding, excessive weight loss, jaundice, and other problems may be identified in a timely manner.

In-person follow-up visits afford the perinatal nurse an opportunity to carefully assess maternal and infant well-being and provide the family with continuing education and support. When in-person follow-up visits are not offered, a postdischarge phone call gives families another opportunity to ask questions and receive important information and referrals. The perinatal nurse can use a standardized assessment tool to ask the family about infant feeding and elimination patterns, cord care, infant appearance and behavior maternal comfort, lochia flow, perineal care, breast care, and maternal emotional well-being (Display 17–9). The nurse should ask the mother if she has any concerns about herself or her infant and reminds the mother about specific situations that would warrant a telephone call to the healthcare provider. Medical complications identified during the visit are immediately referred to the primary healthcare provider. Other issues or concerns

are addressed during the visit or referred to an appropriate resource. This assessment visit can take place in a home or clinic setting as long as the nurse examining the infant is competent in newborn assessment and the results of the follow-up visit are reported to the infant's physician or his or her designees on the day of the visit. The visit should include the following:

- Infant weight, general health, hydration, and degree of jaundice (if present)
- Identification of any new problems
- Review of feeding patterns and technique, including observation of breastfeeding for adequacy of position, latch-on, and swallowing
- Historical evidence of adequate urination and stool patterns
- Assessment of quality of mother–infant interaction and infant behavior
- Reinforcement of maternal or family education in infant care, particularly regarding infant feeding
- Review of outstanding results of laboratory tests performed before discharge
- Performance of screening tests in accordance with state regulations and other tests that are clinically indicated, such as serum bilirubin
- Verification of the plan for healthcare maintenance, including a method for obtaining emergency services, preventive care and immunizations, periodic evaluations and physical examinations, and necessary screenings (AAP & ACOG, 2017)

Maternal postpartum care should be consistent, comprehensive, and organized to ensure that all women and their infants receive the care and support they need (ACOG, 2018a). Ideally, all women should receive a postdischarge visit or telephone call. If resources are limited, the following criteria define circumstances where postdischarge follow-up is essential:

- LOS less than 24 hours after a vaginal birth
- LOS less than 48 hours after a cesarean birth
- Limited or no prenatal care
- Infant feeding problems identified during hospital stay
- Infant gestational age less than 37 completed weeks
- Multiple birth
- Risk factors for developing hyperbilirubinemia
- Maternal or infant health conditions putting mother or infant at risk for complications
- Lack of adequate support system
- Women who express or show they feel overwhelmed, very anxious, or depressed
- Discharge evaluation indicates need for further teaching.

The nurse providing postdischarge follow-up should have access to essential patient information including maternal age, health history, birth information, newborn

DISPLAY 17–9

Postpartum Follow-up Telephone Call Report

Mother: Age _____   G/P _____   Vaginal birth _____   Cesarean birth _____

Marital status: S M W   Discharge date: _____

Baby: Sex: M F   Gestational age: _____

Newborn birth weight _____   Discharge weight: _____

Breast _____   Formula _____   Person making call: _____

BABY CARE	NO CONCERNS	PROBLEM IDENTIFIED	SUGGESTION MADE
Circumcision assessment			
Cord assessment			
Jaundice			
Changes in newborn:			
Behavior			
Feeding			
Temperature			
Breastfeeding:			
No. of wet diapers			
No. of and character of stools			
Latch-on/positioning			
Frequency of feeding/24 hours			
Breast and nipple assessment:			
Sore nipples			
Cracked nipples			
Breast fullness			
Suck/swallow assessment			
Other concerns			
Formula feeding:			
No. of wet diapers			
No. of and characteristics of stools			
Ounces/feedings			
Frequency of feedings			
Skin appearance			
Sleep patterns			
Ability to care for newborn			
MATERNAL CARE	NO CONCERNS	PROBLEM IDENTIFIED	SUGGESTION MADE
Lochia			
Episiotomy			
Incision			
Discomforts:			
Breast			
Perineal			
Incisional			
Cramping			

(continued)

DISPLAY 17-9
Postpartum Follow-up Telephone Call Report (Continued)

MATERNAL CARE	NO CONCERNS	PROBLEM IDENTIFIED	SUGGESTION MADE
Calf/leg tenderness			
Hemorrhoids			
Postbirth warning signs			
Voiding:			
Frequency			
Dysuria			
Bowel movement			
Emotional:			
Weepy			
Fatigue			
Sadness			
Onset of feelings			
Adequate rest:			
Taking naps			
Sleeps well when baby sleeps			
Other			
Ability to care for self			
REFERRALS	DATE	PROBLEM IDENTIFIED	SUGGESTION MADE
Lactation consultant			
Social services			
Physician			
Clinical specialist			
Home healthcare			
WIC			
Other			

assessment, infant weight, method of infant feeding, and name of the infant's and mother's healthcare providers. The nurse's assessment is documented and maintained as part of the permanent medical record.

Maternal postpartum assessments should include physiologic and psychological aspects. Regardless of when the new mother is seen, providers should assess for potential complications such as those outlined in the Postbirth Warning Signs educational handout that can be offered to all women before postpartum discharge (Display 17–10) (Bingham, Suplee, Morris, McBride, 2018; Suplee, Kleppel, Santa-Donato, & Bingham, 2017). Additional information should include education about nutrition, weight loss, self-image, exercise, sexual activity, activity, rest, and birth control. See Display 17–11 for examples of a Postpartum Discharge Education Checklist with detailed information to be shared with the new mother prior

to discharge from the hospital that is supplemental to the patient handout on POST-BIRTH Warning Signs (Suplee et al., 2017).

Since significant maternal morbidity and mortality are known to occur in the first few weeks postpartum, ACOG (2018a) has made substantial recommendations for changes to routine postpartum care. They are summarized as follows:

• Postpartum care must be an ongoing process, rather than a single visit, with services and support individualized for each woman
• A plan for postpartum care that covers the transition to parenthood and well-woman care should be developed in partnership with the woman during the prenatal period.
• The woman's reproductive life plans, including desire for and timing of any future pregnancies should be

DISPLAY 17–10
Postbirth Warning Signs: Handout for Patients

SAVE YOUR LIFE:

Get Care for These POST-BIRTH Warning Signs

Most women who give birth recover without problems. **But any woman can have complications after giving birth.** Learning to recognize these POST-BIRTH warning signs and knowing what to do can save your life.

POST-BIRTH WARNING SIGNS

Call 911 if you have:

- ❑ **Pain in chest**
- ❑ **Obstructed breathing or shortness of breath**
- ❑ **Seizures**
- ❑ **Thoughts of hurting yourself or someone else**

Call your healthcare provider if you have:

(If you can't reach your healthcare provider, call 911 or go to an emergency room)

- ❑ **Bleeding, soaking through one pad/hour, or blood clots, the size of an egg or bigger**
- ❑ **Incision that is not healing**
- ❑ **Red or swollen leg, that is painful or warm to touch**
- ❑ **Temperature of 100.4°F or higher**
- ❑ **Headache that does not get better, even after taking medicine, or bad headache with vision changes**

Trust your instincts. ALWAYS get medical care if you are not feeling well or have questions or concerns.

Tell 911 or your healthcare provider:

"I gave birth on _____ and
(Date)

I am having _____."
(Specific warning signs)

These post-birth warning signs can become life-threatening if you don't receive medical care right away because:

- **Pain in chest, obstructed breathing or shortness of breath** (trouble catching your breath) may mean you have a blood clot in your lung or a heart problem
- **Seizures** may mean you have a condition called eclampsia
- **Thoughts or feelings of wanting to hurt yourself or someone else** may mean you have postpartum depression
- **Bleeding (heavy)**, soaking more than one pad in an hour or passing an egg-sized clot or bigger may mean you have an obstetric hemorrhage

- **Incision that is not healing, increased redness or any pus** from episiotomy or C-section site may mean you have an infection
- **Redness, swelling, warmth, or pain** in the calf area of your leg may mean you have a blood clot
- **Temperature of 100.4°F or higher, bad smelling vaginal blood or discharge** may mean you have an infection
- **Headache (very painful), vision changes, or pain in the upper right area of your belly** may mean you have high blood pressure or post birth preeclampsia

GET HELP

My Healthcare Provider/Clinic: _____   Phone Number: _____

Hospital Closest To Me: _____

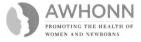

AWHONN
PROMOTING THE HEALTH OF WOMEN AND NEWBORNS

This program is supported by funding from Merck, through Merck for Mothers, the company's 10-year, $500 million initiative to help create a world where no woman dies giving life. Merck for Mothers is known as MSD for Mothers outside the United States and Canada.

Adapted from Association of Women's Health, Obstetric and Neonatal Nurses. Suplee, P. D., Kleppel, L., Santa-Donato, A., & Bingham, D. (2016). Improving postpartum education about warning signs of maternal morbidity and mortality. *Nursing for Women's Health, 20*(6), 552–567.

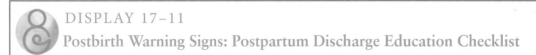

DISPLAY 17–11

Postbirth Warning Signs: Postpartum Discharge Education Checklist

POST-BIRTH WARNING SIGNS:

POSTPARTUM DISCHARGE EDUCATION CHECKLIST

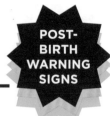

POST-BIRTH WARNING SIGNS

This checklist is a teaching guide for nurses to use when educating all women about the essential warning signs that can result in maternal morbidity and/or mortality.

Instructions:

- Instruct ALL women about all of the following potential complications. All teaching should be documented on this form or in your facility's electronic health record.
- Focus on risk factors for a specific complication first; then review all warning signs.
- Emphasize that women do not have to experience ALL of the signs in each category for them to seek care.
- Encourage the woman's significant other or her designated family members to be included in education whenever possible.

The information included on this checklist is organized according to complications that can result in severe maternal morbidity or maternal mortality. Essential teaching points should be included in all postpartum discharge teaching.

The parent handout, "Save Your Life", is designed to reinforce this teaching. This handout is organized according to AWHONN's acronym, POST-BIRTH, to help everyone remember the key warning signs and when to call 911 or a health provider. A portion of this handout is below for reference.

Call 911 if you have:	❑ **Pain in chest** ❑ **Obstructed breathing or shortness of breath** ❑ **Seizures** ❑ **Thoughts of hurting yourself or your baby**
Call your healthcare provider if you have: (If you can't reach your healthcare provider, call 911 or go to an emergency room)	❑ **Bleeding, soaking through one pad/hour, or blood clots, the size of an egg or bigger** ❑ **Incision that is not healing** ❑ **Red or swollen leg, that is painful or warm to touch** ❑ **Temperature of 100.4°F or higher** ❑ **Headache that does not get better, even after taking medicine, or bad headache with vision changes**

Below is a suggested conversation-starter:

"*Although most women who give birth recover without problems, any woman can have complications after the birth of a baby. Learning to recognize these POST-BIRTH warning signs and knowing what to do can save your life. I would like to go over these POST-BIRTH warning signs with you now, so you will know what to look for and when to call 911 or when to call your healthcare provider.*

Please share this with family and friends and post the "Save Your Life" handout in a place where you can get to it easily (like your refrigerator)."

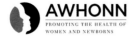

AWHONN PROMOTING THE HEALTH OF WOMEN AND NEWBORNS

This program is supported by funding from Merck, through Merck for Mothers, the company's 10-year, $500 million initiative to help create a world where no woman dies giving life. Merck for Mothers is known as MSD for Mothers outside the United States and Canada.

©2017 Association of Women's Health, Obstetric, and Neonatal Nurses. All rights reserved. Requests for permission to use or reproduce should be directed to permissions@awhonn.org.

(continued)

DISPLAY 17–11
Postbirth Warning Signs: Postpartum Discharge Education Checklist (*Continued*)

POST-BIRTH Warning Signs:
Postpartum Discharge
Education Checklist

Pulmonary Embolism	Essential Teaching for Women
What is Pulmonary Embolism?	Pulmonary embolism is a blood clot that has traveled to your lung.
Signs of Pulmonary Embolism	• Shortness of breath at rest (e.g., tachypneic shallow, rapid respirations) • Chest pain that worsens when coughing • Change in level of consciousness
Obtaining Immediate Care	Call 911 or go to nearest emergency room **RIGHT AWAY**.

RN initials_____ Date_____ Family/support person present? YES / NO

Cardiac (Heart) Disease	Essential Teaching for Women
What is Cardiac Disease?	Cardiac disease is when your heart is not working as well as it should and can include a number of disorders that may have different signs and symptoms.
Signs of Potential Cardiac Emergency	• Shortness of breath or difficulty breathing • Heart palpitations (feeling that your heart is racing) • Chest pain or pressure
Obtaining Immediate Care	Call 911 or go to nearest emergency room **RIGHT AWAY**.

RN initials_____ Date_____ Family/support person present? YES / NO

Hypertensive Disorders of Pregnancy	Essential Teaching for Women
What is Severe Hypertension?	Hypertension is when your blood pressure is much higher than it should be.
Signs of Severe Hypertension	• Severe constant headache that does not respond to over-the-counter pain medicine, rest, and/or hydration
What is Preeclampsia/Eclampsia?	Preeclampsia is a complication of pregnancy that includes high blood pressure and signs of damage to other organ systems. Eclampsia is the convulsive phase of preeclampsia, characterized by seizures.
Signs of Preeclampsia	• Severe constant headache that does not respond to pain medicine, rest, and/or hydration • Changes in vision, seeing spots, or flashing lights • Pain in the upper right abdominal area • Swelling of face, hands, and/or legs more than what you would expect • Change in level of consciousness
Signs of Eclampsia	• Seizures
Obtaining Immediate Care	Call 911 for seizures. Call healthcare provider immediately for any other signs. If symptoms worsen or no response from provider/clinic, call 911 or go to nearest emergency room.

RN initials_____ Date_____ Family/support person present? YES / NO

Obstetric Hemorrhage	Essential Teaching for Women
What is Obstetric Hemorrhage?	Obstetric hemorrhage is when you have an excess amount of bleeding after you have delivered your baby.
Signs of Obstetric Hemorrhage	• Bleeding through more than 1 sanitary pad/hour • Passing 1 or more clots the size of an egg or bigger • Character of clots/differentiation of bright red bleeding from dark with clots
Obtaining Immediate Care	Call healthcare provider immediately for signs of hemorrhage. If symptoms worsen or no response from provider/clinic, call 911 or go to nearest emergency room.

RN initials_____ Date_____ Family/support person present? YES / NO

(continued)

DISPLAY 17–11
Postbirth Warning Signs: Postpartum Discharge Education Checklist (*Continued*)

POST-BIRTH Warning Signs: Postpartum Discharge Education Checklist

Venous Thromboembolism	Essential Teaching for Women
What is Venous Thromboembolism?	Venous thromboembolism is when you develop a blood clot usually in your leg (calf area).
Signs of Venous Thromboembolism	• Leg pain, tender to touch, burning. or redness, particularly in the calf area • Swelling of one leg more than the other
Obtaining Immediate Care	Call healthcare provider immediately for above signs of venous thromboembolism. If symptoms worsen or no response from provider/clinic, call 911 or go to nearest emergency room.

RN initials_____ Date_____ Family/support person present? YES / NO

Infection	Essential Teaching for Women
What is Infection?	An infection is an invasion of bacteria or viruses that enter and spread through your body, making you ill.
Signs of Infection	• Temp is ≥100.4°F (≥38°C) • Bad smelling blood or discharge from the vagina • Increase in redness or discharge from episiotomy or C-Section site or open wound not healing
Obtaining Immediate Care	Call healthcare provider immediately for above signs. If symptoms worsen or no response from provider/clinic, call 911 or go to nearest emergency room.

RN initials_____ Date_____ Family/support person present? YES / NO

Postpartum Depression	Essential Teaching for Women
What is Postpartum Depression (PPD)?	Postpartum depression is a type of depression that occurs after childbirth. PPD can occur as early as one week up to one year after giving birth.
Signs of Postpartum Depression	• Thinking of hurting yourself or your baby • Feeling out of control, unable to care for self or baby • Feeling depressed or sad most of the day every day • Having trouble sleeping or sleeping too much • Having trouble bonding with your baby
Obtaining Immediate Care	Call 911 or go to nearest emergency room if you feel you might harm yourself or your baby. Call healthcare provider immediately for other signs of depression (sadness, withdrawn, difficulty coping with parenting).

RN initials_____ Date_____ Family/support person present? YES / NO

	Essential Teaching for Women
Follow-Up Appointment	• Discuss importance of follow-up visit with doctor, nurse practitioner or midwife in 4–6 weeks (or sooner if health status warrants it) • Provide correct phone number for appointment • Emphasize importance to notifying all healthcare providers of delivery date up to one year after birth of baby • Confirm date for postpartum appointment prior to discharge

RN initials_____ Date_____ Family/support person present? YES / NO

I have received and understand the POST-BIRTH Warning Signs education and handout.
Patient Signature: _____ Date/Time: _____

The patient received the POST-BIRTH Warning Signs education and a copy of the "Save Your Life" handout.
Nurse Initials and Signature: _____ Date/Time:_____

Adapted from Association of Women's Health, Obstetric and Neonatal Nurses. Suplee, P. D., Kleppel, L, Santa-Donato, A., & Bingham, D. (2016). Improving postpartum education about warning signs of maternal morbidity and mortality. *Nursing for Women's Health, 20*(6), 552–567.

discussed prenatally, including shared decision making on contraceptive options.

- The first contact between the new mother and the maternity care provider should occur within the first 3 weeks after birth (either by phone, virtually, or in person), and then followed with ongoing care as needed including a thorough postpartum visit no later than 12 weeks after birth. This thorough postpartum visit should include a full assessment of physical, social, and psychological well-being.
- Women with pregnancies complicated by preterm birth, gestational diabetes, or hypertensive disorders of pregnancy need to be told and understand that these disorders are associated with a higher lifetime risk of maternal cardiometabolic disease.
- Women with chronic medical conditions, such as hypertensive disorders, obesity, diabetes, thyroid disorders, renal disease, mood disorders, and substance use disorders, should be aware of the importance of timely follow-up with their obstetrician–gynecologists or primary care providers for ongoing coordination of care.
- Women who have had a miscarriage, stillbirth, or neonatal death, must be aware of the importance of follow-up with an obstetrician–gynecologist or other obstetric care provider.

SUMMARY

The postpartum period is a time of transition and change for the new mother and her family. Physiologic and psychological changes occur immediately and over time, necessitating careful planning to meet the needs of the new family. Timely, frequent assessments and appropriate interventions require clinical skills and adequate knowledge about these processes. Supportive care that includes education for the woman and her family about what to expect in the first few weeks facilitates the transition from the inpatient setting to home. Partnering with the woman and her family is essential for individualized care. Being present during this period is a responsibility and a privilege that can affect society as a whole, one family at a time.

Resources are available from AWHONN (https://www.awhonn.org/page/PPH) and ACOG on postpartum care (https://www.acog.org/-/media/Departments/Toolkits-for-Health-Care-Providers/Postpartum-Toolkit/2018-Postpartum-Toolkit.pdf?dmc=1&ts=20190502T2359349801).

REFERENCES

Agency for Healthcare Research and Quality. (2014). *Designing and delivering whole-person transitional care: The hospital guide to reducing Medicaid readmissions.* Rockville, MD: Author.

American Academy of Pediatrics. (2015). Hospital stay for healthy term newborn infants. *Pediatrics, 135*(5), 1105–1106. doi:10.1542/peds.2015-0699

American Academy of Pediatrics. (2016). Safe sleep and skin-to-skin care in the neonatal period for healthy term newborns. *Pediatrics, 138*(3), e20161889.

American Academy of Pediatrics & American College of Obstetricians and Gynecologists. (2017). *Guidelines for perinatal care* (8th ed.). Elk Grove Village, IL: Author.

American College of Obstetricians and Gynecologists. (2014). *reVITALize: Obstetric data definitions* (version 1.0). Washington, DC: Author.

American College of Obstetricians and Gynecologists. (2015). *Physical activity and exercise during pregnancy and the postpartum period* (Committee Opinion No. 650; Reaffirmed, 2017). Washington, DC: Author.

American College of Obstetricians and Gynecologists. (2016a). *Management of preterm labor* (Practice Bulletin No. 171). Washington, DC: Author.

American College of Obstetricians and Gynecologists. (2016b). *Prevention and management of obstetric lacerations at vaginal delivery* (Practice Bulletin No. 165). Washington, DC: Author.

American College of Obstetricians and Gynecologists. (2017). *Postpartum hemorrhage* (Practice Bulletin No. 183). Washington, DC: Author.

American College of Obstetricians and Gynecologists. (2018a). *Optimizing postpartum care* (Committee Opinion No. 736). Washington, DC: Author.

American College of Obstetricians and Gynecologists. (2018b). *Postpartum pain management* (Committee Opinion No. 742). Washington, DC: Author.

American College of Obstetricians and Gynecologists. (2019). *Gestational hypertension and preeclampsia* (Practice Bulletin No. 202). Washington, DC: Author.

American Society of Anesthesiologists. (2016). Practice guidelines for obstetric anesthesia: An updated report by the American Society of Anesthesiologists Task Force on Obstetric Anesthesia and the Society for Obstetric Anesthesia and Perinatology. *Anesthesiology, 124,* 270–300. doi:10.1097/ALN.0000000000000935

Association of Women's Health, Obstetric and Neonatal Nurses. (2010). *Guidelines for professional registered nurse staffing for perinatal units.* Washington, DC: Author.

Association of Women's Health, Obstetric and Neonatal Nurses. (2015). *Quantification of blood loss* (AWHONN Practice Brief No. 1). Washington, DC: Author.

Association of Women's Health, Obstetric and Neonatal Nurses. (2016). Immediate and sustained skin-to-skin contact for the healthy term newborn after birth (AWHONN Practice Brief Number 5). *Nursing for Women's Health, 20*(6), 614–616. doi:10.1016/S1751-4851(16)30331-2

Association of Women's Health, Obstetric and Neonatal Nurses. (2018). *Obstetric patient safety classroom course for postpartum hemorrhage.* Washington, DC: Author.

Association of Women's Health, Obstetric and Neonatal Nurses. (2019a). *Perioperative care of the pregnant woman* (Evidence-Based Clinical Practice Guideline, 2nd ed.). Washington, DC: Author.

Association of Women's Health, Obstetric and Neonatal Nurses. (2019b). *Standards and guidelines for professional nursing practice in the care of women and newborns* (8th ed.). Washington, DC: Author.

Baby-Friendly USA. (2019). *The ten steps to successful breastfeeding.* Albany, NY: Author.

Bateman, B. T., Berman, M. F., Riley, L. E., & Leffert, L. R. (2010). The epidemiology of postpartum hemorrhage in a large, nationwide sample of deliveries. *Anesthesia and Analgesia, 110*(5), 1368–1373. doi:10.1213/ANE.0b013e3181d74898

Beck, C. T. (2001). Predictors of postpartum depression: An update. *Nursing Research, 50*(5), 275–285.

Beck, C. T. (2002). Revision of the Postpartum Depression Predictors Inventory. *Journal of Obstetric, Gynecologic, and Neonatal Nursing, 31*(4), 394–402. doi:10.1111/j.1552-6909.2002.tb00061.x

Beck, C. T. (2006). Postpartum depression: It isn't just the blues. *The American Journal of Nursing, 106*(5), 40–50.

Beck, C. T. (2008). State of the science on postpartum depression: What nurse researchers have contributed-part 2. *MCN: The American Journal of Maternal Child Nursing, 33*(3), 151–156. doi:10.1097/01.NMC.0000318349.70364.1c

Beck, C. T., & Gable, R. K. (2005). *Postpartum Depression Screening Scale manual*. Los Angeles, CA: Western Psychological Services.

Beck, C. T., & Indman, P. (2005). The many faces of postpartum depression. *Journal of Obstetric, Gynecologic, and Neonatal Nursing, 34*(5), 569–576. doi:10.1177/0884217505279995

Beck, C. T., Records, K., & Rice, M. (2006). Further development of the Postpartum Depression Predictors Inventory-Revised. *Journal of Obstetric, Gynecologic, and Neonatal Nursing, 35*(6), 735–745. doi:10.1111/j.1552-6909.2006.00094.x

Bingham, D., Suplee, P., Morris, M. H., & McBride, M. (2018). Healthcare strategies for reducing pregnancy-related morbidity and mortality in the postpartum period. *The Journal of Perinatal & Neonatal Nursing, 32*(3), 241–249. doi:10.1097/JPN .0000000000000344

Blackburn, S. T. (2017). *Maternal, fetal, & neonatal physiology: A clinical perspective* (5th ed.). Maryland Heights, MO: Elsevier.

Centers for Disease Control and Prevention. (2011). *Update to CDC's U.S. Medical Eligibility Criteria for Contraceptive Use, 2010: Revised recommendations for the use of contraceptive methods during the postpartum period*. Atlanta, GA: Author.

Centers for Disease Control and Prevention. (2018). *Contraception*. Atlanta, GA: Author.

Côté-Arsenault, D. (2011). *Loss and grief in the childbearing period*. White Plains, NY: March of Dimes.

Cox, J. L., Holden, J. M., & Sagovsky, R. (1987). Detection of postnatal depression. Development of the 10-item Edinburgh Postnatal Depression Scale. *The British Journal of Psychiatry, 150*, 782–786.

Cunningham, F. G., Leveno, K. J., Bloom, S., Spong, C. Y., Dashe, J. S., Hoffman, B. L., & Casey, B. M. (2018). The puerperium. In *Williams obstetrics* (25th ed., pp. 652–665). New York, NY: McGraw-Hill.

Douketis, J. D. (2018). *Deep vein thrombosis (DVT)*. Retrieved from https://www.merckmanuals.com/professional/cardiovascular -disorders/peripheral-venous-disorders/deep-venous-thrombosis-dvt

Driscoll, J. W. (2006a). Postpartum depression. How nurses can identify and care for women grappling with this disorder. *AWHONN Lifelines, 10*(5), 400–409.

Driscoll, J. W. (2006b). Postpartum depression: The state of the science. *The Journal of Perinatal & Neonatal Nursing, 20*(1), 40–42.

Duff, W. P. (2014). Maternal and fetal infections. In R. K. Creasy, R. Resnik, J. D. Iams, C. J. Lockwood, T. R. Moore, & M. Greene (Eds.), *Creasy & Resnik's maternal-fetal medicine: Principles and practice* (7th ed., pp. 802–851). Philadelphia, PA: Saunders.

English, C. L., Alden, K. R., Zomorodi, M., Travers, D., & Ross, M. S. (2018). Evaluation of content on commonly used web sites about induction of labor and pain management during labor. *MCN: The American Journal of Maternal Child Nursing, 43*(5), 271–277. doi:10.1097/NMC.0000000000000455

Friel, L. A. (2018). *Thromboembolic disorders in pregnancy*. Retrieved from https://www.merckmanuals.com/professional /gynecology-and-obstetrics/pregnancy-complicated-by-disease /thromboembolic-disorders-in-pregnancy

Ghadery-Sefat, A., Abdeyazdan, Z., Badiee, Z., & Zargham-Boroujeni, A. (2016). Relationship between parent–infant attachment and parental satisfaction with supportive nursing care. *Iranian Journal of Nurse Midwifery Research, 21*(1), 71–76.

Giraldo-Isaza, M. A., Jaspan, D., & Cohen, A. W. (2011). Postpartum endometritis caused by herpes and cytomegaloviruses. *Obstetrics and Gynecology, 117*(2, Pt. 2), 466–467. doi:10.1097 /AOG.0b013e3181f73805

Gracia, S. R., Muñuzuri, A. P., López, E. S., Castellanos, J. L., Fernández, I. B., Campillo, C. W., . . . Luna, M. S. (2016). Criteria for hospital discharge of the healthy term newborn after delivery. *Anales de Pediatría (English Edition), 86*(5), 289.e1–289.e6.

Grobman, W. A., Rice, M. M., Reddy, U. M., Tita, A. T. N., Silver, R. M., Mallett, G., . . . Macones, G. A. (2018). Labor induction versus expectant management in low-risk nulliparous women. *The New England Journal of Medicine, 379*(6), 513–523. doi:10.1056/NEJMoa1800566

Groër, M., Davis, M., Casey, K., Short, B., Smith, K., & Groër, S. (2005). Neuroendocrine and immune relationships in postpartum fatigue. *MCN: The American Journal of Maternal Child Nursing, 30*(2), 133–138.

Henry, J., & Sherwin, B. B. (2012). Hormones and cognitive functioning during late pregnancy and postpartum: A longitudinal study. *Behavioral Neuroscience, 126*(1), 73–85.

Hoyte, L., Wyman, A., & Hahn, L. (2015). *Vaginal delivery and the pelvic floor: Outcomes of levator ani injury*. Retrieved from http:// www.contemporaryobgyn.net/obstetrics-gynecology-womens-health /vaginal-delivery-and-pelvic-floor-outcomes-levator-ani-injury

Kilpatrick, S. J. (2014). Anemia and pregnancy. In R. K. Creasy, R. Resnik, J. D. Iams, C. J. Lockwood, T. R. Moore, & M. Greene (Eds.), *Creasy & Resnik's maternal-fetal medicine: Principles and practice* (7th ed., pp. 918–931). Philadelphia, PA: Saunders.

Ladewig, P. W., London, M. L., & Davidson, M. R. (2017). *Contemporary maternal-newborn nursing care* (9th ed.). Upper Saddle River, NJ: Prentice Hall.

Lawrence, R. M., & Lawrence, R. A. (2014). The breast and the physiology of lactation. In R. K. Creasy, R. Resnik, J. D. Iams, C. J. Lockwood, T. R. Moore, & M. Greene (Eds.), *Creasy & Resnik's maternal-fetal medicine: Principles and practice* (7th ed., pp. 112–130). Philadelphia, PA: Saunders.

Leung, A. N., & Lockwood, C. J. (2014). Thromboembolic disease. In R. K. Creasy, R. Resnik, J. D. Iams, C. J. Lockwood, T. R. Moore, & M. Greene (Eds.), *Creasy & Resnik's maternal-fetal medicine: Principles and practice* (7th ed., pp. 906–917). Philadelphia, PA: Saunders.

Lewallen, L. P. (2011). The importance of culture in childbearing. *Journal of Obstetric, Gynecologic, and Neonatal Nursing, 40*(1), 4–8. doi:10.1111/j.1552-6909.2010.01209.x

Lyndon, A., Lagrew, D., Shields, L., Main, E., & Cape, V. (2015). *Improving health care response to obstetric hemorrhage*. (Toolkit). Stanford, CA: California Maternal Quality Care Collaborative.

Maìn, E. K., Goffman, D., Scavone, B. M., Low, L. K., Bingham, D., Fontaine, P. L., . . . Levy, B. S. (2015). National partnership for maternal safety: Consensus bundle on obstetric hemorrhage. *Anesthesia and Analgesia, 121*(1), 142–148. doi:10.1097/AOG .0000000000000869

Maloni, J. A. (2010). Antepartum bed rest for pregnancy complications: Efficacy and safety for preventing preterm birth. *Biological Research for Nursing, 12*(2), 106–124.

March of Dimes. (2016). *Maternal, infant, and child health in the United States 2016*. White Plains, NY: Author.

March of Dimes. (2017). *Baby blues after pregnancy*. White Plains, NY: Author.

March of Dimes. (2018). *Postpartum hemorrhage*. White Plains, NY: Author.

Markham, K. B., & Funai, E. F. (2014). Pregnancy-related hypertension. In R. K. Creasy, R. Resnik, J. D. Iams, C. J. Lockwood, T. R. Moore, & M. Greene (Eds.), *Creasy & Resnik's maternal-fetal medicine: Principles and practice* (7th ed., pp. 756–784). Philadelphia, PA: Saunders.

Martin, J. A., Hamilton, B. E., Osterman, M. J., Driscoll, A. K., & Drake, P. (2018). Births: Final data for 2017. *National Vital Statistics Reports, 67*(8), 1–50.

Mercer, R. (1986). *First-time motherhood: Experiences from teens to forties*. New York, NY: Springer.

Mercer, R. T. (1995). *Becoming a mother: Research on maternal identity from Rubin to the present*. New York, NY: Springer.

Meyer, I., & Richter, H. E. (2015). Impact of fecal incontinence and its treatment on quality of life in women. *Womens Health, 11*(2), 225–238.

Moldenhauer, J. S. (2018). *Puerperal endometritis.* Retrieved from https://www.merckmanuals.com/professional/gynecology-and -obstetrics/postpartum-care-and-associated-disorders/puerperal -endometritis#v1075923

Monga, M., & Matrobattista, J. M. (2014). Maternal cardiovascular, respiratory, and renal adaptation to pregnancy. In R. K. Creasy, R. Resnik, J. D. Iams, C. J. Lockwood, T. R. Moore, & M. Greene (Eds.), *Creasy & Resnik's maternal-fetal medicine: Principles and practice* (7th ed., pp. 93–99). Philadelphia, PA: Saunders.

Nader, S. (2014). Thyroid disease and pregnancy. In R. K. Creasy, R. Resnik, J. D. Iams, C. J. Lockwood, T. R. Moore, & M. Greene (Eds.), *Creasy & Resnik's maternal-fetal medicine: Principles and practice* (7th ed., pp. 1022–1037). Philadelphia, PA: Saunders.

National Conference of State Legislatures. (2018). *Maternity length of stay rules.* Denver, CO: Author.

Padayachee, C., & Coombes, J. S. (2015). Exercise guidelines for gestational diabetes mellitus. *World Journal of Diabetes, 6*(8), 1033–1044.

Park, S. C., Yeom, S. R., Han, S. K., Jo, Y. M., & Kim, H. B. (2017). Recombinant activated factor VII as a second line treatment for postpartum hemorrhage. *Korean Journal of Critical Care Medicine, 32*(4), 333–339.

Peragallo Urrutia, R., Polis, C. B., Jensen, E. T., Greene, M. E., Kennedy, E., & Stanford, J. B. (2018). Effectiveness of fertility awareness-based methods for pregnancy prevention: A systematic review. *Obstetrics and Gynecology, 132*(2), 591–604. doi:10.1097/AOG.0000000000002784

Petersen, M. R. (2011). Review of interventions to relieve postpartum pain from perineal trauma. *MCN: The American Journal of Maternal Child Nursing, 36*(4), 241–245. doi:10.1097/NMC .0b013e3182182579

Records, K., Rice, M. J., & Beck, C. T. (2007). Psychometric assessment of the Postpartum Depression Predictors Inventory-Revised. *Journal of Nursing Measurement, 15*(3), 189–202.

Rhodes, M. A. (2017). Postpartum. In M. C. Brucker & T. L. King (Eds.), *Pharmacology for women's health* (2nd ed., pp. 1095–1116). Burlington, MA: Jones & Bartlett Learning.

Robbins, K. S., Martin, S. R., & Wilson, W. C. (2014). Intensive care considerations for the critically ill parturient. In R. K. Creasy, R. Resnik, J. D. Iams, C. J. Lockwood, T. R. Moore, & M. Greene (Eds.), *Creasy & Resnik's maternal-fetal medicine: Principles and practice* (7th ed., pp. 1182–1214). Philadelphia, PA: Saunders.

Rubin, R. (1961a). Puerperal change. *Nursing Outlook, 9,* 753–755.

Rubin, R. (1961b). Puerperal change. *Nursing Outlook, 11,* 828–831.

Rubin, R. (1977). Binding-in in the postpartum period. *Maternal-Child Nursing Journal, 6,* 67–75.

Schaffer, J. I., Bloom, S. L., Casey, B. M., McIntire, D. D., Nihira, M. A., & Leveno, K. J. (2005). A randomized trial of the effects of coached vs uncoached maternal pushing during the second stage of labor on postpartum pelvic floor structure and function. *American Journal of Obstetrics and Gynecology, 192*(5), 1692–1696. doi:10.1016/j.ajog.2004.11.043

Shepherd, R., & Pizzarello, M. (2017). Secondary postpartum hemorrhage and endometritis. In D. J. Angelini & D. LaFontaine (Eds.), *Obstetric triage and emergency care protocols* (2nd ed., pp. 357–364). New York, NY: Springer.

Simpson, K. R. (2015). Nurse staffing and care during the immediate postpartum recovery period. *MCN: The American Journal of Maternal Child Nursing, 40*(6), 403. doi:10.1097/NMC.0000000000000182

Simpson, K. R. (2017a). Avoiding adverse events after postpartum hospital discharge. *MCN. The American Journal of Maternal Child Nursing, 42*(2), 124. doi:10.1097/NMC.0000000000000319

Simpson, K. R. (2017b). Sudden unexpected postnatal collapse and sudden unexpected infant death. *MCN: The American Journal of Maternal Child Nursing, 42*(6), 368. doi:10.1097/NMC .0000000000000376

Stotland, N. E., Boonar, L. M., & Abrams, B. (2014). Maternal nutrition. In R. K. Creasy, R. Resnik, J. D. Iams, C. J. Lockwood, T. R. Moore, & M. Greene (Eds.), *Creasy & Resnik's maternal-fetal medicine: Principles and practice* (7th ed., pp. 131–138). Philadelphia, PA: Saunders.

Suplee, P. D., Kleppel, L., Santa-Donato, A., & Bingham, D. (2017). Improving postpartum education about warning signs of maternal morbidity and mortality. *Nursing for Women's Health, 20*(6), 552–567.

Tähtinen, R. M., Cartwright, R., Tsui, J. F., Aaltonen, R. L., Aoki, Y., Cárdenas, J. L., . . . Tikkinen, K. A. O. (2016). Long-term impact of mode of delivery on stress urinary incontinence and urgency urinary incontinence: A systematic review and meta-analysis. *European Urology, 70,* 148–158.

Tapson, V. F. (2018). *Pulmonary embolism (PE).* Retrieved from https://www.merckmanuals.com/professional/pulmonary -disorders/pulmonary-embolism-pe/pulmonary-embolism-pe

The Joint Commission. (2004). *Preventing infant death and injury during delivery* (Sentinel Event Alert No. 30). Oakbrook Terrace, IL: Author.

The Joint Commission. (2010). *Preventing maternal death* (Sentinel Event Alert No. 44). Oakbrook Terrace, IL: Author.

The Joint Commission. (2018). *Preventing newborn falls and drops* (Advisory on Safety & Quality Issues No. 40). Oakbrook Terrance, IL: Author.

Thorpe, J. M., & Laughon, S. K. (2014). Clinical aspects of normal and abnormal labor. In R. Resnik, R. K. Creasy, J. D. Iams, C. J. Lockwood, T. R. Moore, & M. Greene (Eds.), *Creasy & Resnik's maternal-fetal medicine: Principles and practice* (7th ed., pp. 673–706). Philadelphia, PA: Saunders.

U.S. Department of Health and Human Services. (2018). *Maternal, infant, and child health.* Retrieved from https://www.healthy people.gov/2020/topics-objectives/topic/maternal-infant-and -child-health/objectives

Van Eerden, P. (2017). *Some of the benefits and risks of bed rest during pregnancy.* Retrieved from https://news.sanfordhealth.org /health/womens/are-there-benefits-to-bed-rest/

Webster, J., Pritchard, M. A., Creedy, D., & East, C. (2003). A simplified predictive index for the detection of women at risk for postnatal depression. *Birth, 30*(2), 101–108.

Whitty, J. E., & Dombrowski, M. P. (2014). Respiratory diseases in pregnancy. In R. K. Creasy, R. Resnik, J. D. Iams, C. J. Lockwood, T. R. Moore, & M. Greene (Eds.), *Creasy & Resnik's maternal-fetal medicine: Principles and practice* (7th ed., pp. 965–987). Philadelphia, PA: Saunders.

Williamson, C., Mackillop, L., & Heneghan, M. A. (2014). Diseases of the liver, biliary system, & pancreas. In R. K. Creasy, R. Resnik, J. D. Iams, C. J. Lockwood, T. R. Moore, & M. Greene (Eds.), *Creasy & Resnik's maternal-fetal medicine: Principles and practice* (7th ed., pp. 1075–1091). Philadelphia, PA: Saunders.

World Health Organization & United Nations Children's Fund. (2018). *Revised BFHI Guidance and 10 Steps to Successful Breastfeeding.* Geneva, Switzerland: Author.

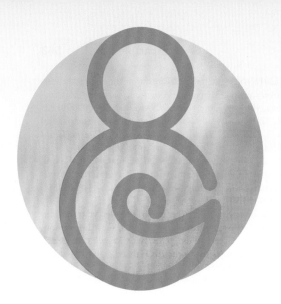

CHAPTER 18

Newborn Adaptation to Extrauterine Life

Debbie Fraser

INTRODUCTION

Transition from fetal to newborn life is a critical period involving diverse physiologic changes. The newborn moves quickly from an organism completely dependent on another for life-sustaining oxygen and nutrients to an independent being, something that requires intense adjustment carried out over a period of minutes to days. Normal physiologic tasks of transition are complicated in some neonates by congenital abnormalities, birth injury, or underlying disease processes. Careful assessment and nursing care are needed during the period of transition to ensure that the neonate who is experiencing problems with transition is recognized and that appropriate interventions are initiated.

This chapter focuses on those factors influencing adaptation and physiologic changes during the early newborn period. These factors include the maternal history and medical and obstetric conditions, intrapartum status, delivery issues, and nursing assessment and interventions during transition, such as resuscitative needs and interventions facilitating maternal–newborn attachment.

MATERNAL MEDICAL AND OBSTETRIC CONDITIONS INFLUENCING NEWBORN ADAPTATION

A thorough review of the mother's prenatal and intrapartum history is essential to identify factors with the potential to compromise transition. Table 18–1 lists maternal risk factors and potential fetal and neonatal complications. In addition to identification of current pregnancy complications, it is important to review prior obstetric history. Complications of a prior pregnancy may recur in subsequent pregnancies (Display 18–1).

Intrapartum risk factors may also influence adaptation (Table 18–2).

Intrapartum fetal assessment provides important data about the fetal response to labor. Electronic fetal heart rate (FHR) monitoring or intermittent auscultation provides documentation of fetal well-being. Requisite perinatal nursing skills include knowledge of the physiologic basis for monitoring, an understanding of FHR patterns, and the initiation of appropriate nursing interventions based on data from the monitor or from auscultation. The FHR reflects the fetal response to labor. The perinatal nurse focuses on discriminating between normal and atypical patterns. If the FHR pattern is atypical, intrauterine resuscitation procedures such as maternal position change, oxygen therapy, and intravenous fluids are initiated. Oxytocin should be decreased or discontinued if infusing, or the next dose of Prepidil, Cervidil, or Cytotec should be delayed. Safe passage through the labor and birth process sets the stage for successful transition to extrauterine life.

UNIQUE MECHANISMS OF NEWBORN PHYSIOLOGIC ADAPTATION

The respiratory, cardiovascular, thermoregulatory, and immunologic systems undergo significant physiologic changes and adaptations during transition from fetal to neonatal life. Successful transition requires a complex interaction among these systems.

Respiratory Adaptations

Critical to the neonate's transition to extrauterine life is the ability to clear fetal lung fluid and establish respirations, allowing the lungs to become the organ of gas exchange after separation from maternal

TABLE 18–1. Maternal Risk Factors and Potential Fetal and Neonatal Complications

Risk factors	Potential complications
Maternal substance use	
Illicit substance exposure	Small for gestational age (SGA); neonatal abstinence syndrome (NAS); neonatal HIV; hepatitis B and C
Opioid use	NAS
Alcohol use	Fetal alcohol spectrum disorder
Smoking/Vaping	SGA; polycythemia
Maternal nutritional status	
Maternal weight <100 lb	SGA
Maternal weight >200 lb	SGA; large for gestational age (LGA), neonatal hypoglycemia
Maternal medical complications	
Hereditary nervous system disorders	Inherited nervous system disorder
Seizure disorders requiring medication	Anomalies (e.g., result of medication [Dilantin] use)
Chronic hypertension	Intrauterine growth restriction (IUGR); asphyxia; SGA
Congenital heart disease with congestive heart failure	Preterm birth; inherited cardiac defects
Anemia <10 g/dL (100 g/L)	Preterm birth; low birth weight
Sickle cell disease	IUGR; fetal demise
Hemoglobinopathies	IUGR; inherited hemoglobinopathies
Immune thrombocytopenia (ITP)	Transient thrombocytopenia; intracranial hemorrhage
Chronic glomerulonephritis, renal insufficiency	IUGR; SGA; preterm birth; asphyxia
Recurrent urinary tract infection	Preterm birth
Uterine malformation	Preterm birth; fetal malposition
Cervical insufficiency	Preterm birth
Diabetes	LGA; hypoglycemia and hypocalcemia; anomalies; respiratory distress syndrome
Thyroid disease	Hypothyroidism; CNS defects; hyperthyroidism; goiter
Current pregnancy complications	
Pregnancy-induced hypertension	IUGR; SGA
Intrauterine infections	IUGR; SGA; active infection; anomalies
Sexually transmitted disease(s)	Ophthalmia neonatorum; congenital syphilis, chlamydial pneumonia
Hepatitis	Hepatitis
AIDS or HIV seropositive	Neonatal HIV
Multiple gestation	Preterm birth; asphyxia; IUGR; SGA, twin-to-twin transfusion, birth trauma
Fetal malposition	Prolapsed cord; asphyxia; birth trauma
Maternal blood group antibodies	Anemia, hyperbilirubinemia, immune-mediated hydrops fetalis
Prolonged pregnancy	Postmaturity; meconium aspiration; IUGR; asphyxia
Intra-amniotic infection	Newborn sepsis; preterm birth
Group B streptococcal colonization/infection	Newborn sepsis; preterm birth

DISPLAY 18–1

Previous Pregnancy Complications that May Recur in Subsequent Pregnancies

Fetal loss beyond 28 weeks' gestation

Preterm birth

Abnormal fetal position or presentation

Previous neonate with group B streptococcal infection

Rh sensitization

Fetal compromise of unknown origin

Birth of newborn with anomalies

Birth of newborn weighing more than 10 lb

Birth of postterm newborn

Neonatal death

uteroplacental circulation. Pulmonary fluid, secreted by the lung epithelium, is essential to the normal growth and development of the alveoli (Morton & Brodsky, 2016). Toward the end of gestation, production of lung fluid gradually diminishes. The catecholamine surge that occurs just before the onset of labor has been shown to correspond to a more rapid drop in fetal lung fluid levels. Those infants who are born by cesarean section without labor are more likely to develop transient tachypnea of the newborn because of lower levels of serum catecholamine combined with the loss of the mechanical effects of labor (Riviere, McKinlay, & Bloomfield, 2017).

Initiation of breathing is a complex process that involves the interplay of biochemical, neural, and mechanical factors. Pulmonary blood flow, surfactant production, and respiratory musculature also influence respiratory adaptation to extrauterine life. Establishment of independent breathing and oxygen–carbon dioxide exchange depends on these physiologic factors.

TABLE 18–2. Intrapartum Risk Factors and Potential Fetal and Neonatal Complications

Risk factors	Potential complications
Umbilical cord	
Prolapsed umbilical cord	Asphyxia
True knot in cord	Asphyxia
Velamentous insertion	Intrauterine blood loss; shock; anemia
Vasa previa	Intrauterine blood loss; shock; anemia
Rupture or tearing of cord	Blood loss; shock; anemia
Membranes	
Premature rupture of membranes	Infection; respiratory distress syndrome; prolapsed cord; asphyxia
Prolonged rupture of membranes	Infection
Amnionitis	Infection
Amniotic fluid	
Oligohydramnios	Congenital anomalies; pulmonary hypoplasia
Polyhydramnios	Congenital anomalies; prolapsed cord
Meconium-stained fluid	Asphyxia; meconium aspiration syndrome
Placenta	
Placenta previa	Preterm birth; asphyxia
Abruptio placenta	Preterm birth; asphyxia
Placental insufficiency	Intrauterine growth restriction; small for gestational age; asphyxia
Abnormal fetal presentations	
Breech birth	Asphyxia; birth injuries (central nervous system [CNS], skeletal)
Face or brow presentation	Asphyxia; facial trauma
Transverse lie	Asphyxia; birth injuries; cesarean birth; umbilical cord prolapse
Birth complications	
Forceps-assisted birth	Nervous system trauma; cephalhematoma; asphyxia; facial trauma
Vacuum extraction	Cephalhematoma; subgaleal hemorrhage
Manual version or extraction	Asphyxia; birth trauma; prolapsed cord
Shoulder dystocia	Asphyxia; brachial plexus injury; fractured clavicle
Precipitous birth	Asphyxia; birth trauma
Undiagnosed multiple gestation	Asphyxia; birth trauma
Administration of drugs	
Oxytocin	Complications of uterine hyperstimulation (asphyxia)
Magnesium sulfate	Hypermagnesemia; CNS and respiratory depression
Analgesics	CNS and respiratory depression
Anesthetics	CNS and respiratory depression; bradycardia

Chemical Stimuli

A number of factors have been implicated in the initiation of breathing at birth: decreased oxygen concentration, increased carbon dioxide concentration, and a decrease in pH, all of which may stimulate fetal aortic and carotid chemoreceptors, triggering the respiratory center in the medulla to initiate respiration. Some researchers have questioned the influence of these factors and suggest instead that factors secreted by the placenta may inhibit breathing and that regular breathing is initiated with the clamping of the cord (Alvaro & Rigatto, 2017).

Mechanical Stimulation

In utero, the fetal lungs are filled with fluid. Mechanical compression of the chest during vaginal birth forces approximately one third of this fluid out of fetal lungs. As the chest is delivered through the birth canal, it re-expands, creating negative pressure and drawing air into the lungs. This passive inspiration of air replaces fluid that previously filled the alveoli. Further expansion and distribution of air throughout the alveoli occurs when the newborn cries. Crying creates positive intrathoracic pressure that keeps alveoli open and forces the remaining fetal lung fluid into pulmonary capillaries and the lymphatic circulation.

Sensory Stimuli

The newborn is exposed to tactile, visual, auditory, and olfactory stimuli during and immediately after birth. Tactile stimulation begins in utero as the fetus experiences uterine contractions and descent through the pelvis and birth canal. Stimulation to initiate breathing continues after birth as the neonate is exposed to light, sound, touch, smell, and pain. Vigorously drying the newborn immediately after birth provides significant tactile stimulation.

Contributing Factors

Pulmonary Blood Flow

In utero, the placenta is the organ of gas exchange for the fetus. Oxygenated blood is delivered from the placenta through the umbilical vein and the ductus venosus into the inferior vena cava where it is preferentially directed across the foramen ovale into the left atrium for distribution to the systemic circulation. Some of the oxygenated blood from the placenta moves into the right atrium where it mixes with blood returning from the systemic circulation. Much of this blood is diverted away from pulmonary circulation to the aorta through the ductus arteriosus which connects the pulmonary artery and the aorta.

The fluid-filled lungs of the fetus create a state of alveolar hypoxia. Fetal pulmonary arterioles, which are very sensitive to oxygen, have thick musculature because of low oxygen tension in utero (Steinhorn, 2015). This results in constriction of pulmonary arterioles, which increases pulmonary vascular resistance (PVR) and decreases pulmonary blood flow. After birth, pulmonary vasodilatation occurs when oxygen, a potent pulmonary vasodilator, enters the lungs. This significantly decreases PVR. Normal postnatal pulmonary blood flow is established as PVR decreases with changes in arterial partial pressure of oxygen (PaO_2), alveolar partial pressure of oxygen (PAO_2), acid–base status, and the removal of vasoactive substances such as prostaglandin and bradykinin which are produced by the placenta. Adequate pulmonary blood flow is crucial for newborn gas exchange and successful transition. After the onset of breathing, fluid in the lungs is replaced by air.

Surfactant Production

Pulmonary surfactant is necessary to maintain expanded alveoli. Surfactant lowers surface tension, preventing alveolar collapse during inspiration and expiration. By approximately 34 to 36 weeks' gestation, there is adequate surfactant production to support respiration and protect against development of respiratory distress syndrome (Gardner, Enzman-Hines, & Nyp, 2016). Surfactant deficiency results in atelectasis and requires greater than normal breathing efforts. Oxygen and metabolic needs increase as the newborn uses more energy to maintain respirations. Preterm newborns are at high risk for surfactant deficiency, which may significantly jeopardize respiratory adaptation to extrauterine life.

Respiratory Musculature

Intercostal muscles support the rib cage and assist with inspiration by creating negative intrathoracic pressure. Intercostal muscles may not be fully developed at birth, increasing risk of respiratory compromise by increasing breathing effort.

Cardiovascular Adaptations

Transition from fetal to neonatal circulation is a major cardiovascular change and occurs simultaneously with respiratory system adaptation. To appreciate hemodynamic changes, an understanding of structural and blood-flow differences between fetal and neonatal circulation is necessary. Figure 18–1 illustrates fetal circulation.

Fetal Circulation

In utero, oxygenated blood flows to the fetus from the placenta through the umbilical vein. Although a small amount of oxygenated blood is delivered to the liver, most blood bypasses the hepatic system through the ductus venosus. The ductus venosus is a vascular structure that forms a connection between the umbilical vein and the inferior vena cava. Oxygenated blood from the inferior vena cava enters the right atrium, and most of it is directed through the foramen ovale to the left atrium, then to the left ventricle, and on to the ascending aorta, where it is primarily directed to the fetal heart and brain. The foramen ovale is a flap-like structure between the right and left atria. Blood flows through the foramen ovale because pressure in the right atrium is greater than that in the left atrium. In addition, the superior vena cava drains deoxygenated blood from the head and upper extremities into the right atrium, where it mixes with oxygenated blood from the placenta. This blood enters the right ventricle and pulmonary artery where again increased resistance in the pulmonary vessels causes 60% of this blood to be shunted across the ductus arteriosus and into the descending aorta. This mixture of oxygenated and deoxygenated blood continues through the descending aorta, oxygenating the lower half of the fetal body and eventually draining back to the placenta through the two umbilical arteries. The remaining 40% of the blood coming from the right ventricle perfuses lung tissue to meet metabolic needs. The blood that actually reaches the lungs represents about 8% to 10% of fetal cardiac output (Blackburn, 2018; Steinhorn 2015).

Neonatal Circulation

During fetal life, the placenta is an organ of low vascular resistance. Diminished blood flow through the umbilical cord at birth eliminates the placenta as a reservoir for blood, causing increased systemic vascular resistance (SVR), an increase in blood pressure, and increased pressures in the left side of the heart. Removal of the placenta also eliminates the need for blood flow through the ductus venosus, causing functional elimination of this fetal shunt. Systemic venous blood flow is then directed through the portal system for hepatic circulation. Umbilical vessels constrict, with functional closure occurring immediately.

Several other significant events must also take place for successful transition to neonatal circulation. With the infant's first breath and exposure to increased oxygen levels, the pulmonary blood flow must increase, allowing the lungs to become the organ for exchange of oxygen and carbon dioxide, the foramen ovale must close (this occurs because left atrial pressures exceed right atrial pressures due to the increased pulmonary venous return) (Lott, 2014), and the ductus arteriosus must close. In utero, shunting of blood from the pulmonary artery through the ductus arteriosus to the

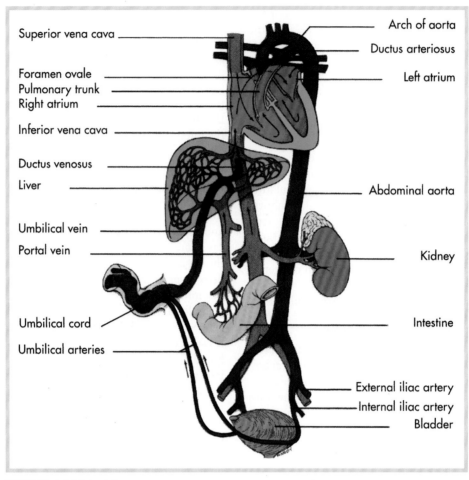

Superior vena cava

Foramen ovale
Pulmonary trunk
Right atrium

Inferior vena cava

Ductus venosus

Liver

Umbilical vein

Portal vein

Umbilical cord

Umbilical arteries

Arch of aorta

Ductus arteriosus

Left atrium

Abdominal aorta

Kidney

Intestine

External iliac artery
Internal iliac artery
Bladder

FIGURE 18–1. Fetal circulation.

aorta occurs as a result of high PVR. After birth, SVR rises and PVR falls, causing a reversal of blood flow through the ductus. As the PaO$_2$ level increases after birth, the ductus arteriosus begins to constrict. In utero, elevated prostaglandin levels helped maintain ductal patency. Removal of the placenta decreases prostaglandin levels, further influencing closure (Goldberg & Krasuski, 2012; Lott, 2014). Constriction of the ductus arteriosus is a gradual process, permitting bidirectional shunting of blood after birth. PVR may be higher than the SVR, allowing some degree of right-to-left shunting, until the SVR rises above PVR and blood flow is directed left to right. Smooth muscle constriction in the wall of the ductus arteriosus narrows the diameter of the ductal wall within 18 hours of birth. Permanent anatomic closure of the ductus arteriosus is usually complete within 14 to 21 days (Goldberg & Krasuski, 2012). Any clinical situation that causes hypoxia, with pulmonary vasoconstriction and subsequent increased PVR, potentiates right-to-left shunting (Lott, 2014). Successful transition and closure of fetal shunts creates a neonatal circulation where deoxygenated blood returns to the heart through the inferior and superior vena cava. It enters the right atrium to the right ventricle and travels through the pulmonary artery to the

pulmonary vascular bed. Oxygenated blood returns through pulmonary veins to the left atrium, the left ventricle, and through the aorta to systemic circulation.

Relationship between Respiratory and Cardiovascular Adaptation

Successful initiation of respirations and transition from fetal to neonatal circulation are essential to maintain life after birth. Conditions that lead to sustained elevated PVR such as hypoxia, acidosis, sepsis, or congenital heart defects can interrupt the normal sequence of events. Closure of fetal shunts depends on oxygenation and pressure changes within the cardiovascular system as described in the previous section. Foramen ovale and ductus arteriosus closure occurs only if PVR drops with the onset of respiration and subsequent oxygenation. The pulmonary vascular bed is very reactive to low oxygen levels. If the neonate experiences significant hypoxia, PVR will remain elevated with resultant decreased pulmonary blood flow and right-to-left shunting across the foramen ovale and ductus arteriosus. These events may induce a state of hypoxia as deoxygenated blood bypasses the lungs through the patent fetal shunts to be mixed with oxygenated blood entering the systemic circulation. The result is persistent pulmonary hypertension of the newborn, requiring aggressive cardiorespiratory support.

Thermoregulation

The newborn's ability to maintain temperature control after birth is determined by external environmental factors and internal physiologic processes. Characteristics of newborns that predispose them to heat loss include a large body surface area in relation to body mass and a limited amount of subcutaneous fat. Newborns attempt to regulate body temperature by nonshivering thermogenesis, increased metabolic rate, and increased muscle activity. Peripheral vasoconstriction also decreases heat loss through the skin surface. Mechanisms of heat loss including evaporation, conduction, convection, and radiation play an integral part in newborn adaptation to extrauterine life. Nursing care is critical in supporting thermoregulation through ongoing assessments and environmental interventions to decrease heat loss.

Mechanisms of Heat Production

Nonshivering Thermogenesis

Newborns have a limited capacity to shiver and, therefore, must generate heat through nonshivering thermogenesis. Heat is produced by metabolism of brown fat, a unique process present only in newborns. This highly vascular adipose tissue is located in the neck, scapula, axilla, and mediastinum, and around kidneys and adrenal glands. Production of brown fat begins around 26 to 28 weeks' gestation and continues for 3 to 5 weeks after birth (Blackburn, 2018). When exposed to cold stress, thermal receptors in skin transmit messages to the central nervous system, activating the sympathetic nervous system and triggering metabolism of brown fat, a process that utilizes glucose and oxygen and produces acids as a byproduct (Brand & Boyd, 2015). Once utilized, brown fat stores are not replaced (Brand & Boyd, 2015).

Voluntary Muscle Activity

Heat produced through voluntary muscle activity is minimal in the newborn. Flexion of the extremities and maintaining a fetal position decreases heat loss to the environment. Term newborns have the ability to maintain this flexed posture, whereas preterm and compromised newborns may lack the muscle tone for this posturing, making them more vulnerable to cold stress (Brand & Boyd, 2015).

Mechanisms of Heat Loss

Evaporation

Evaporation and heat loss occur as amniotic fluid on skin is converted to a vapor. Drying the newborn immediately after birth and removing wet blankets decrease evaporative losses and prevent further cooling.

The amount of insensible water loss from the skin is inversely related to gestational age. Skin of a preterm newborn is more susceptible to evaporative losses because the keratin layer of the skin has not matured (Brand & Boyd, 2015; Gardner & Hernandez, 2016). Because the newborn's head is the largest surface area of the body, covering the head with a knit cap after birth when not under the radiant warmer greatly conserves heat. Under the radiant warmer, use of a cap prevents heat from reaching the newborn's head and may contribute to cold stress. Adding humidity to the environment may also decrease evaporative heat loss. To avoid hypothermia, it is recommended that low-birth-weight infants be placed directly in a sterile food or medical grade plastic bag or wrapped with occlusive wrap after delivery (Gardner & Hernandez, 2016).

Conduction

Conductive heat loss occurs when two solid objects of different temperatures come in contact. Heat loss occurs if the newborn is placed in direct contact with a cold scale, mattress, X-ray plate, or blanket. Mechanisms for preventing conductive heat loss immediately after birth include using a preheated radiant warmer, warm blankets for drying, and covering scales and X-ray plates with warm blankets. Preheating the radiant warmer is necessary because it may take 15 to 30 minutes to warm the mattress.

Providing skin-to-skin contact between mother and newborn after birth helps prevent conductive heat loss and enhances maternal–newborn attachment (Gardner & Hernandez, 2016). Skin-to-skin care has been shown to reduce the risk of mortality, decrease risk of sepsis, increase the rate of exclusive breastfeeding, and improve growth (Conde-Agudelo & Díaz-Rossello, 2016). Preterm newborns provided with opportunities for skin-to-skin contact with their mothers maintained normal oxygen saturation levels and thermal stability (Lorenz et al., 2017).

Convection

Convection is the transfer of heat from a solid object to surrounding air. Heat is lost from newborn skin as cooler air passes over it. Convective heat loss depends on the amount of exposed skin surface, temperature of air, and amount of air turbulence created by drafts. Interventions that prevent convective heat loss in the newborn include dressing or bundling the infant, using a hat, and eliminating source of drafts. If oxygen therapy is needed, the gas should be heated and humidified (Blackburn, 2018).

Radiation

Radiant heat loss occurs when heat is transferred between two objects not in contact with each other. The newborn loses heat by radiation to nearby cooler surfaces such as the incubator walls, windows, or

TABLE 18–3. Mechanisms of Heat Loss and Nursing Interventions that Prevent Cold Stress	
Type of heat loss	Nursing interventions
Evaporation	Dry late preterm or term infant thoroughly.
	Place low-birth-weight infants in a food grade plastic bag immediately after delivery.
	Remove wet linen.
	Place knit cap on infant's head when not under radiant warmer.
	Bathe infant under radiant heat source after temperature stabilizes.
Convection	Move infant away from drafts, open windows, vents, and traffic patterns.
	When necessary, use humidified, warmed oxygen.
	Avoid using ceiling fans in birthing room.
	Move infant in prewarmed transport incubator.
	Place low-birth-weight infants in an incubator.
Conduction	Preheat radiant warmer.
	Place infant skin-to-skin with mother.
	Use warmed blanket.
	Warm stethoscope and your hands.
	Place cover between newborn and metal scale or X-ray plate.
Radiation	Place stabilizing unit on an interior wall of the birthing room (away from cold windows).
	Use a double-wall incubator.
	Preheat radiant warmer or transport incubator.

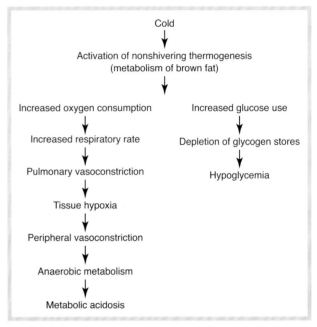

FIGURE 18–2. Effects of cold stress in the newborn.

other objects. Some of the more common and efficient methods for preventing radiant heat loss are use of a radiant warmer after birth, moving the crib or incubator away from a cold window, and use of a double wall or heat shield inside an incubator (for small, preterm newborns), creating an additional warmer barrier between skin and incubator wall.

Effects of Cold Stress

Thermal management of the newborn during the first few hours of age is critical to prevent detrimental effects of cold stress and hypothermia. Table 18–3 summarizes nursing interventions that support the newborn and prevent cold stress. Because heat production requires oxygen and glucose, persistent hypothermia may deplete these stores, leading to metabolic acidosis; hypoglycemia; decreased surfactant production; increased caloric requirements; and, if chronic, impaired weight gain (Blackburn, 2018; Gardner & Hernandez, 2016). This process is illustrated in Figure 18–2.

Immune System Adaptation

Newborns are vulnerable to infection because their immune systems are immature and they lack immunity that normally develops from exposure to organisms. Neonates depend on passive immunity acquired from their mother through active transport via the placenta of immunoglobulin (Ig) G during the third trimester (Jennewein, Abu-Raya, Jiang, Alter, & Marchant, 2017). Preterm

newborns are at greater risk for infection because they may not have received this passive immunity and because the immaturity of the immune system is even more pronounced than in term infants.

Immunity is conferred through immunoglobulins, antibodies secreted by lymphocytes, and plasma cells. There are three main classes of immunoglobulins responsible for immunity: IgG, IgA, and IgM. Because of their small molecular size, only IgG antibodies are capable of crossing the placenta. Maternally transmitted IgG provides protection for the newborn against bacterial and viral infections for which the mother already has antibodies (e.g., diphtheria, tetanus, smallpox, measles, mumps, poliomyelitis).

IgM and IgA immunoglobulins do not cross the placenta. If elevated levels of IgM are found in the newborn, it may indicate the presence of an intrauterine infection caused by organisms traditionally known by the acronym TORCH (i.e., *Toxoplasma gondii* [toxoplasmosis]; other agents such as *Treponema pallidum* [syphilis], varicella virus, HIV; rubella virus; cytomegalovirus; and herpesvirus). The use of the TORCH acronym has largely been abandoned because of the recognition of additional agents capable of causing intrauterine infections. These include viruses such as West Nile and Zika. IgA, found in colostrum, is thought to contribute to passive immunity for breast-fed newborns and may also play an important role in the development of the neonate's immune system (Blackburn, 2018).

Immature leukocyte function in the newborn inhibits the ability to destroy pathogens. Deficiencies are also present in the processes of chemotaxis (movement of leukocytes toward site of infection), opsonization (altering or preparing the cells for ingestion), and phagocytosis (ingestion of cells) from occurring. Low levels of immunoglobulin and complement components (i.e., plasma proteins that assist the immune system) leave newborns, especially preterm newborns, vulnerable to infection.

Lymphocytes are responsible for the specific response in the immune system that involves antibody production. When lymphocytes are exposed to pathogens, they become sensitized to them. If repeated exposure occurs, lymphocytes will recognize and attempt to destroy the pathogen. Because newborns lack exposure to most common organisms, any action by lymphocytes is delayed.

Weak newborn defenses against infection make it imperative for the perinatal nurse and anyone coming in contact with newborns to follow careful handwashing practices and use of aseptic technique. Promoting skin integrity is essential for preventing neonatal infections. Newborn skin is thin and delicate, making it susceptible to alterations in integrity. Fetal scalp electrodes, fetal scalp pH sampling, and skin abrasions create portals for the entry of organisms. Umbilical cord and circumcision sites are also potential sites of infection.

Preterm newborns, with more fragile skin, are at a greater risk for infection. Invasive procedures, performed during the early hours after birth, further challenge the immune system. Treatments such as vitamin K injection, intravenous starts, and heel-stick blood samples predispose newborns to infection if proper aseptic technique is not maintained.

Although most births result in a healthy newborn making the transition to extrauterine life without difficulty, perinatal nurses must anticipate and prepare for complications. This includes ensuring immediate availability of functioning resuscitation equipment and knowledge of equipment operation. The American Academy of Pediatrics (AAP) recommend that someone trained in neonatal resuscitation be available for all births, with an experienced team available in cases with significant risk factors (Wyckoff et al., 2015). Display 18–2 identifies equipment that should be available in every birthing room.

The Neonatal Resuscitation Program developed by the American Heart Association (AHA) and the AAP (Wyckoff et al., 2015) has become the standard for educating healthcare providers involved in newborn stabilization. Figure 18–3 illustrates steps used to evaluate and establish airway, breathing, and circulation as a basis for stabilization of the newborn immediately after birth. Although most newborns respond successfully to tactile stimulation, 10% may require additional interventions and 1% extensive resuscitation, including ventilation by bag and mask or endotracheal intubation, chest compressions, and administration of resuscitative medications (Wyckoff et al., 2015).

Good communication among health team members is essential in anticipating and preparing for high-risk

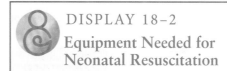

DISPLAY 18–2

Equipment Needed for Neonatal Resuscitation

Clock with second hand

Preheated radiant warmer

Firm, padded resuscitation surface

Warmed blankets

Neonatal stethoscope

Bulb syringe

Gloves and appropriate personnel protection

Pulse oximeter and probe

Mechanical suction with manometer and tubing

Oxygen source, flow meter (flow rate up to 10 L/min), tubing and blender

Resuscitation bag capable of delivering 90%–100% oxygen and pressure gauge

Face masks (newborn and preemie size)

Laryngoscope with size 0 and 1 blades (extra batteries; extra laryngoscope bulbs)

Endotracheal tubes (sizes 2.5, 3.0, 3.5, and 4.0 mm)

Carbon dioxide detector or capnograph

Laryngeal mask airway (optional)

Suction catheters (sizes 5, 8, 10, 12, or 14 Fr)

Meconium aspirator device

8-Fr feeding tube and 20-mL syringe

Syringes (sizes 1, 3, 5, 10, 20, and 50 mL)

Needles 25-, 21-, 18-gauge, or puncture device for needleless system

Umbilical vessel catheterization supplies

Cord clamp

Tape

Scissors

Resuscitative drugs

    Epinephrine 1 mg/10 ml (0.1 mg/ml) (formerly available as 1:10,000)

    Volume expanders

        Normal saline solution

        Lactated Ringer solution 100 or 250 mL

Normal saline for flushes

births. Communicating the details of the maternal and family history that will affect the resuscitation and treatment of the newborn is particularly important. After airway, breathing, and circulation have been established, a thorough assessment of the newborn is performed. This assessment includes Apgar scoring, evaluation of vital signs, physical examination, and measurements. Ideally, all aspects of transitional assessments are performed in the presence of parents in the birthing room. Only if significant maternal or newborn complications occur should parents and newborns be separated.

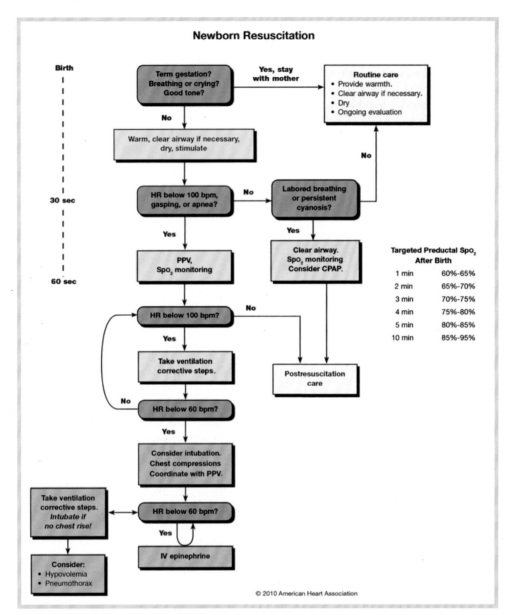

FIGURE 18–3. Resuscitation in the birthing room. CPAP, continuous positive airway pressure; IV, intravenous; HR, heart rate; PPV, positive pressure ventilation; SpO$_2$, oxygen saturation. (From American Academy of Pediatrics & American Heart Association. [2016]. *Textbook of neonatal resuscitation* [7th ed.]. Elk Grove Village, IL: American Academy of Pediatrics.)

APGAR SCORE

The Apgar score was introduced in 1952 by Dr. Virginia Apgar, an anesthesiologist. It provides a simple method to evaluate the condition of the newborn at 1 and 5 minutes of age (Apgar, 1966). Five assessment criteria (i.e., heart rate, respiratory rate, muscle tone, reflex irritability, and color) are scored from 0 to 2. The highest total possible score is 10. The AAP and American College of Obstetricians and Gynecologists (ACOG) (2017) recommend continuing assessment every 5 minutes until the Apgar score is greater than 7. When used to evaluate preterm newborns, the Apgar score may have less validity. Findings common in the preterm newborn such as irregular respirations, decreased muscle tone, and decreased reflex irritability affect the overall score (Cavaliere & Sansoucie, 2014). The Apgar score should not be used as an indication for resuscitation (AHA & AAP, 2016).

PHYSICAL ASSESSMENT

A care provider skilled in newborn assessment should perform a physical assessment within the first 2 hours after birth (AAP & ACOG, 2017). This examination gives the perinatal nurse an opportunity to evaluate overall newborn well-being and transition to extrauterine life. Chapter 19 describes a comprehensive physical examination, including normal and abnormal findings. During the initial examination in the birthing room, all systems are evaluated using inspection, auscultation, and palpation. During the transitional period after birth, temperature, heart rate, skin color, peripheral circulation, respiration, level of consciousness, tone, and activity are monitored and recorded at least once every 30 minutes until the newborn's condition has remained stable for 2 hours (AAP & ACOG, 2017).

Skin

An overall visual assessment of the newborn is performed noting any obvious defects (e.g., neural tube defects, abdominal wall defects, extra digits) or trauma (e.g., bruising, petechiae, puncture wound from fetal scalp electrode). Skin is observed for color, texture, birthmarks, rashes, jaundice, and meconium staining. The newborn's back is inspected, noting a closed vertebral column or presence of abnormalities, such as masses and dimple or tuft of hair along the spine.

Head and Neck

Symmetry of the head and face is noted as well as the presence of molding, caput succedaneum, and bruising. Fontanels are palpated. Although it is not uncommon for eyelids to be edematous, drainage from the eye is not normal during this period. Subconjunctival hemorrhage is sometimes seen and resolves spontaneously. The neck is palpated for masses and full range of motion. The examiner assesses the position of the ears and looks for skin tags or evidence of a sinus on or around the ears. While assessing the mucous membrane of the mouth for a normal pink color, the lips and palate are inspected for a cleft.

Respiratory System

Inspection of the chest includes observing the shape, symmetry, and equality of chest movement. Asymmetry in chest movement may indicate pneumothorax or congenital defect. Respirations should be unlabored at a rate of 30 to 60 breaths per minute. Retractions, grunting, and nasal flaring are abnormal findings indicating respiratory distress. Breath sounds should be equal bilaterally. Initially, moist sounds may be heard as fluid is cleared from the lungs by absorption through pulmonary capillaries and by drainage through the nose and mouth. Special attention is paid to newborns when meconium-stained amniotic fluid is present. Because meconium aspiration is a risk, careful assessment of the respiratory rate, quality of breath sounds, and color determines the need for interventions such as suctioning and supplemental oxygen. In the presence of significant secretions, the newborn's mouth and nose are suctioned with a bulb syringe after delivery.

Cardiovascular System

Inspection of the cardiovascular system includes observation of the color of the skin and mucous membranes and location of the point of maximal impulse. Although acrocyanosis (blueness of the hands and feet) is a normal finding, central cyanosis indicates inadequate oxygenation and the need for supplemental oxygen. Heart rate, rhythm, and normal heart sounds and murmurs are best identified when auscultated using a newborn stethoscope.

Cardiovascular assessment also includes palpation for the presence and equality of femoral pulses. Pulses should be equal and nonbounding. Bounding pulses may indicate patent ductus arteriosus, whereas absent or decreased pulses may occur with coarctation of the aorta (Lott, 2014). Depending on the condition of the newborn, a baseline blood pressure may be recorded. Taking the blood pressure in all four extremities is usually reserved for a newborn showing signs of distress. Routine blood pressure screening for newborns in the absence of risk factors and without complications is not routine practice.

Abdomen

The examiner assesses the shape, symmetry, and consistency of the abdomen. The umbilical cord stump is inspected for the presence of three vessels (i.e., two arteries and one vein). The umbilical cord of a newborn exposed to meconium in utero for an extended period has a yellowish-brown discoloration. The abdomen is auscultated to detect bowel sounds.

Musculoskeletal System

Extremities are assessed for symmetry, range of motion, and the presence of extra or missing digits. While moving the newborn's arm, clavicles are palpated for crepitus, which may indicate a fracture. The newborn's hips are evaluated for "clunks," which may indicate dislocation. Normal muscle tone is noted during this part of the examination and while evaluating the Apgar score.

Genitalia

The presence of normal male or female genitalia is evaluated. Male newborns are assessed for location of the urethral meatus and presence of a hydrocele. The scrotum is palpated to detect the testes.

Neurologic System

A complete neurologic assessment is usually reserved for newborns that are born with or develop complications. A brief neurologic assessment is performed by evaluating reflexes such as Moro, grasp, and suck.

In addition to ongoing physical assessments of the newborn, procedures such as newborn identification, instillation of eye prophylaxis, and administration of vitamin K are performed soon after birth. Ideally, each perinatal unit develops policies and procedures outlining expected newborn care. *Guidelines for Perinatal Care* (AAP & ACOG, 2017) is a resource for developing unit standards.

NEWBORN IDENTIFICATION

One of the first procedures after birth is newborn identification. Perinatal nurses must be meticulous when recording the identification band number and applying identification bands to mothers and newborns (AAP & ACOG, 2017). Some hospitals use a four-band system that includes a band for the support person or father of the newborn in addition to the band for the mother and two bands for the newborn, with one placed on an ankle and one on a wrist. Newborn footprinting and fingerprinting are not adequate methods of identification (AAP & ACOG, 2017). Some hospitals have abandoned these practices altogether, whereas others continue to do footprinting and fingerprinting but give the prints to the parents as a birth souvenir.

Statistics for newborn abductions from hospital facilities are found in Table 18–4. Abductions and attempted abductions remain a threat to infant safety. Between 1965 and May 2019 there were 140 hospital abductions (National Center for Missing & Exploited Children [NCMEC], 2019). Infant abductions can be successfully prevented through a comprehensive safety program that may include alarm systems, video surveillance, and education of both staff and parents (Miller, 2007; York & MacAlister, 2015). The NCMEC in cooperation with the Association of Women's Health, Obstetric and Neonatal Nurses and the National Association of Neonatal Nurses (NCMEC, 2009) offer *Guidelines on Prevention of and Response to Infant Abductions*. Staff education should be combined with the development and testing of critical incident response procedures including mock infant abductions.

Newborn safety and security, including unit visiting policies, should be discussed with parents and family members. Parents should be made aware of what the hospital is doing to ensure the safety of every newborn and should understand what they can do to increase safety. Discussion with the parents should include directions not to leave their newborn unattended and information about identification of caregivers who may transport the newborn to and from the nursery or other hospital departments. Display 18–3 is an example of information that might be reviewed with parents, increasing their awareness of the need for vigilance and what they can do to support hospital systems designed to keep infants secure.

The efficacy of electronic newborn security systems in preventing newborn abductions remains controversial. No one method is superior; the key issue is that there must be some systematic newborn safety program in place known to the parents and perinatal healthcare providers to decrease the risk of newborn abduction. Nothing replaces vigilance on the part of parents, perinatal nurses, and other hospital employees.

VITAMIN K

One of the most important causes of a bleeding syndrome in an otherwise healthy newborn is hemorrhagic disease caused by vitamin K deficiency (Manco-Johnson, McKinney, Knapp-Clevenger, & Hernandez, 2016). During the first week of age, newborns are at risk for bleeding disorders because of an immature liver that is unable to produce several coagulation factors and a gastrointestinal tract that has not begun producing vitamin K. Consumption of breast milk and formula causes colonization of bacteria in the gastrointestinal tract, which is necessary for vitamin K production. Vitamin K stimulates the liver to synthesize coagulation factors II, VII, IX, and X (DeMarini & Rath, 2014). A single dose of 0.5 mg for newborns weighing less than 1.5 kg and 1 mg for newborns weighing more than 1.5 kg is administered intramuscularly within the first hour of age (AAP Committee on Fetus and Newborn, 2003, reaffirmed 2014).

EYE PROPHYLAXIS

Most states in the United States mandate that every newborn receive prophylaxis against eye infections. Erythromycin ointment is the drug of choice because of its effectiveness against gonococcal and chlamydial infections. To facilitate breastfeeding, ointment application

---

TABLE 18–4. Infant Abductions from Healthcare Facilities between January 1, 1965, and May 29, 2019, Organized by Specific Location within Healthcare Facilities

Specific Location of Abduction within Healthcare Facilities	Total January 1965 to May 2019
From mother's room	82 (58.57%)
From "on premises"	22 (15.71%)
From nursery	19 (13.57%)
From pediatrics	17 (12.14%)

Adapted from National Center for Missing & Exploited Children. (2019). *Analysis of infant abduction trends. Data collected: 1965 through May 2019.* Alexandria, VA: Author.

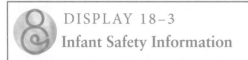

DISPLAY 18–3

Infant Safety Information

We, the nursing staff, welcome you and hope your family's stay here is a safe and pleasurable experience. During your stay, we ask for your cooperation to ensure your infant's safety.

1. If you are feeling weak, faint, or unsteady on your feet, do not lift your baby. Instead, call for assistance from the nurse.
2. Place your baby in the crib when you become drowsy, plan on sleeping, or are using the bathroom. Please call a nurse if you need help. Never leave your baby alone on your bed.
3. Never leave your baby alone in your room. If you walk in the halls or take a shower, please have a family member watch your baby, or return your baby to the nursery.
4. Always keep an eye and hand on your baby when the baby is out of the crib.
5. When walking in the corridor, your baby should be pushed in a crib, lying flat and supine (on the back).
6. Newborns possess some immunity from infections, but we still must protect them. Please ask your visitors to leave if they have any of the following: diarrhea, sore that has a discharge, or cold/contagious disease.
7. The only personnel that should be handling your baby or taking him or her from your room are employees wearing hospital scrubs and a picture ID tag. If you don't know the staff person, call for your nurse to help you.
8. Please call the nurse any time a situation arises with your baby where you do not feel proficient in providing care. We wish to give you as much teaching and information as possible to make your transition to parenthood as easy as possible.
9. There is an association between sudden infant death syndrome (SIDS) and prone (tummy-lying) sleeping in infants. The American Academy of Pediatrics recommends that normal infants be positioned wholly on their back to sleep. It should be stressed that the actual risk of SIDS for an infant placed on his or her stomach is still extremely low.
10. If your new baby's siblings visit, please keep a watchful eye on them so that they do not get hurt.

I understand the above information:

Date:_____

Mother's signature:_____

Date:_____

*Significant other:_____

*If available at the time of admission.

---

can be delayed up to 1 hour after birth (AAP & ACOG 2017). When administering eye prophylaxis, care should be taken to instill the ointment throughout the conjunctival sac. Excessive medication can be wiped away with a sterile cotton ball 1 minute after instillation (AAP & ACOG, 2017).

UMBILICAL CORD CARE

As part of the initial newborn assessment in the birthing room, the umbilical cord is examined for the presence of two arteries and a vein. Because a moist cord is vulnerable to pathogens, measures should be taken to promote drying of the cord, including exposing the cord to air. Over the years, a variety of methods of cord care have been used including alcohol, triple dye, and other antimicrobial agents. Research has shown that use of sterile water or air drying results in cords separating more quickly than those treated with alcohol (Quattrin et al., 2016). The cord should be observed for the presence of serous, purulent, or sanguineous drainage.

PSYCHOLOGICAL ADAPTATION

After addressing physiologic adaptation to extrauterine life, the focus of nursing interventions is psychological adaptation. Perinatal nurses are in a position to promote early maternal–newborn attachment. Early and extended contact between mother and newborn facilitates development of a positive relationship (Crenshaw, 2014). In a Cochrane review, Moore, Bergman, Anderson, and Medley (2016) identified positive benefits of early skin-to-skin contact on breastfeeding duration, infant crying, and early mother–infant attachment. The perinatal nurse assists in the attachment process by encouraging parents to see, touch, and hold their newborn. Providing uninterrupted time for them to be together gives parents the opportunity to recognize and identify unique behavioral and physical characteristics of their newborn.

Practices used to promote attachment usually do not interfere with transition to extrauterine life. Infants who require positive-pressure ventilation at birth or those with low Apgar score or other medical complications may require continuous monitoring. For stable infants, the perinatal nurse can make a positive contribution to enhancing the attachment process by modifying practices that separate mothers and newborns immediately after birth. Stable newborns should be placed skin-to-skin with the mother immediately after birth. If both are covered with a blanket, neonatal thermoregulation is not interrupted. Application of ophthalmic antibiotics may safely occur within the first hour of age, enhancing maternal–newborn eye contact (AAP & ACOG, 2017). Close observation during this initial period of skin-to-skin care must be maintained. A rare complication, sudden unexpected postnatal collapse (SUPC), has been reported in otherwise healthy term infants with the majority of cases occurring in the first 2 hours of age (Feldman-Winter & Goldsmith, 2016). Some cases of SUPC have been attributed to suffocation or entrapment, whereas in other cases, the etiology is unknown.

Maternal attachment is also supported when women are provided the opportunity to breast-feed immediately after birth. Breastfeeding is more than a feeding method; it is an intimate relationship between a mother and her newborn. Early opportunities for uninterrupted contact between mother and newborn increase breastfeeding duration (Moore et al., 2016).

COMPLICATIONS AFFECTING TRANSITION

Infection with group B streptococci (GBS) was one of the leading causes of morbidity and mortality in newborn infants before labor prophylaxis was instituted (Stoll, 2016). It is estimated that 25% to 30% of women are GBS carriers (Donders et al., 2016). Pregnant women colonized with GBS are mostly asymptomatic but may experience urinary tract infections and amnionitis. The incidence of early-onset GBS infection is 0.8 to 1.0 cases per 1,000 live births when prenatal screening and a program of intrapartum antimicrobial prophylaxis (IAP) are in place compared to a rate of 2.0 to 2.5 cases per 1,000 live births prior to the introduction of universal screening and treatment (Benitz, Wynn, & Polin, 2015).

Early-onset GBS infection can occur in the first 7 days of age but most commonly manifests in the first 24 hours after birth. Early-onset infection presents as bacteremia, meningitis, or pneumonia. The mortality rate associated with early-onset GBS infection is 7% to 9% (Shane & Stoll, 2014). Risk factors for the development of GBS infection include gestational age less than 37 weeks, rupture of membranes more than 18 hours before birth, intrapartum fever of 38°C (99.4°F) or higher, a previous GBS-infected newborn, and GBS bacteriuria during pregnancy.

Late-onset GBS infections occur between 1 week and 3 months of age. Sepsis is the most common manifestation of both early- and late-onset GBS; however, meningitis is more common in late-onset than in early-onset disease. The mortality rate for late-onset GBS is 1% to 6% (Leonard & Dobbs, 2015).

In 2010, the Centers for Disease Control and Prevention (CDC), (Verani, McGee, & Schrag) revised previous guidelines (CDC, 2005) and recommended universal screening for GBS in pregnant women between 35 and 37 weeks' gestations. In 2019, ACOG issued updated guidelines. The recommendations for Antibiotic Prophylaxis are presented in Table 18–5 (ACOG, 2019). See Chapter 8 for full details of these guidelines as they apply to the woman in labor. AAP also published updated guidelines in 2019 (Puopolo, Lynfield, Cummings, & AAP, 2019). See Chapter 21

TABLE 18–5. Indications for Intrapartum Antibiotic Prophylaxis to Prevent Neonatal Group B Streptococcal Early-Onset Disease*

Intrapartum GBS Prophylaxis Indicated	Intrapartum GBS Prophylaxis Not Indicated

Maternal history
  Previous neonate with invasive GBS disease
Current pregnancy
  Positive GBS culture obtained at 36 weeks and 0 days of gestation or more during current pregnancy (unless a cesarean birth is performed before onset of labor for a woman with intact amniotic membranes)
  GBS bacteriuria during any trimester of the current pregnancy
Intrapartum
  Unknown GBS status at the onset of labor (culture not done or results unknown) and any of the following:
    Birth at less than 37 weeks and 0 days of gestation
    Amniotic membrane rupture 18 hours or more
    Intrapartum temperature 100.4°F (38.0°C) or higher*
    Intrapartum NAAT result positive for GBS
    Intrapartum NAAT result negative but risk factors develop (i.e., less than 37 weeks and 0 days of gestation, amniotic membrane rupture 18 hours or more, or maternal temperature 100.4°F [38.0°C] or higher)
    Known GBS-positive status in a previous pregnancy
	Colonization with GBS during a previous pregnancy (unless colonization status in current pregnancy is unknown at onset of labor at term)
	Negative vaginal–rectal GBS culture obtained at 36 weeks and 0 days of gestation or more during the current pregnancy
	Cesarean birth performed before onset of labor on a woman with intact amniotic membranes, regardless of GBS colonization status or gestational age
	
	Negative vaginal–rectal GBS culture obtained at 36 weeks and 0 days of gestation or more during the current pregnancy, regardless of intrapartum risk factors
	Unknown GBS status at onset of labor, NAAT result negative and no intrapartum risk factors present (i.e., less than 37 weeks and 0 days of gestation, amniotic membrane rupture 18 hours or more, or maternal temperature 100.4°F [38°C] or higher)

GBS, group B *Streptococcus*; NAAT, nucleic acid amplification test.
*If intraamniotic infection is suspected, broad-spectrum antibiotic therapy that includes an agent known to be active against GBS should replace GBS prophylaxis.
From American College of Obstetricians and Gynecologists. (2019). *Prevention of group B streptococcal early-onset disease in newborns* (Committee Opinion No. 782). Washington, DC: Author. Modified from Verani, J. R., McGee, L., & Schrag, S. J. (2010). Prevention of perinatal group B streptococcal disease: Revised guidelines from CDC, 2010. *Morbidity and Mortality Weekly Report Recommendations and Reports, 59*(RR-10), 1–32.

for full details of these guidelines as they apply to the newborn. Cases of early-onset GBS disease continue to occur despite the new guidelines and affected infants incur significant morbidity and mortality. Inaccurate screening results, improper implementation of IAP, or antibiotic failure all may contribute to persistent disease. This highlights the importance of continued vigilance for signs of infection in the newborn. The assessment and care of a newborn after birth should be based on knowledge of maternal risk factors for GBS sepsis, maternal GBS status if known, and the timing and number of doses of antibiotic administered during labor. After delivery, it is important to evaluate the newborn for signs and symptoms of infection, including respiratory distress, apnea, tachycardia, hypotension, pallor, temperature instability, lethargy, and hypotonia. The Kaiser Sepsis Risk Prediction tool (Kaiser Permanente Research, 2019) for predicting sepsis in the newborn has been tested and validated and is available at https://neonatalsepsis calculator.kaiserpermanente.org/.

HEPATITIS B

Each year in the United States, about 25,000 infants are born to hepatitis B virus (HBV)-positive women (Barbosa et al., 2014). Universal vaccination and prenatal testing for HBV have decreased the incidence of new HBV infections by over 90% (AAP Committee on Infectious Diseases & Committee on Fetus and Newborn, 2017).

An estimated one third of chronic infections worldwide are believed to have resulted from perinatal or early childhood transmission (Nelson, Jamieson, & Murphy, 2014). The spectrum of HBV infection ranges from asymptomatic seroconversion through general malaise, anorexia, nausea, and jaundice to fetal hepatitis. Development of a chronic infection is inversely proportional to the age at which the infection was acquired. Ninety percent of newborns infected in utero or at the time of birth develop chronic infection; in contrast, only 5% of adults develop chronic HBV infection after acute illness (Nelson et al., 2014). The immunologic response to infection leads to the development of cirrhosis, liver failure, or hepatocellular carcinoma in up to 40% of patients (Nelson et al., 2014). Routine screening of pregnant women for hepatitis B surface antigen (HBsAg) should be carried out when the hepatitis status is unknown. HBsAg can be detected in individuals with acute or chronic hepatitis B viral infection.

The AAP recommends universal HBV immunization for all newborns. Newborns born to HBsAg-negative mothers should receive the first dose of vaccine at birth (before hospital discharge), with the second dose 1 to 2 months later and the third dose by 6 to 18 months of age (AAP Committee on Infectious Diseases, 2015). Babies born to HBsAg-positive mothers should receive one dose of hepatitis vaccine within 12 hours of birth, and hepatitis B immunoglobulin (HBIG) should be given concurrently (AAP Committee on Infectious Diseases, 2015). HBIG provides temporary protection in postexposure situations, and HBV vaccine provides long-term protection. Newborns born to women with unknown HBsAg status should receive the first dose of HBV vaccine within 12 hours of birth (AAP & ACOG, 2017; AAP Committee on Infectious Diseases, 2015). Because the vaccine is highly effective in preventing infection in this population, further prophylaxis with HBIG can be delayed up to 7 days while awaiting maternal laboratory results.

SUMMARY

Most newborns need minimal support to make the transition to extrauterine life. Diverse and complex system adaptations make it a critical time for newborns. Strong desires to interact with their newborn make this a significant time for parents. The perinatal nurse must be knowledgeable about normal physiologic changes during the period of newborn transition to extrauterine life. Caring for newborns during this time requires the ability to recognize alterations from normal and becoming proficient at the skills necessary for conducting a newborn resuscitation.

REFERENCES

Alvaro, R. E., & Rigatto, H. (2017). Control of breathing in fetal life and onset and control of breathing in the neonate. In R. Polin, S. Abman, D. Rowitch, W. Benitz, & W. Fox (Eds.), *Fetal and neonatal physiology* (5th ed., pp. 737–747). Philadelphia, PA: Elsevier.

American Academy of Pediatrics & American College of Obstetricians and Gynecologists. (2017). *Guidelines for perinatal care* (8th ed.). Elk Grove Village, IL: Author.

American Academy of Pediatrics & American Heart Association. (2016). *Textbook of neonatal resuscitation* (7th ed.). Elk Grove Village, IL: American Academy of Pediatrics.

American Academy of Pediatrics Committee on Fetus and Newborn. (2003). Controversies concerning vitamin K and the newborn. *Pediatrics*, 112(1, Pt. 1), 191–192.

American Academy of Pediatrics Committee on Infectious Diseases. (2015). *Red book: 2015 Report of the Committee on Infectious Diseases* (30th ed.). Elk Grove Village, IL: Author.

American Academy of Pediatrics Committee on Infectious Diseases & Committee on Fetus and Newborn. (2017). Elimination of perinatal hepatitis B: Providing the first vaccine dose within 24 hours of birth. *Pediatrics*, 140(3), e20171870. doi:10.1542/peds.2017-1870

American College of Obstetricians and Gynecologists. (2019). *Prevention of Group B Streptococcal early-onset disease in newborns* (Committee Opinion No. 782). Washington, DC: Author.

Apgar, V. (1966). The newborn (Apgar) scoring system. Reflections and advice. *Pediatric Clinics of North America*, 13(3), 645–650.

Barbosa, C., Smith, E., Hoerger, T., Fenlon, N., Schillie, S., Bradley, C., & Murphy, T. (2014). Cost-effectiveness analysis of the National Perinatal Hepatitis B Prevention Program. *Pediatrics*, *133*(2), 243–253. doi:10.1542/peds.2013-0718

Benitz, W. E., Wynn, J. L., & Polin, R. A. (2015). Reappraisal of guidelines for management of neonates with suspected early-onset sepsis. *The Journal of Pediatrics*, *166*(4), 1070–1074. doi:10.1016/j.jpeds.2014.12.023

Blackburn, S. T. (2018). *Maternal, fetal, & neonatal physiology: A clinical perspective* (5th ed.). Philadelphia, PA: Saunders.

Brand, M. C., & Boyd, H. (2015). Thermoregulation. In T. Verklan & M. Walden (Eds.), *Core curriculum for neonatal intensive care nursing* (5th ed., pp. 95–109). St. Louis, MO: Elsevier Saunders.

Cavaliere, T., & Sansoucie, D. (2014). Assessment of the newborn and infant. In C. Kenner & J. W. Lott (Eds.), *Comprehensive neonatal care: An interdisciplinary approach* (5th ed., pp. 71–112). Philadelphia, PA: Saunders.

Centers for Disease Control and Prevention. (2005). Early-onset and late-onset neonatal group B streptococcal disease–United States, 1996–2004. *Morbidity and Mortality Weekly Report*, *54*(47), 1205–1208.

Conde-Agudelo, A., & Díaz-Rossello, J. (2016). Kangaroo mother care to reduce morbidity and mortality in low birthweight infants. *Cochrane Database of Systematic Reviews*, (8), CD002771. doi:10.1002/14651858.CD002771.pub4

Crenshaw, J. T. (2014). Healthy birth practice #6: Keep mother and baby together—It's best for mother, baby, and breastfeeding. *The Journal of Perinatal Education*, *23*(4), 211–217. doi:10.1891/1058-1243.23.4.211

DeMarini, S., & Rath, L. L. (2014). Fluids, electrolytes, vitamins, and minerals. In C. Kenner & J. W. Lott (Eds.), *Comprehensive neonatal care: An interdisciplinary approach* (5th ed., pp. 509–529). Philadelphia, PA: Saunders.

Donders, G. G., Halperin, S. A., Devlieger, R., Baker, S., Forte, P., Wittke, F., . . . Dull, P. M. (2016). Maternal immunization with an investigational trivalent group B streptococcal vaccine: A randomized controlled trial. *Obstetrics and Gynecology*, *127*(2), 213–221. doi:10.1097/AOG.0000000000001190

Feldman-Winter, L., & Goldsmith, J. (2016). Safe sleep and skin-to-skin care in the neonatal period for healthy term newborns. *Pediatrics*, *138*(3), e20161889. doi:10.1542/peds.2016-1889

Gardner, S., Enzman-Hines, M., & Nyp, M. (2016). Respiratory diseases. In S. L. Gardner, B. S. Carter, M. I. Enzman-Hines, & J. A. Hernandez (Eds.), *Merenstein & Gardner's handbook of neonatal intensive care* (8th ed., pp. 565–643). St. Louis, MO: Mosby Elsevier.

Gardner, S., & Hernandez, J. (2016). Heat balance. In G. B. Merenstein & S. L. Gardner (Eds.), *Handbook of neonatal intensive care* (8th ed., pp. 105–125). St. Louis, MO: Mosby.

Goldberg, A., & Krasuski, R. (2012). Patent ductus arteriosus and coarctation of the aorta. In B. Griffin (Ed.), *Manual of cardiovascular medicine* (4th ed., pp. 526–536). Philadelphia, PA: Lippincott Williams & Wilkins.

Jennewein, M., Abu-Raya, B., Jiang, Y., Alter, G., & Marchant, A. (2017). Transfer of maternal immunity and programming of the newborn immune system. *Seminars in Immunopathology*, *39*(6), 605–613. doi:10.1007/s00281-017-0653-x

Kaiser Permanente Research. (2019). *Neonatal sepsis risk calculator*. Oakland, CA: Author. Retrieved from https://neonatalsepsiscalculator.kaiserpermanente.org/

Leonard, E., & Dobbs, K. (2015). Postnatal bacterial infections. In R. Martin, A. Fanaroff, & M. Walsh (Eds.), *Fanaroff and Martin's neonatal-perinatal medicine* (10th ed., pp. 734–750). Philadelphia, PA: Saunders.

Lorenz, L., Dawson, J. A., Jones, H., Jacobs, S. E., Cheong, J. L., Donath, S. M., . . . Kamlin, C. O. (2017). Skin-to-skin care in preterm infants receiving respiratory support does not lead to physiological instability. *Archives of Disease in Childhood. Fetal and Neonatal Edition*, *102*(4), F339–F344.

Lott, J. W. (2014). Cardiovascular system. In C. Kenner & J. W. Lott (Eds.), *Comprehensive neonatal care: An interdisciplinary approach* (5th ed., pp. 152–188). Philadelphia, PA: Saunders.

Manco-Johnson, M., McKinney, C., Knapp-Clevenger, R., & Hernandez, J. (2016). Newborn hematology. In G. B. Merenstein & S. L. Gardner (Eds.), *Handbook of neonatal intensive care* (8th ed., pp. 479–510). St. Louis, MO: Mosby.

Miller, R. S. (2007). Preventing infant abduction in the hospital. *Nursing*, *37*(10), 20, 22.

Moore, E. R., Bergman, N., Anderson, G., & Medley, N. (2016). Early skin-to-skin contact for mothers and their healthy newborn infants. *Cochrane Database of Systematic Reviews*, (11), CD003519.

Morton, S., & Brodsky, D. (2016). Fetal physiology and the transition to extrauterine life. *Clinics in Perinatology*, *43*(3), 395–407. doi:10.1016/j.clp.2016.04.001

National Center for Missing and Exploited Children. (2009). *Guidelines on prevention of and response to infant abductions*. Alexandria, VA: Author.

National Center for Missing and Exploited Children. (2019). *Analysis of infant abduction trends. Data collected: 1965 through May 2019*. Alexandria, VA: Author.

Nelson, N. P., Jamieson, D. J., & Murphy, T. V. (2014). Prevention of perinatal hepatitis B virus transmission. *Journal of the Pediatric Infectious Diseases Society*, *3*(Suppl. 1), S7–S12. doi:10.1093/jpids/piu064

Puopolo, K., Lynfield, R., & Cummings, J. J., & American Academy of Pediatrics, Committee on Fetus and Newborn, Committee on Infectious Diseases. (2019). Management of infants at risk for group B streptococcal disease. *Pediatrics*, *144*(2), pii:e20191881. doi:10.1542/peds.2019-1881

Quattrin, R., Iacobucci, K., De Tina, A. L., Gallina, L., Pittini, C., & Brusaferro, S. (2016). 70% Alcohol versus dry cord care in the umbilical cord care: A case-control study in Italy. *Medicine (Baltimore)*, *95*(14), e3207. doi:10.1097/MD.0000000000003207

Riviere, D., McKinlay, C. J., & Bloomfield, F. H. (2017). Adaptation for life after birth: A review of neonatal physiology. *Anaesthesia & Intensive Care Medicine*, *18*(2), 59–67.

Shane, A. L., & Stoll, B. J. (2014). Neonatal sepsis: Progress towards improved outcomes. *Journal of Infection*, *68*(Suppl. 1), S24–S32. doi:10.1016/j.jinf.2013.09.011

Steinhorn, R. H. (2015). Pulmonary vascular development. In R. J. Martin, A. A. Fanaroff, & M. C. Walsh (Eds.), *Fanaroff and Martin's neonatal-perinatal medicine: Diseases of the fetus and infant* (10th ed., pp. 1198–1209). St. Louis, MO: Saunders.

Stoll, B. J. (2016). Early-onset neonatal sepsis: A continuing problem in need of novel prevention strategies. *Pediatrics*, *138*(6), e20163038.

Verani, J. R., McGee, L., & Schrag, S. J. (2010). Prevention of perinatal group B streptococcal disease—Revised guidelines from CDC, 2010. *MMWR. Recommendations and Reports*, *59*(RR-10), 1–36.

Wyckoff, M. H., Aziz, K., Escobedo, M. B., Kapadia, V. S., Kattwinkel, J., Perlman, J. M., . . . Zaichkin, J. G. (2015). Part 13: Neonatal resuscitation: 2015 American Heart Association guidelines update for cardiopulmonary resuscitation and emergency cardiovascular care. *Circulation*, *132*(18 Suppl. 2), S543–S560. doi:10.1161/CIR.0000000000000267

York, T., & MacAlister, D. (2015). *Hospital and healthcare security* (6th ed.). Oxford, United Kingdom: Butterworth-Heinemann.

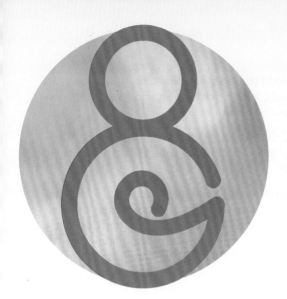

CHAPTER 19

Newborn Physical Assessment

Annie J. Rohan

INTRODUCTION

Perinatal and neonatal nurses frequently perform the first head-to-toe physical assessment of the newborn. Ideally, this examination occurs in the presence of the parents. Conducting the examination while parents observe allows the nurse to use this time to identify and discuss normal newborn characteristics and note variations. It also provides an opportunity for parents to ask questions about the newborn's physical appearance and condition. The focus of this chapter is the physical assessment and findings that the perinatal/neonatal nurse may observe during the time the newborn is in the hospital or birthing center. Home care nurses may also find the information pertinent during early postpartum home visits. Although some references are made to preterm newborns, that subject is not the intended focus of this chapter. It is also assumed that the reader has basic knowledge of physical assessment skills and terminology. Normal findings and common variations for each body system are identified in the text. Tables describe pathologic findings and their causes.

Physical assessment skills of observation, palpation, and auscultation are used frequently throughout the examination. Percussion is not commonly used in the newborn exam. When performing a physical assessment, the following equipment should be available: scale, tape measure, tongue blades, stethoscope with a neonatal diaphragm and bell, and an ophthalmoscope. The initial physical assessment may be conducted with the infant under a radiant warmer, in the crib, or while skin-to-skin with mother. Regardless of the location, attention should be given to avoiding hypothermia and cold stress. Adequate lighting is also essential but should be employed methodically, so as not to startle or irritate the infant.

The sequence in which the nurse conducts the physical assessment is a matter of personal preference and most often depends on the cooperation of the newborn. Although the newborn assessment is presented in this chapter as a sequential examination covering one system at a time, the exam is commonly and appropriately conducted by examining multiple systems in tandem.

It is important to note that many infant disorders and conditions present with varied and nonspecific abnormalities across multiple systems of the physical examination. For example, neonatal abstinence syndrome, and other drug toxicities or withdrawals, may present with a broad range of physical examination findings reflecting dysfunction of autonomic regulation, state control, and sensory or motor functioning (Clark & Rohan, 2015). It is important to not only be able to conduct the examination of multiple systems concurrently but to also consider findings of the individual systems collectively, as the examination progresses.

STATE, WEIGHT, AND GESTATIONAL AGE ASSESSMENT

The general examination of the infant should begin with as many noninvasive assessments as possible, beginning with observation of breathing pattern, overall skin color and perfusion, general state or level of alertness, posture, and muscle tone. The newborn's *state* refers to general level of alertness and is a reflection of a group of characteristics that occur together. In the newborn, these characteristics include body activity, eye movement, facial movements, breathing pattern, and level of response to internal and external stimuli. Understanding the differences in state provides information about how the newborn will respond to the nurse or parents and about the condition of the newborn's health, and it has implications for parent education. Appendix 19–A describes newborn states (deep sleep, light sleep, drowsy, quiet alert, active alert, and crying) and the implications these states have for caregivers.

The size of a newborn is dependent on genetic, environmental, placental, and maternal factors. Every fetus is thought to have inherent growth potential that, under normal circumstances, is closely associated with newborn health. There are standards for weight, as well as for linear measurements (e.g., length, head circumference, abdominal circumference, femur length), for the fetus at all gestational ages as well as for neonates and infants. Actual fetal or infant measurements are compared to these standards, which are found in the form of "growth charts" in most any perinatal setting.

When a fetus does not reach its intrauterine potential for growth and development, usually as a result of compromised placental function, we say that there is *fetal growth restriction* (FGR) (American College of Obstetrics and Gynecologists [ACOG] & Society for Maternal-Fetal Medicine, 2019). The term *intrauterine growth restriction (IUGR)* and *intrauterine growth retardation* have been previously used to characterize this entity, but such nomenclature has fallen out of favor. FGR affects 5% to 10% of pregnancies and is positioned as an obstetrical diagnosis. FGR is generally described as a fetal weight below the 10th percentile of a reference population, occurring either early or late in pregnancy, and often with associated placental insufficiency (Nardozza et al., 2017).

The newborn is weighed and measured. It is normal for newborns to lose up to 10% of their birth weight during the first few days of life. Figure 19–1 illustrates the technique for obtaining accurate measurements. The Centers for Disease Control and Prevention recommends that healthcare providers use growth standards provided by the World Health Organization to monitor neonatal/infant growth (World Health Organization, n.d.). According to these standards, a term newborn should have the following approximate measurements:

- Weight, 2,500 to 4,100 g (5.5 to 9 lb)
- Head circumference, 32 to 36 cm (12.5 to 14 inches)
- Length, 46 to 52 cm (18 to 20.5 inches)

The American Academy of Pediatrics (AAP) and ACOG recommend that the gestational age of newborns be established by incorporating both obstetric and the initial physical and neurologic findings of the newborn (AAP & ACOG, 2017). If indicated, a gestational age assessment, evaluating physical and neuromuscular characteristics, is usually performed as part of the initial physical examination. Although some hospitals make gestational age assessment of all newborns a routine practice, other institutions have established criteria for performing gestational age assessment such as birth weight less than 2,500 g, suspected FGR, respiratory distress in a "term" infant, or upon request by the primary care provider (and then often conducted by this provider). Identifying newborns that are preterm, term, or postterm, those who are small for gestational age (SGA), appropriate for gestational age, or large for gestational age (LGA), and those identified with FGR, increases the likelihood of early identification and timely interventions for potential complications associated with weight and age during the immediate newborn period.

The original tool used for gestational assessment was the Dubowitz Scoring System. It contained 20 items combining neurologic and physical parameters that successfully estimated gestational age in infants older than 34 weeks (Dubowitz, Dubowitz, & Goldberg, 1970). The tool was revised in 1999, increasing the number of items on the neurologic exam. The test expanded the neurologic exam to include behavior states, tone, primitive reflexes, motility, and some aspects of behavior (Dubowitz, Ricciw, & Mercuri, 2005).

The Ballard Maturational Score (BMS) was developed in the late 1970s (Ballard, Novak, & Driver, 1979) for determining gestational age. As more low-birthweight infants were born and survived the initial neonatal period, the BMS was reevaluated and expanded, resulting in the development of a New Ballard Score (Fig. 19–2). The New Ballard has broadened criteria to provide greater accuracy when evaluating extremely premature neonates (Ballard et al., 1991). Use of the New Ballard is now recommended in perinatal clinical practice guidelines (Association of Women's Health, Obstetric and Neonatal Nurses, 2017).

The BMS is conducted by comparing the individual newborn's characteristics with the pictures on the form and assigning a number for each characteristic. Appendix 19–B describes each characteristic evaluated. Controversy has existed about the best timing of this assessment, particularly in more premature newborns. The BMS seems to be most accurate if performed between 10 and 36 hours

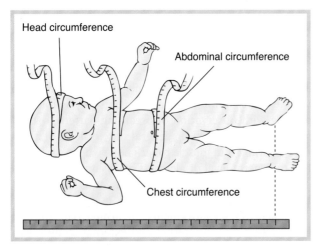

FIGURE 19–1. Newborn measurements. (Adapted from Wong, D. L. [Ed.]. [1997]. *Whaley & Wong's nursing care of infants and children* [6th ed., p. 139]. St. Louis, MO: Mosby-Year Book.)

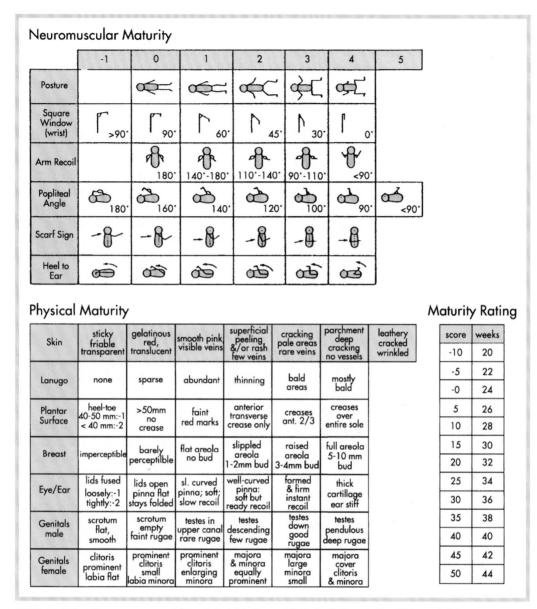

Neuromuscular Maturity

	-1	0	1	2	3	4	5
Posture							
Square Window (wrist)	>90°	90°	60°	45°	30°	0°	
Arm Recoil		180°	140°-180°	110°-140°	90°-110°	<90°	
Popliteal Angle	180°	160°	140°	120°	100°	90°	<90°
Scarf Sign							
Heel to Ear							

Physical Maturity

Skin	sticky friable transparent	gelatinous red, translucent	smooth pink, visible veins	superficial peeling &/or rash few veins	cracking pale areas rare veins	parchment deep cracking no vessels	leathery cracked wrinkled
Lanugo	none	sparse	abundant	thinning	bald areas	mostly bald	
Plantar Surface	heel-toe 40-50 mm:-1 < 40 mm:-2	>50mm no crease	faint red marks	anterior transverse crease only	creases ant. 2/3	creases over entire sole	
Breast	imperceptible	barely perceptilble	flat areola no bud	slippled areola 1-2mm bud	raised areola 3-4mm bud	full areola 5-10 mm bud	
Eye/Ear	lids fused loosely:-1 tightly:-2	lids open pinna flat stays folded	sl. curved pinna; soft; slow recoil	well-curved pinna: soft but ready recoil	formed & firm instant recoil	thick cartilage ear stiff	
Genitals male	scrotum flat, smooth	scrotum empty faint rugae	testes in upper canal rare rugae	testes descending few rugae	testes down good rugae	testes pendulous deep rugae	
Genitals female	clitoris prominent labia flat	prominent clitoris small labia minora	prominent clitoris enlarging minora	majora & minora equally prominent	majora large minora small	majora cover clitoris & minora	

Maturity Rating

score	weeks
-10	20
-5	22
-0	24
5	26
10	28
15	30
20	32
25	34
30	36
35	38
40	40
45	42
50	44

FIGURE 19–2. Gestational age assessment. (From Ballard, J. L., Khoury, J. C., Wedig, K., Wang, L, Eilers-Walsman, B. L., & Lipp, R. [1991]. New Ballard Score, expanded to include extremely premature infants. *Journal of Pediatrics, 119*[3], 417–423.)

of age. Assessment of newborns younger than 26 weeks' gestation is best conducted within the first 12 hours (Gagliardi, Brambilla, Bruno, Martinelli, & Console, 1993). The examination is separated into two parts: neuromuscular maturity assessment and physical maturity assessment. Scores from both sections are added together to determine gestational age (Ballard et al., 1991).

SKIN ASSESSMENT

The newborn's entire body, as well as skin folds and scalp, should be inspected and palpated for changes in texture and the presence of masses that are not visible. Color, birth marks, rashes, skin lesions, texture, and turgor are noted. At birth, newborn skin may be covered with *vernix*, an odorless, white, cheesy, protective coating produced by sebaceous glands. Vernix develops during the third trimester and increases with gestational age. At about 37 weeks, the amount of vernix begins to decrease, and at term, it is present only in the creases of the arms, legs, and neck.

Color

Skin color reflects circulation, oxygenation, and hemoglobin saturation. Color is best observed in a well-lit room while the newborn is quiet. At birth, color ranges from pale to plethoric, depending on hematocrit and general perfusion. Skin pigmentation depends on ethnic origin and deepens over time. Caucasian newborns have pinkish red skin tones a few hours after birth, and African American newborns have a reddish-brown skin color. Hispanic and Asian newborns have an olive or yellow skin tone. Changes in the skin color of Caucasian new-borns may be the first sign of illness such as sepsis, cardio-pulmonary disorders, or hematologic diseases. Variations in skin color indicating illness may be more difficult to evaluate in African American and Asian newborns.

Generalized or *central cyanosis* may be seen initially at the time of birth as the newborn transitions from fetal to neonatal circulation. Central cyanosis occurring beyond the initial minutes following birth refers to blu-ish color of the tongue, skin, lips and nail beds in the newborn and when seen requires urgent attention by a physician or advanced practice nurse because it usually indicates a pathologic condition. It is usually seen when there is less than 5 g of unsaturated hemoglobin per 100 mL of blood or a saturation of <85% (Hernandez & Glass, 2005). *Acrocyanosis*, the blue discoloration of newborn hands and feet and *circumoral cyanosis*, a blu-ish color seen around the newborn's mouth, are normal findings and are often seen in the first 24 to 48 hours of life. Acrocyanosis is related to vasomotor instability and tends to worsen if the newborn becomes cold.

Jaundice

Jaundice, a bright yellow or orange discoloration of the skin, results from deposits of unconjugated bilirubin. Up to 60% of healthy term, newborns develop some degree of jaundice (Kaplan, Wong, Sibley, & Steven-son, 2011). Jaundice results from the reduced ability of the newborn's liver to conjugate bilirubin. An elevated direct bilirubin level is never normal and suggests some pathology involving the liver. The skin color change as-sociated with an elevated direct bilirubin has a green-ish hue (Gomella, Cunningham, & Eyal, 2009a). A mild to moderately elevated indirect bilirubin level is considered normal in the first few days of age. Jaundice associated with indirect hyperbilirubinemia is associ-ated with a distinctive yellow hue that generally moves in a cephalocaudal fashion. Seen first on the head and face, jaundice progresses downward to the trunk and extremities and then to the sclera of the eye. When gentle pressure is applied to skin over cartilage or a bony prominence, skin blanches to a yellow hue on the face when bilirubin levels are 5 mg/dL, on the upper chest when levels are about 10 mg/dL, on the abdo-men when levels are 12 mg/dL, and on the palms and soles of the feet when levels are greater than 15 mg/dL (Gomella, Cunningham, & Eyal, 2009b). Newborns with a positive Coombs test result almost certainly de-velop jaundice. In dark-skinned newborns, jaundice is more easily observed in the sclera and buccal mucosa.

Bruising

Ecchymosis may occur over the head or buttocks if for-ceps or a vacuum extractor was applied or after a breech or face presentation. *Petechiae* (small pinpoint-sized, reddish-to-purple spots on the skin) are common over the presenting part, especially when there has been a rapid descent during second stage of labor, but general-ized or widespread petechiae are abnormal, may signify low platelet counts, and should be further investigated. Bruising may also result from a tight nuchal cord or an umbilical cord wrapped tightly around the upper body.

Variations Related to Vasomotor Instability

Cutis marmorata, mottling, or a lace-like pattern on the skin is a vasomotor response to chilling. Parents should be aware that this may continue after dis-charge. The *harlequin sign* occurs when some new-borns are positioned on their sides. The dependent side of the body becomes pink, and the superior half of the body is pale. This phenomenon is considered benign. The color change lasts 1 to 30 minutes and disappears gradually when the infant is placed on the abdomen or back (Witt, 2019).

Hemangiomas

Hemangiomas are vascular soft tissue tumors. They may be present at birth and may begin as a pale macule with threadlike markings and develop into a bright-red elevated tumor that ranges in size. They can also develop in the first several weeks of life. One percent to 3% of newborns have hemangiomas, and they are more likely to occur in females than in males (Fig. 19–3). They are generally benign and self-limiting in that they often initially grow but then involute with-out treatment. However, they may ulcerate, become cavernous, and cause disfigurement or may require in-tervention (Hoath & Narendran, 2011).

Capillary Lesions

Capillary-composed lesions are also common. *Nevus simplex* ("stork bites") are flat, irregularly shaped reddish-colored patches that blanch with pressure and become darker when the newborn cries. They are most often seen at the back of the neck, on the forehead, on eyelids, on the bridge of the nose, and over the base of the occipital bones. Nevus simplex are among the most common of skin lesions, occurring in up to 70% of newborns, and typically lasting 1 to 2 years (Hoath & Narendran, 2011). *Port wine stains* are ir-regularly shaped flat pink to reddish markings that are most often present at birth, but less common than nevus simplex. Color varies from pink in Caucasian infants to black or deep purple in African American newborns or newborns of color. Port wine stains have discrete borders, do not blanch when pressure is ap-plied, and do not lighten as the child ages (Witt, 2019). These lesions are most often seen on the head and neck and are generally benign unless they occur along the trigeminal nerve root, in which case they may be as-sociated with glaucoma or optic atrophy, seizures, and

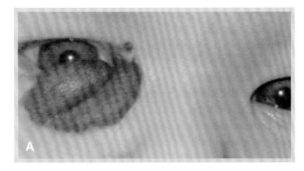
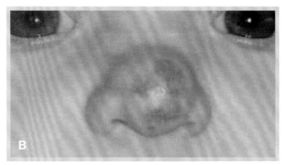
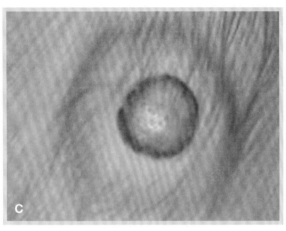

FIGURE 19–3. Hemangioma. Complications of infantile hemangioma: visual obstruction **(A)** and disfiguring facial hemangioma (so-called Cyrano nose) **(B)**. Infantile hemangioma according to anatomical location: mixed type of bright red, intracutaneous hemangioma and bluish, deep hemangioma **(C)**. (From Léauté-Labrèze, C., Harper, J. I., & Hoeger, P. H. [2017]. Infantile haemangioma. *Lancet, 390*[10089], 2017. doi:10.1016/S0140-6736(16)00645-0)

mental retardation (Hoath & Narendran, 2011). Certain types of lasers effectively remove port wine stains.

Mongolian Spots

Mongolian spots are large, nonblanching, blue-gray lesions resembling a bruise that are most often seen over the sacrum and flanks but may be present on the posterior thighs, legs, back, and shoulders (Fig. 19–4). They occur frequently in African American, Asian, and Native American infants, but can be observed in Caucasian infants (Hoath & Narendran, 2011). Mongolian spots are caused by infiltration of melanin-forming cells into the dermal skin layer rather than the epidermis. Mongolian spots may persist into early childhood but usually fade.

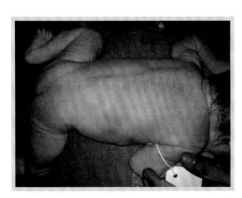

FIGURE 19–4. Mongolian spot. (From Gupta, D., & Thappa, D. M. [2013]. Mongolian spots. *Indian Journal of Dermatology, Venereology, and Leprology, 79*[4], 469–478. doi:10.4103/0378-6323.11307)

Erythema Toxicum and Milia

Erythema toxicum ("newborn rash") and *milia* are benign skin conditions usually limited to the first weeks of age. *Erythema toxicum* generally occurs within 5 days of birth in approximately 50% of term newborn infants (Lund & Kuller, 2007). In preterm newborns, the rash may not develop for several days or weeks. Erythema toxicum is composed of small, yellow papules surrounded by an erythematous margin. The rash continues to appear and disappear over various parts of the body—most commonly the face, trunk, and limbs—for several days to weeks (Witt, 2019). *Milia*, are clogged sebaceous glands that appear as tiny, white, pinhead-sized papules presenting at birth over the chin, cheeks, forehead, and nose. They are benign and disappear during the first month of life (Lund & Kuller, 2007).

Texture

Skin is evaluated for texture surface findings, during the physical examination and as part of the gestational age assessment. Texture ranges from smooth to cracked and peeling. Shortly after birth, most term newborns have dry, flaky skin. Peeling, leathery skin with deep cracks indicates postmaturity. *Lanugo*, a fine, downy hair that covers the body, begins to develop around 12 weeks and is abundant by 17 to 20 weeks' gestation (Moore & Persaud, 2008). It is seen in abundance on premature infants. However, it becomes less abundant as gestation increases and is rarely on newborns who are post 40 weeks. At term, lanugo is usually confined to the shoulders, ears, and forehead.

Turgor

Skin turgor is the natural rebound elasticity of the skin. It can be assessed anywhere on the body by pinching the skin between the examiners thumb and index finger and then quickly releasing it. Skin turgor is best assessed on the abdomen. Healthy, elastic tissue rapidly resumes its normal position without creases or tenting. Skin that remains tented indicates poor hydration and nutritional status.

Table 19–1 identifies skin findings during the physical assessment that are abnormal and their related pathology.

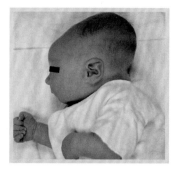

FIGURE 19–5. Temporarily elongated head in cranial molding following vertex vaginal delivery. (From American Journal of Obstetrics and Gynecology. [2012]. Progesterone and preterm birth prevention: Translating clinical trials data into clinical practice. *American Journal of Obstetrics and Gynecology, 206*[5], 376–386.)

TABLE 19–1. Integument

Assessment	Pathology
Pallor	Anemia
	Asphyxia
	Shock
	Sepsis
	Twin-to-twin transfusion
	Cardiac disease
Central cyanosis	Respiratory disorder
	Persistent pulmonary hypertension
	Neurologic disease
	Congenital heart disease
	Sepsis
Plethora	Polycythemia
	Overheated
Gray color	Sepsis
	Shock
Jaundice within 24 hr of birth	Liver disease
	Sepsis
	Maternal ingestion of drugs (e.g., aspirin)
	Blood incompatibilities
Generalized petechiae	Thrombocytopenia
	Clotting disorders
	Sepsis
Pustules	*Staphylococcus*
	Beta-hemolytic *Streptococcus*
	Varicella
Greenish, yellow vernix	Meconium staining
	Hemolytic disease
Generalized edema	Erythroblastosis fetalis
	Renal failure
	Turner syndrome
"Blueberry muffin" spots (purpura)	Congenital viral infection
Multiple tan or light brown macules (café au lait spots)	Neurofibromatosis
Cutis marmorata	Hypovolemia
	Sepsis
	Chromosomal abnormalities
Extensive Mongolian spots	Inborn errors of metabolism (Silengo, Battistoni, & Spada, 1999)

From Silengo, M., Battistoni, G., & Spada, M. (1999). Is there a relationship between extensive mongolian spots and inborn errors of metabolism? *American Journal of Medical Genetics, 87*(3), 276–277. Retrieved from https://www.ncbi.nlm.nih.gov/pubmed/12881938

HEAD ASSESSMENT

The newborn head is examined using inspection and palpation and assessed for size, shape, and symmetry. To measure the newborn's head, a tape measure is placed just above the eyebrows and continues around to the occipital prominence at the back of the skull (see Fig. 19–1). Vaginal birth may cause the cranial bones to overlap as the fetus descends through the birth canal or as a result of the application of vacuum or forceps, giving the head an elongated, asymmetric appearance (Fig. 19–5). The overlapping cranial bones can be palpated along the suture lines. This *molding* may last several days and may result in head circumference being unrepresentative of baseline immediately after birth. The circumference returns to normal within 2 to 3 days after birth. Newborns delivered by cesarean section, especially due to breech position, have a more rounded, symmetric head.

Distinction is made between transiently diminished head circumference due to molding, and true *microcephaly*. In microcephaly, the infant's head is smaller than expected due to poor brain growth (Fig. 19–6). Microcephaly may be an isolated condition, or it can occur as part of a syndrome or in combination with other major birth defects. Microcephaly may be

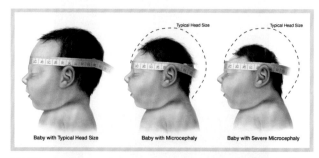

FIGURE 19–6. Normocephaly, microcephaly, and severe microcephaly. (From National Center on Birth Defects and Developmental Disabilities, Centers for Disease Control and Prevention.)

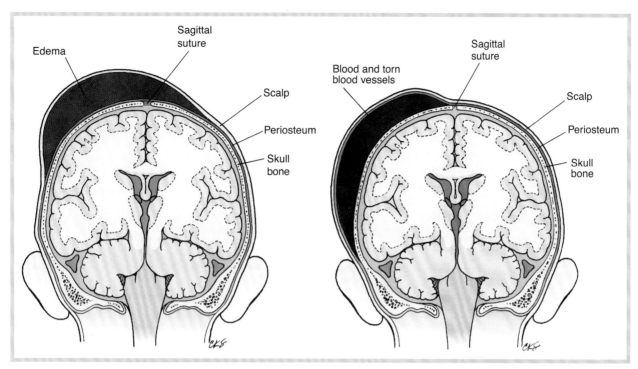

FIGURE 19–7. Comparison of caput succedaneum (*left*) and cephalohematoma (*right*).

associated with fetal alcohol syndrome; Zika virus; Down syndrome; or with maternal infection with cytomegalovirus, rubella, or varicella. There is no known treatment for microcephaly that can return a child's head to normal size.

Examination of the newborn head may reveal evidence of birth trauma such as bruising or swelling. A *cephalohematoma* is a common finding following vaginal delivery. It is a collection of blood between the skull and periosteum which causes a distinct swelling on the newborn head. Cephalohematomas have clearly demarcated edges and are restricted by suture lines. Common locations for cephalohematomas are the occipital and parietal bones. If large, they can contribute to hyperbilirubinemia and jaundice but in general will resolve in several weeks or months.

Caput succedaneum, edema under the scalp, is caused by pressure over the presenting part of the newborn's head against the cervix during labor. Caput feels soft and spongy, crosses suture lines, and resolves within a few days. Figure 19–7 pictorially compares the location of caput succedaneum and cephalohematoma.

The newborn's head is palpated for the presence of all suture lines and fontanelles (Fig. 19–8). Suture lines feel like soft depressions between the cranial bones. If instead a ridge of bone is felt, the examiner should determine whether it is the result of molding or premature closure of the suture. Normal mobility of the cranial bones is determined by placing each thumb on opposite sides of the suture and alternately pushing in slightly on each side. Lack of mobility of cranial bones may indicate premature closure or absence of a suture, a condition, known as *craniosynostosis*. In craniosynostosis, skull growth is hampered along the affected suture, which fosters compensatory growth along another open suture (Rohan, Golombek, & Rosenthal, 1999). This aberrant growth causes the skull to become misshapen in a predictable way (Fig. 19–9). Synostosis involving more than one suture is often associated with a syndrome (e.g., Crouzon syndrome, Fig. 19–10) for which surgery is usually indicated not just to achieve a cosmetic goal but to alleviate brain growth restriction.

The skull is palpated for masses and assessed for *craniotabes*. Craniotabes is a softening of cranial bones caused by pressure of the fetal skull against the bony pelvis. When pressure is exerted with the examiner's fingers at the margins of the parietal or occipital bones, a popping sensation similar to indenting a ping-pong ball is felt. Craniotabes is primarily seen in breech presentations and usually disappears within a few weeks.

Anterior and posterior fontanelles, the soft membranous coverings where two sutures meet, are palpated and measured. Fontanelles are measured diagonally from bone to bone rather than from suture to suture. They vary in size. The anterior fontanelle is diamond shaped and generally measures 1 to 4 cm and closes around 18 months of age. The posterior fontanelle is triangular, generally measures less than a fingertip up to 1.5 cm, and closes between 2 and 4 months (Gardner & Hernandez, 2011). Fontanelles are best palpated when the newborn is quiet and positioned upright.

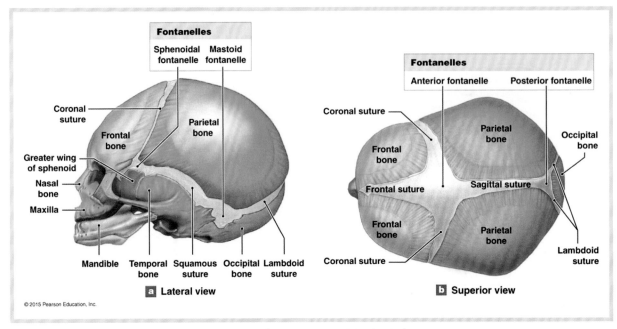

FIGURE 19–8. Bones, sutures, and fontanelles of the infant skull. (From 2015 Pearson Education, Inc.)

The anterior area should be soft, often is depressed slightly, and may bulge with crying. Arterial pulsations may be felt over the anterior fontanelle. Molding may make it impossible to palpate fontanelles in the first few hours of life. Large fontanelles may be associated with various disorders (such as congenital hypothyroidism) and are a notable finding.

The scalp is examined for distribution, amount, and texture of hair. Hair is silky and may be straight, curly, or kinky, depending on ethnic origin. Bruising, lacerations, and bleeding are frequently seen as the result of the application of a scalp electrode or vacuum extractor.

Table 19–2 identifies findings during the physical assessment of the head that are abnormal and their related pathology.

EYE ASSESSMENT

The newborn's eyes are assessed using inspection and an ophthalmoscope. This can be done early in the

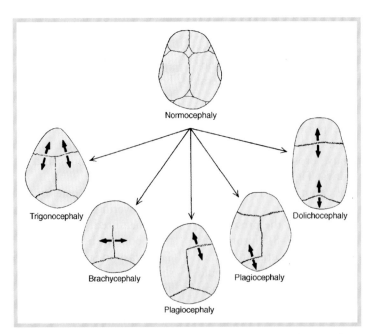

FIGURE 19–9. Craniosynostosis. Skulls that become misshapen by sutural synostosis. (Courtesy of Cohen, M. M., Jr., Halifax, Nova Scotia, Canada.)

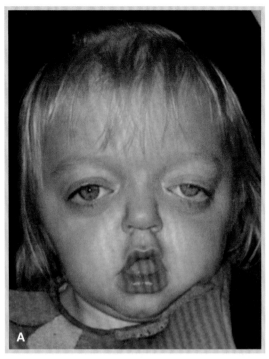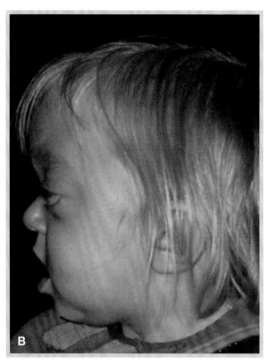

FIGURE 19-10. Crouzon syndrome in a young female. Note the midface hypoplasia, shallow orbits, and ocular proptosis. **A**, Frontal view. **B**, Profile view. (From Chung, K. C. [2013]. *Grabb and Smith's plastic surgery* [8th ed.]. Philadelphia, PA: Wolters Kluwer Health.)

examination as part of the assessment of the head or whenever the newborn spontaneously opens his or her eyes. Although rarely accomplished, it is best done prior to insertion of prophylaxis. Eyes should be symmetric in size and shape. Lids may be edematous and

TABLE 19-2. Head

Assessment	Pathology
The following assessments may indicate increased intracranial pressure:	Hydrocephalus
Sutures separated more than 1 cm	Hypothyroidism
Bulging, tense anterior fontanelle	Tumor
Head circumference greater than 90th percentile for gestational age	Meningitis
Head circumference below 10th percentile for gestational age	Genetic disorder
	Congenital infection
	Maternal drug or alcohol ingestion
Depressed anterior fontanelle	Dehydration
Cephalhematoma: swelling due to bleeding between periosteum and skull bone; does not cross suture line; may not be evident until 1 day after birth and take several weeks to resolve (see Fig. 19-7)	Head trauma during birth
Texture of hair is fine, woolly, sparse, coarse, brittle	Prematurity
	Endocrine disorder
	Genetic disorder
Increased quantity of hair, low-set hairline	Genetic disorder
Limited forward growth of the skull; skull appears broad	Brachycephaly (fused coronal suture)
Limited lateral growth of the skull; skull appears long and narrow	Scaphocephaly (fused sagittal suture)

puffy at birth. The distance between the eyes, measured from the inner canthus of each, is 1.5 to 2.5 cm (Hernandez & Glass, 2005). Eyes spaced closer (i.e., hypotelorism) or farther apart (i.e., hypertelorism) may be a variation of normal or associated with other anomalies. Eyes with small palpebral fissures (i.e., eye openings) may also be normal or associated with other anomalies.

The colors of eye structures are observed. The iris is usually slate gray, brown, or dark blue. Eye color becomes permanent at about 6 months of age. The normally blue-white sclera may contain *subconjunctival hemorrhages*, the result of ruptured capillaries during the birth process. Subconjunctival hemorrhages usually resolve within a week. A yellow sclera indicates hyperbilirubinemia. Years ago when silver nitrate was the standard of care for prophylaxis against ophthalmia neonatorum, the conjunctiva would frequently become inflamed. Today, most hospitals are using erythromycin ointment, which usually does not cause this complication.

Tears are usually absent in the newborn until the lacrimal duct becomes fully patent at about 4 to 6 months of age. Prominent *epicanthal folds* (i.e., Mongolian slant) is a normal finding in Asian infants but may suggest Down syndrome in other ethnic groups (Fig. 19–11).

Blink reflex, size, and reactivity of pupils are evaluated in a darkened room with a pen light or light from the ophthalmoscope. In a normal exam, pupils are equal and reactive to light. When a light is shined at an angle toward the eye, the lens should be clear.

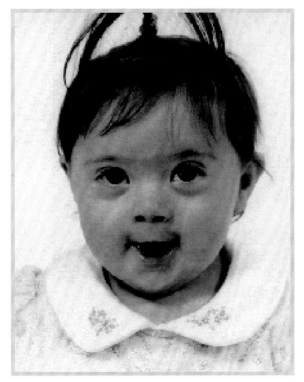

FIGURE 19–11. Infant with Down syndrome showing epicanthal folds of the upper eyelid covering the inner angle of the eye.

TABLE 19–3. Eye

Assessment	Pathology
Persistent purulent discharge	Ophthalmia neonatorum
	Chlamydial conjunctivitis
	Blocked lacrimal duct (dacryocystitis)
Blue sclera	Osteogenesis imperfecta
Sclera visible above iris (sunset eyes)	Hydrocephalus
Black or white spots on periphery of iris (Brushfield spots)	Benign or associated with Down syndrome
Pupils not equal, nonreactive, fixed	Neurologic insult
Keyhole-shaped pupil (coloboma)	Usually associated with other anomalies
Upward slant of palpebral fissures (opening between the upper and lower eyelids)	Down syndrome

Nystagmus (i.e., constant, rapid, involuntary movement of the eye) may occur and usually disappears by 4 months of age. Newborns are nearsighted at birth and respond to bright or primary colors and to high contrast between colors such as black and white. They see objects clearly 8 to 10 inches in front of them.

Table 19–3 identifies findings during the physical assessment of the eye that are abnormal and their related pathology.

EAR ASSESSMENT

The newborn ear is assessed by inspection and palpation. External structures are examined for position, presence of abnormal structures, and injury, which may have occurred during the birth process. The pinna normally lies on or above an imaginary line drawn from the inner to the outer canthus of the eye, back toward the ear (Fig. 19–12). Low-set ears, those that

Equal color, intensity, and clarity of the red reflex in both eyes without opacities or white spots within either red reflex is considered a normal exam (AAP, 2008). Presence of and clarity of the red reflex indicates an intact cornea and lens. Lack of a red reflex suggests congenital glaucoma or cataracts. Pale red reflexes are a normal variation in dark-skinned newborns.

Movement of the eye is observed. *Strabismus*, a crosseyed appearance, is often seen in newborns because of weak eye musculature and lack of coordination.

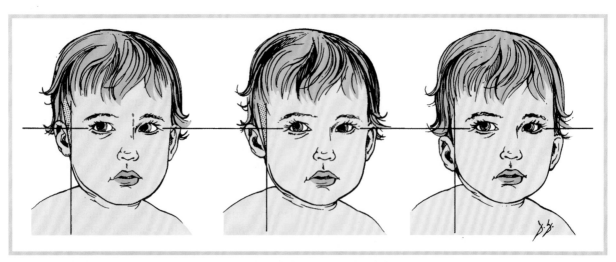

FIGURE 19–12. Normal ear position (*left*). Abnormally angled ear (*middle*). Low-set ears (*right*). (From Reeder, S. J., Martin, L. L., & Koniak-Griffin, D. [1997]. *Maternity nursing: family, newborn, and women's health* [18th ed., p. 706]. Philadelphia, PA: Lippincott-Raven.)

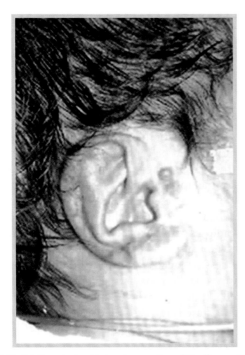

FIGURE 19–13. Preauricular skin tags in a newborn. (http://www.adhb.govt
.nz/newborn/TeachingResources/Dermatology/PreauricularSinus/Preauricular
Sinus.JPG)

fall below this line, may be associated with genetic syndromes. Temporary asymmetry of the ears can result from intrauterine position. *Skin tags* (Fig. 19–13) and small *pits* (Fig. 19–14) located anterior to the ear are usually benign, may be familial, but can also be associated with hearing loss and renal abnormalities. Malformation of the ears may be associated with renal abnormalities, chromosomal abnormalities and other congenital problems (Gardner & Hernandez, 2011). Presence of ecchymosis, swelling, abrasions, or lacerations may be the result of pressure during the birth process, application of forceps or vacuum, or injury during cesarean section.

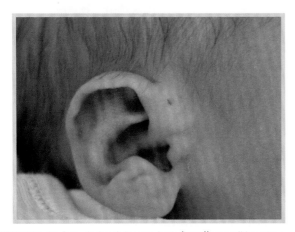

FIGURE 19–14. Preauricular pit in a newborn. (http://www.adhb.govt.nz
/newborn/TeachingResources/Dermatology/PreauricularSinus/Preauricular
Sinus.JPG)

The ear is palpated as part of the gestational assessment to determine the presence and firmness of cartilage. By 38 to 40 weeks' gestation, the pinna is firm and well formed by cartilage, and incurving is present over two thirds of the ear. A soft pinna lacking cartilage is seen in premature newborns. At term, folding the pinna of the ear inward and releasing should result in brisk recoil. The more premature a newborn is, the slower the pinna will be to return to its normal position. The pinna of an extremely premature infant may remain folded.

The ear canal is inspected for patency. Use of the otoscope is limited because newborn ear canals contain vernix, mucus, and cellular debris. The ear canals clear spontaneously several days after birth. At this time, the tympanic membrane is visualized by pulling the pinna back and down. The tympanic membrane appears gray-white and highly vascular. If a neonatal ear infection is suspected, otoscopic examination of the ear is indicated.

Although hearing is well developed at birth, it becomes more acute as the ear canals clear. The AAP currently recommends that all newborns should receive hearing screening using a physiologic measure by 1 month of age, and preferably before hospital discharge (AAP, 2019; Muse et al., 2013). Two technologies are available for hearing screening: evoked otoacoustic emissions (OAE) and auditory brainstem response (ABR). Both methods are noninvasive, quick, and easy to perform. However, OAEs reflect only the status of the peripheral auditory system up to the cochlear outer hair cells, whereas ABRs can also detect neural dysfunction. It is for this reason that infants who have been hospitalized in the neonatal intensive care unit for greater than 5 days are to have ABR screening rather than OAE screening, so that neural hearing loss can be identified (AAP, 2019; Muse et al., 2013).

Support for universal newborn hearing screening (UNHS) is based on the premise that if identification and intervention occur by 6 months of age for newborns who are hard of hearing or deaf, the infants will perform significantly higher on vocabulary, articulation, and other school-related measures because of the ability for language development (AAP, 2019; Muse et al., 2013).

Table 19–4 identifies findings during the physical assessment of the ear that are abnormal and their related pathology.

NOSE ASSESSMENT

The newborn's nose is assessed using inspection. The nose should be symmetric and midline but may be misshapen at birth because of the neonate's positioning in utero. If the septum cannot be easily straightened and the nose remains asymmetric, treatment

TABLE 19–4. Ear

Assessment	Pathology
Low-set ears	Genetic disorder
	Kidney abnormality
Poorly formed external ear	Genetic disorder
Skin tags located on the ear lobe or the skin surface surrounding the ear (see Fig. 19–13)	Familial variation
	Alteration in normal embryologic development
	Genetic disorder associated with urinary tract abnormalities
Preauricular sinuses are connections between the skin surface and cysts. If they close before birth, all that is present is a "pit" or pinpoint size indentation located in front of the ear (see Fig. 19–14).	Familial variation
	Alteration in normal embryologic development
	Genetic disorder associated with deafness and renal abnormalities
Absence of Moro reflex	Hearing loss—if sound was used to stimulate the Moro—if positional change was used, this would not be true
Microtia—abnormally small, underdeveloped external ear	Associated with inner ear malformations and hearing loss

may be required. A flattened or bruised nose may result from passage through the birth canal.

Nasal stuffiness and thin, white mucus is not an uncommon finding immediately after birth. Newborns sneeze to clear the upper respiratory tract. Bilateral nasal patency should be established in all newborns because they are obligatory nose breathers. Patency should be determined by either obstructing one naris and observing breathing through the opposite naris, or passing a 5 French catheter down each naris. If a newborn is breathing comfortably and patency is established by obstructing one naris, there is no need to pass a catheter. This should be done only if naris patency cannot be established with the less intrusive method.

Table 19–5 identifies findings during the physical assessment of the nose that are abnormal and their related pathology.

TABLE 19–5. Nose

Assessment	Pathology
Flat nasal bridge	Down syndrome
Pink when crying; chest retractions and cyanosis at rest; difficulty feeding	Choanal atresia
Stuffy nose and thin, watery discharge	Neonatal drug withdrawal
"Sniffles" persistent; profuse mucopurulent or bloody discharge (Green, 1998)	Congenital syphilis

MOUTH ASSESSMENT

The newborn mouth is assessed using inspection and palpation. In the sequence of the total examination, this assessment is frequently left until last. If the newborn's mouth is forced open, crying may result, altering aspects of the respiratory or cardiac assessments. The lips are observed for location, color, and symmetry. The mouth should be centrally located along the midline. At rest, the lips appear symmetric. Depending on skin color, the lips are pink or more darkly pigmented. Sucking blisters, centrally located on the upper lip, may be filled with fluid or have the consistency of a callus. Calluses may also be found on the hand as a result of vigorous sucking in utero or after birth. Muscle weakness or facial paralysis is best observed when the infant is sucking or crying; both conditions may be missed altogether if the infant is observed only in a quiet, alert state (Fig. 19–15). Rooting, suck, and gag reflexes are evaluated during this portion of the examination or during feeding.

The mucous membrane and internal structures of the mouth are inspected. If the mouth does not open spontaneously while the newborn cries, it can be gently opened by a downward pressure on the chin or with a pediatric tongue blade. In a healthy newborn, the mucous membrane is pink. Increased amounts of mucus during the first 1 to 2 days of life are removed with a bulb syringe. This is especially common in newborns born by elective cesarean section without labor because they do not benefit from the cessation of lung fluid production during labor. The tongue is mobile and prominent within the mouth. Occasionally, the

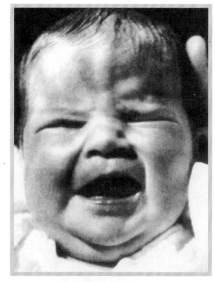

FIGURE 19–15. Facial nerve paralysis. Notice the asymmetry of the mouth during crying. (From Reeder, S. J., Martin, L. L., & Koniak-Griffin, D. [1997]. *Maternity nursing: Family, newborn, and women's health* [18th ed., p. 1205]. Philadelphia, PA: Lippincott-Raven.)

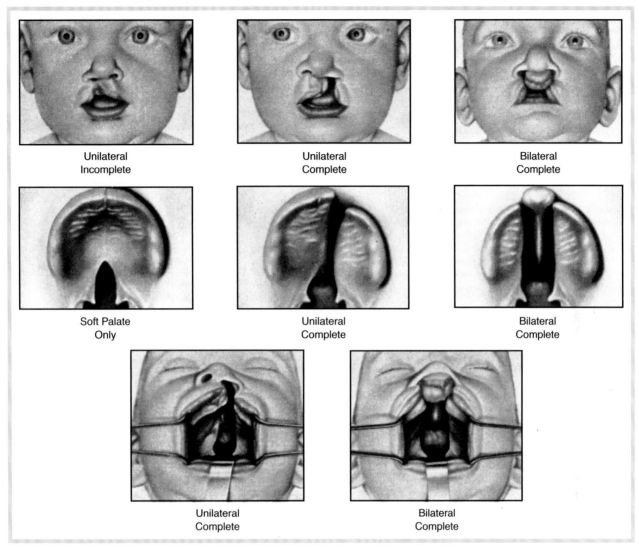

Unilateral
Incomplete

Unilateral
Complete

Bilateral
Complete

Soft Palate
Only

Unilateral
Complete

Bilateral
Complete

Unilateral
Complete

Bilateral
Complete

FIGURE 19–16. Cleft lip and cleft palate (redrawn from drawings by Ross Laboratories). (From Reeder, S. J., Martin, L. L., & Koniak-Griffin, D. [1997]. *Maternity nursing: Family, newborn, and women's health* [18th ed., p. 1108]. Philadelphia, PA: Lippincott-Raven.)

frenulum is short, causing a notch at the tip of the tongue. True congenital *ankyloglossia* (i.e., tongue tie) is rare.

Using adequate lighting, the hard and soft palates are examined. The uvula is midline and located at the posterior soft palate. Some practitioners use an index finger to palpate the hard and soft palates for the presence of clefts (Fig. 19–16). Whitish-yellow cysts (i.e., *Epstein's pearls*) containing epithelial cells may be present on the hard palate at birth, but they disappear within a few weeks. Some newborns are born with one or two *natal teeth*. These immature caps of enamel and dentin have poor root formation and are usually loose. These teeth may be aspirated if dislodged and make breastfeeding difficult, or cause lacerations on the mucosa, lips, or tongue. They are usually removed during the neonatal period.

Table 19–6 identifies findings during the physical assessment of the mouth that are abnormal and their related pathology.

NECK ASSESSMENT

The neck is inspected for symmetry and range of motion and palpated along the midline to identify abnormal masses. The thyroid gland is difficult to palpate unless it is enlarged, an unusual finding during the newborn period. A potential for infection exists within all the cystic structures and abnormal sinuses arising around the newborn's neck.

Newborns have short, thick necks with multiple skin folds. A predominant fat pad in the back of the neck, redundant skin, and webbing are findings associated

TABLE 19–6. Mouth

Assessment	Pathology
Mucous membranes dry	Dehydration
Cyanotic mucous membranes (central cyanosis)	Poor oxygenation, congenital heart disease or respiratory condition
Asymmetric movement of mouth	Facial nerve injury
Cleft lip and/or palate (see Fig. 19–16)	Teratogenic injury Genetic disorder Multifactorial inheritance
Hypertrophied tongue	Down syndrome Beckwith-Wiedemann syndrome Hypothyroidism
Protrusion of tongue	Genetic disorder
Weak, uncoordinated suck and swallow	Prematurity Neuromuscular disorder Asphyxia Maternal analgesia during labor Inborn error of metabolism
Frantic sucking	Infant of drug-addicted mother
Excessive drooling and salivating; unable to pass a nasogastric tube	Esophageal atresia
Circumoral cyanosis	Respiratory distress
Thin upper lip, smooth philtrum, short palpebral fissures	Fetal alcohol syndrome
Translucent, bluish swelling on either side of the frenulum under the tongue	Mucous or salivary gland retention cyst
Bifid uvula	Genetic disorder
Small lower jaw (micrognathia)	Pierre Robin syndrome Treacher Collins syndrome De Lange syndrome
Patches of white on tongue and mucous membrane	*Candida albicans*

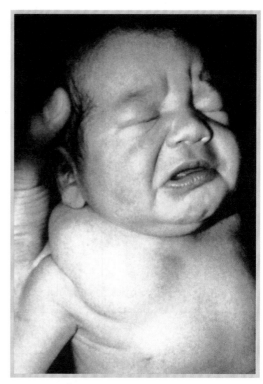

FIGURE 19–17. Cystic hygroma.

with genetic syndromes. The newborn's head should be able to turn completely to face each shoulder. *Torticollis* refers to a postural positioning abnormality that presents on physical exam with the head twisted and turned to one side. Torticollis is most commonly acquired prenatally and results in asymmetry in the length or strength of the sternocleidomastoid muscle (Kuo, Tritasavit, Graham, 2014). As many as 16% of newborns have evidence of torticollis at birth, making it the most common congenital muscular abnormality (Stellwagen, Hubbard, Chambers, & Jones, 2008). On physical exam, interstitial fibrosis of the injured muscle is sometimes palpable as a fusiform fibrous mass that becomes more evident in the first 3 weeks after birth and reaches maximum size by 1 month of age. The head is typically tilted toward the side of the affected muscle and rotated toward the opposite side. Skull (e.g., plagiocephaly), ear, eye, and facial asymmetry is common. Most cases of torticollis can be successfully treated with neck-stretching exercises and physical therapy (Kuo et al., 2014). Surgery to lengthen the tightened muscle is generally reserved if significant asymmetry persists beyond a year of age.

Cystic hygroma is one of the most common neck lesions (Fig. 19–17). This particular cystic structure occurs due to lymph channels that are sequestered and then dilate and become large cysts. Cystic hygroma most commonly occurs in the lateral neck (Johnson, 2019). The lesions vary in size from a few millimeters to large enough to deviate the trachea, cause respiratory distress, or interfere with feeding. A large cystic hygroma usually requires surgical excision.

The neck is palpated along the midline for the trachea and abnormal masses. The thyroid gland is difficult to palpate unless it is enlarged, an unusual finding during the newborn period. A potential for infection exists within all the cystic structures and abnormal sinuses arising around the newborn's neck.

Table 19–7 identifies additional findings during the physical assessment of the neck that are abnormal and their related pathology.

CHEST AND LUNG ASSESSMENT

Auscultation and inspection are used to assess the newborn's chest and respiratory status. The newborn's chest is cylindrical. Measured at the nipple line, its circumference is approximately 2 to 3 cm less than the infant's head (see Fig. 19–1). The xiphoid process is sometimes seen as a small protuberant area at the end of the sternum. Respirations are shallow and irregular. Chest movement should be symmetric and not labored. An accurate respiratory rate is obtained by counting for 1 full minute,

TABLE 19–7. Neck

Assessment	Pathology
Multiple skin folds in the lateral, posterior region of the neck (webbing)	Down syndrome
	Turner syndrome
Enlarged thyroid	Hyperthyroidism
	Hypothyroidism
Absence of head control	Prematurity
	Genetic disorder
	Asphyxia
	Neuromuscular disorder
Abnormal opening along the anterior surface of the sternocleidomastoid muscle	
Brachial sinus leads to a blind pouch or communicates with deeper structures	
Mass high in the neck at midline extending to the base of the tongue; often, thyroglossal duct cyst appears after an upper respiratory infection	
Palpable cystic mass may open onto the skin surface or drain into the pharynx	
Brachial cleft cyst	

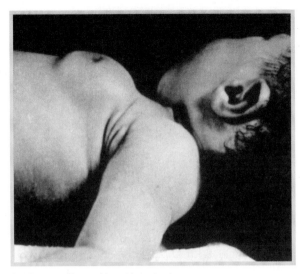

FIGURE 19–18. Neonatal breast hypertrophy.

preferably when the newborn is quiet. Newborns have an average respiratory rate of 30 to 60 breaths per minute, and with each respiration, synchronous abdominal movement occurs. The color of the newborn's skin and mucous membranes is evaluated simultaneously. Presence of cyanosis may be a sign of respiratory distress or congenital cardiac disease.

Tachypnea (i.e., respiratory rate >60 breaths per minute) may be one of the first symptoms of morbidity in the newborn. If tachypnea is present, the respiratory rate may reach 120 breaths per minute. The primary healthcare provider should be notified when respiratory rates are increased, and oral feedings should be withheld if an infant is tachypneic because of the risk of aspiration.

Other signs of respiratory distress include *retractions*, *nasal flaring*, and *grunting*. Retractions are the drawing inward or shortening of small muscles in the chest wall. Retractions occur when more energy is needed to assist respiratory effort. Retractions are seen between the ribs (intercostal), below the rib cage (subcostal), above the sternum (tracheal tug), below the xiphoid process, and surrounding the clavicles. Flaring of the nares occurs with inspiration. It is a compensatory mechanism used by the newborn in respiratory distress. Flaring of the nares widens the upper airway, decreasing airway resistance, and making breathing easier. Grunting is a sound produced on expiration when air passes through a partially closed glottis. The partially closed glottis is a compensatory mechanism that traps air in the alveoli, increasing the time that gas exchange can occur. Grunting may be audible or heard only with a stethoscope.

Inspection of the newborn's chest includes placement, shape, and amount of palpable breast tissue.

Hypertrophy of breast tissue, with or without secretion of milky fluid, may be present by the second or third day of life because of maternal hormones (Fig. 19–18). This condition lasts approximately 1 week. Supernumerary nipples (i.e., accessory nipples) are considered a benign congenital anomaly. They are often seen below and medial to the normal nipples.

Auscultation of the anterior and posterior chest proceeds in an orderly fashion from top to bottom, comparing from side to side for equality of breath sounds and the presence of abnormal sounds such as grunting and rales. The term *crackles* may be used in place of the traditional term *rales* for the fine cracking, bubbling, or fine rustling noises heard when air passes fluid. Rhonchi and wheezing are less common in the newborn period. These lower pitched sounds result from obstruction or narrowing of larger airways.

Newborns have a periodic breathing pattern resulting from the immaturity of their respiratory and central nervous systems. It is common to observe brief pauses in respiratory effort. Pauses lasting 20 seconds or longer and associated with color change or bradycardia are considered apneic periods and should be reported to the primary healthcare provider.

Apnea (i.e., pauses in respirations lasting 20 seconds or longer) or other signs of respiratory distress may occur in almost all illnesses in the newborn period. The list of differential diagnoses for respiratory distress and apnea in the newborn is extensive (Table 19–8).

Table 19–9 identifies findings during the respiratory assessment that are abnormal and their related pathology.

CARDIOVASCULAR ASSESSMENT

The cardiovascular system is assessed using inspection, auscultation, and palpation. The examination begins with inspection of the newborn's color as one

TABLE 19–8. Differential Diagnosis of Respiratory Distress in the Newborn

Respiratory	Extrapulmonary
Respiratory distress syndrome	Congenital heart disease
Transient tachypnea	Patent ductus arteriosus
Meconium aspiration	Hypothermia
Primary pulmonary hypertension	Metabolic acidosis
	Hypoglycemia
Pneumonia	Septicemia
Pulmonary hemorrhage	Ventricular hemorrhage
Pneumothorax	Edema
Airway obstruction	Drugs
Diaphragmatic hernia	Trauma
Hypoplastic lung	Hypovolemia
	Twin-to-twin transfusion

Adapted from Askin, D. F. (1997). *Acute respiratory care of the newborn* (p. 32). Petaluma, CA: NICU INK.

indication of oxygenation and perfusion. As the newborn transitions from intrauterine to extrauterine life, skin color changes occur. At birth, the newborn or neonate may be pale or cyanotic, becoming pink as respirations are established, fetal circulation is reversed, and blood is oxygenated by the lungs and circulated by the strength of the heart muscle.

TABLE 19–9. Respiratory System

Assessment	Pathology
Cessation of breathing for more than 20 sec (apnea)	Hypothermia/hyperthermia
	Infection
	Prematurity
	Respiratory disorders
	Cardiovascular disorders
	Neurologic disorders
	Maternal medications
	Metabolic disorders
	Gastroesophageal reflux
	Vigorous suctioning
	Passage of feeding tube
	Airway obstruction
Tachypnea	Retained lung fluid (transient tachypnea of the newborn)
	Meconium aspiration
	Respiratory distress syndrome
	Pneumonia
	Hyperthermia
	Pulmonary edema
	Sepsis
	Metabolic disorders
Decreased or absent breath sounds	Meconium aspiration
	Atelectasis
	Pneumothorax
	Diaphragmatic hernia
	Hypoplastic lungs
	Diaphragmatic hernia
Bowel sounds heard in place of breath sounds	Diaphragmatic hernia

The precordium (i.e., area on the anterior chest over the heart) is inspected and palpated for movement. In a term newborn, very little movement should be observed in this area (except during the first few hours of life as transition occurs). An active precordium could indicate patent ductus arteriosus or other left-to-right-shunt lesions or occur as a variation of normal in preterm or SGA newborns who are thin and have minimal subcutaneous tissue. After the first few hours or days of life, the point of maximal impulse (PMI) is normally auscultated or palpated in the third to fourth intercostal space at or just left of the midclavicular line. Displacement of the PMI can occur with cardiac enlargement, diaphragmatic hernia, dextrocardia, or pneumothorax. Three additional sensations—*heave, tap,* and *thrill*—may be felt as the chest is palpated. A heave is a diffuse pulsation that can occur with ventricular volume overload. A tap is a pronounced localized pulsation of the PMI. A thrill is a palpated vibration (similar to a purring cat) that is associated with a murmur.

Heart rate and rhythm are best auscultated using the bell and diaphragm of a small neonatal stethoscope while the newborn remains quiet. The diaphragm of the stethoscope can detect high-pitched murmurs, whereas the bell is better for detecting low-pitched murmurs. The stethoscope should be warmed before placement so the newborn is not startled. The apical rate is counted for 1 full minute. The normal heart rate is 100 to 160 beats per minute. In deep sleep, the heart rate may be 80 to 110 beats per minute but should increase quickly if the newborn is disturbed. Auscultation begins at the mitral area (PMI) and proceeds systematically to the tricuspid, pulmonic, and aortic areas using the diaphragm of the stethoscope. The process is then repeated across specific areas of the chest using the bell of the stethoscope (Fig. 19–19).

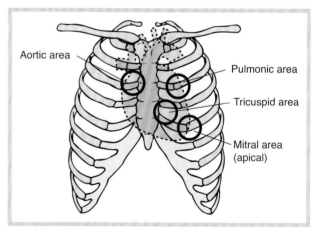

FIGURE 19–19. Auscultatory areas of the heart. (From Tappero, E. P., & Honeyfield, M. E. [Eds.]. [2009]. *Physical assessment of the newborn: A comprehensive approach to the art of physical examination* [4th ed., p. 87]. Petaluma, CA: NICU Ink.)

Heart sounds are louder in newborn infants because of the thin chest wall.

Heart sounds become clearer over the first few hours of life as fetal circulation transitions to extrauterine circulation and the pulmonary vascular resistance lowers. Rapid heart rates often make it difficult to auscultate specific heart sounds. The first heart sound, S_1, is caused by the closure of the tricuspid and mitral valves at the beginning of systole. It is heard best at the apex of the heart, in the fourth intercostal space. S_1 is usually loudest at birth, decreasing in intensity over 24 to 48 hours. The second heart sound, S_2, is caused by the closure of the pulmonic and aortic valves and is heard best at the base of the heart. Splitting of S_2 with inspiration is common after the first 72 hours of life.

Heart murmurs in newborns are common during the neonatal period and are caused by turbulence of blood flow. Murmurs are evaluated for loudness or intensity of sound (i.e., grade), timing in the cardiac cycle (i.e., systolic or diastolic), location of the murmur's maximum intensity, radiation, and pitch or quality of sound. Most murmurs in the newborn are benign and transient in nature and are called innocent murmurs. These murmurs are usually grade I or II (Table 19–10), occur in the first 48 hours of life, and are not associated with any other abnormalities in the physical exam and evaluation. Pathologic murmurs are related to underlying cardiac problems. Pathologic murmurs are generally louder than grade I to II, may begin or persist after 48 hours of age, and may be associated with other symptoms (Vargo, 2019).

The classic presentation of cyanotic congenital heart disease (CHD) is that of a cyanotic term infant with a murmur, normal blood pressure (BP), and a paucity of other respiratory symptoms. Although cyanosis and a murmur are the typical presenting signs, they are by no means defining. If pulmonary circulatory overload is present, cyanotic CHD can present with respiratory distress. Many serious cyanotic lesions are not accompanied by louder than grade II murmurs or may have no murmur (Rohan & Golombek, 2009).

Peripheral pulses (i.e., brachial, radial, femoral, popliteal, and dorsalis pedis) are evaluated for presence, equality, and strength. Femoral pulses may be difficult to palpate but should be present in all infants. It is very important to note an absence or diminishment of the femoral pulses, and this should be further investigated by a physician or advanced practice nurse.

Routine BP screening is not recommended for all newborns (AAP & ACOG, 2017). Evaluating the BP is usually reserved for newborns with signs of distress, persistent murmurs, or abnormal pulses. BP varies depending on birth weight, gestational age, cuff size, and state of alertness. BPs should be taken when the infant is quiet and reserved for the end of the assessment because the pressure of the cuff inflating may cause the newborn to cry. An appropriate size of BP cuff is necessary to ensure an accurate measurement. Cuffs that are too small will produce elevated BP values and cuffs that are too large can produce values that are too low. Using limb length only to determine cuff size used can be misleading. It is important to also consider cuff width when determining BP accurately. The width of the cuff should be 25% to 55% wider than the diameter of the extremity being measured with the bladder entirely circling the extremity (but not overlapping) (Park, 2008). At term, the normal BP range is 65 to 95 mm Hg systolic and 30 to 60 mm Hg diastolic. BP in the lower extremities is usually higher than that in the upper extremities. When there is concern for a potential cardiac abnormality, BP should be measured in all four extremities. The primary caregiver should be notified if the systolic BP in the upper extremities is more than 20 mm Hg higher than that in the systolic BP in the lower extremities (Park, 2008). Table 19–11 identifies findings during the cardiovascular assessment that are abnormal and their related pathology.

ABDOMINAL ASSESSMENT

The abdomen is assessed using inspection, auscultation, and palpation. The abdomen is inspected for size and symmetry and is normally rounded, symmetric, protuberant, and soft because of weak abdominal musculature with a slightly greater diameter above the umbilicus than below. The subcutaneous blood vessels in the abdomen may appear distended and blue (Hernandez & Glass, 2005). Abdominal movements correspond to respirations because newborns use the muscle of the diaphragm, rather than intercostal muscles, to assist with breathing. Movement of the diaphragm causes the abdomen to move. If abdominal distention is suspected, the circumference of the abdomen is periodically measured at the level of the umbilicus (see Fig. 19–1). The umbilical cord is examined for number of vessels, color, and condition. The cord should be opaque to white-blue and contain two thick-walled arteries and one thin-walled vein. Variations include a thin, dry cord associated with *FGR* or

TABLE 19–10. Grading of Murmurs	
Grade	Examination findings
Grade I	Soft, requires extended listening
Grade II	Soft, heard immediately
Grade III	Moderate intensity, no thrill
Grade IV	Loud, often with a thrill or palpable vibration at the murmur site
Grade V	Loud, thrill present; audible with the stethoscope partially off the chest
Grade VI	Loud, audible with the stethoscope off the chest

TABLE 19–11. Cardiovascular System

Assessment	Pathology
Tachycardia (heart rate >160 bpm)	Anemia
	Congestive heart failure
	Shock or hypovolemia
	Respiratory distress
	Supraventricular tachycardia
	Sepsis
	Congenital heart anomalies
	Hyperthermia
Persistent bradycardia (heart rate <100 bpm)	Congenital heart block
	Sepsis
	Asphyxia
	Hypoxemia
	Increased intracranial pressure
Persistent murmurs	Pulmonary hypertension
	Congenital heart defects
	Peripheral pulmonic stenosis
Muffled heart sounds	Pneumothorax
	Pneumopericardium
	Diaphragmatic hernia
	Pneumomediastinum
Heart sound muffled on left side, loud on right side	Dextrocardia
	Pneumothorax with mediastinal shift
Decrease in intensity or absence of femoral pulses	Hip dysplasia
	Coarctation of the aorta
Bounding peripheral pulses; active precordium	Patent ductus arteriosus
	Fluid overload
	Congestive heart failure
	Ventricular septal defect
Difference of systolic blood pressure >20 mm Hg in upper extremities vs. systolic blood pressure in lower extremities	Coarctation of aorta
Central cyanosis	Congenital heart disease
	Hypertension
	Lung disease
	Sepsis
Pulmonary hypertension	
Cyanosis that does not improve with 100% oxygen	Congenital heart disease
Cyanosis that worsens with crying	Congenital heart disease

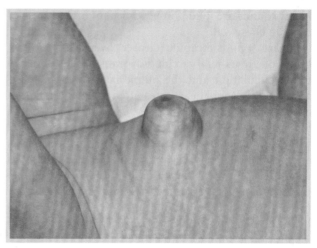

FIGURE 19–20. Umbilical hernia. (From BabyCenter.com. 1997–2019.)

not uncommon and is the result of the newborn's weak abdominal muscles.

The perianal region is inspected for the presence of a patent anus. Most newborns pass meconium within the first 24 hours of life but may go as long as 48 hours occasionally. Failure to pass meconium beyond this time may indicate a gastrointestinal obstruction and necessitates further evaluation.

Bowel sounds are normally present within the first hour of life as the newborn swallows air with crying and the sympathetic nervous system stimulates peristalsis. Bowel sounds are auscultated in all four quadrants.

Most perinatal/neonatal nurses conduct a limited assessment of the abdomen using light palpation for consistency and the presence of masses. A more detailed examination is conducted by the primary healthcare provider. The lower border of the liver is firm soft and palpated in the right upper quadrant 1 to 3 cm below the costal margin. The spleen, located in the left upper quadrant, may be palpable in preterm newborns but rarely in term newborns. The spleen should not be palpated more than 1 cm below the left costal margin (Goodwin, 2009). Kidneys are 4 to 5 cm long and are usually only palpable during the first 1 to 2 days of life (Hernandez & Glass, 2005). After this time, the bowel and stomach become distended with fluid and air, making this assessment difficult. With the newborn's legs flexed against the abdomen, kidneys are located using deep palpations at the level of the umbilicus, lateral to the midclavicular line (Fig. 19–21). The right kidney may be lower than the left.

Inspection and palpation of the femoral region is conducted during this portion of the examination or as part of the cardiovascular assessment. A soft, compressible swelling in the groin may indicate an *inguinal hernia* in males or females, *undescended testes*, or an ovary within the hernia (Fig. 19–22). Bowel sounds

a thick cord seen in LGA newborns. A greenish-yellow discoloration of the cord sometimes occurs with relaxation of the anal sphincter and subsequent passage of meconium prior to birth. The area surrounding the umbilical cord is observed for masses or the herniation of abdominal contents (Fig. 19–20). *Umbilical hernias* occur when the abdominal muscles do not close completely around the umbilicus during embryologic development. They are more common in low-birth-weight, African American, and male newborns. Some hernias are observable only when the newborn is crying. Separation of the abdominorectus muscle (i.e., *diastasis recti*) 0.5 to 2 inches wide may occur along the midline from the xiphoid to umbilicus, occasionally extending to the symphysis pubis. Separation of this muscle is

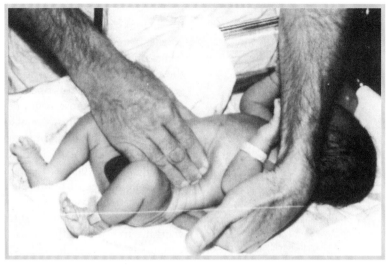

FIGURE 19–21. Examiner demonstrating technique for palpation of the left kidney.

can be auscultated in the testis if swelling is caused by herniation of the bowel.

Table 19–12 identifies findings during the physical assessment of the abdomen that are abnormal and their related pathology.

GENITOURINARY ASSESSMENT

The genitourinary system is assessed using inspection and palpation. External genitalia are evaluated as part of the physical examination and gestational age assessment. Newborns should void within 24 hours of birth. A rust-colored stain on the diaper, which in some instances can be flaked off, is a normal variation caused by uric acid crystals in the urine. Bruising and edema of the genitalia and buttocks can occur in newborns that had a breech presentation.

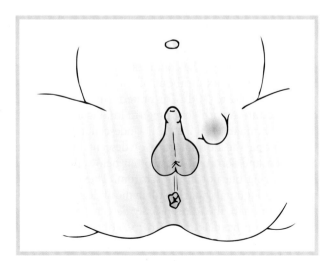

FIGURE 19–22. Left inguinal hernia producing a bulge in the groin of the affected side.

Female Newborns

In term newborns, the clitoris and labia minora are covered by the labia majora. The urinary meatus is located beneath the clitoris. The labia majora and clitoris are enlarged because of maternal hormones circulated to the fetus in utero. Bruising and swelling of the external genitalia may be present after a vaginal birth. In preterm female newborns, the labia majora does not cover the labia minora and clitoris.

In some newborns, when the introitus is gently separated, a hymenal tag is seen in the vagina. This tissue, which developed from the hymen and labia minora, disappears within a few weeks (Cavaliere, 2019). A white mucous discharge from the vagina is not uncommon during the first week of life. *Pseudomenstruation*, caused by withdrawal of maternal hormones, is a pink-tinged mucous discharge lasting 2 to 4 weeks.

The labia majora are palpated for masses that could indicate a hernia or ectopic glands. Palpating a suprapubic mass or mass between the labia majora suggests an *imperforate hymen*. An imperforate hymen causes secretions to pool within the vagina.

Male Newborns

In term male newborns, the external genitalia are observed for a normal penis, with a length of 2.5 to 5 cm (Shulman, Palmert, & Wherrett, 2011), the urethral opening located on the tip of the glans, and the glans covered by the prepuce or foreskin. The foreskin may need to be retracted slightly to accurately determine the location of the meatus. A physiologic *phimosis* (i.e., inability to retract the prepuce or foreskin) is present at birth. By 3 years of age, the foreskin usually can be retracted in 90% of uncircumcised males because

TABLE 19–12. Abdomen

Assessment	Pathology
Scaphoid	Diaphragmatic hernia
	Malnutrition
"Prune belly" flabby, wrinkled abdominal wall (see Fig. 19–23)	Congenital absence of abdominal musculature; associated with other GI or GU anomalies
Asymmetric abdomen	Abdominal mass
	GI/GU anomalies
Abdominal distention	Obstruction
	Masses
	Enlargement of abdominal organs
	Infection (Hernandez & Glass, 2005)
Distention in left upper quadrant	Pyloric stenosis
	Duodenal or jejunal obstruction
Ascites	Hydrops fetalis
	Viral infections (congenital)
Umbilical cord with one artery and one vein	Associated with GI/GU anomalies
Thin membrane covering herniation of abdominal contents through a defect in the umbilical ring	Omphalocele
Uncovered protrusion of abdominal contents, usually to the right of the umbilicus	Gastroschisis
Red, oozing, or foul-smelling cord	Infection (omphalitis)
Persistently moist umbilicus; clear discharge from umbilical cord stump	Granuloma of the umbilical cord (Hernandez & Glass, 2005)
	Umbilical urinary fistula—urachus, embryologic connection between the bladder and umbilicus remains patent
	Urachus cyst
	Omphalomesenteric duct—connection between the umbilicus and ileum (Goodwin, 2009)
Failure to pass meconium stool	Imperforate anus
	Meconium ileus
	Hirschsprung disease
	Meconium plug syndrome
Passage of sticky, thick, small plugs of meconium	Meconium ileus
	Cystic fibrosis
Bruit	Arteriovenous malformation (liver)
	Renal artery stenosis
Partial or complete herniation of the bladder through the abdominal wall	Bladder exstrophy—absence of muscle and connective tissue in the abdominal wall occurring during embryologic development
Hepatomegaly	Congenital heart disease
	Infection
	Hemolytic disease (Hernandez & Glass, 2005)

GI, gastrointestinal; GU, genitourinary.

The second most common genitourinary abnormality in male newborns is *hypospadias*, the placement of the urinary meatus on the ventral surface of the penis anywhere along a line extending from the tip of the penis, penile shaft, scrotum, or perineum. In more severe cases, the meatus opens on the lower penile shaft, junction of the penoscrotum or perineum. Up to 15% of severe hypospadias are associated with endocrine problems, chromosomal or intersex problems (Shulman et al., 2011). Because of the point in embryologic development that the defect occurs, it is usually associated with some degree of failure of the foreskin to develop completely or excessive foreskin on the dorsal surface and absent foreskin on the ventral surface, and *chordee*, ventral curvature of the penis (Shulman et al., 2011). Circumcision, when desired, is delayed when an abnormally located urinary meatus is observed. If repair of the hypospadias is necessary, the foreskin removed during circumcision may be used for urethroplasty or penile shaft skin coverage (Shulman et al., 2011).

The scrotum is more darkly pigmented than the skin surrounding it. This color variation is especially prominent in darker skinned newborns such as African American, Indian, and Hispanic newborns. The scrotum is palpated with the thumb and forefinger for the presence of the testes. Placing a finger between the scrotum and the inguinal canal area while palpating will minimize movement of the testes within the scrotum. Rugae (i.e., ridges or creases) begin to appear on the surface of the scrotum around 36 weeks' gestation, and by term, the entire surface of the scrotum is covered. The scrotum may be enlarged because of the effects of maternal hormones. Rugae and a pendulous scrotum usually indicate descent of the testes. Before 28 weeks' gestation, the testes lie within the abdomen. Migration through the inguinal canal to the scrotum occurs as a result of the effect of testosterone on the genitofemoral nerves. Stimulation of these nerves is postulated to cause the gubernaculum testis, a fetal ligament connecting the testes to the scrotum, to guide the movement of the testes to the scrotum (Moore & Persaud, 2008). Undescended testes (i.e., *cryptorchidism*) is the most common male genital abnormality. The condition may be unilateral or bilateral and occurs in about 3.7% of term newborns and up to 21% to 100% of preterm males depending on the gestation with very preterm infants approaching 100% (Shulman et al., 2011). Undescended testes are found along the normal path of descent between the abdomen and scrotum, most often below the external inguinal ring but not in the scrotum. They can also be within the inguinal canal or still in the abdomen. If undescended at birth, the testes usually descend by 9 months of age, 3 months of age in up to 75% of term males, and 90% of preterm males without intervention (Shulman et al., 2011). It is possible for one testis or both testes to migrate to an ectopic location, away from the normal path to the scrotum, if the gubernaculum ligament is in

adhesions between the prepuce and glans lyse and the distal phimotic ring loosens (Elder, 2007). Small, white cysts filled with epithelial cells may be transiently present on the distal portion of the prepuce. *Smegma*, a whitish-yellow, cheesy substance from sebaceous glands, collects between the glans and the prepuce.

TABLE 19–13. Genitourinary System

Assessment	Pathology
Ambiguous genitalia	Genetic disorder
Decreased or no urination within 24 hr of birth	Urinary tract obstruction
	Potter syndrome
	Polycystic kidney
	Hydronephrosis
	Renal failure
Female	
Urinary meatus near or just inside vagina (hypospadias)	Genitourinary anomaly
Fecal discharge from vagina	Fistula between rectum and vagina
Male	
Epispadias—meatus on dorsal surface of glans	Genitourinary anomaly
Hypospadias—meatus on ventral surface of glans	Genitourinary anomaly
	Congenital syndromes
Scrotal mass which does not transilluminate	Inguinal hernia (see Fig. 19–22)
Red to bluish-red scrotal sac; swelling or small mass palpable (Cavaliere, 2019)	Twisting of the testes and spermatic cord (testicular torsion)
Urinary stream not straight; weak urinary stream	Stenosis of the urethral meatus
	Urinary malformation

40 weeks, the nails may extend beyond the fingertips. Newborns exposed to meconium in utero have yellow discoloration of their nails.

Arms and legs are inspected for flexion and symmetry. Extremities should be flexed and move symmetrically through full range of motion. Clavicles are assessed for fractures that may have occurred during the birth process. This assessment is performed by palpating along the entire length of the clavicle, feeling for a mass. The newborn's arm is moved through passive range of motion while the examiner uses his or her other hand to palpate the newborn's clavicle on that same side. *Crepitus*, produced when the bone slides against itself, may be felt over the clavicle if a fracture exists.

Legs appear slightly bowed with everted feet. A persistent breech presentation in utero may result in abducted hips and extended knees (Fig. 19–23). Positional deformities in the newborn period are often caused by intrauterine positioning and may continue to be present for a few days or weeks. Passive range of motion should correct positional deformities.

Hips

Early detection and management of hip instability, and timely referral, increases the effectiveness of treatment. *Developmental dysplasia of the hip* (DDH) encompasses the spectrum of hip abnormalities involving the relationship between the femoral head and the acetabulum (Auriemma & Potisek, 2018). DDH may

an abnormal location. Either or both of the testes can be classified as *retractile*. A testis is referred to as retractile if, when stimulated by palpation or cold, the cremasteric reflex causes it to move to the upper scrotum or as far as the external inguinal ring. This condition differs from the classification of undescended because gentle pressure can bring the testis completely down into the scrotum. To prevent stimulation of the cremasteric reflex during examination, a finger can again be placed between the scrotum and the inguinal canal area while palpating to minimize movement of the testes within the scrotum. Surgical intervention for undescended or ectopic testes occurs when the child is 6 months to 1 year old.

An enlarged scrotum is evaluated for the presence of a hydrocele, which is an accumulation of fluid. Fluid accumulates during fetal development when sexual differentiation occurs. This fluid is usually reabsorbed in utero. If a hydrocele is present at birth, it should disappear within 3 months. The ability to transilluminate a hydrocele differentiates it from a solid or blood-filled mass. Table 19–13 identifies the findings of the physical assessment of male and female newborns that are abnormal and their related pathology.

MUSCULOSKELETAL ASSESSMENT

Inspection and palpation are used to assess the musculoskeletal system. Examination begins by observing the newborn at rest, noting position, symmetry, and presence of abnormal movements. The hands and feet are inspected for the number of digits. Nails are soft and cover the entire nail bed. In a newborn who is post

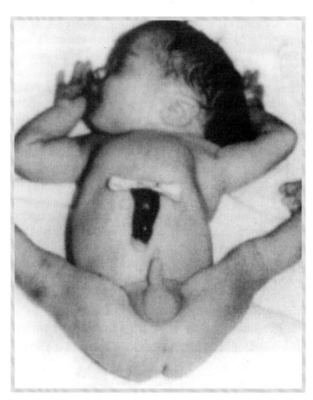

FIGURE 19–23. Typical positioning of newborn following delivery after frank breech in-utero positioning, with abducted hips and extended knees.

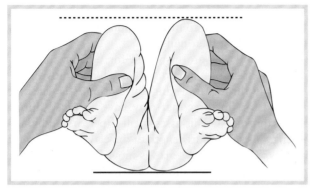

FIGURE 19–24. Asymmetry in number of thigh skin folds and uneven knee level. (From Ballock, R. T., & Richards, B. S. [1997]. Hip dysplasia: Early diagnosis makes a difference. *Contemporary Pediatrics, 14*[7], 110.)

be present at birth, or progress to dislocation later in infancy or childhood. Hip instability occurs in 1% to 2% of full-term newborns, although up to 15% have instability or immaturity detectable with imaging studies (AAP, 2016). DDH is the most common cause of arthritis in women younger than 40 years and accounts for 5% to 10% of all total hip replacements in the United States (AAP, 2016).

Evaluating the newborn's hips requires the infant to be in a quiet state. Crying causes increased muscle tone that could prevent the examiner from identifying an unstable hip. Assessing the newborn for DDH begins with inspection. Position the newborn on his or her back, with diaper off, hips and knees flexed at 90-degree angles, and feet level (Fig. 19–24). The presence of more skin folds on the medial aspect of the thigh or one knee noticeably lower than the other knee (Galeazzi sign) may indicate the femoral head is dislocated or no longer positioned within the acetabulum.

To further determine the presence of an unstable or dislocated hip, the newborn's hips are put through three maneuvers. With the newborn's hips and knees still flexed at 90-degree angles, the hips are simultaneously abducted gently toward the examination table. Normal hips should abduct almost 90 degrees (i.e., thighs resting on the table). This is followed by the *Ortolani maneuver*. To perform the Ortolani maneuver, the examiner stabilizes one hip while the thigh of the hip being tested is abducted and gently pulled anteriorly. If the hip is dislocated, a palpable and sometimes audible "clunk" will be detected as the femoral head moves over the posterior rim of the acetabulum and back into position (Fig. 19–25). The traditional *Barlow maneuver*, performed by adducting the hip while palpating for the head falling out of the back of the acetabulum, has not been shown to have predictive value. If performed forcefully, the Barlow maneuver can itself create instability. The AAP recommends that, if the Barlow test is performed, no posterior-directed force be applied (AAP, 2016). If the hip is dislocated

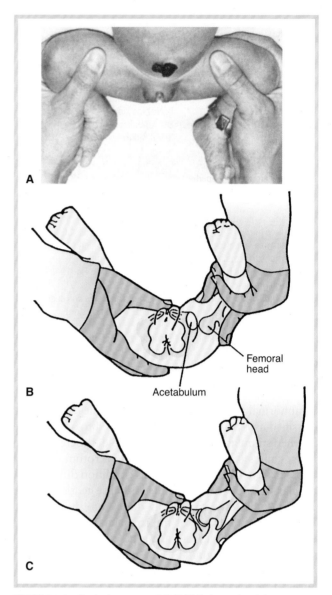

FIGURE 19–25. Ortolani maneuver. **A & B**, With the newborn's legs flexed, the thumb is over the femur and the fingers are on the trochanter. The femur is lifted forward as the thighs are abducted toward the bed. **C**, A "click" is heard or felt as the head of the femur moves into the acetabulum.

by this maneuver, it is relocated by performing the Ortolani maneuver. Hip "clicks" without sensation of instability are clinically insignificant.

Ultrasonographic imaging is recommended either to clarify suspicious physical exam findings at 3 to 4 weeks of age, or to detect clinically silent DDH in high-risk infants from 6 weeks to 6 months of age (AAP, 2016). The continuum of DDH from dysplasia to dislocation is depicted in Figure 19–26.

Early identification of DDH increases the possibility that conservative treatment with bracing and casting can be initiated, and reconstructive surgery avoided (Cooperman & Thompson, 2011). The primary indications for referral in a newborn include an unstable

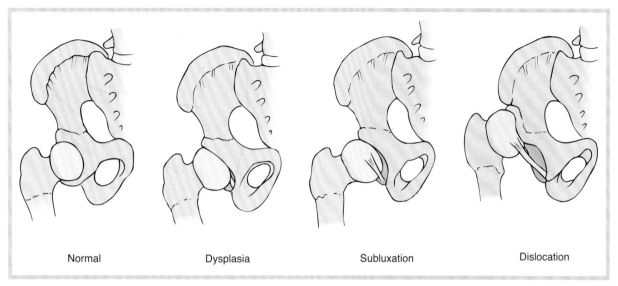

| Normal | Dysplasia | Subluxation | Dislocation |

FIGURE 19-26. Relationship of structures in developmental dysplasia of the hip. (Modified from Wong, D. L. [Ed.]. [1997]. *Whaley & Wong's essentials of pediatric nursing* [5th ed., p. 1137]. St. Louis, MO: Mosby.)

(positive Ortolani test result) or dislocated hip on clinical examination (AAP, 2016).

Feet

Feet are examined to determine whether deformities are positional abnormalities versus structural malformations. Positional abnormalities are temporary, do not involve bone, and refer to alterations in shape and contour of a normally formed foot. Structural malformations usually involve bone and generally form during the 4th to 8th weeks of the embryonic period (Moore & Persaud, 2008). Feet are inspected for 10 digits.

Metatarsus adductus (inward turning of the front one third of the foot with a widening of the space between the first and second toe) is a common positional abnormality occurring in utero due to uterine positioning. Treatment depends on the severity of the abnormality, which progresses along a continuum. The least severe is a foot that returns to the midline spontaneously by stroking the lateral side and usually requires no intervention. Moderately severe is where the examiner is able to easily manipulate the foot into correct position. Exercises performed by parents will usually correct this abnormality. The most severe is the foot that resists correction by the examiner and requires serial casting during infancy.

Talipes calcaneovalgus is a positional deformity caused by the sole of the foot being positioned against the uterine wall. Dorsiflexion of the ankle causes contact between the dorsal surface of the foot and the anterior aspect of the leg (tibia). The leg and foot form the shape of a check mark (✓) rather than the shape of an "L" (Fig. 19–27).

Talipes equinovarus ("clubfoot") involves a deformity of the foot that involves the anklebone and lower leg. In this pathologic deformity, the sole of the foot turns medially and the foot is inverted. There is also mild ankle atrophy. Because of the unusual position, the deformity does not allow weight bearing (Moore & Persaud, 2008). It develops more frequently in males and is bilateral in about half of cases. Treatment may include serial casting; however, if clinical and radiologic correction is not achieved by casting at 3 months of age, surgery is often indicated (Cooperman & Thompson, 2011). A comparison of talipes equinovarus and metatarsus adductus is depicted in Figure 19–28.

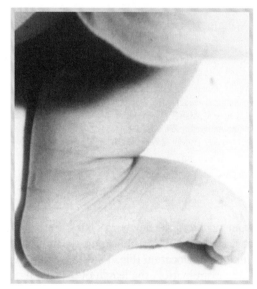

FIGURE 19-27. Talipes calcaneovalgus.

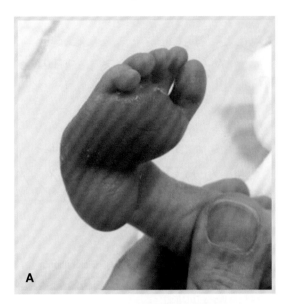

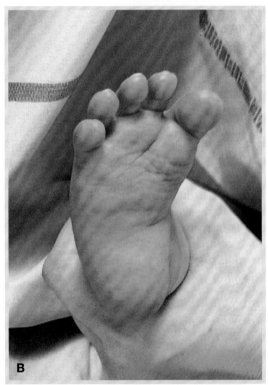

FIGURE 19–28. Congenital foot abnormalities: talipes equinovarus **(A)** and metatarsus adductus **(B)**. (Reproduced from Delpont, M., Lafosse, T., Bachy, M., Mary, P., Alves, A., & Vialle, R. [2015]. Congenital foot abnormalities. *Archives de Pédiatrie, 22*[3], 331–336. doi:10.1016/j .arcped.2014.11.009. Elsevier Masson SAS. All rights reserved.)

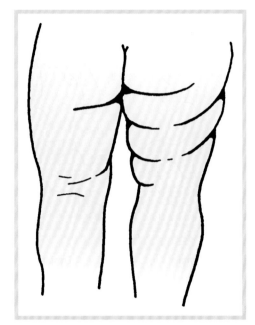

FIGURE 19–29. Asymmetric gluteal folds.

Back

In a prone position, the newborn's back is examined for asymmetric gluteal folds, indicating the presence of a congenital hip dislocation (Fig. 19–29). During this portion of the examination, the length of the spinal column is palpated for masses and abnormal curvatures. The sacral area is inspected for the presence of a *pilonidal*

dimple (Fig. 19–30), tuft of hair, skin lesion, or increased pigmentation that could indicate pathology. Table 19–14 identifies findings of the musculoskeletal assessment that are abnormal and their related pathology.

NEUROLOGIC ASSESSMENT

Assessment of the central nervous system is integrated throughout the physical examination and includes evaluation of posture, cry, muscle tone, and movement; evaluation of most cranial nerves; and evaluation of all developmental reflexes. Findings during the neurologic assessment are influenced by the gestational age and physical health of the newborn.

At rest, a term newborn's posture is flexed, with extremities tight against the trunk. The neuromuscular portion of the gestational age assessment demonstrates the increasing muscle tone that the newborn develops as gestational age progresses. Scarf sign, popliteal angle, and heel-to-ear movements have less range of motion as gestational age increases. Leg and arm recoil also demonstrates how muscle tone normally becomes stronger as gestational age advances.

It is important to evaluate for *weakness* and *hypotonia* in the newborn. The weak infant has an overall reduction of power generated with movements. The hypotonic (or "floppy") infant is unable to sustain postural control and movement against gravity and exhibits poor control of movement. Weak infants are always hypotonic, but hypotonic infants do not all have weakness (Peredo & Hannibal, 2009). Reflexes may be increased, normal or decreased in the hypotonic infant, and muscle mass may be decreased, even at birth.

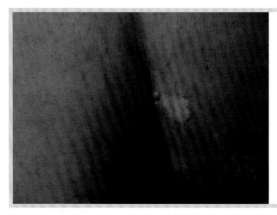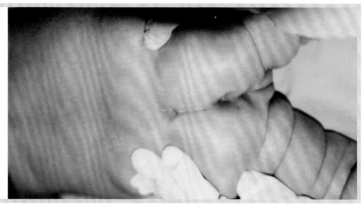

FIGURE 19–30. Sacral skin tag (*left*) and pilonidal dimple (*right*) in a newborn. (Sacral skin tag: From Chung, E., Atkinson-McEvoy, L., Terry, M., & Lai, N. [2014]. *Visual diagnosis and treatment in pediatrics*. Philadelphia, PA: Lippincott Williams & Wilkins. Pilonidal dimple: From Salimpour, R. R., Salimpour, P., & Salimpour, P. [2013]. *Photographic atlas of pediatric disorders and diagnosis*. Philadelphia, PA: Lippincott Williams & Wilkins.)

A healthy newborn's cry is strong and loud. Newborns cry for a variety of reasons. They cry in response to unpleasant environmental stimuli such as fatigue, hunger, cold, or discomfort or because they want the attention of another person. Crying helps the parents develop parenting skills as they become more alert to interpreting their newborn's needs. Responding to a newborn cry helps facilitate attachment between parent and child and increases the newborn's feeling of security. A weak cry is associated with prematurity or illness; a high-pitched cry occurs with drug withdrawal, neurologic abnormalities, metabolic abnormalities, or meningitis.

All of the cranial nerves, with the exception of the olfactory nerve (CN I), should be routinely assessed in the newborn. The advent of UNHS programs has increased the sensitivity of evaluations of the acoustic nerve (CN VIII). Table 19–15 describes how to illicit a response to determine the integrity of each cranial nerve.

TABLE 19–14. Musculoskeletal System

Assessment	Pathology
Weak or absent muscle tone	Neurologic disorder Prematurity Genetic disorder
Extra digit (polydactyly)	Inherited as dominant trait
Partial or complete fusion of digits, more often in feet than hands (syndactyly)	Inherited as dominant trait
Short fingers, incurving of fifth finger, fusion or palmar creases (simian crease), wide space between big toe and second toe	Down syndrome
Jitteriness	Hypoglycemia Hypocalcemia
Arm extended and limp, hand rotated inward, absence of normal movement, absent Moro reflex on affected side	Brachial plexus palsy
Club foot—sole of the foot pointed medially, toes pointed downward and heel pointing upward, upper third of the foot curved downward (can classify as congenital, teratologic, or positional)	Environmental factors in utero which decrease the ability of the fetus to move and/or increase the size of the fetus (i.e., oligohydramnios, maternal diabetes, maternal obesity may cause positional deformities) Exposure to teratogens and maternal smoking may cause teratologic deformities Genetic factors may cause congenital form (Furdon & Donlon, 2002)

From Furdon, S. A., & Donlon, C. R. (2002). Examination of the newborn foot: Positional and structural abnormalities. *Advances in Neonatal Care, 2*(5), 248–258.

TABLE 19–15. Assessing the Integrity of Cranial Nerves

Cranial nerve (CN)	Method of assessment
CN I, olfactory	Not assessed in the neonate
CN II, optic	Newborn follows brightly colored or contrasting object or face; blinks in response to light
CN III, oculomotor CN IV, trochlear CN VI, abducens	Pupils constrict equally in response to light; as newborn's head is moved to face one side or the other, eyes move in the opposite direction (dolls' eyes maneuver)
CN V, trigeminal	Presence of rooting and sucking reflexes; biting
CN VII, facial	Symmetry of facial movement while crying or smiling
CN VIII, acoustic	Positive Moro reflex or movement in the direction of sound; quiets to voice; hearing screening using brainstem auditory evoked response
CN IX, glossopharyngeal CN X, vagus CN XII, hypoglossal	Coordination of suck and swallow; presence of gag reflex; tongue remains midline when mouth is open
CN XI, accessory	Head turns easily to either side; newborn attempts to move head back from side to midline; height of shoulders equal

TABLE 19–16. Neurologic System

Assessment	Pathology
Persistent fisting	Brain lesions, asphyxia
Abnormal position of hands or feet	
Tremors	
Clonus	
Abnormal eye movements	
Poor suck	Neuromuscular disorders
	Basal ganglia or brainstem abnormalities
Altered state of consciousness and seizures	Asphyxia
	Perinatal infections
	Inborn error of metabolism

Reflexes are involuntary neuromuscular responses that provide protection from harm. Whether a specific reflex is present depends on the gestational age of the newborn. Newborns demonstrate two types of reflexes. The first type is protective in nature (i.e., blink, cough, sneeze, and gag). The second type, which disappears during the first year of life, is a result of the neurologic immaturity of newborns. These reflexes are sometimes referred to as developmental or primitive reflexes. Developmental reflexes are all present at birth in the healthy term newborn. Appendix 19–C describes how to elicit these reflexes, defines normal and abnormal responses, and explains at what age they disappear.

Table 19–16 identifies findings during the neurologic assessment that are abnormal and their related pathology.

SUMMARY

A formal assessment of all body systems is completed by the perinatal/neonatal nurse soon after birth and repeated at intervals established by institutional protocol throughout the newborn's hospitalization. Informal assessments are ongoing and occur during caregiving activities. Performing the physical assessment provides a picture of how the newborn is adapting to extrauterine life. The development of keen physical assessment skills allows the nurse to detect subtle changes in the newborn's condition, identify or anticipate the development of problems, and intervene immediately to prevent or minimize these problems.

REFERENCES

American Academy of Pediatrics. (2008). Red reflex examination in neonates, infants, and children. *Pediatrics*, 122(6), 1401–1404. doi:10.1542/peds.2008-2624

American Academy of Pediatrics. (2016). Evaluation and referral for developmental dysplasia of the hip in infants. *Pediatrics*, 13(6), e20163107. doi: https://doi.org/10.1542/peds.2016-3107

American Academy of Pediatrics. (2019). *Program to Enhance the Health & Development of Infants and Children (PEHDIC)*, Elk Grove Village, IL: Author.

American Academy of Pediatrics & American College of Obstetricians and Gynecologists. (2017). *Guidelines for perinatal care* (8th ed.). Washington, DC: Author.

American College of Obstetrics and Gynecologists and Society for Maternal-Fetal Medicine. (2019). Fetal growth restriction (Practice Bulletin No. 204). Washington, DC: Author.

Association of Women's Health, Obstetric and Neonatal Nurses. (2017). *Assessment and care of the late preterm infant* (Evidence-Based Clinical Practice Guideline, 2nd ed.). Washington, DC: Author.

Auriemma, J. & Potisek, N. M. (2018). Developmental dysplasia of the hip. *Pediatrics in Review*, 39(11), 570–572. doi:10.1542/pir.2017-0239.

Ballard, J. L., Khoury, J. C., Wedig, K., Wang, L., Eilers-Walsman, B. L., & Lipp, R. (1991). New Ballard Score, expanded to include extremely premature infants. *Journal of Pediatrics*, 119(3), 417–423.

Ballard, J. L., Novak, K. K., & Driver, M. (1979). A simplified score for assessment of fetal maturation of newly born infants. *Journal of Pediatrics*, 95(5, Pt. 1), 769–774.

Cavaliere, T. A. (2019). Genitourinary assessment. In E. P. Tappero & M. E. Honeyfield (Eds.), *Physical assessment of the newborn: A comprehensive approach to the art of physical examination* (6th ed., pp. 121–138). New York, NY: Springer Publishing Company.

Clark, L., & Rohan, A. J. (2015). Identifying and assessing the substance-exposed infant. *MCN: The American Journal of Maternal Child Nursing*, 40(2), 87–95. doi:10.1097/NMC.0000000000000117

Cooperman, D. R., & Thompson, G. H. (2011). Congenital abnormalities of the upper and lower extremities and spine. In R. J. Martin, A. A. Fanaroff, & M. C. Walsh (Eds.), *Neonatal-perinatal medicine: Diseases of the fetus and newborn* (9th ed., pp. 1782–1801). St. Louis, MO: Elsevier.

Dubowitz, L. M. S., Dubowitz, V., & Goldberg, C. (1970). Clinical assessment of gestational age in the newborn infant. *Journal of Pediatrics*, 77(1), 1–10. doi:10.1016/s0022-3476(70)80038-5

Dubowitz, L. M. S., Ricciw, D., & Mercuri, E. (2005). The Dubowitz neurological examination of the full-term newborn. *Mental Retardation and Developmental Disabilities Research Reviews*, 11(1), 52–60.

Elder, J. S. (2007). Urologic disorders in infants and children. In R. E. Behrman, R. M. Kliegman, & H. B. Jenson (Eds.), *Nelson's textbook of pediatrics* (18th ed., pp. 2253–2260). Philadelphia, PA: Saunders.

Furdon, S. A., & Donlon, C. R. (2002). Examination of the newborn foot: Positional and structural abnormalities. *Advances in Neonatal Care*, 2(5), 248–258.

Gagliardi, L., Brambilla, C., Bruno, R., Martinelli, S., & Console, V. (1993). Biased assessment of gestational age at birth when obstetric gestation is known. *Archives of Disease in Childhood*, 68(1), 32–34.

Gardner, S. L., & Hernandez, J. A. (2011). Initial nursery care. In S. L. Gardner, B. S. Carter, M. Enzman-Hines, & J. A. Hernandez (Eds.), *Handbook of neonatal intensive care* (7th ed., pp. 78–112). St. Louis, MO: Mosby/Elsevier.

Gomella, T. L., Cunningham, M. D., & Eyal, F. G. (2009a). Hyperbilirubinemia, direct (conjugated hyperbilirubinemia). In *Neonatology: Management, procedures, on-call problems, diseases and drugs* (6th ed., pp. 288–293). New York, NY: McGraw-Hill.

Gomella, T. L., Cunningham, M. D., & Eyal, F. G. (2009b). Hyperbilirubinemia, indirect (unconjugated hyperbilirubinemia). In *Neonatology: Management, procedures, on-call problems, diseases and drugs* (6th ed., pp. 293–301). New York, NY: McGraw-Hill.

Goodwin, M. (2009). Abdomen assessment. In E. P. Tappero & M. E. Honeyfield (Eds.), *Physical assessment of the newborn: A comprehensive approach to the art of physical examination* (4th ed., pp. 105–114). Santa Rosa, CA: NICU Ink.

Green, M. (1998). *Pediatric diagnosis: Interpretation of symptoms and signs in infants, children and adolescents* (6th ed.). Philadelphia, PA: Saunders.

Hernandez, P. W., & Glass, S. M. (2005). Physical assessment of the newborn. In P. J. Thureen, J. Deacon, P. J. Hernandez, & D. M. Hall (Eds.), *Assessment and care of the well newborn* (pp. 119–172). Philadelphia, PA: Saunders.

Hoath, S. B., & Narendran, V. (2011). The skin. In R. J. Martin, A. A. Fanaroff, & M. C. Walsh (Eds.), *Neonatal-perinatal medicine: Diseases of the fetus and newborn* (9th ed., pp. 1705–1736). St. Louis, MO: Elsevier.

Johnson, P. (2019). Head, eyes, ears, nose, mouth and neck assessment. In E. P. Tappero & M. E. Honeyfield (Eds.), *Physical assessment of the newborn: A comprehensive approach to the art of physical examination* (6th ed., pp. 61–78). New York, NY: Springer Publishing Company.

Kaplan, M., Wong, R. J., Sibley, E., & Stevenson, D. K. (2011). Neonatal jaundice and liver disease. In R. J. Martin, A. A. Fanaroff, & M. C. Walsh (Eds.), *Neonatal-perinatal medicine: Diseases of the fetus and newborn* (9th ed., pp. 1443–1496). St. Louis, MO: Elsevier.

Kuo, A. A., Tritasavit, S., & Graham, J. M., Jr. (2014). Congenital muscular torticollis and positional plagiocephaly. *Pediatrics in Review*, 35(2), 79–87. doi:10.1542/pir.35-2-79

Lund, C. H., & Kuller, J. M. (2007). Integumentary system. In C. Kenner & J. W. Lott (Eds.), *Comprehensive neonatal care* (4th ed., pp. 65–91). St. Louis, MO: Saunders Elsevier.

Moore, K. L., & Persaud, T. V. N. (2008). *The developing human* (8th ed.). Philadelphia, PA: Saunders/Elsevier.

Muse, C., Harrison, J., Yoshinaga-Itano, C., Grimes, A., Brookhouser, P. E., Epstein, S., . . . Martin, B. (2013). Supplement to the JCIH 2007 position statement: principles and guidelines for early intervention after confirmation that a child is deaf or hard of hearing. *Pediatrics*, 131(4), e1324–e1349. doi:10.1542/peds.2013-0008

Nardozza, L. M. M., Caetano, A. C. R., Zamarian, A. C. P., Mazzola, J. B., Silva, C. P., Marçal, V. M., . . . Araujo Júnior, E. (2017). Fetal growth restriction: Current knowledge. *Archives of Gynecology and Obstetrics*, 295(5), 1061–1077. doi:10.1007/s00404-017-4341-9

Park, M. K. (2008). *Pediatric cardiology for practitioners* (5th ed.). Philadelphia, PA: Mosby.

Peredo, D. E., & Hannibal, M. C. (2009). The floppy infant: Evaluation of hypotonia. *Pediatrics in Review*, 30(9), e66–e76. doi:10.1542/pir.30-9-e66

Rohan, A. J., & Golombek, S. G. (2009). Hypoxia in the term newborn infant: Part 1. Cardio-pulmonary physiology and assessment. *MCN: The American Journal of Maternal/Child Nursing*, 34(2), 106–112. doi:10.1097/01.NMC.0000347304.70208.eb

Rohan, A. J., Golombek, S. G., & Rosenthal, A. D. (1999). Infants with misshapen skulls: When to worry. *Contemporary Pediatrics*, 16(2), 47–73.

Shulman, R. M., Palmert, M. R., & Wherrett, D. K. (2011). Disorders of sex development. In R. J. Martin, A. A. Fanaroff, & M. C. Walsh (Eds.), *Neonatal-perinatal medicine: Diseases of the fetus and newborn* (9th ed., pp. 1584–1620). St. Louis, MO: Elsevier.

Silengo, M., Battistoni, G., & Spada, M. (1999). Is there a relationship between extensive mongolian spots and inborn errors of metabolism? *American Journal of Medical Genetics*, 87(3), 276–277.

Stellwagen, L., Hubbard, E., Chambers, C., & Jones, K. L. (2008). Torticollis, facial asymmetry and plagiocephaly in normal newborns. *Archives of Disease in Childhood*, 93(10), 827–831. doi:10.1136/adc.2007.124123

Vargo, L. (2019). Cardiovascular assessment. In E. P. Tappero & M. E. Honeyfield (Eds.), *Physical assessment of the newborn: A comprehensive approach to the art of physical examination* (6th ed., pp. 93–110). New York, NY: Springer Publishing Company.

Witt, C. (2019). Skin assessment. In E. P. Tappero & M. E. Honeyfield (Eds.), *Physical assessment of the newborn: A comprehensive approach to the art of physical examination* (4th ed., pp. 45–60). New York, NY: Springer Publishing Company.

World Health Organization. (n.d.). *WHO growth standards are recommended for use in the U.S. for infants and children 0 to 2 years of age*. Geneva, Switzerland: Author.

APPENDIX 19–A. Characteristics of Infant State

Infant states	Body activity	Eye movements	Facial movements	Breathing pattern	Level of response	Implications for caregiving
Sleep states						
Deep sleep (or quiet sleep)	Nearly still, except for occasional startle or twitch	None	Without facial movements, except for occasional sucking at regular intervals	Smooth and regular	Threshold to stimuli very high so that only very intense or disturbing stimuli will arouse infants	Caregivers trying to feed infants in deep sleep will probably find the experience frustrating. Infants will be unresponsive even if caregivers use disturbing stimuli (flicking feet) to arouse infants. Infants may arouse only briefly and then become unresponsive as they return to deep sleep. If caregivers wait until infants move to a higher, more responsive state, feeding or care giving will be much more pleasant.
Light sleep (or active sleep)	Some body movements	Rapid eye movements (REM); fluttering of eyes beneath closed eyelids	May smile and make brief fussy or crying sounds	Irregular	More responsive to internal and external stimuli. When stimuli may occur, infant may remain in light sleep, return to deep sleep, or arouse to drowsy.	Light sleep makes up the highest proportion of newborn sleep and usually precedes wakening. The brief fussy or crying sounds made during this state may make caregivers who are not aware that these sounds occur normally think it is time for feeding, and they may try to feed infants before they are ready to eat.
Awake states						
Drowsy	Activity level variable, with mild startles interspersed from time to time; movement usually smooth	Eyes open and close occasionally and are heavy lidded with dull, glazed appearance	Some facial movements possible	Irregular	React to sensory stimuli although responses are delayed	From the drowsy state, infants may return to sleep or awaken further. To facilitate waking, caregivers can provide something for infants to see, hear, or suck. This may arouse them to a quiet alert state, a more responsive state. Infants left alone without additional stimulation from caregiver will progress to quiet alert state.
Quiet alert	Minimal	Brightening and widening of eyes	Face bright, shining, sparkling	Regular	Most attentive to environment, focusing attention on any stimuli that are present	Infants in quiet, alert state provide much pleasure and positive feedback for caregivers. Providing something for infants to see, hear, or suck will often maintain this state. In the first few hours after birth, most newborns commonly experience a period of intense alertness before going into a long sleeping period.
Active alert	Much body activity; periods of fussiness possible	Eyes open with less brightening	Much facial movement; face not as bright as quiet alert state	Irregular	Increasingly sensitive to disturbing stimuli (hunger, fatigue, noise, excessive handling)	Caregivers may intervene at this stage to console and to bring infants to a lower state.
Crying	Increased motor activity, with color changes	Eyes tightly closed or open	Grimaces	More irregular	Extremely responsive to unpleasant external or internal stimuli	Crying is the infant's communication signal. It is a response to unpleasant stimuli from the environment or from within (fatigue, hunger, discomfort). Crying tells us the infant's limits have been reached. Sometimes infants can console themselves and return to lower states. At other times, they need help from caregivers.

From Pearson, J. (1999). Crying and calming: Important information and effective techniques to teach parents of full-term newborns. *Mother Baby Journal, 4*(5), 39–42.

APPENDIX 19-B. Characteristics of the Ballard Gestation Age Assessment Tool

Posture

Observe the newborn lying quietly. Flexion of arms and legs increases with gestational age. The premature newborn lies with arms and legs extended. As gestational age increases, the more flexed the newborn's arms and legs are against the body.

Square Window (Wrist)

The angle that is created when the newborn's palm is flexed toward the forearm. A preterm newborn's wrist exhibits poor flexion and makes a 90-degree angle with the arm. An extremely preterm newborn has no flexor tone and cannot achieve even 90-degree flexion. A term newborn's wrist can flex completely against the forearm.

Arm Recoil

After first flexing the arms at the elbows against the chest, then fully extending and releasing them, term newborns resist extension and quickly return arms to the flexed position. Very preterm newborns do not resist extension and respond with weak and delayed flexion.

Popliteal Angle

With the newborn supine and his or her pelvis flat, flex the thigh to the abdomen and hold it there while extending the leg at the knee. The angle at the knee is estimated. The preterm newborn can achieve greater extension.

Scarf Sign

While the newborn is supine, move his or her arm across his or her chest toward the opposite shoulder. A term newborn's elbow does not cross midline. It is possible to bring the preterm newborn's elbow much farther.

Heel to Ear

Without holding the knee and thigh in place, move the newborn's foot as close to the ear as possible. A preterm newborn is able to get his or her foot closer to his or her head than a term baby.

Skin

Assess for thickness, transparency, and texture. Preterm skin is smooth and thin with visible vessels. Extremely preterm skin is sticky and transparent. Term skin is thick, veins are difficult to see, and peeling may occur.

Lanugo

Fine hair seen over the back of premature newborns by 24 weeks' gestation. It begins to thin over the lower back first and disappears last over the shoulders.

Plantar Creases

One or two creases over the pad of the foot at approximately 32 weeks' gestation. At 36 weeks, creases cover the anterior two thirds of the foot; at term, the whole foot. At very early gestations, the length from the tip of the great toe to the back of the heel is measured.

Breast Tissue

Examined for visibility of nipple and areola and size of bud when grasped between thumb and forefinger. The very premature newborn does not have visible nipples or areolae. These become more defined and then raised by 34 weeks, with a small bud appearing at 36 weeks and growing to 5 to 10 mm by term.

Ear Formation

Lack of cartilage in earlier gestation results in the ear folding easily and retaining this fold. As gestation progresses, soft cartilage provides increasing resistance to folding and increasing recoil. The pinnae are flat in very preterm newborns. Incurving proceeds from the top down toward the lobes as gestation advances.

Genitalia

In males, rugae become visible at 28 weeks. By 36 weeks, the testes are in the upper scrotum, and rugae cover the anterior portion of the scrotum. At term, rugae cover the scrotum, and when postmature, the testes are pendulous. In preterm females, the clitoris is prominent, and the labia minora are flat. By 36 weeks, the labia majora are larger, nearly covering the clitoris.

APPENDIX 19–C. Developmental (Primitive) Reflexes

Reflex	How elicited	Normal response	Abnormal response	Duration of reflex
Rooting and sucking	Touch cheek, lip, or corner of mouth with finger or nipple.	Newborn turns head in direction of stimulus, opens mouth, and begins to suck. In the term newborn, suck is coordinated and strong.	Weak or absent response is seen with prematurity, neurologic deficit, or CNS depression from maternal drug ingestion.	Rooting disappears by 3 to 4 months; sucking disappears by 1 year.
Swallowing	Place fluid on back.	Newborn swallows in coordination with sucking.	Gagging, coughing, or regurgitation of fluid; possibly associated with cyanosis secondary to prematurity, neurologic deficit, or injury.	Does not disappear.
Extrusion	Touch tip of tongue with finger or nipple.	Newborn pushes tongue outward.	Continuous extrusion of tongue or repetitive tongue thrusting is seen with CNS abnormalities or seizures.	Disappears by 6 months.
Moro	Holding the newborn's head off the mattress slightly, let it drop quickly several inches into your hand.	Bilateral symmetric extension and abduction of all extremities, with thumb and forefinger forming characteristic "C," followed by adduction of extremities and return to relaxed flexion.	Asymmetric response is seen with peripheral nerve injury (brachial plexus), fracture of clavicle or long bone of arm or leg, or birth trauma such as skull fracture.	Disappears by 6 months.
Truck incurvature (Galant's reflex)	Use one hand to lift the prone newborn off a flat surface (ventral suspension). With a finger from the free hand, use some pressure to draw a line down the length of the back about an inch from the spinal column.	Newborn flexes pelvis toward the side stimulated.	Absence indicates spinal cord lesion or CNS depression.	Disappears by 4 months.
Tonic neck (fencing)	Turn the newborn's head to one side when infant is resting in the supine position.	Extremity on the side to which the head is turned extends and opposite extremities flex. Response may be absent or incomplete immediately after birth.	Persistent response after 4 months may indicate neurologic injury.	Diminishes by 4 months.
Moro	Expose the newborn to sudden movement or loud noise.	Newborn abducts and flexes all extremities and may begin to cry.	Absence of response may indicate neurologic deficit or deafness. Response may be absent or diminished during sleep.	Diminishes by 4 months.
Crossed extension	Place the newborn in the supine position and extend one leg while stimulating the bottom of the foot.	Newborn's opposite leg flexes and extends rapidly as if trying to deflect stimulus to the other foot.	Weak or absent response is seen with peripheral nerve injury or fracture of a long bone.	Disappears by 6 months.
Palmar grasp	Place a finger in the newborn's palm and apply slight pressure.	Newborn grasps finger; attempting to remove the finger causes newborn to tighten his or her grasp.	Weak or absent grasp is seen in the presence of CNS deficit or nerve or muscle injury.	Does not disappear.

CNS, central nervous system.

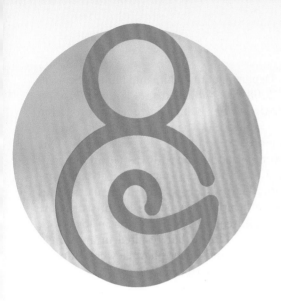

CHAPTER 20

Newborn Nutrition

Jill Janke

OVERVIEW

This chapter offers information and guidelines for the perinatal nurse caring for new mothers and infants during the initiation and early days of infant feeding. The chapter emphasizes that breast milk is the ideal food for the newborn and provides helpful information for nurses working with families who choose to breast-feed. Guidelines are suggested for helping families who choose to formula-feed their newborn.

INFANT FEEDING DECISION

The decision about what to feed a newborn is frequently made by the mother long before giving birth (American Academy of Family Physicians [AAFP], 2015; Asiodu, Waters, Dailey, & Lyndon, 2017; Association of Women's Health Obstetric and Neonatal Nursing [AWHONN], 2015a, 2015b; Labbock & Taylor, 2008; Rollins et al., 2016; Swanson, Power, Kaur, Carter, & Shepherd, 2007). A woman's selection of an infant feeding method is more than just a lifestyle choice; it should be based on current scientific evidence. Perinatal nurses have the responsibility to make sure a woman has the needed information to make an informed decision. However, once an informed decision is made, the mother's choice should be respected by all healthcare professionals (American College of Obstetricians and Gynecologists, 2018; AWHONN, 2015a).

A mother's infant feeding decision is influenced by many factors, including her education (Callen & Pinelli, 2004; Labbock & Taylor, 2008; Lutsiv et al., 2013; Phares et al., 2004; Radzyminski & Callister, 2016); age (Labbock & Taylor, 2008; Lutsiv et al., 2013; Phares et al., 2004; Radzyminski & Callister, 2016); income (Lutsiv et al., 2013); previous breastfeeding experience

(Bailey & Wright, 2011; Lutsiv et al., 2013); prenatal breastfeeding education (Dyson, Green, Renfrew, McMillan, & Woolridge, 2010; Kervin, Kemp, & Pulver, 2010; Lutsiv et al., 2013; Patnode, Henninger, Senger, Perdue, & Whitlock, 2016); health problems, smoking, or drug use status (Lutsiv et al., 2013); and the attitudes, knowledge, and type of healthcare professionals (Britton, McCormick, Renfrew, Wade, & King, 2007; Kervin et al., 2010; Lutsiv et al., 2013; Patnode et al., 2016; Ryan & Zhou, 2006). Sources of personal support also influence the infant feeding decision, including encouragement from the husband, significant others, and extended family, including grandmothers and peers (AAFP, 2015; Rosen-Carole & Hartman, 2015). Roll and Cheater (2016) did a mixed method systematic review and reported that key influences included perceptions of the mothering role and paternal attachment, strength of views toward feeding methods, personal views of the breasts for feeding, female role models, partner/father opinions, professional support versus pressure, health myths versus facts, perceived convenience of the feeding options, and embarrassment and public feeding. Knowledge of factors influencing infant feeding decisions is critical to designing interventions to promote breastfeeding.

BENEFITS OF BREASTFEEDING

Human milk is a dynamic food, meeting the infant's needs to build an immune system, to grow and develop the brain, and to form attachments with other human beings. Research has produced compelling data about the short- and long-term health benefits of breastfeeding for the mother and newborn. Numerous economic advantages of breastfeeding have also been identified (Victora et al., 2016).

Newborn Health Benefits

There is substantial scientific evidence that newborns who are breastfed, or who are given breast milk, are healthier than those who receive formula. Several integrated reviews and meta-analyses have quantified neonatal health benefits (Binns, Lee, & Low, 2016; Ip et al., 2007; Victora et al., 2016). During the first year of age, breastfed infants have decreased their risk for severe respiratory illness by 33% to 72%, otitis media by 50%, gastrointestinal illness by 50% to 64%, necrotizing enterocolitis (NEC) by 58%, and sudden infant death syndrome (SIDS) by 36% to 58%. The long-term neonatal health benefits of breastfeeding have also been identified. Table 20–1 lists long- and short-term medical problems that have been associated with not breastfeeding.

Maternal Health Benefits

Maternal health benefits also are associated with breastfeeding. In the immediate postpartum period, breastfeeding enhances mother–infant attachment. It also stimulates uterine involution resulting in less blood loss and reducing the risk for anemia and infection. Long-term maternal health benefits are also related with breastfeeding. The actual risk reduction will depend on cumulative time spent breastfeeding over a woman's life. The more breastfeeding a woman does, the greater the health benefits. Known benefits include reduced risk for developing breast cancer, ovarian cancer, and type II diabetes (Chowdhury et al., 2015; Ip et al., 2007; Schwarz et al., 2010; Stuebe & Schwarz, 2010; Victora et al., 2016). Other associations have been found between breastfeeding and reduced risk for developing metabolic syndrome (Gunderson et al., 2010), hypertension, hyperlipidemia, and cardiovascular disease (Natland Fagerhaug et al., 2013; Schwarz et al., 2009); rheumatoid arthritis (Adab et al., 2014); and thyroid cancer (Yi, Zhu, Zhu, Liu, & Wu, 2016).

Economic Benefits

Exclusive use of formula and its consequent increased neonatal morbidity is responsible for substantial expenditures of healthcare dollars. Bartick and Reinhold (2010) estimated there would be an annual healthcare cost savings of $13 billion if 90% of new mothers in the U.S. breastfed exclusively for the first 6 months. Rollins et al. (2016) did an economic cost analysis of infant morbidity of breastfeeding, based on treatment costs of otitis media, diarrhea, NEC, pneumonia, asthma, obesity, type 1 diabetes, and leukemia. They estimated there would be a $312 million savings in healthcare costs if the United States increased its exclusive breastfeeding rate by 10%.

The U.S. Department of Health and Human Services (USDHHS, 2008) has published a toolkit, the *Business Case for Breastfeeding*, which includes reports from various companies that have implemented breastfeeding support programs in the workplace. One organization reported increased breastfeeding rates at 6 months (72.5%) after implementation of their support program. They also reported an annual savings of $240,000 in healthcare expenses for breastfeeding mothers and children; a 72% reduction in lost work time due to infant illness that resulted in an annual savings of $60,000; and lower pharmacy costs due to a 62% reduction in prescriptions.

Contraindications to Breastfeeding

The American Academy of Pediatrics (AAP, 2012) and AAFP (2015) maintain that with few exceptions human milk is preferred for all infants, including premature and sick newborns. Contraindications to breastfeeding are rare and include a mother who has human T-cell lymphotropic virus type I or II infection; needs cancer treatment with antimetabolites, chemotherapeutic agents, or radiation; has untreated active tuberculosis; uses illicit drugs; has herpes simplex lesions on the breast; or who is seropositive for the HIV. Breastfeeding is also contraindicated when infants have certain types of inborn errors of metabolism, such as galactosemia (AAP Section on Breastfeeding, 2012).

INCIDENCE OF BREASTFEEDING

Healthy People Goals

Given the importance of breast milk and breastfeeding to mothers, newborns, and society, one of the Healthy People national goals is to increase initiation and duration rates of breastfeeding. The target initiation and duration rates have been altered over the last three decades as more information about infant feeding practices became available. The *Healthy People 2020* target for *any* breastfeeding is that 81.9% of women will initiate breastfeeding, 60.6% will be breastfeeding at 6 months, and 34.1% will still be breastfeeding until the infant is 12 months of age. The *Healthy People 2020* target for *exclusive* breastfeeding is that 46.2% of women who initiated breastfeeding will exclusively breast-feed through the first 3 months and 25.5% will exclusively breastfeed for 6 months (USDHHS, 2011). As we move closer to 2020, the *Healthy People 2030* committee will be reviewing and revising these goals.

Although breastfeeding rates have steadily increased since the 1990s, more work is needed to meet the *Healthy People 2020* goals. According to a national survey conducted on 2014 data, 82.5% of mothers

TABLE 20–1. Infant Risk of Specific Medical Conditions that May Be Associated with Not Breastfeeding

Disease or condition	Study	Result
Asthma	Ip et al. (2007)	Meta-analysis found a significant association between breastfeeding and a 27% reduced risk of asthma in subjects without family history of asthma. Subjects younger than 10 years of age who were breast-fed and had positive family history of asthma also had reduced risk.
	Bener, Ehlayel, Alsowaidi, and Sabbah (2007)	Exclusive breastfeeding prevents development of asthma and allergic diseases in children.
	Ogbuanu, Karmaus, Arshad, Kurukulaaratchy, and Ewart (2009)	Using lung function as a measure of susceptibility to asthma, children breastfed for at least 4 months had increased lung volume suggesting a decreased susceptibility to asthma.
	Victora et al. (2016)	Reported a 9% reduction in risk with breastfeeding; however, more research is needed with better control over potentially confounding variables.
Otitis media	Ip et al. (2007)	Meta-analysis showed breastfeeding was associated with a significant reduction (50%) in the risk of otitis.
	Victora et al. (2016)	Strong evidence breastfeeding protects against otitis for children younger than 2 years of age.
Respiratory conditions	Ip et al. (2007)	Meta-analysis found a 72% reduction in the risk of being hospitalized with a lower respiratory tract disease in infants who were exclusively breastfed for 4 months or longer.
	Victora et al. (2016)	Meta-analysis found 33% of respiratory infections could be prevented by breastfeeding; it could prevent 57% of hospital admissions for acute respiratory infections.
	Mihrshahi, Oddy, Peat, and Kabir (2008)	Exclusive or predominant breastfeeding can reduce rates of respiratory infection.
GI infection	Ip et al. (2007)	Evidence from three primary studies that breastfeeding was associated with 64% reduction in the risk for GI infection during first year of age.
	Victora et al. (2016)	Meta-analysis found 50% of diarrhea episodes could be prevented with breastfeeding and 72% of hospital admissions for diarrhea could be avoided.
	Mihrshahi et al. (2008)	Exclusive or predominant breastfeeding can reduce rates of diarrhea.
	Monterrosa et al. (2008)	Predominantly, breastfed infants had lower risk for GI infection during the first 6 months when compared to formula fed and partially breastfed infants.
Cognitive development	Ip et al. (2007)	Meta-analysis included preterm and term infants; results inconclusive because no studies controlled for maternal IQ
	Victora et al. (2016)	Meta-analysis of controlled studies showed a 3.4 to 7 points increase in IQ with longer breastfeeding.
	Kramer et al. (2008)	Randomized controlled trial with 17,046 infants (81.5% were followed to age 6.5 years); reported strong evidence that prolonged and exclusive breastfeeding is associated with children's cognitive development
	Bartels, van Beijsterveldt, and Boomsma (2009)	Significant positive effect of breastfeeding found on cognitive abilities after controlling for differences in maternal education.
	Rees and Sabia (2009)	A study of siblings concluded breastfeeding is associated with cognitive ability.
	Sloan, Stewart, and Dunne (2010)	Study of 137 infants, concluded breastfeeding over a month may have a beneficial effect on cognitive development.
Obesity	Ip et al. (2007)	Meta-analysis concluded there is an association between breastfeeding and reduced risk of obesity later in life.
	Victora et al. (2016)	Meta-analysis found infants' breastfed for longer durations was associated with a 13% reduction in overweight or obesity later in life, however, the studies failed to control for confounding variables.
	Butte (2009)	Breastfeeding had small but consistent protective effect against childhood obesity. Author noted that genetic and environmental variables may pose greater risk, such as socioeconomic status, parental obesity, parental smoking, and birth weight and rapid weight gain during infancy.
	Griffiths, Smeeth, Hawkins, Cole, and Dezateux (2009)	Initiating and prolonging breastfeeding may reduce excessive weight gain during the preschool years.

(continued)

TABLE 20–1. Infant Risk of Specific Medical Conditions that May Be Associated with Not Breastfeeding *(Continued)*

Disease or condition	Study	Result
Diabetes	Ip et al. (2007)	Evidence suggests that breastfeeding for >3 months is associated with reduced risk of developing type 1 and type 2 diabetes (39%).
	Victora et al. (2016)	Meta-analysis concluded the evidence that breastfeeding protects against later development of diabetes is growing; however, researchers need better control over confounding variables.
	Taylor, Kacmar, Nothnagle, and Lawrence (2005)	Systematic review concluded that being breastfed for at least 2 months might lower the risk of diabetes in children.
NEC	Ip et al. (2007)	Evidence supports an association between breastfeeding and reduced risk of NEC in preterm infants.
	Victora et al. (2016)	Meta-analysis of a 58% reduction in NEC when the infant received breast milk
	Henderson, Craig, Brocklehurst, and McGuire (2009)	Subjects who did not develop NEC were significantly more likely to have received human breast milk when compared to those who did develop NEC (91% vs. 75%).
	Chauhan, Henderson, and McGuire (2008)	Concluded that feeding preterm infants human milk versus formula can reduce the risk of NEC threefold
Allergies	Ip et al. (2007) Victora et al. (2016)	Results equivocal; more research needed
SIDS	Ip et al. (2007) Victora et al. (2016)	Meta-analysis showed a significant reduction in the incidence of SIDS (36%) when infant was breastfed.
Cardiovascular disease	Ip et al. (2007) Victora et al. (2016)	Results inconclusive on the relationship between breastfeeding and adult cholesterol and between breastfeeding and mortality from cardiovascular disease. However, there was a significant association between breastfeeding and a small reduction in adult blood pressure.
Childhood leukemia and lymphomas	Ip et al. (2007)	Meta-analysis concluded there was a significant association between breastfeeding for at least 6 months and a reduced risk for acute lymphocytic leukemia (ALL) and acute myelogenous leukemia (AML).
	Victora et al. (2016)	Meta-analysis concluded there was a 19% reduced risk of developing leukemia
Dental malocclusions	Victora et al. (2016)	Meta-analysis showed a 68% reduction in malocclusions when the infant was breastfed.

GI, gastrointestinal; NEC, necrotizing enterocolitis; SIDS, sudden infant death syndrome.

in the United States initiated breastfeeding; of those, 46.6% were exclusively breastfeeding at 3 months. At 6 months, 55.3% continued to do some breastfeeding, with 24.9% breastfeeding exclusively. At 1 year, 33.7% of women continued doing some breastfeeding, and at 18 months, 13.5% were still breastfeeding (Centers for Disease Control and Prevention [CDC], 2017).

The AAP (2012), AAFP (2015), and the Academy of Nutrition and Dietetics (Lessen & Kavanagh, 2015) recommend that women continue to breast-feed longer than 12 months if mutually desired. The World Health Organization (WHO, 2011a) extends that recommendation to 2 years or longer. Researchers have reported distinct benefits to extending breastfeeding past the first year. Given that the immune components of breast milk are maintained into the second year of lactation, breastfeeding continues to protect against infection and allergies. An older study reported that

breastfeeding toddlers between the ages of 16 and 30 months had fewer illnesses and when they did get sick, their illnesses were of shorter duration when compared to nonnursing toddlers (Gulick, 1986). More recently, there is growing evidence that the benefits of breastfeeding are dose dependent. Extended breastfeeding is reported to have long-term health benefits for mother and infant (Brockway & Venturato, 2016; Ip et al., 2007; Jansen, Mallan, Byrne, Daniels, & Nicholson, 2016).

Despite research identifying the benefits of giving breast milk to preterm infants, no national goal has been set for this high-risk population. It is unknown what the U.S. breastfeeding rates are for preterm infants, but we do know they are lower than for term infants. Between 2003 and 2004, breastfeeding rates in Philadelphia's neonatal intensive care units (NICUs) ranged from 36.9% to 50% (Castrucci, Hoover, Lim, & Maus, 2007). Hospitals that used lactation consultants

TABLE 20–2. Healthy People Breastfeeding Goals

Goal	2010 target	2020 target	National immunization study 2014 (CDC, 2017)	
			Overall United States average	Range (state disparity)
Initiate any breastfeeding	75%	81.9%	82.5%	57.5% to 93.2%*
At 6 months any breastfeeding	50%	60.6%	55.3%	29.2% to 70%†
At 12 months any breastfeeding	25%	34.1%	33.7%	15.3% to 52.8%†
At 3 months exclusive breastfeeding	40%	44.3%	46.6%	25.2% to 62.7%**
At 6 months exclusive breastfeeding	17%	25.5%	24.9%	11.1% to 38.3%††

*Thirty-five states have exceeded *Healthy People 2020* goal for initiating any breastfeeding.
†Fifteen states have exceeded *Healthy People 2020* goal for any breastfeeding at 6 months.
†Twenty states have exceeded *Healthy People 2020* goal for any breastfeeding at 12 months.
**Thirty-four states have exceeded *Healthy People 2020* goal for exclusive breastfeeding at 3 months.
††Twenty-five states have exceeded *Healthy People 2020* goal for exclusive breastfeeding at 6 months.

were noted to have the higher rates. A 2015 report by Kachoria and Oza-Frank reported an upward trend in NICU breastfeeding in the state of Ohio. It went from 53.3% in 2006 to 63.8% in 2012, with the largest absolute increase seen in the extremely preterm infants (43.8% to 70.6%). The authors suggested the trend reflected growing awareness of the benefits of breast milk to preterm infants, the Baby Friendly Hospital Initiative (BFHI), and the development of *Ten Steps to Successful Breastfeeding* tailored for NICUs.

Although overall breastfeeding rates have improved, there is ongoing disparity in breastfeeding initiation and duration between geographic areas and various population groups, with some states reporting much higher rates (CDC, 2017). See Table 20–2 for a comparison of *Healthy People 2010* and *Healthy People 2020* goals, the average U.S. breastfeeding rates as well as the range disparities in rates between states.

Profile of Women Who Breast-feed

Knowing the characteristics of women who are less likely to initiate and continue breastfeeding can help the perinatal nurse target at-risk populations for more education and support. Researchers have reported consistently that breastfeeding is lowest among women who are African American, had less than or equal to a high school education, were single and younger than 20 years of age, lived in the Southern United States, and were enrolled in the Women, Infants, and Children (WIC) program (Anstey, Chen, Elam-Evans, & Perrine, 2017; CDC, 2017; Lee, Edmunds, Cong, & Sekhobo, 2017; Sriraman & Kellams, 2016; Ziol-Guest & Hernandez, 2010). In contrast, women who were more likely to initiate and continue breastfeeding tended to be Caucasian or Hispanic, at least 30 years of age, married, college educated, not enrolled in the WIC program, and living in the Mountain or Pacific regions of the United States (Anstey et al., 2017; CDC, 2017; Lee et al., 2017; Sriraman & Kellams, 2016).

Since the association between WIC and reduced breastfeeding rates was identified, federal regulations were passed that offered incentives to WIC women who exclusively breastfed. Examples of incentives included receiving larger maternal food packages over a longer time period (1 year). By comparison, mothers who used formula received free formula and smaller maternal food packages for a shorter time (6 months). These incentives, in addition to the breastfeeding education and support from WIC counselors, resulted in a small but significant increase in breastfeeding. In addition, they reported that the prevalence of exclusive breastfeeding at 3 and 6 months doubled (Langellier, Chaparro, Wang, Koleilat, & Whaley, 2014).

Barriers to Breastfeeding

Researchers have identified barriers to breastfeeding that are responsive to interventions (Display 20–1). The *Healthy People 2020* national plan addresses several of those interventions including increased worksite support, reduced hospital supplementation rates, and improved hospital practices (USDHHS, 2011).

It is well documented that hospital policies can adversely impact breastfeeding. In 1991, the WHO and the United Nations International Children's Emergency Fund (UNICEF) published the *Baby Friendly Hospital Initiative* (WHO & UNICEF Joint Statement, 1989). This document included the *Ten Steps to Successful Breastfeeding* that was designed to eliminate counterproductive hospital practices (Display 20–2). Researchers have reported that implementation of the *Ten Steps to Successful Breastfeeding* facilitates successful breastfeeding by all women (Abrahams & Labbock, 2009; Bartick, Stuebe, Shealy, Walker, & Grummer-Strawn, 2009; DiGirolamo, Grummer-Strawn, & Fein, 2008; Forster & McLachlan, 2007; Munn, Newman, Mueller, Phillips, & Taylor, 2016; Murray, Rickets, & Dellaport, 2007; Pérez-Escamilla,

DISPLAY 20-1

Barriers to Breastfeeding that are Responsive to Interventions

- Healthcare professionals
  - Apathy
  - Misinformation
  - Professional education that lacks information on breastfeeding
  - Outdated clinical practices
- Hospital practices
  - Failing to provide skilled support (i.e., lactation experts)
  - Routine separation of mother–infant dyad
  - Delay of first feeding
  - Routine formula or water supplementation
  - Use of pacifiers
  - Lack of staff training
  - Lack of a breastfeeding policy
  - Inappropriate interventions (i.e., supplemental feeding, pacifiers, overuse of nipple shields)
  - Disruptions of breastfeeding
  - Discharge packs that include formula samples and/or coupons for formula
  - Lack of discharge policy
  - Lack of follow-up after discharge
  - Lack of support
    - From partner, peers, and family
    - From workplace
    - From healthcare professionals
- Societal attitudes
  - Media portrayal of bottle feeding as normal
  - Commercial pressures on mothers to bottle feed or supplement with formula
  - Formula club sign-up sheets in obstetric offices and clinics
  - Prenatal formula starter kits
  - Coupons for free formula
  - Formula ads in parent magazines
  - Formula ads on Internet sites of interest to parents
  - Discounted formula available through the Internet

DISPLAY 20-2

Ten Steps to Successful Breastfeeding

1. Have a written breastfeeding policy that is routinely communicated to all healthcare staff (see Philipp, 2010).
2. Educate healthcare providers in skills necessary to implement this policy.
3. Inform all pregnant women about the benefits and management of breastfeeding.
4. Help mothers initiate breastfeeding within 1 hr of birth.
5. Show mothers how to breast-feed and how to maintain lactation even when they are separated from their newborns.
6. Give newborns no food or drink other than breast milk, unless medically indicated.
7. Practice "rooming-in"—allow mothers and newborns to remain together 24 hr each day.
8. Encourage unrestricted breastfeeding.
9. Give no artificial nipples or pacifiers to breastfeeding newborns.
10. Foster the establishment of breastfeeding support groups and refer mothers to them on discharge from the hospital or clinic.

World Health Organization & United Nations International Children's Emergency Fund Joint Statement. (1989). *Protecting and supporting breastfeeding: The special role of maternity services.* Geneva, Switzerland: World Health Organization.

Martinez, & Segura-Perez, 2016; Rosenberg, Stull, Adler, Kasehagen, & Crivelli-Kovach, 2008).

Some hospitals have sought official "Baby Friendly Hospital" certification. In 2006, there were 52 Baby Friendly hospitals and birthing centers in the United States. As of 2017, this has increased to 476 facilities, resulting in 22.75% of annual births occurring in Baby Friendly hospitals. Although not all hospitals have sought Baby Friendly certification, many have modeled their policies and protocols after the *Ten Steps to Successful Breastfeeding* with similar improvements in breastfeeding rates.

Nationwide, the percentage of hospitals who have implemented over five of the Baby Friendly steps increased from 28.7% in 2007 to 53.9% in 2013 (Perrine et al., 2015). Hospitals did best the steps related to encouraging breastfeeding on demand (87.3%), teaching breastfeeding techniques (92.2%), and educating parents on the benefits and managements of breastfeeding (91.1%). More work is needed on staff training (60.2%) and initiating breastfeeding within 1 hour of birth (64.8%). The steps needing the most work include having a written breastfeeding policy (26.3%), limiting non–breast milk feeds to healthy full term infants (26.4%), and 24-hour rooming-in (44.8%).

Perinatal nurses have a significant role in promoting breastfeeding. AWHONN (2015a) identifies the professional responsibilities of perinatal nurses who care for breastfeeding women and newborns in the prenatal and postpartum periods (Display 20–3). Nurses are responsible to be knowledgeable about breastfeeding and demonstrate the competence to provide evidence-based breastfeeding support through the preconception, prenatal, and postpartum periods. The United States Breastfeeding Committee (USBC) has developed core competencies that detail what health professionals should know (USBC, 2010). Additional recommendations were made for the education and curricular content for pediatric nurse practitioners (Boyd & Spatz, 2013).

DISPLAY 20-3

Breastfeeding and the Role of the Nurse in the Promotion of Breastfeeding

- Attain knowledge about the benefits of breastfeeding including anatomy and physiology of lactation, initiation of lactation, and management of common concerns and problems.
- Provide preconception and antenatal counseling on the benefits of breastfeeding.
- Provide breastfeeding education to all women during prenatal period including exploration of concerns, fears, and myths that may inhibit successful breastfeeding.
- Work in collaboration with lactation specialists and other healthcare providers to optimize the breastfeeding experience for the mother and infant.
- Integrate culturally appropriate and sensitive information into all breastfeeding education.
- Ensure that breastfeeding is initiated in the immediate postpartum period whenever possible.
- Promote nonseparation of mother and baby during the postpartum period.
- Provide information about breastfeeding resources in the community at the time of hospital or birthing center discharge.
- Use and conduct research related to breastfeeding.

From Association of Women's Health, Obstetric and Neonatal Nursing. (2015a). Breastfeeding (Position Statement). *Journal of Obstetric, Gynecologic, and Neonatal Nursing, 44*(1), 145–150. doi:10.1111/1552-6909.12530

It is important to educate women, so they can make an informed decision regarding infant feeding. We should provide culturally sensitive breastfeeding promotion and support. In the event a woman chooses to or is required to formula feed, nurses are equally responsible for providing education and resources on how to safely formula feed.

BREASTFEEDING PROMOTION

Several systematic reviews were published on interventions designed to increase breastfeeding initiation, exclusivity, and duration in term infants (Balogun et al., 2016; Chapman, Morel, Anderson, Damio, & Pérez-Escamilla, 2010; Chung, Raman, Trikalinos, Lau, & Ip, 2008; Hannula, Kaunonen, & Tarkka, 2008; Haroon, Das, Salam, Imdad, & Bhutta, 2013; Patnode et al., 2016; Rollins et al., 2016; Sinha et al., 2015). The most effective intervention to improve rates of any breastfeeding was following the Baby Friendly initiative (Munn et al., 2016; Sinha et al., 2015). The first step of the initiative is to have a written breastfeeding policy. The Academy of Breastfeeding Medicine

(ABM) has published a model breastfeeding policy that addresses steps of the Baby Friendly initiative (Phillipp, 2010). Consistently, studies have concluded that multiple interventions, using a variety of educational methods and sources of professional and peer support were more effective over any single intervention. In addition, programs that spanned the prenatal, intrapartal, and postpartal periods were more successful than interventions that focused on a single period. A systematic review on breastfeeding promotion in NICU found the following interventions to be effective in promoting preterm breastfeeding: skin-to-skin contact, peer support, breast milk pumping on both breasts simultaneously, staff training across all disciplines, and Baby Friendly accreditation (Munn et al., 2016; Renfrew et al., 2009; Sinha et al., 2015). The authors concluded it was unlikely any single intervention made a difference; rather it was the combination of multiple interventions.

PHYSIOLOGY OF MILK PRODUCTION

Perinatal nurses need to understand the science of milk production. This knowledge is essential to help women breast-feed successfully.

Mammogenesis

Mammogenesis refers to growth of the mammary glands. It occurs in two stages as the gland responds to the hormones of puberty and later during the first half of pregnancy. During pregnancy, estrogen and progesterone prepare the breasts for lactation. Numerous external changes occur. The breasts enlarge; the skin stretches and appears thinner making veins more visible. The nipples enlarge, and the Montgomery glands become prominent and start to secrete a substance that lubricates and protects the nipples and areola. The areola grows in diameter and darkens. Internal changes in the breast also occur and include growth and differentiation of the mammary ducts as well as development of the lobules and alveoli. Sometime in the second trimester, lactogenesis I begins (Buckley, 2015; Lauwers & Swisher, 2016; Lawrence & Lawrence, 2015).

Lactogenesis I

Lactogenesis I starts around midpregnancy and lasts until 1 to 2 days postpartum. During this time, further cell differentiation occurs and the lactocytes that are capable of secreting milk components proliferate. Prolactin levels rise during pregnancy and stimulate production of colostrum, which is present from midpregnancy, forward (Lauwers & Swisher, 2016; Lawrence & Lawrence, 2015).

Lactogenesis II

Lactogenesis II is defined as the onset of copious milk production that occurs 48 to 72 hours after the birth. Prolactin levels rise higher in the postpartum period when levels of progesterone drop after the placenta is expelled. The higher prolactin levels, along with infant suckling, stimulate the breast to synthesize and secrete milk (Lauwers & Swisher, 2016; Lawrence & Lawrence, 2015).

Delayed onset of lactogenesis II can occur. In one study, 44% of the 431 subjects experienced delayed onset of lactation (Nommsen-Rivers, Chantry, Peerson, Cohen, & Dewey, 2010; Truchet & Honvo-Houéto, 2017). It is important that perinatal nurses know the risk factors for delayed onset and monitor and intervene accordingly. Common risk factors for delayed onset of lactogenesis II are listed in Display 20–4.

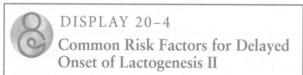

DISPLAY 20–4

Common Risk Factors for Delayed Onset of Lactogenesis II

Primiparity

Maternal age ≥30 years

Cesarean birth

Prolonged labor

Obesity

High levels of stress during the birth

Premature delivery (including late preterm)

Insulin-dependent diabetes mellitus

Birth weight >3,600 g

Retained placenta

Surgical procedures on breast

Insufficient mammary tissue

Breast hypoplasia

Polycystic ovarian syndrome

Sheehan's syndrome (postpartum pituitary gland necrosis)

Delay with first feeding

Hypothyroid

Hypertension

From Hurst, N. M. (2007). Recognizing and treating delayed or failed lactogenesis II. *Journal of Midwifery & Women's Health, 52*(6), 588–594; Parker, L. A., Sullivan, S., Krueger, C., & Mueller, M. (2015). Association of timing of initiation of breastmilk expression on milk volume and timing of lactogenesis stage II among mothers of very low-birth-weight infants. *Breastfeeding Medicine, 10*(2), 84–91. doi:10.1089/bfm.2014.0089; Preusting, I., Brumley, J., Odibo, L., Spatz, D. L., & Louis, J. M. (2017). Obesity as a predictor of delayed lactogenesis II. *Journal of Human Lactation, 33*(4), 684–691; and Scott, J. A., Binns, C. W., & Oddy, W. H. (2007). Predictors of delayed onset of lactation. Maternal & Child Nutrition, 3(3), 186–193. doi:10.1111/j.1740-8709 .2007.00096.x

Lactogenesis III

Lactogenesis III is the phase when a woman has established a mature milk supply. Production of milk changes from the hormonal endocrine control that exists in the first few days after birth to autocrine control when the milk supply is more established. With autocrine control, prolactin continues to be produced in response to infant suckling and emptying of the breasts. Oxytocin is also released in response to suckling. This occurs numerous times during a feeding. Oxytocin stimulates the cells around the alveoli to contract and eject milk down the ducts, making it accessible when the newborn suckles. The sensation that accompanies the release of oxytocin on breast tissue is referred to as the letdown reflex or the milk ejection reflex. Some mothers feel this as a heaviness or tingling sensation in the breast. Other mothers never feel the milk letdown but observe milk leaking from the other breast or hear the newborn swallowing milk (Walker, 2017; Wambach & Riordan, 2016).

Oxytocin also stimulates uterine contractions that control postpartum bleeding and promote involution. Mothers, especially multiparous women, feel these "after-birth pains" during feedings for several days after the birth. The discomfort can create a distraction that inhibits milk letdown. It is important to make the mother comfortable prior to and during the feeding. To minimize discomfort from afterpains, mothers should be encouraged to keep their bladder empty because a full bladder contributes to cramping. An analgesic prior to feeding should be considered. Ibuprofen is often effective, but in some cases, a mother might need something stronger. Nurses should reassure the mother that afterpains are normal and help limit blood loss; they are also self-limiting, lasting a few days (Walker, 2017; Wambach & Riordan, 2016).

Oxytocin-producing neurons throughout the brain are thought to be associated with social behavior and attachment (Feldman & Bakermans-Kranenburg, 2017). In addition to being released in the maternal brain tissue, oxytocin is released into the newborn brain by means of milk transfer and is thought to modulate attachment behaviors between mother and newborn. Oxytocin also is partially responsible for the calmness women exhibit while breastfeeding and has been linked to a decreased response to stressors and pain in the breastfeeding woman (Buckley, 2015; Goer, Davis, & Hemphill, 2002).

Milk production is a supply and demand system; as milk is removed from the breast, prolactin triggers the breast to produce more milk. For most women, milk production closely matches the needs of the newborn. The more efficiently the newborn nurses, the faster the rate of milk synthesis (Lawrence & Lawrence, 2015).

Leaving milk in the breasts for long periods can contribute to slower and lower amounts of milk production. A whey protein, feedback inhibitor of lactation (FIL), inhibits milk secretion as alveoli become distended and milk is not removed. The longer the period of time milk is left in the breast, the greater the concentrations of FIL. This mechanism works independently, and each breast will synthesize milk at different rates depending on the frequency and degree of drainage (Lawrence & Lawrence, 2015).

BIOSPECIFICITY OF HUMAN MILK

Human milk is a species-specific fluid. The composition is not static or uniform. Breast milk is designed to meet the needs of newborns for brain development and growth, protect the immature gut, be a substitute for an immature immune system, and assist in developing attachment behavior. The composition of human milk changes over time. Colostrum (1 to 5 days postpartum) evolves to transitional milk (6 to 13 days postpartum) and then into mature milk (14 days and beyond). During any given feeding, foremilk changes to hindmilk the longer the infant breastfeeds. Milk composition also fluctuates over the course of the entire lactation. Milk of preterm mothers differs from that of term mothers to meet the nutritional needs based on gestational age. For example, during the first 3 to 5 days after birth, term milk contains 1.85 g/dL of protein, whereas preterm milk contains 3.00 g/dL (Walker, 2017).

Colostrum is present in the breast from about 12 to 16 weeks of pregnancy. This first milk is thick and has a yellowish color. Average energy value is about 18 kcal/oz, compared with mature milk, which contains 21 kcal/oz (AAP, 2014). The volume of colostrum is low (measured in teaspoons), which assures the infant will want to nurse frequently. This frequent nursing is what stimulates the transition to milk. Compared with mature milk, colostrum is higher in protein, sodium, chloride, potassium, and fat-soluble vitamins. It is rich in antioxidants, antibodies, interferon, fibronectin, and immunoglobulins, especially secretory immunoglobulin A (IgA). Secretory IgA is antigen specific. When mothers come in contact with microbes, antibodies are synthesized in her milk, targeting pathogens in the newborn's immediate environment. These antibodies are passed to the newborn. Separating the mother and newborn interferes with this defense mechanism. Colostrum begins the establishment of normal bacterial flora in the newborn's gastrointestinal tract and exerts a laxative effect that begins elimination of meconium, decreasing the potential reabsorption of bilirubin (Walker, 2017; Wambach & Riordan, 2016).

Mature milk composition changes during the feeding. Foremilk is produced initially; it is more watery and has lower fat content. Later in the feeding on a given breast, cell membranes release fat globules and protein, which forms hindmilk (Lawrence & Lawrence, 2015). Hindmilk is high in calories and fat and is critical to growth and brain development. To make sure infants get adequate hindmilk, the baby should be allowed to finish on one side before offering the other breast. Babies are done feeding on a breast when the baby lets go of the nipple, falls asleep, or ceases to actively suck and swallow (Lawrence & Lawrence, 2015).

NUTRITIONAL COMPONENTS

Water

Human milk is composed of 87.5% water, in which all other components are dissolved, dispersed, or in suspension (Walker, 2017; Wambach & Riordan, 2016). Infants receiving adequate amounts of breast milk do not need additional water, even in hot climates (AAP, 2012; WHO, 2014).

Fat (Lipids)

Fat content of human milk ranges from 3.5% to 4.5% and contributes 50% of the calories (Walker, 2017). It varies during a feeding; hindmilk has almost double the fat content when compared to levels in foremilk (O. Ballard & Morrow, 2013; Saarela, Kokkonen, & Koivisto, 2005). Fat content increases over the first days of lactation and shows diurnal rhythms. Total fat content is reduced in mothers who smoke (Napierala, Macela, Merritt, & Florek, 2016) and increases when women breastfeed more frequently. The long-chain polyunsaturated fatty acids docosahexaenoic acid and arachidonic acid contained in breast milk are found in the brain, retina, and central nervous system of newborns and are necessary for the growth of these structures during the first year of age (Wambach & Riordan, 2016). The absence of these fatty acids in formula may contribute to differences in cognitive development that has been reported in the literature (Ip et al., 2007; Walker, 2017).

Protein

Protein concentration is high in colostrum and settles to 0.8% to 1.0% in mature milk. The whey-to-casein ratio in human milk changes from 90:10 in the early milk, to 60:40 in mature milk, and 50:50 in late lactation (AAP, 2014; Walker, 2017). The whey protein that predominates in human milk forms soft curds that are easily digested and supply the infant with most of the nutrients in human milk. One of the components of the whey protein, lactoferrin, is important in the immunologic effects of human milk. The bacteriostatic effect of lactoferrin makes iron unavailable to pathogens that require the mineral to proliferate (Wambach & Riordan, 2016).

Carbohydrate

The principal carbohydrate in human milk is lactose. Lactose supports colonization of the gut with microflora that increases the acidity of the intestine. The increased acidity decreases growth of pathogens and ensures a supply of galactose and glucose, which are necessary for brain development. Calcium absorption is also enhanced in the acidic environment (Walker, 2017; Wambach & Riordan, 2016).

Vitamins and Minerals

Breast milk contains the vitamins and minerals needed by most term infants for about the first 6 months of age. However, in recent years, lifestyle changes and the use of sunscreen has contributed to a rise in vitamin D insufficiency and rickets. AAP (2012) now recommends that all breastfed infants receive 400 IU of vitamin D daily beginning at hospital discharge. It is important to note that human milk does have an estimated 26 IU/mL of vitamin D. Although adequate for some infants, this quantity is inadequate in cases where infants lack sun exposure (due to climate or use of sunscreen) or when the mother is deficient in vitamin D during pregnancy (AAP, 2012).

Other supplementation may be necessary based on gestational age and infant's iron stores. After 6 months of exclusive breastfeeding iron supplementation is recommended (AAP, 2012). Infants living in communities where the fluoride concentration in the water is <0.3 ppm should receive supplemental fluoride from age 6 months to 3 years.

Mothers consuming a vegan diet with no dairy products may need supplemental vitamin B_{12} or an acceptable source in their diet to have it present in breast milk. AAP published a policy statement (Rogan et al., 2014) recommending iodine supplementation for breastfeeding women. In recent decades, the United States has seen a rise in iodine deficiency. This is mainly due to our increased consumption of processed foods, which use non-iodized salt. Iodine is needed to produce thyroid hormone, which is essential for brain development in children (Rogan et al., 2014).

PRETERM MILK AND LACTATION

Differences between Preterm and Term Milk

Like milk produced by mothers of term infants, milk produced by mothers of preterm infants changes to meet the infant's growth needs. Composition differs from term milk with higher levels of immune factors, energy, lipids, protein, nitrogen, and fatty acids (Walker, 2017; Wambach & Riordan, 2016). AAP (2012) recommends premature infants receive both a multivitamin and oral iron supplement.

Benefits of Human Milk for Preterm Infants

The preterm infant benefits from receiving human milk with lower rates of sepsis, necrotizing enterocolitis, and hospital readmissions. In addition, preterm infants who receive breast milk have improved feeding tolerance, enhanced neurodevelopment, and lower rates of severe retinopathy of prematurity. Long-term benefits of feeding human milk to premature infants are still being discovered. There is evidence that it is associated with increased scores on cognitive and developmental tests, closer family attachment, lower rates of metabolic syndrome, lower blood pressures in adolescent, low-density lipoprotein, and improved leptin and insulin metabolism. Mothers who breast-feed or provide breast milk for their preterm infants demonstrated increased self-esteem and maternal role attainment. Although these benefits are similar for term infants, they have far greater impact on the vulnerable preterm infant (AAP, 2012; Merewood, Brooks, Bauchner, MacAuley, & Mehta, 2006). The benefits of human milk are so compelling that AAP recommends all preterm infants receive human milk (AAP, 2012). When the mothers' own milk is insufficient or unavailable, AAP (2017) recommends the use of carefully regulated donor human milk with high-risk infants when the mothers own milk is insufficient or unavailable.

Preterm Breastfeeding Barriers

Mothers of preterm infants face the same barriers to breastfeeding as do mothers of term infants. They also have unique barriers, such as the need to use hand expression or a breast pump for a prolonged period and possible limited contact with their infant. Reduced mother–infant contact may be due to the infant's condition or due to the mother being discharged from the hospital. In some large regional centers, mothers may live a distance from the facility. Stress is also known to inhibit milk production (Walker, 2017). The NICU environment contributes to maternal stress with all its machines, monitoring devices, and alarms (AAFP, 2015). Other sources of stress for NICU mothers often include fear for their infant, separation from their infant, or concerns about the cost of intensive care.

Promoting Preterm Breastfeeding

Nurses play a major role in promoting breastfeeding for preterm infants. Certain practices have proven helpful: early discussion of breastfeeding; written materials; early promotion of hand expression along with simultaneous pumping of both breasts with a

DISPLAY 20–5

Resources and Guidelines for Preterm Breastfeeding

Organization	Resources
Academy of Breastfeeding Medicine (ABM)	"ABM Clinical Protocol #10: Breastfeeding the Late Preterm Infant (34 0/7 to 36 6/7 Weeks Gestation) and Early Term Infants (37-3 6/7 Weeks of Gestation), 2nd Revision 2016" (Boies & Vaucher, 2016)
	"ABM Clinical Protocol #16: Breastfeeding the Hypotonic Infant, Revision 2016" (Thomas & Marinelli, 2016)
	"ABM Clinical Protocol #22: Guidelines for Management of Jaundice in Breastfeeding Infant 35 Weeks or More Gestation—Revised 2017" (Flaherman & Maisels, 2017)
AWHONN	*Breastfeeding Support: Preconception Care through the First Year Guideline* (3rd ed.) (AWHONN, 2015b)
	Assessment & Care of the Late Preterm Infant Guideline (2nd ed.) (AWHONN, 2017)
California Perinatal Quality Care Collaborative (2008)	*Care and Management of the Late Preterm Infant Toolkit* (Zlotnik, 2013)
Centers for Disease Control and Prevention	Proper storage and preparation of breast milk. (2010).
Cochrane Review	"Avoidance of Bottles during the Establishment of Breast Feeds in Preterm Infants" (Collins, Gillis, McPhee, Suganuma, & Makrides, 2016)
	"Cup Feeding Versus Other Forms of Supplemental Enteral Feeding for Newborn Infants Unable to Fully Breastfeed" (Flint, New, & Davies, 2016)
March of Dimes	Prematurity Awareness Campaign
Oklahoma Infant Alliance	*Caring for the Late Preterm Infant: A Clinical Practice Guideline* (2010)
University of California San Diego Health	Supporting Premature Infant Nutrition (SPIN). Provides resources for parents and NICU staff
World Health Organization	*Feeding of Low-Birth-Weight Infants in Low- and Middle-Income Countries* (2011b)

hospital grade electric pump; breast massage; encouraging skin-to-skin contact (kangaroo care) to facilitate attachment, milk production, and subsequent establishment of breastfeeding; and use of an alternate feeding method, such as cup feeding, instead of an artificial nipple (AAFP, 2015). Mothers also need to learn about storage methods for expressed milk. Display 20–5 provides a list of guidelines and resources for preterm breastfeeding.

BREASTFEEDING PROCESS

Preparation for Breastfeeding

Physical Preparation

There is no research supporting physical preparation of the breasts during pregnancy. Prenatal nipple rolling, application of creams, and expression of colostrum have not been shown to decrease pain or nipple trauma during the postpartum period. Use of methods to improve nipple erectility, such as Hoffman exercises and breast shells, may decrease a woman's desire and motivation to breast-feed by conveying the message that her nipples are inferior and need correcting (Johnson & Strube, 2011; Wambach & Riordan, 2016).

Prenatal Education

Women should be encouraged to attend prenatal breastfeeding classes. The short postpartum hospital stay puts pressure on the nurse, the mother, and the newborn to demonstrate effective breastfeeding before some mother–baby couples are ready. The fast learning pace in the inpatient setting and the mother's cognitive sluggishness for verbal instructions during the first 24 hours postpartum suggest that there would be a benefit in providing breastfeeding information before birth. Prenatal breastfeeding education programs have been shown to increase the knowledge levels of pregnant women and their partners, increase the support women perceive from their partners around the decision to breast-feed, and increase breastfeeding initiation and duration rates (Lauwers & Swisher, 2016; Patnode et al., 2016; Sikorski, Renfrew, Rindoria, & Wade, 2002; Wambach & Riordan, 2016). The ABM (Rosen-Carole & Hartman, 2015) has a clinical protocol for breastfeeding promotion in the prenatal setting. It addresses the need for breastfeeding-friendly healthcare offices and communities; sensitivity to the background, ethnicity, and culture of prenatal women and their families; and integration of breastfeeding promotion, education, and support throughout the prenatal care period.

Positioning for Breastfeeding

A variety of positions are used for breastfeeding. It is important that the mother assume a relaxed, comfortable position with her back and arms well supported. If she is seated in a chair, placing a footstool beneath her feet decreases strain on her back and may discourage her from leaning forward over the baby. Some mothers benefit from a pillow on the lap or use of a commercially available nursing pillow. These can be especially helpful when nursing twins. If the mother is lying on her side, a pillow behind her back will help with support (Walker, 2017; Wambach & Riordan, 2016).

The newborn and mother should face each other while breastfeeding. The mother should not lean forward over the newborn but instead concentrate on bringing the baby toward her. The newborn should be loosely wrapped or not wrapped at all so the nurse and mother can clearly see the infant's position on the breast. There is no need to be concerned about keeping the newborn warm because mother and baby generate body heat during breastfeeding. Skin-to-skin contact is useful for increasing a low temperature in a newborn during the transitional period. As the feeding progresses, if necessary, a light blanket may be placed over both for privacy (Walker, 2017; Wambach & Riordan, 2016).

Cradle Hold

With the mother comfortably seated, the newborn is held in a side-lying position with its entire body completely facing the mother. Held on a slight incline, the newborn's lower arm is tucked around the outside of the breast. The newborn's body is in complete contact with the mother; the newborn's legs are wrapped around her waist. If the newborn is wrapped in a

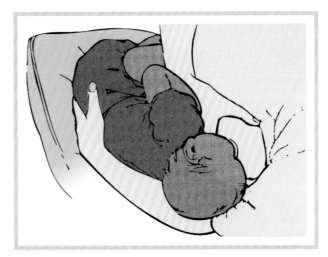

FIGURE 20–1. Cradle hold.

blanket, it should be loosened to permit the newborn to move its arms and legs. Avoid covering the infant's hands with the undershirt cuffs. The newborn's head should rest on the mother's forearm, which along with her wrist and hands supports the baby's back and bottom (Fig. 20–1).

Cross-Cradle Hold

The cradle position can be modified by having the woman alter the position of her arms, using what is called the cross-cradle hold. This is a good position to use for preterm infants and infants with fractured clavicles. The newborn is placed in the same position as the cradle hold but held with the opposite arm such that the head is in the mother's hand and her forearm is supporting the back. This gives the mother much more control over positioning and, along with the clutch hold, may be easier to learn (Fig. 20–2).

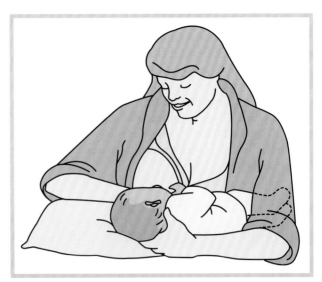

FIGURE 20–2. Cross-cradle hold.

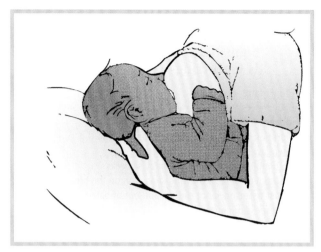

FIGURE 20–3. Clutch hold.

Clutch Hold

The clutch position (i.e., football hold) is useful for feeding preterm infants or twins and for mothers who have had a cesarean birth. The newborn is positioned to the mother's side. Placing a pillow under the newborn raises the infant slightly and decreases the weight the mother needs to lift. The newborn's head is in her hand, and its feet are positioned toward her back. Care should be taken to ensure that the full weight of the breast does not rest on the newborn's chest (Fig. 20–3).

Side Lying

The side-lying position works well after a cesarean birth or for a woman with a painful perineum. In this position, the newborn and mother lay on their sides facing each other. A small rolled blanket can be placed behind the newborn's back, or the mother can support the infant with her free arm (Fig. 20–4).

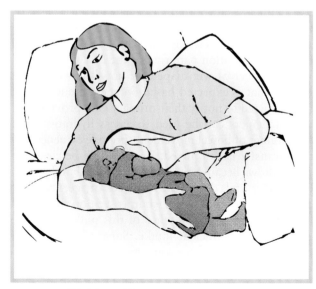

FIGURE 20–4. Side-lying position.

Laid Back Breastfeeding

Laid-back breastfeeding is based on the concept of biologic nurturing (BN). Central to BN is the assumption that breastfeeding initiation is intrinsic for both mother and baby and not something they need to learn. BN stresses the fact that no one posture is right for everyone. Women are capable of finding a position of comfort, and positions can change and evolve over time (Colson, 2012; Colson, Meek, & Hawdon, 2008; Schafer & Genna, 2015).

Many women choose a semireclined position. Once the mother is comfortable, the baby is placed prone on the mother's front with the baby's face near the breast. Skin-to-skin should be optional based on the mother's preference. Although the traditional positions (see above) may work for some women, the BN approach allows women more options and is much less prescriptive.

Supporting the Breast

Historically, mothers have been encouraged to support their breasts using a variety of techniques (scissor hold, C-hold, etc.). The current approach is to let the mother decide what works best for her. In some cases, and in some positions, there is no need to hold the breast. In the event the breast is being held, a variety of techniques could be used as long as the mother's fingers do not compress the ducts or impede the infant from a correct latch (Colson et al., 2008).

Figure 20–1 shows the commonly used C-hold. With this technique, the mother supports her breast with her thumb on top and fingers below and against the chest wall. The thumb and fingers are away from the areola. This hold makes it easy for the mother to direct her nipple toward the center of the mouth during latch-on. Mothers are encouraged to use whichever hand is more comfortable. Pressure should not be applied to the breast with the thumb. The newborn's pug-shaped nose allows breathing through the grooves along the sides of the nares during breastfeeding, even when the nose is touching the breast. In all breastfeeding positions, pulling the newborn's buttocks closer to the mother's body or gently lifting the breast causes the newborn's head to drop back slightly, providing room for breathing (Walker, 2017; Wambach & Riordan, 2016).

Latch-On

Proper attachment of the newborn at the breast is necessary for pain-free and effective milk transfer. Once positioned comfortably, the mother moves the newborn's lips to the nipple; when the newborn's mouth is wide open, she draws the newborn toward her. The lower lip and chin contact the breast first.

DISPLAY 20–6
Observations Indicating Correct Latch-On

- Lips are rolled outward (flared).
- Clicking or smacking sounds are absent.
- Dimpled cheeks are absent.
- Muscles above and in front of the ear move.
- Both cheeks are equally close to the breast.
- Chin and nose are touching the breast.
- All of the nipple and part of the areola is covered by the newborn's mouth.
- More of the areola is visible above the upper lip than below it.
- Angle at the corner of the mouth is wide.
- When the lower lip is gently pulled away from the breast, the tongue is visible over the lower gum line.

From Lauwers, J., & Swisher, A. (2016). *Counseling the nursing mother: A lactation consultant's guide* (6th ed.). Burlington, MA: Jones & Bartlett; Lawrence, R. A., & Lawrence, R. M. (2015). *Breastfeeding: A guide for the medical profession* (8th ed.). Philadelphia, PA: Elsevier; and Wambach, K., & Riordan, J. M. (2016). *Breastfeeding and human lactation* (enhanced 5th ed.). Burlington, MA: Jones & Bartlett Learning.

DISPLAY 20–7
Signs that Milk Transfer Is Occurring

- Proper latch-on
- Baby moves from short rapid sucks to slow deep sucks early in feed
- Vibration on the occipital region of the head
- Deep jaw excursion
- No dimpling or puckering of baby's cheeks
- Mother verbalizes a drawing sensation on the breast
- Breast tissue does not slide in and out of baby's mouth when baby sucks or pauses
- No smacking or clicking sounds with sucking which indicate that the tongue has lost contact with the nipple and areola
- Mother notices letdown
- Audible swallows (usually heard after onset of copious milk production)
- Mother's breast softens (noted after stage II lactogenesis)
- Baby spontaneously unlatches and is satiated
- Mother's nipple does not appear blanched or compressed
- Adequate newborn weight gain of 4 to 6 oz/week
- Baby stooling and voiding appropriate for age
- Baby content between most feedings

From Lauwers, J., & Swisher, A. (2016). *Counseling the nursing mother: A lactation consultant's guide* (6th ed.). Burlington, MA: Jones & Bartlett; Lawrence, R. A., & Lawrence, R. M. (2015). *Breastfeeding: A guide for the medical profession* (8th ed.). Philadelphia, PA: Elsevier; and Wambach, K., & Riordan, J. M. (2016). *Breastfeeding and human lactation* (enhanced 5th ed.). Burlington, MA: Jones & Bartlett Learning.

The newborn should grasp the nipple and areola, pulling it as a unit forward and deep into his or her mouth. The tongue is cupped and thrust forward over the lower gum. When the jaw lowers and creates negative pressure, milk moves into the trough of the tongue and is channeled to the back of the mouth, where the swallow reflex is triggered. Display 20–6 lists observations made when the newborn is latched on to the breast correctly.

For women with very large breasts, a rolled receiving blanket or small towel can be placed under the breast, so the baby does not drag down on the nipple. Care should be taken to avoid pushing the newborn's head into the breast. Pressure on the occipital region of the head causes extension of the neck. Tilting, squeezing, or distorting the nipple or areola should also be avoided because doing so can cause pain and skin damage. If the mother feels a pinching or biting sensation while nursing, she should be instructed to pull down gently on the newborn's chin. This causes his mouth to open wider so that more of the areola is drawn into his mouth. If this does not work, have the mother insert her little finger into the side of the newborn's mouth to release the suction (Walker, 2017; Wambach & Riordan, 2016). She should begin again to achieve a better latch-on.

Milk Transfer

When the newborn suckles effectively, the breast releases milk and milk transfer occurs. Even though a newborn may suck at the breast for 15 minutes with its jaw moving up and down, it does not mean that there has been a transfer of milk. Display 20–7 lists the signs that are observed when milk transfer occurs.

Signs of Adequate Intake

Evaluating the newborn for adequate intake is based on elimination patterns, behavioral observations, moist mucous membranes, and weight gain. Table 20–3 outlines elimination patterns for the first week of age. If the number of wet diapers or bowel movements is below what is expected based on age, parents should be instructed to notify their primary care provider.

Wet diapers can be used to assess hydration, and the number of bowel movements provide evidence that milk transfer has occurred. Urine should be clear and pale yellow. Because urine contains an abundance of uric acid crystals during the first week of age, occasionally, a pink or rust-colored stain is seen on the diaper. After the first week, presence of this pink stain is an indicator of insufficient intake. Super absorbent diapers make it difficult for some parents to tell when the diaper is wet. Parents can place a soft, dry paper towel, tissue, or square of toilet paper inside the diaper with each change to more easily tell when the diaper is wet.

TABLE 20–3. Breastfeeding Infant Elimination Patterns during the First Week

Infant's age (days)	Number of wet diapers	Number of bowel movements	Baby stool (color and texture)
1	1 to 2	1	Meconium:
2	2 to 3	2	greenish-black tarry
3	3 to 4	3 to 4	Transitional: lighter,
4	4 to 5	3 to 4	less sticky, more liquid
5	4 to 5	3 or more	Breast milk stool:
6	6 to 8	3 or more	green-yellow to
7	8 or more	3 or more	bright yellow, soft and loose, small curds

Other signs that the newborn is sufficiently hydrated include moist mucous membranes and skin that does not remain tented when lightly pinched. Stools change from meconium to transitional stools to yellow, seedy liquid. Yellow stool should be present by the end of the first week. Some infants stool as frequently as every feeding for the first 4 to 6 weeks. Other indications of adequate intake are earlier transition to yellow bowel movements, earlier return to birth weight, and increased weight at 14 days of age (Walker, 2017; Wambach & Riordan, 2016).

Observation of newborn behaviors also provide clues regarding adequacy of intake. The newborn should demonstrate a range of behaviors during the day, including being alert, acting hungry, being fussy, and acting satisfied after feeding (Walker, 2017; Wambach & Riordan, 2016).

Newborns should regain their birth weight by 2 weeks of age and continue to gain 4 to 7 oz weekly or at least 1 lb per month (Lawrence & Lawrence, 2015). According to Benitz (2015), newborns discharged before 48 hours should be seen by their healthcare practitioner within 48 hours, and according to AAP (2012) all breastfed newborns should be assessed by a healthcare provider 3 to 5 days after birth (or sooner if indicated) to assure there is adequate intake. An infant who has lost more than 7% of their birth weight may have breastfeeding problems that need addressing (Walker, 2017; Wambach & Riordan, 2016).

Researchers are currently looking at iatrogenic neonatal weight loss that is unrelated to breastfeeding problems. In 2011, researchers reported that excessive neonatal weight loss was associated with mothers who received large quantities of intravenous (IV) fluids in labor (Chantry, Nommensen-Rivers, Peerson, Cohen, & Dewey, 2011). They hypothesized that the IV fluids resulted in fetal volume expansion, which increased birth weight. They reported that newborns of mothers who had large amounts of IV fluids had more voids when compared to newborns of mothers who did receive large amounts of IV fluids. Although these are preliminary findings, the authors proposed that increased number of voids resulted in greater weight loss (Chantry et al., 2011). Other researchers have suggested that weight loss >7% is a normal phenomenon among breastfeeding newborns. DiTomasso and Paiva (2018) studied 151 mother–infant breastfeeding pairs and reported 56% of the newborns lost >7% of their birth weight. Their findings were similar to Thulier (2017) who reported 58% of 286 newborns lost >7% of their birth weight. They also reported many of the infants who had weight loss >7% had been supplemented with formula. More research is needed to establish an accurate range of expected neonatal weight loss.

BREASTFEEDING MANAGEMENT

Getting Started

Early and frequent breastfeeding along with skin-to-skin contact promotes optimal breastfeeding (Forster et al., 2018; Merten, Dratva, & Ackermann-Liebrich, 2005; Wambach & Riordan, 2016). Breastfeeding should be initiated within an hour of birth. This is an ideal time because the infant demonstrates sucking movements that peak 45 minutes after birth and decline over the next 2 hours. Early feedings are associated with mothers who breast-feed for a longer duration (Chaves, Lamounier, & César, 2007; Ekström, Widström, & Nissen, 2003; Hake-Brooks & Anderson, 2008; Moore, Bergman, Anderson, & Medley, 2016). Skin-to-skin contact following the birth (vaginal and cesarean) has been correlated with exclusive breastfeeding (Aghdas, Talat, & Sepideh, 2014; Brown, Kaiser, & Nailon, 2014; Guala et al., 2017; Hughes, Rodriguez-Carter, Hill, Miller, & Gomez, 2015; Linares et al., 2017). A dose-response relationship was found with the odds of exclusive breastfeeding increasing the longer the initial skin-to-skin contact lasted. Women who experienced skin-to-skin contact for 15 minutes were 1.3 times more likely to exclusively breast-feed, whereas those who had skin-to-skin contact for an hour or longer were 3.15 times more likely to exclusively breast-feed (Bramson et al., 2010).

It is recommended that the healthy newborn be placed skin-to-skin on the mother's chest and given the opportunity to seek and find the nipple. Nonsedated babies follow a predictable pattern of prefeeding behavior when held on the mother's chest immediately after birth. This enhances bonding and elicits newborn feeding behavior such as bringing hands to mouth, nuzzling, and licking the breast (Colson, 2012; Colson et al., 2008; Righard, 2008). Successful latch-on and suckling at this time greatly reduces sucking disorganization or dysfunction later and contributes to increased breastfeeding duration (Chaves et al., 2007; Wiklund, Norman, Uvnäs-Moberg, Ransjö-Arvidson, & Andolf, 2009). It also lowers the risk of hypothermia (Galligan, 2006), hyperbilirubinemia and hypoglycemia, all of which can adversely influence breastfeeding initiation and duration (McCall, Alderdice, Halliday, Jenkins, & Vohra, 2010; Walker, 2017; Walters, Boggs, Ludington-Hoe, Price, & Morrison, 2007). A recent study by Vittner et al. (2018) reported an increase in oxytocin levels in parents and their preterm infants when they engaged in skin-to-skin contact. They also noted a significant decrease in cortisol levels in the infants during skin-to-skin contact. They concluded that skin-to-skin contact might have the added advantage of reducing parent and infant stress in the NICU.

There is some evidence that drug exposure during labor may have an adverse effect on newborn breastfeeding, including epidurals, analgesics, and exogenous oxytocin. However, the results are conflicting due to many study limitations (D. L. Bai, Wu, & Tarrant, 2013; Brimdyr et al., 2015; Erickson & Emeis, 2017; French, Cong, & Chung, 2016; Jordan, Emery, Bradshaw, Watkins, & Friswell, 2005; Lind, Perrine, & Li, 2014; Mauri et al., 2015; Ransjö-Arvidson et al., 2001; Zuppa et al., 2014). A systematic review by French et al. (2016) of 23 articles found 12 studies reported a negative association between breastfeeding and labor epidural; 10 studies showed no effect, and 1 showed a positive association. There are many differences in the studies that made comparison difficult. Ultimately, practitioners should recognize labor medications have potential risk factors for breastfeeding. It has been suggested that side effects of labor medications could be minimized by allowing the mother–infant dyad unlimited skin-to-skin, encouraging early initiation of breastfeeding, and providing good breastfeeding support. This can be facilitated by keeping the mother and newborn together and teaching the mother to recognize hunger cues (Brimdyr et al., 2015; Lauwers & Swisher, 2016).

Sustained Maternal–Newborn Contact

Twenty-four-hour rooming-in supports breastfeeding and is an integral component of family-centered maternity care. However, the practice of rooming-in needs to be flexible, and its implementation needs to be respectful of the needs and desires of new mothers. Rooming-in enables a woman to recognize and respond to her newborn's needs and begin to develop confidence in her mothering role. If the mother and newborn are together when the newborn demonstrates

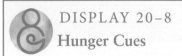

DISPLAY 20–8
Hunger Cues

- Rapid eye movements under the eyelids
- Sucking movements of the mouth and tongue
- Hand-to-mouth movements
- Body movements
- Small sounds (soft cooing or sighing sounds)
- Rooting
- Mouth opening in response to tactile stimulation
- Smacking of lips
- Wide-open eyes, quiet alert state
- Restlessness

Note: Crying is a late feeding cue and may interfere with effective breastfeeding.
From Lauwers, J., & Swisher, A. (2016). *Counseling the nursing mother: A lactation consultant's guide* (6th ed.). Burlington, MA: Jones & Bartlett; Lawrence, R. A., & Lawrence, R. M. (2015). *Breastfeeding: A guide for the medical profession* (8th ed.). Philadelphia, PA: Elsevier; and Wambach, K., & Riordan, J. M. (2016). *Breastfeeding and human lactation* (enhanced 5th ed.). Burlington, MA: Jones & Bartlett Learning.

early hunger cues (Display 20–8), she can begin feeding. If the newborn is in a nursery, feeding is delayed until a healthcare professional witness the hunger cues and transports the newborn to the mother's room. During this delay, the newborn may become increasingly agitated, self-console, and return to sleep or become exhausted from crying and return to sleep. By the time the newborn reaches his mother, the optimal feeding opportunity is missed.

Hunger cues can be observed for up to 30 minutes before the newborn begins a sustained cry for food. Feeding is most successful if initiated while the newborn is in a quiet, alert state. Crying is a late hunger cue and may interfere with effective breastfeeding. It is often necessary to console the newborn before he or she will settle and feed well. Feeding before the newborn begins a sustained cry reduces stress and some of the accompanying undesirable physiologic side effects such as glycogen depletion, increased intracranial pressure, resumption of fetal circulation within the heart, disorganized sucking, and poor feeding (Walker, 2017; Wambach & Riordan, 2016).

Extended contact with the newborn may facilitate a feeding pattern that includes clustered feedings (i.e., 5 to 10 feedings over 2 to 3 hours, followed by 4 to 5 hours of deep sleep). Parents need to understand that cluster feedings are normal and that they often occur in the evenings. Many mothers interpret the increased feeding demands as an inadequate supply of breast milk and it undermines their confidence. Cluster feedings often occur in the evening (6 to 10 pm), which results in the deep sleep occurring when parents also want to sleep. Despite the many benefits of rooming-in, the CDC reported less than 45% of hospitals kept mothers and babies together throughout the entire hospital stay (CDC, 2015).

Feeding Frequency and Duration

Historically, fixed breastfeeding schedules were thought to be more scientific, safer because the stomach had to be emptied before allowing a refill, a way to prevent sore nipples, less disruptive for the family if the newborn was on a schedule, and more efficient on a maternity unit. Current understanding of this practice is that restricting breastfeeding in the early days after birth can increase the incidence of sore nipples, engorgement, and perceived need to supplement. In addition, fixed schedules were associated with women discontinuing breastfeeding by 6 weeks postpartum (Renfrew, Lang, Martin, & Woolridge, 2000). Breastfeeding patterns, however, vary widely between mother–baby pairs, over each 24-hour period, and during the lactation. When no artificial time limits are placed on breastfeeding, the number of feedings during each 24 hours range from 8 to 12. The number of feedings depends on age, physiologic capacity of the stomach, ability of the newborn, and storage capacity of the breasts (Walker, 2017; Wambach & Riordan, 2016).

Frequency and duration of feedings is different for breastfed and formula-fed newborns. Formula-fed infants have a mean gastric half-emptying time of 65 minutes, with a range of 27 to 98 minutes; breastfed infants have a mean gastric half-emptying time of 47 minutes, with a range of 16 to 86 minutes (Van Den Driessche et al., 1999). The shorter emptying time means breastfed newborns can be hungry 30 to 60 minutes after a feeding, and parents need to know this is normal and expected. They also need to know that newborns who nurse frequently are learning to feed and that the amount of colostrum available for initial feedings is ideal to meet the current physiologic stomach capacity of the newborn. In a typical feeding, the newborn should feed on the first breast until satiated. The feeding ends when the newborn comes off the breast on its own after swallowing for most of the feeding. If the mother is uncertain whether the newborn is satisfied, she can use hand/manual expression (Display 20–9) and/or alternate massage (Display 20–10). Alternate massage is recommended when infant's swallowing is slowing down. This technique increases the volume and fat content of the milk. There are no time limits on the duration of feedings. In the first days after birth, some newborns nurse from only one breast at a feeding. The other side is offered at the next feeding, usually within 1 or 2 hours. Feeding frequently encourages an abundant milk supply, minimizes engorgement and sore nipples, enhances weight gain, reduces jaundice and hypoglycemia, and increases breastfeeding duration. Display 20–11 lists behavioral signs that indicate

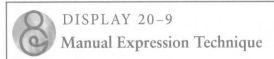

DISPLAY 20–9
Manual Expression Technique

Preparation

Wash hands.

Have a clean container to collect expressed milk (or a towel if not saving the milk).

Promote flow of milk, for example.

Gently massage breasts prior to and throughout manual expression.

Take warm shower or bath.

Apply warm moist cloth before expressing milk or take a shower.

Try relaxation techniques, picture of baby, etc.

Find comfortable position, nipple aimed at collection container.

Technique*

Position hands on breast:

1. Place thumb behind areola, above nipple, usually 2 to 3 cm behind areola.[†]
2. Place index finger behind areola, usually 2 to 3 cm behind areola.[†]
3. Some women choose a two-handed technique, especially if hands are small relative to breast size.

Expression

1. Press thumb and index finger directly back toward chest wall.
2. Then gently compress ducts with thumb and finger together.
3. Maintain compression while moving thumb and finger back toward the nipple in a milking action (this is a rolling motion, caution the mother not to slide the thumb or fingers along the skin—this will quickly make her sore).
4. Repeat steps 1 through 3 while rotating fingers around the breast (e.g., think of the nipple as a clock, begin with thumb at 12 and finger at 6, and then move to 1 and 7, 2 and 8, 3 and 9, etc.).

---

*Many mothers find a variation of the above method that works equally well or better. Encourage experimentation until they find what works best for them. There is no one correct way.
[†]This is the same position where baby's gums should be during efficient latch-on.
From Lauwers, J., & Swisher, A. (2016). *Counseling the nursing mother: A lactation consultant's guide* (6th ed.). Burlington, MA: Jones & Bartlett; Lawrence, R. A., & Lawrence, R. M. (2015). *Breastfeeding: A guide for the medical profession* (8th ed.). Philadelphia, PA: Elsevier; and Wambach, K., & Riordan, J. M. (2016). *Breastfeeding and human lactation* (enhanced 5th ed.). Burlington, MA: Jones & Bartlett Learning.

the newborn is satiated after feeding. Observing these cues provides new parents with positive feedback that increases their confidence (Walker, 2017; Wambach & Riordan, 2016).

Assessment

Nursing History

Breastfeeding assessments may be brief or comprehensive, depending on where in the perinatal period

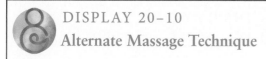

DISPLAY 20–10

Alternate Massage Technique

Purpose
- Encourages sucking in a sleepy baby or poor feeder
- Increases volume of fat content per feeding
- Increases the volume of milk ingested

Technique
- Massage when infant pauses between sucking bursts; massage should be downward and inward to deliver milk into baby's mouth.
- Compress milk ducts with thumb above and your fingers below.
- Gently massage breast with flat surface of middle fingers.
- Rotate massage around breasts.

From Lauwers, J., & Swisher, A. (2016). *Counseling the nursing mother: A lactation consultant's guide* (6th ed.). Burlington, MA: Jones & Bartlett; Lawrence, R. A., & Lawrence, R. M. (2015). *Breastfeeding: A guide for the medical profession* (8th ed.). Philadelphia, PA: Elsevier; and Wambach, K., & Riordan, J. M. (2016). *Breastfeeding and human lactation* (enhanced 5th ed.). Burlington, MA: Jones & Bartlett Learning.

the mother is encountered and on whether she or the newborn are having problems. An initial assessment includes a thorough history. Information should be elicited about any surgery or breast trauma as well as previous experiences with breastfeeding such as problems with latch-on, sore nipples, engorgement, and newborn weight gain. Other information that may be useful includes the amount and quality of social support, the mothers' knowledge regarding the mechanics of breastfeeding, how long the mother exclusively breastfed other children, when or if she introduced

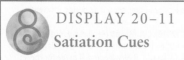

DISPLAY 20–11

Satiation Cues

- Gradual decrease in number of sucks over course of feeding
- Pursed lips followed by pulling away from the breast and releasing the nipple
- Relaxed body
- Legs extended
- Absence of hunger cues
- Sleep
- Small amount of milk drools from mouth
- Contented state

From Lauwers, J., & Swisher, A. (2016). *Counseling the nursing mother: A lactation consultant's guide* (6th ed.). Burlington, MA: Jones & Bartlett; Lawrence, R. A., & Lawrence, R. M. (2015). *Breastfeeding: A guide for the medical profession* (8th ed.). Philadelphia, PA: Elsevier; and Wambach, K., & Riordan, J. M. (2016). *Breastfeeding and human lactation* (enhanced 5th ed.). Burlington, MA: Jones & Bartlett Learning.

pacifiers and/or bottles, how satisfied she was with the feeding experience, and how long she plans to breast-feed this newborn. It is also important to review a list of all current medications to determine what effect, if any, they may have on lactation. This comprehensive history provides insight into potential problem areas. Without proper evaluation, the wrong nursing interventions may be used.

Physical Assessment

A thorough physical assessment should be performed at the time breastfeeding is initiated. Some abnormal physical findings are risk factors for breastfeeding difficulties and should alert the nurse of the need for more help with breastfeeding initiation. Some observations to be aware of include inverted nipples, hypoplastic breasts, and scars.

Women with inverted nipples can breast-feed successfully but may need extra help from a lactation expert. Protraction of the nipple often increases with breastfeeding and becomes more pronounced with subsequent pregnancies (Walker, 2017; Wambach & Riordan, 2016).

Another finding indicative of potential breastfeeding problems is hypoplastic breasts. Hypoplastic breasts appear tubular, flat or empty, small, and are usually spaced far from each other. The nipple and areola appear enlarged and bulging at tip. Women with hypoplastic breasts may have difficulty producing milk due to the diminished breast tissue. Initiation of lactation will require frequent on demand feedings as well as pumping or hand expression (see Display 20–9) in-between feedings to stimulate milk production. When milk supply is still inadequate to meet the neonate's needs, referral to a lactation expert should be made and other feeding options should be considered, such as a supplementary feeding device (Walker, 2017; Wambach & Riordan, 2016).

Presence of scars on the breasts should be explored to determine their origin whether surgical or traumatic. Many factors determine if a woman with a history of trauma or surgery can breastfeed. In most cases, they are encouraged to initiate breastfeeding. With the nurses' help and support, many are quite successful in fully or partially breastfeeding.

Assessment Tools

Common methods of documenting breastfeeding interactions do not always provide useful information. Subjective words such as well, fair, and poor do not capture the data needed to assess adequate intake or effectively identify problem areas. Similarly, the phrase "breast-feeding well" does not capture information regarding latch-on, audible swallow, time frames, or satiation.

TABLE 20–4. Latch: Breastfeeding Charting System			
System component	0	1	2
L Latch	Too sleepy or reluctant No latch achieved	Repeated attempts Hold nipple in mouth Stimulate to suck	Grasps breast Tongue down Lips flanged Rhythmic sucking
A Audible swallowing	None	A few with stimulation	Spontaneous and intermittent <24 hr old Spontaneous and frequent <24 hr old
T Type of nipple	Inverted	Flat	Everted (after stimulation)
C Comfort (breast/nipple)	Engorged Cracked, bleeding, large blisters or bruises Severe discomfort	Filling Reddened small blisters or bruises Mild or moderate discomfort	Soft Nontender
H Hold (positioning)	Full assist (staff holds infant at breast)	Minimal assist (i.e., place pillows for support, elevate head of bed) Teach one side; mother does other Staff holds and then mother takes over	No assist from staff Mother able to position and hold baby

From Jensen, D., Wallace, S., & Kelsey, P. (1994). LATCH: A breastfeeding charting system and documentation tool. *Journal of Obstetric, Gynecologic, and Neonatal Nursing, 23*(1), 27–32.

Numerous breastfeeding assessment tools assist the perinatal nurse by providing consistent guidelines for evaluating individual feeding events, ensuring continuity of care and communication between healthcare professionals, and providing a clear record in the chart of breastfeeding progress. One example of a breastfeeding assessment tool, the LATCH-5 item tool, is displayed in Table 20–4 (Jensen, Wallace, & Kelsey, 1994). Like an Apgar score, this tool assists the perinatal nurse to perform and document a thorough assessment and to identify areas where assistance and support are needed. A 4-item version of the LATCH was recently tested. It eliminated the "comfort" ("C") item. The psychometric properties improved slightly, providing a shorter version of the tool and making it more amenable to clinical use (Lau, Htun, Lim, Ho-Lim, & Klainin-Yobass, 2016).

Another clinical instrument, the Preterm Infant Breastfeeding Behavior Scale (PIBBS) was developed specifically for assessment of preterm infants. The instrument measures rooting, alveolar grasp, duration of latch, sucking, and swallowing (Hedberg Nyqvist & Ewald, 1999; Nyqvist, Rubertsson, Ewald, & Sjödén, 1996). A new instrument, the Bristol Breastfeeding Assessment Tool (BBAT) was developed in 2015 by Ingram, Johnson, Copeland, Churchill, and Taylor. The tool evaluates positioning, attachment, sucking, and swallowing and had an initial reliability rating of .668. The authors not only acknowledge the instrument has potential for clinical use but also recommend more research. Selection of an assessment tool should be based on what it measures and whether it is appropriate for a given population. Many facilities use a combination of tools. It is important to monitor the literature, because new instruments are being developed and there is ongoing refinement of existing ones. See Table 20–5 for a list of tools currently in use.

Supplemental Feedings

Supplemental feedings for term, healthy, breastfed newborns are seldom necessary except for medical indications (AAP, 2012). If supplementation is being considered, a thorough assessment of the mother and infant should be conducted by a lactation expert. Illnesses in the mother or newborn that may require supplementation include inborn errors of metabolism, very low-birth-weight infants, preterm infants, and certain medications being taken by the mother. Use of supplements without a medical indication is associated with decreased rates of breastfeeding duration and exclusivity (Asole, Spinelli, Antinucci, & Di Lallo, 2009; Chantry, Dewey, Peerson, Wagner, & Nommsen-Rivers, 2014; Chezem, Friesen, & Boettcher, 2003; Forde & Miller, 2010; Hauck, Fenwick, Dhaliwal, & Butt, 2010; Pincombe et al., 2008; Rodríguez-García & Acosta-Ramírez, 2008). Placing formula or water bottles in the bassinet or at the bedside of a breastfeeding mother sends a negative message about her ability to successfully breast-feed. Despite the known adverse effect of routine supplementation, more effort is needed to change practice. In 2007, 20.6% of U.S. birth facilities reported limiting non–breast milk

TABLE 20–5. Breastfeeding Assessment Instruments

Name of instrument	Assessment parameters	Reference
Infant Breastfeeding Assessment Tool (IBFAT)	Readiness to feed Rooting Fixing (latch-on) Sucking pattern	Matthews (1988)
Latch Assessment Documentation Tool	Baby's gum line placement Flanged lips Complete jawbone movement Tongue under areola Adequate suction	Jenks (1991)
Systematic Assessment of the Infant at Breast (SAIB)	Alignment Areolar grasp Areolar compression Audible swallowing	Shrago and Bocar (1990)
Mother Baby Assessment (MBA)	Signaling Positioning Fixing Milk transfer Ending	Mulford (1992)
LATCH-5 item Scoring System	Latch Audible swallowing Type of nipple Comfort (breast/nipple) Hold	Jensen et al. (1994)
LATCH-4 item Scoring System	Latch Audible swallowing Type of nipple Hold	Lau et al. (2016)
Breastfeeding Assessment Score	Maternal age Previous breastfeeding experience Latching difficulty Breastfeeding interval Number of bottles of formula	Hall et al. (2002)
H & H Lactation Scale	Maternal confidence/commitment to breastfeeding Perceived infant breastfeeding satiety Maternal/infant breastfeeding satisfaction	Hill and Humenick (1996)
Neonatal Oral-Motor Assessment Scale	29 characteristics of sucking Diagnoses disorganized and dysfunctional sucking	Palmer (1993)
Preterm Infant Breastfeeding Behavior Scale (PIBBS)	Rooting Areolar grasp Duration of latch while sucking Longest sucking episode Swallowing Scores range from 1 to 20.	Nyqvist, Rubertsson, Ewald, and Sjödén (1996)
Mother–Infant Breastfeeding Progress Tool	Mother responds to feeding cues. Mother goes ≤3 hr between feeding attempts. Mother independently positions self for feeding. Mother independently latches infant onto breast. No nipple trauma is present. No negative comments about breastfeeding.	Johnson, Mulder, and Strube (2007)
United Nations International Children's Emergency Fund United Kingdom Baby Friendly Initiative	Breastfeeding tools and forms for health professionals, including a breastfeeding assessment instrument.	United Nations International Children's Emergency Fund United Kingdom (n.d.)
Bristol Breastfeeding Assessment Tool	Instrument evaluates positioning, attachment, sucking, swallowing, and comfort	Ingram et al. (2015)

TABLE 20–5. Breastfeeding Assessment Instruments *(Continued)*		
Name of instrument	Assessment parameters	Reference
Supportive Needs of Adolescents Breastfeeding Scale (SNAB)	Nurses can use to evaluate the breastfeeding support they offer adolescent mothers and to ultimately improve the breastfeeding support offered to adolescent mothers	Grassley, Spencer, and Bryson (2013)
Breastfeeding Self-Efficacy Scale-Short Form (BSES-SF)	Perceived self-efficacy in breastfeeding (14 Likert scale items with anchors of 1—not at all confident to 5—always confident)	Dennis (2003)
Iowa Infant Feeding Attitude Scale (IIFAS)	Strong predictor of breastfeeding intention, initiation, and duration	De la Mora, Russell, Dungy, Losch, and Dusdieker (1999)

feedings to breastfed infants. In 2013, that had only increased to 26.4% (Perrine et al., 2015).

When supplementation is indicated, the following supplements should be considered, in order of preference: refrigerated mother's milk, frozen mother's milk, pasteurized donor banked human milk, and hypoallergenic infant formula (AAP, 2012). Once the supplement is chosen, a decision must be made about its delivery. It is better to avoid using an artificial nipple because it requires a different sucking technique when compared to breastfeeding and may create problems when the infant is transitioned back to the breast. Using other devices may be preferable to avoid nipple confusion. Some options include tube feeding, cup feeding, finger feeding, spoon feeding, or using a dropper or syringe. All these methods have strengths and limitations that must be considered (Walker, 2017).

The AAP (2017) recommends the use of carefully regulated donor human milk with high-risk infants when the mothers' own milk is insufficient or unavailable. The nonprofit Human Milk Banking Association of North American has over 25 milk banks in the United States and Canada. The milk is carefully tested, pasteurized, and retested before freezing. The frozen milk is then shipped overnight to recipients.

Use of Pacifiers and Artificial Nipples

Artificial nipples and pacifiers have been associated with incorrect sucking techniques at the breast (Lauwers & Swisher, 2016), decreased total duration of breastfeeding (Buccini, Pérez-Escamilla, & Venancio, 2016; Howard et al., 2003; Kramer et al., 2001; Kronborg & Vaeth, 2009; Lauwers & Swisher, 2016; E. A. Nelson, Yu, & Williams, 2005), and fewer feeds in 24 hours (Aarts, Hörnell, Kylberg, Hofvander, & Gebre-Medhin, 1999; Howard et al., 1999; Victora, Behague, Barros, Olinto, & Weiderpass, 1997). Use of the artificial nipple may not

be the cause of breastfeeding problems; rather their use may be an indicator of breastfeeding difficulties (Benis, 2002; Kramer et al., 2001; Kronborg & Vaeth, 2009; Lauwers & Swisher, 2016). Mothers who request bottles or pacifiers may be doing so because they lack appropriate knowledge about the effects of artificial nipples and pacifiers and lack confidence in their ability to successfully breast-feed. These women may benefit from contact with a skilled perinatal nurse or lactation consultant to assess the situation and provide appropriate support and education for the breastfeeding mother–infant dyad (Walker, 2017; Wambach & Riordan, 2016).

In the past, concerns were raised that use of pacifiers or artificial nipples could interfere with breastfeeding by causing nipple confusion. A recent Cochrane Review meta-analysis of pacifier use in 1,302 healthy term breastfeeding infants found no significant effect on duration of exclusive breastfeeding (Jaafar, Ho, Jahanfar, & Angolkar, 2016). However, caregivers are cautioned that early pacifier use may be an indicator of possible breastfeeding difficulties (Benis, 2002; Kramer et al., 2001; Kronborg & Vaeth, 2009; Lauwers & Swisher, 2016). To address this potential problem, the AAP (2012) recommends avoiding pacifiers until breastfeeding is fully established at around 3 to 4 weeks of age. At that time, they suggest offering the pacifier to the infant at onset of sleep to reduce the incidence of SIDS. Multiple case-controlled studies have shown a 50% to 90% reduction in SIDS rates with pacifier use. Because SIDS typically occurs in infants over 2 months of age, delaying introduction of the pacifier 1 month should not pose a risk (Moon, 2016). The exact mechanism of protection is unknown, although some speculate it may be due to the pacifier protecting the airway, or perhaps it lessens the likelihood of sleep apnea. At no time should an infant be forced to take a pacifier, nor should the pacifier be reinserted into the mouth if it falls out while the infant is asleep. To decrease risk of infection, pacifiers should be cleaned (boiling or dishwasher) often and replaced regularly. It is also recommended to avoid pacifiers made from latex, given the risk of allergies and to avoid pacifier clips with strings long enough to wrap around the baby's neck (Walker, 2017; Wambach & Riordan, 2016). Parents should be cautioned that pacifier use be reduced or stopped after 6 months to reduce the risk of otitis media and dental malocclusions (Sexton & Natale, 2009).

Milk Expression and Breast Pumps

In some situations, a woman may not be able to breast-feed early and frequently enough to stimulate and sustain lactation. When there is a delay, perinatal nurses should teach hand expression (see Display 20–9) and advise the mother to use a breast pump. A Cochrane Systematic Review (Becker, Smith, & Cooney, 2016) noted the best method for milk expression will vary based on time since birth, reason for expression, and individual characteristics of the mother and infant. They also reported that in some circumstances, low-cost interventions such as relaxation, massage, warming the breasts, and hand expression can be as effective as electric pumps. However, when a pump is needed, these same techniques can enhance its effectiveness.

Practitioners should be able to justify the use of a pump for an individual mother prior to recommending it use (Becker et al., 2016). Others maintain the practitioner should assess the mother's breast pump dependency when recommending pumps (Meier, Patel, Hoban, & Engstrom, 2016). Women who are partially or completely dependent on a pump to remove milk and regulate lactation (as opposed to the infant) require a pump that is effective, efficient, comfortable, and convenient. Hospital grade electric pumps meet these requirements. Women who are minimally dependent on a breast pump are those whose infant is at the breast for at least half of the daily feedings. Manual, battery operated, or mini electric pumps are intended for brief separations from a healthy infant, whereas double electric pumps are recommended when the mother returns to full-time work or when the mother needs to be away from the baby for 1 to 2 days.

Meier et al. (2016) stressed that when recommending a pump, the phase of lactation be taken into consideration. The transition from lactogenesis I to lactogenesis II (the first 72 hours postbirth) is a critical time to the establishment of human milk synthesis. Timing of breast pump initiation is critical to subsequent establishment of lactation. Women who gave birth to very LBW (VLBW) infants who pumped in the first hour postbirth resulted in significantly more human milk production at 1 and 3 weeks when compared to mothers whose first use of the breast pump was later (Parker, Sullivan, Krueger, & Mueller, 2015). The hospital grade electric breast pump was recommended for these circumstances.

Nurses should be aware of the following evidence-based recommendations and allow them to guide practice:

- If an infant is unable to breast-feed after birth, early (first hour, if possible) milk expression should be initiated.
- Greater milk volume results when the mother warms the breasts, has the correct size breast shield/flange, uses a relaxation technique (such as listening to music), and begins early and frequent pumping.
- Mothers who use breast massage while pumping will have higher fat content in their milk (Becker et al., 2016).
- Breast milk obtained with a large electric pump has higher protein content than a manual pump.
- A recent article (Meier et al., 2016) recommended an evidence-based approach to individualizing breast pump technology.

Nurses should know how to correctly size the shield/flange of the breast pump. Shields that are too big or too small can lead to nipple soreness, cracks, and excoriation. A shield that is too big can result in a loss of suction, which leads to inadequate stimulation and lower milk volume (Becker et al., 2016; Jones & Hilton, 2008). It has been estimated that 30% to 50% of mothers using a breast pump need a larger shield (Jones, Dimmock, & Spencer, 2001; Jones & Spencer, 2007).

Women need education on the correct use of breast pumps and storage of breast milk. Aseptic technique should be used, starting with clean hands and clean equipment. Many women begin a pumping session by warming the breasts, massaging them, and expressing a few drops of milk. This does a better job at stimulating letdown than starting immediately with the pump. To stimulate lactation, women should pump at least 8 to 12 times every 24 hours, no matter how high the milk volume. Pumping at night may produce larger quantities of milk because of the higher prolactin levels at that time of day; mothers should be encouraged to pump at least once during the night. Based on the circumstances, a mother may pump to stimulate initiation of lactation, in place of a missed feeding, between feedings, on one breast while feeding the baby on the other breast, or at the end of a feeding. Table 20–6 describes proper breast milk storage.

Hospital Discharge

Birth facilities should have a discharge protocol to ensure ongoing successful breastfeeding after mothers

TABLE 20–6. Proper Handling and Storage of Human Milk for Healthy Term Infants

Cautions	Do not add fresh milk to already frozen milk.
	Do not save milk from a used bottle for use at another feeding.
	Do not refreeze breast milk once it is thawed.
	Milk should be labeled with date and time.
	Store in 1 to 4 oz portions to avoid waste and allow faster thawing; you can add portions together (always using oldest milk first).
Thawing	Transfer to refrigerator or thaw in warm water.
	Do not use microwave: heats unevenly and could scald baby or damage milk (Heat will destroy up to 30.5% of IgA.)
Milk storage for term infants (Centers for Disease Control and Prevention, 2010)	Human milk can be kept in the back of the refrigerator for 3 to 5 days (less temperature fluctuation).
	Milk can be stored in a refrigerator freezer for 6 months (don't store near ice maker or on door because temperature fluctuates).
	Milk can be stored in deep freezer for up to 1 year.
Storage containers	Plastic bags designed specifically for freezing human milk. These bags are sturdier than those used in baby bottles and have self-closures that are easier to seal and label. Avoid using ordinary plastic storage bags or formula bottle bags because these could easily leak or spill.
	Glass or clear hard plastic bottles with single component top (Cloudy plastic bottles may have been made with BPA, which can leach into the milk.)
Labeling	Clearly label the milk with the date it was expressed to facilitate using the oldest milk first.
	If delivering breast milk to a child care provider, clearly label the container with the child's name and date.

BPA, bisphenol A; IgA, immunoglobulin A.
From Centers for Disease Control and Prevention. (2010). *Proper storage and preparation of breast milk.* Atlanta, GA: Author; Wambach, K., & Riordan, J. M. (2016). *Breastfeeding and human lactation* (enhanced 5th ed.). Burlington, MA: Jones & Bartlett Learning.

go home. General recommendations include formal documentation of breastfeeding effectiveness prior to discharge; identification of possible breastfeeding problems based on maternal and/or infant risk factors and a plan of action to address them; ongoing encouragement to breastfeed exclusively for 6 months, followed by ongoing breastfeeding combined with appropriate complimentary foods through the first year of age and if desired, for the first 2 years; and provision of noncommercial breastfeeding educational materials. Additional discharge recommendations can be found in the *Guideline for Hospital Discharge* (Evans, Marinelli, Taylor, 2014). Newborns should demonstrate at least two effective breast-feed before discharge.

Historically, women in the United States come to the hospital expecting to receive some type of discharge "gift bag." The dilemma for perinatal nurses who supported breastfeeding was that frequently, these packs contained formula samples. It has been established that receipt of formula samples has an adverse impact on breastfeeding duration and exclusivity (J. M. Nelson, Li, & Perrine, 2015; Rosenberg, Eastham, Kasehagen, & Sandoval, 2008). Between 2007 and 2013, the percentage of hospitals in the United States handing out formula samples decreased from 72.6% to 31.6%. Ideally, a discharge pack given to breastfeeding women would not contain formula samples or coupons but have products that support breastfeeding, such as instructions for manual expression, chemical cold packs, and breast pads. In a 2013 study, researchers tested this hypothesis and reported an average exclusive breastfeeding rate of 8.28 weeks for women who received a breastfeeding product bag that included a pump. Women who received a breastfeeding product bag without a pump had an average exclusive breastfeeding rate of 7.87 weeks, although the group that got a commercial bag with formula samples had an average rate of 6.12 weeks, which was significantly lower than the other two groups receiving breastfeeding supplies and information (Y. Bai, Wunderlich, & Kashdan, 2013).

The International Code on Marketing of Breastmilk Substitutes states hospitals and birthing centers should not accept free or low-cost infant formula or should they provide free samples of infant formula to families or advertise breast milk substitutes. This code was adopted by WHO in 1981 and is supported by the BFHI.

POTENTIAL BREASTFEEDING PROBLEMS

Reluctant Nurser

Newborns are described as reluctant nursers when they latch on only after many attempts, move their head from side to side without latching on, fall asleep or aggressively push away from the breast and arch their back, prefer nursing only on one side, do not latch on, or latch on but feed ineffectively. Numerous factors can contribute to a newborn being reluctant to nurse (Display 20–12). Managing this situation requires that the nurse and parents be very patient and not give up on the newborn's ability to eventually latch on correctly and nurse efficiently. Table 20–7 identifies

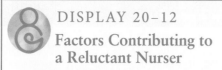

DISPLAY 20–12

Factors Contributing to a Reluctant Nurser

- Poor position at the breast
- Interruption of the organized sequence of prefeeding behaviors immediately after birth
- Use of medications during labor that may prolong the period of state disorganization
- Hypertonia (i.e., jaw clenching, pursed lips, neck and back hyperextension, and tongue retraction or elevation)
- Infrequent feeds leading to an overly hungry newborn baby
- Excessive or prolonged crying resulting in behavioral disorganization
- Interference with imprinting on the breast from separation, artificial nipples, pacifiers, or inappropriate use of nipple shields
- Excessive pressure on the occipital region of the baby's head from pushing the head forward into the breast
- Vigorous or deep suctioning or intubation causing swelling or pain in the mouth or throat
- Ankyloglossia (tongue-tie)

From Lauwers, J., & Swisher, A. (2016). *Counseling the nursing mother: A lactation consultant's guide* (6th ed.). Burlington, MA: Jones & Bartlett; Wambach, K., & Riordan, J. M. (2016). *Breastfeeding and human lactation* (enhanced 5th ed.). Burlington, MA: Jones & Bartlett Learning.

interventions that the nurse can use to encourage the newborn to latch on successfully (Lauwers & Swisher, 2016; Walker, 2017). In the event the reluctance continues, the mother will need to express milk (manual or pump) in-between attempts to stimulate lactogenesis II (Lauwers & Swisher, 2016; Walker, 2017). Care should be taken to ensure early follow-up after discharge, within 24 hours (Lauwers & Swisher, 2016).

Ankyloglossia (Tongue-Tie)

Ankyloglossia refers to a lingual frenulum that is excessively short and restricts movement of the tongue. The incidence of ankyloglossia in newborns ranges from 3.2% (J. L. Ballard, Auer, & Khoury, 2002) to 11% (Hogan, Wescott, & Griffiths, 2005) with a male-to-female ratio of 2:1 (Hong, 2013). In some cases, it can lead to breastfeeding difficulties such as problems with latch-on, nipple pain, trauma, poor milk transfer, low weight gain, and ultimately to premature weaning (Francis, Krishnaswami, & McPheeters, 2015; Geddes et al., 2008). When there is clinically significant ankyloglossia, a frenotomy is the preferred treatment (Forlenza, Paradise Black, McNamara, & Sullivan, 2010). Rowan-Legg (2015) and Francis et al. (2015) did systematic reviews and reported a small to moderate body of evidence associating a frenotomy with maternal reports of improved breastfeeding and less nipple pain. Perinatal nurses should routinely

assess the frenulum at birth and reassess should problems with latch-on and pain develop (ABM Protocol Committee, 2004). Specifically, they should look for a tongue that does not extrude past the lips, a tongue tip that cannot touch the roof of the mouth, a tongue that cannot be moved sideways, a tongue tip that may look flat, square, or heart shaped instead of pointy when the tongue is extruded.

Nipple Pain

Transient tender nipples are a common concern in the early postpartum period. The reported incidence of nipple pain and trauma varies widely from 34% to 96% (Buck, Amir, Cullinane, & Donath, 2014; Dennis, Jackson, & Watson, 2014; Wagner, Chantry, Dewey, & Nommsen-Rivers, 2013). Pain can range from mild tenderness to major discomfort. Nipple pain is one of the primary reasons women stop breastfeeding, and nurses should routinely assess for sore nipples. Pain or tenderness may occur in the following situations:

- When the newborn first latches on, disappearing after the newborn begins swallowing
- Periodically during the feeding
- Throughout an entire feeding
- After and/or in-between feedings

Obtaining a thorough history of the pain characteristics, observing a feeding, and doing a physical assessment can help identify the cause of nipple pain and guide interventions. Physical findings include vertical or horizontal red or white lines on the breast; fissures, cracks, or bleeding from the nipple; and blisters or scabs on one or both nipples. Display 20–13 outlines factors that contribute to nipple pain. Transient nipple pain usually peaks between postpartum days 3 and 6. Prolonged or severe soreness beyond the first week requires intervention (Lauwers & Swisher, 2016; Lawrence & Lawrence, 2015; Wambach & Riordan, 2016).

Perinatal nurses need to be aware that a common misconception is that limiting time on the breast will prevent sore nipples. In reality, it only delays the onset of soreness and causes additional feeding complications such as delay in lactogenesis II, insufficient milk for the baby, increased nipple soreness due to breaking the suction to remove the baby from the breast, and inadequate emptying of the breast (Lauwers & Swisher, 2016; Lawrence & Lawrence, 2015; Wambach & Riordan, 2016).

Systematic reviews of the literature concluded the most important way to prevent sore nipples was to provide prenatal and early postnatal education related to proper breastfeeding techniques and latch-on as well as anticipatory guidance (Dennis et al., 2014; Dias, Vieira, & Vieira, 2017; Kent et al., 2015).

TABLE 20–7. Techniques to Encourage Latch-On

Management	Rationale
Keep the mother and baby together.	
After birth, allow the newborn time to seek and find the nipple.	This approach provides the opportunity for the prefeeding sequence of behaviors to occur, which increases the likelihood of proper attachment to the breasts.
Place baby skin-to-skin on mother's chest.	This approach reestablishes or repatterns the initial sucking sequence that may not have occurred immediately after birth. It often calms the baby.
Try laid-back breastfeeding (biologic nursing).	Encourages mothers and babies to do what they know how to do instinctually
	Stresses that mother positions for her comfort, often in a semireclined position. Mother places baby "tummy down" on chest and lets gravity keep baby in position. Infant's cheek is rested somewhere near the breast. The baby can lie across the mother in many positions (e.g., vertical, horizontal, at an angle). Using skin-to-skin while doing laid-back nursing also helps.
Help mother recognize feeding cues.	
Instruct the mother to feed her baby on cue (see Display 20–8).	The mother who recognizes and responds to early feeding cues by offering the breast is more likely to achieve successful latch-on.
Check positioning at the breast.	
Newborn should completely face the mother with head, neck, and spine aligned.	Poor positioning increases the number of latch attempts needed before obtaining milk, which can frustrate the mother and newborn.
Mother reclined back comfortably and not leaning forward	Incorrect position increases the chances that the newborn will not latch correctly, leading to sore nipples, engorgement, insufficient milk production, and slow weight gain.
Mother stabilizes breast if needed and avoids doing so in a way that interferes with milk flow (e.g., scissor hold, fingers touching areola).	Compressing the breast may block ducts slowing or preventing milk flow.
If the newborn needs help with attachment:	Avoid pushing on the back of the head; this can stimulate some newborns to arch away.
• Support head by putting your palm behind baby's shoulders and your index finger and thumb behind the ear.	
• Cradle head in hand and direct newborn toward breast with heel of hand.	
• Use forearm to support shoulders.	
Bring newborn's nose near nipple with chin touching breast under areola.	Gentle touch of chin on breast triggers reflex to open wide (approximately 140-degree angle)
With mouth opens wide bring newborn onto breast chin first; lower lip should cover more of the areola than upper lip.	This places the nipple at the back of the mouth and allows the tongue and jaw to work smoothly to remove the milk.
Provide latch and sucking incentives.	
Place newborn skin-to-skin.	Helps to calm newborn; stimulates instinctive feeding efforts
Have mother express colostrum into a spoon and let newborn lap it up.	Provides nutrients and calms newborn if hungry
A syringe or soft clinic dropper with expressed colostrum can be used to elicit sucking and guide baby to breast.	
After crying hard for a while, the newborn may not be able to organize himself or herself to feed.	
Place skin-to-skin.	These interventions can calm the newborn and allow him or her to have a little food in his or her stomach so he or she is not so hungry.
Allow newborn to suck on a finger.	
Try spoon, cup, or finger feeding with a little colostrum.	

There is anecdotal support for other treatments; however, the scientific evidence is inconclusive for the use of expressed breast milk, breast shells, breast shields, aerosol spray, hydrogel dressing, film dressing, modified lanolin, collagenase, peppermint water/gel, tea bag compresses, and dexpanthenol. The only treatment found to be detrimental was a glycerin-based hydrogel dressing, which was associated with infection in one study (Dennis et al., 2014; Jackson & Dennis, 2017; Lochner, Livingston, & Judkins, 2009; Melli et al., 2007; Morland-Schultz & Hill, 2005). A recent student evaluated the effect of low-level laser therapy on reducing nipple pain (Coca et al., 2016). They concluded it was effective in reducing pain and prolonging breastfeeding. However, the use of other treatments concurrently such as antifungals and antibiotics were potential confounders and more research is needed. Perinatal nurses need to closely monitor the literature on this topic as more research is being conducted on the older treatments as well as some new treatments.

Once the skin is broken around the nipple, there is increased risk of infection. It has been suggested that putting expressed colostrum/breast milk on the nipple helps to prevent infection and assist healing. This is

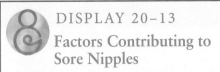

Factors Contributing to Sore Nipples

- Poor latch
- Candida pain (yeast infection of breast) causes a burning or stabbing pain that continues during the feeding
- Vasospasm caused by infant compressing the nipple so that blood flow is interrupted.
- Natural oils being removed from nipple or keratin layers broken down by drying agents (e.g., soap)
- Nipples not being allowed to dry
- Delayed letdown resulting in unrelieved negative pressure
- Manipulation of the nipple and areola such as squeezing it, tilting or pointing it up or down, or pushing it into the mouth
- Mother leaning over to "insert" the breast into the newborn's mouth instead of bringing the baby to the breast
- Not enough of the nipple and areola in the mouth
- Lips curled under rather than flared out
- Tongue behind lower gum and pinching or biting of the nipple
- Breast pushed sideways into the mouth rather than centered over where the nipple points naturally
- Nipple confusion (i.e., mouth configured for feeding on an artificial nipple or pacifier)
- Disorganized or dysfunctional sucking pattern
- Flat or retracted nipples
- Mouth not opened wide enough to encompass areola
- Ankyloglossia (tongue-tie)
- Incorrect use of breast pump or shield/flange not correct size for breast

From Lauwers, J., & Swisher, A. (2016). *Counseling the nursing mother: A lactation consultant's guide* (6th ed.). Burlington, MA: Jones & Bartlett; Lawrence, R. A., & Lawrence, R. M. (2015). *Breastfeeding: A guide for the medical profession* (8th ed.). Philadelphia, PA: Elsevier; and Wambach, K., & Riordan, J. M. (2016). *Breastfeeding and human lactation* (enhanced 5th ed.). Burlington, MA: Jones & Bartlett Learning.

based on knowledge of its bacteriostatic qualities, the antibodies, and anti-inflammatory factors present in colostrum and breast milk. Antibiotic ointment has also been used to prevent bacterial infection once the integrity of the skin is broken. Oral antibiotics are recommended if there is an active infection. Using a thin silicone nipple shield when the skin is broken to prevent further damage may also help; a lactation expert should be consulted whenever a shield is considered to assure its proper use (Wambach & Riordan, 2016).

Engorgement

Women experience a sense of full breasts during the transition to full milk production. This is a physiologic process that is expected and normal. Engorgement is different and results in painful swelling that occurs when the breasts become overfull (Lauwers &

Swisher, 2016). Three elements contribute to breast engorgement: congestion and vascularity, accumulation of milk, and edema caused by the swelling and obstruction of drainage of the lymphatic system. Engorgement can involve the areola, the body of the breast, or both areas (Lawrence & Lawrence, 2015).

Areolar Engorgement

Areolar engorgement may reflect edema from large amounts of IV fluids infused during labor or may be due to distention from milk production. If IV fluids cause areolar engorgement, the areola may appear puffy and is responsive to cold-pack application. If distended with milk, the areola may envelop the nipple, and the whole unit becomes difficult for the newborn to grasp. When this occurs, the mother should hand express some milk (see Display 20–10) before putting the baby to breast to avoid tissue damage and pain (Lawrence & Lawrence, 2015).

Peripheral Engorgement

Peripheral engorgement usually does not develop until 2 to 3 days after birth. Some swelling of the entire breast is normal, but if the breasts become hard, red, hot, shiny, and throbs, physiologic engorgement has changed to pathologic engorgement. This can be extremely painful, and the mother needs to breast-feed frequently using gentle, alternate massage (see Display 20–10). Hand expression (see Display 20–9) may provide relief, and some women are made more comfortable by using cold packs wrapped around the breast (a bag of frozen peas works well). It is important to breast-feed even when engorged because milk stasis can increase the risk of mastitis (Amir, 2014); is a major cause of insufficient milk production; and contributes to sore nipples, poor latch-on, reduced milk transfer, and slow weight gain by the infant. Separating mothers and babies, especially at night, giving unnecessary supplements, skipping night feedings, and long intervals between feedings exacerbates the problem of engorgement. It is vital to maintain frequent and thorough drainage of the breasts when the breasts become engorged because backpressure in the ducts can lead to atrophy of the milk secreting cells (Lawrence & Lawrence, 2015; Mangesi & Zakarija-Grkovic, 2016).

Hypoglycemia

Hypoglycemia in a term newborn usually refers to a blood glucose level below 40 mg/dL. This is a common and usually transient occurrence in the immediate postbirth period. Routine monitoring of blood glucose in healthy term newborns is unnecessary (Adamkin, 2011). For at-risk newborns (such as large for gestational age [LGA], small for gestational age [SGA], growth restricted, or an infant of a diabetic mother) specific protocols for screening and treatment are recommended (Adamkin, 2011, 2017; Wright & Marinelli, 2014).

Hypoglycemia in breastfed newborns can be prevented or greatly reduced by hospital policies that support breastfeeding (Adamkin, 2011; Holmes, McCleod, & Bunik, 2013; Wright & Marinelli, 2014):

- Breastfeeding within 30 to 60 minutes of birth
- Skin-to-skin contact between mother and newborn to prevent cold stress and use of glucose stores
- Breastfeeding 8 to 12 times per day
- Feeding in response to readiness cues and not on a predetermined schedule
- Not leaving the newborn to cry because prolonged crying rapidly depletes glycogen stores and can contribute to a steep drop in blood sugar levels
- Continuous mother–baby rooming-in

Hypoglycemia that recurs or persists longer than 48 to 72 hours of age may be caused by hyperinsulinemia, an underlying medical condition that is not related to feeding. Hypoglycemia in an asymptomatic newborn that does not respond to oral feeding or in a symptomatic newborn usually necessitates IV glucose infusions. The mother should be encouraged to pump or hand express colostrum into a spoon or cup for the newborn that is unable or reluctant to suckle at the breast. This will help stimulate and maintain the milk supply. If the medical condition permits, the newborn should be fed colostrum every 1 to 2 hours until able to feed effectively at the breast (Wambach & Riordan, 2016).

Jaundice

Clinical signs of hyperbilirubinemia are present in up to 84% of all term newborns in their first week and in nearly all preterms (Bhutani et al., 2013; Flaherman & Maisels, 2017; Muchowski, 2014). Untreated severe hyperbilirubinemia can result in kernicterus. This rare condition causes brain damage due to high levels of bilirubin. It can lead to several neurologic conditions. Some are minor, like learning disabilities, whereas others are serious, like cerebral palsy. There are several types of jaundice and the perinatal nurse should be able to differentiate between them because the treatment depends on early detection and the etiology.

Physiologic Jaundice

Physiologic jaundice, also known as normal newborn jaundice, appears after 24 hours of age, peaks on the third or fourth day of age, and steadily declines through the first month to normal levels. It occurs when bilirubin production exceeds the liver's ability to process it. This results in unbound, unconjugated bilirubin circulating in the blood stream and then being deposited in the skin (AAP, 2004; Flaherman & Maisels, 2017; Lauer & Spector, 2011; Lauwers & Swisher, 2016).

Breastfeeding-Associated Jaundice or Suboptimal Intake Jaundice

Breastfeeding-associated jaundice or suboptimal intake jaundice (Flaherman & Maisels, 2017) results from iatrogenic causes such as maternal–newborn separation, delayed or scheduled feedings, pacifier use, labor medications resulting in sleepy babies, and unnecessary supplementation. Elevated bilirubin in breastfeeding-associated jaundice is due to inadequate caloric intake and subsequent decreased stooling that allows the high levels of bilirubin in meconium to be reabsorbed. It typically resolves in 1 to 2 weeks, with treatment. Hospital policies based on the *Ten Steps to Successful Breastfeeding* (see Display 20–2) helps eliminate practices that lead to this type of jaundice (Flaherman & Maisels, 2017; Lauwers & Swisher, 2016; Muchowkski, 2014).

Prolonged Physiologic Jaundice (Breast Milk Jaundice; Late-Onset Jaundice)

Prolonged physiologic jaundice in healthy term infants, beyond the second or third week, is also known as breast milk jaundice or late onset jaundice. Bilirubin levels peak during the second or third week and may continue for 2 to 3 months. The etiology is unknown; however, experts agree it is related to suboptimal feeding. Around 10% to 18% of exclusively breastfed infants in the United States lose more than 10% of their birth weight and reduced caloric intake leads to increased concentrations of bilirubin (Flaherman & Maisels, 2017).

Optimal breastfeeding practices can decrease the incidence and severity of this type of jaundice. However, once identified it is important to closely monitor bilirubin levels in the event it rises to toxic levels. In a few cases, it might require treatment. Treatment can include phototherapy and/or short-term supplementation or replacement of breast milk with formula feedings. Supplementation is more supportive of breastfeeding but results in a slower drop in bilirubin levels. When supplementing breastfeeding, excessive amounts of formula should be avoided so the mother can maintain frequent breastfeeding. Another option is to stop breast milk totally for 24 hours and substitute formula. Mothers will need support to maintain breast milk production if they need to supplement or replace breast milk. Care needs to be taken to help mothers understand there is nothing wrong with their breast milk. Rather it is believed that formulas produced from cow's milk inhibit the intestinal absorption of bilirubin (Wambach & Riordan, 2016).

Pathologic Jaundice

Jaundice is considered pathologic if it occurs in the first 24 hours of age, the total serum bilirubin rises 5 mg/dL, or it rises to 17 dL or higher. The most common causes of pathologic jaundice include conditions that increase bilirubin production (ABO or Rh incompatibility; birth trauma leading to bruising or cephalohematoma; polycythemia). Conditions that impair bilirubin conjugation or decrease bilirubin excretion are rarer. Additional risk factors have been identified, such as prematurity, low birth weight, certain metabolic disorders, and sepsis (Lauer & Spector, 2011).

Jaundice Prevention

The following steps are recommended to prevent high levels of bilirubin (AAP, 2004; Flaherman et al., 2017; Lauer & Spector, 2011; Lauwers & Swisher, 2016; Maisels et al., 2009; Muchowski, 2014):

- Early initiation of breastfeeding, as early as possible, preferably within 1 hour of birth
- Frequent on demand breastfeeding (8 to 12 times per 24 hours)
- Hand expression of colostrum in-between feedings to provide extra milk and help establish lactogenesis II
- Implementation of protocols for the identification and evaluation of hyperbilirubinemia
  - Assessment of jaundice at least every 8 to 12 hours
  - Provider education stressing that visual inspection is not reliable as the sole method for assessing jaundice
  - Giving nurses independent authority to obtain a TSB (total serum bilirubin) or TcB (transcutaneous bilirubin) level
- Exclusive breastfeeding (no test feedings or supplementation)
- Optimization of breastfeeding management from birth: position, latch, observation of feeding, presence of expert help (i.e., healthcare provider trained in breastfeeding management)
- Maternal education on early hunger cues and satiation cues
- Identification of at-risk infants (so close surveillance/early interventions occur)
- Parental education (written and verbal) on jaundice
- Follow-up care and screening based on time of discharge and risk assessment

Insufficient Milk

Real or perceived insufficient milk supply is the most common reason for premature weaning (Gatti, 2008; Li, Fein, Chen, & Grummer-Strawn, 2008; Neifert & Bunik, 2013). An estimated 5% of mothers have true insufficient milk production; however, this number may be increasing (Stuebe et al., 2014) due to older women giving birth, the increased incidence of obesity, and its subsequent association with other health conditions.

Perceived insufficient milk is often related to a mother's lack of confidence or a lack of knowledge on typical newborn behavior (Lauwers & Swisher, 2016). In the early postpartum period, most women who think they do not have enough milk, have a problem with ineffective breastfeeding. This is an ideal time for perinatal nurses to educate the mother on ways to ensure adequate supply, to recognize infant hunger (see Display 20–8) and satiety cues (see Display 20–11) as well as signs of milk transfer (see Display 20–7), and signs of adequate intake. Mothers also need to know what "normal newborn behavior" is regarding infant feeding. Many women report they have insufficient milk when the infant wants to eat every 1 to 2 hours or will not sleep through the night; they need to know these are normal and expected behaviors. Anticipatory guidance should include the normality of cluster feeds, and the sudden increased demand to feed during growth spurts, which typically occur around 2 to 3 weeks, 6 weeks, 3 months, and 6 months. The mother should understand that by feeding frequently, milk supply increases.

A small percentage of women produce insufficient milk for psychological, physiologic, or pathologic reasons. These reasons can lead to decreased production and ejection of milk (Wambach & Riordan, 2016). Psychological factors include stress, embarrassment, and pain, all of which may increase production of epinephrine, which causes blood vessels to constrict resulting in reduced milk synthesis. Epinephrine also decreases production of oxytocin, which is needed for letdown to occur. Physiologic factors include maternal illness such as diabetes, hypothyroidism, anemia, retained placenta, smoking over 15 cigarettes per day, severe postpartum bleeding, past breast surgery (i.e., reduction and augmentation), and some medications. Conditions that interfere with the early, effective, and consistent stimulation of the breasts may also result in insufficient milk. Examples include restrictions on frequency and duration of feedings, more than 3 hours between feedings, skipping night feedings, and use of supplements. Pathologic factors that negatively affect milk production are related to endocrine problems.

Mothers often describe perceived insufficient milk when they experience one or more of the following:

- Baby does not settle or fusses after a feeding.
- Baby wants to feed more frequently (usually associated with growth spurt).
- Baby takes formula from a bottle directly after breastfeeding (artificial nipples stimulate the sucking reflex even when the infant is satiated).
- Mother is unable to express much milk.

- Baby does not sleep through the night or is awake much of the day.
- Breasts are smaller and softer than they should be.
- Initial weight loss of a healthy term baby exceeds 7% (Lauwers & Swisher, 2016; Lawrence & Lawrence, 2015; Wambach & Riordan, 2016).

Strategies to handle real or perceived insufficient milk depend on the cause of the problem. Mismanagement of breastfeeding is the most common contributor to low milk production. This problem is usually revealed during a feeding history. Mothers should be breastfeeding 8 to 12 times each 24 hours with no supplements or pacifiers. A feeding observation is necessary to confirm whether the newborn is swallowing milk or simply engaging in nonnutritive sucking. Mothers should perform alternate massage (see Display 20–10) and feed at closer intervals to increase milk production. Refer mothers to a lactation consultant for a thorough breastfeeding assessment and follow-up.

Candida albicans

If the mother complains of burning pain on the nipple or burning and shooting pains in the breast, a fungal infection (i.e., thrush) may be present. This is usually caused by *Candida albicans*. Positive predictive symptoms of Candida include complaints of soreness, burning, pain on nipple/areola, nonstabbing pain of the breast, stabbing pain in the breast, and/or skin changes of the nipple/areola that look shiny and flaky. Common predisposing factors for mothers include women who tested positive for vaginal *C. albicans*, who used broad-spectrum antibiotics, who have nipple damage, whose infant has oral thrush, or whose infant uses a pacifier and/or bottle. Certain oral contraceptives and asthma medications are also risk factors, along with maternal conditions such as diabetes, obesity, or poor endocrine function (Walker, 2017; Wambach & Riordan, 2016). Treatment can be challenging because women often present with Candida and *Staphylococcus aureus*, especially if there are nipple fissures. Treatment can be topical or systemic. Every treatment plan should include both mother and infant. Early diagnosis and treatment for Candida of the nipple and/or breast is critical to supporting successful long-term breastfeeding (Walker, 2017; Wambach & Riordan, 2016; Wiener, 2006).

The newborn with *C. albicans* presents with white patches (i.e., "crumbling curds") on the buccal mucosa, gums, or tongue that can travel to the hard and soft palate and down to the tonsils. It may also appear as pearly white or gray patches. An infant can have the infection in the intestines and stools, which contributes to a *Candida*-caused diaper rash. Some newborn's mouths are colonized with *C. albicans*, but it is not clinically apparent. Infected infants may be fussy, have a poor appetite, breast-feed poorly, and experience general discomfort (Walker, 2017; Wambach & Riordan, 2016).

The treatment of the fungal infection depends on the location and severity of the infection. Treatment of the mother and newborn simultaneously is important, even if only one has clinical symptoms. Women or infants with suspected *C. albicans* infection should be referred to their primary care provider.

Plugged Duct

Plugged ducts are small, tender breast lumps, the size of a pea. Symptoms include tenderness, heat, possible redness, or a palpable lump with generalized fever. Sometimes, the plug can be seen at the opening of the nipple duct (Wambach & Riordan, 2016). Milk stasis or a component of the milk may contribute to this. The application of hot packs and massaging the lump while the baby is sucking helps move this blockage. Other treatments include breast massage, altering infant position for feeding, and avoiding constrictive clothing. Some women experience plugged ducts repeatedly and describe fatty strings being expressed from the breast. Continued milk stasis increases the risk for mastitis (Wambach & Riordan, 2016).

Mastitis

Mastitis is an inflammatory condition of the breast that may or may not lead to an infection. The incidence of mastitis is between 3% and 30%, and onset is typically in the first 6- week-postpartum, although it can occur at anytime. The inflammation tends to be unilateral. Symptoms include fever >38°C (100.4°F), aching, chills, swelling, and pain. The site may also be red, hot, and hard; have tenderness under the arm; and red streaks from lump toward axilla. Common risk factors include cracked or bleeding nipples, inefficient removal of milk, engorgement, stress or getting run down, missed feedings, longer intervals between feedings, rapid weaning, and pressure on the breast (i.e., tight bra) (Amir, 2014; Lawrence & Lawrence, 2015).

Treatment of mastitis includes nursing frequently on both breasts, starting on the unaffected breast until letdown occurs and then switching. The affected breast should be emptied at each feeding, and the mother should get plenty of rest and adequate nutrition. If symptoms become severe, most clinicians treat with antibiotics. Although antibiotics treat the infection, they do not address the underlying cause of the mastitis. Antibiotic therapy must be accompanied by interventions to identify and correct the cause. Early identification of the cause and the use of appropriate interventions may halt the inflammatory process and prevent progression of an infection. Pain and inflammation at this point can be treated with a nonsteroidal anti-inflammatory drug such as ibuprofen. If there is no improvement within 8 to 24 hours and the mother has signs of a bacterial infection such as a discharge of pus from the nipple, continued fever, or a sudden spike of fever, she should contact her primary care provider immediately. Because *S. aureus* is most commonly associated with breast infections, choices of antibiotics are generally penicillinase-resistant penicillins or cephalosporins. These antibiotics are safe for the infant, and the mother should continue breastfeeding frequently from the affected side (Amir, 2014; Lawrence & Lawrence, 2015).

LATE PRETERM

Late preterm infants (34 to 36 weeks and 6 days' gestation) and early term (37 to 38 weeks and 6 days' gestation) are often treated the same as term infants. However, they have a high risk for breastfeeding problems. These infants tend to be sleepy, tire easily, have problems latching on, and may struggle with coordinating their suck-swallow-breathe pattern. In addition, they are at increased risk for dehydration, hypothermia, respiratory distress, hypoglycemia, and jaundice. These problems, along with possible separation of mother and infant secondary to the problems, increase the risk for delayed lactogenesis, which can lead to excessive weight loss (Ahmed, 2010; Boies & Vaucher, 2016; Hamilton, Martin, & Ventura, 2007; Meier, Furman, & Degenhardt, 2007). Interventions should concentrate on establishment of milk supply. The following actions are recommended for stable newborns:

- Have immediate and extended skin-to-skin contact at birth.
- Breast-feed within 1 hour of birth.
- Monitor closely in the first 12 to 24 hours for physiologic stability (temperature, apnea, tachypnea, hypoglycemia).
- Have mother room-in and use frequent skin-to-skin contact.
- Breast-feed on demand, at least 8 times in 24 hours and preferably more.
- Offer breast if the newborn does not show feeding cues within 2 to 3 hours.
  - To wake a sleepy newborn who needs to feed try some of the following: unwrap, place skin to skin, dim the lights, talk to him or her and try to make eye contact, hold him or her upright, rub his or her back in a circular motion from shoulder blades down and back up, stroke his or her scalp in gentle but firm circles, change his or her diaper, wipe his or her face with a cool, damp cloth.

- Avoid dehydration or excessive weight loss (weight loss >3% by day 1 or >7% by day 3).
  - Begin using breast pump and/or hand expression if the newborn cannot sustain 15 minutes of effective sucking at least 8 times per 24 hours OR within 4 hours of birth if not breastfeeding well; this provides needed stimulation for milk production. Pumping and hand expression can be after a feeding or in-between feeding.
  - If ineffective breastfeeding continues, there may be a need to supplement with pumped milk using a supplemental feeding device. Cup feeding has been associated with a protective effect on exclusive breastfeeding (Yilmaz, Caylan, Karacan, Bodur, & Gokcay, 2014) and should be used if possible. Other options include finger, spoon, syringe, dropper, or bottle.
- Consider an ultrathin silicone nipple shield if there is difficulty with latch or evidence of ineffective milk transfer. If a nipple shield is used, the mother and infant should be assessed and followed by lactation specialist/expert.
- Assess and document breastfeeding at least 2 times per day by two different healthcare professionals using standardized tool, such as LATCH score, Infant Breastfeeding Assessment Tool (IBFAT), or Mother–Baby Assessment Tool (see Table 20–5).

There are numerous protocols and guidelines on breastfeeding preterm infants available to perinatal nurses. Some are specific to late preterm infants (see Display 20–5).

MEDICATIONS AND BREASTFEEDING

Interruption of breastfeeding for women who are taking medications is usually an unnecessary and potentially damaging recommendation. Most medications have few side effects because the dose received by the newborn is usually less than 1% of the maternal dose and may have low bioavailability to the newborn. Antimetabolites and therapeutic doses of radiopharmaceuticals are examples of medications where breastfeeding is contraindicated. If such medication is needed for a short time period, women can be assisted to pump and dispose of their milk until it is safe for the newborn to nurse (Hale & Rowe, 2017). Ideally, newborns can be syringe or cup fed during this time. There are several excellent sources providing information on the safe use of medications for breastfeeding women (Display 20–14).

Galactagogues are a group of drugs and herbal remedies used to help induce or increase milk production (ABM Protocol Committee, 2011; Bazzano, Hofer, et al., 2016; Bazzano, Littrell, et al., 2016). The most common drugs are the off-label use of metoclopramide (Reglan)

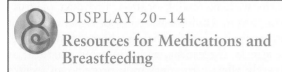

and domperidone (Motilium). The most widely used herbal remedy is fenugreek. Although there is little scientific evidence to support their use, there are anecdotal reports from the woman using the substances. Rigorous research is needed to determine the efficacy and safety of using these remedies.

POSTPARTUM SURGERY AND BREASTFEEDING

Occasionally, a woman needs surgery while still breastfeeding. When this occurs, she may be advised to stop breastfeeding for a variety of reasons such as the mother's condition, the mother's medications, the lack of caregiver knowledge, or the inability to room in with the infant. Ideally, everything should be done to help the woman continue breastfeeding if that is her choice. Lactating women admitted to a medical or surgical unit should be seen by a lactation consultant. The staff and the mother often need education on use of the breast pump and the recommended schedule for

pumping. If the milk is still safe for the infant, additional education is needed on the storage of the milk. The perinatal nurse and lactation experts have the responsibility of letting other units and physicians know of their availability for consultation.

FORMULA FEEDING

Use of a commercially prepared, iron-fortified infant formula is another method of providing nutrition during the first year of age. Although there is formula available without iron, its use should be discouraged. Parents should be told that the amount of iron in formula is what the baby needs and contrary to common belief, it does not cause stomach upset or constipation. Use of formula is indicated for newborns in the following situations (AAP, 2014):

- When a mother chooses not to breast-feed or not to breast-feed exclusively
- In the presence of maternal infections caused by organisms that may be transmitted through human milk (such as HIV)
- If the newborn is diagnosed with an inborn error of metabolism causing intolerance to components of human milk, such as galactosemia
- When the mother has been exposed to foods, medications, or environmental agents that are excreted in human milk and may be harmful to the newborn (i.e., drugs of abuse, antineoplastics, mercury, lead)
- After exposure to radioactive compounds requiring temporary cessation of breastfeeding
- As supplementation to breast milk when the newborn does not demonstrate adequate weight gain

Parents may benefit from an understanding that newborns fed formula have a greater risk of acute and chronic illness in the immediate newborn period as well as later in life. Cow's milk; goat's milk; 1%, 2%, or fat-free milk; and evaporated milk are not recommended during the first year of age. These milk products do not contain adequate iron; they increase the renal solute load because of the amount of protein, sodium, potassium, and chloride and may result in deficiencies in essential fatty acids, vitamin E, and zinc (AAP, 2014). This important information should be provided to the women in an objective manner. The purpose of the discussion is not to make women feel guilty about their choices but to make sure they have made an informed choice.

Composition of Formula

Commercially prepared formula can never totally duplicate the hormones, immunologic agents, enzymes, and live cells found in human milk. In 1980, Congress passed the first Infant Formula Act, which was revised in 2010, and has addressed some of the differences between breast milk and formula (Infant Formula Nutrient Specifications, 2010). This legislation sets minimum and maximum levels of certain nutrients and requires that manufacturers analyze all batches of formula and state on the labels the concentration of specific nutrients.

The concentrations of nutrients in formula vary slightly between manufacturers and are usually slightly higher in formula than in breast milk to compensate for the possible lower bioavailability (AAP, 2014). Although formula companies may be able to provide a rationale for their individual differences, large randomized clinical trials supporting their conclusions do not exist. Most formulas use cow's milk as the protein base. Because some newborns develop formula intolerance and some families are aware of existing milk intolerance, formula companies manufacture alternative formulas of special composition for newborns with gastrointestinal or metabolic disturbances.

Milk-Based Formula

Formula development and improvement is an ongoing challenge. Recent changes have been made to make the formulas more closely resemble breast milk. For example, there have been changes in the whey-casein ratio, the quantity of nucleotides, and the addition of long-chain polyunsaturated fatty acids (Guo, 2014). Animal fat in cow's milk has been replaced with vegetable oils to improve digestibility and absorption, eliminate cholesterol, increase the concentration of essential fatty acids, and reduce environmental pollutants (AAP, 2014). The major source of carbohydrate in human milk and formula is lactose. The presence of lactose in the bowel is responsible for proliferation of acidophilic bacterial flora necessary to prevent the growth of pathogenic organisms. Most formulas are fortified with iron, minerals, and electrolytes such as calcium, phosphorus, magnesium, sodium, potassium, and chloride. Cow's milk is the source of most minerals and electrolytes, although some are added as inorganic salts.

Milk-based formulas are available for newborns with special needs. Newborns requiring a lower renal solute load, such as those with cardiovascular or renal disease, can use formulas containing low levels of minerals and electrolytes. Newborns that experience lactose intolerance or have a family history of lactose intolerance can be given a lactose-free formula in which glucose rather than lactose is the carbohydrate source. Because this formula contains very small amounts of lactose, it should not be given to newborns with galactosemia. There are also milk-based formulas in which the fat content has been lowered for

newborns with fat malabsorption, bile duct obstruction, or severe cholestasis. Newborns who cannot digest protein (i.e., cystic fibrosis, short gut syndrome, biliary atresia, cholestasis, and protracted diarrhea) or are severely allergic to cow's milk protein can receive formula in which the protein has been treated with heat and enzymes, decreasing the potential allergic response (Guo, 2014).

Soy Formulas

According to AAP (2014), soy formula is recommended for term infants with galactosemia, congenital or transient lactase deficiency, or documented immunoglobulin E–associated allergy to cow's milk who are not allergic to soy protein. Soy formulas may also be used by strict vegan families who want to avoid animal protein. Preterm infants should not be given soy protein because there is significantly less weight gain with soy and an increase in osteopenia of prematurity (AAP, 2014).

Preterm Human Milk Modifiers

Preterm and VLBW infants may need to supplement breast milk with a human milk fortifier. The AAP Policy Statement on Breastfeeding and the Use of Human Milk (AAP, 2012) recommends the use of human milk fortifiers containing protein, minerals, and vitamins to ensure preterm human milk meets the nutritional needs for VLBW newborns.

Mechanics of Formula Feeding

The perinatal nurse should ensure that parents who choose to use commercially prepared formula have sufficient information and are doing so safely. Unfortunately, this is not always done. In one study, using the 2005 to 2007 Infant Feeding Practices Study II data, 77% of the participants reported they had not received instruction from healthcare professionals on how to prepare formula and 73% did not receive instruction on formula storage (Labiner-Wolf, Fein, & Shealy, 2008). Errors in formula preparation do occur. In one trial, less than half of the mothers mixed the feeding correctly, and 26% offered overly concentrated feedings, with the potential for serious consequence such as diarrhea (Lucas, Lockton, & Davies, 1992). Oral water intoxication can be the outcome of mixing too much water with the formula to stretch its availability or accidentally adding water to read-to-feed formula. These babies may present to the emergency room with seizures and apnea (Keating, Schears, & Dodge, 1991). Parents need to read labels carefully for expiration dates and preparation instructions. This may be a problem if the adult cannot read or does not speak English (Lauwers & Swisher, 2016).

Types of Formula

Formula is available as ready-to-feed, liquid concentrate, or as a powder. Ready-to-feed is the most expensive but safest in terms of risk for contamination. No water is needed for dilution and it is sterilized during manufacturing. Liquid concentrate is also sterilized during manufacturing but must be mixed with equal parts of water (1:1 ratio). Powdered formula requires one level scoop added to every 2 oz of water. Unlike the liquid forms of formula, powdered formula is not sterile and carries a small risk of being contaminated with *Enterobacter sakazakii*. The risk can be minimized when parents follow preparation and storage guidelines. Premature and low-birth-weight infants are more likely to become infected if exposed to *E. sakazakii*, and many providers recommend using ready-to-feed or concentrated formula with vulnerable populations, especially during the first 3 months of age (AAP, 2014; Lauwers & Swisher, 2016; WHO & Food and Agriculture Organization of the United Nations, 2007). The WHO, in collaboration with the Food and Agriculture Organization of the United Nations (2007), has published guidelines on safe preparation, storage, and handling of powdered infant formula and how to prepare formula for bottlefeeding at home that may help perinatal nurses when teaching about formula safety.

Formula Reconstitution

Water safety should be reviewed with parents. Typically, water for reconstitution comes from the tap or is bottled. With tap water, higher levels of impurities are found in hot water and water that has sat in pipes for a while. Therefore, it is best to run cold water from the tap for a few minutes before filling the bottle. If parents are unsure about water quality they can use bottled water or bring cold tap water to a full boil for 1 minute, allowing it to cool before using (AAP, 2014). Parents should talk with their healthcare provider about the most appropriate source of water, because this may vary based on water source and locale.

Tap water from most municipal systems in the United States is safe because it must meet federal standards. However, water must pass through various fixtures to get to the tap and can absorb lead; copper; or other contaminants from the fixtures and pipes, especially in older buildings. Most municipal water sources fluoridate the water. Too much fluoride (0.7 mg/L or higher) puts the baby at risk for enamel fluorosis, which can result in faint white lines or white areas on the permanent teeth. Parents can check with their water utility to find out how much fluoride is present. Parents can test their water for lead, arsenic, pesticides, and bacteria using a home test kit. They should read and follow the directions carefully to get accurate results.

Bottled water is filtered so impurities are removed, but it is not sterilized. By law, bottled water must meet the U.S. Food and Drug Administration's Standard of Water Quality, which is at least as stringent as the Environmental Protection Agency's standards for tap water. Low fluoride bottled water will be labeled as purified, deionized, demineralized, distilled, or prepared by reverse osmosis. Most grocery stores sell these types of low fluoride water.

Parents should be cautioned to mix formula as directed by the manufacturer. Remind them not to add extra water because it can slow growth and development; it may also lead to seizures due to an electrolyte imbalance (AAP, 2014). Bottles of reconstituted powder formula may be refrigerated for 24 hours; bottles of liquid concentrate or ready-to-feed formula are good for 48 hours in the refrigerator. Caution parents to follow directions on the formula container for proper storage.

New bottles, nipples, caps and rings should be washed in warm soapy water and then sterilized by placing them in a pan of boiling water for 5 minutes. After initial sanitizing, subsequent cleaning can be done with warm soapy water, using a bottle and nipple brush to remove dried formula (Alden, 2012; AAP, 2014). Dishwashers are usually safe; however, parents should follow their caregiver and manufacturer instructions before cleaning equipment in a dishwasher.

Frequency of Feeding

Standard commercially prepared formula contains 20 kcal/oz and can be offered to newborns on demand. During the first 3 months of age, intake is approximately 150 to 200 mL/kg/day (AAP, 2009). This provides 100 to 135 kcal/kg/day. Weight gain should be approximately 25 to 30 g/day. Infants receiving formula do not need additional water in their diet.

Parents can begin feeding ½ to 1 oz of formula at each feeding during the first 24 hours of age. During the next 24 hours, the feedings can be increased by ½ oz increments, feeding the same volume for two to three feedings before increasing. Parents should not force the baby to finish the bottle and should feed on cue when the baby shows signs of hunger. The newborn should be burped halfway through the feeding. During a feeding, the infant should be held at about a 45-degree angle, and the bottle should be held so that the nipple is full of formula to avoid sucking air.

Once a bottle is prepared it should be used or remain in the refrigerator until needed. Any formula remaining in the bottle when the infant is done eating should be discarded because it is an excellent medium for bacterial growth. To avoid waste, smaller amounts of formula should be prepared for the early postbirth period, gradually increasing until the infant is eating 6 to 8 oz per feeding. Formula should be fed at room temperature. A bottle from the refrigerator can be warmed by placing it in a pan of warm water. Microwaves should never be used to warm formula as it heats unevenly, and the infant may be burned.

Hunger and Satiety Cues

Parents who formula feed need to recognize and respond to infant cues. The cues are the same as for infants who are breastfed (see Display 20–8 and 20–11). Like breastfeeding, parents should watch for and respond to early signs of hunger and not wait until the infant is upset or crying. Some infants eat less than what is in the bottle. It is important that the infant not be forced to finish a bottle or should the parents keep the bottle to use at the next feeding.

Feeding Positions

There is evidence that feeding position contributes to the increased incidence of otitis media in bottle fed newborns. Supine feeding, positioning the newborn in a horizontal position, or propping the bottle for feeding has been associated with reflux of milk into the Eustachian tubes. Researchers have identified a significant difference in the number of abnormal postfeeding tympanogram results when infants were fed in the supine position compared with those fed in the semi-upright position (Tully, Bar-Haim, & Bradley, 1995). Propping bottles can also lead to dental caries (bottle mouth syndrome), choking, or aspiration. This information should be shared with parents choosing to bottle feed along with the following recommendations:

- Hold infant during feedings. The newborn needs human contact and this provides an ideal time for socialization and bonding. Avoid feeding while infant is in an infant seat.
- Sit in a comfortable armchair while feeding to reduce arm fatigue; use pillows to support arm as needed.
- Rest newborn's head in the crook of the elbow, with head slightly higher than the rest of his body so he faces caregiver's face (a position similar to the breastfeeding newborn).
- Keep upright after feeding for about 15 minutes before placing the infant in a supine position to sleep.
- Never put the newborn to bed with a bottle or prop bottles.
- Refrigerated bottles should be placed in warm water for no longer than 15 minutes. Prior to feeding, shake the bottle, and test the temperature by sprinkling a few drops on the inside of the wrist. Never use a microwave because it does not heat evenly and there may be hot spots in the milk.

Equipment for Bottle Feeding

There are many different types of bottles and nipples. Each has advantages and disadvantages. Some parents may need to try several to find one that works best for their infant. If feeding does not go smoothly, some experimentation may be necessary.

Nipple holes should allow a few drops to come out when the bottle is inverted. If holes are too big, formula flows too fast and if too small, the infant gets frustrated and ingests air. Nipples come in three standard flow variations with different size holes. Typically, smaller babies prefer slower flows, whereas older babies prefer faster flow. Avoid latex nipples due to allergy risks; instead use nipples made from silicone.

Bottles come in a variety of shapes: standard bottles (classic shape), angle-neck bottles, disposable liner bottles, and natural flow bottles. Several are designed to prevent air ingestion (angle neck, line bottles, and natural flow bottles). Caution parents about bisphenol A (BPA). BPA is used to harden plastics, keep bacteria from contaminating foods and prevent cans from rusting. In 2008, concern was raised that it can leach into food. Bottles or bag inserts that have a recycle code of "7" and the letters "PC" or those that are certified or identified on the labeling as BPA free are safe options.

LACTATION SUPPRESSION

In postpartum women who are not breastfeeding, milk leakage and breast pain begins 1 to 3 days after the birth and engorgement begins between 1 and 4 days after the birth. Considerable pain may be experienced during this time. Over the years, a variety of interventions have been suggested to decrease milk leakage and pain associated with lactation suppression, but few interventions are supported by randomized, controlled clinical research. Some techniques that may help include:

- Wearing a well-fitting bra or sport bra 24 hours each day until the breasts are soft and nontender
- Applying cold packs to the breasts. These may be commercial cold packs or bags of frozen peas. If the woman does not want to use cold for cultural reasons, warmth may also provide comfort.
- Using mild over-the-counter analgesics, taken according to manufacturers' recommendations
- Avoiding nipple or breast stimulation; however, when discomfort is severe, hand expressing, or pumping a small amount of milk may provide relief; taking a warm shower and letting the water run over the breasts may stimulate milk leakage. This type of stimulation is not enough to prolong the time needed to stop producing milk.

Restricting fluids is neither necessary nor desirable. The breasts return to normal and tenderness decreases within 48 to 72 hours after engorgement occurs.

SUMMARY

The abundance of research on breastfeeding and human lactation clearly shows the importance of breastfeeding, the adverse effects of newborn formula use, and the evidence that many traditional newborn feeding practices have no scientific or physiologic validity. Parents and health professionals should be aware of this information. Healthcare professionals have an obligation to support changes in practice that have been shown to remove institutional barriers to breastfeeding. Clinical nurse specialists, advance practice nurses, educators, nurse managers, lactation consultants, hospital administrators, and physicians can take steps to see that breastfeeding is supported in their community, clinic, and institution.

Many national organizations have policies that support breastfeeding. For example, AWHONN (2015a) supports breastfeeding as the optimal method of feeding and challenges its membership to foster environments that support breastfeeding. In 2010, the Joint Commission (2010) included exclusive breast milk feeding rates as part of its perinatal care core measures for maternity hospitals seeking accreditation.

The choice of infant feeding method has a significant effect on the health and development of the newborn, health of the mother, and cost of illness to the healthcare system. The perinatal nurse's interactions with families should reflect promotion, protection, and support of breastfeeding as the normal and natural way to feed a newborn. Perinatal nurses also are responsible to provide support and education for women who choose to formula feed. Making sure parents clearly understand formula preparation is critical to the health and well-being of the newborn.

REFERENCES

Aarts, C., Hörnell, A., Kylberg, E., Hofvander, Y., & Gebre-Medhin, M. (1999). Breastfeeding patterns in relation to thumb sucking and pacifier use. *Pediatrics, 104*(4), e50.

Abrahams, S. W., & Labbok, M. H. (2009). Exploring the impact of the Baby-Friendly Hospital Initiative on trends in exclusive breastfeeding. *International Breastfeeding Journal, 4,* 11. doi:10.1186/1746-4358-4-11

Academy of Breastfeeding Medicine Protocol Committee. (2004). ABM Clinical Protocol #11: *Guidelines for the evaluation and management of neonatal ankyloglossia and its complications in the breastfeeding dyad.* New Rochelle, NY: Author.

Academy of Breastfeeding Medicine Protocol Committee. (2011). ABM Clinical Protocol #9: Use of galactagogues in initiating or augmenting the rate of maternal milk secretion (first revision January 2011). *Breastfeeding Medicine, 6*(1), 41–50.

Adab, P., Jiang, C. Q., Rankin, E., Tsang, Y. W., Lam, T. H., Barlow, J., . . . Cheng, K. K. (2014). Breastfeeding practice, oral contraceptive use and risk of rheumatoid arthritis among Chinese women: The Guangzhou Biobank cohort study. *Rheumatology (Oxford, England), 53*(5), 860–866. doi:10.1093/rheumatology/ket456

Adamkin, D. H. (2011). Clinical report: Postnatal glucose homeostasis in late-preterm and term infants. *Pediatrics, 127*(3), 575–579. doi:10.1542/peds.2010-3851

Adamkin, D. H. (2017). Neonatal hypoglycemia. *Seminars in Fetal & Neonatal Medicine, 22*(1), 36–41. doi:10.1016/j.siny.2016.08.007

Aghdas, K., Talat, K., & Sepideh, B. (2014). Effect of immediate and continuous mother-infant skin-to-skin contact on breastfeeding self-efficacy of primiparous women: A randomised control trial. *Women and Birth, 27*(1), 37–40. doi:10.1016/j.wombi.2013.09.004

Ahmed, A. H. (2010). Role of the pediatric nurse practitioner in promoting breastfeeding for late preterm infants in primary care settings. *Journal of Pediatric Health Care, 24*(2), 116–122. doi:10.1016/j.pedhc.2009.03.005

Alden, K. R. (2012). Newborn nutrition and feeding. In D. L. Lowdermilk, S. E. Perry, K. Cashion, & K. R. Alden (Eds.), *Maternity and women's health care* (10th ed., pp. 606–636). St. Louis, MO: Mosby.

American Academy of Family Physicians. (2015). *Breastfeeding, family physicians supporting* (Position paper). Retrieved from https://www.aafp.org/about/policies/all/breastfeeding-support.html

American Academy of Pediatrics. (2004). Management of hyperbilirubinemia in the newborn infant 35 or more weeks of gestation. *Pediatrics, 114*(1), 297–316.

American Academy of Pediatrics. (2009). *Pediatric nutrition handbook* (6th ed.). Elk Grove Village, IL: Author.

American Academy of Pediatrics. (2012). Breastfeeding and the use of human milk. *Pediatrics, 129*(3), e827–e841. doi:10.1542/peds.2011-3552

American Academy of Pediatrics. (2014). *Pediatric nutrition handbook* (7th ed.). Elk Grove Village, IL: Author.

American Academy of Pediatrics. (2017). Donor human milk for the high-risk infant: Preparation, safety, and usage options in the United States. *Pediatrics, 139*(1), e20163440. doi:10.1542/peds.2016-3440

American College of Obstetricians and Gynecologists. (2018). *Optimizing support of breastfeeding as part of obstetric practice* (Committee Opinion No. 756). Washington, DC: Author.

Amir, L. H. (2014). ABM Clinical Protocol #4: Mastitis. *Breastfeeding Medicine, 9*(5), 239–243.

Anstey, E. H., Chen, J., Elam-Evans, L. D., & Perrine, C. G. (2017). Racial and geographic difference in breastfeeding—United States, 2011-2015. *MMWR Morbidity and Mortality Weekly Report, 66*(27), 723–727. doi:10.15585/mmwr.mm6627a3

Asiodu, I. V., Waters, C. M., Dailey, D. E., & Lyndon, A. (2017). Infant feeding decision-making and the influences of social support persons among first-time African American mothers. *Maternal and Child Health Journal, 21*(4), 863–872. doi:10.1007/s10995-016-2167-x

Asole, S., Spinelli, A., Antinucci, L. E., & Di Lallo, D. (2009). Effect of hospital practices on breastfeeding: A survey in the Italian region of Lazio. *Journal of Human Lactation, 25*(3), 333–340.

Association of Women's Health Obstetric and Neonatal Nursing. (2015a). Breastfeeding (Position Statement). *Journal of Obstetric, Gynecologic, and Neonatal Nursing, 44*(1), 145–150. doi:10.1111/1552-6909.12530

Association of Women's Health Obstetric and Neonatal Nursing. (2015b). *Breastfeeding support: Preconception care through the first year* (Evidence-Based Clinical Practice Guideline, 3rd ed.). Washington, DC: Author.

Association of Women's Health Obstetric and Neonatal Nursing. (2017). *Assessment & care of the late preterm infant* (Evidence-Based Clinical Practice Guideline, 2nd ed.). Washington, DC: Author.

Bai, D. L., Wu, K. M., & Tarrant, M. (2013). Association between intrapartum interventions and breastfeeding duration. *Journal of Midwifery & Women's Health, 58*(1), 25–32. doi:10.1111/j.1542-2011.2012.00254.x

Bai, Y., Wunderlich, S. M., & Kashdan, R. (2013). Alternative hospital gift bags and breastfeeding exclusivity. *ISRN Nutrition, 2013,* 560810. doi:10.5402/2013/560810

Bailey, B. A., & Wright, H. N. (2011). Breastfeeding initiation in a rural sample: Predictive factors and the role of smoking. *Journal of Human Lactation, 27*(1), 33–40. doi:10.1177/0890334410386955

Ballard, J. L., Auer, C. E., & Khoury, J. C. (2002). Ankyloglossia: Assessment, incidence, and effect of frenuloplasty on the breastfeeding dyad. *Pediatrics, 110*(5), e63.

Ballard, O., & Morrow, A. L. (2013). Human milk composition: Nutrients and bioactive factors. *Pediatric Clinics of North America, 60*(1), 49–74. doi:10.1016/j.pcl.2012.10.002

Balogun, O. O., O'Sullivan, E. J., McFadden, A., Ota, E., Gavine, A., Garner, C. D., . . . MacGillivray, S. (2016). Interventions for promoting the initiation of breastfeeding. *Cochrane Database of Systematic Reviews,* (11), CD001688. doi:10.1002/14651858.CD001688.pub3

Bartels, M., van Beijsterveldt, C. E. M., & Boomsma, D. I. (2009). Breastfeeding, maternal education and cognitive function: A prospective study of twins. *Behavior Genetics, 39*(6), 616–622. doi:10.1007/s10519-009-9293-9

Bartick, M., & Reinhold, A. (2010). The burden of suboptimal breastfeeding in the United States: A pediatric cost analysis. *Pediatrics, 125*(5), e1048–e1056. doi:10.1542/peds.2009-1616

Bartick, M., Stuebe, A., Shealy, K. R., Walker, M., & Grummer-Strawn, L. M. (2009). Closing the quality gap: Promoting evidence-based breastfeeding care in the hospital. *Pediatrics, 124*(4), e793–e802. doi:10.1542/peds.2009-0430

Bazzano, A. N., Hofer, R., Thibeau, S., Gillispie, V., Jacobs, M., & Theall, K. P. (2016). A review of herbal and pharmaceutical galactagogues for breast-feeding. *The Ochsner Journal, 16*(4), 511–524.

Bazzano, A. N., Littrell, L., Brandt, A., Thibeau, S., Thriemer, K., & Theall, K. P. (2016). Health provider experiences with galactagogues to support breastfeeding: A cross-sectional survey. *Journal of Multidisciplinary Healthcare, 9,* 623–630.

Becker, G. E., Smith, H. A., & Cooney, F. (2016). Methods of milk expression for lactating women. *Cochrane Database of Systematic Reviews,* (9), CD006170. doi:10.1002/14651858.CD006170.pub5

Bener, A., Ehlayel, M. S., Alsowaidi, S., & Sabbah, A. (2007). Role of breast feeding in primary prevention of asthma and allergic diseases in traditional society. *European Annals of Allergy and Clinical Immunology, 39*(10), 337–343.

Benis, M. M. (2002). Are pacifiers associated with early weaning from breastfeeding? *Advances in Neonatal Care, 2*(5), 259–266.

Benitz, W. E. (2015). Hospital stay for healthy term newborn infants. *Pediatrics, 135*(5), 948–953. doi:10.1542/peds.2015-0699

Bhutani, V. K., Stark, A. R., Lazzeroni, L. C., Poland, R., Gourley, G. R., Kazmierczak, S., . . . Stevenson, D. K. (2013). Predischarge screening for severe neonatal hyperbilirubinemia identifies infants who need phototherapy. *The Journal of Pediatrics, 162*(3), 477.e1–482.e1. doi:10.1016/j.jpeds.2012.08.022

Binns, C., Lee, M., & Low, W. Y. (2016). The long-term public health benefits of breastfeeding. *Asia-Pacific Journal of Public Health, 28*(1), 7–14. doi:10.1177/1010539515624964

Boies, E. G., & Vaucher, E. (2016). ABM Clinical Protocol #10: Breastfeeding the late preterm infant (34 0/7 to 36 6/7 weeks gestation) and early term infants (37-3 6/7 weeks of gestation), 2nd revision 2016. *Breastfeeding Medicine, 11*(10), 494–500. doi:10.1089/bfm.2016.29031.egb

Boyd, A. E., & Spatz, D. L. (2013). Breastfeeding and human lactation: Education and curricular issues for pediatric nurse practitioners. *Journal of Pediatric Health Care, 27*(2), 83–90. doi:10.1016/j.pedhc.2011.03.005

Bramson, L., Lee, J. W., Moore, E., Montgomery, S., Neish, S., Bahjri, K., & Melcher, C. (2010). Effect of early skin-to-skin mother-infant contact during the first 3 hours following birth on exclusive breastfeeding during the maternity hospital stay. *Journal of Human Lactation, 26*(2), 130–137. doi:10.1177/0890334409355779

Briggs, G. G., Freeman, R. K., Towers, C. V., & Forinash, A. B. (Eds.). (2017). *Drugs in pregnancy and lactation: A reference guide to fetal and neonatal risk* (11th ed.). Philadelphia, PA: Wolters Kluwer.

Brimdyr, K., Cadwell, K., Widström, A., Svensson, K., Neumann, M., Hart, E. A., . . . Phillips, R. (2015). The association between common labor drugs and suckling when skin-to-skin during the first hour after birth. *Birth, 42*(4), 319–328. doi:10.1111/birt.12186

Britton, C., McCormick, F. M., Renfrew, M. J., Wade, A., & King, S. E. (2007). Support for breastfeeding mothers. *Cochrane Database of Systematic Reviews,* (1), CD001141. doi:10.1002/14651858.CD001141.pub3

Brockway, M., & Venturato, L. (2016). Breastfeeding beyond infancy: A concept analysis. *Journal of Advanced Nursing, 72*(9), 2003–2015. doi:10.1111/jan.13000

Brown, P. A., Kaiser, K. L., & Nailon, R. E. (2014). Integrating quality improvement and translational research models to increase exclusive breastfeeding. *Journal of Obstetrics, Gynecologic, and Neonatal Nursing, 43*(5), 545–553. doi:10.1111/1552-6909.12482

Buccini, G. D. S., Pérez-Escamilla, R., & Venancio, S. I. (2016). Pacifier use and exclusive breastfeeding in Brazil. *Journal of Human Lactation, 32*(3), NP52–NP60. doi:10.1177/0890334415609611

Buck, M. L., Amir, L. H., Cullinane, M., & Donath, S. M. (2014). Nipple pain, damage, and vasospasm in the first 8 weeks postpartum. *Breastfeeding Medicine, 9*(2), 56–62. doi:10.1089/bfm.2013.0106

Buckley, S. J. (2015). *Hormonal physiology of childrearing: Evidence and implications for women babies, and maternity care.* Washington, DC: Childbirth Connection Programs, National Partnership for Women and Families.

Butte, N. F. (2009). Impact of infant feeding practices on childhood obesity. *Journal of Nutrition, 139*(2), 412S–416S. doi:10.3945/jn.108.097014

California Perinatal Quality Care Collaborative. (2008). *Nutritional support of the VLBW infant* (Toolkit). Stanford, CA: Author.

Callen, J., & Pinnelli, J. (2004). Incidence and duration of breastfeeding for term infants in Canada, United States, Europe, and Australia: A literature review. *Birth, 31*(4), 285–292.

Castrucci, B. C., Hoover, K. L., Lim, S., & Maus, K. C. (2007). Availability of lactation counseling services influences breastfeeding among infants admitted to neonatal intensive care units. *American Journal of Health Promotion, 21*(5), 410–415.

Centers for Disease Control and Prevention. (2010). *Proper storage and preparation of breast milk.* Atlanta, GA: Author.

Centers for Disease Control and Prevention. (2015). *Hospital actions affect breastfeeding.* Atlanta, GA: Author.

Centers for Disease Control and Prevention. (2017). *Breastfeeding among U.S. children born 2002-2014, CDC National Immunization Survey.* Atlanta, GA: Author.

Chantry, C. J., Dewey, K. G., Peerson, J. M., Wagner, E. A., & Nommsen-Rivers, L. A. (2014). In-hospital formula use increases early breastfeeding cessation among first-time mothers intending to exclusively breastfeed. *The Journal of Pediatrics, 164*(6), 1339e.5–1345.e5. doi:10.1016/j.jpeds.2013.12.035

Chantry, C. J., Nommensen-Rivers, L. A., Peerson, J. M., Cohen, R. J., & Dewey, K. G. (2011). Excess weight loss in first-born breastfed newborns related to maternal intrapartum fluid balance. *Pediatrics, 127*(1), e171–e179. doi:10.1542/peds.2009-2663

Chapman, D. J., Morel, K., Anderson, A. K., Damio, G., & Pérez-Escamilla, R. (2010). Breastfeeding peer counseling: From efficacy through scale-up. *Journal of Human Lactation, 26*(3), 314–326. doi:10.1177/0890334410369481

Chauhan, M., Henderson, G., & McGuire, W. (2008). Enteral feeding for very low birth weight infants: Reducing the risk of necrotising enterocolitis. *Archives of Disease in Childhood. Fetal and Neonatal Edition, 93*(2), F162–F166. doi:10.1136/adc.2007.115824

Chaves, R., Lamounier, J. A., & César, C. C. (2007). Factors associated with duration of breastfeeding. *Jornal de Pediatria, 83*(3), 241–246.

Chezem, J., Friesen, C., & Boettcher, J. (2003). Breastfeeding knowledge, breastfeeding confidence, and infant feeding plans: Effects on actual feeding practices. *Journal of Obstetric, Gynecologic, and Neonatal Nursing, 32*(1), 40–47.

Chowdhury, R., Sinha, B., Sankar, M. J., Taneja, S., Bhandari, N., Rollins, N., . . . Martines, J. (2015). Breastfeeding and maternal health outcomes: A systematic review and meta-analysis. *Acta Paediatrica, 104*(467), 96–113. doi:10.1111/apa.13102

Chung, M., Raman, G., Trikalinos, T., Lau, J., & Ip, S. (2008). Interventions in primary care to promote breastfeeding: An evidence review to the U.S. Preventive Services Task Force. *Annals of Internal Medicine, 149*(8), 565–582.

Coca, K. P., Marcacine, K. O., Gamba, M. A., Corrêa, L., Aranha, A. C. C., & Abrão, A. C. (2016). Efficacy of low-level laser therapy in relieving nipple pain in breastfeeding women: A triple-blind, randomized, controlled trial. *Pain Management Nursing, 17*(4), 281–289. doi:10.1016/j.pmn.2016.05.003

Collins, C. T., Gillis, J., McPhee, A. J., Suganuma, H., & Makrides, M. (2016). Avoidance of bottles during the establishment of breast feeds in preterm infants. *Cochrane Database of Systematic Reviews*, (10), CD005252. doi:10.1002/14651858.CD005252.pub4

Colson, S. D. (2012). Biological nurturing: The laid-back breastfeeding revolution. *Midwifery Today, 101*, 9–11, 66.

Colson, S. D., Meek, J. H., & Hawdon, J. M. (2008). Optimal positions for the release of primitive neonatal reflexes stimulating breastfeeding. *Early Human Development, 84*(7), 441–449.

De la Mora, A., Russell, D. W., Dungy, C. I., Losch, M., & Dusdieker, L. (1999). The Iowa Infant Feeding Attitude Scale: Analysis of reliability and validity. *Journal of Applied Social Psychology, 29*(11), 2362–2380.

Dennis, C. (2003). The breastfeeding self-efficacy scale: Psychometric assessment of the short form. *Journal of Obstetric, Gynecologic, and Neonatal Nursing, 32*(6), 734–744.

Dennis, C., Jackson, K., & Watson, J. (2014). Interventions for treating painful nipples among breastfeeding women. *Cochrane Database of Systematic Reviews*, (12), CD007366. doi:10.1002/14651858.CD007366.pub2

Dias, J. S., Vieira, T. O., & Vieira, G. O. (2017). Factors associated to nipple trauma in lactation period: A systematic review. *Revista Brasileira de Saúde Materno Infantil, 17*(1), 27–42.

DiGirolamo, A. M., Grummer-Strawn, L. M., & Fein, S. B. (2008). Effect of maternity-care practices on breastfeeding. *Pediatrics, 122*, S43–S49. doi:10.1542/peds.2008-1351e

DiTomasso, D., & Paiva, A. L. (2018). Neonatal weight matters: An examination of weight changes in full-term breastfeeding newborns during the first 2 weeks of life. *Journal of Human Lactation, 34*(1), 86–92. doi:10.1177/0890334417722508

Dyson, L., Green, J. M., Renfrew, M. J., McMillan, B., & Woolridge, M. (2010). Factors influencing the infant feeding decision for socioeconomically deprived pregnant teenagers: The moral dimension. *Birth, 37*(2), 141–149. doi:10.1111/j.1523-536X.2010.00394.x

Ekström, A., Widström, A. M., & Nissen, E. (2003). Duration of breastfeeding in Swedish primiparous and multiparous women. *Journal of Human Lactation, 19*(2), 172–178.

Erickson, E. N., & Emeis, C. L. (2017). Breastfeeding outcomes after oxytocin use during childbirth: An integrative review. *Journal of Midwifery & Women's Health, 62*(4), 397–417. doi:10.1111/jmwh.12601

Evans, A., Marinelli, K. A., & Taylor, J. S. (2014). ABM Clinical Protocol #2: Guidelines for hospital discharge of the breastfeeding term newborn and mother: "The going home protocol," revised 2014. *Breastfeeding Medicine, 9*(1), 3–8. doi:10.1089/bfm.2014.9996

Feldman, R., & Bakermans-Kranenburg, M. J. (2017). Oxytocin: A parenting hormone. *Current Opinion in Psychology, 15*, 13–18. doi:10.1016/j.copsyc.2017.02.011

Flaherman, V. J., & Maisels, J. (2017). ABM Clinical Protocol #22: Guidelines for management of jaundice in breastfeeding infant 35 weeks or more gestation—Revised 2017. *Breastfeeding Medicine, 12*(5), 250–257. doi:10.1089/bfm.2017.29042.vjf

Flint, A., New, K., & Davies, M. W. (2016). Cup feeding versus other forms of supplemental enteral feeding for newborn infants unable to fully breastfeed. *Cochrane Database of Systematic Reviews*, (8), CD005092. doi:10.1002/14651858.CD005092.pub3

Forde, K. A., & Miller, L. J. (2010). 2006-07 North Metropolitan Perth breastfeeding cohort study: How long are mothers breastfeeding? *Breastfeeding Review, 18*(2), 14–24.

Forlenza, G. P., Paradise Black, N. M., McNamara, E. G., & Sullivan, S. E. (2010). Ankyloglossia, exclusive breastfeeding, and failure to thrive. *Pediatrics, 125*(6), e1500–e1504. doi:10.1542/peds.2009-2101

Forster, D. A., Johns, H. M., McLachlan, H. L., Moorhead, A. M., McEgan, K. M., & Amir, L. H. (2018). Feeding infants directly at the breast during the postpartum hospital stay is associated with increased breastfeeding at 6 months postpartum: A prospective cohort study. *BMJ Open, 5*, e007512. doi:10.1136/bmjopen-2014-007512

Forster, D. A., & McLachlan, H. L. (2007). Breastfeeding initiation and birth setting practices: A review of the literature. *Journal of Midwifery & Women's Health, 52*(3), 273–280.

Francis, D. O., Krishnaswami, S., & McPheeters, M. (2015). Treatment of ankyloglossia and breastfeeding outcomes: A systematic review. *Pediatrics, 135*(6), e1458–e1466. doi:10.1542/peds.2015-0658

French, C. A., Cong, X., & Chung, K. S. (2016). *Labor epidural analgesia and breastfeeding: A systematic review.* Los Angeles, CA: Sage. doi:10.1177/0890334415623779

Galligan, M. (2006). Proposed guidelines for skin-to-skin treatment of neonatal hypothermia. *MCN: The American Journal of Maternal Child Nursing, 31*(5), 298–306.

Gatti, L. (2008). Maternal perceptions of inadequate milk supply in breastfeeding. *Journal of Nursing Scholarship, 40*(4), 355–363.

Geddes, D. T., Langton, D. B., Gollow, I., Jacobs, L. A., Hartman, P. E., & Simmer, K. (2008). Frenulotomy for breastfeeding infants with ankyloglossia: Effect on milk removal and sucking mechanism as imaged by ultrasound. *Pediatrics, 122*(1), e188–e194. doi:10.1542/peds.2007-2553

Goer, M. W., Davis, M. W., & Hemphill, J. (2002). Postpartum stress: Current concepts and the possible protective role of breastfeeding. *Journal of Obstetric, Gynecologic, and Neonatal Nursing, 31*(4), 411–417.

Grassley, J. S., Spencer, B. S., & Bryson, D. (2013). The development and psychometric testing of the Supportive Needs of Adolescents Breastfeeding Scale. *Journal of Advanced Nursing, 69*(3), 708–716. doi:10.1111/j.1365-2648.2012.06119.x

Grey Bruce Health Services—Owen Sound. (2007). *Adapted LAT.*

Griffiths, L. J., Smeeth, L., Hawkins, S. S., Cole, T. J., & Dezateux, C. (2009). Effects of infant feeding practices on weight gain from birth to 3 years. *Archives of Diseases in Childhood, 94*(8), 577–582. doi:10.1136/adc.2008.137554

Guala, A., Boscardini, L., Visentin, R., Angellotti, P., Grugni, L., Barbaglia, M., . . . Finale, E. (2017). Skin-to-skin contact in cesarean birth and duration of breastfeeding: A cohort study. *The Scientific World Journal*, *2017*, 1940756. doi:10.1155 /2017/1940756

Gulick, E. E. (1986). The effects of breast-feeding on toddler health. *Pediatric Nursing*, *12*(1), 51–54.

Guo, M. (Ed.). (2014). *Human milk biochemistry and infant formula manufacturing technology*. Cambridge, United Kingdom: Woodhead.

Gunderson, E. P., Jacobs, D. R., Chiang, V., Lewis, C. E., Feng, J., Quesenberry, C. P., Jr., & Sidney, S. (2010). Duration of lactation and incidence of the metabolic syndrome in women of reproductive age according to gestational diabetes mellitus status: A 20-year prospective study in CARDIA (Coronary Artery Risk Development in Young Adults). *Diabetes*, *59*(2), 495–504.

Hake-Brooks, S. J., & Anderson, G. C. (2008). Kangaroo care and breastfeeding of mother-preterm infant dyads 0-18 months: A randomized, controlled trial. *Neonatal Network*, *27*(3), 151–159.

Hale, T., & Rowe, H. E. (2017). *Medications and mothers' milk* (17th ed.). New York, NY: Springer.

Hall, R. T., Mercer, A. M., Teasley, S. L., McPherson, D. M., Simon, S. D., Santos, S. R., & Hipsh, N. E. (2002). A breast-feeding assessment score to evaluate the risk for cessation of breast-feeding by 7 to 10 days of age. *Journal of Pediatrics*, *141*(5), 659–664.

Hamilton, B. E., Martin, J. A., & Ventura, S. J. (2007). Births: Preliminary data for 2006. *National Vital Statistics Reports*, *56*(7), 1–18.

Hannula, L., Kaunonen, M., & Tarkka, M. T. (2008). A systematic review of professional support interventions for breastfeeding. *Journal of Clinical Nursing*, *17*(9), 1132–1143. doi:10.1111 /j.1365-2702.2007.02239.x

Haroon, S., Das, J. K., Salam, R. A., Imdad, A., & Bhutta, Z. A. (2013). Breastfeeding promotion interventions and breastfeeding practices: A systematic review. *BMC Public Health*, *13*(Suppl. 3), S20. doi:10.1186/1471-2458-13-S3-S20

Hauck, Y., Fenwick, J., Dhaliwal, S., & Butt, J. (2010). A Western Australian survey of breastfeeding initiation, prevalence and early cessation patterns. *Maternal and Child Health Journal*, *15*(2), 260–268. doi:10.1007/s10995-009-0554-2

Healthy Children Project. (2000). *Latch-on Assessment Tool (LAT)*. East Sandwich, MA: Author.

Hedberg Nyqvist, K., & Ewald, U. (1999). Infant and maternal factors in the development of breastfeeding behaviour and breastfeeding outcome in preterm infants. *Acta Paediatrica*, *88*(11), 1194–1203.

Henderson, G., Craig, S., Brocklehurst, P., & McGuire, W. (2009). Enteral feeding regimens and necrotizing enterocolitis in preterm infants: A multicentre case-control study. *Archives of Disease in Childhood. Fetal and Neonatal Edition*, *94*(2), F120–F123.

Hill, P., & Humenick, S. (1996). Development of the H & H Lactation Scale. *Nursing Research*, *45*(3), 136–140.

Hogan, M., Westcott, C., & Griffiths, M. (2005). Randomized, controlled trial of division of tongue-tie in infants with feeding problems. *Journal of Paediatrics and Child Health*, *41*(5–6), 246–250.

Holmes, A. V., McLeod, A. Y., & Bunik, M. (2013). ABM Clinical Protocol #5: Peripartum breastfeeding management for the healthy mother and infant at term, revision 2013. *Breastfeeding Medicine*, *8*(6), 469–473. doi:10.1089/bfm.2013.9979

Hong, P. (2013). Ankyloglossia (tongue-tie). *CMAJ*, *185*(2), E128. doi:10.1503/cmaj.120785

Howard, C. R., Howard, F. M., Lanphear, B., deBlieck, E. A., Eberly, S., & Lawrence, R. A. (1999). The effects of early pacifier use on breastfeeding duration. *Pediatrics*, *103*(3), E33.

Howard, C. R., Howard, F. M., Lanphear, B., deBlieck, E. A., Oakes, D., & Lawrence, R. A. (2003). Randomized clinical trial of pacifier use and bottle-feeding or cupfeeding and their effect on breastfeeding. *Pediatrics*, *111*(3), 511–518.

Hughes, K. N., Rodriguez-Carter, J., Hill, J., Miller, D., & Gomez, C. (2015). Using skin-to-skin contact to increase exclusive breastfeeding at a military medical center. *Nursing for Women's Health*, *19*(6), 478–489. doi:10.1111/1751-486X.12244

Hurst, N. M. (2007). Recognizing and treating delayed or failed lactogenesis II. *Journal of Midwifery & Women's Health*, *52*(6), 588–594.

Infant Formula Nutrient Specifications, 21 C.F.R. § 107.100 (2010). Retrieved from http://www.accessdata.fda.gov/scripts/cdrh/cfdocs /cfcfr/CFRSearch.cfm

Ingram, J., Johnson, D., Copeland, M., Churchill, C., & Taylor, H. (2015). The development of a new breast feeding assessment tool and the relationship with breast feeding self-efficacy. *Midwifery*, *31*, 132–137. doi:10.1016/j.midw.2014.07.001

Ip, S., Chung, M., Raman, G., Chew, P., Magula, N., DeVine, D., & Lau, J. (2007). *Breastfeeding and maternal and infant health outcomes in developed countries* (Evidence Report/Technology Assessment No. 153; AHRQ Publication No. 007-E007). Rockville, MD: Agency for Healthcare Research and Quality.

Jaafar, S. H., Ho, J. J., Jahanfar, S., & Angolkar, M. (2016). Effect of restricted pacifier use in breastfeeding term infants for increasing duration of breastfeeding. *Cochrane Database of Systematic Reviews*, (8), CD007202. doi:10.1002/14651858.CD007202.pub4

Jackson, K. T., & Dennis, C. L. (2017). Lanolin for the treatment of nipple pain in breastfeeding women: A randomized controlled trial. *Maternal & Child Nutrition*, *13*(3). doi:10.1111/mcn.12357

Jansen, E., Mallan, K. M., Byrne, R., Daniels, L. A., & Nicholson, J. M. (2016). Breastfeeding duration and authoritative feeding practices in first-time mothers. *Journal of Human Lactation*, *32*(3), 498–506. doi:10.1177/0890334415618669

Jenks, M. (1991). Latch assessment documentation in the hospital. *Journal of Human Lactation*, *7*(1), 19–20.

Jensen, D., Wallace, S., & Kelsey, P. (1994). LATCH: A breastfeeding charting system and documentation tool. *Journal of Obstetric, Gynecologic, and Neonatal Nursing*, *23*(1), 27–32.

Johnson, T. S., Mulder, P. J., & Strube, K. (2007). Mother-infant breastfeeding progress tool: A guide for education and support of the breastfeeding dyad. *Journal of Obstetric, Gynecologic, and Neonatal Nursing*, *36*(4), 319–327.

Johnson, T. S., & Strube, K. (2011). Breast care during pregnancy. *Journal of Obstetric, Gynecologic, and Neonatal Nursing*, *40*(2), 144–148. doi:10.1111/j.1552-6909.2011.01227.x

Joint Commission. (2010). *Specifications manual for Joint Commission National Quality Measures* (v2011A). Oakbrook Terrace, IL: Author.

Jones, E., Dimmock, P. W., & Spencer, S. A. (2001). A randomised controlled trial to compare methods of milk expression after preterm delivery. *Archives of Disease in Childhood. Fetal and Neonatal Edition*, *85*, F91–F95.

Jones, E., & Hilton, S. (2008). Correctly fitting breast shields are the key to lactation success for pump dependent mothers following preterm delivery. *Journal of Neonatal Nursing*, *15*, 14–17. doi:10.1016/j.jnn.2008.07.011

Jones, E., & Spencer, S. A. (2007). The physiology of lactation. *Paediatrics and Child Health*, *17*(6), 244–248.

Jordan, S., Emery, S., Bradshaw, C., Watkins, A., & Friswell, W. (2005). The impact of intrapartum analgesia on infant feeding. *BJOG*, *112*(7), 927–934.

Kachoria, R., & Oza-Frank, R. (2015). Trends in breastfeeding initiation in the NICU by gestational age in Ohio, 2006-2012. *Birth*, *42*(1), 56–61. doi:10.1111/birt.12146

Keating, J. P., Schears, G. J., & Dodge, P. R. (1991). Oral water intoxication in infants. An American epidemic. *American Journal of Diseases of Children (1960)*, *145*(9), 985–990.

Kent, J. C., Ashton, E., Hardwick, C. M., Rowan, M. K., Chia, E. S., Fairclough, K. A., . . . Geddes, D. T. (2015). Nipple pain in breastfeeding mothers: Incidence, causes and treatments. *International Journal of Environmental Research and Public Health*, *12*(10), 12247–12263. doi:10.3390/ijerph121012247

Kervin, B. E., Kemp, L., & Pulver, L. J. (2010). Types and timing of breastfeeding support and its impact on mothers' behaviours. *Journal of Paediatrics and Child Health*, *46*(3), 85–91.

Kramer, M. S., Aboud, F., Mironova, E., Vanilovich, I., Platt, R. W., Matush, L., . . . Shapiro, S. (2008). Breastfeeding and child cognitive development: New evidence from a large randomized trial. *Archives of General Psychiatry*, *65*(5), 578–584. doi:10.1001/archpsyc.65.5.578

Kramer, M. S., Barr, R. G., Dagenais, S., Yang, H., Jones, P., Ciofani, L., & Jané, F. (2001). Pacifier use, early weaning, and cry/fuss behavior: A randomized controlled trial. *JAMA*, *286*(3), 322–326.

Kronborg, H., & Vaeth, M. (2009). How are effective breastfeeding technique and pacifier use related to breastfeeding problems and breastfeeding duration? *Birth*, *36*(1), 34–42. doi:10.1111/j.1523-536X.2008.00293.x

Labbock, M., & Taylor, E. (2008). *Achieving exclusive breastfeeding in the United States: Findings and recommendations*. Washington, DC: United States Breastfeeding Committee.

Labiner-Wolfe, J., Fein, S. B., & Shealy, K. R. (2008). Infant formula-handling education and safety. *Pediatrics*, *122*, S85–S90. doi:10.1542/peds.2008-1315k

Langellier, B. A., Chaparro, M. P., Wang, M. C., Koleilat, M., & Whaley, S. E. (2014). The new food package and breastfeeding outcomes among women, infants, and children participants in Los Angeles County. *American Journal of Public Health*, *104*(Suppl. 1), S112–S118. doi:10.2105/AJPH.2013.301330

Lau, Y., Htun, T. P., Lim, P. I., Ho-Lim, S., & Klainin-Yobas, P. (2016). Psychometric evaluation of 5- and 4-item versions of the LATCH Breastfeeding Assessment Tool during the initial postpartum period among a multiethnic population. *PLoS One*, *11*(5), e0154331. doi:10.1371/journal.pone.0154331

Lauer, B. J., & Spector, N. D. (2011). Hyperbilirubinemia in the newborn. *Pediatrics in Review*, *32*(8), 341–349. doi:10.1542/pir.32-8-341

Lauwers, J., & Swisher, A. (2016). *Counseling the nursing mother: A lactation consultant's guide* (6th ed.). Burlington, MA: Jones & Bartlett.

Lawrence, R. A., & Lawrence, R. M. (2015). *Breastfeeding: A guide for the medical profession* (8th ed.). Philadelphia, PA: Elsevier.

Lee, F., Edmunds, L. S., Cong, X., & Sekhobo, J. (2017). Trends in breastfeeding among infants enrolled in the special supplemental nutrition program for women, infants, and children—New York, 2002-2015. *MMWR Morbidity and Mortality Weekly Report*, *66*(23), 610–614.

Lessen, R., & Kavanagh, K. (2015). Position of the Academy of Nutrition and Dietetics: Promoting and supporting breastfeeding. *Journal of the Academy of Nutrition and Dietetics*, *115*(3), 444–449. doi:10.1016/j.jand.2014.12.014

Li, R., Fein, S. B., Chen, J., & Grummer-Strawn, L. M. (2008). Why mothers stop breastfeeding: Mothers' self-reported reasons for stopping during the first year. *Pediatrics*, *122*(Suppl. 2), S69–S76. doi:10.1542/peds.2008-1315i

Linares, A. M., Wambach, K., Rayens, M. K., Wiggins, A., Coleman, E., & Dignan, M. B. (2017). Modeling the influence of early skin-to-skin contact on exclusive breastfeeding in a sample of Hispanic immigrant women. *Journal of Immigrant and Minority Health*, *19*(5), 1027–1034. doi:10.1007/s10903-016-0380-8

Lind, J. N., Perrine, C. G., & Li, R. (2014). Relationship between use of labor pain medications and delayed onset of lactation. *Journal of Human Lactation*, *30*(2), 167–173. doi:10.1177/0890334413520189

Lochner, J. E., Livingston, C. J., & Judkins, D. Z. (2009). Clinical inquiries: Which interventions are best for alleviating nipple pain in nursing mothers? *The Journal of Family Practice*, *58*(11), 612a–612c.

Lucas, A., Lockton, S., & Davies, P. S. (1992). Randomised trial of a ready-to-feed compared with powdered formula. *Archives of Disease in Childhood*, *67*(7), 935–939.

Lutsiv, O., Pullenayegum, E., Foster, G., Vera, C., Giglia, L., Chapman, B., . . . McDonald, S. (2013). Women's intentions to breastfeed: A population-based cohort study. *BJOG*, *120*, 1490–1498. doi:10.1111/1471-0528.12376

Maisels, M. J., Bhutani, V. K., Bogen, D., Newman, T. B., Stark, A. R., & Watchko, J. F. (2009). Hyperbilirubinemia in the newborn infant > or =35 weeks' gestation: An update with clarifications. *Pediatrics*, *124*(4), 1193–1198. doi:10.1542/peds.2009-0329

Mangesi, L., & Zakarija-Grkovic, I. (2016). Treatments for breast engorgement during lactation. *Cochrane Database of Systematic Reviews*, (6), CD006946. doi:10.1002/14651858.CD006946.pub3

Matthews, M. K. (1988). Developing an instrument to assess infant breastfeeding behaviour in the early neonatal period. *Midwifery*, *4*(4), 154–165.

Mauri, P. A., Contini, N. N. G., Giliberti, S., Barretta, F., Consonni, D., Negri, M., & Di Benedetto, I. (2015). Intrapartum epidural analgesia and onset of lactation: A prospective study in an Italian birth centre. *Maternal and Child Health Journal*, *19*(3), 511–518. doi:10.1007/s10995-014-1532-x

McCall, E., Alderdice, F., Halliday, H. L., Jenkins, J. G., & Vohra, S. (2010). Interventions to prevent hypothermia at birth in preterm and/or low birthweight infants. *Cochrane Database of Systematic Reviews*, (1), CD004210. doi:10.1002/14651858.CD004210.pub3

Meier, P. P., Furman, L. M., & Degenhardt, M. (2007). Increased lactation risk for late preterm infants and mothers: Evidence and management strategies to protect breastfeeding. *Journal of Midwifery & Women's Health*, *52*, 579–587.

Meier, P. P., Patel, A. L., Hoban, R., & Engstrom, J. L. (2016). Which breast pump for which mother: An evidence-based approach to individualizing breast pump technology. *Journal of Perinatology*, *36*(7), 493–499. doi:10.1038/jp.2016.14

Melli, M. S., Rashidi, M. R., Nokohoodchi, A., Tagavi, S., Farzadi, L., Sadaghat, K., . . . Sheshvan, M. K. (2007). A randomized trial of peppermint gel, lanolin ointment and placebo gel to prevent nipple crack in primiparous breastfeeding women. *Medical Science Monitor*, *13*(9), CR406–CR411.

Merewood, A., Brooks, D., Bauchner, H., MacAuley, L., & Mehta, S. D. (2006). Maternal birthplace and breastfeeding initiation among term and preterm infants: A statewide assessment for Massachusetts. *Pediatrics*, *118*(4), e1048–e1054.

Merten, S., Dratva, J., & Ackermann-Liebrich, U. (2005). Do baby-friendly hospitals influence breastfeeding duration on a national level? *Pediatrics*, *116*(5), e702–e708. doi:10.1542/peds.2005-0537

Mihrshahi, S., Oddy, W. H., Peat, J. K., & Kabir, I. (2008). Association between infant feeding patterns and diarrhoeal and respiratory illness: A cohort study in Chittagong, Bangladesh. *International Breastfeeding Journal*, *3*, 28. doi:10.1186/1746-4538-3-28

Monterroso, E. C., Frongillo, E. A., Vásquez-Garibay, E. M., Romero-Velarde, E., Casey, L. M., & Willows, N. D. (2008). Predominant breast-feeding from birth to six months is associated with fewer gastrointestinal infections and increased risk for iron deficiency among infants. *Journal of Nutrition*, *138*(8), 1499–1504.

Moon, R. (2016). SIDS and other sleep-related infant deaths: Evidence base for 2016 updated recommendations for a safe infant sleeping environment. *Pediatrics*, *138*(5), e1–e34. doi:10.1542/peds.2016-2940

Moore, E. R., Bergman, N., Anderson, G. D., & Medley, N. (2016). Early skin-to-skin contact for mothers and their healthy newborn infants. *Cochrane Database of Systematic Reviews*, (11), CD003519. doi:10.1002/14651858.CD003519.pub4

Morland-Schultz, K., & Hill, P. (2005). Prevention of and therapies for nipple pain: A systematic review. *Journal of Obstetric, Gynecologic, and Neonatal Nursing*, *34*(4), 428–443. doi:10.1177/0884217505276056

Muchowski, K. E. (2014). Evaluation and treatment of neonatal hyperbilirubinemia. *American Family Physician*, *89*(11), 873–878.

Mulford, C. (1992). The Mother-Baby Assessment (MBA): An "Apgar score" for breastfeeding. *Journal of Human Lactation*, *8*(2), 79–82.

Munn, A. C., Newman, S. D., Mueller, M., Phillips, S. M., & Taylor, S. N. (2016). The impact in the United States of the Baby-Friendly Hospital Initiative on early infant health and breastfeeding outcomes. *Breastfeeding Medicine*, *11*, 222–230. doi:10.1089/bfm.2015.0135

Murray, E. K., Ricketts, S., & Dellaport, J. (2007). Hospital practices that increase breastfeeding duration: Results from a population-based study. *Birth*, *34*(3), 202–211.

Napierala, M., Mazela, J., Merritt, T. A., & Florek, E. (2016). Tobacco smoking and breastfeeding: Effect on the lactation process, breast milk composition and infant development. A critical review. *Environmental Research*, *151*, 321–338. doi:10.1016/j.envres.2016.08.002

Natland Fagerhaug, T., Forsmo, S., Jacobsen, G. W., Midthjell, K., Andersen, L. F., & Ivar Lund Nilsen, T. (2013). A prospective population-based cohort study of lactation and cardiovascular disease mortality: The HUNT study. *BMC Public Health*, *13*(1), 1070. doi:10.1186/1471-2458-13-1070

Neifert, M., & Bunik, M. (2013). Overcoming clinical barriers to exclusive breastfeeding. *Pediatric Clinics of North America*, *60*(1), 115–145. doi:10.1016/j.pcl.2012.10.001

Nelson, E. A., Yu, L., & Williams, S. (2005). International child care practices study: Breastfeeding and pacifier use. *Journal of Human Lactation*, *21*(3), 289–295.

Nelson, J. M., Li, R., & Perrine, C. G. (2015). Trends of US hospitals distributing infant formula packs to breastfeeding mothers, 2007 to 2013. *Pediatrics*, *135*(6), 1051–1056. doi:10.1542/peds.2015-0093

Nommsen-Rivers, L. A., Chantry, C. J., Peerson, J. M., Cohen, R. J., & Dewey, K. G. (2010). Delayed onset of lactogenesis among first-time mothers is related to maternal obesity and factors associated with ineffective breastfeeding. *American Journal of Clinical Nutrition*, *92*(3), 574–584. doi:10.3945/ajcn.2010.29192

Nyqvist, K. H., Rubertsson, C., Ewald, U., & Sjödén, P. O. (1996). Development of the Preterm Infant Breastfeeding Behavior Scale (PIBBS): A study of nurse-mother agreement. *Journal of Human Lactation*, *12*(3), 207–219.

Ogbuanu, I. U., Karmaus, W., Arshad, S. H., Kurukulaaratchy, R. J., & Ewart, S. (2009). Effect of breastfeeding duration on lung function at age 10 years: A prospective birth cohort study. *Thorax*, *64*(1), 62–66. doi:10.1136/thx.2008.101543

Palmer, M. M. (1993). Identification and management of the transitional suck pattern in premature infants. *The Journal of Perinatal & Neonatal Nursing*, *7*(1), 66–75.

Parker, L. A., Sullivan, S., Krueger, C., & Mueller, M. (2015). Association of timing of initiation of breastmilk expression on milk volume and timing of lactogenesis stage II among mothers of very low-birth-weight infants. *Breastfeeding Medicine*, *10*(2), 84–91. doi:10.1089/bfm.2014.0089

Patnode, C. D., Henninger, M. L., Senger, C. A., Perdue, L. A., & Whitlock, E. P. (2016). Primary care interventions to support breastfeeding: Updated evidence report and systematic review for the US Preventive Services Task Force. *JAMA*, *316*(16), 1694–1705. doi:10.1001/jama.2016.8882

Pérez-Escamilla, R., Martinez, J. L., & Segura-Perez, S. (2016). Impact of the Baby-Friendly Hospital Initiative on breastfeeding ad child health outcomes: A systematic review. *Maternal & Child Nutrition*, *12*(3), 402–417. doi:10.1111/mcn.12294

Perrine, C. G., Galuska, D. A., Dohack, J. L., Shealy, K. R., Murphy, P. E., Grummer-Strawn, L. M., & Scanlon, K. S. (2015). Vital signs: Improvements in maternity care policies and practices that support breastfeeding—United States, 2007-2013. *MMWR Morbidity and Mortality Weekly Report*, *64*(39), 1112–1117.

Phares, T. M., Morrow, B., Lansky, A., Barfield, W. D., Prince, C. B., Marchi, K. S., . . . Kinniburgh, B. (2004). Surveillance for disparities in maternal health-related behaviors—Selected states, Pregnancy Risk Assessment Monitoring Systems (PRAMS), 2000-2001. *Morbidity and Mortality Weekly Report Surveillance Summaries*, *53*(4), 1–13.

Philipp, B. L. (2010). ABM Clinical Protocol #7: Model breastfeeding policy (revision 2010). *Breastfeeding Medicine*, *5*(4), 173–177. doi:10.1089/bfm.2010.9986

Pincombe, J., Baghurst, P., Antoniou, G., Peat, B., Henderson, A., & Reddin, E. (2008). Baby-Friendly Hospital Initiative practices and breast feeding duration in a cohort of first-time mothers in Adelaide, Australia. *Midwifery*, *24*(1), 55–61.

Preusting, I., Brumley, J., Odibo, L., Spatz, D. L., & Louis, J. M. (2017). Obesity as a predictor of delayed lactogenesis II. *Journal of Human Lactation*, *33*(4), 684–691. doi:10.1177/0890334417727716

Radzyminski, S., & Callister, L. C. (2016). Mother's beliefs, attitudes, and decision making related to infant feeding choices. *The Journal of Perinatal Education*, *25*(1), 18–28. doi:10.1891/1058-1243.25.1.18

Ransjö-Arvidson, A. B., Matthiesen, A. S., Lilja, G., Nissen, E., Widström, A. M., & Uvnäs-Moberg, K. (2001). Maternal analgesia during labor disturbs newborn behavior: Effects on breastfeeding, temperature, and crying. *Birth*, *28*(1), 5–12.

Rees, D. I., & Sabia, J. J. (2009). The effect of breastfeeding on educational attainment: New evidence from siblings. *Journal of Human Capital*, *3*(1), 43–72.

Renfrew, M. J., Craig, D., Dyson, L., McCormick, F., Rice, S., King, S. E., . . . Williams, A. F. (2009). Breastfeeding promotion for infants in neonatal units: A systematic review and economic analysis. *Health Technology Assessment*, *13*(40), 1–146.

Renfrew, M. J., Lang, S., Martin, L., & Woolridge, M. W. (2000). Feeding schedules in hospitals for newborn infants. *Cochrane Database of Systematic Reviews*, (2), CD000090.

Righard, L. (2008). The baby is breastfeeding—Not the mother. *Birth*, *35*(1), 1–2.

Rodríguez-García, J., & Acosta-Ramírez, N. (2008). Factors affecting how long exclusive breastfeeding lasts. *Revista de Salud Publica (Bogota, Colombia)*, *10*(1), 71–84.

Rogan, W. J., Paulson, J. A., Baum, C., Brock-Utne, A. C., Brumberg, H. L., Campbell, C. C., . . . Trasande, L. (2014). Iodine deficiency, pollutant chemicals, and the thyroid: New information on an old problem. *Pediatrics*, *133*(6), 1163–1166. doi:10.1542/peds.2014-0900

Roll, C. L., & Cheater, F. (2016). Expectant parents' views of factors influencing infant feeding decisions in the antenatal period: A systematic review. *International Journal of Nursing Studies*, *60*, 145–155. doi:10.1016/j.ijnurstu.2016.04.011

Rollins, N. C., Bhandari, N., Hajeebhoy, N., Horton, S., Lutter, C. K., Martines, J. C., . . . Victoria, C. G. (2016). Why invest, and what it will take to improve breastfeeding practices? *Lancet*, *387*(10017), 491–504. doi:10.1016/S0140-6736(15)01044-2

Rosenberg, K. D., Eastham, C. A., Kasehagen, L. J., & Sandoval, A. P. (2008). Marketing infant formula through hospitals: The impact of commercial hospital discharge. *American Journal of Public Health*, *98*(2), 290–295.

Rosenberg, K. D., Stull, J. D., Adler, M. R., Kasehagen, L. J., & Crivelli-Kovach, A. (2008). Impact of hospital policies on breastfeeding outcomes. *Breastfeeding Medicine*, *3*(2), 110–116.

Rosen-Carole, C., & Hartman, S. (2015). ABM Clinical Protocol #19: Breastfeeding promotion in the prenatal setting, revision 2015. *Breastfeeding Medicine*, *10*(10), 451–457. doi:10.1089/bfm.2015.29016.ros

Rowan-Legg, A. (2015). Ankyloglossia and breastfeeding. *Paediatrics & Child Health*, 20(4), 209–213.

Ryan, A., & Zhou, W. (2006). Lower breastfeeding rates persist among the special supplemental nutrition program for women, infants, and children participants, 1978-2003. *Pediatrics*, 117(4), 1136–1142.

Saarela, T., Kokkonen, J., & Koivisto, M. (2005). Macronutrient and energy content of human milk fractions during the first six months of lactation. *Acta Paediatrica*, 94(9), 1176–1181.

Schafer, R., & Genna, C. W. (2015). Physiologic breastfeeding: A contemporary approach to breastfeeding initiation. *Journal of Midwifery & Women's Health*, 60(5), 546–553. doi:10.1111/jmwh.12319

Schwarz, E. B., Brown, J. S., Creasman, J. M., Stuebe, A., McClure, C. K., Van Den Eeden, S. K., & Thom, D. (2010). Lactation and maternal risk of type 2 diabetes: A population-based study. *The American Journal of Medicine*, 123(9), 863.e1–863.e6. doi:10.1016/j.amjmed.2010.03.016

Schwarz, E. B., Ray, R. M., Stuebe, A. M., Allison, M. A., Ness, R. B., Freiberg, M. S., & Cauley, J. A. (2009). Duration of lactation and risk factors for maternal cardiovascular disease. *Obstetrics & Gynecology*, 113(5), 974–982. doi:10.1097/01.AOG.0000346884.67796.ca

Scott, J. A., Binns, C. W., & Oddy, W. H. (2007). Predictors of delayed onset of lactation. *Maternal & Child Nutrition*, 3(3), 186–193. doi:10.1111/j.1740-8709.2007.00096.x

Sexton, S., & Natale, R. (2009). Risks and benefits of pacifiers. *American Family Physician*, 79(8), 681–685.

Shrago, L., & Bocar, D. (1990). The infant's contribution to breastfeeding. *Journal of Obstetric, Gynecologic, and Neonatal Nursing*, 19, 209–215.

Sikorski, J., Renfrew, M. J., Rindoria, S., & Wade, A. (2002). Support for breastfeeding mothers. *Cochrane Database of Systematic Reviews*, (2), CD001141.

Sinha, B., Chowdhury, R., Sankar, M. J., Martines, J., Taneja, S., Mazumder, S., . . . Bhandari, N. (2015). Interventions to improve breastfeeding outcomes: A systematic review and meta-analysis. *Acta Paediatrica*, 104(467), 114–134. doi:10.1111/apa.13127

Sloan, S., Stewart, M., & Dunne, L. (2010). The effect of breastfeeding and stimulation in the home on cognitive development in one-year-old infants. *Child Care in Practice*, 16(2), 101–110.

Sriraman, N. K., & Kellams, A. (2016). Breastfeeding: What are the barriers? Why women struggle to achieve their goals. *Journal of Women's Health*, 25(7), 714–722. doi:10.1089/jwh.2014.5059

Stuebe, A. M., Horton, B. J., Chetwynd, E., Watkins, S., Grewen, K., & Meltzer-Brody, S. (2014). Prevalence and risk factors for early, undesired weaning attributed to lactation dysfunction. *Journal of Women's Health*, 23(5), 404–412. doi:10.1089/jwh.2013.4506

Stuebe, A. M., & Schwarz, E. B. (2010). The risks and benefits of infant feeding practices for women and children. *Journal of Perinatology*, 30(3), 155–162. doi:10.1038/jp.2009.107

Swanson, V., Power, K., Kaur, B., Carter, H., & Shepherd, K. (2007). The impact of knowledge and social influences on adolescents' breast-feeding beliefs and intentions. *Public Health Nutrition*, 9(3), 297–305.

Taylor, J. S., Kacmar, J. E., Nothnagle, M., & Lawrence, R. (2005). A systematic review of the literature associating breastfeeding with type 2 diabetes and gestational diabetes. *Journal of the American College of Nutrition*, 24(5), 320–326.

Thomas, J., & Marinelli, K. A. (2016). ABM Clinical Protocol #16: Breastfeeding the hypotonic infant, revision 2016. *Breastfeeding Medicine*, 11(6), 271–276. doi:10.1089/bfm.2016.29014.jat

Thulier, D. (2017). Challenging expected patterns of weight loss in full-term breastfeeding neonates born by cesarean. *Journal of Obstetric, Gynecologic, and Neonatal Nursing*, 46, 18–28.

Truchet, S., & Honvo-Houéto, E. (2017). Physiology of milk secretion. *Best Practice & Research. Clinical Endocrinology & Metabolism*, 31(4), 367–384. doi:10.1016/j.beem.2017.10.008

Tully, S. B., Bar-Haim, Y., & Bradley, R. L. (1995). Abnormal tympanography after supine bottle feeding. *The Journal of Pediatrics*, 126(6), S105–S111.

United Nations International Children's Emergency Fund United Kingdom. (n.d.). *The Baby Friendly Initiative: Breastfeeding Assessment Tools*. London, UK: Author.

United States Breastfeeding Committee. (2010). *Core competencies in breastfeeding care and services for all health professionals*. Washington, DC: Author.

U.S. Department of Health and Human Services. (2008). *The Business Case for Breastfeeding: Steps for creating a breastfeeding friendly workplace*. Washington, DC: Author.

U.S. Department of Health and Human Services. (2011). *Healthy People 2020*. Washington, DC: Author.

Van Den Driessche, M., Peeters, K., Marien, P., Ghoos, Y., Devlieger, H., & Veereman-Wauters, G. (1999). Gastric emptying in formula-fed and breastfed infants measured with the 13C-octanoic acid breath test. *Journal of Pediatric Gastroenterology and Nutrition*, 29(1), 46–51.

Victora, C. G., Bahl, R., Barros, A., França, G., Horton, S., Krasevec, J., . . . Rollins, N. C. (2016). Breastfeeding in the 21st century: Epidemiology, mechanisms, and lifelong effect. *Lancet*, 387(10017), 475–490. doi:10.1016/S0140-6736(15)01024-7

Victora, C. G., Behague, D. P., Barros, F. C., Olinto, M. T., & Weiderpass, E. (1997). Pacifier use and short breastfeeding duration: Cause, consequence, or coincidence? *Pediatrics*, 99(3), 445–453.

Vittner, D., McGrath, J., Robinson, J., Lawhon, G., Cusson, R., Eisenfeld, L., . . . Cong, X. (2018). Increase in oxytocin from skin-to-skin contact enhances development of parent–infant relationship. *Biological Research for Nursing*, 20(1), 54–62. doi:10.1177/1099800417735633

Wagner, E. A., Chantry, C. J., Dewey, K. G., & Nommsen-Rivers, L. A. (2013). Breastfeeding concerns at 3 and 7 days postpartum and feeding status at 2 months. *Pediatrics*, 132(4), e865–e875. doi:10.1542/peds.2013-0724

Walker, M. (2017). *Breastfeeding management for the clinician: Using the evidence* (4th ed.). Burlington, MA: Jones & Bartlett.

Walters, M. W., Boggs, K. M., Ludington-Hoe, S., Price, K. M., & Morrison, B. (2007). Kangaroo care at birth of full term infants: A pilot study. *MCN: The American Journal of Maternal Child Nursing*, 32, 375–381.

Wambach, K., & Riordan, J. M. (2016). *Breastfeeding and human lactation* (enhanced 5th ed.). Burlington, MA: Jones & Bartlett Learning.

Wiener, S. (2006). Diagnosis and management of Candida of the nipple and breast. *Journal of Midwifery & Women's Health*, 51(2), 125–128.

Wiklund, I., Norman, M., Uvnäs-Moberg, K., Ransjö-Arvidson, A. B., & Andolf, E. (2009). Epidural analgesia: Breast-feeding success and related factors. *Midwifery*, 25(2), e31–e38.

World Health Organization. (2011a). *Exclusive breastfeeding for six months best for babies everywhere*. Geneva, Switzerland: Author.

World Health Organization. (2011b). *Feeding of low-birth-weight infants in low- and middle-income countries*. Geneva, Switzerland: Author.

World Health Organization. (2014). *Why can't we give water to a breastfeeding baby before the 6 months, even when it is hot?* Geneva, Switzerland: Author.

World Health Organization & Food and Agriculture Organization of the United Nations. (2007). *Safe preparation, storage and handling of powdered infant formula guidelines*. Geneva, Switzerland: World Health Organization.

World Health Organization & United Nations International Children's Emergency Fund Joint Statement. (1989). *Protecting and supporting breastfeeding: The special role of maternity services*. Geneva, Switzerland: World Health Organization.

Wright, M., & Marinelli, K. A. (2014). ABM Clinical Protocol #1: Guidelines for blood glucose monitoring and treatment of hypoglycemia in term and late-preterm neonates, revised 2014. *Breastfeeding Medicine*, 9(4), 173–179. doi:10.1089/bfm.2014.9986

Yi, X., Zhu, J., Zhu, X., Liu, G. J., & Wu, L. (2016). Breastfeeding and thyroid cancer risk in women: A dose-response meta-analysis of epidemiological studies. *Clinical Nutrition (Edinburgh, Scotland)*, 35, 1039–1046. doi:10.1016/j.clnu.2015.12.005

Yilmaz, G., Caylan, N., Karacan, C. D., Bodur, I., & Gokcay, G. (2014). Effect of cup feeding and bottle feeding on breastfeeding in late preterm infants: A randomized controlled study. *Journal of Human Lactation*, 30(2), 174–179. doi:10.1177/0890334413517940

Ziol-Guest, K. M., & Hernandez, D. C. (2010). First- and second-trimester WIC participation is associated with lower rates of breastfeeding and early introduction of cow's milk during infancy. *Journal of the American Dietetic Association*, 110(5), 702–709. doi:10.1016/j.jada.2010.02.013

Zlotnik, P. (2013). *Care and management of the late preterm infant (toolkit)*. Stanford, CA: California Perinatal Quality Care Collaborative.

Zuppa, A. A., Alighieri, G., Riccardi, R., Cavani, M., Iafisco, A., Cota, F., & Romagnoli, C. (2014). Epidural analgesia, neonatal care and breastfeeding. *Italian Journal of Pediatrics*, 40(1), 82. doi:10.1186/s13052-014-0082-6

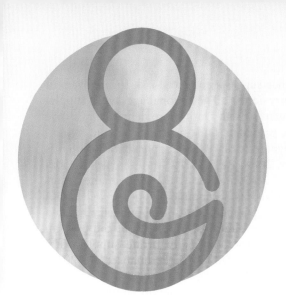

CHAPTER 21

Common Neonatal Complications

Annie J. Rohan

INTRODUCTION

Most newborns with complications are identified and cared for in community hospitals or Level II perinatal centers (American Academy of Pediatrics [AAP], 2012). Perinatal and neonatal nurses at these facilities must have a thorough understanding of pathophysiology and clinical signs of illness during the immediate newborn period. Brief length of stay limits the time to identify behavioral cues or subtle changes that could potentially compromise newborn well-being.

Complications discussed in this chapter include common conditions such as respiratory distress, congenital heart disease (CHD), hypoglycemia, hyperbilirubinemia, and sepsis. Less common but important topics covered include neonatal resuscitation, perinatal HIV-1 exposure, neonatal substance exposure, and hypoxic ischemic encephalopathy (HIE).

NEONATAL RESUSCITATION AND STABILIZATION

Most newborns transition from fetal to extrauterine life uneventfully. However, approximately 1 in 10 will require some assistance after delivery to initiate or sustain respiratory effort, and 1% will require extensive measures to survive. In keeping with the "ABCs" of resuscitation, providers must ensure that the airway is clear and unimpeded, breathing is spontaneous and unassisted, and that circulation is maintained to adequately perfuse tissues and organs. Both the American Heart Association (AHA) and the AAP recommend that all births be attended by someone capable of initiating resuscitation and those resources for sustained resuscitation efforts be available as needed (AAP & AHA, 2016).

Prior to birth, the fetus receives oxygen by diffusion from the mother's blood across the placental membranes. Because the fetal lungs do not participate in oxygenation, only a small fraction of fetal blood passes through them. The fetal alveoli, although round and expanded, are fluid filled and the surrounding arterioles are constricted. The increase in pulmonary vascular resistance (PVR) favors blood flow in a manner, which bypasses the lungs through a series of fetal shunts, allowing delivery of optimally oxygenated blood through the ductus arteriosus to the body. After birth, the placenta no longer supports fetal needs, and the newborn must quickly establish ventilation, clear fluid from the alveoli, and dilate the pulmonary vasculature to support ongoing oxygenation. Failure to do so results in hypoxemia and acidosis. The newborn may respond briefly to hypoxia with compensatory tachypnea, although this is quickly followed by primary apnea and a fall in heart rate. If breathing is not quickly established, secondary apnea occurs and assisted ventilation must be provided to reverse the process (AAP & AHA, 2016).

Certain antepartum and intrapartum risk factors are associated with the need for resuscitation. Maternal factors may be chronic or acute and include such conditions as diabetes, hypertension, cardiopulmonary disease, substance exposure, late trimester bleeding, and infection. Intrapartum factors may also complicate fetal transition, including assisted vaginal birth, cesarean birth, abnormal fetal lie, presence of meconium, and placental complications. Newborns who are postterm, who are premature, or who have size-dates discrepancy pose additional risks for poor transition. An anticipated compromised birth warrants the presence of personnel who can initiate and sustain resuscitation, including use of ventilatory support, chest compressions, and selected medications. However, risk factors are not always apparent and providers must be able to anticipate and intervene quickly to support the compromised newborn. Four assessment prompts will assist with quick identification of newborns who will require support: Is the baby term? Is the amniotic fluid clear? Is the baby breathing? Is there good muscle tone (AAP & AHA, 2016)?

The neonatal resuscitation program (NRP) is an education program endorsed by the AAP to provide a systematic method for managing the compromised newborn. It supports consistent and appropriate actions to address ventilation and circulation needs, which are continually evaluated using an algorithm containing action blocks. The resuscitation sequence begins with positioning the newborn infant on his or her back or side to open the airway and then proceeding to drying and stimulating. It is important to ensure resuscitation occurs in a warm environment. If the infant responds adequately with sustained breathing or crying, additional measures are unnecessary. However, an infant who does not establish sustained breathing is presumed to be exhibiting secondary apnea, and resuscitation commences with assisted ventilation. The infant is continually assessed, and additional interventions are applied according to infant response (AAP & AHA, 2016).

Effective neonatal resuscitation for at-risk infants requires not only dexterity with maneuvers such as ventilation and compressions but also collaboration among a neonatal team to ensure timely and organized support. Poor communication and lack of teamwork have been identified as factors in poor outcomes following neonatal resuscitation (Perlman et al., 2010; Zaichkin & Weiner, 2011). Accordingly, NRP recommendations include a focus on team building and collaboration skills and support learning strategies including use of simulation and debriefing (AAP & AHA, 2016).

NRP guidelines are continually evaluated and updated using best evidence. Since 2006, for example, the NRP has posed updated recommendations for management of meconium-exposed infants based on evidence showing little or no benefit to suctioning—and at least some evidence of potential harm—even in depressed infants (Chettri, Adhisivam, & Bhat, 2015). Therefore, routine immediate suctioning is no longer recommended for any meconium-exposed infant (AAP & AHA, 2016). Data regarding use of supplemental oxygen during neonatal resuscitation is also evolving and the ideal concentration of oxygen during resuscitation is unknown (Rabi, 2010). The use of room air for initial resuscitation of the term infant is currently recognized as acceptable practice if well monitored (AAP & AHA, 2016; Zaichkin & Weiner, 2011).

Data regarding use of supplemental oxygen during neonatal resuscitation is evolving, and the ideal concentration of oxygen during resuscitation is unknown.

Some evidence suggests enhanced risk for inadvertent oxidant injury across all gestational ages when supplemental oxygen is used. Until more definitive evidence is available, providers must attempt to avoid hypoxemia and hyperoxemia when supplemental oxygen is applied (Bry, 2008; Rabi, 2010), and the use of room air for initial resuscitation of the term infant is currently recognized as acceptable practice if well monitored. It is recommended that pulse oximetry be used for neonatal resuscitations, especially of the preterm population, to more optimally titrate supplemental oxygen (AAP & AHA, 2016; Perlman et al., 2010; Zaichkin & Weiner, 2011).

An additional education program endorsed by the AAP is S.T.A.B.L.E., which reinforces key stabilization skills via an acronym: *Sugar, Temperature, Airway, Blood pressure, Lab work assessment, and Emotional support of families*. This program supports birth attendants and nursery staff who participate in postresuscitation/pretransport stabilization of the sick neonate and encourages a systematic approach to management (Taylor & Price-Douglas, 2008). Both S.T.A.B.L.E. and the NRP have been disseminated worldwide as stabilization programs for at-risk neonates.

RESPIRATORY DISTRESS

Respiratory distress is a major cause of neonatal morbidity and mortality despite significant technologic and pharmacologic advances during the past 30 years. Respiratory distress is one of the most common neonatal complications seen by the perinatal and neonatal nurse and is a principal indication for neonatal transfer to tertiary-care units. The pathophysiology and etiology of respiratory distress varies, but the result is decreased ability to exchange the oxygen and carbon dioxide necessary to ensure delivery of well-oxygenated blood to vital organs. Respiratory distress may be an isolated finding or occur in association with other medical or systemic problems. It may be due to structural or functional abnormality, or as a consequence of acute lung injury, and result in prolonged transition to extrauterine life. Five of the most common respiratory diseases occurring during the neonatal period are respiratory distress syndrome (RDS), meconium aspiration syndrome (MAS), pneumonia, transient tachypnea of the newborn (TTNB), and persistent pulmonary hypertension of the newborn (PPHN).

Respiratory Distress Syndrome

RDS primarily occurs in preterm newborns. In the United States, approximately 24,000 newborns each year develop RDS; the incidence of RDS is inversely related to gestational age: 60% of infants born at less than 28 weeks, 30% of those born at 28 to 34 weeks' gestation, and less than 5% of those born after 34 weeks are affected (Warren & Anderson, 2009). The mortality rate for RDS across all gestational ages is currently about 10%, attributable to improved prenatal and postnatal management (Dudell & Stoll, 2007; Warren & Anderson, 2009). RDS is caused by insufficient amounts of surfactant or delayed or impaired surfactant synthesis. Surfactant is a mixture of phospholipids and proteins synthesized, packaged, and excreted by alveolar type II cells that lowers surface tension in the alveoli and functions as a stabilizer to prevent atelectasis and alveolar collapse at end-expiration (Cole, Nogee, & Hamvas, 2006). Without surfactant, atelectasis (alveolar collapse) occurs, resulting in a series of events that progressively increase disease severity. These events include hypoxemia (decreased concentration of oxygen), hypercapnea (increased concentration of carbon dioxide), mismatch of ventilation with perfusion, acidosis, pulmonary vasoconstriction, alveolar endothelial and epithelial damage, and subsequent protein-rich interstitial and alveolar edema. This cascade of events further decreases surfactant synthesis, storage, and release and leads to pulmonary failure (Dudell & Stoll, 2007; Warren & Anderson, 2009).

Meconium Aspiration Syndrome

Passage of meconium in utero or perinatally is primarily seen in term and postterm infants, and those experiencing stress such as growth restricted infants or those with cord complications compromising uteroplacental circulation (Dudell & Stoll, 2007). Meconium passage occurs as a response to hypoxia, because relaxation of the anal sphincter allows passive escape of meconium into the amniotic fluid. Under normal intrauterine conditions, amniotic fluid does not enter the fetal lung. However, when the fetus experiences hypoxemia, gasping may result in aspiration of meconium-stained amniotic fluid. Eight percent to 20% of newborns are exposed to amniotic fluid stained by meconium; of these, 5% to 10% will go on to develop MAS (American College of Obstetricians and Gynecologists [ACOG], 2006; Dudell & Stoll, 2007; van Ierland & de Beaufort, 2009).

Preventive strategies have been evaluated for cases at risk for MAS, including amnioinfusion and direct tracheal suctioning of the neonate. Although amnioinfusion appears to be a reasonable treatment for repetitive variable decelerations, its sole use as a technique to prevent MAS is not warranted (ACOG, 2006; Xu, Wei, & Fraser, 2008). When aspirated by the fetus before or during birth, meconium can obstruct the airways, leading to severe hypoxia, inflammation, and infection, and cause significant respiratory difficulties. Past evidence suggested that intrapartum suctioning before the first breath would decrease the risk of MAS; however, subsequent evidence from a large multicentered randomized trial did not show benefit from routine intrapartum oropharyngeal and nasopharyngeal suctioning (van Ierland & de Beaufort, 2009; Velaphi & Vidyasagar, 2006). Currently, the NRP no longer recommends that all meconium-stained babies routinely receive intrapartum suctioning (AAP & AHA, 2016; Vain, Szyld, Prudent, & Aguilar, 2009).

Pneumonitis is an inflammatory response likely secondary to bile salts present in aspirated meconium. Pneumonitis results in acute lung injury with protein-rich interstitial and alveolar edema. In situations where meconium only partially obstructs the airway, a ball-valve effect results. Air enters the lower airways on inspiration but cannot escape on expiration. This causes overdistention of alveoli, leading to alveolar rupture and pulmonary air leaks. Pneumonitis and airway obstruction result in hypoxemia and acidosis, which cause increased PVR and subsequent PPHN (Steinhom & Farrow, 2007).

Pneumonia

Enteric organisms such as *Escherichia coli* and Group B *Streptococcus* (GBS) are the frequent causative bacterial agents of congenital pneumonia, and viruses are increasingly recognized as culprits for this infection. Rarely, a postnatally acquired pneumonia is observed in the early newborn. The diagnosis of neonatal pneumonia is typically an imprecise science. It is generally based on the history, physical examination, chest X-ray results, and lab data. Although pneumonia in newborns is relatively rare, premature infants have at least a 10-fold increased incidence of infections when compared to term infants. Mothers with intrapartum fever and prolonged rupture of membranes have a greater risk of transmitting infections to their infants. Symptoms of pneumonia in a neonate, which often present within 48 hours of delivery, include vital signs instability and respiratory distress. Laboratory data often suggests infection. Chest radiograph typically depicts unilateral or bilateral streaky densities of the perihilar region in bilateral lung fields. Like RDS, symptoms are highly variable and dictate the degree of supportive care (Rohan & Golombek, 2009b).

Transient Tachypnea of the Newborn

TTNB occurs in approximately 0.3% to 0.5% of newborns, although the exact incidence is unknown (Yurdakök, 2010). Generally, TTNB is a mild, self-limiting disorder of term and near-term infants, lasting from 12 to greater than 72 hours. Fetal lungs are fluid-filled during gestation, although production of lung fluid decreases at birth with the onset of breathing and secondary to other influences of labor. Fluid is then absorbed from the air spaces through blood vessels, lymphatics, and upper airways (Yurdakök, 2010).

In certain infants, however, the residual fluid in the alveoli persists, alters oxygen exchange, and increases work of breathing. Several pathophysiology mechanisms have been suggested for TTNB. Historically, this condition was thought to be related to delayed reabsorption of lung fluid by the pulmonary lymphatic system. Retained fluid causes bronchiolar collapse with air trapping or hyperinflation of the alveoli. Hypoxia results when poorly ventilated alveoli are perfused, and hypercarbia results from mechanical interference with alveolar ventilation by fluid. Decreased lung compliance results in tachypnea and increased energy needed to do the work of breathing. It is known that stimuli during labor and at the time of birth cause active transport of chloride from plasma into the fetal lung fluid to cease. As the concentration of chloride becomes higher in the plasma, fetal lung fluid begins to be reabsorbed. Two thirds of the fetal lung fluid is absorbed before birth. Newborns without the benefit of labor and those born prematurely do not have the same amount of time to reabsorb lung fluid as those born after a normal course of labor. Infants delivered by elective cesarean section (CS) also have a higher incidence of TTNB (L. Jain & Dudell, 2006; L. Jain & Eaton, 2006). Some also suggest that TTNB may result from mild immaturity of the surfactant system, which may explain cases of TTNB in late preterm infants (Yurdakök, 2010).

Persistent Pulmonary Hypertension of the Newborn

PPHN is a disorder in which the newborn infant cannot transition from fetal circulation (high PVR and low pulmonary blood flow) to newborn circulation (low PVR and high pulmonary blood flow) (Rohan & Golombek, 2009b). The exact mechanisms that cause the progression to PPHN remain unclear, but PPHN mimics many signs and symptoms of structural heart disease, and distinction between the two is a clinical challenge. PPHN may be a primary problem with little precursory history or coexisting parenchymal lung disease, or it may occur together with MAS, diaphragmatic hernia, infections, RDS, CHD, or perinatal asphyxia (Dudell & Stoll, 2007; Lapointe & Barrington, 2011; Stayer & Lui, 2010; Steinhorn & Farrow, 2007). The disease, however, is uniformly characterized by marked pulmonary vascular hypertension that causes right heart to left heart shunting of blood, decreased pulmonary blood flow, and resultant hypoxemia. This extrapulmonary shunting of blood can occur at the level of the patent foramen ovale (PFO) and/or at the level of the patent ductus arteriosus (PDA). PPHN must be considered whenever a late preterm, term, or postdated neonate presents with hypoxia (Rohan & Golombek, 2009a). Infants with PPHN are typically extremely labile, with frequent desaturation episodes, and blood pressure that may rapidly fluctuate

(Rohan & Golombek, 2009a). A small percentage with refractory hypoxemia may require extracorporeal membrane oxygenation (ECMO) for survival (Dudell & Stoll, 2007). Administration of surfactant or inhaled nitric oxide therapy at a lower acuity of illness can decrease the risk of ECMO/death, progression of disease, and duration of hospital stay (Steinhorn, 2016).

Assessment of Respiratory Distress

Clinical signs of respiratory distress may be present at birth or occur at any time in the early neonatal period. These signs include tachypnea, grunting, retractions, nasal flaring, and cyanosis. Tachypnea is defined as a sustained respiratory rate greater than 60 to 70 breaths per minute. Tachypnea develops when the newborn attempts to improve ventilation. Because of the very compliant chest wall, especially in the preterm newborn, it is more energy efficient for the newborn to increase the respiratory rate, rather than the depth of respirations. However, persistent tachypnea results in muscular fatigue and, over time, further compromises pulmonary status.

On exhalation, a grunting sound is sometimes heard in newborns with respiratory distress. Grunting is the result of forceful closure of the glottis in an attempt to increase intrapulmonary pressure, keep alveoli open, and create residual lung gas volume (functional residual capacity). Keeping alveoli open during exhalation is a compensatory response to decreased partial pressure of oxygen (PO_2) and allows more time for gas exchange to occur (Gardner, Enzman-Hines, & Dickey, 2011). Retractions are depressions observed between the ribs, above the sternum, or below the xiphoid process during inhalation. Retractions are the result of a very compliant chest wall and noncompliant lung. As the amount of negative intrathoracic pressure increases on inspiration, the rib cage expands until the soft tissue of the thorax and weak intercostal muscles are pulled inward toward the spine. The result is worsening atelectasis with marked oxygenation and ventilation abnormalities (Cifuentes, Segars, & Carlo, 2003; Gardner et al., 2011). Nasal flaring may also occur with respiratory distress as the newborn attempts to decrease airway resistance and increase the inflow of air through dilation of the alae nasi (Cifuentes et al., 2003; Gardner et al., 2011).

Cyanosis results from inadequate oxygenation caused by atelectasis, poor lung compliance, and right-to-left shunting at the level of the PDA, or PFO. Although the newborn's color may be an indicator of oxygenation, variables such as skin temperature and perfusion affect the accuracy of this finding. Precise measurement of oxygen and acid–base status may be necessary for the management of respiratory distress using tools such as pulse oximetry and blood gases (Gardner et al., 2011; Rohan & Golembek, 2009a).

Interventions for Respiratory Distress

Care for newborns with respiratory distress focuses on oxygenation and ventilation as well as controlling factors that increase oxygen demands such as hypothermia or stress. Adequate oxygenation and ventilation requires supportive mechanisms ranging from supplemental oxygen only to application of assisted ventilation with techniques such as continuous positive airway pressure or mechanical ventilation. Pulse oximetry and direct arterial blood gas monitoring are methods used to ensure adequate gas exchange. In a preterm newborn, delivery of oxygen should be sufficient to maintain arterial oxygen tension at 50 to 70 mm Hg, corresponding to a pulse oximetry reading of approximately 85% to 95% (Dudell & Stoll, 2007). Because oxygen may be toxic to some tissue, care should be taken to avoid excessive tissue oxygenation, which might have toxic effects such as chronic lung disease or retinopathy of prematurity. In a term newborn at risk for PPHN, oxygen delivery should be sufficient to maintain normoxemia yet avoid hypoxia, which is a potent stimulus for vasoconstriction (Lapointe & Barrington, 2011). Infants with suspected PPHN will need to be transferred to a tertiary-care center for further evaluation and management including potential use of high-frequency ventilation (HFOV), inhaled nitric oxide, or ECMO for severe hypoxemia (Stayer & Liu, 2010; Steinhom & Farrow, 2007).

Select pharmacologic agents may be used in the prevention or management of neonatal respiratory distress. Prenatally, at-risk mothers may receive antenatal steroids to stimulate surfactant synthesis in an effort to prevent RDS. Postnatally, commonly used preparations include airway-instilled surfactant (for RDS prophylaxis or treatment), antibiotics (for pneumonia prophylaxis or treatment), and inhaled or vascularly delivered pulmonary vasodilators (for PPHN treatment) (Konduri & Kim, 2009; Warren & Anderson, 2009).

A neutral thermal environment is crucial in the care of a newborn with respiratory distress. Hypothermia or hyperthermia both increase metabolic demands, leading to decreased oxygenation, metabolic acidosis, and worsening respiratory distress (Cifuentes et al., 2003). Newborns with respiratory distress are cared for under a radiant warmer or in an incubator.

Adequate nutrition frequently requires the administration of intravenous (IV) fluids during the early neonatal period. Care is taken to prevent hypoglycemia that may occur from respiratory distress and increased metabolic demands (Rohan & Golombek, 2009a).

CONGENITAL HEART DISEASE

Cardiovascular System

The cardiovascular system begins to develop in the third week of gestation and is fully developed by the end of the eighth week. It is the first major organ system to develop in the embryo. In the United States, an estimated minimum of 40,000 infants (between 4 and 10 per 1,000 live births) are expected to be affected by CHD annually. Of these, approximately 25%, or 2.4 per 1,000 live births, will require invasive treatment in the first year of age (AHA, 2018). Heart defects are among the most common birth defects and are the leading cause of birth defect–related deaths. However, the overall mortality has significantly declined over the past few decades (AHA, 2018). The cause of CHD cannot be ascribed to any single factor. Most cases are multifactorial, involving genetic predisposition, familial recurrence, and environmental factors. A family history of CHD is significant; if the mother has a history of a child with CHD, her risk of recurrence increases by threefold (Kenney, Hoover, Williams, & Iskersky, 2011). CHD can also be associated with chromosomal abnormalities (e.g., trisomy 21, 18, 13; chromosome deletion syndromes; DiGeorge deletion 22q; Turner syndrome; and Cornelia de Lange) and maternal–environmental factors, such as drug (e.g., thalidomide, anticonvulsants, lithium, retinoic acid) and alcohol exposures or diseases (insulin-dependent diabetes or maternal lupus erythematosus) or infections (e.g., rubella, coxsackie B, and enteroviruses; Kenney et al., 2011).

Cardiac lesions are classified as cyanotic, acyanotic, or according to the hemodynamic characteristics related to pulmonary blood flow. Five of the most commonly occurring cardiac lesions presenting in the early neonatal period include ventricular septal defect (VSD), tetralogy of Fallot (TET), PDA, atrial septal defect (ASD), and transposition of the great arteries (TGA).

The assessment to exclude CHD includes the following:

- Close observation of cardiorespiratory status
- Palpation of peripheral pulses
- Blood pressures of the four extremities
- Chest radiograph to evaluate heart size and pulmonary vascularity
- Blood gas determinations to evaluate oxygenation and metabolic status
- Echocardiography to visualize the structure and function of the heart

Historically, a hyperoxia test was used to distinguish CHD and other causes of cyanosis (Rohan & Golombek, 2009a). However, in many centers, echocardiography is performed if CHD is suspected in lieu of the hyperoxia test because of the potential harmful effects of 100% oxygen, especially in preterm infants. Hyperoxia may still be used if echocardiography is not immediately available. The classic presentation of CHD is that of a cyanotic term infant with a murmur, no significant perinatal history, and a paucity of other respiratory symptoms. Although cyanosis and a murmur are the typical presenting signs, they are by no means definitive. If pulmonary circulatory overload is present, cyanotic cardiac disease can present with respiratory distress (Rohan & Golombek, 2009a). Both the severity of hypoxemia and the hemoglobin concentration determine the degree of cyanosis (Kenney et al., 2011). It is important to differentiate central cyanosis from acrocyanosis (cyanosis of the extremities is commonly seen in newborns because of reduced blood flow through the small capillaries), which is considered a normal finding (Kenney et al., 2011; Lott, 2007).

The newborn with certain types of CHD may also present shortly after birth or within the first weeks of age with symptoms of congestive heart failure (CHF). Infants with CHF typically present with significant respiratory distress. Common clinical signs associated with CHF include (Kenney et al., 2011; Lott, 2007)

- Tachypnea (due to pulmonary edema)
- Respiratory distress
- Gallop rhythm (caused by dilation of the ventricles)
- Decreased peripheral pulses and mottling of the extremities (decrease in peripheral tissue perfusion)
- Tachycardia (in an attempt to compensate for a decrease in cardiac output, the heart either increases the rate or the stroke volume)
- Hepatomegaly (right ventricle does not adequately empty leading to an elevated right atrium pressure resulting in hepatic venous congestion)
- Poor feeding (due to high respiratory rate and increases in basal metabolic rate demands)

Many serious cyanotic lesions are not accompanied by holosystolic or diastolic murmurs (Rohan & Golombek, 2009a). A murmur, if present, varies in quality and intensity, depending on the particular cardiac lesion present. If a VSD or an ASD is present, allowing mixing of oxygenated and unoxygenated blood, only mild cyanosis may occur in the setting of CHD. If there is no intracardiac shunt, severe cyanosis can be observed.

Ventricular Septal Defect

Pathophysiology

The partitioning of the embryonic heart into chambers of the atria and ventricles begins near the fourth week of gestation and is completed by the end of the seventh week (Auckland, 2010). A VSD is present when there is incomplete division of the right and left ventricles. VSDs are classified by their anatomic location; perimembranous and muscular are the two most common types. A perimembranous VSD is located just below the aortic valve and accounts for 80% of all VSDs. A muscular VSD is located in the muscular septum. Seventy-five percent to 80% of membranous and muscular VSDs close spontaneously. A VSD is considered an acyanotic lesion with increased pulmonary

blood flow. The size and location of the defect, as well as the pulmonary-to-systemic vascular resistance ratio, determine the degree of left-to-right shunt. The timing of the onset of symptoms is directly related to the normal fall in the PVR after birth (Kenney et al., 2011).

Assessment

The onset of symptoms resulting from a VSD is related to the size of the defect and PVR. A newborn with a small defect has minimal left-to-right shunting at the ventricular level and may appear well with few or no symptoms other than a holosystolic systolic murmur heard best at the lower left sternal border. The murmur develops as the PVR falls. A newborn with a large defect may present with symptoms of CHF but not until approximately 2 to 4 weeks of age. As with the smaller defects, the murmur is holosystolic and heard over the left lower sternal border. Preterm newborns with large VSDs may present sooner and be more symptomatic compared to their term counterparts because preterm infants have lower PVR at birth resulting in greater left-to-right shunting (Kenney et al., 2011).

Tetralogy of Fallot

Pathophysiology

TET consists of a large perimembranous VSD, pulmonary artery stenosis, an overriding aorta, and right ventricle hypertrophy (Kenney et al., 2011). This lesion is a result of disordered embryonic cardiac functioning. TET occurs during the embryonic stage of development, when some unknown factor influences functioning of the heart at the cellular level. This alteration in cellular function is partly responsible for determining development. TET is generally considered a cyanotic lesion with decreased pulmonary blood flow, but the hemodynamics vary widely, depending on the severity of pulmonary stenosis, the size of the VSD, and the pulmonary and systemic vascular resistance. Most newborns with TET present with cyanosis because of the right-to-left intracardiac shunt. However, if the intracardiac shunt is mainly left to right, due to a mild or moderate right ventricular outflow obstruction, the infant will not be cyanotic (Kenney et al., 2011). Typically, the course worsens over the first year of age.

Assessment

TET is the most common cyanotic heart disease seen in the first year of age. Newborns with TET are most often diagnosed in the first few weeks of age due to either a loud murmur or cyanosis. Newborns with TET often present with cyanosis, hypoxia, and dyspnea. However, newborns that are symptomatic typically have severe right ventricular outflow tract obstruction (Kenney et al., 2011). The timing and degree of cyanosis depend on the severity of the pulmonary stenosis and may not be noticed until closure of the ductus arteriosus. In the case of pulmonary atresia and hypoplasia of the pulmonary arteries, marked cyanosis may be observed immediately after birth. The clinical signs of right-sided heart failure, resulting from right ventricular outflow tract obstruction, include hepatomegaly, tricuspid valve regurgitation, and a grade II to IV/VI harsh systolic murmur best heard over the mid to upper left sternal border.

Patent Ductus Arteriosus

Pathophysiology

The ductus arteriosus is a normal pathway of fetal circulation. The ductus arteriosus connects the pulmonary artery to the aorta, allowing blood to bypass the lungs directly into the placenta. During fetal life, PVR is greater than systemic vascular resistance. After birth, with spontaneous respiration, the arterial oxygen level increases and PVR decreases, causing the ductus to close. Functionally, the PDA closes within hours to several days after birth, but closure is often delayed in premature infants. If the ductus arteriosus does not close, blood begins to flow left to right through the patent ductus as the PVR decreases. A PDA is an acyanotic lesion with increased pulmonary blood flow. It presents with signs and symptoms of CHF. It occurs much more commonly in preterm newborns, with the incidence inversely proportional to gestational age (Kenney et al., 2011).

Assessment

The manifestation of PDA depends on the gestational age and the degree of lung disease. Preterm newborns generally develop signs associated with CHF at 3 to 7 days of age, but it can develop sooner in the smaller preterm newborn treated with surfactant. The development of clinical signs is related to the normal fall in the PVR resulting in increased blood flow to the pulmonary circulation and volume overload of the left ventricles. In newborns, a grade I to III systolic ejection murmur will likely develop, if left untreated, a classic machinery-like continuous murmur may result in older infants and children. PDA murmurs are best heard at the upper left sternal border (over the first and second intercostal spaces to the left of the sternum) and may radiate to the back, between the scapulae. However, with a right-to-left shunt, a murmur may be absent (Kenney et al., 2011).

Atrial Septal Defect

Pathophysiology

The separation of the atrium begins near the middle of the fourth week of gestation and is completed by the sixth week, leaving the foramen ovale open between the two atria. An abnormality occurring during atrial separation can result in an ASD. An ASD is considered an acyanotic lesion with increased pulmonary blood flow. Approximately 10% of newborns with very large ASDs develop CHF as the PVR decreases and a left-to-right shunt develops with concomitant right ventricular volume overload and hypertrophy (Sadowski, 2010). Three major types of ASDs occur and are differentiated from each other by whether they involve other structures of the heart and how they are formed during fetal development (Lott, 2007). The first type is ostium secundum, the most common yet least serious type of ASD, is caused when a part of the atrial septum fails to close completely while the heart is developing. The second type is an ostium primum defect, part of the spectrum of atrioventricular canal defects that is often associated with a cleft in the leaflet of the mitral valve. The third type is the sinus venosus defect, which occurs at the superior vena cava and right atrium junction and is most often associated with partial anomalous pulmonary venous connection.

Assessment

Newborns with an uncomplicated ASD are generally asymptomatic. However, about 10% present with signs of CHF, poor feeding, and poor growth. These symptoms develop as the PVR falls over the first few weeks of age. Associated with an ASD is a soft, systolic murmur best heard over the second intercostal space at the left upper sternal border.

d–Transposition of the Great Arteries

Pathophysiology

The truncus arteriosus begins to divide during the fifth week of gestation. As the cardiac tube folds, the vessel twists on itself and divides into two separate vessels. The exact etiology of transposition remains unknown. Historically, transposition was thought to occur because of a failure of the aorticopulmonary septum to grow in a spiral fashion, resulting in inappropriate migration of the vessels. However, additional causes continue to be explored (Sankaran & Brown, 2007). A dextro-transposition of the great arteries (d-TGA) occurs when the aorta arises from the right ventricle, and the pulmonary artery arises from the left ventricle, resulting in pulmonary and systemic circulations functioning in parallel. When these two arteries are transposed, unoxygenated blood returning from the body enters the right side of the heart and returns to the body, and oxygenated blood returning from the lung enters the left side of the heart and returns to the lungs. d-TGA is considered a cyanotic lesion with increased pulmonary blood flow. d-TGA can occur in isolation or can be associated with other defects (e.g., PDA, ASD,

VSD, pulmonary stenosis). The degree of cyanosis depends on the amount of mixing of oxygenated and unoxygenated blood between the parallel systemic and pulmonary circulations through the associated lesions (e.g., PFO, VSD, ASD, PDA) or collateral circulation (Kenney et al., 2011).

Assessment

d-TGA is the most common cyanotic heart lesion that presents in the newborn period and is more prevalent in males (Kenney et al., 2011). The newborn with d-TGA presents with cyanosis typically within the first hours after birth, and the degree of cyanosis varies depending on the amount of intracardiac mixing. For instance, if the mixing occurs through a large VSD or PDA, the cyanosis may be mild. If the ventricular septum is intact or the PDA is closing, the cyanosis is profound because there is no intracardiac shunt. With the exception of cyanosis, the physical examination findings are often otherwise unremarkable. With a large VSD or ASD, signs of CHF develop over time as the PVR falls and the pulmonary blood flow increases. In the absence of an intracardiac shunt, severe hypoxemia and metabolic acidosis develop, followed by a rapid demise if emergency measures are not instituted.

Interventions for Congenital Heart Disease

Newborns with known or suspected CHD usually require transfer to a tertiary center for treatment and follow-up. The complete diagnostic workup and subsequent repairs or palliative surgery are performed in centers with pediatric cardiac capabilities. Pulse oximetry on asymptomatic newborns may detect some cases on CHD (Mahle et al., 2009). Nursing care for newborns with known or suspected CHD includes the following:

- Cardiorespiratory monitoring
- Pulse oximetry
- Blood work, including blood gas determinations
- Ongoing assessment of color, perfusion, and degree of respiratory distress
- Maintaining a neutral thermal environment
- IV hydration and nutrition
- Oxygen therapy, if appropriate, and mechanical ventilation, if required

Metabolic acidosis is treated with sodium bicarbonate, pulmonary edema with respiratory distress is treated with diuretics, and shock is treated with vasopressors and calcium gluconate. A lesion such as d-TGA without an intracardiac shunt is treated with prostaglandin E1 to maintain patency of the ductus arteriosus until surgical correction takes place (Kenney et al., 2011).

HYPOGLYCEMIA

Current evidence does not support a specific concentration of glucose that can discriminate normal from abnormal or can potentially result in acute or chronic irreversible neurologic damage (Adamkin & Committee on Fetus and Newborn, 2011). Blood glucose concentrations as low as 30 mg/dL are common in healthy neonates within 1 to 2 hours after birth, and usually are transient, free from clinical signs, and considered to be part of normal adaptation to postnatal life (Adamkin & Committee on Fetus and Newborn, 2011; A. F. Williams, 2005). There is no absolute threshold applicable to all babies, and there is no glucose concentration, which absolutely determines clinical risk or predicts sequelae. Rather than identifying strict definitions of hypoglycemia, most authors suggest the use of *operational thresholds*. A glucose value must be assessed in conjunction with other clinical data, and treatment based on this integrated input.

Early feeding may possibly contribute to stabilization of newborn blood sugar and is currently a mainstay of treatment for the infant that presents with hypoglycemia (Adamkin & Committee on Fetus and Newborn, 2011). This practice is hardly free from controversy. Other researchers have concluded that glucose concentrations of normal newborns during the transitional period are "remarkably stable and relatively unaffected by the timing of initial feeding or interval between feedings (Thornton et al., 2015).

Pathophysiology

During fetal life, insulin is secreted by the fetal pancreas in response to glucose that readily crosses the placenta. At birth, the newborn's blood glucose level is approximately 70% to 80% that of the mother. After removal of placental circulation, the newborn must maintain glucose homeostasis. This requires initiation of various metabolic processes, including gluconeogenesis (e.g., forming glucose from noncarbohydrate sources such as protein and fat) and glycogenolysis (e.g., conversion of glycogen stores to glucose), as well as an intact regulatory mechanism and an adequate supply of substrate (Kayiran & Gürakan, 2010; Sperling & Menon, 2004). Although this is effective for the well term infant, the sick or preterm infant is constrained in effectively mobilizing or using fuel sources.

Assessment

Identification of those infants at risk for developing hypoglycemia facilitates planning and implementation of appropriate nursing care. This process begins with a review of maternal prenatal and intrapartum history for risk factors associated with neonatal hypoglycemia and a careful physical examination. Factors predisposing

TABLE 21–1. Recognizing Neonates at Increased Risk for Early and Persistent Hypoglycemia

Neonates at increased risk for hypoglycemia and require glucose screening

1. Symptoms of hypoglycemia
2. Large for gestational age (even without maternal diabetes)
3. Perinatal stress
   a. Birth asphyxia/ischemia; cesarean delivery for fetal distress
   b. Maternal preeclampsia/eclampsia or hypertension
   c. Fetal growth restriction or small for gestational age
   d. Meconium aspiration syndrome, erythroblastosis fetalis, polycythemia, hypothermia
4. Premature or postmature delivery
5. Infant of diabetic mother
6. Family history of a genetic form of hypoglycemia
7. Congenital syndromes (e.g., Beckwith-Wiedemann), abnormal physical features (e.g., midline facial malformations, microphallus)

Neonates in whom to exclude persistent hypoglycemia before discharge

1. Severe hypoglycemia (e.g., episode of symptomatic hypoglycemia or need for IV dextrose to treat hypoglycemia)
2. Inability to consistently maintain preprandial PG concentration >50 mg/dL up to 48 hr of age and >60 mg/dL after 48 hr of age
3. Family history of a genetic form of hypoglycemia
4. Congenital syndromes (e.g., Beckwith-Wiedemann), abnormal physical features (e.g., midline facial malformations, microphallus)

IV, intravenous; PG, plasma glucose.
From Thornton, P. S., Stanley, C. A., De Leon, D. D., Harris, D., Haymond, M. W., Hussain, K., . . . Wolfsdorf, J. I. (2015). Recommendations from the Pediatric Endocrine Society for evaluation and management of persistent hypoglycemia. *Journal of Pediatrics, 167*(2), 238–245. doi:10.1016/j.jpeds.2015.03.057

infants to early or persistent hypoglycemia can be found in Table 21–1. Symptoms of hypoglycemia are nonspecific and not easily differentiated from many other common neonatal conditions (Display 21–1). Neuroglycopenic signs and symptoms are caused by brain dysfunction resulting from a deficient glucose supply to sustain brain energy metabolism. Findings common in older children—such as confusion—are not identifiable

DISPLAY 21–1
Symptoms of Hypoglycemia

Jitteriness, tremors

Tachypnea, grunting

Diaphoresis

Cyanosis

Lethargy

Hypotonia

Irritability

Temperature instability

Apnea

Seizures, coma

in patients who are unable to communicate their symptoms. Neonatal signs of hypoglycemia are nonspecific and not easily differentiated from many other common neonatal conditions. These include irritability or somnolence, pallor, diaphoresis, tachycardia, jitteriness or shakiness, and clammy skin.

Universal blood glucose screening before clinical signs develop is not currently recommended by the AAP or Pediatric Endocrine Society (Adamkin & Committee on Fetus and Newborn, 2011; Thornton et al., 2015). Selective screening of at-risk newborns is more appropriate and does not appear to decrease quality of care or result in adverse outcomes.

Newborns at risk should be screened within 30 minutes of the first feed, which should occur within an hour of birth (Adamkin & Committee on Fetus and Newborn, 2011). Point-of-care testing (POCT) provides an expedient estimation of glucose values using a capillary whole blood sample. Accuracy of POCT screening depends on the hematocrit, blood source, and operator's skill. There is no point-of-care method that is sufficiently reliable and accurate in the low range of blood glucose to allow it to be used as the sole method for screening for hypoglycemia. Venous blood samples have glucose levels that are approximately 10% less than capillary specimens (Deshpande & Ward Platt, 2005). Failure to run the venous blood sample tests promptly after sampling may result in red blood cell oxidation of glucose and produce falsely low values. Venous blood samples should be transported on ice and analyzed quickly.

Interventions

At-risk newborns with asymptomatic hypoglycemia should be fed immediately and then retested. Invasive interventions on the basis of low values detected by screening are not warranted as long as infants are assessed and are found to be without clinical findings attributable to hypoglycemia. A low glucose in the asymptomatic newborn may initially be managed by offering a breastfeeding or providing expressed breast milk or formula. The infant should be refed within 2 to 3 hours and, if the glucose remains low for a second measurement, should be refed or have IV therapy started. Clinical practice guidelines are available to assist providers in decision making surrounding glucose homeostasis screening. One such algorithm outlining AAP recommendations for screening and management of postnatal glucose homeostasis in at-risk infants can be found in Figure 21–1.

Newborns with symptomatic hypoglycemia, particularly those with neurologic signs and low POCT bedside blood glucose, should be treated immediately with an IV infusion of glucose, and a blood sample should be drawn and sent to the laboratory for glucose evaluation. Infusion rates should be similar to that

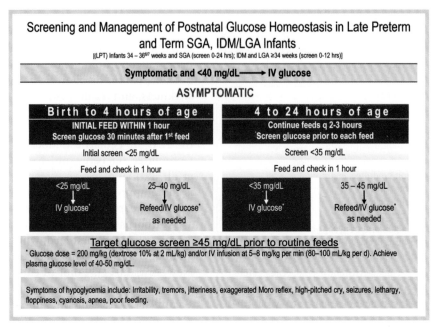

Screening and Management of Postnatal Glucose Homeostasis in Late Preterm and Term SGA, IDM/LGA Infants

[(LPT) Infants 34 – 36⁶ᐟ⁷ weeks and SGA (screen 0-24 hrs); IDM and LGA ≥34 weeks (screen 0-12 hrs)]

Symptomatic and <40 mg/dL ⟶ IV glucose

ASYMPTOMATIC

Birth to 4 hours of age	4 to 24 hours of age
INITIAL FEED WITHIN 1 hour	Continue feeds q 2-3 hours
Screen glucose 30 minutes after 1ˢᵗ feed	Screen glucose prior to each feed
Initial screen <25 mg/dL	Screen <35 mg/dL
Feed and check in 1 hour	Feed and check in 1 hour

<25 mg/dL	25–40 mg/dL	<35 mg/dL	35 – 45 mg/dL
IV glucose*	Refeed/IV glucose* as needed	IV glucose*	Refeed/IV glucose* as needed

Target glucose screen ≥45 mg/dL prior to routine feeds
* Glucose dose = 200 mg/kg (dextrose 10% at 2 mL/kg) and/or IV infusion at 5–8 mg/kg per min (80–100 mL/kg per d). Achieve plasma glucose level of 40-50 mg/dL.

Symptoms of hypoglycemia include: Irritability, tremors, jitteriness, exaggerated Moro reflex, high-pitched cry, seizures, lethargy, floppiness, cyanosis, apnea, poor feeding.

FIGURE 21–1. Use glucose algorithm. (From Adamkin, D. H., & Committee on Fetus and Newborn. [2011]. Clinical report: Postnatal glucose homeostasis in late preterm and term infants. *Pediatrics, 127*[3], 575–579.)

expected with endogenous hepatic glucose production (approximately 5 mg/kg/min depending on maturity and weight for gestation—equivalent to 10% dextrose at approximately 70 to 80 mL/kg/day or 3 mL/kg/hr and titrated based on response; A. F. Williams, 2005). Gradual increases in glucose infusion rate should not exceed 2 mg/kg/min each hour. Newborns who are unable to nipple feed and those whose blood glucose levels do not respond to oral feedings or have very low glucose levels (e.g., <20 mg/dL) should receive a 200 mg/kg (2 mL/kg) bolus of 10% dextrose in water intravenously over 1 minute, followed by a continuous infusion at the rates given above until the blood glucose is stabilized (Rozance & Hay, 2010). Correction of hypoglycemia should result in resolution of the symptoms. IV administration is tapered off slowly and the blood glucose level is monitored frequently, every 1 to 2 hours, initially and then intermittently before feedings until stable (A. F. Williams, 2005).

Newborns that experience persistent hypoglycemia may require an increased concentration of glucose, such as 12.5%, 15%, or 20%; dextrose solutions with concentrations greater than 12.5% require placement of a central line because of the risk of tissue extravasation. Other treatments for persistent or refractory hypoglycemia include glucagon, which promotes glycogenolysis and requires adequate stores; and corticosteroids, which induce gluconeogenic enzyme activity (A. Jain et al., 2010).

Hypoglycemia severe enough to warrant IV therapy, or which persists or recurs, requires further investigation to rule out underlying pathology, particularly infection or metabolic and endocrine disease

(Deshpande & Ward Platt, 2005). The focus of nursing care is to prevent hypoglycemia when possible. Care should be taken to avoid cold stress and to recognize signs of respiratory distress or sepsis that can increase the newborn's risk for developing hypoglycemia.

HYPERBILIRUBINEMIA

Hyperbilirubinemia resulting in clinical jaundice is detected in up to 60% of term and 80% of preterm newborns (Juretschke, 2005; Piazza & Stoll, 2007). Typically, healthy newborns are discharged from the hospital before the usual peak of total serum bilirubin (TSB) (72 to 120 hours). Most jaundice is benign and resolves within 7 to 10 days in term newborns. However, severe hyperbilirubinemia develops in up to 9% of all newborns during the first postnatal week (Kamath, Thilo, & Hernandez, 2011). Jaundice is a common indication for hospital readmission, especially among late preterm infants (Alkalay, Bresee, & Simmons, 2010). Because of the potential for bilirubin to be toxic to the newborn brain at high levels, newborns require assessment to identify those at risk for severe hyperbilirubinemia, so as to prevent the rare cases of bilirubin encephalopathy or kernicterus. Unconjugated hyperbilirubinemia results from physiologic mechanisms (Display 21–2) or pathologic causes (Display 21–3).

Pathophysiology

Bilirubin is produced from the breakdown of heme-containing proteins (Cohen, Wong, Stevenson, 2010; Juretschke, 2005). The major heme-containing protein

DISPLAY 21–2

Mechanisms Attributing to Physiologic Hyperbilirubinemia

Increased bilirubin related to relative polycythemia and short (80 to 90 days) life span of fetal red blood cells

Decreased uptake of bilirubin by the liver

Decreased enzyme activity and ability to conjugate bilirubin

Decreased ability to excrete bilirubin

Breastfeeding

is hemoglobin, which is the source of approximately 75% of the bilirubin produced. Heme is acted on by the enzyme heme oxygenase, releasing carbon monoxide and biliverdin. Biliverdin is then reduced to bilirubin through the activity of the enzyme biliverdin reductase. The degradation of every 1 g of hemoglobin produces 34 to 35 mg of bilirubin. Bilirubin binds with albumin for transport to the liver. Bilirubin, but not albumin, diffuses into the liver cytoplasm, where it is transported to the endoplasmic reticulum for conjugation. Bilirubin combines with glucuronate with the help of glucuronyl transferase, the conjugating enzyme. Conjugated bilirubin is water soluble and excreted into bile and subsequently into the small intestine through the common bile duct. In the gut, conjugated bilirubin is excreted from the body through stool or converted to unconjugated bilirubin by a gut enzyme (β-glucuronidase) that renders it reabsorbable. In fetal life, this reabsorption facilitates transport of bilirubin to the placenta for maternal excretion; however, postnatally, this pathway adds to the infant's bilirubin load (Kamath et al., 2011; Piazza & Stoll, 2007; Thilo, 2005).

Excretion of conjugated bilirubin is facilitated by bacteria in the gut. Meconium contains large amounts of bilirubin, but excretion is inhibited in the newborn because of the sterility of the gut. Normal colonization of bacteria occurs over time and is facilitated by

early and frequent feeding. Feeding introduces bacteria into the gut. Lack of bacterial flora allows conversion of conjugated bilirubin back to an unconjugated form. This, along with greater red cell mass per kilogram in the newborn than in the adult and a shortened red cell life span, sets the stage for development of physiologic unconjugated hyperbilirubinemia. Newborns produce twice as much bilirubin as adults (Halamek & Stevenson, 2002; Piazza & Stoll, 2007; Thilo, 2005).

In a term newborn, physiologic unconjugated hyperbilirubinemia is characterized by a progressive increase in serum bilirubin to a peak of 6 to 8 mg/dL at 72 hours of age, and steady decline over the next week. In a preterm newborn, bilirubin continues to rise until the fourth to seventh postnatal day, reaching a peak of 8 to 12 mg/dL and decreasing thereafter as the processes of metabolism and excretion mature (Halamek & Stevenson, 2002). When jaundice is evident within the first 24 to 36 hours of age, bilirubin levels rise >5 mg/dL/day or peak in excess of 12 to 14 mg/dL, or jaundice persists beyond 2 weeks of age, it is less likely to represent a physiologic process and warrants assessment (Burgos, Flaherman, & Newman, 2011; Piazza & Stoll, 2007).

Hyperbilirubinemia may result from three mechanisms: (1) increased bilirubin production, (2) increased bilirubin reabsorption, or (3) decreased bilirubin excretion. In addition, hyperbilirubinemia may be attributed to *physiologic* or *pathologic* causes. Conditions contributing to physiologic, unconjugated hyperbilirubinemia include normal bilirubin load from a large, short–life span fetal red blood cell mass as well as delayed stooling. Breastfed infants may experience exaggerated jaundice related to initial decreased caloric intake, decreased stooling with subsequent increase of enterohepatic circulation, or effects of substances within the milk which interfere with conjugation and excretion (Kamath et al., 2011). Physiologic conditions are exaggerated in the near-term, late preterm, and preterm infant. Pathologic hyperbilirubinemia is most commonly associated with conditions that acutely increase the bilirubin load, such as isoimmune hemolytic disease in cases of RH, ABO, or other minor blood group incompatibility between fetus and mother. Other pathologic causes contributing to excess bilirubin load or impaired excretion include extravascular blood, polycythemia, intestinal obstruction, infection, maternal diabetes, and rare metabolic or inherited conditions (Kamath et al., 2011; Juretschke, 2005). Table 21–2 lists maternal and newborn risks for hyperbilirubinemia.

Unconjugated bilirubin is a potent antioxidant that may be useful for protecting against oxidative injuries, but it becomes a potent neurotoxin once it crosses the blood–brain barrier. Unconjugated bilirubin can damage most types of brain cells, thereby affecting

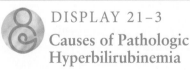

DISPLAY 21–3

Causes of Pathologic Hyperbilirubinemia

Hemolytic disease of the newborn

Bruising, extravascular blood

Polycythemia

Intestinal obstruction

Metabolic conditions

Prematurity

Infection

Respiratory distress

TABLE 21–2. Risk Factors for Hyperbilirubinemia

Newborn	Maternal
Birth weight <1,500 g	Oxytocin, Valium
Preterm delivery	Forceps or vacuum delivery
Male	Diabetes
Hypothermia	East Asian heritage
Asphyxia	Native American heritage
Hypoalbuminemia	Hypertensive disorders of pregnancy
Sepsis	Family history of jaundice, liver
Meningitis	disease, anemia, or splenectomy
Polycythemia (Hct >65%)	Blood incompatibilities
Drugs that affect albumin	
binding	
Birth trauma (e.g.,	
cephalhematoma, bruising)	
Congenital hypothyroidism	
Bruising	
Poor feeding	
Inborn error of metabolism	
Intestinal obstruction	
Erythrocyte disorders	
(e.g., G6PD deficiency)	

G6PD, glucose-6-phosphate dehydrogenase; Hct, hematocrit.

brain circuits or loops that influence cognition, learning, behavior, sensory, and language (Amin, Smith, & Timler, 2018). Although rare, bilirubin-induced brain injury in the neonatal period has detrimental effects on neurodevelopment that persist into childhood and adulthood, contributing to childhood developmental disorders (Amin et al., 2018).

During the early phase of acute bilirubin-induced brain injury, severely jaundiced infants become lethargic and hypotonic and have a poor suck. An intermediate phase is characterized by moderate stupor, hypertonia, and irritability. The infant may also develop a fever and high-pitched cry that alternates with drowsiness and hypotonia. This hypertonia is characterized by backward arching of the trunk (opisthotonos) and of the neck (retrocollis). CNS damage may in some cases be reversed during this phase with a combination of intensive phototherapy and an emergent exchange transfusion. The advanced phase of bilirubin encephalopathy is characterized by pronounced retrocollis and opisthotonos, shrill cry, inability to feed, apnea, fever, deep stupor to coma, seizures, and death. In the chronic form, kernicterus, surviving infants may develop severe athetoid cerebral palsy, auditory dysfunction, dental-enamel dysplasia, paralysis of upward gaze, as well as intellectual and other handicaps (Bhutani, Johnson, & Shapiro, 2004). There is no absolute level at which bilirubin encephalopathy occurs in all newborns. Gestational age, postnatal age, clinical condition, and the pathophysiologic process involved all play a part in determining what level of unconjugated bilirubin causes encephalopathy in a particular newborn (Juretschke, 2005).

Assessment

Clinical jaundice is apparent at serum bilirubin levels of 5 to 7 mg/dL (Juretschke, 2005; Kamath et al., 2011) and progresses cephalocaudal from head to the lower extremities. A careful physical examination of any newborn presenting with jaundice aids in determining the cause of hyperbilirubinemia. The newborn should be assessed for risks including prematurity; low birth weight; indicators of bleeding or extravascular blood collections such as bruising, cephalohematoma, or petechiae; and hepatosplenomegaly. Visual recognition of jaundice is inaccurate, unreliable, and unsafe and varies with the experience and level of training of the observer. Therefore, in conjunction with the clinical examination, transcutaneous bilirubin (TcB) assessment or laboratory testing including serum bilirubin may be done to quantify the bilirubin level and determine potential causes (Display 21–4). Any infant with jaundice presenting within the first 24 hours of age should have a bilirubin assessment (Burgos et al., 2011).

There are numerous resources for providers who care for infants at risk for hyperbilirubinemia. The AAP established guidelines in 2004 for the management of hyperbilirubinemia in the newborn infant ≥35 weeks' gestation (AAP, 2004a). These guidelines stress the importance of universal systematic assessment while the newborn is hospitalized, close follow-up, and prompt intervention when indicated. The key elements of the recommendation suggest that the clinician should do the following:

- Promote and support successful breastfeeding.
- Establish nursery protocols for the identification and evaluation of hyperbilirubinemia.
- Measure the total TSB or TcB level on infants jaundiced in the first 24 hours.
- Recognize that visual estimation of the degree of jaundice can lead to errors, particularly in darkly pigmented infants.

DISPLAY 21–4

Laboratory Tests to Evaluate the Cause of Jaundice

Total and direct bilirubin

Blood type

Coombs test

Hematocrit

Peripheral smear for red blood cell morphology

Liver enzymes

Viral and/or bacterial cultures

pH

Serum albumin

- Interpret all bilirubin levels according to the infant's age in hours.
- Recognize that infants at less than 38 weeks' gestation, particularly those who are breast-fed, are at higher risk of developing hyperbilirubinemia and require closer surveillance and monitoring.
- Perform a systematic assessment on all infants before discharge for the risk of severe hyperbilirubinemia.
- Provide parents with written and verbal information about newborn jaundice.
- Provide appropriate follow-up based on the time of discharge and the risk assessment.
- Treat newborns, when indicated, with phototherapy or exchange transfusion.

Interventions

In supporting adequate breastfeeding, clinicians should instruct mothers to nurse their infants 8 to 10 times per day over the first several days (Thilo, 2005). This not only promotes adequate hydration and caloric intake but also decreases the likelihood of subsequent significant hyperbilirubinemia. Nurseries should have established protocols for the assessment of jaundice. Newborns should be assessed with vital signs, but no less than every 8 to 12 hours. Assessment should be done in a well-lit room; however, it is important to remember that visual assessment of jaundice is unreliable and potentially unsafe (Piazza & Stoll, 2007; Watchko & Maisels, 2010). A low threshold should be used for assessing bilirubin. Noninvasive TcB devices have proven to be very useful as screening tools. It has also been recommended that protocols allow nurses access to bilirubin testing either TcB or TSB, without a physician's order.

Every newborn should be assessed for the risk of developing severe hyperbilirubinemia before discharge. As serum bilirubin rises >19 mg/dL, the risk of kernicterus increases disproportionately (Smitherman, Stark, & Bhutani, 2006). In the Pilot Kernicterus Registry, causes for kernicterus are attributed to the following three categories in equal proportions: hemolytic disorders (mostly ABO immunization); G6PD deficiency (associated with hemolysis and impaired bilirubin conjugation); and idiopathic causes (presumably from delayed or impaired function of the glucuronyl transferase enzyme system), coupled with breastfeeding and inadequate nutritional intake (Bhutani et al., 2004). All nurseries should establish protocols for assessing this risk. This is particularly important if the infant is discharged before 72 hours of age. This risk can be assessed by predischarge measurement of bilirubin and/or assessment of clinical risk factors. Regardless of how risk is assessed, appropriate follow-up is essential. An hour-specific nomogram is a useful tool for determining the need for and appropriate timing of repeated TcB or TSB measurements. The assigned low- intermediate- or high-risk zone in which the individual bilirubin level falls (Fig. 21–2) will indicate the risk for developing clinically significant hyperbilirubinemia (Bhutani, Johnson, & Sivievri, 1999).

There are several risk factors associated with severe hyperbilirubinemia. Among these are: jaundice in the first 24 hours of age, predischarge TcB or TSB levels in the high-risk zone of the nomogram, jaundice within the first 24 hours of age, blood group incompatibility or other known hemolytic disease with a positive direct antiglobulin test, gestational age 35 to 36 weeks, previous sibling who received phototherapy, cephalhematoma or significant bruising, East Asian race, and exclusive

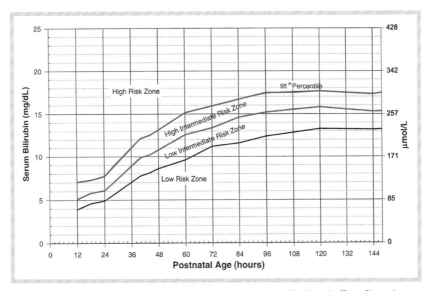

FIGURE 21–2. Nomogram for designation of risk of developing hyperbilirubinemia. (From Bhutani, V. K., Johnson, L. H., & Sivievri, E. M. [1999]. Predictive ability of a predischarge hour-specific serum bilirubin for subsequent significant hyperbilirubinemia in healthy term and near-term newborns. *Pediatrics, 103*[1], 6–14.)

breastfeeding, particularly if nursing is not going well and weight loss is excessive (AAP, 2004a; Burgos et al., 2011).

Written and verbal information must be provided to parents at discharge. This should include an explanation of jaundice, the need to monitor infants for jaundice, and advice on how monitoring should be done. Newborn jaundice resource materials are available for parents in multiple languages (English, Spanish, Chinese, and Italian) and include a frequently asked question sheet from the AAP (2004b). All infants should be examined by a qualified healthcare professional in the first days after discharge, and those with jaundice should be evaluated within twenty-four hours (AAP, 2004a).

In the late 1940s, exchange transfusion was the only available treatment for newborns with hyperbilirubinemia. In the mid-1950s, an observant nurse noticed that newborns exposed to sunlight had less clinical jaundice over exposed areas and decreased serum bilirubin levels. This observation led to the use of phototherapy, which remains the primary treatment for hyperbilirubinemia. In nearly all newborns, phototherapy decreases or blunts the rise in serum-unconjugated bilirubin regardless of gestational age, race, or presence or absence of hemolysis. Phototherapy is used for treatment and prophylaxis of hyperbilirubinemia. No serious long-term side effects have been reported. Recommendations for treatment in infants born at ≥35 weeks' gestation are found in Figure 21–3. There is no consensus or recommendation regarding the discontinuation of phototherapy (Watchko & Maisels, 2010).

The goal of phototherapy is to decrease the level of unconjugated bilirubin. Phototherapy accomplishes this goal by means of the following:

- Absorption of light by bilirubin molecule;
- Photoconversion of bilirubin by photochemical reaction, restructuring the molecule into an isomer;
- Excretion of bilirubin through urine and bile, bypassing the conjugation process (Maisels & McDonagh, 2008).

Effectively used phototherapy can decrease bilirubin levels by 0.5 to 1 mg/dl per hour (Kamath et al., 2011).

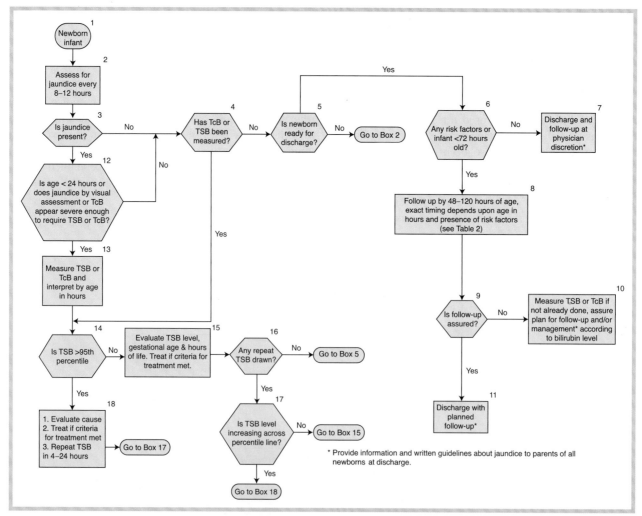

FIGURE 21–3. Algorithm for the management of jaundice in the newborn nursery. (From American Academy of Pediatrics. [2004a]. Management of hyperbilirubinemia in the newborn infant 35 or more weeks' gestation. *Pediatrics*, *114*[1], 297–316.)

For phototherapy to be effective, there must be illumination of an adequate area of exposed skin at a sufficiently short distance. Factors to consider in prescribing and implementing phototherapy are (1) emission range of the light source, (2) the light intensity (irradiance), (3) the exposed ("treatable") body surface area illuminated, and (4) the decrease in total bilirubin concentration (Bhutani & Committee on Fetus and Newborn, 2011). Although any light source with irradiance between 400 and 500 nm can be used, devices with maximum emission within the 460- to 490-nm (blue-green) region of the visible spectrum are probably the most effective for treating hyperbilirubinemia (Bhutani & Committee on Fetus and Newborn, 2011). There is a direct relationship between the irradiance used and the rate of bilirubin decline with phototherapy. Irradiance should be monitored and is measured with a radiometer as $\mu W/cm^2/nm$. Currently, however, no single method is in general use for measuring phototherapy dosages. In addition, the calibration methods, wavelength responses, and geometries of instruments are not standardized. Consequently, different radiometers may show different values for the same light source (Bhutani & Committee on Fetus and Newborn, 2011).

AAP has recommended that the irradiance for intensive phototherapy be at least $30\ \mu W \cdot cm^{-2} \cdot nm^{-1}$ over the waveband interval 460 to 490 nm (AAP, 2004a). Devices that emit lower irradiance may be supplemented with auxiliary devices to achieve this target. To expose the maximum surface area of the infant, for example, overhead phototherapy can be used with a fiberoptic blanket. The newborn is placed naked under the phototherapy light, atop the blanket, and repositioned at least every 2 hours to ensure adequate light exposure to all areas, but within the dosing range. Much higher doses of phototherapy ($>65\ \mu W \cdot cm^{-2} \cdot nm^{-1}$) might have (as-yet-unidentified) adverse effects.

Although phototherapy has not been associated with any serious long-term effects, important short-term side effects include temperature instability, increased insensible fluid losses, and rash. The focus of nursing care is to prevent or minimize side effects. Newborns receiving phototherapy from phototherapy lamps are placed in a bassinet or under a radiant heat source, and axillary temperature is monitored frequently to assess for hyperthermia. Loose stools are a common effect of phototherapy and can also result in increased insensible water loss. A generalized macular rash frequently develops and resolves spontaneously when phototherapy is discontinued (Stokowski, 2006).

The newborn's eyes are covered at all times while under phototherapy lamps to prevent potential retinal damage. An advantage of the fiberoptic blanket is that eye protection is unnecessary. Eye patches should be removed during feedings to observe for drainage and to promote social stimulation and visual development. Corneal injury can result from eye patches that apply excessive pressure to the eyes or which are loose enough to allow eye opening under the patch (Piazza & Stoll, 2007; Thilo, 2005). Although human studies have not confirmed irradiance effects on the developing gonads, diapers or small diaper-like devices are used as a shield for the testicles or ovaries during phototherapy (Stokowski, 2006).

For infants with severe hyperbilirubinemia, treatment may also include use of a double-volume exchange transfusion to directly remove excess unconjugated bilirubin from the bloodstream. This procedure is reserved for severe cases in whom phototherapy or other treatments have proven ineffective, or whose rate of bilirubin production is escalating rapidly. This procedure involves vascular access and vigilant monitoring, necessitating transfer to the intensive care nursery setting (Kamath et al., 2011).

NEONATAL SEPSIS

The incidence of neonatal sepsis has decreased substantially in the last two decades and is now approximately 0.5 cases per 1,000 live births (Centers for Disease Control and Prevention [CDC], 2017). The clinical signs of neonatal sepsis are nonspecific and often camouflaged or associated with other neonatal diseases such as RDS, metabolic disorders, intracranial hemorrhage, and asphyxia (Rohan & Golombek, 2009c). As such, infection is considered and empirically treated with nearly all unexpected events of hypoxia in the term newborn. Diagnosis of neonatal sepsis is based on clinical signs and supported by a positive blood culture (Bentlin, Suppo, & Rugolo, 2010). Risks for sepsis at birth include factors such as adequacy of perinatal care, infant gestational age, and presence of chorioamnionitis. Table 21–3 identifies these and other factors that may pose risk for neonatal sepsis.

Pathophysiology

Many microorganisms are responsible for infection during the neonatal period. The most common causative bacterial agents are GBS and *E. coli* (Puopolo, Benitz, & Zaoutis, 2018). Infection occurs as a result of the following conditions:

- Intrauterine exposure by means of ascending infection from one or more of the endogenous flora of the cervix or vagina or, less commonly, by a transplacental route from maternal circulation
- Cutaneous transmission as the fetus passes through the birth canal
- Environmental contamination after the birth

TABLE 21–3. Maternal and Perinatal Factors Predisposing Newborns to Sepsis

Maternal factors	Intrapartum factors	Neonatal factors
Low parity	Internal monitoring/ increased duration of internal monitoring	Low Apgar score/ perinatal depression
Recent urinary tract infection	Premature or prolonged rupture of membranes	Low birth weight
Insufficient prenatal care	Maternal infection (e.g., UTI, sepsis)	Premature delivery (including late preterm delivery)
Prior birth of infant with GBS sepsis	Greater duration of labor	Indwelling devices (e.g., umbilical catheter)
History of GBS UTI during pregnancy	Maternal fever >38°C	Male sex
GBS colonization of cervix (especially without chemoprophylaxis)	Chorioamnionitis	Disease/disorder affecting skin integrity
	Difficult delivery/ instrumented delivery	
	Meconium staining/ nonreassuring fetal heart tracing	

GBS, group B *Streptococcus*; UTI, urinary tract infection.
Adapted from Rohan, A. J., & Golombek, S. G. (2009). Hypoxia in the term newborn infant: Part three: Sepsis and hypotension, neurologic, hematologic and metabolic disorders. *MCN: The American Journal of Maternal Child Nursing, 34*(4), 224–233. doi:10.1097/01 .NMC.0000357914.95358.be

Two presentations of infection, early versus late onset, are observed in neonates. Early-onset sepsis occurs within the first 72 hours of age, although clinicians define early infections as those occurring within the first week of age (Wynn et al., 2014). Frequently, inoculation occurred in utero. If symptoms are not present immediately after birth, most newborns become symptomatic within 12 hours with respiratory distress and nonspecific findings such as feeding intolerance, abdominal distension, apnea, or bradycardia (Ohlin, Björkqvist, Montgomery & Schollin, 2010). Late-onset sepsis presents beyond 3 to 7 days of age (Bentlin et al., 2010; Shane, Sanchez, & Stoll, 2017). Late-onset sepsis is likely due to exposure during the birth process or nosocomial transmission after birth from caregivers or invasive procedures and results in findings such as septicemia, pneumonia, and meningitis. Unrecognized sepsis may progress rapidly to hypotension and septic shock.

GBS is the most common gram-positive organism causing sepsis in the newborn and is still a leading infectious etiology of infant mortality and morbidity in the United States (Verani, McGee, & Schrag,

2010; CDC, 2017). Twenty percent to 30% of pregnant women are colonized with GBS; 50% of their infants will be colonized with GBS and 1 in 200 will develop invasive disease (Verani et al., 2010). Most of these infections are now prevented by use of prophylactic antimicrobials in at-risk women. The CDC, AAP, American College of Nurse Midwives, American Academy of Family Physicians, and ACOG endorse protocols to prevent early-onset sepsis. Summary points from the 2018 AAP clinical report for management of early-onset sepsis in neonates born at ≥35 0/7 weeks' gestation (Puopolo et al., 2018) are as follows:

- The epidemiology of early-onset sepsis differs substantially between term and/or late preterm infants and very preterm infants.
- Infants born at ≥35 0/7 weeks' gestation can be stratified by the level of risk for early-onset sepsis. Acceptable approaches to risk stratification include the following:
  ○ Categorical algorithms in which threshold values for intrapartum risk factors are used
  ○ Multivariate risk assessment based on both intrapartum risk factors and infant examinations
  ○ Serial physical examination to detect the presence of clinical signs of illness after birth
- Birth centers should consider the development of locally tailored, documented guidelines for early-onset sepsis risk assessment and clinical management. Ongoing surveillance once guidelines are implemented is recommended.
- The diagnosis of early-onset sepsis is made by using blood or cerebrospinal fluid (CSF) cultures. Early-onset sepsis cannot be diagnosed by using laboratory tests, such as a complete blood cell (CBC) count or C-reactive protein (CRP) or by using surface cultures, gastric aspirate analysis, or urine culture.
- The combination of ampicillin and gentamicin is the appropriate empirical antibiotic regimen for most infants who are at risk for early-onset sepsis. The empirical administration of additional broad-spectrum agents may be indicated in term infants who are critically ill until appropriate culture results are known.
- When blood cultures are sterile, antibiotic therapy should be discontinued by 36 to 48 hours of incubation unless there is clear evidence of site-specific infection.

Assessment

As with all neonatal complications, early identification of newborns at risk and prompt recognition of developing signs decreases morbidity and increases the chances of survival. Recognizing multiple risk factors is the first step in identifying newborns whose early days may be complicated by infection. Risk factors can be categorized as maternal, neonatal, and environmental. A thorough review of antepartum and intrapartum history should specifically look for conditions that increase the risk of early-onset sepsis. If different nurses care for the mother and newborn, communication among healthcare team members is essential to ensure that maternal complications with potential impact on the newborn are not overlooked. The nurse caring for the mother during the postpartum period should notify the neonatal care provider if fever or other symptoms of infection develop.

The primary neonatal factors influencing development of early-onset sepsis are gestational age and birth weight. Gestational age and birth weight vary inversely with morbidity and mortality from sepsis. Preterm newborns may be exposed to the same organisms as term newborns, but their ability to fight infection is lessened. Other factors associated with increased risk of sepsis are resuscitation at birth and low Apgar scores. Congenital anomalies in which the skin or mucous membrane is not intact increase the risk of sepsis because a cutaneous port of entry is available for microorganisms. A history of a nonreassuring fetal heart rate pattern during labor, with or without meconium in the amniotic fluid, may identify fetuses at risk for infection. Maternal risk factors include premature rupture of membranes, chorioamnionitis, intrapartal fever, and GBS colonization (Puopolo et al., 2018). In the case of early-onset sepsis related to GBS, approximately 95% of cases are diagnosed within 48 hours of birth (Nanduri et al., 2019).

The most obvious environmental risk for developing late-onset sepsis is admission to a newborn intensive care unit (NICU). Newborns in the NICU are compromised because of the original reason for admission along with being subjected to manipulation and invasive procedures that frequently puncture the skin, the first line of defense against infection. Environmental risks of nosocomial infection include use of equipment; indwelling catheters and chest tubes; inadequate handwashing or cleaning procedures; breaks in skin integrity, oxygen therapy, mechanical ventilation, surgical procedures, and possibly cohorting. Hand contamination is the most common source of late-onset sepsis in infants in the hospital, underscoring the importance of hand hygiene (Shane et al., 2017).

In addition to reviewing antepartum and intrapartum history, identifying the newborn with neonatal sepsis requires a thorough physical examination, evaluation of vital signs and laboratory data, and recognition of signs consistent with the diagnosis of sepsis. The clinical signs of neonatal sepsis are nonspecific and often camouflaged or associated with other neonatal diseases such as RDS, metabolic disorders, intracranial

hemorrhage, and asphyxia. As such, infection is considered and empirically treated with nearly all unexpected events of hypoxia in the term newborn (Rohan & Golombek, 2009c).

A diagnostic evaluation typically includes a CBC count with a differential cell count, aerobic and anaerobic blood cultures, and supportive cultures such as tracheal aspirate, cerebral spinal fluid, or urine as clinically indicated. For best yield, cultures should be obtained before the initiation of antibiotic therapy from any newborn suspected of being septic. A positive blood culture remains the gold standard for the diagnosis of septicemia. Other studies may include evaluation of acute-phase reactants such as CRP.

Interventions

Many institutions have developed protocols for evaluations to exclude sepsis, including laboratory data and frequency of vital signs and clinical assessment. Such protocols should incorporate evidence, such as AAP (Puopolo, Lynfield, & Cummings [2019]), or ACOG (2019b) published recommendations for the prevention of early-onset sepsis in neonates. In particular, updated AAP (Puopolo et al., 2019) recommendations address challenges that clinicians faced in establishing the obstetric diagnosis of maternal infection and vague definition of newborn clinical illness. The new guidelines describe three current approaches to risk assessment in the term or near term infant: (1) categorical risk assessment, (2) multivariate risk assessment (the Neonatal Early-Onset Calculator), or risk-assessment based on newborn clinical condition. Figure 21–4 elaborates on these three options for early-onset sepsis risk assessment. The new AAP recommendations also consider separately the management of infants born at or near term (Fig. 21–4) and those born preterm (see Fig. 21–6).

After the diagnostic evaluation has been completed in a symptomatic neonate, antibiotic agents are initiated. For early-onset sepsis, ampicillin, a broad-spectrum antimicrobial that is bactericidal for gram-positive and gram-negative bacteria, is used in combination with an aminoglycoside such as gentamicin. The usual dosage of ampicillin used to treat sepsis is 50 to 100 mg/kg every 8 to 12 hours for 7 to 10 days. When sepsis is complicated by meningitis, the dosage is increased and the duration of treatment is extended to 14 days. The choice of antibiotics is ultimately determined by the particular sensitivity of a recovered organism.

PERINATAL HIV INFECTION

Despite great strides in the prevention of perinatal and early childhood transmission of HIV infection, it remains an important source of mortality worldwide.

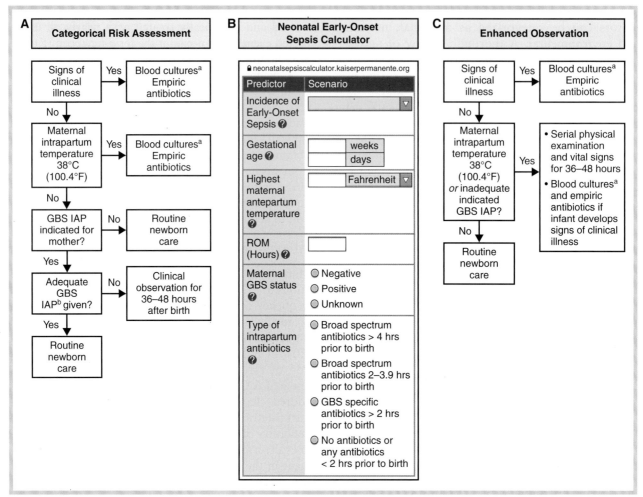

FIGURE 21–4. Options for early-onset sepsis risk assessment among infants born ≥35 weeks' gestation. **A**, Categorical risk assessment. **B**, Neonatal Early-Onset Sepsis Calculator. The screenshot of the Neonatal Early-Onset Sepsis Calculator (https://neonatalsepsiscalculator.kaiserpermanente.org/) was used with permission from Kaiser-Permanente Division of Research. **C**, Enhanced observation. [a]Consider lumbar puncture and CSF culture before initiation of empiric antibiotics for infants who are at the highest risk of infection, especially those with critical illness. Lumbar puncture should not be performed if the infant's clinical condition would be compromised, and antibiotics should be administered promptly and not deferred because of procedure delays. [b]Adequate GBS IAP is defined as the administration of penicillin G, ampicillin, or cefazolin ≥4 hours before delivery. GBS, Group B streptococcal; IAP, intrapartum antibiotic prophylaxis. (From Puopolo, K. M., Lynfield, R., & Cummings, J. J. [2019]. Management of infants at risk of group B streptococcal disease. *Pediatrics, 144*[2], e20191881. doi:10.1542/peds.2019-1881)

Accounting for both developed and developing countries, it is estimated that 1,800 children will become infected with HIV daily, primarily from maternal-to-child transmission. In developed countries, however, the rate of maternal–child transmission has fallen from 15% to 30% to as low as 2%, attributable to the use of preventive strategies including antiretroviral therapy and restricted breastfeeding (Thorne & Newell, 2007).

ACOG and the CDC recommend offering all women of childbearing age the opportunity for preconception counseling and care as a component to routine medical care (ACOG, 2019a; Branson et al., 2006). ACOG, AAP, and the Canadian Paediatric Society recommend HIV testing and counseling, with consent, for all pregnant women in North America and

advocate preconception counseling as part of a comprehensive healthcare program for all women (ACOG, 2019a; Branson et al., 2006; Havens, Mofenson, & AAP Committee on Pediatric AIDS, 2009). HIV testing must be voluntary and free from coercion. No woman should be tested without her knowledge, and each woman has the option to decline or opt out of the HIV screening (Branson et al., 2006). Early identification of the HIV-infected pregnant woman is essential for her health and that of her exposed infant (Panel on Antiretroviral Therapy and Medical Management of HIV-Infected Children, 2010).

Many women with HIV infection enter pregnancy with a known diagnosis and are already receiving antiretroviral therapy, although adjustment to their regimen may be necessary (ACOG, 2018). Decisions regarding therapy should be the same for pregnant and nonpregnant women with HIV infection, with the additional consideration of the potential impact of therapy on the fetus and infant. A chemoprophylaxis regimen such as zidovudine-Nevirapine-lamivudine (ZDV-NVP-3TC) alone or in combination with other antiretroviral drugs should be discussed and offered. Discussions regarding the treatment of HIV should not be coercive, and the woman is ultimately responsible for the final decision.

Chemoprophylaxis for Perinatal HIV Transmission

Perinatal transmission is largely preventable, and studies show nearly a 70% reduction in HIV transmission in infants whose mothers received chemoprophylaxis. The mechanism by which ZDV reduces transmission is not fully defined; protection is likely multifactorial but may be unique to ZDV due to the fact that is metabolized within the placenta itself. The current recommendations for use of antiretroviral chemoprophylaxis to reduce the risk of perinatal transmission of the HIV infection are guidelines only, and flexibility should be exercised according to individual circumstances.

The patient who presents in labor without documented HIV status should receive rapid HIV antibody testing; and those with positive antibody results should commence antiretroviral prophylaxis promptly. Repeat testing is recommended in the third trimester for the pregnant woman with a previous negative HIV antibody test if she remains in a high-risk category (e.g., engages in risky behavior or lives in a high-prevalence area). For the patient in whom acute infection is suspected, virologic testing (e.g., plasma HIV RNA assay) should be obtained because serologic testing may be negative at early stages of infection (Panel on Antiretroviral Therapy and Medical Management of HIV-Infected Children, 2010).

If a woman does not receive ZDV as a component of her antenatal antiretroviral regimen, intrapartum and newborn ZDV is still recommended. If a woman has not received prior therapy, initiation of an antiretroviral regimen may be delayed until after the first trimester, due to the potential of teratogenic effects related to therapy. If a woman is already on drug therapy, ZDV should be added in the first trimester whenever possible followed by a 6-week newborn course of ZDV. There are several recommendations for HIV-infected women who present in labor and have had no prior therapy (ACOG, 2018; Havens et al., 2009).

- Intrapartum IV ZDV followed by 6 weeks of PO ZDV for the newborn
- PO ZDV and 3TC during labor followed by 1 week of PO ZDV-3TC for the newborn

- A single dose of nevirapine at the onset of labor followed by a single dose of nevirapine for the newborn at 48 hours of age
- A single dose of nevirapine at the onset of labor combined with intrapartum IV ZDV and 6 weeks PO ZDV for the newborn

Although intrapartum antiretroviral therapy will not prevent perinatal transmission that occurs before labor, most transmission occurs near or during labor and delivery. Therefore, preexposure prophylaxis is recommended to give antiretroviral drug levels in the fetus during the intensive exposure to HIV-1 in maternal genital secretions and blood during birth (ACOG, 2018).

Mode of Birth

Optimal medical management should focus on minimizing the risk of both perinatal transmission of HIV-1 and the potential for maternal and neonatal complications. A meta-analysis found that the rate of perinatal HIV-1 transmission in women undergoing elective CS was significantly lower than in those women undergoing non-elective CS or vaginal delivery regardless of whether they received ZDV prophylaxis (Andiman et al., 1999). ACOG (2018) recommends considering an elective CS for HIV-1-infected women with HIV-1 RNA levels >1,000 copies per milliliter near the time of delivery (ACOG, 2018). If an elective cesarean delivery is performed, it is recommended that to be done at 38 weeks' gestation; IV ZDV should begin 3 hours before surgery.

Care of the Newborn

HIV-exposed infants should be identified early. Viral diagnostic testing is recommended at birth for infants at high risk for HIV infection, including those born to HIV-positive mothers without prenatal care, those without prenatal antiretroviral prophylaxis, and those with an HIV viral load ≥1,000 copies per milliliter near the time of delivery. Repeated viral testing should occur at 14 to 21 days, 1 to 2 months, and 4 to 6 months postnatally (Panel on Antiretroviral Therapy and Medical Management of HIV-Infected Children, 2010).

Immediate care of the newborn should limit exposure to maternal fluids. A bath should be given once the infant's temperature is stable. Infants born to HIV-infected mothers should have an HIV polymerase chain reaction (PCR) test and CBC with manual differential as part of their admission labs (Havens et al., 2009). Chemoprophylaxis should begin within 8 to 12 hours after birth and continue for 6 weeks (Table 21–4). The recommended ZDV dosage for infants relates to their ability to clear the drug and differs between preterm and term. Infants born at ≥35

TABLE 21–4. Neonatal Antiretroviral (ARV) Drug Dosing for Prevention of Mother-to-Child Transmission of HIV

ARV drug and dose	Duration
Zidovudine should be given to ALL HIV-exposed newborns and should be started as soon after birth as possible, preferably within 6 to 12 hr of delivery.	
≥35 weeks' gestation at birth: 4 mg/kg orally twice daily (if unable to tolerate oral agents, 3 mg/kg/dose intravenously, beginning within 6 to 12 hr of delivery, then every 12 hr)	Birth through 6 week
≥35 to <35 weeks' gestation at birth: 2 mg/kg orally (or 1.5 mg/kg intravenously) every 12 hr, advanced to 3 mg/kg orally (or 2.3 mg/kg intravenously) every 12 hr after age 4 week	Birth through 6 week
Nevirapine administered in addition to zidovudine to newborns of HIV-infected women who received no antepartum ARV prophylaxis	
Weight band closing	Three doses in the first week of age
Birth weight 1.5 to 2 kg: 8 mg for each dose[*]	First dose within 48 hr of birth (as soon after birth as possible)
Birth weight >2 kg: 12 mg for each dose[*]	Second dose 48 hr after first
	Third dose 96 hr after second

From Havens, P. L., & Mofenson, L. M. (2009). Evaluation and management of the infant exposed to HIV-1 in the United States. *Pediatrics, 123*(1), 175–187. doi:10.1542/peds.2008-3076; Siberry, G. K. (2014). Preventing and managing HIV infection in infants, children, and adolescents in the United States. *Pediatrics in Review, 35*(7), 268-286. doi:10.1542/pir.35-7-268

weeks' gestation should receive 1.5 mg/kg/dose every 12 hours IV or 2 mg/kg/dose (syrup) PO every 12 hours, advancing to every 8 hours at 2 weeks of age if ≥30 weeks' gestation at birth or at 4 weeks of age if <30 weeks' gestation at birth. The dosing for full-term infants is 2 mg/kg/dose (syrup) PO every 6 hours or 1.5 mg/kg/dose IV every 6 hours.

In developed countries, including the United States and Canada where access to formula is assured, HIV-infected women should be counseled to avoid breastfeeding regardless of whether they are receiving antiretroviral therapy (Havens et al., 2009).

Anemia is a primary complication of the 6-week course of ZDV in the neonate (Branson et al., 2006). Therefore, at a minimum, a hemoglobin level should be obtained at the end of the treatment course. Infants with negative virologic test results during the first 6 weeks of age should have a repeat HIV DNA PCR after completion of antiretroviral treatment. Routine infant immunizations should be administered to HIV-exposed infants, using disease-specific guidelines (Havens et al., 2009). To prevent *Pneumocystis carinii* pneumonia, all infants born to HIV-infected mothers should also begin prophylaxis after completion of the ZDV prophylaxis regimen.

NEONATAL SUBSTANCE EXPOSURE

Neonatal withdrawal syndrome is a term that was introduced into the literature over two decades ago to describe the variable spectrum of signs of neonatal neurologic and behavioral dysregulation that occurs as a result of withdrawal from certain psychoactive drugs, particularly those that cause addiction in adults (Clark & Rohan, 2015). The neurobehavioral findings associated specifically with opioid withdrawal at birth, following in utero exposure, has been termed the *neonatal abstinence syndrome* (NAS) (Hudak & Tan, 2012). These nonspecific signs may also be associated with non-opioid drug toxicity (Clark & Rohan, 2015).

As the rate of opioid prescription grows, so does fetal exposure to opioids in pregnancy. Between 2000 and 2009, it was estimated that prenatal maternal opiate use increased from 1.2 to 5.6 per 1,000 live hospital births per year (Patrick et al., 2012). In the United States, methadone and heroin are the most common opioids implicated in prenatal exposure, although incidence of fetal exposure to hydrocodone and buprenorphine is increasing (Manchikanti, Fellows, Ailinani, & Pampati, 2010). Between 2000 and 2009, the incidence of NAS among newborns increased from 1.2 to 3.4 per 1,000 hospital births per year, with iatrogenic NAS accounting for only 5% of all cases (Patrick et al., 2012). With increasing fetal exposure to both prescription and nonprescription drugs, there has been a concurrent increase in the identification of abstinence and adaptation difficulties after birth. In addition, the extended use of opioids, barbiturates, and benzodiazepines in neonatal intensive care has resulted in iatrogenic toxicities and abstinence syndromes.

Other in utero substance exposures have presented a challenge to newborn providers, but not necessarily because of withdrawal. For example, the impact of alcohol exposure on the fetus ranges from growth reduction to a spectrum of fetal effects known as the *fetal alcohol syndrome*. Use of cocaine by pregnant women has been implicated as a factor in long-term learning and behavioral difficulties (Cain, Bornick, & Whiteman, 2013). Cigarette smoking has been long recognized to increase the risk fetal growth restriction (Caputo, Wood, & Jablour, 2016).

PATHOPHYSIOLOGY

Maternal drug use in pregnancy has been associated with higher rates of fetal distress and demise, lower Apgar scores, growth retardation, adverse neurodevelopmental outcomes that may not manifest until later in infancy, and acute withdrawal during the neonatal period (Rosen & Bateman, 2002). It is difficult to know whether substance abuse alone or (more likely) the multifactorial influence of drug abuse and social problems is responsible. Many pregnant women who use one substance also use others. The general physical and mental health of these women may be poor, predisposing them to suboptimal weight gain, anemia, or risky behaviors.

Complete information on transmission of illicit drugs to the fetus is unavailable, but most appear to pass easily through the placenta. Increased maternal blood flow in later gestation appears to increase transport of substances to the fetus. The vasoconstricting effects of many of these substances can cause abruptio placentae, elevated blood pressure, precipitous labor, inadequate contraction patterns, decreased fetal oxygenation, and decreased length and head circumference (Rosen & Bateman, 2002). Cocaine is also thought to increase fetal vasoconstricting hormones, leading to increased blood pressure and heart rate in the neonate. These physiologic responses increase risk of cerebral ischemia and hemorrhagic lesions (Rosen & Bateman, 2002).

Although addressed less extensively in substance abuse literature, there can be effects on the fetus and neonate from cigarette tobacco exposure during pregnancy. Thirteen percent to 20% of pregnant women admit to smoking during pregnancy, which poses risks to the parturient as well. Maternal smoking during pregnancy causes a range of negative pregnancy outcomes including miscarriage, low birth weight, preterm birth, and perinatal death (Li, Saad, Oliver, & Chen, 2018). Furthermore, there have also been links between maternal smoking and adverse neurobehavioral, cardiovascular, respiratory, endocrine, and metabolic outcomes in the offspring, which can persist into adulthood (Li et al., 2018). It has been suggested that smoking cessation among childbearing women would reduce stillbirths more than 10% and newborn death by approximately 5% (Rogers, 2008).

The popularity of marijuana and e-cigarettes has been recently increasing, including during pregnancy. E-cigarettes heat e-liquids containing carcinogens and toxins (such as formaldehyde, diacetyl, heavy metals, and nitrosamines) to produce a vapor that delivers flavorings and nicotine. These compounds can accumulate in the developing fetus, affecting intrauterine development. Recent animal studies suggest that maternal e-vapor exposure during pregnancy could cause respiratory and neurologic disorders in the offspring (Li et al., 2018). In a recent study conducted in Colorado, a state with legalized medical and recreational marijuana, the self-reported prevalence of cannabis use at any time during pregnancy was 5.7%, and prenatal cannabis use was found to result in a 50% increased likelihood of low birth weight (Crume et al., 2018).

Assessment

There remains a lack of evidence to support the use of any one specific evaluation strategy to identify NAS (Hudak & Tan, 2012). Maternal fear, guilt and shame related to drug use limit truthful dialogue between women and their healthcare providers (Murphy-Oikonen, Montelpare, Southon, Bertoldo, & Persichino, 2010). Selective newborn toxicology screening using biologic samples is another identification method, but also limited by testing sensitivity, timing requirements, and the application of screening criteria (Murphy-Oikonen et al., 2010). It is important for providers to acknowledge that there has been a changing face of drug addiction in the United States, whereby the illicit use of prescription psychotherapeutics and opioids now overshadows the use of nonprescription illicit drugs (Manchikanti et al., 2010). Selective screening criteria should be regularly reviewed to assure that they address dynamic risk factors for prenatal drug use and addiction (Clark & Rohan, 2015). Toxicology testing obtained using restricted screening criteria (e.g., limited prenatal care, teen parent, child protective agency involvement) may overshadow identification of other important risk factors for NAS (e.g., history of pain syndrome) (Clark & Rohan, 2015). In addition, providers need to be aware that negative newborn toxicology screening does not rule out maternal substance abuse nor does positive screening confirm abuse or addiction (Farst, Valentine, & Hall, 2011).

In NAS, the newborn experiences withdrawal from exposure to a dependency-producing substance, which results in a broad array of clinical signs (Table 21–5). Most commonly, the multisystem impact involves the central nervous and gastrointestinal (GI) systems. Although the most severe withdrawal symptoms are seen in the newborn exposed to opioids, signs of withdrawal or toxicity can also occur after exposure to other drugs. There has been increasing interest in the association between maternal antidepressants and withdrawal signs in the newborn. Selective serotonin

TABLE 21–5. Signs of Neonatal Abstinence and Drug Toxicity

Feeding and gastrointestinal	Autonomic and metabolic	Respiratory and vasomotor	State, tone, and CNS	Other
Uncoordinated suck	Fever	Tachypnea	Lethargy	Skin excoriation
Weak/poor suck	Temperature instability	Retractions	Hypotonia	Poor weight gain
Excessive sucking	Mottling	Nasal stuffiness	Hypertonia	Excessive weight loss
Watery/loose stools	Piloerection	Sneezing	Tone regulation difficulty	High pain scores
Vomiting/reflux	Diaphoresis	Yawning	Hyperreflexia	
Projectile vomiting	Hypoglycemia	Nasal flaring	Seizure/convulsion	
Hyperphagia		Bradycardia	Tremor/jitteriness	
Abdominal tenderness		Tachycardia	Myoclonus/clonus	
"Poor feeding/colic"		Hypertension	Opisthotonus	
			Agitation/irritability	
			Increased wakefulness	
			Hyperactivity	
			Restlessness	
			Poor sleeping pattern	
			Frequent/excessive crying	
			High-pitched crying	

CNS, central nervous system.
From Clark, L., & Rohan, A. J. (2015). Identifying and assessing the substance-exposed infant. *MCN: The American Journal of Maternal Child Nursing, 40*(2), 87–95. doi:10.1097/NMC.0000000000000117

reuptake inhibitors (SSRIs) are frequently used to treat depression in pregnant women. Third trimester exposure to SSRI antidepressants has been associated with a constellation of neonatal signs that are similar to those observed in NAS (Jansson & Velez, 2012). Although SSRI antidepressants have the potential to cause NAS, it has been postulated that some of these cases may in fact represent serotonin toxicity, or a combination of withdrawal and toxicity. It can be difficult to distinguish between withdrawal and toxicity because signs are nonspecific and similar, although plasma concentrations of psychotropic drugs are generally low in withdrawal and high in toxicity. A compilation of drugs that have been associated with signs of withdrawal/toxicity in neonates, or that have properties implicated in NAS, can be found in Table 21–6.

Opioid therapy exceeding 5 to 7 days in length has been consistently implicated as a risk factor for NAS (Cramton & Gruchala, 2013). Early researchers reported rates of withdrawal from prenatal opioids of 55% to 94% (Fricker & Segal, 1978; Harper, Solish, Feingold, Gersten-Woolf, & Sokal, 1977). Researchers acknowledged, however, difficulties in determining actual prenatal opioid usage rates. In one recent study, researchers have demonstrated that NAS occurred in only 5.6% of neonates whose mothers used prescription narcotics in pregnancy (Kellogg, Rose, Harms, & Watson, 2011).

The timing of NAS symptoms can be anticipated based on knowledge of the half-life of drugs to which the fetus was prenatally exposed. Infants can experience withdrawal symptoms within 6 hours of birth for short-acting opioids (such as heroin), whereas long-acting opiates (such as methadone) typically produce withdrawal symptoms after 36 hours (Lugo,

Satterfield, & Kern, 2005). The severity of the abstinence syndrome is affected by the drug or combination of drugs used, although it may not correlate predictably with dose or duration of substance exposure (Burgos & Burke, 2009).

Gestational age appears to affect the severity of NAS, with milder signs developing in more premature infants. The reason for this blunted presentation may be central nervous system immaturity or lower fat deposits in the premature infant, or decreased total drug exposure (Jansson, Dipietro, Elko, & Velez, 2010; Logan, Brown, & Hayes, 2013). It is difficult to accurately assess the severity of abstinence in preterm newborns because the tools available were originally developed for use with term newborns. Many of the characteristics seen in neonatal drug withdrawal are common in preterm newborns, such as tremors, high-pitched cry, tachypnea, and poor feeding.

Interventions

The goals of therapy for NAS are to ensure that the infant receives adequate nutrition and sleep in order to achieve adequate weight gain and integrate into the social environment (Hudak & Tan, 2012). This is accomplished with both nonpharmacologic and pharmacologic therapies. The threshold for initiating pharmacologic therapies is widely variable among institutions (Kellogg et al., 2011; Kuschel, 2007). All substance-exposed neonates should receive individualized supportive, nonpharmacologic care. This necessitates a thorough evaluation of the infant's state, behaviors, and responses to stimuli. Nonpharmacologic interventions or "comfort care" may include targeted positioning (swaddling, therapeutic

TABLE 21–6. Substances Associated with Signs of Neonatal Withdrawal or Toxicity

Opioids/narcotics	CNS stimulants	CNS depressants	Hallucinogens	Other psychotropics
Buprenorphine	Amphetamine	Alcohol	Dextromethorphan	Cyclic antidepressants
Codeine	Caffeine	Barbiturates	Inhalants (solvents/	Amitriptyline
Fentanyl	Cocaine	Amobarbital	aerosols)	Amoxapine
Heroin	Dexamphetamine	Butabarbital	Ketamine	Clomipramine
Hydrocodone	Dextroamphetamine	Butalbital	Lysergic acid	Desipramine
Hydromorphone	Fenfluramine	Methohexital	Diethylamide	Doxepin
Meperidine	Gamma-hydroxybutyric acid	Pentobarbital	Mescaline	Imipramine
Methadone	Methamphetamine	Phenobarbital	Nitrous oxide	Nortriptyline
Morphine	Methylphenidate	Secobarbital	Phencyclidine	Protriptyline
Naloxone	Nicotine	Thiopental	Phenylisopropylamine	Trimipramine
Naltrexone	Pemoline	Benzodiazepines	MDA	Hydroxyzine
Opium	Phencyclidines	Alprazolam	MDEA	Lamotrigine
Oxycodone	Phendimetrazine	Chlordiazepoxide	MDMA	Lithium
Oxymorphone	Phentermine	Clonazepam	Synthetic cathinones	Meprobamate
Pentazocine	Phenylpropanolamine	Diazepam	(bath salts)	SSRI antidepressants
Propoxyphene	Pseudoephedrine	Flurazepam		Citalopram
Tapentadol		Lorazepam		Escitalopram
Tramadol		Midazolam		Fluoxetine
		Oxazepam		Fluvoxamine
		Temazepam		Paroxetine
		Triazolam		Sertraline
		Cannabinoids		Viibryd
		Chlordiazepoxide		
		Chloral hydrate		
		Ethchlorvynol		
		Glutethimide		
		Hashish		
		Marijuana		
		Methaqualone		

CNS, central nervous system; SSRI, selective serotonin reuptake inhibitor.
From Clark, L., & Rohan, A. J. (2015). Identifying and assessing the substance-exposed infant. *MCN: The American Journal of Maternal Child Nursing, 40*(2), 87–95. doi:10.1097/NMC.0000000000000117

tucking), soothing techniques (nonnutritive sucking, gentle rocking, massage), and interaction modifications (minimal stimulation environment). Nonpharmacologic techniques are routinely implemented prior to the initiation of pharmacologic therapies for NAS, and as an adjunct to pharmacologic therapies (Display 21–5). Breastfeeding is the preferred method of feeding for almost all term infants. For infants with methadone- or buprenorphine-dependent mothers, breastfeeding has been identified as safe, and even beneficial, regardless of dose (Pritham, 2013). In addition, the use of IV hydration or small, hypercaloric feedings has been used to minimize the effects of GI disruption, improve nutrition, and prevent dehydration (Hudak & Tan, 2012).

Newborns who do not respond to symptomatic treatment alone may need medication. Ideally, the decision to begin medication is based on an objective assessment of symptoms such as a Modified Finnegan Scoring System (Fig. 21–5). The newborn is assessed and scored every 2 hours for the first 48 hours and then every 8 hours while symptoms of withdrawal persist. Points are given for all behaviors or symptoms observed during the scoring interval. The newborn must be awake and calm to assess muscle tone, respirations, and Moro reflex. Observations should be made after feeding whenever possible because hunger can mimic withdrawal. If, despite nursing interventions, scores exceed the scoring tool threshold, medications are initiated (Kuschel, 2007). A simplified scoring system, the Neonatal Withdrawal Inventory, has been

DISPLAY 21–5

Nonpharmacologic Interventions to Support the Newborn Experiencing Withdrawal

Swaddling

Rocking

Decrease tactile stimulation

Dark room

Decrease environmental noise and stimulation

Water bed

Small, frequent feedings

Use of a pacifier

A modified Finnegan scoring system for assessment of neonatal abstinence syndrome

System	Signs and symptoms	Score	Date and time									
Central nervous system disturbances	High-pitched cry	2	...	...	...	...	...	...	...	...	...	...
	Continuous high-pitched cry	3	...	...	...	...	...	...	...	...	...	...
	Sleeps <1 h after feeding	3	...	...	...	...	...	...	...	...	...	...
	Sleeps <2 h after feeding	2	...	...	...	...	...	...	...	...	...	...
	Sleeps <3 h after feeding	1	...	...	...	...	...	...	...	...	...	...
	Mild tremors when disturbed	1	...	...	...	...	...	...	...	...	...	...
	Moderate–severe tremors when disturbed	2	...	...	...	...	...	...	...	...	...	...
	Mild tremors–undisturbed	3	...	...	...	...	...	...	...	...	...	...
	Moderate–severe tremors–undisturbed	4	...	...	...	...	...	...	...	...	...	...
	Increased muscle tone	2	...	...	...	...	...	...	...	...	...	...
	Excoriation (specify are)	1	...	...	...	...	...	...	...	...	...	...
	Myoclonic jerks	3	...	...	...	...	...	...	...	...	...	...
	Generalized convulsions	5	...	...	...	...	...	...	...	...	...	...
Metabolic, vasomotor, respiratory disturbances	Sweating	1	...	...	...	...	...	...	...	...	...	...
	Fever (37.5–38.3 °C)	1	...	...	...	...	...	...	...	...	...	...
	Fever (38.4 °C and higher)	2	...	...	...	...	...	...	...	...	...	...
	Frequent yawning (>3–4 times)	1	...	...	...	...	...	...	...	...	...	...
	Nasal stuffiness	1	...	...	...	...	...	...	...	...	...	...
	Sneezing (>3-4 times)	1	...	...	...	...	...	...	...	...	...	...
	Nasal flaring	2	...	...	...	...	...	...	...	...	...	...
	Respiratory rate >60/min	1	...	...	...	...	...	...	...	...	...	...
	Respiratory rate >60/min with retractions	2	...	...	...	...	...	...	...	...	...	...
Gastrointestinal disturbances	Excessive sucking	1	...	...	...	...	...	...	...	...	...	...
	Poor feeding	2	...	...	...	...	...	...	...	...	...	...
	Regurgitation	2	...	...	...	...	...	...	...	...	...	...
	Projectile vomiting	3	...	...	...	...	...	...	...	...	...	...
	Loose stools	2	...	...	...	...	...	...	...	...	...	...
	Watery stools	3	...	...	...	...	...	...	...	...	...	...
	Total score	...	...	...	...	...	...	...	...	...	...	...
	Scorer's initials	...	...	...	...	...	...	...	...	...	...	...

Consider treatment if scores are >8.

FIGURE 21–5. A Modified Finnegan Scoring System. (From Kuschel, C. [2007]. Managing drug withdrawal in the newborn infant. *Seminars in Fetal and Neonatal Medicine, 12*, 128.)

developed based on the Finnegan and other more complex scoring systems (Zahorodny et al., 1998).

A variety of medications are used to treat NAS, and the choice of medication varies with individual nurseries. The AAP recommends the use of pharmacologic treatments for NAS to relieve moderate-to-severe signs and to prevent complications (fever, weight loss) in an infant who does not respond to nonpharmacologic therapies (Hudak & Tan, 2012) while recognizing that opioids generally increase length of hospital stay (Osborn, Jeffery, & Cole, 2010). The most common single agent used in NAS is oral morphine, although methadone and buprenorphine are acceptable first-line choices (Cramton & Gruchala, 2013; Hudak & Tan, 2012).

Whether infants exhibiting signs of NAS or at risk for NAS receive inpatient or outpatient management varies across settings, and according to case-specific risk factors. Discharge from the hospital for older infants who have received opioids for NAS can be individualized in consideration of the infant's age, overall status, stability of home environment, and availability of support and follow-up. For younger infants, it is prudent to delay hospital discharge until neurobehavioral assessments are free from signs of withdrawal for a period of 24 to 48 hours following discontinuation of opioids (Clark & Rohan, 2015; Hudak & Tan, 2012).

LATE PRETERM INFANTS

Prematurity is the major determinant of neonatal mortality and morbidity. The preterm birth rate in the United States rose to 9.93% in 2017, a 1% rise from 2016 (9.85%), and the third straight year of increase in this rate (9.57% in 2014). The preterm birth rate (percentage of all births delivered at less than 37 completed weeks of gestation) had declined steadily from 2007 to 2014. Most of the increase in the total preterm birth rate for 2016 to 2017 was among infants born late preterm (34 to 36 weeks), up from 7.09% to 7.17%. The early preterm birth rate (less than 34 weeks) was 2.76% in 2017, unchanged since 2015 but down from 2.93% in 2007 (Martin, Hamilton, Osterman, Driscoll, & Drake, 2018).

Late preterm births present a unique challenge to healthcare providers. These infants are often treated like full-term newborns. However, they have many of the same risks of complications as infants born prematurely. Professional organizations including the Association of Women's Health, Obstetric and Neonatal Nurses (AWHONN), the National Institute of Child Health and Human Development (NICHD) of the National Institutes of Health, and the AAP have led the way in defining and educating healthcare providers and the public on the distinct needs of the late preterm infant.

In 2005, the NICHD convened a multidisciplinary task force, which summarized the current state of knowledge on late preterm births and published a special, two-part supplement summarizing the findings from the meetings in Seminars in Perinatology (National Institute of Child Health and Human Development Workshop, 2005; Raju, Higgins, Stark, & Leveno, 2006). This multidisciplinary team of experts discussed the definition and terminology, epidemiology, etiology, biology of maturation, clinical care, surveillance, and public health aspects of late preterm infants. Knowledge gaps were identified and research priorities listed. The NICHD panel recommended that births between 34 completed weeks (34 0/7 weeks or day 239) and less than 37 completed weeks (36 6/7 weeks or day 259) of gestation be referred to as late preterm (Raju et al., 2006). Also in 2005, AWHONN (Medoff-Cooper, Bakewell-Sachs, Buus-Frank, & Santa-Donato, 2005) launched a multiyear initiative to address the unique physiologic and developmental needs of the late preterm infant that resulted in the development of a conceptual framework for optimizing the health of late preterm infant. In 2010, AWHONN released an evidence-based clinical practice guideline to provide nurses and other healthcare professionals with state-of-the-science recommendations to accurately assess and manage this high-risk population. Since its initial release, this guideline has been updated to reflect new evidence (AWHONN, 2017). Additionally, in a clinical report defining and describing late preterm infants and their unique characteristics, the AAP has published guidelines for care of these at-risk infants (Engle, Tomashek, Wallman, & Committee on Fetus and Newborn, 2007).

Obstetrical and Neonatal Issues

Obstetricians face many challenges when managing a woman in preterm labor (Hankins & Longo, 2006; Lee, Cleary-Goldman, & D'Alton, 2006; Sibai, 2006). Continuous assessment of anticipated risks for both the mother and the fetus is crucial. Although a baby born prematurely increases neonatal morbidity and mortality, a fetus left in a suboptimal intrauterine environment can lead to fetal demise. There are specific medical indications for delivering prior to 39 weeks' gestation (placental abruption, placenta previa, bleeding, infection, hypertension, preeclampsia, idiopathic preterm labor, preterm premature rupture of membranes, fetal growth restriction, and multiple gestation); however, up to 15% of all births in the United States are currently performed electively (without identifiable medical or obstetric indication) (Clark, Frye, et al., 2010; Clark, Knox, Simpson, & Hankins, 2010; Clark et al., 2009). Early elective induction of labor and elective primary and repeat cesarean delivery resulting in late preterm births has contributed to the overall neonatal morbidity (Clark et al., 2009; Tita et al., 2009). Providers have been cautioned against elective delivery prior to 39 weeks' gestation (Tita et al., 2009). Nursing and medical leadership need to adopt strategies to reduce elective deliveries prior to 39 completed weeks. Specific evidence-based strategies and resources are available for clinicians to use in discouraging elective births prior to 39 completed weeks with the goal of improving both perinatal and infant mortality (March of Dimes, 2010a, 2010b).

Pathophysiology

Late preterm births present a unique challenge to healthcare providers. Although it is encouraging that the overall rate of preterm birth has declined, late preterm birth continues to comprise over 70% of all preterm births in the United States. Late preterm infants, compared to term infants, have a higher rate of respiratory distress, temperature instability, hypoglycemia, hyperbilirubinemia, apnea, seizures, feeding difficulties, rehospitalization, and long-term behavior and learning problems (Engle et al., 2007; Raju et al., 2006; Wang, Dorer, Fleming, & Catlin, 2004). Compared to term infants, late preterm infants have not only significantly more medical problems but also increased hospital costs (Bird et al., 2010; McLaurin, Hall, Jackson, Owens, & Mahadevia, 2009).

Although late preterm infants have many of the same risks of complications as infants born prematurely, they often masquerade as term newborns in size. Subtle signs of a difficult transition to extrauterine life may result in many of these challenged infants being triaged to the newborn nursery where policies, staffing, and care models focus on normal term newborns.

Guidelines for caring for the late preterm infant population is now based on a growing body of evidence. Among these guidelines are recommendations for providing a safe and supported institutional environment in which parents can learn to care for their higher need newborn in the days following birth. In particular, AAP and AWHONN guidelines provide the foundation for recommendations that follow in this section.

Hypothermia and Hypoglycemia

Cold stress and hypoglycemia are very common in late preterm infants during the early transitional period of adaptation (Engle et al., 2007; Laptook & Jackson, 2006; Vachharajani & Dawson, 2009). Late preterm infants have less brown fat compared to term newborns, resulting in a higher risk of developing hypothermia. These infants are poorly prepared to deal with the increased energy demands of cold stress because metabolic reserves are low (Garg & Devaskar, 2006; Laptook & Jackson, 2006). Accordingly, the risk of hypoglycemia is exponentially increased for late preterm infants as they face this and other high-metabolic states.

Hyperbilirubinemia

Late preterm infants are more prone to developing hyperbilirubinemia and its sequelae and to require hospital readmission for treatment (Engle et al., 2007; Wang et al., 2004). These vulnerable infants are 2.4 times more likely to develop significant hyperbilirubinemia and have significantly higher TSB levels. Elevated bilirubin levels are primarily due to immature liver function and diminished capacity for bilirubin conjugation. These physiologic risks, coupled with more difficult feeding patterns and lower oral intake, exacerbate increased enterohepatic recirculation of bilirubin and may explain the correlation among decreased postmenstrual age, hyperbilirubinemia, and the increased risk for kernicterus (Sarici et al., 2004). Although the incidence of kernicterus in late preterms is unknown, compared to term infants, these infants are at increased risk for bilirubin neurotoxicity and kernicterus (Bhutani et al., 2004; Sarici et al., 2004).

Respiratory Distress

Studies have shown the high incidence of respiratory distress and NICU admissions in the late preterm infants (Clark, 2005; Escobar et al., 2005; Hibbard et al., 2010; Roth-Kleiner, Wagner, Bachmann, & Pfenninger, 2003). These infants have a higher incidence of TTNB, pneumonia, RDS, PPHN, and hypoxic respiratory failure than term infants (Hibbard et al., 2010). Nearly 50% of infants born at 34 weeks gestation require intensive care; this number drops to 15% at 35 weeks and 8% at 36 weeks gestation (Dudell & Jain, 2006). The last few weeks of gestation are critical for fetal development and maturation specifically related to surfactant and lung maturity. Biochemical and hormonal changes that accompany spontaneous labor and vaginal delivery also play an important role in the newborn's ability to transition smoothly to an extrauterine environment (Dudell & Jain, 2006). For effective gas exchange to occur, alveolar spaces must be cleared of excess fluid and ventilated, and pulmonary blood flow must be increased to match ventilation with perfusion. Failure of either of these events may jeopardize neonatal transition and cause respiratory distress. A significant number of late preterm infants are delivered by CS, which is a factor that contributes to the already comparatively high CS rate of over 30% in the United States (Betrán et al., 2016). A higher occurrence of respiratory morbidity in late preterm and term infants delivered by CS has been observed (Hansen, Wisborg, Uldbjerg, & Henriksen, 2007; L. Jain & Dudell, 2006; Levine, Ghai, Barton, & Strom, 2001). These infants are known to develop PPHN and become seriously ill and require significant clinical interventions such as inhaled nitric oxide, HFOV, vasopressor support, and ultimately may progress to ECMO (Ramachandrappa & Jain, 2008). The inability to clear lung fluid, the relative deficiency of pulmonary surfactant, and birth in the absence of labor all contribute to pulmonary dysfunction (L. Jain & Eaton, 2006; Ramachandrappa & Jain, 2008).

Apnea of Prematurity

Late preterm infants are three times more likely to experience apnea than their term counterparts (Engle et al., 2007). Between 32 and 34 weeks of gestation, the fetus develops synchrony and control of breathing. This period of breathing pattern maturation decreases the risk of apnea of prematurity. The pathogenesis of apnea is multifactorial and includes immature lung volume and upper airway control, ventilatory responses to hypoxia and carbon dioxide, and feeding as well as physiologic and iatrogenic anemia (Darnall, Ariagno, & Kinney, 2006). It is important to remember that infants born between 33 and 38 weeks' gestation continue to have apnea and are at risk for the resulting periods of bradycardia and hypoxia and are at higher risk for sudden infant death syndrome (SIDS) (Hunt, 2006; Ramanathan et al., 2001).

Brain and Long-term Outcomes

Compared to term newborns, late preterm infants have a more immature brain. It is estimated that an infant at 35 weeks' gestation has fewer sulci and that the weight of the brain is approximately 65% that of the term infant. Periventricular leukomalacia is a known predictor of adverse neurologic outcomes in preterm infants. Late preterm infants are at risk for developing periventricular leukomalacia; however, the exact incidence is unknown (Kinney, 2006). Brainstem development of infants born between 33 and 38 weeks' gestation is less mature than that of a term newborn, although more research on this specific population of infants is needed (Darnall et al., 2006). There is a paucity of data on the long-term neurodevelopmental outcome in late preterm infants. Few studies have examined the long-term neurodevelopmental status of late preterm infants and the prevalence rates for subtle neurologic abnormalities, learning and behavioral difficulties, and scholastic achievement (Raju et al., 2006). However, there is growing concern that these infants are more vulnerable to brain injury and long-term neurologic sequelae (Adams-Chapman, 2006; Chyi, Lee, Hintz, Gould, & Sutcliffe, 2008; Morse, Zheng, Tang, & Roth, 2009; Petrini et al., 2009) and are at more than a threefold increased risk for developing cerebral palsy compared to term newborns (Wang et al., 2004). In contrast to these studies, no significant differences in neurologic outcomes were found in school age children (between the ages of 4 and 15 years) who were born late preterm compared to children born at term (Gurka, LoCasale-Crouch, & Blackman, 2010).

Feeding Challenges

The GI tract continues to develop throughout gestation, but the late preterm infant adapts quickly to enteral feedings, including the digestion and absorption of lactose, protein, and fats (Neu, 2006). However, peristaltic functions and sphincter controls in the esophagus, stomach, and intestines are less likely to be mature and fully functional in late preterm infants, which may lead to difficulty in coordinating suck and swallowing, gastroesophageal reflux, a delay in successful breastfeeding, poor weight gain, and dehydration during early postnatal weeks (Escobar et al., 2002; Neu, 2006; Tomashek et al., 2006).

The physiologic organization of sucking is almost fully organized by 36 weeks' gestation, whereas swallow rhythm is established by 32 weeks' gestation (Gewolb, Vice, Schweiter-Kenney, Taciak, & Bosma, 2001). Precise timing for the activation of several upper airway muscles is critical for suck–swallow coordination, but unlike sucking, swallowing interrupts breathing, allowing protection of the airway and decreasing the risk for aspiration (Thach, 2005; Walker, 2008). It is likely that the etiology of the frequent feeding issues encountered by late preterm infants stems from the immaturity of the coordination of sucking, swallowing, and breathing (Darnall et al., 2006; Walker, 2008). It is important to remember that less energy is required to feed from the breast than from the bottle, because the peristaltic activity of the tongue provokes the peristaltic movement of the GI tract and stimulates swallowing (Aguayo, 2001).

Sepsis

Late preterm infants do have unique susceptibilities to infection including the closed setting of a NICU, and the immunologic immaturity of premature infants sets the stage for development of nosocomial infections (Benjamin & Stoll, 2006). Late preterm infants are more likely to be evaluated for sepsis and treated with a 7-day course of antibiotics compared to term newborns (Wang et al., 2004). There are little data on the host-defense capabilities of late preterm infants. Recent advances provide a framework for understanding the mechanisms underlying the propensity of infections in this at-risk population. Compared with term and extremely preterm infants, late preterm infants are intermediate with regard to immunologic maturity (Clapp, 2006). A current approach to managing early-onset sepsis in preterm infants—particularly GBS disease—is based on circumstances surrounding birth. Although many of these infants have been exposed to intrapartum antibiotic prophylaxis (IAP), the most reasonable approach is often to obtain a blood culture and start on empiric antibiotics (Fig. 21–6).

Care Environment

Late preterm infants masquerade as term newborns, making it difficult to determine their potential immediately following delivery. Pathologic signs and symptoms of late preterm infants transitioning to extrauterine life may be subtle or may be considered normal transition. Depending on their presentation at delivery, an astute assessment of the late preterm infant is critical because many of these infants may be triaged to the newborn nursery and/or room in with their parents where policies, staffing, and care models focus on normal term newborns. This may result in suboptimal time for nurses to perform vigilant assessments, establish lactation, and provide detailed discharge instruction (Pappas & Walker, 2010).

Parent Education, Family Support, and Discharge Planning

Discharge teaching should include information about SIDS prevention. Compared to term infants, late preterm infants are at a twofold higher risk of developing SIDS (Darnall et al., 2006). Healthcare providers need to educate families about infants' increased risk for SIDS and demonstrate appropriate SIDS prevention strategies within the nurseries prior to discharge so families can mimic appropriate caregiving behaviors. The AAP (2016) recommends infants be placed supine (wholly on the back) for every sleep, the use of firm sleep surfaces (soft materials or objects should not be placed under a sleeping infant), keeping soft objects and loose bedding out of crib, avoiding maternal smoking during pregnancy and newborn exposure to secondhand smoke, and a separate sleep surface that is close to the parents' bed. Additional considerations should include the following: offering a pacifier at bed time or nap time once breastfeeding has fully been established, avoiding overheating and

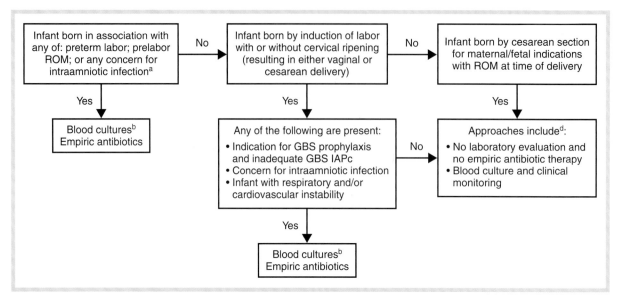

FIGURE 21–6. Early-onset sepsis risk assessment among infants born ≤34 weeks' gestation. [a]Intraamniotic infection should be considered when a pregnant woman presents with unexplained decreased fetal movement and/or there is sudden and unexplained poor fetal testing. [b]Lumbar puncture and CSF culture should be performed before initiation of empiric antibiotics for infants who are at the highest risk of infection unless the procedure would compromise the infant's clinical condition. Antibiotics should be administered promptly and not deferred because of procedural delays. [c]Adequate GBS IAP is defined as the administration of penicillin G, ampicillin, or cefazolin ≥4 hours before delivery. [d]For infants who do not improve after initial stabilization and/or those who have severe systemic instability, the administration of empiric antibiotics may be reasonable but is not mandatory. CSF, cerebrospinal fluid; GBS, Group B streptococcal; IAP, intrapartum antibiotic prophylaxis. (From Puopolo, K. M., Lynfield, R., & Cummings, J. J. [2019]. Management of infants at risk of group B streptococcal disease. *Pediatrics, 144*[2], e20191881. doi:10.1542/peds.2019-1881)

commercial products inconsistent with safe sleep recommendations, not using home monitors as a strategy to reduce the incidence of SIDS, and encouraging "tummy time" when the infant is awake and observed to minimize development of positional plagiocephaly (i.e., assymetrical skull) (AAP, 2016).

The AAP has established specific criteria for discharging late preterm infants (Engle et al., 2007). According to these guidelines, late preterm infants must be medically stable and able to spontaneously breathe room air without apnea, bradycardia, or episodes of significant desaturation prior to be discharged. These infants must be able to maintain a normal body temperature without the use of adjunctive heating devices and should be assessed closely for immature feeding behaviors. Parents need to be confident and competent in their ability to care for their baby prior to discharge and need to be equipped and empowered with the knowledge to appropriately and effectively care for this population of infants and their potential risks after discharge. Specifically, parent education needs to include the increased risk that their child has hyperbilirubinemia, feeding difficulties, apnea, sepsis, respiratory problems, and hypothermia. It is imperative that a follow-up visit 24 to 48 hours after discharge is scheduled with an identified primary care provider prior to discharge.

Readmission Risk and Newborn Follow-up

Late preterm infants are two to three times more likely to be readmitted to the hospital compared to term newborns (Burgos, Schmitt, Stevenson, & Phibbs, 2008; McLaurin et al., 2009; Tomashek et al., 2006). Hospital readmission risk factors include maternal complications during labor and delivery, families receiving support from a public payer, parents who are of Asian/Pacific Islander ethnicity, a firstborn infant, male gender, use of assisted ventilation, and an infant being breast-fed at discharge (Escobar, Clark, & Green, 2006; Escobar et al., 2002; Nanduri et al., 2019; Shapiro-Medoza et al., 2006; Tomashek et al., 2006). Jaundice, proven or suspected infections, feeding and respiratory difficulties (including gastroesophageal reflux disease), sepsis, and failure to thrive were the most common diagnoses at readmission (Escobar et al., 2006; S. Jain & Cheng, 2006).

Despite gains in the overall rate of premature birth in the United States, late preterm birth continues to impact overall child health outcomes, including hospital admission and readmission rates (Burgos et al., 2011). The use of standardized evidence-based protocols such as those developed by AWHONN (2017) reduces the burden of disease for late preterm infants. A summary of these guidelines is presented in Table 21–7.

TABLE 21–7. Assessment and Care of the Late Preterm Infant

Goal	Nursing assessment and care interventions
Determine accurate gestational age	• Review prenatal records to confirm gestational age from prenatal assessment. • Perform postnatal gestational assessment within 12 hr of age (e.g., New Ballard Score). • Obtain infant's length, weight, and head circumference and plot on validated growth curve to determine size/dates (i.e., AGA, SGA, or LGA).
Cardiopulmonary stability	• VS within 30 min of age, every 30 min until 2 hr of age, and then every 2 to 4 hr as stable • Assess respiratory rate (normal 30 to 60 breaths/min); note: LPI may exhibit periodic breathing or brief tachypnea during transition. • Assess and document signs of respiratory distress; note: Normal newborns may exhibit grunting during the first 2 postnatal hr. • If work of breathing is increased, implement appropriate interventions: Notify healthcare provider, apply pulse oximeter probe to determine saturation, and consider supplemental oxygen (monitored and heated/humidified) to achieve pulse oximetry target of 85% to 95% saturation. • Assess heart rate (normal 120 to 160 bpm) and perfusion (normal capillary refill time up to 3 sec). • Assess muscle tone and overall activity as indicator of oxygenation. • If infant is without distress, may initiate kangaroo care (KC)
Thermal stability	• Assess temperature within 30 min of age, followed by every 30 min until 2 hr of age, and then every 2 to 4 hr as stable. • Review perinatal history to identify risks for heat loss/cold stress. • Thoroughly dry infant; provide prewarmed linens and dry cap for head. • Preheat radiant warmer or incubator and use temperature controls. • Target infant temperature: 97.7° to 99.3°F (36.5° to 37.4°C) • Avoid heat loss through conduction, convection, evaporation, and radiation. • Initiate measures to support thermoneutrality, such as KC or swaddling. • Postpone bath until thermal and cardiopulmonary stabilities are evident (typically 2 to 4 hr after birth), then bathe, incorporating measures such as short bath duration, sponge or swaddled bath, bath water temperature of 100° to 104°F, minimized room drafts, room temperature set between 79°F and 81°F, prewarmed towels for drying, immediate cap and wrap in warm blankets. • If infant becomes hypothermic, place in KC, incubator, or under radiant warmer and monitor temperature every 30 min until normalized; review history for risk factors or other indicators of illness.
Glucose stability	• Review antenatal/perinatal history to identify risks for glucose instability. • Perform screening point-of-care glucose assessment within the first 2 hr of life and thereafter as indicated if infant is displaying symptoms suggesting hypoglycemia. • Provide early, frequent feedings on demand, with interval between feedings no longer than 2 to 3 hr if breastfed and 3 to 4 hr if formula fed. • If hypoglycemia is suspected, immediately assess glucose level; in general, for glucose <40 to 45 mg/dL (2.2 to 2.6 mmol/L), immediately send confirmatory serum glucose; note: No exact definition of hypoglycemia exists. • For plasma glucose ≥40 to 45 mg/dL (2.2 to 2.6 mmol/L), establish frequent feedings and follow clinically. • For plasma glucose <40 to 45 mg/dL, immediately feed per breast or formula per gavage or bottle and repeat glucose level within 30 min of feeding. • If the infant exhibits signs of hypoglycemia and the glucose is <40 to 45 mg/dL and feedings are not tolerated, provide IV bolus of 10% dextrose in water (2 mL/kg) and establish IV maintenance at 4 to 6 mg/kg/min; repeat glucose testing within 30 min of bolus and thereafter every 1 to 2 hr until stabilized. • For persistent hypoglycemia, consider transferring infant to a higher acuity unit or facility for supportive care.
Feeding readiness and tolerance	• Assess readiness for feeding prior to initiating oral feedings, including infant's ability to coordinate sucking/swallowing and breathing; LPI may have weak suck, immature feeding pattern, and limited ability to display robust feeding cues. • Monitor for stability during feedings; LPI may easily fatigue and lose stamina during feedings at bottle and breast. • Evaluate maternal position for breastfeeding, latch, and milk transfer. • Facilitate early and frequent breastfeeding (8 to 12 times/day). • Observe, educate, and validate maternal knowledge about feeding behaviors seen in the LPI, including need to wake before feedings, feeding frequently, and continually assessing coordination of sucking/swallowing/breathing. • Encourage adequate milk supply and transfer with strategies such as prepumping breast prior to breastfeeding attempt and using support of lactation consultant; extended lactation support, education, and frequent follow-up are warranted in this population to ensure successful lactation and to avoid potentially dangerous complications related to insufficient lactation (Radtke, 2011).

(continued)

TABLE 21–7. Assessment and Care of the Late Preterm Infant *(Continued)*

Goal	Nursing assessment and care interventions
Recognition of potential complications	• Recognize that the late preterm is at increased risk for sepsis and identify maternal, perinatal, and neonatal risks. • Identify and address presenting signs of infection, including, but not limited to, temperature instability, behavioral changes, poor feeding, or cardiopulmonary instability. • Recognize that the late preterm is at increased risk for significant hyperbilirubinemia and identify maternal and neonatal risks. • Note presence of clinical jaundice within the first 24 hr of life and initiate immediate screening of total serum bilirubin if visible jaundice exists; plot bilirubin level on hour-specific nomogram and initiate phototherapy for levels above threshold. • Evaluate bilirubin level prior to discharge using serum or transcutaneous assessment. • If the planned postdischarge primary provider visit does not coincide with the anticipated peak of bilirubin (e.g., 5 to 7 days of age), plan additional follow-up visit.
Developing and supporting parental role	• Provide parent support to establish their new role. • Encourage KC and prioritize care to support uninterrupted periods for parent/infant bonding. • Help parents identify infant behaviors, especially alertness and hunger/satiety cues; develop and model appropriate responses to infant cues. • Encourage parents to room-in prior to discharge. • Assess level of emotional distress in parents, with attention to depression and post-traumatic stress symptoms and refer as needed. • Ensure that parents identify primary care provider and community follow-up resources prior to discharge; first provider visit should occur within 24 to 48 hr of discharge. • Document and clearly communicate all outpatient provider appointments.
Discharge planning	• *Discharge should not be considered prior to 48 hr of age.* • Conduct and document complete health assessment within 24 hr of discharge. • Teach parents how to assess for signs of distress and intervene appropriately. • Counsel parents about environmental risks, including secondhand smoke exposure. • Reinforce supine positioning for sleep and avoidance of soft blankets, pillows, and crib toys. • Assess for risks for *respiratory syncytial virus* (RSV) including <35 weeks' gestational age at birth, childcare attendance, preschool-aged siblings, exposure to environmental pollutants, male gender, household having more than five persons, SGA. • Confirm pediatric care provider (PCP) follow-up visit is planned within 24 to 48 hr of discharge. • Ensure that car seat safety test is performed prior to discharge. • Confirm infant's ability to sustain normal temperature in open crib with appropriate clothing. • Teach proper procedures for determining axillary temperature and performing bath. • Complete teaching and assess learning about infant safety and indications for seeking assistance from PCP, including elevated temperature, signs of dehydration, poor feeding, lethargy, or irritability and provide supportive written information.

AGA, appropriate for gestational age; IV, intravenous; LGA, large for gestational age; LPI, late preterm infant; SGA, small for gestational age; VS, vital signs. Adapted from Association of Women's Health, Obstetric and Neonatal Nurses. (2017). *Assessment and care of the late preterm infant* (Evidence-Based Clinical Practice Guideline, 2nd ed.). Washington, DC: Author.

There remains great opportunity for research and policy to guide strategies to further reduce the incidence and impact of late preterm birth, thereby diminishing its economic and social costs to society.

HYPOXIC ISCHEMIC ENCEPHALOPATHY

HIE is the leading cause of neonatal encephalopathy in term and late-preterm newborns and is a major cause of death and disability (Pfister & Soll, 2010). Typically, HIE ensues after a disruption in cerebral blood flow and oxygen delivery to the brain, secondary to insufficient placental blood flow and gas exchange. The progression of HIE and degree of injury are dependent on the timing, duration, and severity of the insult (Pfister & Soll, 2010). The incidence of HIE ranges from 1 to 8 per 1,000 live births in developed countries and is as high as 26 per 1,000 live births in underdeveloped countries (Kurinczuk, White-Koning, & Badawi, 2010). Perinatal factors associated with the risk of HIE include maternal diabetes, morbid obesity, chorioamnionitis, placental abruption, umbilical cord prolapsed, uterine rupture, tight nuchal cord, or acute blood loss (Rutherford et al., 2005; Selway, 2010).

Pathophysiology

Adequate blood flow helps the fetal brain maintain homeostasis and meet cellular energy demands. Perinatal factors that result in hypoxia to the fetus eventually lead to a decrease in fetal cardiac output, which reduces cerebral blood flow. If cerebral blood flow is only moderately decreased, the cerebral arteries shunt blood flow from the anterior circulation to the posterior circulation to maintain adequate perfusion of the brainstem, cerebellum, and basal ganglia (Douglas-Escobar & Weiss, 2015). As a result, damage is restricted to the cerebral cortex and watershed areas of the cerebral hemispheres. On the other hand, acute hypoxia causes an abrupt and more severe decrease in cerebral blood flow, which produces injury to the basal ganglia and thalami (Harteman et al., 2013).

Physiologic consequences of hypoxic ischemia evolve over hours to days, resulting in a biphasic pattern of energy failure leading to brain injury, separated by a brief recovery or "latent phase" (Douglas-Escobar & Weiss, 2015; Gluckman et al., 2005). In the acute phase, decreased cerebral blood flow reduces the delivery of oxygen and glucose to the brain, which leads to anaerobic metabolism. As a result, production of adenosine triphosphate decreases and that of lactic acid increases. The depletion in adenosine triphosphate reduces transcellular transport and leads to intracellular accumulation of sodium, water, and calcium (Perlman, 2006; Selway, 2010; Wassink, Gunn, Drury, Bennet, & Gunn, 2014). When the membrane depolarizes, the cell releases the excitatory amino acid glutamate, and calcium flows into the cell via N-methyl-D-aspartate–gated channels. This cascade of events perpetuates injury in a process termed *excitotoxicity*. The peroxidation of free fatty acids by oxygen free radicals leads to more cellular damage (Ferriero, 2004). The culmination of energy failure, acidosis, glutamate release, lipid peroxidation, and the toxic effects of nitric oxide leads to primary cell death (necrosis) and activates apoptotic cascades if the oxygen deprivation is not corrected (Douglas-Escobar & Weiss, 2015; Ferriero, 2004).

Depending on the timing of injury and intervention, a partial recovery occurs during 30 to 60 minutes after the acute insult or the primary phase of injury and introduces a latent phase of injury (Bennet et al., 2012). During this latent phase period of reperfusion, complete recovery or development of a secondary phase may occur. The latent phase thereby constitutes a "therapeutic window"; may last from 1 to 6 hours; and is characterized by recovery of oxidative metabolism, inflammation, and continuation of the activated apoptotic cascades (Perlman, 2006; Selway, 2010; Wassink et al., 2014). A secondary deterioration follows the latent phase in neonates with moderate-to-severe injury, and in whom reversal does not occur. This secondary phase occurs approximately 6 to 15 hours after the injury. Cytotoxic edema, excitotoxicity, and secondary energy failure with nearly complete failure of mitochondrial activity characterize this phase, which leads to further cell death and clinical deterioration (Bennet et al., 2012; Cooper, 2011; Douglas-Escobar & Weiss, 2015; Mathur, Smith, & Donze, 2008; Shankaran & Laptook, 2007). Seizures typically occur during this secondary phase (Mathur et al., 2008; Perlman, 2006; Selway, 2010).

TABLE 21–8. Clinical Stages of Encephalopathy

Stage I	**Duration of the stage:** <24 hr after injury **Level of consciousness:** hyperalertness **Neuromuscular:** normal tone with mild distal flexion, myoclonus, overactive stretch reflexes **Reflexes:** hyperreflexia, weak suck, strong Moro (startle) reflex **Activation of sympathetic nervous system:** dilated pupils, increased heart rate, decreased secretions, normal or decreased GI motility **EEG:** absence of seizures, normal awake EEG **Outcome at 6 to 12 mo of age:** good, if infant did not progress to stage II and III
Stage II	**Duration of the stage:** 2 to 14 d **Level of consciousness:** lethargy **Neuromuscular:** hypotonia with strong distal flexion, myoclonus, overactive stretch reflexes **Reflexes:** hyperreflexia, weak suck, and Moro reflex **Activation of parasympathetic nervous system:** constricted pupils, decreased heart rate, increased secretions, increased GI motility **EEG:** low voltage early, with multifocal seizures later **Outcome at 6 to 12 mo of age:** good if clinical exam and EEG become normal within 5 d
Stage III	**Duration of the stage:** hours to weeks **Level of consciousness:** stupor **Neuromuscular:** flaccidity with intermittent decerebrate posturing, absent myoclonus, decreased or absent stretch reflexes **Reflexes:** absent such and Moro reflex **Suppression of sympathetic and parasympathetic nervous system:** pupils small to midposition and often unequal, weak pupillary response to light; hypothermia; variable heart rate, secretions, and GI motility **EEG:** is potential EEG or with infrequent periodic discharges; rare seizures **Outcome at 6 to 12 mo of age:** poor

EEG, electroencephalogram; GI, gastrointestinal.
Adapted from Sarnat, H. B., & Sarnat, M. S. (1976). Neonatal encephalopathy following fetal distress: A clinical and electroencephalographic study. *Archives of Neurology, 33*(10), 696–705.

Neonates with suspected HIE are classified according to the Sarnat staging of encephalopathy criteria (Sarnat & Sarnat, 1976) (Table 21–8). These criteria describe the evolution of the clinical encephalopathy over the first several days of age and emphasize that this encephalopathy is a dynamic clinical state that warrants close monitoring.

Intervention: Therapeutic Hypothermia

Until recently, supportive care and anticonvulsants for seizure control has been the management of choice for these infants. However, both large and small randomized controlled trials have demonstrated the efficacy and safety of instituting therapeutic hypothermia (whole-body cooling or selective head cooling) to reduce death and disability in infants with moderate-to-severe HIE (Azzopardi et al., 2009; Eicher et al.,

2005; Gluckman et al., 2005; Lin et al., 2006; Shankaran et al., 2005). Induced hypothermia initiated within 6 hours of birth is significantly associated with fewer deaths and less neurodevelopmental disability at 18-month follow-up in infants born at highest risk for brain injury (as defined by specific protocols) (Edwards et al., 2010). Both total body and selective head cooling methods have been shown to be effective (Jacobs, Hunt, Tarnow-Mordi, Inder, & Davis, 2007).

According to the AAP's and the AHA's NRP, therapeutic hypothermia is the treatment of choice in the delivery room for term or late preterm infants with evolving moderate encephalopathy (Perlman et al., 2010). Whole body or selective head cooling should be initiated and conducted in the context of rigorous and clearly defined protocols within neonatal intensive care facilities with provisions for monitoring side effects and long-term follow-up.

Intervening with a neuroprotective intervention, such as therapeutic hypothermia (cooling), prior to the secondary phase of energy failure is the single most promising intervention for infants with HIE (Fairchild, Sokora, Scott, & Zanelli, 2010; Mathur et al., 2008; Pfister & Soll, 2010). Although the exact mechanism by which hypothermic neuroprotection works is unknown, it does seem to attenuate the secondary phase of neuronal injury. Most clinical trials have induced therapeutic hypothermia for hypoxic-ischemic neonates within 6 hours of birth. However, evidence that the duration of the latent phase is inversely proportional to the severity of the ischemic insult, suggests that the therapeutic window for starting hypothermia therapy may be much shorter, within 2 hours of the suspected insult and no later than 6 hours (Iwata et al., 2007; Pfister & Soll, 2010). Therefore, early identification of hypoxic-ischemic neonates who meet the criteria for hypothermia therapy is critical. These infants have complex needs and are typically managed in tertiary centers with the availability of subspecialty evaluation and treatment. However, many of these at-risk infants are born in hospitals that do not provide neonatal intensive care, requiring transports that often take hours. Additionally, the timing of the onset of injury is often unclear and because the therapeutic window for neuroprotection is limited, early initiation of cooling is often warranted. Induced hypothermia should be only provided under strict protocols in nontertiary centers under guidance of the regional neonatal intensive care unit and transport team. If a cooling protocol is not available, every effort to avoid overheating the infant should be made. Cooling protocols may vary, typically, passive cooling is initiated (if portable cooling equipment is unavailable) and achieved by turning off the radiant warmer and the infant is cooled to a rectal temperature between 34°C and 35°C. Close monitoring of the rectal or esophageal temperature is required with the appropriate probe or low reading thermometer (at least every 15 minutes or continuously, if possible) (Azzopardi et al., 2009; Fairchild et al., 2010; Kendall, Kapetanakis, Ratnavel, Azzopardi, & Robertson, 2010). Potential adverse effects of passive overcooling have been reported, highlighting the need for vigilant continuous or intermittent rectal temperature monitoring, ongoing education, and continuous collaboration among all members of the healthcare team (Hallberg, Olson, Bartocci, Edqvist & Blennow, 2009; Thoresen, 2008).

Criteria for Cooling

Criteria for cooling should be discussed between the referring center and the neonatologist who is accepting the responsibility of the infant's care. Cooling criteria are fairly consistent among clinical practice guidelines for therapeutic hypothermia and generally include (1) gestational age at least 36 weeks or more; (2) ≥1,800 g; (3) ≤6 hours of age at time of cooling; (4) pH ≤7 or base deficit >12 mEq/L within 1 hour of delivery or umbilical cord blood gas showing a pH 7.01 to 7.15; (5) moderate-to-severe electroencephalogram (EEG) amplitude reduction (lower margin <5 microvolts and/or upper margin <10 microvolts) on a 20-minute aEEG, or evidence of seizures. Exclusion criteria generally targets infants with major congenital defects such as diaphragmatic hernia requiring ventilation, suspected major chromosomal anomalies, uncontrolled active bleeding, or parental decline of the therapy (Cooper, 2011; Mathur et al., 2008). Exclusion criteria include infants with major congenital defects such as diaphragmatic hernia requiring ventilation, suspected chromosomal anomalies (e.g., trisomies 13 or 18), congenital disorders of the central nervous system, uncontrolled active bleeding, or parental refusal (Cooper, 2011; Mathur et al., 2008). It's extremely important to investigate other causes of neonatal encephalopathy, including infection and metabolic disorders and institute specific treatment.

Care and Assessment

Nurses are key to early identification of infants who are at risk for developing HIE as a result of an acute perinatal event. Nurses in the delivery room need to be knowledgably astute of the clinical signs associated with neonatal asphyxia, seizures, and the criteria for therapeutic hypothermia. Using a standard checklist for the neurologic examination provides optimal documentation of the stage and evolution of encephalopathy. Supportive nursing care is an essential element of cooling. Continuous monitoring of oxygenation, ventilation, perfusion, cardiac output, strict intake and output, and glucose levels is essential to avoid additional adverse effects. Infants who are cooled typically have lower heart rates (e.g., heart rate <100 beats per minute); however, prolonged bradycardia (e.g., <80 beats per minute) may indicate the need for slight warming (Selway, 2010). It is important to remember that vigilant monitoring and documentation of body temperatures are essential in these high-risk infants. Additionally, infants who are cooled need to be monitored and assessed closely for pain and appropriate pharmacologic and nonpharmacologic therapies should be implemented (Cooper, 2011). Nurses are also key providing parents' emotional support. Parents and family members need to know what to expect over the course of the next hours and days, the rationale for implementing therapeutic hypothermia, and the importance of further evaluation and management at a tertiary center with subspecialty availability.

TRANSPORT AND RETURN TRANSPORT

Many conditions complicating the neonatal period do not begin with dramatic clinical symptoms. Experience and well-developed assessment skills allow perinatal nurses to recognize subtle changes and intervene before the newborn's condition worsens. Occasionally, the condition of the newborn and services available at a particular perinatal center require transport to a level III NICU. The goal of neonatal transport is to bring a sick newborn to a tertiary-care center in stable condition. The availability of neonatal intensive care has improved outcomes in high-risk newborns, although no standard definitions exist for graded levels of complexity of care that NICUs provide, thus making it difficult to compare outcomes (AAP, 2012). However, a uniform definition and classification of neonatal resources according to the different levels of care as recommended by AAP provides a framework for the development and implementation of consistent standards of service provided (AAP, 2012). Stabilization is an ongoing process, which begins with the referring hospital through consultation with the tertiary center as needed until the arrival and eventual departure of the transport team. Because of the diversity in the disease process and gestational age, stabilization takes on many forms. Basic care needs of newborns requiring transport to a tertiary center include adequate oxygenation, prevention of hypothermia, prevention of hypoglycemia, conservation of energy, and maintenance of physiologic integrity.

After the newborn's condition is no longer critical, in the event that an extended hospitalization is anticipated, the decision may be made to move the newborn back to the hospital in which he or she was born. This decision is made with input from neonatology staff at the level III center, the newborn's primary care provider, and nursing staff in the level II hospital, and the parents. The decision also is influenced by the parents' insurance carrier or managed care providers. In order to make informed decision, the healthcare team and individual families need to consider the advantages and disadvantages associated with transporting convalescing infants back to their community hospital before return transport (Bowen, 2010). Return transport offers many advantages to family members of the high-risk newborn, although it requires involvement of personnel from the transferring and the receiving hospital as well as adequate parent preparation to be successful. Family involvement is essential to success of return transport. Ideally, the prospect of a return transport is introduced when the infant is initially transferred to the level III center. Return transports should be celebrated as a milestone and a positive step toward discharge.

To provide newborns with the best care possible, healthcare professionals within the referring hospital and between the referring hospital and the tertiary center must communicate and work together as a team. The decision to transport back to the level II hospital first depends on whether the care needs of the newborn can be met at that institution. Communication between the level III and the level II hospitals when a return transport is anticipated should begin several days before the actual transfer. This assists in preparing the parents, and the receiving hospital has time to anticipate staffing and equipment needs. Using a formal documentation system provides the receiving hospital with information about the current condition of the newborn.

SUMMARY

Most newborns are born in level II hospitals. They are healthy at birth, develop no complications during the neonatal period, and are discharged to their homes with their mothers. A small group of newborns are born with complications or develop complications immediately after birth. It is the newborn who develops complications that poses the challenge to the perinatal nurse. The nurse in a level II hospital must strive to identify complications in a timely fashion, care for the infant appropriately, stabilize the infant before transport to a level III facility, and be prepared to accept the patient as a return transfer when he or she is no longer in need of intensive care.

REFERENCES

Adamkin, D. H., & Committee on Fetus and Newborn. (2011). Postnatal glucose homeostasis in late-preterm and term infants. *Pediatrics*, 127(3), 575–579. doi:10.1542/peds.2010-3851

Adams-Chapman, I. (2006). Neurodevelopmental outcome of the late preterm infant. *Clinics in Perinatology*, 33(4), 947–964.

Aguayo, J. (2001). Maternal lactation for preterm newborn infants. *Early Human Development, 65*(Suppl.), S19–S29.

Alkalay, A. L., Bresee, C. J., & Simmons, C. F. (2010). Decreased neonatal jaundice readmission rate after implementing hyperbilirubinemia guidelines and universal screening for bilirubin. *Clinical Pediatrics, 49*(9), 830–833. doi:10.1177/0009922810363728

American Academy of Pediatrics. (2004a). Management of hyperbilirubinemia in the newborn infant 35 or more weeks of gestation. *Pediatrics, 114*(1), 297–316.

American Academy of Pediatrics. (2004b). *Questions and answers on jaundice and your newborn.* Washington, DC: Author.

American Academy of Pediatrics. (2012). Levels of neonatal care. *Pediatrics, 130*(3), 587–597. doi:10.1542/peds.2012-1999

American Academy of Pediatrics. (2016). SIDS and other sleep-related infant deaths: Updated 2016 recommendations for a safe infant sleeping environment. *Pediatrics, 138*(5), e20162938. doi:10.1542/peds.2016-2938

American Academy of Pediatrics & American Heart Association. (2016). *Textbook of neonatal resuscitation* (7th ed.). Elk Grove Village, IL: American Academy of Pediatrics.

American College of Obstetricians and Gynecologists. (2006). *Amnioinfusion does not prevent meconium aspiration syndrome* (Committee Opinion No. 346). Washington, DC: Author.

American College of Obstetricians and Gynecologists. (2018). *Labor and delivery management of women with human immunodeficiency virus infection* (Committee Opinion No. 751). Washington, DC: Author.

American College of Obstetricians and Gynecologists. (2019a). *Prepregnancy Counseling* (Committee Opinion No. 762). Washington, DC: Author.

American College of Obstetricians and Gynecologists. (2019b). *Prevention of Group B Streptococcal early onset disease in newborns* (Committee Opinion No. 782). Washington, DC: Author.

American Heart Association. (2018). *Heart disease and stroke statistics—2018 Update. A report from the American Heart Association Statistics Committee and Stroke Statistics Subcommittee.* Dallas, TX: Author.

Amin, S. B., Smith, T., & Timler, G. (2018). Developmental influence of unconjugated hyperbilirubinemia and neurobehavioral disorders. *Pediatric Research, 85*(2), 191–197. doi:10.1038/s41390-018-0216-4

Andiman, W., Bryson, Y., de Martino, M., Fowler, M., Harris, D., Hutto, C., . . . Tuomala, R. (1999). The mode of delivery and the risk of vertical transmission of human immunodeficiency virus type 1—A meta-analysis of 15 prospective cohort studies. *The New England Journal of Medicine, 340*, 977–987.

Auckland, A. K. (2010). Ventricular septal defects. In J. A. Drose (Ed.), *Fetal echocardiography* (2nd ed., pp. 105–118). St. Louis, MO: Saunders.

Association of Women's Health, Obstetric and Neonatal Nurses. (2017). *Assessment and care of the late preterm infant* (Evidence-Based Clinical Practice Guideline, 2nd ed.). Washington, DC: Author.

Azzopardi, D. V., Strohm, B., Edwards, A. D., Dyet, L., Halliday, H. L., Juszczak, E., . . . Brocklehurst, P. (2009). Moderate hypothermia to treat perinatal asphyxial encephalopathy. *The New England Journal of Medicine, 361*(14), 1349–1358. doi:10.1056/NEJMoa0900854

Benjamin, D. K., & Stoll, B. J. (2006). Infection in late preterm infants. *Clinics in Perinatology, 33*(4), 871–882. doi:10.1016/j.clp.2006.09.005

Bennet, L., Tan, S., Van den Heuij, L., Derrick, M., Groenendaal, F., van Bel, F., . . . Gunn, A. J. (2012). Cell therapy for neonatal hypoxia-ischemia and cerebral palsy. *Annals of Neurology, 71*(5), 589–600. doi:10.1002/ana.22670

Bentlin, M. R., Suppo, L. M., & Rugolo, S. (2010). Late-onset sepsis: Epidemiology, evaluation, and outcome. *NeoReviews, 11*(8), e426–e435.

Betrán, A. P., Ye, J., Moller, A. B., Zhang, J., Gülmezoglu, A. M., & Torloni, M. R. (2016). The increasing trend in caesarean section rates: Global, regional and national estimates: 1990-2014. *PLoS One, 11*(2), e0148343. doi:10.1371/journal.pone.0148343

Bhutani, V. K., Johnson, L. H., & Shapiro, S. M. (2004). Kernicterus in sick and preterm infants (1999–2002): A need for an effective preventive approach. *Seminars in Perinatology, 28*(5), 319–325.

Bhutani, V. K., Johnson, L. H., & Sivieri, E. M. (1999). Predictive ability of a predischarge hour-specific serum bilirubin for subsequent significant hyperbilirubinemia in healthy term and near-term newborns. *Pediatrics, 103*(1), 6–14.

Bhutani, V. K., & Committee on Fetus and Newborn. (2011). Phototherapy to prevent severe neonatal hyperbilirubinemia in the newborn infant 35 or more weeks of gestation. *Pediatrics, 128*(4), e1046–e1052. doi:10.1542/peds.2011-1494

Bird, T. M., Bronstein, J. M., Hall, R. W., Lowery, C. L., Nugent, R., & Mays, G. P. (2010). Late preterm infants: Birth outcomes and health care utilization in the first year. *Pediatrics, 126*(2), e311–e319. doi:10.1542/peds.2009-2869

Bowen, S. L. (2010). Intrafacility and interfacility neonatal transport. In M. T. Verklan & M. Walden (Eds.), *Core curriculum for neonatal intensive care nursing* (4th ed., pp. 415–433). St. Louis, MO: Saunders.

Branson, B. M., Handsfield, H. H., Lampe, M. A., Janssen, R. S., Taylor, A. W., Lyss, S. B., & Clark, J. E. (2006). Revised recommendations for HIV testing of adults, adolescents, and pregnant women in health-care settings. *MMWR. Morbidity and Mortality Weekly Report, 55*(RR-14), 1–17.

Bry, K. (2008). Newborn resuscitation and the lung. *NewReviews, 9*(11), e506–e512.

Burgos, A. E., & Burke, B. L. (2009). Neonatal abstinence syndrome. *NeoReviews, 19*(5), e222–e229.

Burgos, A. E., Flaherman, V. J., & Newman, T. B. (2011). Screening and follow-up of neonatal hyperbilirubinemia: A review. *Clinical Pediatrics, 5*(1), 7–16. doi:10.1177/0009922811398964

Burgos, A. E., Schmitt, S. K., Stevenson, D. K., & Phibbs, C. S. (2008). Readmission for neonatal jaundice in California, 1991–2000: Trends and implications. *Pediatrics, 121*(4), e864–e869. doi:10.1542/peds.2007-1214

Cain, M. A., Bornick, P., & Whiteman, V. (2013). The maternal, fetal, and neonatal effects of cocaine exposure in pregnancy. *Clinics in Obstetrics and Gynecology, 56*(1), 124–132. doi:10.1097/GRF.0b013e31827ae167

Caputo, C., Wood, E., & Jabbour, L. (2016). Impact of fetal alcohol exposure on body systems: A systematic review. *Birth Defects Research. Part C, Embryo Today: Reviews, 108*(2), 174–180. doi:10.1002/bdrc.21129

Centers for Disease Control and Prevention. (2017). *LCWK7: Infant, neonatal, and postneonatal deaths, percent of total deaths, and mortality rates for the 15 leading causes of infant death by race and sex: United States, 1999–2015.* Atlanta, GA: Author.

Chettri, S., Adhisivam, B., & Bhat, B. V. (2015). Endotracheal suction for nonvigorous neonates born through meconium stained amniotic fluid: A randomized controlled trial. *Journal of Pediatrics, 166*(5), 1208.e1–1213.e1. doi:10.1016/j.jpeds.2014.12.076

Chyi, L. J., Lee, H. C., Hintz, S. R., Gould, J. B., & Sutcliffe, T. L. (2008). School outcomes of late preterm infants: Special needs and challenges for infants born at 32 to 39 weeks gestation. *Journal of Pediatrics, 153*(1), 25–31. doi:10.1016/j.jpeds.2008.01.027

Cifuentes, J., Segars, A. H., & Carlo, W. A. (2003). Respiratory system management and complications. In C. Kenner & J. W. Lott (Eds.), *Comprehensive neonatal nursing: A physiologic perspective* (3rd ed., pp. 348–375). St. Louis, MO: Saunders.

Clapp, D. W. (2006). Developmental regulation of the immune system. *Seminars in Perinatology, 30*(2), 48–51. doi:10.1053/j.semperi.2006.02.004

Clark, L., & Rohan, A. J. (2015). Identifying and assessing the substance-exposed infant. *MCN: The American Journal of Maternal Child Nursing, 40*(2), 87–95. doi:10.1097/NMC.0000000000000117

Clark, R. H. (2005). The epidemiology of respiratory failure in neonates born at an estimated gestational age of 34 weeks or more. *Journal of Perinatology, 25*(4), 251–257.

Clark, S. L., Frye, D. R., Meyers, J. A., Belfort, M. A., Dildy, G. A., Kofford, S., . . . Perlin, J. A. (2010). Reduction in elective delivery at <39 weeks of gestation: Comparative effectiveness of 3 different approaches to change and the impact on newborn intensive care admissions and stillbirth. *American Journal of Obstetrics & Gynecology, 203*(5), 449.e1–449.e6. doi:10.1016/j.ajog.2010.05.036

Clark, S. L., Knox, E., Simpson, K. R., & Hankins, G. D. (2010). Quality improvement opportunities in intrapartum care. In March of Dimes (Ed.), *Toward improving the outcome of pregnancy III* (pp. 66–74). New York, NY: March of Dimes.

Clark, S. L., Miller, D. D., Belfort, M. A., Dildy, G. A., Frye, D. K., & Meyers, J. A. (2009). Neonatal and maternal outcomes associated with elective term delivery. *American Journal of Obstetrics & Gynecology, 200*(2), 156.e1–156.e4. doi:10.1016/j.ajog.2008.08.068

Cohen, R. S., Wong, R. J., & Stevenson, D. K. (2010). Understanding neonatal jaundice: A perspective on causation. *Pediatrics and Neonatology, 51*(3), 143–148. doi:10.1016/S1875-9572(10)60027-7

Cole, F. S., Nogee, L. M., & Hamvas, A. (2006). Defects in surfactant synthesis: Clinical implications. *Pediatrics Clinics of North America, 53*(5), 911–927.

Cooper, D. J. (2011). Induced hypothermia for neonatal hypoxic-ischemic encephalopathy: Pathophysiology, current treatment, and nursing considerations. *Neonatal Network, 30*(1), 29–35. doi:10.1891/0730-0832.30.1.29

Cramton, R. E., & Gruchala, N. E. (2013). Babies breaking bad: Neonatal and iatrogenic withdrawal syndromes. *Current Opinion in Pediatrics, 25*(4), 532–542. doi:10.1097/MOP.0b013e328362cd0d

Crume, T. L., Juhl, A. L., Brooks-Russell, A., Hall, K. E., Wymore, E., & Borgelt, L. M. (2018). Cannabis use during the perinatal period in a state with legalized recreational and medical marijuana: The association between maternal characteristics, breastfeeding patterns, and neonatal outcomes. *Journal of Pediatrics, 197*, 90–96. doi:10.1016/j.jpeds.2018.02.005

Darnall, R. A., Ariagno, R. L., & Kinney, H. C. (2006). The late preterm infant and the control of breathing, sleep, and brainstem development: A review. *Clinics in Perinatology, 33*(4), 883–914. doi:10.1016/j.clp.2006.10.004

Deshpande, S., & Ward Platt, M. W. (2005). The investigation and management of neonatal hypoglycaemia. *Seminars in Fetal & Neonatal Medicine, 10*(4), 351–361.

Douglas-Escobar, M., & Weiss, M. (2015). Hypoxic-ischemic encephalopathy: A review for the clinician. *JAMA Pediatrics, 169*(4), 397–403. doi:10.1001/jamapediatrics.2014.3269

Dudell, G. G., & Jain, L. (2006). Hypoxic respiratory failure in the late preterm infant. *Clinics in Perinatology, 33*(4), 803–830. doi:10.1016/j.clp.2006.09.006

Dudell, G. G., & Stoll, B. J. (2007). Respiratory tract disorders. In R. M. Kliegman, R. E. Behrman, H. B. Jensen, & B. F. Stanton (Eds.), *Nelson textbook of pediatrics* (18th ed., pp. 728–753). Philadelphia, PA: Saunders Elsevier.

Edwards, A. D., Brocklehurst, P., Gunn, A. J., Halliday, H., Juszczak, E., Levene, M., & Azzopardi, D. (2010). Neurological outcomes at 18 months of age after moderate hypothermia for perinatal hypoxic ischaemic encephalopathy: Synthesis and meta-analysis of trial data. *BMJ, 34*, 363. doi:10.1136/bmj.c363

Eicher, D. J., Wagner, C. L., Katikaneni, L. P., Hulsey, T. C., Bass, W. T., Kaufman, D. A., . . . Yager, J. Y. (2005). Moderate hypothermia in neonatal encephalopathy: Safety outcomes. *Pediatric Neurology, 32*(1), 18–24. doi:10.1016/j.pediatrneurol.2004.06.015

Engle, W. A., Tomashek, K. M., & Wallman, C., & Committee of Fetus and Newborn. (2007). "Late-preterm" infants: A population at risk. *Pediatrics, 120*, 1390–1401. doi:10.1542/peds.2007-2952

Escobar, G. J., Clark, R. H., & Green, J. D. (2006). Short-term outcomes of infants born at 35 and 36 weeks gestation: We need to ask more questions. *Seminars in Perinatology, 30*(1), 28–33.

Escobar, G. J., Gonzales, V. M., Armstrong, M. A., Flock, B. F., Xiong, B., & Newman, T. B. (2002). Rehospitalization for neonatal dehydration: A nested case-control study. *Archives of Pediatrics & Adolescent Medicine, 156*(2), 155–161.

Escobar, G. J., Greene, J. D., Hulac, P., Kincannon, E., Bischoff, K., Gardner, M. N., . . . France, E. K. (2005). Rehospitalisation after birth hospitalisation: Patterns among infants of all gestations. *Archives of Disease in Childhood, 90*(2), 124–131.

Fairchild, K., Sokora, D., Scott, J., & Zanelli, S. (2010). Therapeutic hypothermia on neonatal transport: 4-Year experience in a single NICU. *Journal of Perinatology, 30*(5), 324–329. doi:10.1038/jp.2009.168

Farst, K. J., Valentine, J. L., & Hall, R. W. (2011). Drug testing for newborn exposure to illicit substances in pregnancy: Pitfalls and pearls. *International Journal of Pediatrics, 2011*, 951616. doi:10.1155/2011/951616

Ferriero, D. M. (2004). Neonatal brain injury. *The New England Journal of Medicine, 351*(19), 1985–1995.

Fricker, H. S., & Segal, S. (1978). Narcotic addiction, pregnancy, and the newborn. *American Journal of Disease of Children, 132*(4), 360–366.

Gardner, S. L., Enzman-Hines, M., & Dickey, L. A. (2011). Respiratory diseases. In S. L. Gardner, B. S. Carter, M. Enzman-Hines, & J. A. Hernandez (Eds.), *Merenstein & Gardner's handbook of neonatal intensive care* (7th ed., pp. 581–677). St. Louis, MO: Mosby.

Garg, M., & Devaskar, S. U. (2006). Glucose metabolism in the late preterm infant. *Clinics in Perinatology, 33*(4), 853–870.

Gewolb, I. H., Vice, F. L., Schweiter-Kenney, E. L., Taciak, V. L., & Bosma, J. F. (2001). Developmental patterns of rhythmic suck and swallow in preterm infants. *Developmental Medicine and Child Neurology, 43*(1), 22–37.

Gluckman, P. D., Wyatt, J. S., Azzopardi, D., Ballard, R., Edwards, A. D., Ferriero, D. M., . . . Gunn, A. J. (2005). Selective head cooling with mild systemic hypothermia after neonatal encephalopathy: Multicentre randomized trial. *Lancet, 365*(9460), 663–670.

Gurka, M. J., LoCasale-Crouch, J., & Blackman, J. A. (2010). Long-term cognition, achievement, socioemotional, and behavioral development of healthy late-preterm infants. *Archives of Pediatrics & Adolescent Medicine, 164*(6), 525–532. doi:10.1001/archpediatrics.2010.83

Halamek, L. P., & Stevenson, D. K. (2002). Neonatal jaundice and liver disease. In A. A. Fanaroff & R. J. Martin (Eds.), *Neonatal-perinatal medicine diseases of the fetus and infant* (7th ed., pp. 1309–1350). St. Louis, MO: Mosby.

Hallberg, B., Olson, L., Bartocci, M., Edqvist, I., Blennow, M. (2009). Passive induction of hypothermia during transport of asphyxiated infants: A risk of excessive cooling. *Acta Paediatrica, 98*(6), 942–946.

Hankins, G. D. V., & Longo, M. (2006). The role of stillbirth prevention and late preterm (near-term) births. *Seminars in Perinatology, 30*(1), 20–23.

Hansen, A. K., Wisborg, K., Uldbjerg, N., & Henriksen, T. B. (2007). Elective caesarean section and respiratory morbidity in the term and near-term neonate. *Acta Obstetricia Gynecologica Scandinavica, 86*(4), 389–394. doi:10.1080/00016340601159256

Harper, R. G., Solish, G., Feingold, E., Gersten-Woolf, N. B., & Sokal, M. M. (1977). Maternal ingested methadone, body fluid methadone, and the neonatal withdrawal syndrome. *American Journal of Obstetrics & Gynecology, 129*(4), 417–424.

Harteman, J. C., Nikkels, P. G., Benders, M. J., Kwee, A., Groenendaal, F., & de Vries, L. S. (2013). Placental pathology in full-term infants with hypoxic-ischemic neonatal encephalopathy and association with magnetic resonance imaging pattern of brain injury. *Journal of Pediatrics, 163*(4), 968.e2–995.e2. doi:10.1016/j.jpeds.2013.06.010

Havens, P. L., Mofenson, L. M., & American Academy of Pediatrics Committee on Pediatric AIDS. (2009). Evaluation and management of the infant exposed to HIV-1 in the United States. *Pediatrics, 123*(1), 175–187. doi:10.1542/peds.2008-3076

Hibbard, J. U., Wilkins, I., Sun, L., Gregory, K., Haberman, S., Hoffman, M., . . . Zhang, J. (2010). Respiratory morbidity in late preterm births. *JAMA, 304*(4), 419–425. doi:10.1001/jama.2010.1015

Hudak, M. L., & Tan, R. C. (2012). Neonatal drug withdrawal. *Pediatrics, 129*(2), e540–e560. doi:10.1542/peds.2011-3212

Hunt, C. E. (2006). Ontogeny of automatic regulation in late preterm infants born at 34–37 weeks postmenstrual age. *Seminars in Perinatology, 30*(2), 73–76.

Iwata, O., Iwata, S., Thornton, J. S., De Vita, E., Bainbridge, A., Herbert, L., . . . Robertson, N. J. (2007). "Therapeutic time window" duration decreases with increasing severity of cerebral hypoxia ischaemia under normothermia and delayed hypothermia in newborn piglets. *Brain Research, 1154*, 173–180.

Jacobs, S., Hunt, R., Tarnow-Mordi, W., Inder, T., & Davis, P. (2007). Cooling for newborns with hypoxic ischaemic encephalopathy. *Cochrane Database of Systematic Reviews*, (4), CD003311.

Jain, A., Aggarwal, R., Jeeva Sankar, M. J., Agarwal, R., Deorari, A. K., & Paul, V. K. (2010). Hypoglycemia in the newborn. *Indian Journal of Pediatrics, 77*(10), 1137–1142. doi:10.1007/s12098-010-0175-1

Jain, L., & Dudell, G. G. (2006). Respiratory transition in infants delivered by cesarean section. *Seminars in Perinatology, 30*, 296–304.

Jain, L., & Eaton, D. C. (2006). Physiology of fetal lung fluid clearance and effect of labor. *Seminars in Perinatology, 30*(1), 34–43.

Jain, S., & Cheng, J. (2006). Emergency department visits and rehospitalizations in late preterm infants. *Clinics in Perinatology, 33*(4), 935–945.

Jansson, L. M., Dipietro, J. A., Elko, A., & Velez, M. (2010). Infant autonomic functioning and neonatal abstinence syndrome. *Drug and Alcohol Dependence, 109*(1–3), 198–204. doi:10.1016/j.drugalcdep.2010.01.004

Jansson, L. M., & Velez, M. (2012). Neonatal abstinence syndrome. *Current Opinions in Pediatrics, 24*(2), 252–258. doi:10.1097/MOP.0b013e32834fdc3a

Juretschke, L. J. (2005). Kernicterus: Still a concern. *Neonatal Network, 24*(2), 7–19.

Kamath, B. D., Thilo, E. H., & Hernandez, J. A. (2011). Jaundice. In S. L. Gardner, B. S. Carter, M. Enzman-Hines, & J. A. Hernandez (Eds.), *Merenstein & Gardner's handbook of neonatal intensive care* (7th ed., pp. 531–552). St. Louis, MO: Mosby.

Kayiran, S. M., & Gürakan, B. (2010). Screening of blood glucose levels in healthy neonates. *Singapore Medical Journal, 51*(11), 853–855.

Kellogg, A., Rose, C. H., Harms, R. H., & Watson, W. J. (2011). Current trends in narcotic use in pregnancy and neonatal outcomes. *American Journal of Obstetrics & Gynecology, 204*(3), 259.e1–254.e1. doi:10.1016/j.ajog.2010.12.050

Kendall, G. S., Kapetanakis, A., Ratnavel, N., Azzopardi, D., & Robertson, N. J. (2010). Passive cooling for initiation of therapeutic hypothermia in neonatal encephalopathy. *Archives of Disease in Childhood. Fetal and Neonatal Edition, 95*(6), F408–F412. doi:10.1136/adc.2010.187211

Kenney, P. M., Hoover, D., Williams, L. C., & Iskersky, V. (2011). Cardiovascular diseases and surgical interventions. In S. L. Gardner, B. S. Carter, M. Enzman-Hines, & J. A. Hernandez (Eds.), *Merenstein & Gardner's handbook of neonatal intensive care* (7th ed., pp. 678–716). St Louis, MO: Mosby.

Kinney, H. C. (2006). The near-term (late preterm) human brain and risk for periventricular leukomalacia: A review. *Seminars in Perinatology, 30*(2), 81–88.

Konduri, G. G., & Kim, U. O. (2009). Advances in the diagnosis and management of persistent pulmonary hypertension of the newborn. *Pediatric Clinics of North America, 56*(3), 579–600. doi:10.1016/j.pcl.2009.04.004

Kurinczuk, J. J., White-Koning, M., & Badawi, N. (2010). Epidemiology of neonatal encephalopathy and hypoxic-ischaemic encephalopathy. *Early Human Development, 86*(6), 329–338. doi:10.1016/j.earlhumdev.2010.05.010

Kuschel, C. (2007). Managing drug withdrawal in the newborn infant. *Seminars in Fetal & Neonatal Medicine, 12*(2), 127–133. doi:10.1016/j.siny.2007.01.004

Lapointe, A., & Barrington, K. J. (2011). Pulmonary hypertension and the asphyxiated newborn. *Journal of Pediatrics, 158*(Suppl. 2), e19–e24. doi:10.1016/j.jpeds.2010.11.008

Laptook, A., & Jackson, G. L. (2006). Cold stress and hypoglycemia in the late preterm ("near-term") infant: Impact on nursery of admission. *Seminars in Perinatology, 30*(1), 24–27.

Lee, Y. M., Cleary-Goldman, J., & D'Alton, M. E. (2006). Multiple gestations and late preterm (near-term) deliveries. *Seminars in Perinatology, 30*(2), 103–112.

Levine, E. M., Ghai, V., Barton, J. J., & Strom, C. M. (2001). Mode of delivery and risk of respiratory disease in newborn. *Obstetrics & Gynecology, 97*(3), 439–442.

Li, G., Saad, S., Oliver, B. G., & Chen, H. (2018). Heat or burn? Impacts of intrauterine tobacco smoke and e-cigarette vapor exposure on the offspring's health outcome. *Toxics, 6*(3). doi:10.3390/toxics6030043

Lin, Z. L., Yu, H. M., Lin, J., Chen, S. Q., Liang, Z. Q., & Zhang, Z. Y. (2006). Mild hypothermia via selective head cooling as neuroprotective therapy in term neonates with perinatal asphyxia: An experience from a single neonatal intensive care unit. *Journal of Perinatology, 26*(3), 180–184.

Logan, B. A., Brown, M. S., & Hayes, M. J. (2013). Neonatal abstinence syndrome: Treatment and pediatric outcomes. *Clinics in Obstetrics and Gynecology, 56*(1), 186–192. doi:10.1097/GRF.0b013e31827feea4

Lott, J. W. (2007). Cardiovascular system. In C. Kenner & J. W. Lott (Eds.), *Comprehensive neonatal care: An interdisciplinary approach* (4th ed., pp. 32–64). St. Louis, MO: Saunders.

Lugo, R. A., Satterfield, K. L., & Kern, S. E. (2005). Pharmacokinetics of methadone. *Journal of Pain & Palliative Care Pharmacotherapy, 19*(4), 13–24.

Mahle, W. T., Newburger, J. W., Matherne, G. P., Smith, F. C., Hoke, T. R., Koppel, R., . . . Grosse, S. D. (2009). Role of pulse oximetry in examining newborns for congenital heart disease: A scientific statement from the AHA and AAP. *Pediatrics, 124*(2), 823–836.

Maisels, M. J., & McDonagh, A. F. (2008). Phototherapy for neonatal jaundice. *The New England Journal of Medicine, 358*, 920–928.

Manchikanti, L., Fellows, B., Ailinani, H., & Pampati, V. (2010). Therapeutic use, abuse, and nonmedical use of opioids: A ten-year perspective. *Pain Physician, 13*(5), 401–435.

March of Dimes. (2010a). *Elimination of non-medically indicated (elective) deliveries before 39 weeks gestation age.* White Plains, NY; Author.

March of Dimes. (2010b). *Toward improving the outcome of pregnancy: Enhancing perinatal health through quality, safety and performance initiatives (TIOP III).* White Plains, NY: Author.

Martin, J. A., Hamilton, B. E., Osterman, M. J. K., Driscoll, A. K., & Drake, P. (2018). Births: Final data for 2017. *National Vital Statistics Reports, 67*(8), 1–50.

Mathur, A. M., Smith, J. R., & Donze, A. (2008). Hypothermia and hypoxic-ischemic encephalopathy: Guideline development using the best evidence. *Neonatal Network, 27*(4), 271–286.

McLaurin, K. K., Hall, C. B., Jackson, E. A., Owens, O. V., & Mahadevia, P. J. (2009). Persistence of morbidity and cost differences between late-preterm and term infants during the first year of life. *Pediatrics, 123*(2), 653–659. doi:10.1542/peds.2008-1439

Medoff-Cooper, B., Bakewell-Sachs, S., Buus-Frank, M. E., & Santa-Donato, A. (2005). The AWHONN near-term infant initiative: A conceptual framework for optimizing health for near-term infants. *Journal of Obstetric, Gynecologic, and Neonatal Nursing, 34*(6), 666–671.

Morse, S. B., Zheng, H., Tang, Y., & Roth, J. (2009). Early school-age outcomes of late preterm infants. *Pediatrics, 123*(4), e622–e629.

Murphy-Oikonen, J., Montelpare, W. J., Southon, S., Bertoldo, L., & Persichino, N. (2010). Identifying infants at risk for neonatal abstinence syndrome: A retrospective cohort comparison study of 3 screening approaches. *Journal of Perinatal & Neonatal Nursing, 24*(4), 366–372. doi:10.1097/JPN.0b013e3181fa13ea

Nanduri, S. A., Petit, S., Smelser, C., Apostol, M., Alden, N. B., Harrison, L.H., . . . Schrag, S. J. (2019). Epidemiology of invasive early-onset and late-onset group B streptococcal disease in the United States, 2006 to 2015: Multistate laboratory and population-based surveillance. *JAMA Pediatrics, 173*(3), 224–233. doi:10.1001/jamapediatrics.2018.4826

National Institute of Child Health and Human Development Workshop. (2005). *Optimizing care and long-term outcome of near-term pregnancy and near-term newborn infant.* Bethesda, MD: Author.

Neu, J. (2006). Gastrointestinal maturation and feeding. *Seminars in Perinatology, 30*(2), 77–80.

Ohlin, A., Björkqvist, M., Montgomery, S. M., & Schollin, J. (2010). Clinical signs and CRP values associated with blood culture results in neonates evaluated for suspected sepsis. *Acta Paediatrica, 99*(11), 1635–1640.

Osborn, D. A., Jeffery, H. E., & Cole, M. J. (2010). Opiate treatment for opiate withdrawal in newborn infants. *Cochrane Database of Systematic Reviews,* (10). doi:10.1002/14651858.CD002059.pub3

Panel on Antiretroviral Therapy and Medical Management of HIV-Infected Children. (2010). *Guidelines for the use of antiretroviral agents in pediatric HIV infection.* Retrieved from http://aidsinfo.nih/gov/ContentFiles/PediatricGuidelines.pdf

Pappas, B. E., & Walker, B. (2010). Care of the late preterm infant. In M. T. Verklan & M. Walden (Eds.), *Core curriculum for neonatal intensive care nursing* (4th ed., pp. 447–452). St. Louis, MO: Saunders.

Patrick, S. W., Schumacher, R. E., Benneyworth, B. D., Krans, E. E., McAllister, J. M., & Davis, M. M. (2012). Neonatal abstinence syndrome and associated health care expenditures: United States, 2000–2009. *JAMA, 307*(18), 1934–1940. doi:10.1001/jama.2012.3951

Perlman, J. M. (2006). Intervention strategies for neonatal hypoxic-ischemic cerebral injury. *Clinical Therapeutics, 28*(9), 1352–1365.

Perlman, J. M., Wyllie, J., Kattwinkel, J., Atkins, D. L., Chameides, L., Goldsmith, J. P., . . . Velaphi, S. (2010). Part 11: Neonatal resuscitation: 2010 International consensus on cardiopulmonary resuscitation and emergency cardiovascular care science with treatment recommendations. *Circulation, 122*(Suppl. 2), S516–S538.

Petrini, J. R., Dias, T., McCormick, M. C., Massolo, M. L., Green, N. S., & Escobar, G. J. (2009). Increased risk of adverse neurological development for late preterm infants. *Journal of Pediatrics, 154*(2), 169–176.

Pfister, R. H., & Soll, R. F. (2010). Hypothermia for the treatment of infants with hypoxic ischemic encephalopathy. *Journal of Perinatology, 30,* S82–S87.

Piazza, A. J., & Stoll, B. J. (2007). Digestive system. In R. M. Kliegman, R. E. Berman, H. B. Jensen, & B. F. Stanton (Eds.), *Nelson textbook of pediatrics* (19th ed., pp. 753–766). Philadelphia, PA: Saunders Elsevier.

Pritham, U. A. (2013). Breastfeeding promotion for management of neonatal abstinence syndrome. *Journal of Obstetric, Gynecologic and Neonatal Nursing, 42*(5), 517–526. doi:10.1111/1552-6909.12242

Puopolo, K. M., Benitz, W. E., & Zaoutis, T. E. (2018). Management of neonates born at >35 0/7 weeks' gestation with sus-

pected or proven early-onset bacterial sepsis. *Pediatrics, 142*(6), e20182894. doi:10.1542/peds.2018-2894

Puopolo, K. M., Lynfield, R., & Cummings, J. J. (2019). Management of infants at risk of group B streptococcal disease. *Pediatrics, 144*(2), e20191881. doi:10.1542/peds.2019-1881

Rabi, Y. (2010). Oxygen and resuscitation of the preterm infant. *NeoReviews, 11*(3), e130–e138.

Radtke, J. V. (2011). The paradox of breastfeeding-associated morbidity among late preterm infants. *Journal of Obstetrics, Gynecologic, and Neonatal Nursing, 40*(1), 9–24. doi:10.1111/j.1552-6909.2010.01211

Raju, T. N., Higgins, R. D., Stark, A. R., & Leveno, K. J. (2006). Optimizing care and outcome for late-preterm (near-term) infants: A summary of the workshop sponsored by the National Institute of Health and Human Development. *Pediatrics, 118*(3), 1207–1214.

Ramachandrappa, A., & Jain, L. (2008). Elective cesarean section: Its impact on neonatal respiratory outcome. *Clinics in Perinatology, 35*(2), 373–393. doi:10.1016/j.clp.2008.03.006

Ramanathan, R., Corwin, M. J., Hunt, C. E., Lister, G., Tinsley, L. R., Baird, T., . . . Keens, T. G. (2001). Cardiorespiratory events recorded on home monitors: Comparison of healthy infants with those at increased risk for SIDS. *JAMA, 285*(17), 2199–2207.

Rogers, J. M. (2008). Tobacco and pregnancy: Overview of exposure and effects. *Birth Defects Research. Part C, Embryo Today: Reviews, 84*(1), 1–15. doi:10.1002/bdrc.20119

Rohan, A. J., & Golembek, S. G. (2009a). Hypoxia in the term newborn: Part 1. Cardiopulmonary physiology and assessment. *MCN: The American Journal of Maternal Child Nursing, 34*(2), 106–112. doi:10.1097/01.NMC.0000347304.70208.eb

Rohan, A. J., & Golombek, S. G. (2009b). Hypoxia in the term newborn: Part 2. Primary pulmonary disease, obstruction, and extrinsic compression of the lung. *MCN: The American Journal of Maternal Child Nursing, 34*(3), 145–151. doi:10.1097/01.NMC.0000351700.12890.da

Rohan, A. J., & Golombek, S. G. (2009c). Hypoxia in the term newborn: Part 3. Sepsis and hypotension, neurologic, hematologic and metabolic disorders. *MCN: The American Journal of Maternal Child Nursing, 34*(4), 224–233. doi:10.1097/01.NMC.0000357914.95358.be

Rosen, T. S., & Bateman, D. A. (2002). Infants of addicted mothers. In A. A. Fanaroff & R. J. Martin (Eds.), *Neonatal-perinatal medicine diseases of the fetus and infant* (7th ed., pp. 661–673). St. Louis, MO: Mosby.

Roth-Kleiner, M., Wagner, B. P., Bachmann, D., & Pfenninger, J. (2003). Respiratory distress syndrome in near-term babies after caesarean section. *Swiss Medical Weekly, 133*(19–20), 283–288.

Rozance, P. J., & Hay, W. W. (2010). Describing hypoglycemia: Definition or operational threshold? *Early Human Development, 86*(3), 275–280. doi:10.1016/j.earlhumdev.2010.05.002

Rutherford, M. A., Azzopardi, D., Whitelaw, A., Cowan, F., Renowden, S., Edwards, A. D., & Thoresen, M. (2005). Mild hypothermia and the distribution of cerebral lesions in neonates with hypoxic-ischemic encephalopathy. *Pediatrics, 116*(4), 1001–1006.

Sadowski, S. L. (2010). Cardiovascular disorders. In M. T. Verklan & M. Walden (Eds.), *Core curriculum for neonatal intensive care nursing* (4th ed., pp. 534–588). St. Louis, MO: Saunders.

Sankaran, V. G., & Brown, D. W. (2007). Congenital heart disease. In L. S. Lilly (Ed.), *Pathophysiology of heart disease* (4th ed., pp. 371–396). Baltimore, MD: Lippincott Williams & Wilkins.

Sarici, S. U., Serdar, M. A., Korkmaz, A., Erdem, G., Oran, O., Tekinalp, G., . . . Yigit, S. (2004). Incidence, course, and prediction of hyperbilirubinemia in near-term and term newborns. *Pediatrics, 113*(4), 775–780.

Sarnat, H. B., & Sarnat, M. S. (1976). Neonatal encephalopathy following fetal distress. A clinical and electroencephalographic study. *Archives of Neurology, 33*(10), 696–705.

Selway, L. D. (2010). State of the science: Hypoxic ischemic encephalopathy and hypothermic intervention for neonates. *Advances in Neonatal Care, 10*(2), 60–66. doi:10.1097/ANC.0b013e3181d54b30

Shane, A. L., Sánchez, P. J., & Stoll, B. J. (2017). Neonatal sepsis. *Lancet (London, England), 390*(10104), 1770–1780. doi:10.1016/S0140-6736(17)31002-4

Shankaran, S., & Laptook, A. R. (2007). Hypothermia as a treatment for birth asphyxia. *Clinical Obstetrics and Gynecology, 50*(3), 624–635.

Shankaran, S., Laptook, A. R., Ehrenkranz, R. A., Tyson, J. E., McDonald, S. A., Donovan, E. F., . . . Jobe, A. H. (2005). Whole-body hypothermia for neonates with hypoxic-ischemic encephalopathy. *The New England Journal of Medicine, 353*(15), 1574–1584.

Shapiro-Mendoza, C. K., Tomashek, K. M., Kotelchuck, M., Barfield, W., Weiss, J., & Evans, S. (2006). Risk factors for neonatal morbidity and mortality among "healthy," late preterm newborns. *Seminars in Perinatology, 30*(2), 54–60.

Sibai, B. M. (2006). Preeclampsia as a cause of preterm and late preterm (near-term) births. *Seminars in Perinatology, 30*(1), 16–19.

Smitherman, H., Stark, A. R., & Bhutani, V. K. (2006). Early recognition of neonatal hyperbilirubinemia and its emergent management. *Seminars in Fetal & Neonatal Medicine, 11*(3), 214–224.

Sperling, M. A., & Menon, R. K. (2004). Differential diagnosis and management of neonatal hypoglycemia. *Pediatric Clinics of North America, 51*(3), 703–723.

Stayer, S. A., & Liu, Y. (2010). Pulmonary hypertension of the newborn. *Best Practices & Research. Clinical Anaesthesiology, 24*(3), 375–386.

Steinhorn, R. H. (2016). Advances in neonatal pulmonary hypertension. *Neonatology, 109*(4), 334–344. doi:10.1159/000444895

Steinhorn, R. H., & Farrow, K. N. (2007). Pulmonary hypertension in the neonate. *NeoReviews, 8*(1), e14–e21.

Stokowski, L. A. (2006). Fundamentals of phototherapy for neonatal jaundice. *Advances in Neonatal Care, 7*(2), 303–312.

Taylor, R. M., & Price-Douglas, W. (2008). The S.T.A.B.L.E. program: Postresuscitation/pretransport stabilization care of sick infants. *Journal of Perinatal & Neonatal Nursing, 22*(2), 159–165.

Thach, B. T. (2005). Can we breathe and swallow at the same time? *Journal of Applied Physiology, 99*(5), 1633.

Thilo, E. H. (2005). Neonatal jaundice. In P. J. Thureen, J. Deacon, J. A. Hernandez, & D. M. Hall (Eds.), *Assessment and care of the well newborn* (2nd ed., pp. 245–254). St. Louis, MO: Saunders Elsevier.

Thoresen, M. (2008). Supportive care during neuroprotective hypothermia in the term newborn: Adverse effects and their prevention. *Clinics in Perinatology, 35*(4), 749–763.

Thorne, C., & Newell, M. (2007). HIV. *Seminars in Fetal & Neonatal Medicine, 12*(3), 174–181.

Thornton, P. S., Stanley, C. A., De Leon, D. D., Harris, D., Haymond, M. W., Hussain, K., . . . Wolfsdorf, J. I. (2015). Recommendations from the Pediatric Endocrine Society for evaluation and management of persistent hypoglycemia in neonates, infants, and children. *Journal of Pediatrics, 167*(2), 238–245. doi:10.1016/j.jpeds.2015.03.057

Tita, A. T., Landon, M. B., Spong, C. Y., Lai, Y., Leveno, K. J., Varner, M. W., . . . Mercer, B. M. (2009). Timing of elective repeat cesarean delivery at term and neonatal outcomes. *The New England Journal of Medicine, 360*(2), 111–120. doi:10.1056/NEJMoa0803267

Tomashek, K. M., Shapiro-Mendoza, C. K., Weisss, J., Kotelchuck, M., Barfield, W., Evans, S., . . . Declerq, E. (2006). Early discharge among late preterm and term newborns and risk of neonatal morbidity. *Seminars in Perinatology, 30*(2), 61–68. doi:10.1053/j.semperi.2006.02.003

Vachharajani, A. J., & Dawson, J. G. (2009). Short-term outcomes of late preterms: An institutional experience. *Clinical Pediatrics, 48*(4), 383–388. doi:10.1177/0009922808324951

Vain, N. E., Szyld, E. G., Prudent, L. M., & Aguilar, A. M. (2009). What (not) to do at and after delivery? Prevention and management of meconium aspiration syndrome. *Early Human Development, 85*(10), 621–626. doi:10.1016/j.earlhumdev.2009.09.013

van Ierland, Y., & de Beaufort, A. J. (2009). Why does meconium cause meconium aspiration syndrome? Current concepts of MAS pathophysiology. *Early Human Development, 85*(10), 617–620. doi:10.1016/j.earlhumdev.2009.09.009

Velaphi, S. V., & Vidyasagar, D. (2006). Intrapartum and post delivery management of infants born to mothers with meconium-stained amniotic fluid: Evidence-based recommendations. *Clinics in Perinatology, 33*(4), 29–42.

Verani, J. R., McGee, L., & Schrag, S. (2010). Prevention of perinatal group B streptococcal disease: Revised guidelines from CDC, 2010. *MMWR. Morbidity and Mortality Weekly Report, 59*(RR-10), 1–36.

Walker, M. (2008). Breastfeeding the late preterm infant. *Journal of Obstetrics, Gynecologic, and Neonatal Nursing, 37*(6), 692–701. doi:10.1111/j.1552-6909.2008.00293.x

Wang, M. L., Dorer, D. J., Fleming, M. P., & Catlin, E. A. (2004). Clinical outcomes of near-term infants. *Pediatrics, 114*(2), 373–376.

Warren, J. B., & Anderson, J. M. (2009). Core concepts: Respiratory distress syndrome. *NeoReviews, 10*(7), e351–e361.

Wassink, G., Gunn, E. R., Drury, P. P., Bennet, L., & Gunn, A. J. (2014). The mechanisms and treatment of asphyxial encephalopathy. *Frontiers in Neuroscience, 8*(40). doi:10.3389/fnins.2014.00040

Watchko, J. F., & Maisels, M. J. (2010). Enduring controversies in the management of hyperbilirubinemia in preterm neonates. *Seminars in Fetal & Neonatal Medicine, 15*, 136–140. doi:10.1016/j.siny.2009.12.003

Williams, A. F. (2005). Neonatal hypoglycaemia: Clinical and legal aspects. *Seminars in Fetal & Neonatal Medicine, 10*(4), 363–368.

Wynn, J. L., Wong, H. R., Shanley, T. P., Bizzarro, M. J., Saiman, L., & Polin, R. A. (2014). Time for a neonatal-specific consensus definition for sepsis. *Pediatric Critical Care Medicine, 15*(6), 523–528. doi:10.1097/PCC.0000000000000157

Xu, H., Wei, S., & Fraser, W. D. (2008). Obstetric approaches to the prevention of meconium aspiration syndrome. *Journal of Perinatology, 28*, S14–S18. doi:10.1038/jp.2008.145

Yurdakök, M. (2010). Transient tachypnea of the newborn: What is new? *Journal of Maternal-Fetal & Neonatal Medicine*, (Suppl. 3), S24–S26. doi:10.3109/14767058.2010.507971

Zahorodny, W., Rom, C., Whitney, W., Giddens, S., Samuel, M., Maichuk, G., & Marshall, R. (1998). The neonatal withdrawal inventory: A simplified score of newborn withdrawal. *Journal of Developmental and Behavioral Pediatrics, 19*(2), 89–93.

Zaichkin, J., & Weiner, G. M. (2011). Neonatal resuscitation program (NRP) 2011: New science, new strategies. *Neonatal Network, 30*(1), 5–13. doi:10.1891/0730-0832.30.1.5

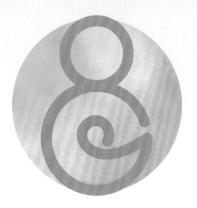

Item Bank Questions and Answer Key

QUESTIONS

Chapter 1 Perinatal Patient Safety and Quality

Multiple Choice

1. Maternal mortality data are collected in the United States by

    a. Centers for Disease Control and Prevention.
    b. National Institutes of Health.
    c. United States Public Health Service.

2. For every maternal death in the United States, how many maternal near-miss events are estimated to have occurred?

    a. 10 to 30
    b. 40 to 60
    c. 70 to 100

3. The most comprehensive analysis of maternal deaths occurs via

    a. professional liability claims reviews.
    b. sentinel event reports.
    c. state maternal mortality review committees.

4. The Centers for Disease Control and Prevention defines pregnancy-related death as death of a woman while pregnant or within

    a. 1 week of the end of pregnancy.
    b. 42 days of the end of pregnancy.
    c. 1 year of the end of pregnancy.

5. The pregnancy-related mortality ratio is an estimate of pregnancy-related deaths for every

    a. 1,000 live births.
    b. 10,000 live births.
    c. 100,000 live births.

6. Findings from analysis of maternal deaths from nine states' maternal mortality review committees suggest what percentage of maternal deaths are likely preventable?

    a. 40%
    b. 50%
    c. 60%

7. The leading cause of maternal death for all women in the United States is

    a. cardiovascular disease.
    b. hemorrhage.
    c. infection.

8. The leading cause of maternal death for non-Hispanic Black women is

    a. cardiomyopathy.
    b. hemorrhage.
    c. preeclampsia/eclampsia.

9. Based on data from the Centers for Disease Control and Prevention, maternal mortality for non-Hispanic Black women is how many times higher than for non-Hispanic White women?

    a. 2 times
    b. 3 times
    c. 4 times

10. The most common complication of childbirth for women having cesarean birth is

    a. hemorrhage requiring a blood transfusion.
    b. unplanned hysterectomy.
    c. ruptured uterus.

11. The cesarean birth rate in the United States rose what percent from 1965 to 2017?

    a. 200%
    b. 400%
    c. 600%

12. The most recent addition to The Joint Commission Perinatal Care Core Measures is

    a. elective induction of labor at 39 completed weeks of gestation.
    b. primary cesarean birth rate.
    c. unexpected complications in term newborns.

13. Which age group of mothers at time of birth has decreased in the United States over the past two decades?

    a. 15 to 19 years
    b. 30 to 34 years
    c. 40 to 44 years

14. Which age group of mothers at time of birth has the highest rates of infant, neonatal, and perinatal mortality?

    a. under 20 years
    b. 30 to 34 years
    c. 40 years and over

15. Which group based on race/ethnicity has the highest infant mortality rate?

    a. Hispanic women
    b. Native American/Native Alaskan women
    c. Non-Hispanic Black women

16. What was the cesarean birth rate in the United States in 1965?

    a. 4.5%
    b. 7.5%
    c. 10.5%

17. The National Quality Forum has a list of serious reportable events in healthcare also known as

    a. adverse events.
    b. never events.
    c. sentinel events.

18. The recommendations in the AIM bundles are formatted based on

    a. assessment, identification, appropriate treatment.
    b. patient, clinician, hospital.
    c. readiness, recognition, and response.

19. Never events include

    a. infant abduction.
    b. maternal admission to the intensive care unit.
    c. transfusion of more than 10 blood products to the mother.

20. Nurses' responsibilities for speaking up to advocate for the rights, health, and safety of patients are outlined in the

    a. American Academy of Nursing Policy Priorities.
    b. American Nurses Association Code of Ethics for Nurses.
    c. American Medical Association Vision on Health Care Reform.

Chapter 2 Integrating Cultural Beliefs and Practices When Caring for Childbearing Women and Families

Multiple Choice

1. A 25-year-old Vietnamese woman admitted to the birthing unit requests that her husband stay in the waiting area until after she gives birth. The appropriate response is based on the nurse's knowledge that

    a. all husbands should be present during labor and birth.
    b. the husband may fear his response to his wife giving birth.
    c. the woman's request should be honored.

2. Wang Din Wah, a Laotian mother who is 24 hours postpartum, rejects the nurse's instructions to bring the newborn back to the clinic by the seventh day of life for a phenylketonuria test. Wang's reasons for this refusal are most likely based on

    a. her lack of recognition of appropriate healthcare for the baby.
    b. the baby's early care being provided largely by the maternal grandmother.
    c. the first month after birth being considered a time for confinement and rest.

3. Berta Wolf Creek is 4 hours postpartum and requests permission to take her placenta home with her. Appropriate instruction by the nurse would include

    a. keeping the placenta in a leakproof container.
    b. keeping the placenta frozen until burial.
    c. requiring disposal of the placenta by internment (burial).

4. Maria Ochoa, a 23-year-old Filipino American, is 18 weeks pregnant. After receiving a prescription for prenatal vitamins, she tells the nurse that her mother has warned her to take only herbal medication during pregnancy. The nurse appropriately

   a. advises Maria that the pills are only vitamins and not considered medication.
   b. assesses the significance of Maria's mother's advice.
   c. reminds her that the vitamins were ordered by the nurse-midwife.

5. The percentage of the U.S. population who are African American or Black is nearly

   a. 6%.
   b. 13%.
   c. 20%.

6. An African American/Black woman who believes she should not swallow her saliva and carries a spit cup with her during pregnancy is most likely from

   a. Barbados.
   b. Haiti.
   c. West Indies.

7. A major cultural group of childbearing women at increased risk for alcoholism, heart disease, cirrhosis of the liver, and diabetes mellitus is the population of women who are

   a. African American/Black.
   b. American Indian/Alaskan native.
   c. Asian American/Pacific Islander.

8. According to the hot/cold theory, pregnancy is thought to be which kind of a condition?

   a. cold
   b. hot
   c. lukewarm

9. The sacred day of worship with observant Muslim women is

   a. Friday at sunset.
   b. Saturday at sunset.
   c. Sunday.

10. Ethnocentrism is the belief that

   a. cultural values are major determiners of one's behavior.
   b. every cultural group has a core or center of common beliefs.
   c. values and practices of one's own culture are superior.

11. A woman whose discharge plan includes her mother-in-law caring for her and her newborn during the postpartum period by tradition is most likely from which of the following cultures?

   a. Korean
   b. Laotian
   c. Tongan

12. What percentage of nurses come from racial or ethnic minority backgrounds?

   a. 9%
   b. 13%
   c. 17%

13. Goals each nurse can set to increase cultural competence while caring for culturally diverse childbearing women and their families are described as

   a. culturally driven.
   b. externally based.
   c. self-generated.

Fill in the Blank

14. Identify three strategies to increase the cultural competence of the nurse.

   a. _____
   b. _____
   c. _____

Chapter 3 Physiologic Changes of Pregnancy

Multiple Choice

1. During a normal pregnancy, plasma volume increases by approximately

   a. 10% to 30%.
   b. 40% to 60%.
   c. 70% to 80%.

2. During pregnancy, maternal cardiac output is optimized in which of the following positions?

   a. lateral
   b. semi-Fowler
   c. supine

3. During labor, maternal cardiac output

   a. decreases slightly.
   b. increases progressively.
   c. remains the same.

4. An intravenous fluid bolus is given before epidural anesthesia to prevent

   a. hypotension.
   b. renal hypoperfusion.
   c. sympathetic blockade.

5. Normally, during pregnancy, maternal sitting and standing diastolic blood pressure readings

   a. decrease and then increase toward baseline levels.
   b. increase progressively to term.
   c. remain unchanged throughout pregnancy.

6. The volume of the maternal autotransfusion immediately after birth is approximately

   a. 600 mL.
   b. 800 mL.
   c. 1,000 mL.

7. What happens to maternal P_aO_2 and P_aCO_2 levels during pregnancy?

   a. both decrease.
   b. both increase.
   c. P_aO_2 increases and P_aCO_2 decreases.

8. The slight increase in pH that occurs during pregnancy is due to a/an

   a. decrease in hemoglobin and hematocrit.
   b. decrease in renal excretion of bicarbonate.
   c. increase in tidal volume/minute ventilation.

9. During pregnancy, serum urea and creatinine levels

   a. decrease.
   b. increase.
   c. remain constant.

10. Heartburn is common during pregnancy due primarily to

   a. decreased gastric motility.
   b. increased secretion of hydrochloric acid.
   c. relaxation of the lower esophageal sphincter.

11. A physical finding that may occur during pregnancy in response to normal cardiovascular and hematologic changes is

   a. decreased heart rate.
   b. dependent edema.
   c. elevated blood pressure.

12. The average blood loss during vaginal birth is less than

   a. 300 mL.
   b. 500 mL.
   c. 700 mL.

13. The average blood loss during cesarean birth is less than

   a. 600 mL.
   b. 800 mL.
   c. 1,000 mL.

14. During pregnancy, cardiac output increases approximately

   a. 10% to 25%.
   b. 30% to 50%.
   c. 60% to 75%.

15. Cardiac output is greatest during which period of the birth process?

   a. first stage, active phase
   b. immediately after birth
   c. second stage

16. A cardiovascular parameter that normally decreases during pregnancy is

   a. heart rate.
   b. stroke volume.
   c. systemic vascular resistance.

17. The usual white blood cell count during labor and the early postpartum may reach

   a. 8,000 to 10,000 mm^3.
   b. 13,000 to 15,000 mm^3.
   c. 20,000 to 30,000 mm^3.

18. Which of the following coagulation factors does not increase during pregnancy?

   a. fibrin
   b. fibrinogen
   c. platelets

19. Which of the following increases during pregnancy?

   a. glomerular filtration rate
   b. serum oncotic pressure
   c. serum osmolality

20. By term, blood flow to the uterus is approximately

   a. 200 to 400 mL/min.
   b. 500 to 800 mL/min.
   c. 900 to 1,200 mL/min.

21. During pregnancy, the pigmented line in the skin that traverses the abdomen longitudinally from the sternum to the symphysis is called the

    a. linea nigra.
    b. spider nevus.
    c. striae gravidarum.

22. Which of the following is a change occurring in the respiratory system during pregnancy?

    a. oxygen consumption increases.
    b. respiratory rate decreases.
    c. tidal volume decreases.

23. A normal finding during pregnancy is increased real excretion of

    a. glucose.
    b. potassium.
    c. sodium.

24. The respiratory system parameter that decreases during pregnancy is the

    a. functional residual capacity.
    b. minute ventilation.
    c. vital capacity.

25. A metabolic change characteristic of late pregnancy is decreased

    a. blood free fatty acid levels.
    b. insulin sensitivity.
    c. serum glucose levels after meals.

Fill in the Blank

26. Metabolic changes are characterized by _____ during the first half of pregnancy and _____ during the second half.

27. The greater increase in plasma volume than in red blood cell volume results in _____.

28. Maternal weight gain during the first half of pregnancy is primarily due to changes in the weight of the _____.

29. Both maternal metabolic rate and thyroid hormone levels _____ during pregnancy.

30. The primary determinant of volume hemostasis is _____.

31. The renal clearance of many substances is increased during pregnancy due to the _____.

32. Normal stretching of the skin and hormonal changes during gestation may produce "stretch marks" that are called _____.

33. The hormone released from the anterior pituitary that is responsible for initiating lactation is _____.

34. The increased maternal intestinal absorption of calcium is due to increased _____.

35. Compared to nonpregnant women, a pregnant woman in the third trimester has a _____ initial fasting blood glucose.

36. The hormone responsible for maintaining progesterone and estrogen production by the ovaries until the placenta is established is _____.

37. Placental production of the hormone _____ requires interaction of the mother, fetus, and placenta.

38. Increases in plasma volume and red cell mass result in an increase in _____ during pregnancy.

39. Cardiac output progressively decreases postpartum and returns to nonpregnant levels by _____.

40. The _____ accommodates one third of the additional maternal blood volume at term.

41. The hormone _____ produces relaxation of smooth muscle and vasodilation.

42. Blood pressure reaches its lowest point at _____ weeks.

43. During pregnancy, the woman becomes resistant to the pressor effects of _____.

44. Pregnancy is considered a _____ state due to the increases of several essential coagulation factors.

45. The pregnant woman is at increased risk for venous thrombus formation due to _____ and _____.

46. _____ are potent vasodilators that affect smooth muscle contractility and play an important role in labor onset, myometrial contractility, and cervical ripening.

47. Irregularly shaped brown blotches on the face are known as _____, or the "mask of pregnancy."

48. The bluish discoloration of the cervix occurring during pregnancy is known as _____ sign.

Chapter 4 Antenatal Care

Multiple Choice

1. Between 2007 and 2014, the preterm birth rate in the United States
   a. declined.
   b. increased.
   c. remained the same.

2. An appropriate recommendation for weight gain for an underweight pregnant woman would be
   a. 20 lb.
   b. 25 lb.
   c. 30 lb.

3. The best time to encourage a woman to stop smoking is
   a. as soon as she knows she is pregnant.
   b. before pregnancy.
   c. by the end of the first trimester.

4. The time during pregnancy when blood pressure is lowest in the normotensive woman is the
   a. first trimester.
   b. second trimester.
   c. third trimester.

5. The time when measurement of fundal height in centimeters should correlate with gestational age is
   a. after 20 weeks' gestation.
   b. before 20 weeks' gestation.
   c. near term.

6. Planning culturally specific care includes
   a. making sure that a translator is available when requested.
   b. noting patterns of decision making in the family.
   c. using a translator at each visit.

7. A nonreactive nonstress test at 39 weeks' gestation is an indication for
   a. expedited birth.
   b. further testing.
   c. reassurance about fetal status.

8. Health promotion and education to improve pregnancy outcomes in the next generation should begin with
   a. health courses in public high schools directed to both genders.
   b. public health awareness activities that young children can understand.
   c. specific prenatal education provided in the first trimester.

9. An appropriate gestational age for a glucose screening test is at
   a. 23 weeks' gestation.
   b. 26 weeks' gestation.
   c. 29 weeks' gestation.

10. Risk assessment for all women during the initial prenatal visit should include a/an
    a. complete health history.
    b. triple screen.
    c. ultrasound for fetal anomalies.

11. Which of the following puts a woman at risk for nutritional problems during pregnancy?
    a. advanced maternal age
    b. cigarette smoking
    c. gravida III, term I, preterm 0, abortion I, living child I

12. An effect of cigarette smoking during pregnancy is increased incidence of
    a. low birth weight and prematurity.
    b. neonatal transient tachypnea of the newborn.
    c. pregnancy-induced hypertension.

13. Maternal serum alpha-fetoprotein specifically screens for
    a. heart defects.
    b. neural tube defects.
    c. placental defects.

14. If both parents are affected by sickle cell disease, the risk of their children being affected by sickle cell disease is
    a. 25%.
    b. 50%.
    c. 100%.

15. A primary method of fetal surveillance during pregnancy is

    a. fetal kick counts.
    b. nonstress testing.
    c. ultrasonography.

16. The most significant food shortages for low-income women occur

    a. at the end of the month, when federal/local resources diminish.
    b. before Women, Infants, and Children (WIC) eligibility is determined.
    c. postpartum, when fatigue prevents appointments with WIC.

17. A key component of preterm birth prevention education is

    a. discussing the hospital admission criteria.
    b. empowering the woman to act on her own instincts and self-knowledge.
    c. involving the significant other in the teaching.

True or False

18. True/False: With low income, the risk of perinatal morbidity increases after the age of 35 years, but with adequate income and healthcare, these women have only a slight increase in gestational diabetes or pregnancy-induced hypertension.

Fill in the Blank

19. The monitoring of fetal activity by kick counts is initiated at _____ weeks' gestation.

20. It is recommended that every woman have an initial serology and gonorrhea culture and that the tests be repeated at _____ weeks.

21. The recommended weight gain for an obese woman during pregnancy is _____.

22. Severe congenital malformations occur in _____% of births.

23. A _____ is an agent that causes congenital malformations.

24. A biophysical profile summative score of _____ or greater is considered a sign of fetal well-being.

25. Ultrasonography prior to _____ weeks' gestation can accurately determine gestational age within ±1 week.

26. Tay-Sachs disease is a recessive disorder common in families of _____ ancestry.

27. _____ use during pregnancy is contraindicated and associated with fetal malformations.

28. Women of childbearing age should take _____ folic acid daily to prevent neural tube defects.

29. List three basic components of prenatal care.

    a. _____
    b. _____
    c. _____

30. Moderate physical activity during an uncomplicated pregnancy maintains _____ and _____ fitness.

31. Diagnosis of gestational diabetes mellitus is made when a glucose tolerance test result has _____.

32. Maternal serum screening is offered between _____ and _____ weeks' gestation.

33. A healthy fetus usually has _____ perceivable movements in 1 hour.

34. List the five parameters assessed in the biophysical profile.

    a. _____
    b. _____
    c. _____
    d. _____
    e. _____

Chapter 5 Hypertensive Disorders of Pregnancy

Multiple Choice

1. A diagnosis of severe preeclampsia is consistent with a 24-hour urine showing protein excretion of

    a. 1 g/L.
    b. 3 g/L.
    c. 5 g/L.

2. An indication of impending magnesium sulfate toxicity in the patient being treated for preeclampsia is the absence of

   a. deep tendon reflexes.
   b. fetal movement.
   c. urine output.

3. The therapeutic range of serum magnesium during magnesium sulfate therapy to prevent eclamptic seizures is

   a. 1 to 4 mg/dL.
   b. 5 to 8 mg/dL.
   c. 9 to 12 mg/dL.

4. Medications used for blood pressure control in severe hypertension include

   a. hydralazine, labetalol, or magnesium sulfate.
   b. hydralazine, labetalol, or nifedipine.
   c. labetalol, magnesium sulfate, or nifedipine.

5. Diagnosis of gestational hypertension requires the presence of hypertension and

   a. edema.
   b. pregnancy.
   c. proteinuria.

6. Severe preeclampsia can be diagnosed in the presence of

   a. excretion of 4,500 g protein in a 24-hour urine collection.
   b. serial diastolic blood pressures of at least 110 mm Hg.
   c. serum blood urea nitrogen of 10 mg/dL with a serum creatinine of 1 mg/dL.

Fill in the Blank

7. _____ disorders are the most common medical complication of pregnancy.

8. A systolic blood pressure of _____ mm Hg or a diastolic blood pressure of _____ mm Hg on two occasions at least 4 hours apart is necessary for diagnosis of preeclampsia.

9. The blood pressure should be recorded with the pregnant woman in the _____ position.

10. _____ is the drug of choice to prevent seizure activity in the woman with preeclampsia.

11. Maternal morbidity from hypertension in pregnancy results from

   a. _____
   b. _____
   c. _____
   d. _____

12. The goals of antihypertensive therapy in the woman with preeclampsia are to _____ and to _____.

13. Laboratory markers for HELLP syndrome are _____, _____, and _____.

14. A leading cause of maternal morbidity following an eclamptic seizure is _____.

Chapter 6 Bleeding in Pregnancy

Multiple Choice

1. Invasion of the trophoblastic cells into the uterine myometrium is termed placenta

   a. accreta.
   b. increta.
   c. percreta.

2. The incidence of abnormal placental adherence is increasing likely due to

   a. better diagnostic tools such as transvaginal ultrasound.
   b. increased rate of cesarean birth.
   c. more women delaying childbirth until they are older.

3. Painless, bright red vaginal bleeding at 28 weeks' gestation is most likely due to

   a. abruptio placentae.
   b. placenta previa.
   c. uterine rupture.

4. A clinical finding associated with a dehiscence of a uterine scar during a trial of labor after cesarean birth is

   a. cessation of uterine contractions.
   b. fetal heart rate abnormality.
   c. sudden decrease of intrauterine pressure.

5. The initial drug of choice for excessive bleeding in the immediate postpartum period is

   a. methylergonovine maleate (Methergine) IM.
   b. oxytocin IV infusion.
   c. prostaglandin 15-MF2α suppository.

6. The most common cause of postpartum hemorrhage is a/an

   a. atonic uterus.
   b. cervical laceration.
   c. placenta accreta.

7. In the last 10 years in the United States, the maternal mortality rate has

   a. decreased.
   b. increased.
   c. stabilized.

8. Which group has the highest maternal mortality rate?

   a. Black women
   b. Hispanic women
   c. Native American women

9. Approximately two thirds of maternal trauma seen in the emergency department is related to

   a. domestic/intimate partner violence.
   b. falls at home or in the workplace.
   c. motor vehicle accidents.

10. The risk of uterine inversion is increased with

    a. a prior uterine scar.
    b. suprapubic pressure.
    c. traction applied to the cord.

11. Cervical lacerations after birth should be suspected if

    a. estimated blood loss exceeds 500 mL.
    b. the mother reports severe cramping pain.
    c. the uterus is well contracted but frank bleeding continues.

Fill in the Blank

12. Vasa previa is the result of a _____ insertion of the cord.

13. For the fetus to maintain adequate oxygenation, the maternal oxygen saturation must be at least _____%.

14. _____ is a late sign of hypovolemia in the woman experiencing bleeding during pregnancy.

15. Active management of the third stage of labor involves _____.

Chapter 7 Preterm Labor and Birth

Multiple Choice

1. Which of the following is not a common symptom of preterm labor?

   a. headache
   b. menstrual-like cramps
   c. pelvic pressure

2. The principal risk factor predictive of preterm birth is

   a. history of preterm birth.
   b. low prepregnancy weight.
   c. smoking during pregnancy.

3. Infants born between 37 weeks and 38 completed weeks of gestation are categorized as

   a. early term births.
   b. late preterm births.
   c. term births.

4. A drug that is used for tocolysis but is not classified as a beta-mimetic is

   a. nifedipine.
   b. ritodrine.
   c. terbutaline.

5. To accurately be considered preterm, an infant must be

   a. born at gestational age <37 weeks.
   b. <10th percentile in weight.
   c. small for gestational age.

6. Teaching pregnant women about the symptoms of preterm labor

   a. has been shown to prevent preterm birth.
   b. should be ongoing throughout pregnancy.
   c. should only be done on a one-to-one basis.

7. When administering intravenous (IV) fluids for a woman with preterm contractions, it is important to consider that

   a. IV hydration has not been shown to be an effective preventative measure for preterm birth.
   b. preterm labor contractions usually diminish within 1 hour of initiation of IV hydration.
   c. the first liter of IV fluid should be administered within the first hour of the admission.

8. Antenatal glucocorticoid administration for acceleration of fetal lung maturation is appropriate

    a. for all women who could give birth preterm before 37 weeks' gestation.
    b. for woman at 24 to 34 weeks' gestation at risk for preterm birth within 7 days.
    c. once a week from the time of significant preterm symptoms until birth or 34 weeks' gestation, whichever comes first.

9. Research has shown that bed rest

    a. allows the pregnant woman to gain appropriate amounts of weight.
    b. increases the risk of developing a venous thromboembolism.
    c. inhibits preterm labor contractions.

10. Researchers believe that at least half of spontaneous preterm births of *unknown origin* may be due to

    a. exercise.
    b. infections/inflammation.
    c. smoking.

Fill in the Blank

11. Preterm birth in the United States is _____ among African American woman than among White women.

12. Women who are battered have _____ rates of preterm birth than women who do not experience intimate partner violence.

13. Mortality rates associated with preterm babies demonstrate that survival rates _____ as gestational age and birth weight decrease.

14. Signs and symptoms of preterm labor include

    a. _____
    b. _____
    c. _____
    d. _____
    e. _____
    f. _____
    g. _____

Chapter 8 Diabetes in Pregnancy

Multiple Choice

1. An indication to initiate insulin in a pregnant woman with gestational diabetes is

    a. fasting blood sugar (FBS) <85 mg/dL on two or more occasions.
    b. FBS = normal but 2-hour postprandial ≥100 mg/dL.
    c. FBS consistently ≥95 mg/dL, a 1-hour postprandial blood glucose ≥140 mg/dL, or a 2-hour postprandial consistently ≥120 mg/dL

2. Hypoglycemia is defined as a plasma blood glucose of

    a. exactly 90 mg/dL.
    b. greater than 80 mg/dL.
    c. less than 60 mg/dL.

3. To assist in controlling blood glucose, the recommendation for pregnant women with gestational diabetes is to exercise

    a. at least three times a week for 20 minutes.
    b. daily for less than 20 minutes.
    c. every other day for 45 minutes.

4. Women with a history of gestational diabetes with a normal postpartum follow-up test should be tested for overt diabetes

    a. before a subsequent pregnancy.
    b. every 1 to 3 years.
    c. a and b.

5. Intensive management of diabetes in women with pregestational diabetes should begin

    a. only if planning to breast-feed.
    b. postpartum.
    c. prior to conception.

6. In women with diabetes, medical nutrition therapy is

    a. a vital component of care.
    b. not effective on glycemic control.
    c. not necessary.

7. For women with diabetes, breastfeeding

    a. can prevent pregnancy.
    b. has been associated with reduced incidence of childhood obesity and diabetes later in life.
    c. is contraindicated; a baby should be bottle-fed.

8. Diagnostic testing for gestational diabetes is accomplished using a

    a. 2-hour 75-g oral glucose tolerance test.
    b. 3-hour 100-g oral glucose tolerance test.
    c. either a or b.

9. Insulin dosage during periods of nausea and vomiting in pregnant women should be

    a. based on a sliding scale.
    b. individualized based on the provider's recommendations.
    c. withheld until nausea is resolved.

10. Weekly nonstress testing should be initiated in women with diabetes beginning at the gestational age of

    a. 26 to 28 weeks.
    b. 30 to 32 weeks.
    c. 34 to 36 weeks.

Fill in the Blank

11. _____ diabetes results due to an autoimmune reaction directed at the pancreas following an environmental trigger.

12. Metabolic changes during the first half of pregnancy characterized by fat storage is called the _____ phase.

13. List five diabetogenic hormones of pregnancy.

    a. _____
    b. _____
    c. _____
    d. _____
    e. _____

14. Preterm labor in women with diabetes should be treated with _____.

15. Three specific symptoms of hyperglycemia are

    a. _____
    b. _____
    c. _____

Chapter 9 Cardiac Disease in Pregnancy

Multiple Choice

1. Congenital cardiac disease occurs in what approximate percentage of live births?

    a. 0.8%
    b. 1.5%
    c. 2.0%

2. Maternal outcomes in pregnancies of women with Marfan syndrome are related to

    a. cardiac dysrhythmias.
    b. degree of aortic root dilation.
    c. hypervolemia of pregnancy.

3. Symptoms indicative of heart disease in pregnancy include

    a. jugular venous distention, tachycardia, pedal edema, grade II/VI systolic murmur.
    b. palpitations, exertional dyspnea, irregular syncope, third heart sound.
    c. severe dyspnea, diastolic murmurs, hemoptysis, chest pain with exertion.

4. In a review of pregnancy-related deaths in the United States from 2011 to 2013, what was the leading cause of indirect mortality?

    a. cardiomyopathy and cardiovascular disease
    b. HIV/AIDS
    c. motor vehicle collisions

5. The peak incidence of peripartum cardiomyopathy is during the

    a. last month of pregnancy or with 5 months of birth.
    b. second trimester of pregnancy.
    c. 6 to 12 month's postpartum.

6. A pregnant woman with New York Heart Association (NYHA) class II cardiac disease is symptomatic with

    a. bed rest.
    b. heavy exertion.
    c. mild exertion.

7. Use of an epidural for labor pain management for women with cardiac disease requires

    a. a hospital pharmacy on the unit for emergency medications if needed.
    b. an anesthesiologist knowledgeable of cardiac disease in pregnancy.
    c. the same criteria as women without cardiac disease.

8. The time during labor and birth when cardiac output increases the most is during

    a. birth.
    b. second stage with fetal descent.
    c. second week of the postpartum period.

9. The physiologic changes of pregnancy that tend to be problematic for women with cardiac disease include

   a. decreased functional residual lung capacity, relaxation of the cardiac sphincter, and hypotension.
   b. increase in blood volume, decrease in systemic vascular resistance, the hypercoagulable state of pregnancy, and fluctuations in cardiac output.
   c. tachycardia and decreased blood volume.

10. An initial sign of inadequate cerebral perfusion is

    a. low pulse oximeter readings.
    b. restlessness.
    c. unequal pupil dilation.

Fill in the Blank

11. _____ system undergoes dramatic change during pregnancy that can impact cardiac disease.

12. Mitral and aortic stenosis are examples of cardiac diseases caused by _____.

13. A diagnostic test often used for diagnosis of myocardial infarction is _____.

14. Current risk counseling for pregnant women with cardiac disease is based on the _____ and the _____.

15. The NYHA classification system for cardiac disease categorizes patients by _____.

Chapter 10 Pulmonary Complications in Pregnancy

Multiple Choice

1. During pregnancy, predicted values of peak expiratory flow rates are

   a. decreased.
   b. increased.
   c. unchanged.

2. The mainstay of asthma pharmacologic therapy is

   a. beta-2 agonists.
   b. corticosteroids.
   c. immunotherapy.

3. Moderate-to-severe asthma is apparent when respiratory rate is greater than

   a. 20 breaths per minute.
   b. 30 breaths per minute.
   c. 40 breaths per minute.

4. During an exacerbation of asthma, there is

   a. decreased functional residual capacity.
   b. increased expiratory airflow.
   c. increased peripheral vascular resistance.

5. A breath sound rarely auscultated in asthmatics is

   a. rale.
   b. rhonchi.
   c. wheeze.

6. The most commonly seen pneumonia of pregnancy is

   a. aspiration.
   b. bacterial.
   c. viral.

7. A complication seen in up to 26% of women with varicella pneumonia in the first 20 weeks of gestation is

   a. intrauterine infection.
   b. pneumothorax.
   c. small-for-gestational-age fetus.

8. When aspiration pneumonia occurs during pregnancy, it is most commonly a result of

   a. bronchitis.
   b. general anesthesia.
   c. smoking.

9. Initial arterial blood gases in the pregnant woman with pneumonia usually reflect significant

   a. acidosis.
   b. hypercapnia.
   c. hypoxia.

10. Hypoxia should be suspected when a pregnant woman is noted to have

    a. hypotension.
    b. increased urine output.
    c. restlessness.

Fill in the Blank

11. Asthma affects up to _____% of women during pregnancy.

12. Maintaining oxygen saturation of greater than _____% by pulse oximetry is vital for a pregnant woman with pneumonia.

13. The underlying _____ of the woman's asthma prepregnancy may be an indicator for exacerbation rates during pregnancy.

14. Lifestyle risk factor that may increase a woman's risk of acquiring pneumonia during pregnancy is _____.

15. The most common bacterial pathogen in pneumonia during pregnancy is _____.

16. The maternal position that best supports maximum oxygenation is _____.

17. Common inhalation irritants for many asthmatics are _____.

18. Markers for potentially fatal asthma are _____.

19. Maternal complications of pneumonia during pregnancy are _____.

20. Amniotic fluid embolism is a rare condition unique to _____.

Chapter 11 Multiple Gestation

Multiple Choice

1. The highest overall multiple birth rates are in which maternal age group?

   a. 25 to 30 years
   b. 30 to 35 years
   c. 45 to 54 years

2. Perinatal risks are greatest in

   a. monochorionic gestations.
   b. multifetal reduction.
   c. older maternal age.

3. The lambda sign, a triangle-shaped ultrasound marker seen at the junction of the chorions and amnions, indicates

   a. dizygotic gestation.
   b. monozygotic gestation.
   c. trizygotic gestation.

4. An itching rash prominent in stretch marks in a woman pregnant with triplets is most likely

   a. herpes gestationis.
   b. pruritic folliculitis of pregnancy.
   c. pruritic urticarial papules and plaques of pregnancy syndrome.

5. The practice shown to be effective in decreasing the risks associated with preterm birth of multiples is

   a. 17-alpha-hydroxyprogesterone caproate administration.
   b. corticosteroid administration between 24 and 34 weeks if delivery is anticipated within 7 days.
   c. serial transvaginal ultrasound cervical assessments.

6. The greatest complication of tocolytic therapy for women with multiple gestations is

   a. hyperreflexia.
   b. maternal tachycardia.
   c. pulmonary edema.

7. The risk of fetal death in twin gestations is highest at

   a. 24 weeks.
   b. 35 weeks.
   c. 40 weeks.

8. The most appropriate treatment for severe twin-to-twin transfusion syndrome is

   a. amniotic membrane septostomy.
   b. expectant management.
   c. fetoscopic laser therapy.

9. The prenatal diagnostic screening test most accurate in multiple gestations is

   a. cell-free fetal DNA.
   b. nuchal translucency assessment.
   c. second trimester maternal serum testing.

10. A woman with a normal body mass index who is pregnant with twins should gain

    a. 25 to 35 lb.
    b. 37 to 54 lb.
    c. unlimited weight.

11. The recommended timing of birth for uncomplicated monoamniotic twins is

    a. 30 0/7 to 32 0/7 weeks.
    b. 32 0/7 to 34 0/7 weeks.
    c. 34 0/7 to 36 0/7 weeks.

12. The optimal delivery route for dichorionic/diamniotic twins (A vertex; B breech) at 35 2/7 weeks is

    a. cesarean birth.
    b. vaginal birth if the obstetrician is experienced in podalic version and vaginal breech delivery.
    c. vaginal birth of twin A and cesarean birth of twin B.

13. While birthing dichorionic twins (A vertex; B transverse), a potential complication during the time between the two births is

    a. maternal hypertension.
    b. shoulder dystocia.
    c. umbilical cord prolapse.

14. The recommendation for safe sleep at home for fraternal boy twins born at 35 weeks' gestation is

    a. each twin should have his own crib.
    b. preterm twins who have cobedded in the neonatal intensive care unit should continue to cobed at home.
    c. wait to start cobedding until after the first month.

15. A sign of abnormal parent–infant interaction with multiples is

    a. alternating eye contact among infants.
    b. initial unit attachment.
    c. ongoing preferential attention.

16. After birth of multiples, breastfeeding or pumping should begin

    a. as soon as possible, within the first hour.
    b. when the mother's milk comes in.
    c. within 48 hours.

17. When part of a set of multiples dies, parents often

    a. begin grieving immediately.
    b. can bond effectively with the survivor.
    c. experience paradoxical feelings.

True or False

18. True/False: Hypertensive disorders in multiple gestations follow a classic pattern of signs and symptoms.

19. True/False: Prenatal education for parents expecting multiples should begin in the early second trimester.

20. True/False: The increased prevalence of cerebral palsy in multiple birth infants is solely explained by the greater proportion of low birth weight and preterm births.

21. True/False: Mothers of multiples should begin simultaneous breastfeeding before hospital discharge.

Fill in the Blank

22. The greatest predictors of infant morbidity and mortality in multiples are _____ and _____.

23. The term for similarity in fetal heart rate accelerations, baseline oscillations, and periodic changes with contractions in healthy twins is _____ _____.

Chapter 12 Obesity in Pregnancy

Multiple Choice

1. Based on the most recent data, what proportion of the U.S. population is estimated to be either overweight or obese?

    a. one third
    b. one half
    c. two thirds

2. Which maternal factor contributes the greatest risk for large-for-gestational-age infants?

    a. excessive weight gain
    b. gestational diabetes
    c. preconception overweight or obesity

3. The World Health Organization and the American College of Obstetricians and Gynecologists recommend which of the following for pregnant women with a body mass index (BMI) ≥30 over the course of their pregnancy?

    a. 1- to 10-lb weight gain
    b. 11- to 20-lb weight gain
    c. weight loss of 0 to 10 lb

4. With increasing BMI, labor proceeds

   a. more quickly.
   b. more slowly.
   c. no change in labor progression.

5. Infants born to obese women have an increased risk for

   a. extra digits on the hand.
   b. gastroschisis.
   c. neural tube defects.

6. Typically, a low transverse incision for cesarean birth is

   a. associated with less pain postoperatively.
   b. easier to accomplish on a mother who is extremely obese.
   c. preferred by most obstetricians for obese women.

7. A common complication of anesthesia encountered with obese pregnant women when compared to normal weight women is

   a. allergic reaction to anesthetic agents.
   b. difficulty with catheter placement.
   c. excessive response to narcotic analgesia.

8. The risk for venous thromboembolism in obese women, compared to normal weight women, is

   a. decreased.
   b. increased.
   c. remains unchanged.

9. Fetal programming refers to the

   a. genetic predisposition of the fetus of an obese woman to develop obesity later in life despite healthy eating habits.
   b. inability of an obese pregnant woman with healthy lifestyle changes to pass these characteristics on to the developing fetus.
   c. process in which an in utero stimulus establishes a permanent fetal response that can lead to increased susceptibility to disease throughout life.

10. Patients are considered eligible for weight-loss surgery if they have a body mass index of

    a. >35 kg/m^2 with other comorbid conditions.
    b. >40 kg/m^2.
    c. either a or b.

Fill in the Blank

11. According to the World Health Organization, obesity is defined as a body mass index of _____ kg/m^2.

12. A mother who is overweight should gain approximately _____ lb during her pregnancy.

13. Obesity before pregnancy is associated with a _____ risk of spontaneous preterm birth.

14. Maternal morbidity and mortality _____ as BMI increases.

15. Following bariatric surgery, most obstetricians recommend women to postpone pregnancy for _____ months.

16. Uterine contractility is often _____ in overweight and obese women.

17. The amount of time from incision to birth may be _____ with obese women.

Chapter 13 Maternal–Fetal Transport

Multiple Choice

1. Which federal agency is responsible for developing the Emergency Medical Treatment and Active Labor Act (EMTALA)?

   a. Centers for Disease Control and Prevention
   b. Centers for Medicare & Medicaid Services
   c. U.S. Public Health Service

2. The primary purpose of the EMTALA regulation is to ensure that

   a. all patients are provided medical treatment regardless of ability to pay or insurance status.
   b. pregnant women will not be transferred to another facility while in labor.
   c. reimbursement for medical services is provided on an equal basis to hospitals.

3. Which organization first recommended regionalization of perinatal care?

   a. American Academy of Pediatrics
   b. American College of Obstetricians and Gynecologists
   c. March of Dimes

4. Regionalization of perinatal care promotes

   a. closure of small perinatal services in rural areas.
   b. limitations on the number of level III neonatal services in each state.
   c. transfer of high-risk mothers to hospitals with appropriate level of care based on the gestational age of their fetus(es).

5. Which national organization recommended using babies under 1,500 g born at a hospital with the appropriate level of care as a quality care indicator?

   a. National Quality Forum
   b. Society for Maternal-Fetal Medicine
   c. The Joint Commission

6. When compared to neonatal transport, maternal transport of babies in utero has been shown to

   a. cause a significant number of babies to be born during transport.
   b. improve neonatal outcomes.
   c. increase costs.

7. A common EMTALA violation is

   a. failure to document patient insurance status prior to transfer.
   b. inaccurate diagnosis by sending physician.
   c. lack of patient stabilization prior to transfer.

Fill in the Blank

8. Common modes of maternal transport include

   a. _____
   b. _____
   c. _____

9. The following equipment is suggested regardless of the method of maternal transport:

   a. _____
   b. _____
   c. _____
   d. _____
   e. _____
   f. _____
   g. _____
   h. _____

Chapter 14 Labor and Birth

Multiple Choice

1. Multiple studies have shown what percent of women attempting trial of labor after cesarean (TOLAC) have successful vaginal births?

   a. 20% to 30%
   b. 50%
   c. 60% to 80%

2. An appropriate lubricant to use for vaginal examinations during labor is

   a. povidone-iodine gel.
   b. sterile water.
   c. water-soluble jelly.

3. According to the American Society of Anesthesiologists Guidelines for Obstetrical Anesthesia, an elective cesarean could be done when the woman has been nothing by mouth for at least

   a. 4 hours.
   b. 5 hours.
   c. 6 hours.

4. An involuntary urge to push is most likely a sign of

   a. low fetal station.
   b. occiput posterior fetal position.
   c. transition.

5. Amnioinfusion during the first stage of labor is an appropriate intervention for

   a. recurrent late decelerations.
   b. recurrent variable decelerations.
   c. thick meconium fluid.

6. According to American College of Obstetricians and Gynecologists (ACOG), elective cesarean birth should be considered for women without diabetes who carry a fetus with suspected macrosomia with an estimated fetal weight of at least

   a. 4,000 g.
   b. 4,500 g.
   c. 5,000 g.

7. The primary factor that would allow second stage of labor to continue beyond 2 hours is

   a. an epidural is in place and the woman is comfortable.
   b. as the presenting part descends, the fetal heart rate does not suggest fetal compromise.
   c. the woman's request to not have a cesarean birth.

8. Clinicians should be aware that most cases of shoulder dystocia occur in

   a. nondiabetic women with normal-sized newborns.
   b. women with gestational diabetes.
   c. women with prolonged second stage of labor.

9. Included in the definition of tachysystole is

   a. contraction duration of >60 seconds.
   b. contraction frequency of >5 in 10 minutes.
   c. contraction intensity of >80 mm Hg.

10. A high probability of successful induction of labor is associated with a Bishop score of

    a. >4.
    b. >6.
    c. >8.

11. Appropriate treatment of uterine tachysystole with fetal intolerance after dinoprostone administration is

    a. IV bolus of D5W.
    b. terbutaline 0.25 mg subcutaneously.
    c. vaginal irrigation with normal saline.

12. In the absence of complications, immediate postpartum maternal vital signs should be assessed every

    a. 5 minutes for 30 minutes.
    b. 15 minutes for 2 hours.
    c. 30 minutes for 2 hours.

13. After administration of misoprostol, ACOG recommends delaying the administration of oxytocin

    a. 2 hours.
    b. 4 hours.
    c. 6 hours.

14. Use of the vacuum extractor increases risk for

    a. medically indicated episiotomy.
    b. neonatal cephalohematoma and retinal hemorrhage.
    c. third- and fourth-degree perineal tears.

15. Uterine response to IV oxytocin occurs in

    a. 1 to 2 minutes.
    b. 3 to 5 minutes.
    c. 6 to 10 minutes.

16. Anesthesia personnel are required to remain with a patient in the post-anesthesia care unit (PACU) until the

    a. monitoring equipment has been applied.
    b. PACU nurse accepts responsibility for the patient.
    c. patient is alert and oriented.

17. The normal length of the pregravid cervix is

    a. 2.5 to 3.0 cm.
    b. 3.5 to 4.0 cm.
    c. 4.5 to 5.0 cm.

18. True labor is characterized by

    a. effacement and/or dilation of the cervix.
    b. painful uterine contractions.
    c. suprapubic discomfort at regular intervals.

19. One liter of D5L/R provides

    a. 150 calories.
    b. 180 calories.
    c. 250 calories.

20. Facilitating a family-centered birth experience involves

    a. allowing immediate family members to participate.
    b. providing a waiting area for siblings.
    c. supporting family as defined by the childbearing woman.

Fill in the Blank

21. Diastolic blood pressure measurements taken from an automatic blood pressure device are typically _____ than diastolic measurements using a stethoscope and a mercury cuff.

22. During the second stage of labor, an alternative to squatting that provides the same benefits is _____.

23. Bearing down efforts accompanied by prolonged breath-holding typifies _____ pushing, which has associated negative maternal and fetal _____ effects.

24. Association of Women's Health, Obstetric and Neonatal Nurses's second-stage labor nursing management protocol for a woman with epidural analgesia encourages rest until the occurrence of _____.

25. The McRoberts maneuver is used to facilitate birth when there is an occurrence of _____.

26. Adverse outcomes associated with episiotomy include

    a. _____
    b. _____
    c. _____
    d. _____
    e. _____
    f. _____
    g. _____

27. Measures to aid perineal stretching and aid in the goal to avoid episiotomy include

    a. _____
    b. _____
    c. _____

28. Women who have a support person with them in labor have been found to have

    a. _____
    b. _____
    c. _____

29. Before the use of a cervical ripening or labor induction agent, the following should be assessed:

    a. _____
    b. _____
    c. _____

30. Normal latent phase labor of nulliparous women can last up to _____ hours

31. An interval of _____ hours is recommended between the final dose of dinoprostone and oxytocin administration.

32. Nursing documentation following amniotomy should include

    a. _____
    b. _____
    c. _____

33. A _____-degree laceration extends into the rectal lumen.

34. The maternal landmarks that must be identified to determine fetal stations are the _____.

35. With a physician or certified nurse-midwife order, nurses with appropriate training may administer the cervical ripening agents _____ and _____.

36. _____ is a contraindication for the use of misoprostol and Cervidil.

37. A nursing measure to use before forceps application to help prevent maternal trauma is _____.

38. Requirements for post-anesthesia recovery care include availability of

    a. _____
    b. _____
    c. _____
    d. _____
    e. _____

39. According to ACOG, selection criteria for women who are candidates for a TOLAC include

    a. _____
    b. _____
    c. _____
    d. _____
    e. _____

40. _____ is the most common sign of uterine dehiscence or rupture in women experiencing a TOLAC.

41. Four maternal factors proposed as being responsible for initiation of labor are

    a. _____
    b. _____
    c. _____
    d. _____

42. If any of the following findings are present in a pregnant woman, the perinatal provider should be notified promptly:

    a. _____
    b. _____
    c. _____
    d. _____
    e. _____
    f. _____

43. The Bishop score evaluates these five parameters:

    a. _____
    b. _____
    c. _____
    d. _____
    e. _____

44. Unnecessary interventions during labor increase the risk of _____.

45. Informed consent for vaginal birth after cesarean birth correctly includes discussion about

    a. _____
    b. _____
    c. _____

Chapter 15 Fetal Assessment during Labor

Multiple Choice

1. For women receiving oxytocin during the first stage of labor, assessment of fetal status using electronic fetal monitoring (EFM) should occur every

   a. 15 minutes.
   b. 30 minutes.
   c. 60 minutes.

2. For women receiving oxytocin while actively pushing, assessment of fetal status using EFM should occur every

   a. 5 minutes.
   b. 15 minutes.
   c. 30 minutes.

3. The normal fetal heart rate (FHR) baseline rate

   a. decreases during labor.
   b. fluctuates during labor.
   c. increases during labor.

4. Bradycardia in the second stage of labor following a previously normal tracing may be caused by fetal

   a. hypoxemia.
   b. rotation.
   c. vagal stimulation.

5. A likely cause of fetal tachycardia with moderate variability is

   a. fetal hypoxemia.
   b. maternal fever.
   c. vagal stimulation.

6. Reduction in FHR variability can result from

   a. fetal scalp stimulation.
   b. medication administration.
   c. vaginal examination.

7. The primary goal in treatment for late decelerations is to

   a. correct cord compression.
   b. improve maternal oxygenation.
   c. maximize uteroplacental blood flow.

8. The most frequently observed type of FHR deceleration is

   a. early.
   b. late.
   c. variable.

9. Amnioinfusion may be useful in alleviating recurrent decelerations that are

   a. early.
   b. late.
   c. variable.

10. Findings indicative of progressive fetal hypoxemia are

    a. late decelerations, moderate variability, and stable baseline rate.
    b. prolonged decelerations recovering to baseline and moderate variability.
    c. recurrent late or variable decelerations and loss of variability.

11. Clinically significant fetal metabolic acidemia is indicated by an umbilical arterial cord gas pH of ≤7.10 and a base deficit of

    a. 3.
    b. 6.
    c. 12.

12. Fetal bradycardia can result during

    a. fetal sleep.
    b. umbilical vein compression.
    c. vagal stimulation.

13. While caring for a 235-lb laboring woman who is HIV-seropositive, the external FHR tracing is difficult to obtain. An appropriate nursing action would be to

    a. apply a fetal scalp electrode.
    b. auscultate for presence of FHR variability.
    c. notify the attending midwife or physician.

14. FHR decelerations that are benign and do not require intervention are

    a. early.
    b. late.
    c. variable.

15. FHR decelerations that result from decreased uteroplacental blood flow are

    a. early.
    b. late.
    c. variable.

16. FHR decelerations that result from umbilical cord occlusion are

    a. early.
    b. late.
    c. variable.

17. FHR pattern associated with severe fetal anemia is

    a. lambda.
    b. saltatory.
    c. sinusoidal.

18. A workup for maternal systemic lupus erythematosus would likely be ordered in the presence of fetal

    a. complete heart block.
    b. premature ventricular contractions.
    c. supraventricular tachycardia.

19. Which intravenous fluid is most appropriate for maternal administration for intrauterine resuscitation?

    a. D5L/R
    b. Lactated Ringer's solution
    c. Normal saline

20. The position/s that best promote/s maternal–fetal exchange is

    a. left lateral.
    b. right lateral.
    c. either right or left lateral.

21. Maternal oxygen for intrauterine resuscitation should be given at

    a. 8 L/min.
    b. 10 L/min.
    c. 12 L/min.

22. The most appropriate equipment for administration of maternal oxygen for intrauterine resuscitation is a

    a. nasal cannula.
    b. nonrebreather face mask.
    c. simple face mask.

23. Accurate determination of baseline FHR requires

    a. at least 2 contiguous minutes of FHR in a 10-minute window.
    b. evaluation of the FHR over at least a 10-minute window.
    c. averaging the FHR over 30 minutes.

24. An electronic fetal monitoring tracing with moderate variability, no accelerations, and early decelerations would be classified as

    a. normal (category I).
    b. indeterminate (category II).
    c. abnormal (category III).

25. An EFM tracing with a sinusoidal pattern would be classified as

    a. normal (category I).
    b. indeterminate (category II).
    c. abnormal (category III).

26. An EFM tracing with marked variability would be classified as

    a. normal (category I).
    b. indeterminate (category II).
    c. abnormal (category III).

27. An EFM tracing with minimal variability and recurrent late decelerations would be classified as

    a. normal (category I).
    b. indeterminate (category II).
    c. abnormal (category III).

28. An EFM tracing with FHR 170 beats per minute and moderate variability would be classified as

    a. normal (category I)
    b. indeterminate (category II)
    c. abnormal (category III)

29. An EFM tracing with absent variability and no decelerations would be classified as

    a. normal (category I).
    b. indeterminate (category II).
    c. abnormal (category III).

30. An EFM tracing with absent variability and recurrent variable decelerations would be classified as

    a. normal (category I).
    b. indeterminate (category II).
    c. abnormal (category III).

31. The predictive value of recurrent late decelerations for fetal acidemia is

    a. high.
    b. low.
    c. variable.

32. Interpretation and classification of FHR patterns are based on predictability of fetal status

    a. at birth.
    b. at the time the pattern is observed.
    c. over the previous hour.

33. Amnioinfusion is an appropriate measure for

    a. oligohydramnios.
    b. recurrent variable decelerations unresolved by position changes.
    c. thick, meconium-stained fluid.

34. Baroreceptors respond to changes in fetal

    a. acid–base status.
    b. blood pressure.
    c. oxygen status.

35. Fetal scalp stimulation is appropriate in the context of

    a. bradycardia.
    b. minimal variability.
    c. prolonged deceleration.

36. The key issue in the management of tachysystole is

    a. absence or presence of associated FHR abnormalities.
    b. the stage of labor in which it occurs.
    c. whether tachysystole is spontaneous or induced.

37. When tachysystole occurs with a category I tracing, the rate of the oxytocin infusion should be

    a. decreased by half.
    b. discontinued.
    c. maintained at the current rate.

38. Oxygen is transferred from the mother to the fetus via the placenta through

    a. active transport.
    b. facilitated diffusion.
    c. passive diffusion.

39. Uterine resting tone and intensity of uterine contractions cannot be assessed by

    a. external tocodynamometer.
    b. intrauterine pressure catheter.
    c. manual palpation.

40. The FHR characteristic most predictive of a well-oxygenated newborn at the time observed is

    a. absence of decelerations.
    b. moderate variability.
    c. stable baseline rate.

41. During an acute episode of fetal hypoxemia, fetal blood flow is shifted primarily to the

    a. brain.
    b. liver.
    c. lung.

42. Baroreceptor-mediated decelerations are

    a. early.
    b. late.
    c. variable.

43. The primary goal in the treatment of variable decelerations is to

    a. correct umbilical cord occlusion.
    b. improve maternal oxygenation.
    c. maximize blood flow to the uterus.

44. Umbilical artery blood gas results reflect the status of the

    a. fetus.
    b. mother.
    c. placenta.

45. An appropriate initial treatment for recurrent late decelerations with moderate variability during first stage labor is

    a. amnioinfusion.
    b. maternal repositioning.
    c. oxygen at 10 L per nonrebreather facemask.

Fill in the Blank

46. A prolonged deceleration lasts greater than or equal to ____ minutes but less than ____ minutes from onset to return to baseline.

47. Variable decelerations are characterized by a/an _____ decrease of FHR below the baseline.

48. Early decelerations are characterized a/an _____ decrease and return to baseline FHR associated with a uterine contraction. In most cases, the onset, nadir, and recovery of the deceleration occur at the same time as the _____, _____, and _____ of the contraction, respectively.

49. Normal (category I) FHR tracings have an absence of late or variable decelerations, _____ variability, and may show accelerations.

50. Most fetal arrhythmias are not life-threatening except for sustained _____, which may lead to fetal congestive heart failure.

51. Minimal baseline variability may be caused by multiple factors including _____, _____, and _____.

52. In the presence of variable decelerations, progressive hypoxemia may be characterized by an increasing _____ and loss of _____.

53. Decelerations are defined as _____ if they occur with greater than or equal to 50% of the uterine contractions in a 20-minute segment.

54. Uterine resting tone and the intensity of contractions are measured in millimeters of mercury only when a/an _____ is being used.

55. A sinusoidal pattern may develop in the Rh-sensitized fetus or the fetus who is _____.

56. In low-risk women not receiving oxytocin, auscultation of the fetal rate should occur every _____ minutes in the active phase of the first stage of labor and every _____ minutes during active pushing in the second stage of labor.

57. Moderate baseline variability is defined as _____ beats per minute.

58. Correcting variable decelerations can best be accomplished by _____.

59. Decelerations are defined as _____ if they occur with less than 50% of the uterine contractions in a 20-minute segment.

60. The presence of FHR accelerations greater than 15 beats per minute above baseline and lasting more than 15 seconds reliably exclude fetal _____ acidemia.

61. To correctly interpret a baseline FHR as tachycardic or bradycardic, the rate must persist for a minimum of _____ minutes.

62. In assessing fetal well-being, the most important FHR characteristic is _____.

63. Intrauterine resuscitation measures to improve fetal oxygen delivery include

    a. _____
    b. _____
    c. _____
    d. _____

64. The normal FHR baseline range is _____ to _____ beats per minute.

65. The National Institute of Child Health and Human Development (2008) expert group recommended _____ categories of FHR tracings.

66. FHR variability that is undetected from baseline is classified as _____.

Chapter 16 Pain in Labor: Nonpharmacologic and Pharmacologic Management

Multiple Choice

1. A woman's pain experienced during the first stage of labor is caused by

    a. cervical and lower uterine segment stretching and traction on ovaries, fallopian tubes, and uterine ligaments.
    b. pressure on the urethra, bladder, and rectum by the descending fetal presenting part.
    c. uterine muscle hypoxia, lactic acid accumulation, and distention of the pelvic floor muscles.

2. The release of maternal catecholamines during labor results in

    a. decreased metabolic rate and oxygen consumption.
    b. fetal bradycardia.
    c. uterine hypoperfusion and decreased blood flow to the placenta.

3. Continuous nursing support for women in labor

    a. improves outcomes compared with women who do not have such support.
    b. increases use of analgesia due to more rapid availability.
    c. lengthens the women's first and second stages of labor.

4. A contraindication for the use of nitrous oxide administered as Entonox (a 50:50 oxygen: nitrous oxide mixture) is

   a. advanced cervical dilatation.
   b. inability to self-administer.
   c. posterior fetal presentation.

5. A medication given to women experiencing a prolonged latent phase to produce a period of rest or sleep is

   a. butorphanol (Stadol).
   b. morphine sulfate.
   c. promethazine hydrochloride (Phenergan).

6. Neonatal respiratory depression may result from the maternal administration of intravenous (IV) opioids if birth occurs within

   a. 1 hour or after 4 hours following administration.
   b. 2 to 3 hours of administration.
   c. 12 hours of administration.

7. Ephedrine is used to correct which side effect of epidural anesthesia/analgesia?

   a. hypotension
   b. nausea and vomiting
   c. pruritus

8. Pain tolerance may be defined as the point at which a laboring woman

   a. describes the pain as severe.
   b. reaches a pain level of 4 on a rating scale of 0 to 10.
   c. requests pharmacologic pain relief or increased comfort measures.

9. Touch/massage is thought to decrease or interrupt the pain of labor by

   a. activating large myelinated nerve fibers.
   b. activating nerve fibers that transmit sensations of pain from the uterus.
   c. interrupting the habituation that occurs when labor is prolonged.

10. Opioids added to continuous epidural infusions

    a. enter the placental space and cause neonatal respiratory depression.
    b. have little if any effect on neonatal respirations.
    c. increase fetal heart rate variability.

11. Advantages of the combined spinal-epidural technique are

    a. decreased hypotension, decreased motor blockade, and increased maternal satisfaction.
    b. decreased hypotension, faster onset of pain relief, and decreased pruritus.
    c. faster onset of pain relief, decreased motor blockade, and increased maternal satisfaction.

12. The greatest hazard of IV opioid administration during labor is

    a. maternal respiratory depression.
    b. neonatal neurobehavioral depression, which may last for several days.
    c. tolerance and continued use of opioids.

13. Mixed agonist-antagonist administration in labor may lead to maternal

    a. drug withdrawal.
    b. hypotension.
    c. respiratory depression.

14. Epidural catheter placement and administration is associated with a

    a. higher rate of cesarean birth.
    b. lower rate of instrumental vaginal birth.
    c. lower rate of spontaneous vaginal birth.

15. Epinephrine may be added to the epidural to

    a. decrease the amount of narcotic needed.
    b. lessen pruritus associated with epidural narcotic.
    c. prevent hypotension.

16. A test dose of a local anesthetic mixed with epinephrine may be injected to determine that the catheter is not in the epidural vein. Injection of epinephrine into an epidural vein causes an almost immediate

    a. decrease in maternal blood pressure.
    b. increase in maternal blood pressure.
    c. increase in maternal heart rate.

17. With standard epidural, a bolus of anesthetic medication is injected. Depending on the specific medications used, women begin to feel relief in

    a. 1 to 2 minutes.
    b. 5 to 10 minutes.
    c. 15 to 20 minutes.

18. Unlike the registered nurse, the doula

 a. has minimal or no contact with the parents after the birth.
 b. meets the woman for the first time in labor.
 c. provides continuous labor support.

19. When hydrotherapy is used during labor, water should be maintained at a temperature of

 a. 34° to 35°C.
 b. 36° to 37°C.
 c. 38° to 39°C.

20. One of the contraindications to neuraxial analgesia is that the woman received her last dose of low-molecular-weight heparin within

 a. 1 hour.
 b. 6 hours.
 c. 12 hours.

21. The initial intervention for a woman experiencing pain on one side during a continuous epidural infusion is to

 a. maintain the woman in a lateral position, off the painful side.
 b. request that an anesthesiologist reevaluate the woman.
 c. turn the woman toward the side with pain.

22. The current recommendation from the American Society of Anesthesiologists regarding nourishment during labor is that solid foods

 a. and liquids do not need to be avoided during labor because of superior anesthesia techniques available today, which do not increase the risk for complications should cesarean section become necessary.
 b. and liquids need to be avoided after the patient has reached 3 cm due to the potential for cesarean section and the potential risk of respiratory complications when any patient receives anesthesia.
 c. should be avoided, but clear liquids increase maternal comfort and satisfaction and do not increase maternal complications.

23. According to Association of Women's Health, Obstetric and Neonatal Nurses, non-anesthetist registered nurses can

 a. increase/decrease the rate of a continuous epidural infusion.
 b. reinitiate an epidural infusion once it has been stopped.
 c. remove an epidural catheter after successfully completing an educational program.

24. Maintaining a horizontal position in labor promotes

 a. descent of the presenting part.
 b. increased perception of pain.
 c. maternal oxygenation and comfort.

25. Pain induces a stress reaction triggering

 a. a parasympathetic response.
 b. a sympathetic response.
 c. increased uteroplacental blood flow.

26. Patient-controlled epidural anesthesia provides

 a. greater sedation than pain relief.
 b. increased satisfaction.
 c. shorter labor duration.

27. A postdural puncture headache may occur after a spinal anesthetic due to

 a. insufficient preloading of intravenous fluids.
 b. leakage of cerebrospinal fluid through the dural hole.
 c. relative intracranial hypertension.

28. In comparing IV opioids, which of the following has the shortest duration of action?

 a. butorphanol (Stadol)
 b. fentanyl (Sublimaze)
 c. morphine sulfate

29. A cutaneous method of nonpharmacologic pain relief is employed by use of

 a. a birthing ball.
 b. acupressure.
 c. guided imagery.

30. Signs of coping in labor include

 a. rhythmic breathing.
 b. tense fists.
 c. wincing.

Fill in the Blank

31. A major limitation for recommending most nonpharmacologic methods of pain relief for use in labor is the lack of large _____.

32. Women who labor with the fetal head in the occiput posterior position report significantly less back pain when using _____ positioning.

33. Counterpressure requires application of enough force to meet the intensity of pressure from the fetal occipital bone against the _____.

34. _____ equalizes the pressure exerted on all parts of the body below the water surface.

Complete questions 35 to 37 with the following: increase or decrease

35. Unrelieved anxiety and stress cause increased production of cortisol, glucagon, and catecholamines which _____ metabolism and oxygen consumption.

36. Labor pain has an indirect effect on the fetus due to the _____ in uteroplacental perfusion.

37. A fluid bolus should be administered before the initiation of regional analgesia/anesthesia to _____ the potential for maternal hypotension.

38. The failure to obtain complete pain relief despite proper placement of the epidural catheter may be due to the presence of _____ in the epidural space, which limit areas of the epidural space that can be reached by the medication infused.

Chapter 17 Postpartum Care

Multiple Choice

1. A normal hemodynamic/hematologic change occurring during the immediate postpartum period is

    a. decreased white blood cell count.
    b. elevated blood pressure.
    c. increased cardiac output.

2. During the postpartum period, normal respiratory and acid–base changes include

    a. decreased base excess.
    b. hypercapnia.
    c. increased PCO_2.

3. Postpartum teaching about sexual activity includes the information that

    a. interest in sexual activity may increase due to hormonal changes.
    b. lubricants will not be needed due to increased vaginal mucus.
    c. sexual intercourse should be avoided until vaginal bleeding has ceased.

4. A normal physiologic finding during the immediate postpartum period is

    a. dizziness when sitting up from a reclining position.
    b. saturation of the peripad every 15 minutes.
    c. urinary output of 20 mL/hr.

5. An appropriate nursing intervention for postpartum hemorrhage is

    a. bimanual pressure.
    b. bladder catheterization.
    c. continuous fundal massage.

6. On the second postpartum/postoperative day following her cesarean delivery, a woman exhibits hypotension, dyspnea, hemoptysis, and abdominal/chest pain. The nurse recognizes these as signs and symptoms of

    a. endometritis.
    b. pulmonary embolism.
    c. sepsis.

7. Normal metabolic changes during the postpartum period include increased levels of

    a. blood glucose.
    b. plasma renin and angiotensin II.
    c. prolactin.

8. The most significant factor influencing a woman's successful transition to motherhood is

    a. emotional support and physical involvement in child care by a significant other.
    b. regular attendance at parent support group meetings.
    c. resumption of a positive and satisfying sexual relationship with her partner.

9. Postpartum endometritis is

    a. associated with internal monitoring, amnioinfusion, prolonged labor, and prolonged rupture of membranes.
    b. effectively treated with a single dose of ampicillin or cephalosporin.
    c. less frequent following cesarean birth due to sterile technique used during surgery.

10. Disruptions in the integrity of the anal sphincter, third-degree tears, and sphincter weakness are

    a. associated with increased incidence of incontinence of flatus/stool.
    b. prevented through the judicious use of operative delivery.
    c. problems freely discussed by women with their healthcare providers.

11. The nurse can positively affect a new mother's self-concept and mothering abilities by encouraging

    a. establishment of a feeding schedule that the mother finds satisfying.
    b. supportive family and friends to participate in learning opportunities and infant care during the mother's hospitalization.
    c. the mother to provide as much of the infant care as possible.

12. Appropriate fundal massage for postpartum uterine atony involves using

    a. continuous two-handed pressure on the uterus until bleeding stops.
    b. firm one-handed pressure on the fundus until clots are expressed.
    c. two hands: one anchors the lower uterine segment and the other gently massages the fundus.

13. Stress incontinence during the postpartum period is more likely to be associated with the techniques used to manage which stage of labor?

    a. first
    b. second
    c. third

14. No more than 800 mL of urine should be removed during postpartum catheterization to minimize the potential for

    a. bladder spasm.
    b. hypertension.
    c. hypotension.

15. The most effective prevention of endometritis is

    a. handwashing.
    b. use of early pericare.
    c. use of intrapartum antibiotics.

16. The most likely cause of a decline in sexual interest/activity during the postpartum period is

    a. bleeding from the vagina.
    b. fatigue.
    c. vaginal dryness.

17. Initial treatment for postpartum hemorrhage is

    a. administration of blood products.
    b. exploratory laparotomy.
    c. uterotonic agents.

18. Peak cardiac output after birth occurs at

    a. 1 to 5 minutes.
    b. 10 to 15 minutes.
    c. 30 minutes.

19. A normal hematologic change during the postpartum period is a/an

    a. drop in hematocrit between days 2 and 4.
    b. increase in the sedimentation rate.
    c. leukocytosis of 25,000 to 30,000/μL.

20. Nutritional counseling for women who breast-feed should include increasing caloric intake by

    a. 300 calories.
    b. 400 calories.
    c. 500 calories.

Fill in the Blank

21. To increase venous return during postpartum hemorrhage, the woman should be positioned with _____.

22. A white blood cell count of 28,000/mm^3 on postpartum day 2 would be considered _____.

23. Vital signs within normal limits do not rule out hypovolemic shock in a woman who has experienced a postpartum hemorrhage because alterations in vital signs do not occur until there is _____.

24. _____ is an assessment technique for identification of deep vein thrombosis.

25. When a postpartum woman displays dyspnea and chest pain, the nurse most appropriately suspects _____.

26. The first blood pressure response to hypovolemia would be decreased _____.

27. Counseling regarding contraceptive methods must include information about the _____, _____, and _____.

28. Symptoms of postpartum blues include

    a. _____
    b. _____
    c. _____
    d. _____
    e. _____

29. During the initial postpartum period, the nurse should assess _____, _____, and _____ every 15 minutes for at least 1 hour, or more often if indicated.

30. Typically, postpartum blues occur at _____ days postpartum and continue for no more than a few days.

31. The normal postpartum physiologic diuresis begins within _____ hours of delivery and continues up to _____ days.

32. The acronym BUBBLERS, used to organize postpartum assessment, stands for

    a. _____
    b. _____
    c. _____
    d. _____
    e. _____
    f. _____
    g. _____
    h. _____

33. For each 500 mL of blood loss, the hematocrit will decrease _____ and the hemoglobin will decrease _____ g/dL.

34. Assessment findings suggesting the development of mastitis include

    a. _____
    b. _____
    c. _____
    d. _____

35. Essential topics to be discussed during postpartum teaching are

    a. _____
    b. _____
    c. _____
    d. _____

36. A major factor affecting emotional adjustment during the postpartum period in low-risk women is _____.

37. The first hour after birth is the time of greatest risk for postpartum hemorrhage because _____.

38. Symptoms indicating the development of postpartum preeclampsia are

    a. _____
    b. _____
    c. _____

39. It is important that the nurse has the drug _____ readily available when patients are receiving heparin therapy for thrombophlebitis.

40. Symptoms of impending postpartum eclamptic seizure are

    a. _____
    b. _____
    c. _____
    d. _____
    e. _____

Chapter 18 Newborn Adaptation to Extrauterine Life

Multiple Choice

1. The newborn's metabolism of brown fat occurs

    a. immediately after birth.
    b. in response to cold stress.
    c. when oxygen saturation is below 90.

2. A 10-minute Apgar is assigned when the

    a. 1-minute Apgar is less than 8.
    b. 5-minute Apgar is less than 7.
    c. newborn has required resuscitation.

3. During the first week of life, newborns are at risk for bleeding because

    a. milk intake is inadequate to supply vitamin K requirements.
    b. several clotting factors are being under-produced by the spleen.
    c. the liver is immature and not yet producing several clotting factors.

4. According to the American Academy of Pediatrics, vitamin K should be administered

    a. after the infant is weighed and measured.
    b. after 2 hours of life.
    c. within 1 hour of birth.

5. After administration of eye prophylaxis, excess erythromycin ophthalmic ointment is correctly

    a. left in place until absorbed.
    b. removed using sterile water.
    c. wiped away after 1 minute.

6. According to research, there is an association between shorter separation time and umbilical cord care using

    a. alcohol.
    b. sterile water.
    c. triple antibiotic dye.

7. The key to infant abduction prevention is a

    a. carefully obtained set of newborn footprints.
    b. state-of-the-art electronic infant abduction alert.
    c. systematic infant safety program.

8. Vitamin K is produced by the newborn as

    a. a normal compensatory mechanism whenever bleeding occurs.
    b. a response to the parenteral administration of vitamin K.
    c. the gastrointestinal tract becomes colonized with bacteria following initiation of feeding.

9. As part of the algorithm for performing neonatal resuscitation, medications are administered when the

    a. code team physician orders them.
    b. heart rate is below 60 beats per minute after positive pressure ventilation (PPV) with 100% oxygen.
    c. heart rate is 60 to 80 beats per minute and not increasing.

10. Initiation of respirations is triggered in the brain by decreased concentration of

    a. carbon dioxide.
    b. oxygen.
    c. surfactant.

11. Fetal pulmonary vascular resistance is

    a. equal to neonatal.
    b. higher than neonatal.
    c. lower than neonatal.

12. In the fetus, blood is shunted into the inferior vena cava through the

    a. ductus arteriosus.
    b. ductus venosus.
    c. foramen ovale.

13. Clamping the umbilical cord at birth causes

    a. decreased blood pressure and decreased systemic vascular resistance.
    b. increased blood pressure and decreased systemic vascular resistance.
    c. increased blood pressure and increased systemic vascular resistance.

14. The major factor contributing to closure of the ductus arteriosus is sensitivity to

    a. decreasing arterial carbon dioxide concentration.
    b. decreasing left ventricular pressure.
    c. increasing arterial oxygen concentration.

15. In most healthy newborns, the ductus arteriosus will be structurally closed by

    a. 3 to 6 days of age.
    b. 7 to 13 days of age.
    c. 14 to 21 days of age.

16. The premature infant is more susceptible to evaporative heat loss because of

    a. decreased body surface area.
    b. decreased muscle tone.
    c. increased permeability of skin.

17. Hemorrhagic disease of the newborn is prevented by administration of

    a. vitamin A.
    b. vitamin D.
    c. vitamin K.

18. To protect newborns from infection with hepatitis B virus, all newborns

    a. born to mothers with unknown hepatitis B surface antigen (HBsAg) status should receive one dose of vaccine within 12 hours of birth.
    b. should be screened for HBsAg within 12 hours of birth.
    c. should receive hepatitis immunoglobulin within the first 72 hours of life.

19. Intrauterine infection should be suspected when the newborn has elevated

    a. immunoglobulin (Ig) A.
    b. IgG.
    c. IgM.

20. An infant born to a group B streptococcus (GBS)–positive mother who did not receive antibiotics during labor is at risk for

    a. hyperbilirubinemia.
    b. hypoglycemia.
    c. pneumonia.

For questions 21 to 24, the following nursing interventions support the newborn's transition to extrauterine life by interrupting what mechanism of heat loss (a to d)?

21. _____ Dry newborn thoroughly; remove wet linen.

   a. evaporation
   b. convection
   c. conduction
   d. radiation

22. _____ When necessary, use humidified, warmed oxygen.

   a. evaporation
   b. convection
   c. conduction
   d. radiation

23. _____ Place cover between newborn and metal scale.

   a. evaporation
   b. convection
   c. conduction
   d. radiation

24. _____ Preheat radiant warmer.

   a. evaporation
   b. convection
   c. conduction
   d. radiation

Fill in the Blank

25. Maternal intrauterine transmission of _____ antibodies protects the newborn from bacterial and viral infections for which the mother has already produced antibodies.

26. The action that best protects newborns from infection is _____.

27. A 2,000-g infant should receive _____ mg of vitamin K.

28. Erythromycin ophthalmic ointment protects newborns from the organisms _____ and _____.

29. Immediately following birth, in the absence of spontaneous respirations, a nurse begins giving the newborn PPV. The second nurse should _____.

30. Respiratory adaptations during the transition to extrauterine life are dependent on _____, _____, and _____ stimuli to the brain.

31. In utero, oxygenated blood flows from the placenta to the fetus through the _____.

32. During fetal life, the placenta is an organ of _____ vascular resistance.

33. The vessels in the umbilical cord are two _____ and one _____.

34. The four main mechanisms of heat loss in the neonate are _____, _____, _____, and _____.

35. Nonshivering thermogenesis generates heat in the newborn through _____ metabolism.

36. Hypothermia in the neonate increases _____ consumption.

37. The action of surfactant is to _____ in the alveoli.

38. In neonatal resuscitation, chest compressions should be initiated if the heart rate is below _____ beats per minute.

39. Women who are positive for GBS infection should be treated with _____ during labor.

40. Postpartum practices that increase breastfeeding duration include _____ and _____.

Chapter 19 Newborn Physical Assessment

Multiple Choice

1. In a newborn with hypospadias, the urinary meatus is located on the

   a. anterior surface of the glans.
   b. posterior surface of the glans.
   c. tip of the glans.

2. A nevus simplex "stork bite"

   a. is usually elevated, rough, and dark red.
   b. most often appears on the neck, forehead, and eyelids.
   c. will not blanch with pressure.

3. Tears are usually absent in a baby until the age of

   a. 2 to 4 weeks.
   b. 2 to 3 months.
   c. 4 to 6 months.

4. Newborn femoral pulses would characteristically be decreased or absent in

   a. congenital heart abnormalities.
   b. hip dysplasia.
   c. sepsis.

5. A persistent newborn heart rate of less than 100 beats per minute is consistent with

   a. congenital heart block.
   b. congestive heart failure.
   c. vagal stimulation.

6. In dark-skinned newborns, jaundice is more easily observed in the

   a. feet and hands.
   b. nail beds.
   c. sclera and buccal mucosa.

7. In the neonate, blood pressure in the lower extremities is usually

   a. higher than in the upper extremities.
   b. lower than in the upper extremities.
   c. no different than in the upper extremities.

8. The normal umbilical cord contains

   a. one artery and one vein.
   b. two arteries and one vein.
   c. two veins and one artery.

9. Jaundice within the first 24 hours of life may be related to

   a. asphyxia.
   b. cardiac disease.
   c. liver disease.

10. Edema over the presenting part of a newborn's head that feels spongy and resolves within a few days of life is characteristic of

    a. caput succedaneum.
    b. cephalohematoma.
    c. trauma during birth.

11. A gestational age assessment indicating the greatest degree of physical maturity is

    a. labia majora covering clitoris and labia minora.
    b. labia majora large and labia minora small.
    c. prominent clitoris and enlarging labia minora.

12. Newborn jaundice appears initially on the

    a. head and face.
    b. trunk and extremities.
    c. sclera.

13. Newborn fontanelles are assessed for size and

    a. color.
    b. depression or bulging.
    c. distribution of overlying hair.

14. A cross-eyed appearance in a newborn is called

    a. hypertelorism.
    b. nystagmus.
    c. strabismus.

15. Bowel sounds are expected to be present in the newborn

    a. after passage of first meconium stool.
    b. immediately after birth.
    c. within 1 hour of birth.

16. A prominent xiphoid process identified during a newborn physical assessment is

    a. a normal finding.
    b. associated with intrauterine growth retardation.
    c. indicative of respiratory distress.

17. The most common finding in assessment of the newborn's skin is a

    a. hemangioma.
    b. Mongolian spot.
    c. nevus simplex.

18. Permanent eye color is present by the age of

    a. 2 months.
    b. 4 months.
    c. 6 months.

19. In a newborn, the skin lesion that has discrete borders and does not blanch to pressure or lighten with age is a

    a. hemangioma.
    b. Mongolian spot.
    c. port wine stain.

20. The presence of the red reflex in the newborn indicates

    a. congenital cataracts.
    b. intact cornea and lens.
    c. weak eye musculature.

21. Umbilical hernias are more commonly seen in newborns who are

    a. African American.
    b. Native American.
    c. Southeast Asian.

22. Screening programs evaluating newborns at high risk for hearing loss will potentially miss what percentage of newborns with hearing loss?

    a. 25%
    b. 50%
    c. 75%

23. The most common abnormal neck finding in newborns is

    a. cystic hygroma.
    b. torticollis.
    c. webbing.

24. The Moro reflex should disappear by the age of

    a. 2 months.
    b. 4 months.
    c. 6 months.

25. A genitourinary finding in a gestational age assessment of a newborn male at 36 weeks' gestation is

    a. rugae becoming visible.
    b. pendulous scrotum.
    c. testes in the upper scrotum.

26. During the first few days of life, the percentage of newborns with developmental hip dysplasia that is identified during physical assessment is

    a. 40%.
    b. 60%.
    c. 80%.

27. A scrotal mass that does not transilluminate is a/an

    a. hydrocele.
    b. inguinal hernia.
    c. testis.

Fill in the Blank

28. When examining the clavicles, _____ is felt by the examiner if there is a fracture present.

29. At birth, newborns are covered with an odorless, white, cheesy substance called _____.

30. Epstein's pearls are composed of _____ cells.

31. Popping sensations (similar to indenting a ping-pong ball) felt when palpating the parietal or occipital bones of a newborn are called _____.

32. The anterior fontanelle normally closes at about _____ months.

33. The posterior fontanelle normally closes at about _____ months.

34. Apnea refers to pauses in respirations that last _____ seconds or longer.

35. Newborns can see an object clearly when the object is _____ inches away.

36. _____ describes the inability to completely retract the foreskin of the penis.

37. _____ is an asymmetric neck deformity in which the head is noted to be pulled toward the affected side, with the chin pointing toward the opposite shoulder, due to injury to the _____ muscle.

38. Acrocyanosis is the result of _____ and tends to worsen if the newborn becomes chilled.

39. _____ is a compensatory mechanism that decreases upper airway resistance, allowing more air to enter the nasal passages.

40. Newborn _____ are involuntary protective neuromuscular responses.

Chapter 20 Newborn Nutrition

Multiple Choice

1. Women at risk for delayed onset of lactogenesis II include those with

    a. hyperthyroidism.
    b. multiparity.
    c. obesity.

2. The onset of milk production in a postpartum woman is triggered by the

    a. periodic stimulation of oxytocin.
    b. rapid rise in prolactin.
    c. sudden decrease in progesterone.

3. A pregnant woman who asks what she should do to prepare her nipples for breastfeeding is correctly informed that nipple exercises

    a. do little to prevent nipple soreness.
    b. improve nipple erectility.
    c. reduce the incidence of engorgement.

4. Which of the following is not a breastfeeding risk factor for a late preterm infant?

    a. dehydration
    b. hyperglycemia
    c. latch problems

5. Breast engorgement in the breastfeeding mother is minimized by

    a. avoiding unnecessary nipple stimulation.
    b. nursing without time limits.
    c. pumping after nursing.

6. Signs that milk transfer is occurring include all except

    a. audible swallows.
    b. dimpling of cheeks.
    c. maternal sensation of letdown.

7. As maternal prolactin levels decline over time, what is responsible for continued milk production?

    a. maternal ingestion of adequate fluids
    b. newborn sucking
    c. return of normal estrogen levels

8. A woman calls the hospital asking what she should do for her 10-day-old breastfeeding newborn who wants to nurse "all the time." The nurse should recommend that the mother

    a. continue breastfeeding based on the newborn's cues.
    b. offer formula if the newborn is still hungry after breastfeeding.
    c. use other comforting techniques to space feedings at least 2 hours apart.

9. A formula-feeding mother asks whether she should give her baby water. The nurse should instruct her to

    a. add a little extra water to the formula on hot days.
    b. feed the newborn properly mixed formula.
    c. give the newborn water between feedings if fussy.

10. The hormone responsible for milk ejection is

    a. oxytocin.
    b. progesterone.
    c. prolactin.

11. Mothers can encourage newborns to open their mouths wider while nursing by

    a. applying a small amount of downward pressure on the newborn's chin.
    b. guiding the newborn's head toward the breast.
    c. leaning the breast forward toward the newborn.

12. Compared to mature milk, colostrum is higher in

    a. fat.
    b. immunoglobulin G.
    c. protein.

13. As human milk matures, the concentration of proteins

    a. decreases.
    b. increases.
    c. remains the same.

14. Formula feeding is recommended for newborns with

    a. galactosemia.
    b. jaundice.
    c. thalassemia.

15. Factors contributing to lactogenesis II, the onset of copious milk production, include the following, except

    a. a rise in progesterone levels.
    b. a rise in prolactin levels.
    c. infant suckling.

16. Benefits of human milk for preterm infants include the following, except

    a. enhanced neurodevelopment.
    b. lower rates of sepsis.
    c. reduced risk of hyperthyroidism.

17. Methods to increase comfort while suppressing lactation include

    a. applying heat to the breast.
    b. limiting fluid intake for 48 hours.
    c. wearing a firm-fitting bra.

18. Which of the following breastfeeding positions is most useful for the mother recovering from a cesarean birth?

    a. Clutch hold
    b. Cradle hold
    c. Cross cradle hold

19. Which of the following statements regarding supplementation of the breastfeeding infant is false?

    a. American Academy of Pediatrics recommends breastfed infants receive a vitamin D supplement.
    b. Most infants need iron supplementation before 6 months of age.
    c. Mothers on a vegan diet, which excludes dairy products, may need supplemental vitamin B_{12}.

20. Promotion of breastfeeding for the stable late preterm infants should include

    a. breastfeeding within 1 hour of birth.
    b. feeding every 2 hours for 30 minutes minimum.
    c. frequent skin-to-skin contact.

21. Which of the following is true about infant hunger cues?

    a. Crying is an early hunger cue.
    b. Feeding is best initiated when the infant is in a quiet, alert state.
    c. Hunger cues can be observed for up to an hour before the newborn begins a sustained cry.

22. All the following statements are true about physiologic jaundice, except it

    a. appears after 24 hours of age.
    b. peaks on the third or fourth day of life.
    c. results from iatrogenic causes.

23. Satiation cues include all the following, except

    a. gradual decrease in number of sucks over the course of feeding.
    b. legs flexed to abdomen.
    c. small amount of milk drool from mouth.

24. Breastfed infants may have inadequate intake if they

    a. fail to regain birth weight by 2 weeks.
    b. have two to three wet diapers by day 2.
    c. have uric acid crystals during the first week.

25. Which of the following is a true statement about pacifier use?

    a. Early introduction has been shown to prevent sore nipples.
    b. Introduction of a pacifier during sleep time, after breastfeeding is established, may prevent sudden infant death syndrome.
    c. Pacifiers effectively correct sucking problems.

26. Ankyloglossia can lead to

    a. nipple pain.
    b. reliance on pacifiers.
    c. yeast infections.

27. Approximately what percentage of U.S. birth facilities have policies to limit non–breast milk feedings to breastfed infants?

    a. 25% to 30%
    b. 45% to 50%
    c. 65% to 70%

28. For a mother who is pumping, which of the following is NOT an evidence-based recommendation?

    a. Breast massage while pumping will result in higher fat content in their milk.
    b. Sterile technique is needed when storing breast milk for later use.
    c. Warming the breasts results in greater milk volume.

Fill in the Blank

29. Healthy People 2020's target for percentage of women who initiate breastfeeding is _____%.

30. Plugged ducts should be treated with _____ and _____.

31. When the breastfeeding baby is correctly latched onto the mother's breast, the tongue covers the _____.

32. A general guideline for newborn weight gain during the first few weeks of life is to regain birth weight by _____ weeks.

33. Newborns often lose _____% of their birth weight in their first few days of life.

34. The best way to prevent sore nipples is to _____.

35. Alternate breast massage is used to _____.

36. Uric acid crystals in the baby's diaper after the first week of life is a sign of _____.

37. Abnormal physical findings of the breast that may be risk factors for breastfeeding difficulties include _____.

38. Use of supplemental feeds without a medical indication is associated with _____.

Chapter 21 Common Neonatal Complications

Multiple Choice

1. Transient tachypnea develops more often in the newborn who is born

   a. after a prolonged first stage of labor.
   b. by cesarean.
   c. small for gestational age.

2. In a newborn, tachypnea is defined as a respiratory rate greater than

   a. 40 breaths per minute.
   b. 60 breaths per minute.
   c. 80 breaths per minute.

3. A cardiac lesion considered to be cyanotic is

   a. atrial septal defect.
   b. patent ductus arteriosus (PDA).
   c. transposition of great arteries.

4. A cardiac lesion that results in decreased pulmonary blood flow is

   a. atrial septal defect.
   b. tetralogy of Fallot.
   c. PDA.

5. A medication used to maintain patency of the ductus arteriosus is

   a. caffeine.
   b. indomethacin.
   c. prostaglandin E1.

6. Hypoglycemia in the infant born to an insulin-dependent diabetic mother occurs after birth between

   a. 1 and 3 hours.
   b. 5 and 7 hours.
   c. 8 and 10 hours.

7. One etiology of hypoglycemia is decreased production of glucose, which should be suspected in the newborn who is

   a. cold stressed.
   b. the infant of a diabetic mother.
   c. small for gestational age.

8. Clinical jaundice is first apparent at serum bilirubin levels of

   a. 1 to 3 mg/dL.
   b. 5 to 7 mg/dL.
   c. 9 to 11 mg/dL.

9. In a full-term newborn, physiologic hyperbilirubinemia is characterized by a progressive increase in serum bilirubin that peaks at

   a. 24 hours.
   b. 48 hours.
   c. 72 hours.

10. A neurologic sign associated with neonatal abstinence syndrome is

    a. decreased muscle tone.
    b. diminished deep tendon reflexes.
    c. high-pitched crying.

11. Which drug, when used alone, is responsible for the most severe withdrawal in the newborn?

    a. cocaine
    b. heroin
    c. methadone

12. When ruling out sepsis in the newborn, broad-spectrum antimicrobial agents most commonly initiated after cultures have been obtained are

    a. ampicillin/cephalosporin.
    b. ampicillin/gentamicin.
    c. penicillin/gentamicin.

13. Intravenous antibiotic treatment for neonatal sepsis should continue for

    a. 3 to 5 days.
    b. 7 to 10 days.
    c. 12 to 14 days.

14. Hypothermia can cause

    a. decreased metabolic demand.
    b. hypoglycemia.
    c. metabolic alkalosis.

15. A sign of hypoglycemia in the newborn is

    a. decreased skin turgor.
    b. increased appetite.
    c. temperature instability.

16. An indication to screen for hypoglycemia is an infant who is

    a. a second twin weighing 3,000 g.
    b. born at 38 weeks' gestation.
    c. small for gestational age.

17. In the newborn, physiologic hyperbilirubinemia is characterized by a progressive increase in serum bilirubin to a peak of

    a. 5 mg/dL at 72 hours of age.
    b. 8 mg/dL at 72 hours of age.
    c. 10 mg/dL at 48 hours of age.

18. Infants undergoing phototherapy should have axillary temperatures monitored at least every

    a. 30 minutes.
    b. 1 hour.
    c. 2 hours.

19. Infants born to cocaine-addicted mothers frequently exhibit

    a. constipation.
    b. feeding difficulties.
    c. lethargy.

20. Which of the following interventions is useful to support an infant experiencing abstinence syndrome?

    a. massage
    b. music
    c. rocking

21. The diagnosis of neonatal sepsis is made in the presence of a positive culture of

    a. blood.
    b. both blood and urine.
    c. urine.

22. ACOG and the American Academy of Pediatrics (AAP) recommend HIV testing and counseling with consent for

    a. all pregnant teenagers.
    b. all pregnant women.
    c. pregnant women in at-risk populations.

Fill in the Blank

23. Surfactant _____ surface tension in the alveoli functions as a stabilizer to prevent collapse during expiration.

24. When meconium only partially obstructs the airway, a _____ effect results in which air enters the lower airways on inspiration but cannot _____ on expiration.

25. The _____ is the first major organ system to function in the embryo.

26. A ventricular septal defect (VSD) is considered to be a(n) _____ lesion with _____ pulmonary blood flow.

27. The three pathophysiologic findings in tetralogy of Fallot are

    a. _____
    b. _____
    c. _____

28. The incidence of the congenital heart defect _____ is inversely proportional to gestational age.

29. An atrial septal defect (ASD) is considered to be a(n) _____ lesion with _____ pulmonary blood flow.

30. Dextro-transposition of the great arteries occurs when the aorta arises from the _____ ventricle, and the pulmonary artery arises from the _____ ventricle, resulting in pulmonary and systemic circulations functioning in _____.

31. Glucose homeostasis requires the initiation of various metabolic processes, including _____ (forming glucose from noncarbohydrate sources), and _____ (conversion of glycogen stores to glucose).

32. As bilirubin levels rise, there is concern that bilirubin encephalopathy, also known as _____, will develop.

33. In nearly all newborns, phototherapy decreases or blunts the rise in serum _____ bilirubin regardless of gestational age, race, or presence or absence of hemolysis.

34. _____ is the one common side effect of all of the medications used to treat neonatal abstinence.

35. The two bacterial agents most commonly associated with neonatal sepsis are _____ and _____.

36. The primary neonatal factors influencing the development of sepsis are _____ and _____.

37. Intrapartum administration of prophylactic antibiotics has proven to be beneficial in preventing _____.

38. Heroin withdrawal in a newborn may last _____ weeks.

39. Skin care is important during phototherapy because the infant often has _____.

40. An infant born to a mother who received tocolytic therapy would be prone to _____.

41. Narcotics used to manage labor pain may result in _____ respiratory effort in the newborn.

42. The mortality rate associated with neonatal sepsis increases as birth weight _____.

43. Studies show a nearly _____ reduction in HIV-1 transmission in infants whose mothers received azidothymidine (ZDV) prophylaxis.

44. ACOG recommends considering an _____ for HIV-1 infected women with HIV-1 RNA levels >1,000 copies per milliliter near the time of delivery.

45. Newborn chemoprophylaxis should begin _____ hours after birth.

46. _____ is the primary complication of the 6-week course of ZDV in the neonate.

47. In the United States, women infected with HIV-1 are counseled not to _____ to avoid postnatal transmission.

ANSWER KEY

Chapter 1 Perinatal Patient Safety and Quality

1. a
2. c
3. c
4. c
5. c
6. c
7. a
8. a
9. b
10. a
11. c
12. c
13. a
14. a
15. c
16. a
17. b
18. c
19. a
20. b

Chapter 2 Integrating Cultural Beliefs and Practices When Caring for Childbearing Women and Families

1. c
2. c
3. a
4. b
5. b
6. b
7. b
8. b
9. a
10. c
11. a
12. a
13. c
14. enhance communication skills; develop linguistic skills; determine who the family decision makers are; understand that agreement may not indicate comprehension; use nonverbal communication; use appropriate names and titles; use culturally appropriate teaching techniques

Chapter 3 Physiologic Changes of Pregnancy

1. b
2. a
3. b
4. a
5. a
6. c
7. c
8. c
9. a
10. c
11. b
12. b
13. c
14. b
15. b
16. c
17. c
18. c
19. a
20. b
21. a
22. a
23. a
24. a
25. b
26. anabolism; catabolism
27. hemodilution
28. mother
29. increase
30. renal sodium
31. increased glomerular filtration rate
32. striae gravidarum
33. prolactin
34. vitamin D (or calciferol)
35. lower
36. human chorionic gonadotropin
37. estriol
38. blood volume
39. 6 to 12 weeks postpartum
40. uterus
41. progesterone
42. 24 to 32
43. angiotensin II
44. hypercoagulable
45. coagulation changes; venous stasis
46. Prostaglandins
47. melasma
48. Chadwick

Chapter 4 Antenatal Care

1. a
2. c
3. b
4. b
5. a
6. b
7. b
8. b
9. b
10. a
11. b

12. a
13. b
14. c
15. a
16. a
17. b
18. True
19. 26 to 28
20. 28
21. 11 to 20 lb
22. 3
23. teratogen
24. 8
25. 14
26. Jewish
27. Statin
28. 0.4 mg
29. early and continuing risk assessment, health promotion, medical and psychosocial intervention
30. cardiorespiratory; muscular
31. two or more abnormally elevated values
32. 15; 20
33. 10
34. fetal tone, fetal reflex movement, fetal breathing, amniotic fluid volume, nonstress test

Chapter 5 Hypertensive Disorders of Pregnancy

1. c
2. a
3. b
4. b
5. b
6. b
7. Hypertensive
8. 140; 90
9. semi-Fowler
10. Magnesium sulfate
11. abruptio placentae, disseminated intravascular coagulation, hepatic failure, acute renal failure
12. prevent maternal cerebral vascular accident; maintain uteroplacental perfusion
13. hemolysis; elevated liver enzymes; low platelets
14. aspiration

Chapter 6 Bleeding in Pregnancy

1. b
2. b
3. b
4. b
5. b
6. a
7. b
8. a
9. c

10. c
11. c
12. velamentous
13. 95
14. Hypotension
15. administering oxytocin with delivery of the anterior shoulder; clamping/cutting the umbilical cord by 2 to 3 minutes of birth; controlling traction of the umbilical cord, with the provider's hand supporting the uterus to prevent uterine inversion; performing vigorous fundal massage for at least 15 seconds

Chapter 7 Preterm Labor and Birth

1. a
2. a
3. a
4. a
5. a
6. b
7. a
8. b
9. b
10. b
11. higher
12. higher
13. worsen
14. uterine cramping (menstrual-like cramps, intermittent or constant); uterine contractions every 10 to 15 minutes or more frequently; low abdominal pressure (pelvic pressure); dull, low backache (intermittent or constant); increase or change in vaginal discharge; feeling that the baby is "pushing down"; abdominal cramping with or without diarrhea

Chapter 8 Diabetes in Pregnancy

1. c
2. c
3. a
4. c
5. c
6. a
7. b
8. c
9. a
10. a
11. Type 1
12. anabolic
13. human placental lactogen; cortisol; estrogen; progesterone; prolactin magnesium sulfate
14. magnesium sulfate
15. polyuria; polyphagia; polydipsia

Chapter 9 Cardiac Disease in Pregnancy

1. a
2. b
3. c
4. a
5. a
6. b
7. b
8. a
9. b
10. b
11. Cardiovascular
12. rheumatic fever
13. cardiac troponin I
14. type of cardiac disorder; secondary complications
15. functional ability

Chapter 10 Pulmonary Complications in Pregnancy

1. c
2. b
3. b
4. c
5. a
6. b
7. a
8. b
9. c
10. c
11. 4 to 8
12. 95
13. severity
14. illicit drug use; cigarette smoking; alcohol abuse
15. *Streptococcus pneumoniae*
16. high Fowler
17. pollens, molds, dust mites, animal dander, cockroach antigens, air pollutants, strong odors, food additives, tobacco smoke
18. systemic steroid therapy >4 weeks; three visits for asthma recently; history of multiple hospitalizations for asthma; history of hypoxic seizure, hypoxic syncope, or intubation; history of admission to intensive care unit for asthma
19. preterm labor, pericardial tamponade, bacteremia, pneumothorax, atrial fibrillation, respiratory failure
20. humans

Chapter 11 Multiple Gestation

1. c
2. a
3. a
4. c
5. b
6. c
7. c
8. c
9. b
10. b
11. b
12. b
13. c
14. a
15. c
16. a
17. c
18. False
19. True
20. False
21. False
22. low birth weight; preterm birth
23. fetal synchrony

Chapter 12 Obesity in Pregnancy

1. c
2. a
3. b
4. b
5. c
6. a
7. b
8. b
9. c
10. c
11. greater than or equal to 30
12. 15 to 25
13. decreased
14. increase
15. 12 to 24
16. decreased
17. increased

Chapter 13 Maternal–Fetal Transport

1. b
2. a
3. c
4. c
5. a
6. b
7. c
8. ambulance; airplane; helicopter
9. vital sign monitoring equipment; Doppler for FHR assessment; IV administration setup; respiratory equipment; medications; emergency birth equipment; infant resuscitation equipment; documentation method

Chapter 14 Labor and Birth

1. c
2. c
3. c
4. a
5. b
6. c
7. b
8. a
9. b
10. c
11. b
12. b
13. b
14. b
15. b
16. b
17. b
18. a
19. b
20. c
21. lower
22. sitting on the toilet
23. closed glottis; hemodynamic
24. spontaneous bearing-down efforts (urge to push)
25. shoulder dystocia
26. blood loss; infection; pain; third- and fourth-degree laceration; delayed healing; sexual dysfunction; scarring.
27. open glottis—gentle pushing; spontaneous rather than directed pushing; upright position in second stage
28. fewer perinatal complications; shorter labors; fewer NICU admissions
29. maternal status; fetal well-being; cervical status
30. 18
31. 6 to 12
32. color and amount of fluid; FHR before procedure; fetal response to procedure
33. fourth
34. ischial spines
35. misoprostol; Cervidil
36. Prior cesarean birth or uterine scar
37. emptying the maternal bladder
38. oxygen delivery system; continuous and intermittent suction; blood pressure monitoring equipment; ECG monitoring equipment; pulse oximeter; adjustable lighting; means to ensure patient privacy
39. one or two prior low transverse cesarean births; clinically adequate pelvis; no prior uterine surgery or rupture; physician immediately available and capable of performing emergent cesarean birth; surgical team and anesthesia personnel available for emergent cesarean birth
40. FHR abnormality (e.g., recurrent variable or late decelerations; prolonged deceleration; bradycardia)
41. stretching of uterine muscles; pressure on the cervix; endogenous oxytocin; change in estrogen: progesterone ratio
42. vaginal bleeding; acute abdominal pain; temperature of 100.4°F or higher; preterm labor; premature preterm rupture of membranes; hypertension
43. dilation; effacement; station; consistency; position
44. iatrogenic injuries to the mother and/or fetus
45. risks; benefits; alternative approaches

Chapter 15 Fetal Assessment during Labor

1. a
2. a
3. b
4. c
5. b
6. b
7. c
8. c
9. c
10. c
11. c
12. c
13. c
14. a
15. b
16. c
17. c
18. a
19. b
20. c
21. b
22. b
23. b
24. a
25. c
26. b
27. b
28. b
29. b
30. c
31. b
32. b
33. b
34. b
35. b
36. a
37. a
38. c
39. a
40. b
41. a
42. c
43. a

44. a
45. b
46. 2; 10
47. abrupt
48. gradual; beginning; peak; ending
49. moderate
50. supraventricular tachycardia
51. three of the following: medications, prematurity, fetal sleep, fetal arrhythmia, anesthetic agents, cardiac anomaly
52. depth of decelerations; variability
53. recurrent
54. intrauterine pressure catheter
55. anemic
56. 15 to 30; 5 to 15
57. 6 to 25
58. changing maternal position (amnioinfusion also acceptable)
59. intermittent
60. metabolic
61. 10
62. variability
63. initiate maternal lateral positioning; reduce uterine contraction frequency; discontinue oxytocin or cervical ripening agents; administer IV fluids; administer maternal oxygen by nonrebreather facemask; modify second-stage pushing efforts
64. 110; 160
65. three
66. absent

Chapter 16 Pain in Labor: Nonpharmacologic and Pharmacologic Management

1. a
2. c
3. a
4. b
5. b
6. a
7. a
8. c
9. a
10. b
11. c
12. a
13. a
14. c
15. a
16. c
17. b
18. c
19. b
20. c
21. c
22. c

23. c
24. b
25. b
26. b
27. b
28. b
29. a
30. a
31. randomized controlled clinical trials
32. hands and knees
33. sacrum
34. Hydrostatic pressure
35. increase
36. decrease
37. decrease
38. connective tissue bands

Chapter 17 Postpartum Care

1. c
2. c
3. c
4. a
5. b
6. b
7. b
8. a
9. a
10. a
11. c
12. c
13. b
14. c
15. a
16. b
17. c
18. b
19. c
20. c
21. legs elevated 20 to 30 degrees
22. nonpathologic leukocytosis
23. a loss of 15% to 20% of the total blood volume
24. Measurement of the affected leg circumference
25. pulmonary embolism
26. pulse pressure to 30 mm Hg or less
27. advantages; disadvantages; prevention of sexually transmitted diseases
28. insomnia; weepiness; anxiety; irritability; poor concentration
29. vital signs; lochia; uterine tone/position
30. 3 to 6
31. 12; 5
32. Breast; uterus; bladder; bowel; lochia; episiotomy/incision; emotional response; Homans sign
33. 2% to 4%; 1 to 1.5
34. fever and chills; localized tenderness; palpable, hard, reddened mass; tachycardia

35. pelvic floor exercises; postpartum exercise; sexuality; contraception
36. fatigue
37. large venous areas are exposed after placental expulsion
38. blood pressure of 140/90 mm Hg; headache; decreased urine output
39. protamine sulfate
40. severe persistent headache; scotomata; blurred vision; photophobia; epigastric or right upper quadrant pain

Chapter 18 Newborn Adaptation to Extrauterine Life

1. b
2. b
3. c
4. c
5. c
6. b
7. c
8. c
9. b
10. b
11. b
12. a
13. c
14. c
15. c
16. c
17. c
18. a
19. c
20. c
21. a
22. b
23. c
24. c
25. IgG
26. hand washing
27. 1
28. chlamydia; gonococcus
29. apply a pulse oximeter to the infant's right wrist
30. chemical; mechanical; sensory
31. umbilical vein
32. low
33. arteries; vein
34. evaporation; convection; conduction; radiation
35. brown fat
36. oxygen
37. lower surface tension
38. 60
39. antibiotics
40. early suckling; uninterrupted contact between mother and newborn

Chapter 19 Newborn Physical Assessment

1. b
2. b
3. c
4. b
5. a
6. c
7. a
8. b
9. c
10. a
11. a
12. a
13. b
14. c
15. c
16. a
17. c
18. c
19. c
20. b
21. a
22. b
23. a
24. c
25. c
26. b
27. b
28. crepitus
29. vernix
30. epithelial
31. craniotabes
32. 18
33. 2 to 4
34. 20
35. 8 to 10
36. Phimosis
37. Torticollis; sternocleidomastoid
38. vasomotor instability
39. Flaring
40. reflexes

Chapter 20 Newborn Nutrition

1. c
2. c
3. a
4. b
5. b
6. b
7. b
8. a
9. b
10. a
11. a
12. c

13. a
14. a
15. a
16. c
17. c
18. a
19. b
20. b
21. b
22. c
23. b
24. a
25. b
26. a
27. a
28. b
29. 81.9
30. hot packs; massage
31. lower gum
32. 2
33. 7
34. correct positioning and latch
35. increase volume and fat content of milk; treat plugged ducts
36. insufficient intake
37. inverted nipples; scars; hypoplastic breasts
38. decreased rates of breastfeeding duration and exclusivity

Chapter 21 Common Neonatal Complications

1. b
2. b
3. c
4. b
5. c
6. a
7. c
8. b
9. c
10. c
11. c
12. b
13. b
14. b
15. c
16. c
17. b
18. c
19. b
20. c
21. a
22. b
23. decreases
24. ball-valve; escape
25. cardiovascular system
26. acyanotic; increased
27. VSD; pulmonary stenosis; overriding aorta and right ventricular hypertrophy
28. patent ductus arteriosus (PDA)
29. acyanotic; increased
30. right; left; parallel
31. gluconeogenesis; glycogenolysis
32. kernicterus
33. unconjugated or indirect
34. Sedation
35. GBS; *Escherichia coli*
36. gestational age; birth weight
37. early-onset GBS sepsis
38. 8 to 16
39. loose stools
40. hypoglycemia
41. poor
42. decreases
43. 70%
44. elective cesarean section
45. 8 to 12
46. Anemia
47. breast-feed

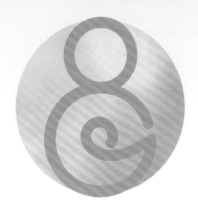

Index

Note: Page numbers followed by "*f*" indicate figures; "*t*" indicates tables; "*d*" indicates displays